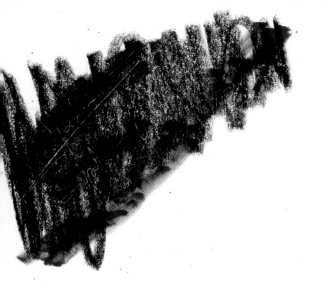

Roenigk & Roenigk's
Dermatologic Surgery
Principles and Practice
Second Edition

edited by
Randall K. Roenigk
Department of Dermatology
Mayo Clinic and Foundation
Mayo Medical School
Rochester, Minnesota

Henry H. Roenigk, Jr.
Department of Dermatology
Northwestern University Medical School
Chicago, Illinois

Marcel Dekker, Inc.   **New York•Basel•Hong Kong**

Library of Congress Cataloging-in-Publication Data

Roenigk & Roenigk's dermatologic surgery : principles and practice /
  edited by Randall K. Roenigk, Henry H. Roenigk, Jr.—2nd ed.
        p.   cm.
    Rev. ed. of: Dermatologic surgery. c1989.
    Includes bibliographical references and index.
    ISBN 0-8247-9503-2 (alk. paper)
    1. Skin—Surgery.   I. Roenigk, Randall K.
  II. Roenigk, Henry H.
        [DNLM: 1. Skin—surgery.   WR 650 R715 1996]
  RD520.D46 1996
  617.4′ 77–dc20
  DNLM/DLC   95-46848
  for Library of Congress   CIP

The Editors would like to acknowledge with grateful appreciation Arielle N. B. Kauvar for the artful cover design for our text.

Material in this text should not be construed as being endorsed by the Mayo Clinic/Foundation.

The publisher offers discounts on this book when ordered in bulk quantities. For more information, write to Special Sales/Professional Marketing at the address below.

This book is printed on acid-free paper.

Marcel Dekker, Inc.
270 Madison Avenue, New York, New York 10016

Current printing (last digit):
10 9 8 7 6 5 4 3 2 1

PRINTED IN THE UNITED STATES OF AMERICA

Dedication

A text such as ours does not come together without many hours of work and dedication by hundreds of people, to all of whom we are grateful. This includes the 108 authors and their support staff, the publishers at Marcel Dekker, Inc., and, in particular, our own staff. Both of us sincerely appreciate our secretaries, nurses, colleagues, and patients at Mayo Clinic/ Foundation and Northwestern University who in one way or another have contributed to this text. Most importantly, we would not have been able to work on this project without the support and love of our families, in particular our wives, Julie and Kathie. We dedicate this book to all of you.
Thank you.

Randall K. Roenigk
Henry H. Roenigk, Jr.

Preface

In the first edition of *Dermatologic Surgery: Principles and Practice*, H. Bryan Neel III, Professor of Otolaryngology at Mayo, wrote a foreword extolling the virtues of the intradisciplinary approach to patient care. Peter McKinney, Professor of Plastic Surgery at Northwestern University, discussed new trends in medical specialties adapting overlapping techniques, and related the story of Dr. Jacques Joseph, who was dismissed from Wolff's Clinic in 1896 for performing an aesthetic procedure. We quoted Dr. William J. Mayo, who in 1910 wrote "The best interest of the patient is the only interest to be considered, . . .". From publication of the first edition in 1989 to the second edition in 1996, the subspecialty of dermatologic surgery has matured. Our acceptance as a subspecialty has not been without growing pains, yet we continue to evolve. The high incidence of cutaneous malignancy, the demand for cosmetic surgery, and socioeconomic pressures to provide quality medical care at the least possible cost have maintained the demand for outpatient-based surgical procedures performed by dermatologists.

The basic template for *Roenigk & Roenigk's Dermatologic Surgery: Principles and Practice, Second Edition* remains the same. We have updated the section on Basic Principles to include new anesthetic techniques, complications, and infectious risks inherent with the AIDS epidemic. The section on surgical management of skin tumors and disease has been slightly reorganized and expanded. Some sections have changed little. The hallmark of a classic procedure is that it becomes standard and difficult to improve upon despite years of practice by many practitioners. Such is the case with Mohs micrographic surgery.

Reconstructive surgery has become a more important part of dermatologic surgery. A decade ago, for example, a cancer excised by the Mohs micrographic technique was normally allowed to heal by second intention. Now it is standard practice for dermatologic surgeons to perform repairs including flaps and grafts, many of which are complex in nature. Therefore, we have expanded this section of the book. In addition, laser technology continues to evolve. In the past seven years, new lasers have been developed and some problems, such as tattoos and hemangiomas, are managed far better now than in the past because of this new technology.

Finally, cosmetic surgery continues to be in strong demand by patients, while physicians are looking for new ways to expand their practice because of the rapidly changing health care market. We have expanded the number of chapters on chemical peel, as techniques have changed significantly. Micrograft hair transplantation has become standard and is aesthetically superior to older techniques. Liposuction is among the most commonly performed operations in the United States, while fat injection is a new method of soft tissue augmentation.

We stated in the preface to our first edition that our goal was to help define dermatologic surgery. Now we can hardly keep up with it. This text will serve as a good resource to complement many other publications that document the rapid evolution of our subspecialty. We hope the pages of your copy of *Roenigk & Roenigk's Dermatologic Surgery: Principles and Practice*, *Second Edition* become wrinkled and the binding cracked from regular use.

Randall K. Roenigk, M.D.
Henry H. Roenigk, Jr., M.D.

Contents

II. Standard Procedures

III. Regional Dermatologic Surgery

Contributors

Rex A. Amonette, M.D.   Clinical Professor of Dermatology, Department of Medicine, University of Tennessee, Memphis, Tennessee

Philip L. Bailin, M.D., M.B.A., and F.A.C.P.   Chairman, Department of Dermatology, The Cleveland Clinic Foundation, Cleveland, Ohio

Abnoeal D. Bakus, Ph.D.   Assistant Director of Laser Research, Department of Dermatology, Northwestern University Medical School, Chicago, Illinois

Mark R. Balle, M.D.   Director, Mohs Surgery Section, Department of Dermatology, Henry Ford Hospital, Detroit, Michigan

Wilma F. Bergfeld, M.D., F.A.C.P.   Head, Section of Dermatopathology, Department of Pathology, and Head, Clinical Research, Department of Dermatology, The Cleveland Clinic Foundation, Cleveland, Ohio

Leonard Bernstein, M.D.   Department of Dermatology, Northwestern University School of Medicine, Chicago, Illinois

Steven C. Bernstein, M.D.   Department of Dermatology, University of Montreal, Montreal, Quebec, Canada

David G. Brodland, M.D.   Assistant Professor of Dermatology, Department of Dermatology, Mayo Clinic/Foundation, Rochester, Minnesota

Harold J. Brody, M.D.   Clinical Associate Professor, Department of Dermatology, Emory University School of Medicine, Atlanta, Georgia

Marc D. Brown, M.D.   Associate Professor of Dermatology, Director, Division of Mohs Surgery and Cutaneous Oncology, Department of Dermatology, University of Rochester, Rochester, New York

Roger I. Ceilley, M.D.   Assistant Clinical Professor, Department of Dermatology, University of Iowa, Iowa City, Iowa

Holly L. F. Christman, M.D.   Assistant Clinical Professor, Department of Dermatology, Dermatologic Surgery Unit, University of California, San Francisco, California

William P. Coleman, III, M.D.   Clinical Professor, Department of Dermatology, Tulane University School of Medicine, New Orleans, Louisiana

Bari B. Cunningham, M.D.   Department of Dermatology, Northwestern University School of Medicine, Chicago, Illinois

Terence M. Davidson, M.D., F.A.C.S.   Department of Otolaryngology, University of California, San Diego, School of Medicine, San Diego, California

James F. Dolezal, R.Ph., M.D.   Assistant Clinical Professor, Creighton University, Omaha, Nebraska

Zoe Diana Draelos, M.D.   Clinical Assistant Professor, Department of Dermatology, Bowman Gray School of Medicine, Winston-Salem, North Carolina

Dirk M. Elston, M.D.   Staff Dermatologist/Dermatopathologist, Department of Dermatology, Brooke Army Medical Center, Fort Sam Houston, Houston, Texas

Neil A. Fenske, M.D., F.A.C.P.   Professor of Medicine and Pathology, Director, Dermatology and Cutaneous Surgery, Department of Internal Medicine, University of South Florida College of Medicine, Tampa, Florida

James E. Fitzpatrick, M.D., COL, MC   Chief, Department of Dermatology Service, Fitzsimons Army Medical Center, Aurora, Colorado

Richard E. Fitzpatrick, M.D.   Assistant Clinical Professor in Dermatology/Medicine, University of California School of Medicine and Dermatology Associates of San Diego County, Inc., San Diego, California

Robert W. Fleming, M.D., F.A.C.S.   Clinical Professor, Department of Otolaryngology–Head and Neck Surgery, Division of Facial Plastic and Reconstructive Surgery, University of Southern California School of Medicine, Los Angeles, California

Robert S. Flowers, M.D.   Department of Otolaryngology, University of Hawaii School of Medicine, and Plastic Surgery Center of the Pacific, Inc., Honolulu, Hawaii

Marc Friedman, M.D.   Private Practice, Kenner, Louisiana

Robert J. Friedman, M.D., M.Sc.   Clinical Assistant Professor, Department of Dermatology, New York University School of Medicine, New York, New York

Jerome M. Garden, M.D.   Associate Professor of Clinical Dermatology, Department of Dermatology, Northwestern University Medical School, Chicago, Illinois

Roy G. Geronemus, M.D. Clinical Associate Professor of Dermatology, New York University Medical Center, and Director, Laser and Skin Surgery Center of New York, New York, New York

Lawrence E. Gibson, M.D. Associate Professor, Department of Dermatology, Mayo Medical School, and Consultant in Dermatology, Mayo Clinic, Rochester, Minnesota

Hugh M. Gloster, Jr., M.D. Assistant Professor, Department of Dermatology, and Director of Dermatologic Surgery, University of Cincinnati, Cincinnati, Ohio

Jeffry A. Goldes, M.D. Dermatologist/Pathologist, Associated Dermatology, Helena, Montana

Mitchel P. Goldman, M.D. Assistant Clinical Professor in Medicine/Dermatology, University of California School of Medicine, and Dermatology Associates of San Diego County, Inc., San Diego, California

Loren E. Golitz, M.D. Professor, Department of Dermatology and Pathology, University of Colorado School of Medicine, Denver, Colorado

William J. Grabski, M.D. Director of Dermatologic Surgery, Department of Dermatology, Brooke Army Medical Center, Fort Sam Houston, Houston, Texas

Donald J. Grande, M.D. Department of Dermatology, Tufts University School of Medicine, Boston, Massachusetts

Hubert T. Greenway, M.D. Head, Dermatologic Surgery, Department of Dermatology and Cutaneous Surgery, Scripps Clinic and Research Foundation, La Jolla, California

Roy C. Grekin, M.D. Director and Associate Professor, Dermatologic Surgery Unit, Department of Dermatology, University of California, San Francisco, California

Robert Haber, M.D. Assistant Professor of Dermatology and Assistant Director, Dermatologic Surgery, Department of Dermatology, University Hospitals of Cleveland, Cleveland, Ohio

C. William Hanke, M.D. Vice-Chairman and Professor of Dermatology, Professor of Pathology and Laboratory Medicine, and Professor of Dermatology, Pathology, and Otolaryngology, Indiana University School of Medicine, Indianapolis, Indiana

Christopher Barry Harmon, M.D. Captain, United States Air Force, and Staff Dermatologist, Department of Internal Medicine (Dermatology), Keesler Medical Center, Keesler Air Force Base, Biloxi, Mississippi

Harry J. Hurley, M.D., D.Sc. Clinical Professor of Dermatology, Department of Dermatology, University of Pennsylvania School of Medicine, Philadelphia, Pennsylvania

Francisco J. Jimenez, M.D. The Stough Clinic, Hot Springs, Arkansas

Grace F. Kao, M.D. Professor of Pathology and Dermatology, University of Maryland School of Medicine, Baltimore, Maryland

Arielle N. B. Kauvar, M.D. Clinical Assistant Professor of Dermatology, Department of Dermatology, New York University Medical Center, and Associate Director, Laser and Skin Surgery Center of New York, New York, New York

Jefferson J. Kaye, M.D.   Department of Dermatology, The Ochsner Clinic, New O.leans, Louisiana

Mark Klingensmith, M.D.   Division of Plastic and Reconstructive Surgery, Department of Otolaryngology–Head and Neck Surgery, University of Illinois Medical Center and St. Joseph Hospital, Chicago, Illinois

Glenn Kolansky, M.D.   Department of Dermatology, University of Iowa Hospitals and Clinics, Iowa City, Iowa

Edward A. Krull, M.D.   Chairman, Department of Dermatology, Henry Ford Hospital, Detroit, Michigan

Emanuel G. Kuflik, M.D.   Clinical Professor, Department of Dermatology, University of Medicine and Dentistry of New Jersey–New Jersey Medical School, Newark, New Jersey

Phillip R. Langsdon, M.D.   Department of Otolaryngology, University of Tennessee College of Medicine, Memphis, Tennessee

Barry Leshin, M.D.   Associate Professor of Dermatology, and Associate Professor of Otolaryngology, Department of Dermatology, Bowman Gray School of Medicine, Wake Forest University, Winston-Salem, North Carolina

Serge M. Letessier, M.D.   Dermatologist, Department of Dermatologic Surgery, L'Hôpital Saint Louis, Paris, France

Patrick J. Lillis, M.D.   Assistant Clinical Professor, Department of Dermatology, University of Colorado Health Sciences Center, Denver, Colorado

Katherine K. Lim, M.D.   Department of Dermatology, Mayo Clinic/Foundation, Rochester, Minnesota

Clifford Warren Lober, M.D., F.A.C.P.   Clinical Associate Professor of Medicine, Department of Internal Medicine, Division of Dermatology and Cutaneous Surgery, University of South Florida College of Medicine, Tampa, Florida

Wesley Low, M.D.   Department of Otolaryngology, University of California, San Diego, School of Medicine, San Diego, California

Brian P. Maloney, M.D., F.A.C.S.   Assistant Clinical Professor, Division of Otolaryngology, University of Alabama Medical School, and the McCollough Plastic Surgery Clinic, P.A., Birmingham, Alabama

Ernest K. Manders, M.D.   Professor of Surgery and Pediatrics, and Chief, Division of Plastic and Reconstructive Surgery, Department of Plastic and Reconstructive Surgery, The Milton S. Hershey Medical Center, Pennsylvania State Hospital, Hershey, Pennsylvania

Toby G. Mayer, M.D.   Clinical Professor, Department of Otolaryngology–Head and Neck Surgery, Division of Facial Plastic and Reconstructive Surgery, University of Southern California School of Medicine, Los Angeles, California

E. Gaylon McCollough, M.D., F.A.C.S.   Clinical Professor, Department of Surgery, University of Alabama Medical School, and McCollough Plastic Surgery Clinic, P.A., Birmingham Alabama

J. Ramsey Mellette, Jr., M.D.   Professor of Dermatology, and Director of Mohs and Cutaneous Surgery, Department of Dermatology, University of Colorado Health Sciences Center, Denver, Colorado

Jeffrey L. Melton, M.D. Assistant Professor and Director of Mohs and Dermatologic Surgery, Department of Dermatology, Loyola University of Chicago, Maywood, Illinois

Romulo Mene, M.D. Private Practice, Rio de Janeiro, Brazil

Lawrence S. Moy, M.D. Assistant Professor, Department of Medicine, Division of Dermatology, University of California, Los Angeles, California

Rhoda S. Narins, M.D. Chief, Liposuction Surgery Unit, and Associate Clinical Professor of Dermatology, Department of Dermatology, New York University Medical Center, New York, New York

Robert Nossa, M.D. Department of Dermatology, New York University School of Medicine, New York, New York

Clark C. Otley, M.D. Department of Dermatology, Mayo Clinic/Foundation, Rochester, Minnesota

Stephen S. Park, M.D. Assistant Professor, Department of Otolaryngology, Head & Neck Surgery and Chief, Section of Facial and Plastic Reconstructive Surgery, University of Virginia Medical Center, Charlottesville, Virginia

Harold O. Perry, M.D. Professor Emeritus, Department of Dermatology, Mayo Clinic/Foundation, Rochester, Minnesota

James Bernard Pinski, M.D., F.A.C.P., F.I.C.S. Associate Professor of Clinical Dermatology, Department of Dermatology, Northwestern University Medical School, Chicago, Illinois

Kevin S. Pinski, M.D. Department of Dermatology, Northwestern University Medical School, Chicago, Illinois

Sheldon V. Pollack, M.D., F.R.C.P.C. Associate Professor of Medicine (Dermatology), Faculty of Medicine, University of Toronto, Toronto, Ontario, Canada

Steven Proper, M.D., J.D. Department of Dermatology, The University of Florida School of Medicine, Tampa, Florida

Henry W. Randle, M.D., Ph.D. Associate Professor of Dermatology and Head, Mohs Micrographic Surgery, Department of Dermatology, Mayo Clinic/Foundation, Jacksonville, Florida

Desiree Ratner, M.D. Department of Dermatology, Tufts University School of Medicine, Boston, Massachusetts

John Louis Ratz, M.D., F.A.C.P. Clinical Associate Professor of Dermatology, Tulane University and Louisiana State University, and Director, Dermatologic Surgery, Department of Dermatology, The Ochsner Clinic, New Orleans, Louisiana

Sorrel S. Resnik, M.D. Clinical Professor of Dermatology, Department of Dermatology and Cutaneous Surgery, University of Miami School of Medicine, Miami, Florida

Darrell S. Rigel, M.D. Clinical Associate Professor, Department of Dermatology, New York University School of Medicine, New York, New York

June K. Robinson, M.D. Professor of Dermatology and Surgery, Department of Dermatology, Northwestern University Medical School, Chicago, Illinois

Henry H. Roenigk, Jr., M.D.   Professor of Dermatology, Department of Dermatology, Northwestern University Medical School, Chicago, Illinois

Randall K. Roenigk, M.D.   Professor of Dermatology, Department of Dermatology, Mayo Clinic/Foundation and Mayo Medical School, Rochester, Minnesota

Thom W. Rooke, M.D.   Division of Cardiovascular Diseases, Department of Internal Medicine, Mayo Clinic/Foundation, Rochester, Minnesota

Timothy J. Rosio, M.D.   Director, Mohs and Laser Surgery, and Associate Clinical Professor, Department of Dermatology and Cutaneous Surgery, Epstein Photomedicine Institute, Marshfield Clinic, Marshfield, Wisconsin

Richard M. Rubenstein, M.D.   Department of Dermatology, Northwestern University Medical School, Chicago, Illinois

Stuart J. Salasche, M.D.   Associate Professor, Department of Dermatology, University of Arizona Health Sciences Center, Tucson, Arizona

Richard K. Scher, M.D., F.A.C.P.   Professor, Department of Dermatology, Columbia University College of Physicians and Surgeons, New York, New York

Bryan C. Schultz, M.D.   Clinical Associate Professor of Medicine, Dermatology Division, Loyola University Stritch School of Medicine, Maywood, Illinois

Robert A. Schwartz, M.D., M.Ph.   Professor and Head of Dermatology, Professor of Medicine, and Professor of Pediatrics, University of Medicine and Dentistry of New Jersey–New Jersey Medical School, Newark, New Jersey

Jack E. Sebben, M.D.   Associate Clinical Professor, Department of Dermatology, University of California, Davis, Medical School, Sacramento, California

Sarah Silverman, M.D.   Department of Dermatology, New York University School of Medicine, New York, New York

Miguel J. Stadecker, M.D., Ph.D.   Professor, Department of Pathology, New England Medical Center and Tufts University School of Medicine, Boston, Massachusetts

Thomas Stasko, M.D.   Assistant Professor of Medicine (Dermatology), Vanderbilt University Medical Center, Nashville, Tennessee

Dow B. Stough, IV, M.D.   Clinical Assistant Professor of Dermatology, University of Arkansas Medical Sciences, Little Rock, and The Stough Clinic, Hot Springs, Arkansas

M. Eugene Tardy, Jr., M.D.   Division of Plastic and Reconstructive Surgery, Department of Otolaryngology–Head and Neck Surgery, University of Illinois Medical Center and St. Joseph Hospital, Chicago, Illinois

Rufus M. Thomas, M.D.   Private Practice, Waynesville, North Carolina

Abel Torres, M.D., J.D.   Assistant Dean for Clinical Education/Associate Professor of Dermatology, Department of Internal Medicine, Section of Dermatology, Loma Linda University School of Medicine, Loma Linda, California

J. Corwin Vance, M.D. Assistant Professor, Department of Dermatology, University of Minnesota; Assistant Chief, Department of Dermatology, Hennepin County Medical Center, Minneapolis, Minnesota

Richard F. Wagner, Jr., M.D., J.D. Department of Dermatology, The University of Texas Medical Branch, Galveston, Texas

Tom D. Wang, M.D. Associate Professor, Department of Otolaryngology–Head and Neck Surgery, Section of Facial Plastic and Reconstructive Surgery, Oregon Health Sciences University, Portland, Oregon

Ronald G. Wheeland, M.D. Professor and Chairman, Department of Dermatology, University of New Mexico, Albuquerque, New Mexico

Duane C. Whitaker, M.D. Professor of Dermatology, Director, Division of Dermatologic Surgery and Cutaneous Laser Surgery, Department of Dermatology, University of Iowa Hospitals and Clinics, Iowa City, Iowa

Gregory J. Wilmoth, M.D. Department of Dermatology, Mayo Clinic/Foundation, Rochester, Minnesota

Dana Wolfe, M.D. Department of Otolaryngology, University of California, San Diego, School of Medicine, San Diego, California

David T. Woodley, M.D. Professor and Chair, Department of Dermatology, Northwestern University School of Medicine, Chicago, Illinois

John M. Yarborough, Jr., M.D. Clinical Professor of Dermatology, Department of Dermatology, Tulane University School of Medicine, New Orleans, Louisiana

Randall J. Yetman, M.D., F.A.C.S. Staff Surgeon, Department of Plastic Surgery, Cleveland Clinic, Cleveland, Ohio

Setrag A. Zacarian, M.D., F.A.C.P. Clinical Professor of Dermatology, Tufts University Medical School, Boston, Massachusetts, and Associate Clinical Professor of Dermatology (Emeritus), Yale University School of Medicine, New Haven, Connecticut

Mark J. Zalla, M.D. Assistant Professor, Department of Dermatology, Mayo Clinic/Foundation and Mayo Medical School, Scottsdale, Arizona

John A. Zitelli, M.D. Shadyside Medical Center, Pittsburgh, Pennsylvania

FOREWORD
The History of Dermatologic Surgery

In the past 25 years, rapid growth of cutaneous surgery has occurred, expanding the scope of the specialty of dermatology to include both medical and surgical aspects. A major step in this "skin care revolution" was the founding of the American Society for Dermatologic Surgery (ASDS) at the American Academy of Dermatology (AAD) Annual Meeting on December 5, 1970, in Chicago. Under the leadership of Drs. Leonard A. Lewis and Sorrel S. Resnik, 29 founding members were organized, and Dr. Norman A. Orentreich was elected as its founding president. The ASDS immediately established working arrangements with the AAD. The ASDS's first course, "Basic Surgical Techniques for Dermatologists" was held in 1972 at the University of Miami School of Medicine during the Annual AAD Convention. This enabled the ASDS to act as the umbrella organization for all aspects of dermatologic surgery. Many more surgical societies have since been formed.

Dermatology has always been considered both a medical and a surgical specialty. Dermabrasion was introduced by Kromayer (1950); chemical peels by MacKee and Karp (1952) and by Ayres (1960); hair transplant surgery by Orentreich (1959); Mohs micrographic surgery by Mohs (1947) and fresh tissue Mohs by Tromovitch (1976); laser surgery by Goldman (1961); and liquid nitrogen cryosurgery by Zacarian (1966). New dermatologic advances have also been introduced in liposuction and fat transplantation, scalp reduction surgery, flaps, and grafts, as well as in blepharoplasty, face-lift surgery, and chemical peeling with trichloroacetic acid (TCA), glycolic acid, phenol, and combination peels.

In 1971, the ASDS had a membership of 120 men and women. Today over 2400 members have made the ASDS the second largest dermatologic society in the United States. From 1972 to 1975, courses and seminars were held in skin grafting, hair transplant surgery, dermabrasion, and chemical peeling, as well as basic surgical procedures. In 1975, the *Journal of Dermatologic Surgery* (later the *Journal of Dermatologic Surgery and Oncology* and now *Dermatologic Surgery*) was founded by Drs. Perry Robins and George Popkin.

The American College of Mohs Micrographic Surgery and Cutaneous Oncology (ACMMSCO) was formed in 1967. In 1977, the American College of Cryosurgery was formed by dermatologists, as well as physicians in several specialties. In 1979, the AAD began cryosurgical courses at its annual meetings.

In 1979, the International Society for Dermatologic Surgery (ISDS) was founded by Dr. Perry Robins to promote education and scholarship in dermatologic surgery on a global basis and it now offers a central meeting point for skin surgery groups from around the world. In 1992, the Council of National Dermatologic Surgery Societies was founded in Paris to establish a dialogue among national societies.

In 1980, the University of Miami Department of Dermatology, under the direction of Dr. Harvey Blank, was the first department in the United States to change its name to the Department of Dermatology and Cutaneous Surgery and in 1982, Florida was the first state to organize a dermatologic surgery society—the Florida Society of Dermatologic Surgeons. Other state surgical societies have been formed in Colorado (1987) and Georgia, North Texas, and Ohio (1992).

Advances have also been made in education and research, with new reference textbooks of dermatologic surgery (such as this one) and the *Yearbook of Dermatologic Surgery* and *Medical and Surgical Dermatology, A Critical Guide to World Literature*. Funding for basic science research in surgery has been provided by the ASDS. The Residency Review Committee for Dermatology, sponsored by the Accreditation Council for Graduate Medical Education, expanded residency requirements in 1990 to include training in laser, complex closures, flaps, and grafts; in addition, a surgical program director for each residency program is now required. In 1988, the Association of Academic Dermatologic Surgeons was formed to represent these surgical program directors. In 1993, the ASDS became the thirteenth sponsoring organization for the Accreditation Association for Ambulatory Health Care (AAAHC), a group that provides the opportunity to upgrade the quality of care in our surgical outpatient facilities.

The medical and surgical aspects of dermatology can be harmoniously blended and taught. We must educate the patient as well as other physicians about the skin, and direct our efforts to improve the quality of care and cost effectiveness. Surgical societies that have concerns about practice parameters in this new subspecialty should arbitrate their differences in an effort to teach and refine the surgical skills of all dermatologists and unify dermatology for the benefit of our patients.

Sorrel S. Resnik

Surgical Preparation, Facilities, and Monitoring

Jack E. Sebben

University of California, Davis, Medical School, Sacramento, California

Prior to the popularity of outpatient surgery, the surgeon could direct nearly all his or her attention to surgical technique and postoperative care. The ancillary tasks such as skin preparation and infection control, instrument sterilization, and facility organization were all managed by other members of the health care team. When surgery is performed in the office setting, however, it is often the surgeon who must see that high standards are maintained.

There are many advantages associated with an office-based surgical facility. The surgery may be performed conveniently with efficient use of time. The surgeon has the advantage of working with personnel specifically trained and experienced to provide the highest quality assistance to the surgeon and attentive care to patients. Scheduling is easier and more flexible. The entire process runs more efficiently since the nursing staff works under the direction of the surgeon rather than answering to a hospital administrator.

Outpatient surgery also offers advantages to the patient, since most prefer to have surgery done outside a hospital. An outpatient facility is less threatening and the atmosphere is more private. Office surgery is also more economical. Frequently, surgery can be performed in an outpatient facility for 40% of the cost at a hospital.

To deliver the highest level of surgical care to the patient in the office setting, there must be adequate preparation prior to surgery. The steps include proper preparation of the skin, appropriate instrument selection and care, and an adequate facility for the procedure as well as to meet any unexpected needs.

SURGICAL PREPARATION OF THE SKIN

The skin must be adequately prepared for surgery to decrease the possibility of wound contamination and subsequent infection. The extent of antiseptic preparation and associated precautions taken varies considerably with the surgical procedure. Simple biopsies and small shave excisions rarely become infected, and the consequence of a minor infection is usually not significant.

Dermatologic surgeons performing complex procedures involving large areas of subcutaneous tissue and major tissue movement must take extra precautions. Wound infections most commonly involve dermis, subcutaneous tissue, and superficial fascial planes. Certain precautions to avoid infection is the standard of care whether surgery is performed in the hospital or office setting.

In the Middle Ages, physicians thought that suppuration ("laudable pus") was a necessary part of the healing process. Girolama Francostora, an Italian physician, believed that contagion was spread by minute bodies capable of self-multiplication. This idea was largely ignored until Louis Pasteur laid the foundation for bacteriology when he confirmed the existence of microorganisms susceptible to heat destruction. Robert Koch established a relationship between bacteria and infection that led to the basic concepts of infectious disease. These concepts were not applied to surgical infection control until Joseph Lister, an English surgeon, applied the principles of asepsis to surgical procedures. This had a profound effect on the success of surgery because prevention was the only reliable means of dealing with the risk of surgical infection.

The development of broad-spectrum antibiotics several decades ago provided a means of dealing with infection. This may have slightly precluded strict attention to antisepsis. In the hospital setting, efforts are directed toward infection control. However, with the shift from the hospital to outpatient surgery, particularly in cutaneous surgery, the burden of responsibility for adequate infection control is on the surgeon.

The goal of surgical preparation is twofold. The surgeon must do everything possible to decrease the chance of wound contamination and subsequent infection, which may lead to complications secondary to the infection. In addition, adequate antisepsis is essential to prevent infection transfer to office personnel, medical equipment, and other patients (Fig. 1).

Bacteriology

It is impossible to sterilize the skin completely. Ten to 20% of the resident flora are found in the deeper layers of the skin, primarily within the pilosebaceous units. Most of the resident flora,

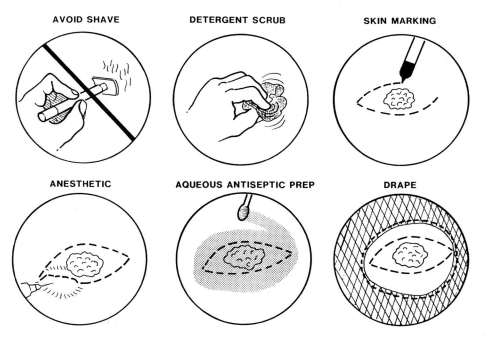

Figure 1 The components for satisfactory skin preparation prior to incisional surgery. Note that shaving is not recommended except when absolutely necessary to remove hair that interferes with the surgery.

however, are in the superficial layers of the skin. The normal flora vary considerably with the anatomic site. Approximately 90% of the resident aerobic bacteria is *Staphylococcus epidermidis*. Additional strains include *Staphylococcus aureus*, micrococci, diphtheroids, streptococci, and some gram-negative bacilli.

The skin may also contain several transient and pathogenic microorganisms. These are the bacteria usually involved in wound infection and, fortunately, are easily removed by adequate surgical preparation. The single most commonly found organism in wound infections is *S. aureus*. Staphylococci and, to a lesser degree, streptococci are the most common offenders in outpatient surgery. In the hospital setting, the majority of pathogens in surgical wounds are gram-negative bacteria. These include *Escherichia coli, Pseudomonas aeruginosa, Klebsiella, Enterobacter*, and *Proteus* species. This difference between the hospital and the private office reflects cross-contamination in the hospital environment.

Antiseptic Agents

The ideal antiseptic agent should rapidly destroy all microorganisms without risk of toxicity, irritation, or allergenicity. It also should be inexpensive, easily applied, and cosmetically acceptable. No one antiseptic agent satisfies all of these criteria, but some come closer than others (Table 1).

Soaps

Ordinary soaps have very little antibacterial effect. However, their mechanical emulsifying action removes a large portion of the superficial transient and pathogenic bacteria. Thus, an adequate scrub with a soap or detergent, preferably combined with the killing power of an antiseptic, is the first and most important step in prepping the skin.

Chlorhexidine

Chlorhexidine gluconate is a biguanide agent that is very effective against a wide range of gram-positive and gram-negative bacteria. It has been used extensively in Europe since 1954 and was introduced to the United States in 1977 as a 4% concentration with 4% alcohol in a sudsing base. The product is marketed as Hibiclens. A combination of chlorhexidine and alcohol for use as a final skin prep was sold as Hibitane but has since been discontinued due to the fire hazard of its high alcohol concentration.

Chlorhexidine produces rapid bacterial destruction and binds with the protein of the stratum corneum to leave some degree of residual action. It is not irritating to the skin and is not absorbed through it. There is no evidence of systemic toxicity. It also appears to be more resistant to contamination than many of the other antiseptic agents.

Chlorhexidine has been shown to be safe for use on the oral mucosa, but the sudsing base can be irritating to the conjunctiva, so it should be kept away from the eyes. It can also be toxic to the middle ear. Therefore, it should not be placed into the auditory canal if there is any possibility that the tympanic membrane is not intact. This precaution applies to many other antiseptic agents. At the present time, chlorhexidine appears to be the agent of choice for a surgical scrub.

Iodophors

Pure iodine is a rapidly acting, powerful antiseptic agent. However, it tends to be unstable and is irritating to the skin. Most of the problems associated with elemental iodine have been solved by the development of iodophors, which are a combination of iodine and a polymer. The water-soluble complex slowly releases free iodine. The lower concentration of iodine is less irritating to the skin and, although less effective than iodine, is still an excellent antiseptic.

Povidone-iodine is one of the most popular iodophor complexes (Betadine). This aqueous solution may be applied as a final skin prep. A detergent base may be added (Betadine Surgi-

Table 1 Antiseptics and Disinfectants

Agent	Spectrum	Indications
Chlorhexidine	Rapidly cidal to gram-positive and gram-negative bacteria; some gram-negative resistance; sporicidal at elevated temperatures; affects some fungi and viruses	Surgical scrub; hand-washing; preoperative prep
Iodophors	Cidal to gram-positive and gram-negative bacteria; fungicidal; viricidal; sporicidal with prolonged exposure; not tuberculicidal	Surgical scrub; hand-washing; preoperative prep
Isopropyl alcohol	Bactericidal to all common pathogenic bacteria; erratic fungicide and viricide; inactive against spores	Prep for needle sticks and simple biopsies; enhancer for chlorhexidine or iodine compounds
Ethyl alcohol	Same as isopropyl but less active above 70% concentration	Same as for isopropyl alcohol
Hexachlorophene	Primarily bacteriostatic against gram-positive bacteria	Skin cleanser
Benzalkonium chloride	Bactericidal to gram-positive and gram-negative bacteria; not effective in *Pseudomonas* or *Mycobacteria*	Skin cleanser; preservative; disinfectant
Mercurials	Weakly bacteriostatic and fungistatic	Preservative for drugs and cosmetics
Hydrogen peroxide	Broad spectrum but weak	Wound cleanser
Glutaraldehyde	Effective on all microorganisms; vegetative forms in 10–15 min and spores in 3–10 hr	Disinfectant; sterilizing solution

Safety	Precautions	Comments
Nontoxic; low irritancy	Avoid conjunctiva and inner ear	Persists in stratum corneum more than 24 hr
Contact dermatitis rare; iodine absorption when used on large denuded areas	Avoid in iodine-sensitive patients: do not apply to raw surfaces	More effective against gram-negatives than chlorhexidine but shorter duration of action
Can be a fire hazard	Do not apply to raw surfaces	Less corrosive to metal than ethanol
Can be a fire hazard	Do not apply to raw surfaces	Odor less offensive than isopropanol
Risk of neurotoxicity and teratogenicity from percutaneous absorption	Avoid repeated use in infants and pregnant women; gram-negative overgrowth may occur	Better choices are available for surgical preparation
Nonirritating; nontoxic	Easily inactivated by blood or purulent matter; prone to contamination	More effective combined with alcohol
Can cause dermatitis; risk of toxic absorption	Easily inactivated by organic matter	Obsolete as antiseptic
Low incidence of irritancy; leaves no residue	Decomposes to pure water with storage	Not for surgical preparation
Not for use on skin; toxic; can cause contact dermatitis	Must be rinsed from instruments before use	The only reliable sterilizing solutions

cal Scrub) to produce a sudsing antiseptic preoperative scrub. These agents have a wide range of antibacterial activity, including the destruction of some bacterial spores.

The iodophors may occasionally cause skin reactions in iodine-sensitive individuals. Although it is of little risk in cutaneous surgery, iodine toxicity can result from absorption when iodophors are applied to large areas of denuded skin.

Aqueous iodine preparations should not be used as wound cleansers because the iodine may have a denaturing effect on the exposed tissues. This can irritate the tissue and increase the incidence of wound infection. There have been a few reports of contamination and lack of effectiveness, but the iodophors still appear to be one of our best antiseptic agents. They are particularly useful as a final skin prep since a nondetergent chlorhexidine skin prep is not currently available.

Alcohols

Alcohols are excellent broad-spectrum antiseptics, but their full effectiveness is not achieved in the usual clinical application. Seventy percent ethyl alcohol can destroy 90% of cutaneous bacteria within 2 min if constant alcohol moisture is maintained during that time period. However, a single wipe with an ethyl alcohol–soaked swab produces a reduction of approximately 75% of the cutaneous bacteria.

Alcohol is effective as an organic solvent that removes oil and debris containing large numbers of bacteria. The effect of a brief wipe is probably no greater than that of ordinary soap and water.

Alcohol should not be applied to an open wound because, like iodine, it denatures and damaged tissue protein. The damaged tissue can then better support bacterial growth. Isopropyl alcohol is somewhat less irritating to the tissues than ethyl alcohol. It can cause some degree of vasodilatation, which may enhance the bleeding of small needle puncture sites.

Alcohols are most useful in conjunction with other antiseptic agents. In the past, antiseptic tinctures were often applied as a final skin prep prior to draping. Because they are flammable and a fire hazard, antiseptic tinctures should not be used in the presence of electrosurgical equipment.

Benzalkonium Chloride

A number of quaternary ammonium compounds are used as antiseptics and preservatives. Benzalkonium chloride (Zephiran) has enjoyed some popularity in the past as a surgical antiseptic. It is now seldom used because it lacks effectiveness. It destroys many gram-positive and some gram-negative bacteria and fungi. However, it is not effective against *Mycobacterium tuberculosis, P. aeruginosa*, spores, and many viruses. It is often contaminated by some of these organisms.

Quaternary ammonium compounds are cationic agents and are easily inactivated by anionic compounds such as soaps, detergents, blood, and other organic materials. These agents are still used as disinfecting solutions but are certainly not adequate for surgical preparation of the skin.

Mercurial Compounds

Over the years, various metal salts have been used as antiseptics, including mercury, silver, and zinc. The organic mercurial compounds have been the most popular for skin antisepsis. Merbromin (Mercurochrome) and thimerosal (Merthiolate) have been used at various times for surgical skin preps. These agents can irritate the skin, are weak antiseptics, and are easily inactivated. They have no role in the surgical preparation of the skin.

Hair Removal

For years it was standard practice to shave the skin around the operative field. This was often done many hours prior to surgery. It has been shown that shaving traumatizes the skin and promotes bacterial growth. This results in an increased incidence of wound infections. Shaving should be avoided if possible. If done, the skin should first be prepped with an antiseptic scrub, then shaved immediately prior to surgery so there is no time for bacterial regrowth.

If hair must be removed, it is preferable to clip away only the hair that interferes with surgery. Small areas may be cut satisfactorily using scissors. Electric clippers are convenient, but small spicules of hair should be removed carefully. Some surgeons have used depilatories for hair removal. These agents are effective but irritating.

Marking Proposed Incision Lines

Most skin surgery is facilitated by drawing proposed incision lines on the skin prior to the actual incision. Traction and contraction often cause tissue distortion, and deviation from the proposed incision can thus be avoided.

The proposed incision lines should be marked prior to injection of local anesthesia. The patient should be sitting up or standing so that pluming may account for gravitational effects on skin tension lines. The skin should first be degreased with an alcohol wipe and dried with a gauze sponge, so the skin markings are not removed with the surgical prep.

The marking agent should be water-resistant. A number of agents are available. Bonney Blue and Berwick's solution are popular compounds that are applied with a small pointed object such as a broken applicator stick. Other dyes such as 2% gentian violet or brilliant green can be applied in the same manner. Many surgeons prefer to use sterile disposable marking pens. These usually contain gentian violet. Because there is no control over the amount of dye saturating the tip, the application is often erratic and unsatisfactory. Superior results are obtained from commercially available indelible marking pens, provided the skin is oil-free and dry, thus resisting smearing from the aqueous antiseptic preps very well.

Draping

The patient is now ready for the sterile surgical drape. Cotton drapes are supple, porous, and more comfortable for the patient. Most office procedures are performed using disposable drapes. These are impermeable to moisture. If a fenestrated paper drape is used, it should be laminated with a layer of plastic between two sheets of paper. Nonlaminated paper drapes are chemically treated to resist moisture. Pure plastic drapes are available with an adhesive margin around the fenestration. This keeps the drape stable and is particularly useful when one is working in anatomic concavities.

Preparation of the Surgeon

The surgeon must also be prepared to enter the now sterile surgical environment in an antiseptic manner. The hands should be covered with sterile surgical gloves. Because gloves are occasionally punctured or are defective, there should be minimal bacteria present on the hands within the gloves. Bacteria multiply very rapidly in the warm, moist environment inside surgical gloves. This may be significant in longer procedures. Standard surgical scrubs have been prescribed for hospital operating rooms; however, studies show that a brief scrub with effective agents may be just as effective. Regular washing with an antiseptic detergent before and between cases should result in a very low degree of bacterial contamination of the hand.

Glove use for infection control extends beyond simple use during complex surgical procedures. The surgeon should wear gloves for any minor procedure. Nonsterile examination gloves may be used for procedures such as ulcer debridement, acne surgery, and cyst incision.

A full surgical outfit consisting of cap, mask, and gown is rarely used for skin surgery. Masks should be used during larger or more prolonged procedures. The operative site may be completely prepped in a sterile fashion, only to be contaminated by oral or nasal material from the surgeon. Increased infection rates have been traced to nasal carriage of staphylococci. Cloth masks are obsolete. Disposable paper masks are far more effective air filters.

PREPARATION AND STERILIZATION OF SURGICAL INSTRUMENTS

All instruments and materials used for incisional surgery should be sterile. When surgical procedures are performed in hospital operating rooms or hospital-based outpatient surgery centers, sterilization is managed by specialists in this field. Hospitals must follow established standards for the maintenance of sterile equipment. In an outpatient facility, the physician may delegate sterile equipment management to an office assistant. However, it is still the responsibility of the physician to see that adequate standards of sterilization are maintained.

There are two basic methods for the maintenance of sterile instruments in the surgical office: the open system and the closed system. The open technique involves the storage of sterile surgical instruments in trays, from which the instruments are removed as needed. These trays may be dry metal containers, or they may contain a disinfecting solution. The closed technique involves placing individual or groups of surgical instruments in containers that are opened only once when the instrument is needed for a specific procedure.

Over the years, there has been a shift from the open to the closed technique in private offices. This is fortunate because instruments stored in open containers are prone to contamination.

Instrument Selection

The first step in instrument maintenance is the selection of top-quality surgical instruments. They must withstand repeated use and abuse. The instruments should be made by a reputable manufacturer. Quality instruments are relatively expensive. Cheap instruments are not worthwhile because they wear rapidly.

Most instruments are made of high-grade stainless steel. Cheaper non–stainless steel instruments are chrome-plated and not recommended. When the plating chips, the exposed surface will rust and small fragments may enter the wound.

Stainless steel instruments are usually available with either a highly polished or a brushed luster surface. The luster finish is recommended because it does not reveal scratches or water spots as easily as the polished finish. Black anodized finishes are available for use with laser surgery; the black surface is nonreflective.

The working or cutting surface of a surgical instrument is usually constructed of the same material as the rest of the instrument. It is desirable to have the working surface constructed of a more durable material. Needle holders and scissors are available with a special tungsten carbide alloy insert along the tips. This material is extremely hard and maintains a precise cutting edge much longer. The alloy is too brittle to be used for construction of the entire instrument. The insert is bonded to the instrument with either adhesive or solder. Some adhesives break down after repeated autoclavings. Silver solder is preferable. Instruments with tungsten carbide inserts are more expensive, but this cost is recovered through increased longevity and decreased maintenance (Fig. 2).

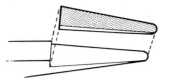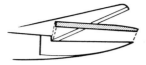

Figure 2 Tungsten carbide inserts in needle holders and scissors greatly increase instrument longevity.

Instrument Cleaning

After instruments have been used, they should be rinsed with warm water to remove debris. If they are soaked, it is best to add a detergent to the water. A detergent used for cleaning instruments should be of neutral pH. Acid detergents will break down the stainless steel surface and result in a black stain. Basic detergents leave a brown, rustlike deposit on the instrument. This appears after autoclaving and may interfere with the operation of the instrument since it is usually retained in the joint areas.

All tissue and foreign material must be carefully removed from the instruments. This material may be removed manually by scrubbing with a stiff plastic brush. A safer and more efficient method would be to use an ultrasonic cleaner. The instruments are placed in ultrasonic cleaner fluid, which consists of water and a neutral pH detergent. The ultrasonic machine is activated for 5–10 min. Sonic energy is produced and is transformed in the fluid to mechanical energy. This creates tiny bubbles on the surface of instruments that release foreign material. Once the cycle is completed, the instruments are lifted from the ultrasonic cleaner in a basket and rinsed with running water. The ultrasonic fluid should be changed frequently, particularly if it appears cloudy (Fig. 3). The ultrasonic cleaner removes only surface debris. It is not a disinfecting or sterilizing process.

After the instruments have been removed from the ultrasonic cleaner and rinsed, they should be dried. Ultrasonic cleaning can remove lubrication in hinged areas. To restore this lubrication, the instruments should be placed in instrument milk. This restores lubrication but may leave a greasy film on the surface. Some physicians prefer to use instrument milk only when the instruments need lubrication. Oils, silicone spray, or grease should not be used as lubrication because they tend to bake when autoclaved and stiffen rather than lubricate the joints (Fig. 4).

Before the instruments are packed, they should be inspected to make sure they are in proper working order. Scissor blades can be tested for sharpness by cutting a piece of tissue paper. The cut should be smooth and without resistance (Fig. 5). The tips of forceps and hemostats should be aligned. The opposing surfaces of needle holders should meet completely and be able to grasp 6–0 nylon suture securely from any angle.

Equipment is available for sharpening instruments in the office. However, many instrument manufacturers will sharpen and repair instruments at a very reasonable cost.

Sterilization

An instrument that is truly sterile is totally free of all microorganisms. Any instrument introduced beneath the body surface must be sterile. Not all medical items must be sterile. Noncritical items such as examination instruments, examination gloves, surgical masks, surgical caps, and similar items of apparel must be free of vegetative pathogens but need not be sterilized.

There are many methods of sterilization. Most very efficiently destroy vegetative forms of bacteria. However, it is important to use a method that will adequately destroy all bacterial spores and viruses.

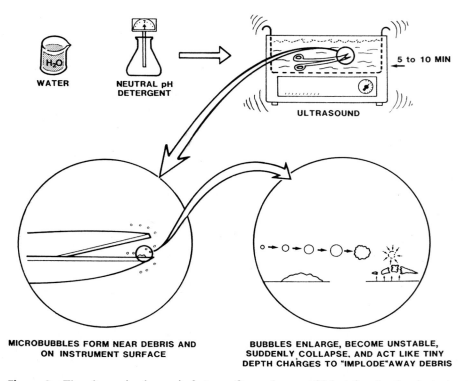

MICROBUBBLES FORM NEAR DEBRIS AND ON INSTRUMENT SURFACE

BUBBLES ENLARGE, BECOME UNSTABLE, SUDDENLY COLLAPSE, AND ACT LIKE TINY DEPTH CHARGES TO "IMPLODE" AWAY DEBRIS

Figure 3 The ultrasonic cleaner is faster, safer, and more efficient for cleaning instruments than scrubbing by hand. This procedure is necessary to remove foreign material prior to instrument sterilization.

Steam Autoclave

Steam at 100°C will destroy the vegetative forms of all bacteria, but many spores will be resistant. The steam autoclave functions as a pressure cooker to increase the pressure by 2 atm. At this pressure, the temperature of steam is 121°C. When this environment is maintained for more than 15 min, all microorganisms are destroyed. The recommended cycle times for most auto-

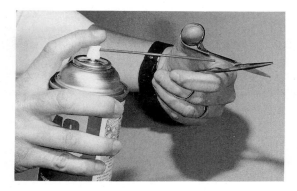

Figure 4 Lubricants such as oils, greases, or silicones should never be applied to surgical instruments. The heat from sterilization bakes these materials into the joints and interferes with their function.

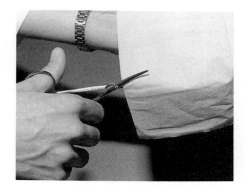

Figure 5 Scissors can be tested for sharpness by cutting tissue paper. If the scissors are sharp and in proper working order, the cut should be clean.

Table 2 Steam Autoclave Exposure Time

Items	Time (min) at 121°C and 15 PSI
Small instrument packs	20
Double-wrapped instruments	30
Unwrapped instruments	15
Wrapped sponges and dressings	30

The time starts after steam penetration and heat transfer have occurred.

claves are somewhat longer. The 15-min exposure time begins when steam has penetrated all areas. This may require an additional 5–15 min, depending on the size of the surgical pack (Table 2).

The steam autoclave may be used for the sterilization of most surgical materials including metal, cloth, paper, glassware, and heat-resistant plastics. Sharp cutting surfaces, particularly those made of high-grade carbon steel, may be dulled by 100% humidity. This is insignificant on the sharp edges of scissors but affects scalpel blades and biopsy and hair-transplant punches.

Steam is the fastest method of sterilization. It is also the easiest, safest, and most reliable, making it the method of choice for the private office.

Chemiclave

The Chemiclave is very similar to the steam autoclave but with much lower humidity, usually less than 15%. The low humidity precludes damage to sharp surgical edges. Instruments are drier at the end of the autoclave cycle. However, instead of distilled water, the Chemiclave uses a special chemical solution that contains formaldehyde, methyl ethyl ketone, acetone, and a mixture of several alcohols. This system is efficient and reliable but does not release a chemical vapor at the end of the autoclave cycle.

Dry Heat

Dry heat autoclaves are small, modified ovens. These units are inexpensive, and, due to the absence of moisture, there is no problem with corrosion or dulling. Dry heat sterilization requires high temperatures and prolonged exposure times (Table 3). The usual instrument-packing materials (cloth, paper, or plastic) cannot be used for dry heat sterilization due to the high temperatures. The instruments must be placed in special containers or sterilized in metal trays or foil packs.

Gas Sterilization

Gas sterilization is an effective alternative for instruments and materials that cannot be exposed to heat. This process requires elaborate equipment and prolonged exposure times. For office use,

Table 3 Minimum Exposure Time for Dry Heat Sterilization

Temperature	Time (hr)
171°C (340°F)	1
160°C (320°F)	2
140°C (285°F)	3
121°C (250°F)	6

small gas sterilization units are available that consist of small canisters or bags into which a vial of ethylene oxide gas is released. Caution is advised with their use because the gas is quite toxic and mutagenic. Ethylene oxide penetrates porous materials and aeration is necessary: 24 hr for paper and thin rubber; 96 hr for plastics; 7 days for polyvinyl chloride and items of plastic or rubber sealed in plastic.

This method is suitable for special mechanical equipment such as a dermabrasion handpiece or dermatome. It may be more convenient and safer to make arrangements with a nearby hospital to perform gas sterilization on special items. Gas sterilization is a complicated process and should involve biologic monitoring for every cycle. Never use gas for any item that can be satisfactorily sterilized by steam.

Chemical (Cold Tray) Sterilization

This method was once popular for the "sterilization" of instruments for limited procedures. Its popularity has declined. Chemical sterilization should not be performed on instruments used for incisional surgery. Many of the agents are effective against the vegetative forms of bacteria and viruses, including hepatitis B, but most are not effective against bacterial spores, and the solutions are prone to contamination during instrument storage.

A variety of disinfectant solutions or germicides are available. Most are a combination of ingredients such as a very low concentration of alcohol, a detergent, an antirust additive, and a quaternary ammonium compound antiseptic. These antiseptic agents are easily inactivated and are not effective against *M. tuberculosis, Pseudomonas,* or bacterial spores.

The glutaraldehyde preparations are the only agents that are reliable for use as cold sterilizing agents. Glutaraldehyde reaches its maximum antibacterial effect when it is buffered to a pH of 8.5. However, it is relatively unstable at this pH and tends to polymerize over a period of weeks. Therefore, activated glutaraldehyde must be renewed frequently. Unbuffered glutaraldehyde antiseptics are also available, and, although they are more stable, studies indicate that the unbuffered forms are less effective. The glutaraldehydes may be the only choice for a tray-sterilizing agent but present many problems. The vegetative forms of bacteria are adequately destroyed within a few minutes, but many hours are required to destroy spores. If tray contamination occurs or a contaminated instrument is replaced in the tray of solution, 8–10 hr must elapse before any instrument in that solution can be considered sterile. Glutaraldehyde can be irritating to the skin and mucosal surfaces. It should be rinsed from the instruments with sterile water prior to use. This introduces an additional contamination factor. Finally, most glutaraldehyde preparations produce a suitable but disagreeable odor. If a number of containers are placed in a single room, the odor may be overbearing.

Even if a superior disinfecting agent is introduced in the future, the real problem is not effectiveness. The problem is that any group of instruments residing in a tray of solution is prone to accidental contamination that may go unrecognized.

Instrument Packing

Cloth

The traditional instrument pack material used in hospitals is cloth, but this is not popular in the private office. Cloth must be laundered and, due to the permeability of the cloth, the instrument storage time is greatly reduced. To be an effective barrier, the cloth wrapping material should be a tight-weave 270–thread count Pima cotton fabric.

Paper

Disposable paper packs are far more convenient than cloth for use in the private office. Crepe paper wraps are available for use as a wrap similar to cloth. Paper envelopes are easier to use.

The most convenient choice is a paper/transparent pack that is self-sealing. The transparent side of the pack allows one to see the contents. A built-in heat-sensitive indicator on the paper surface changes color when it has been exposed to the autoclave cycle. It is important to remember this indicator shows that the pack has been exposed to heat but does not guarantee the adequacy of the sterilization process. For this purpose, special autoclave monitors are available. These are inserted into the packs to check periodically on the thoroughness of sterilization.

Open Containers and Solutions

Some prefer to autoclave instruments unpacked in metal trays. After the sterile trays are removed, the instruments are removed as needed from them. Another variation is to remove the freshly sterilized instruments from the autoclave tray and transfer them to a germicide holding solution. Both of these techniques introduce all the possibilities of storage contamination associated with cold sterilization. All surgical instruments should be compartmentalized into separate packs or containers so that the container is violated only once for a particular procedure. Sterility of the instruments is difficult to maintain with any open technique. This method is often used in the interest of speed and convenience (Fig. 6).

Instrument Storage

After instruments have been autoclaved, they should be stored in a manner that will maintain sterility. Prior to autoclaving, the date should be written on the packs for later reference. Storage time will vary depending upon the packing material used (Table 4).Well-sealed paper/transparent pouches have the longest storage time—up to 12 months. Instruments must be stored away from moisture. Any wet surgical pack must be considered contaminated. Packs should be subjected to limited handling. Handling traumatizes the paper surfaces and may result in breaks in the barrier. An instrument pack filing system should be devised so the office assistant does not have to search through several packs to find the desired item.

Surgical Tray Set-Up

In preparation for surgery, the surgical instruments must be arranged on a sterile tray. This is usually done by placing a sterile barrier drape over a tray such as the Mayo stand (Fig. 7). A

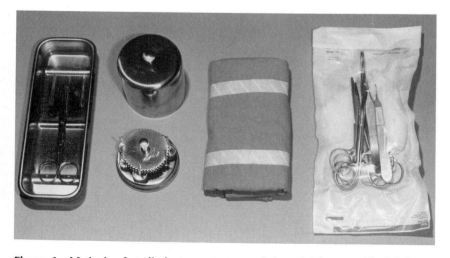

Figure 6   Methods of sterile instrument storage (left to right): tray with disinfectant solution, dry metal-container, cloth pack sealed with autoclave tape, paper/transparent pouch.

Table 4 Instrument Packing and Storage

Method	Advantages	Disadvantages	Safe storage time
Commercially packaged, pre-sterilized, disposable items	Fast and simple	Expensive	Sterile until opened or damaged
Sealed paper transparent pouches	Fast packing and opening; excellent barrier; instruments are visible	Moderately expensive	12 months
Nonwoven synthetic fabric	Disposable; tear resistant	Expensive; moisture retention	3–4 months
Paper wrap	Inexpensive	Tears and punctures easily	3–8 weeks
Muslin wrap	Most economical; lies flat and becomes sterile field drape	Must be laundered; produces lint; short shelf life	3–4 weeks; 6–12 months if immediately sealed in plastic after sterilization
Disinfectant holding solution	Minimal materials required; fast	Unreliable; prone to contamination; skin irritation	Must be replaced and instruments resterilized every 2 weeks or more often

disposable barrier drape consists of a layer of polyethylene film laminated between two layers of paper. This is necessary to provide a moisture barrier. The instruments are then placed on this barrier drape. When the instruments are packed in disposable pouches, the pouch is opened a short distance above the tray. The instruments should be packed in a manner that allows them to fall out handle-first onto the tray. This avoids damage to the delicate instrument tips as well

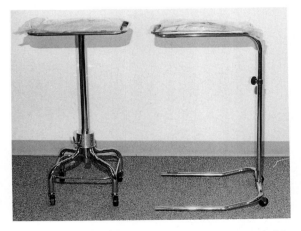

Figure 7 The Mayo table on the left is recommended for office surgery. The four casters allow easy movement of the table with the foot. The base also serves as a handy footrest. The Mayo stand on the right is awkward and requires the help of a nonsterile assistant if it must be moved.

as preventing puncture of the barrier drape. The instruments are then arranged neatly on the tray with transfer forceps. Suture material and scalpel blades may be added last.

SURGICAL FACILITY

Not all offices have space available for a room devoted exclusively to surgical procedures. The largest examination room available should be equipped for minor surgical procedures. The physician who performs only limited minor surgical procedures will not require a fully equipped suite; however, those with a larger surgical practice will require most of the recommended items and perhaps two or three similar surgical rooms.

Surgical Suite

A separate room should be reserved for surgical procedures. Ideally, the surgery room should not be used for routine office visits or for the evaluation or treatment of infected lesions. This minimizes the chance of contamination. The surgical suite will usually contain more equipment than an examination room. Minimizing the patient volume in this room will decrease the chance of damage to delicate and expensive items.

The room size should be at least 160 square feet. For major procedures, 250 square feet are recommended. It is possible to do surgery in a much smaller room, but space will be tight and there will be insufficient room for ancillary and emergency equipment (Fig. 8). A hard-surfaced floor is easiest to keep clean; however, floor contamination is rarely a problem in dermatologic surgery. Although explosive anesthetic agents are no longer used, antiquated laws in some states

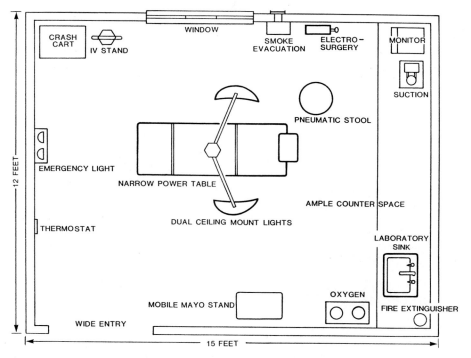

Figure 8 A room designed exclusively for operative procedures should be between 160 and 250 square feet. This example is 180 square feet and provides adequate room for essential items.

require a conductive, hard-surfaced floor for licensed operating rooms. A low-density carpet has a sound-deadening quality and adds warmth to the room. The walls should be covered with a washable material. The ceilings in most offices are constructed of standard suspended acoustic ceiling material. Acoustic tile is satisfactory for office surgery, but not adequate to meet the requirements for a licensed facility. That may require a ceiling of solid, nonporous material, which is easier to clean and is possibly more sanitary. Windows provide some natural lighting and can be opened for better ventilation.

There should be ample counter space with a large, laboratory-style sink (licensing may require the sink to be near, but outside, the operating room) (Fig. 9). Since most dermatologic surgery is performed on the head and neck, the counter and sink are most conveniently located at the head end of the room. There should be adequate cabinet space, while overhead cabinet storage is recommended. The entry doors should be oversized to allow easy passage of a wheelchair or stretcher cart.

The operating room should be situated so there is room for additional storage nearby. Laboratory and sterilizing areas should also be in close proximity.

Lighting

The basic room lighting should be fluorescent. Three to four ceiling modules containing four 48-inch fluorescent lights each should provide adequate basic room light for 160 square feet or less.

There should be two surgical lights. Ceiling or wall-mounted lights are preferred because they do not use valuable floor space and are usually more flexible in their range of coverage (Fig. 10). Wall-mounted lights are easier to install but are better for smaller rooms. Floor lights are best limited to supplemental lighting (Fig. 11).

Single-point source, spotlight-type lights should be avoided. Harsh shadows are produced and make surgical visualization difficult. Single-point lights, such as head-mounted lights, are useful for supplemental lighting. The primary surgical light should come from multiple points or from a light with a large reflector to produce shadowless light. Halogen lights produce a high-intensity natural light with minimal heat production. All surgery lights should have a transparent, protective safety shield to minimize the hazards associated with bulb failure. The light head should be periodically cleaned and inspected to make sure there are no loose or defective parts.

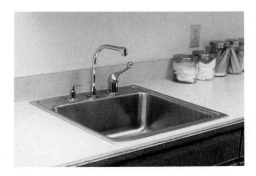

Figure 9 The surgery room sink should be large and have a laboratory-style spout to facilitate thorough hand-washing. Water control should be with either long levers or a foot-operated valve.

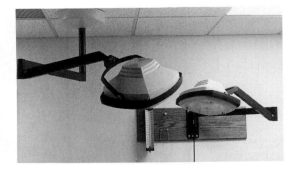

Figure 10 A surgery light mounted on the ceiling is most convenient and provides the widest coverage area. Wall-mounted surgery lights usually have a smaller range of coverage but are easier to install.

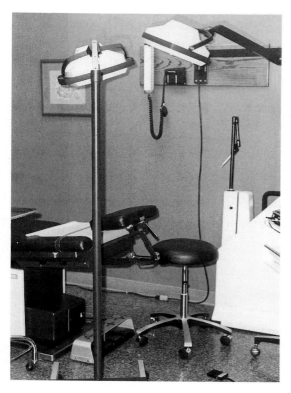

Figure 11 Floor lights are useful for supplementary lighting. They are not the best choice for a primary surgery light because they require additional floor space, which is often at a premium.

Once the surgeon is gloved, the assistant can manipulate the light into the optimal position. Many surgery lights have accessory handles that can be sterilized and attached to the light for manipulation by the gloved surgeon. The sterilized handles should be cuffed to prevent contamination.

Atmosphere

Hospital operating rooms often have laminar flow air systems to minimize contamination. However, there is very little evidence to indicate that these systems alter the rate of infection. Most postoperative infections do not arise from contamination from the inanimate environment. They are usually due to contamination from the patient, surgeon, surgical material, or breaks in sterile technique.

The room should have good temperature control. Preferably, the operating room should have its own temperature-regulating system. The temperature of the room may rise considerably during long procedures performed under warm surgical lights. Some procedures, particularly dermabrasions, are performed more satisfactorily in a cool room.

A sound system providing soothing music serves to distract the patient and minimizes the awareness of strange noises produced during surgery. The use of a television set for patients' comfort during long procedures (i.e., hair transplants) may add to the patients' comfort and relaxation.

Surgical Table

Next to adequate lighting, a good surgical table is one of the most important features of the operating room. The ease of surgery will be greatly facilitated by an adaptable table that allows proper positioning. A power table is highly recommended. However, for those who wish to have a licensed operating room, some codes require the operating table to be ungrounded and have no electrical connection. This is not a significant hazard for outpatient cutaneous surgery.

A wide table may increase patient comfort but may be less convenient for the surgeon working on midline structures. A narrow table, 22–24 inches, is recommended. The table should be relatively thin, particularly at the head end. This allows the surgeon to put his or her legs under the table while seated and working in the head and neck region (Fig. 12).

The table should adapt to several positions. A well-contoured table may be comfortable for the patient lying supine but may not accommodate the patient in the prone or lateral position. The table should be adjustable for Trendelenburg and proctoscopic positions. Side rails are a useful option for attaching armboards or surgical trays.

Surgical Stool

Some procedures can be performed with the surgeon seated. A good surgical stool should be on rollers and have pneumatic height adjustment. The height adjustment is usually hand-controlled, but a foot adjustment is a convenience for the gloved surgeon. Some stools are available with an extended backrest, which can provide valuable arm support.

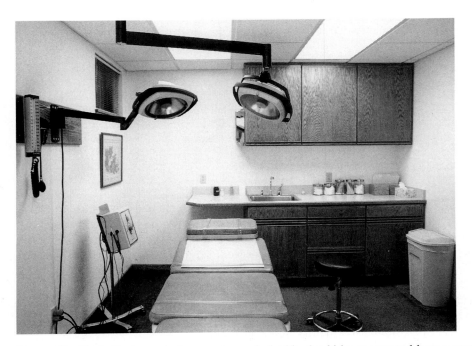

Figure 12 To facilitate surgical access, a surgical table should be narrow and have a recessed base that allows placement of legs under the table. This permits comfortable work in the head and neck region while the surgeon is seated. Surgical lights should be installed to permit coverage at any point on the table.

Surgical Stands

A surgical tray attached to a power table is inflexible and may present problems. It is better to have an independent table that may be moved about the surgical field. The most common choice is a Mayo table or stand. A Mayo table is recommended because it rests on four casters and can be easily shifted with the surgeon's foot. The traditional Mayo stand is constructed with two casters and one or two legs and is not as stable. The advantages of the Mayo stand is the ease of placement directly over the patient (see Fig. 7).

Electrosurgical Equipment

A wide variety of electrosurgical equipment is available. The surgeon must tailor the equipment to the procedures performed. Most surgeons only need to perform coagulation and electro-desiccation. A simple Birtcher Hyfrecator will provide these functions quite well. Bipolar electro-coagulation of blood vessels may easily be performed with optional attachments. Other surgeons may require a higher degree of coagulation and the ability to generate cutting current.

For simple electrocoagulation of bleeding points during incisional surgery, specialized equipment is not necessary. A nonsterile assistant can manipulate an electrosurgical handpiece with a sterile tip to contact the surgeon's forceps to transmit coagulating current. For more complex procedures, the surgeon may prefer to use sterile bipolar forceps or a sterile electrosurgical pencil with a switching handle.

When extensive electrosurgery, particularly cutting current, is used in the course of a procedure, a large amount of smoke and a disagreeable odor is produced. The problem is decreased with adequate ventilation but is better handled by a smoke-evacuation device (Fig. 13).

Laser Equipment

Laser surgery introduces additional hazards to the operating room environment. All occupants of the operating room need eye protection to prevent accidental corneal burns due to stray la-

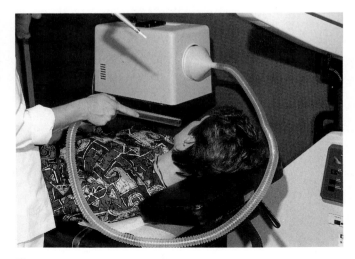

Figure 13   Large amounts of smoke and odor can be produced by electrosurgery or laser surgery. This problem is eliminated by using a filtered smoke-evacuation system.

ser beams. It is recommended that a warning sign be placed outside the door indicating when laser surgery is being performed. Some recommend that the door have an inside lock to prevent people from walking in while the surgeon working. The chance of extraneous laser beams being reflected about the room is minimized by the use of nonreflective instruments. The finish on the instruments is a dark color from blue titanium alloy, black chrome-plated stainless steel, or anodized stainless steel. These finishes defocus and disperse the laser beam.

Laser surgery produces more smoke than electrosurgery. This smoke is both disagreeable and potentially hazardous. The use of a smoke-evacuation device is essential.

Most laser equipment cannot be sterilized in the office. Sterile plastic bags are available to cover the portion of the laser used in a sterile field.

Emergency Equipment

Fire Extinguisher

An often overlooked hazard in the operating room is fire. This is a particular risk with laser surgery, but combustible items may also be easily ignited with electrosurgery. Many of the fire extinguishers supplied with medical offices dispense a fire-retardant powder. This may be effective but is not recommended for spraying in the region of a surgical wound. A gas fire extinguisher should be available.

Resuscitation Equipment

Every office should be equipped with a crash cart or emergency kit to store drugs and equipment for cardiopulmonary resuscitation (Fig. 14).

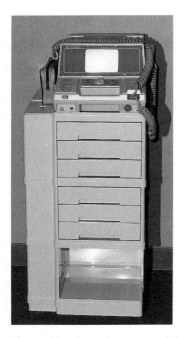

Figure 14 A crash cart containing emergency supplies should be immediately available. This cart is an artist's supply cart, which makes a convenient stand for a cardiac monitor as well as providing ample drawer space for emergency supplies.

Oxygen

An oxygen system is recommended for use with patients in respiratory distress. The physician should be familiar with the indications and contraindications of oxygen administration.

Suction

Suction equipment is a useful addition to any operating room. It may be necessary in some emergencies and also for fluid aspiration during some procedures. For nonemergency suction use, an electrical pump-type suction unit is recommended. Venturi suction attachments are available for use with oxygen tanks. These are satisfactory when a brief period of suction is required for emergency procedures. However, these attachments require a high oxygen flow and deplete the oxygen supply rapidly.

Defibrillator

Although not a common item in private offices, a defibrillator with a cardiac monitor is a useful addition to the office in which advanced surgical procedures are performed, particularly on elderly patients.

Monitoring Equipment

In addition to a cardiac monitor combined with a defibrillator, other forms of patient status monitoring should be considered in a complete surgical facility. Such monitoring devices are useful for unstable patients, but are mandatory for patients who undergo some form of conscious sedation, particularly intravenous sedation.

A digital pulse oximeter provides continuous monitoring of the pulse rate as well as the oxygen saturation level. This allows the physician to readily identify the patient who has significant respiratory depression that interferes with adequate blood oxygenation. Pulse oximeters are useful in all patients, but may be somewhat unreliable in patients with severe chronic obstructive pulmonary disease or significant peripheral vascular disease.

Continuous blood pressure monitoring is essential for sedated patients. An automatic blood pressure–monitoring device is highly recommended.

For any of these monitoring devices, it is recommended to have a machine that prints out a hard copy record of the data. Otherwise, the information should be carefully charted on a flow sheet at regular intervals.

Wheelchair

Some patients may not exit the surgery suite as easily as they entered it. An office wheelchair may prove valuable in dealing with this unexpected occurrence.

Back-Up Equipment

Power failures are not uncommon, and the surgeon should be adequately prepared to deal with them if they occur during the course of a surgical procedure. Emergency lights are available that have a continuous charging battery system (Fig. 15). When a failure to the charging system is detected, the lights are automatically activated. These units will provide adequate ambient lighting for the room.

An auxiliary source of power should be available for the operation of electrosurgical equipment, dermabrasion equipment, and surgical lights. A 600-watt generator will run all of these devices adequately. Storage battery back-up systems with similar outputs are available and may be necessary when the use of a generator is not feasible.

A back-up should be available for any mechanical equipment necessary for the completion of a surgical procedure. This is particularly true for dermabrasion power equipment. An inexpensive Dremel tool with the correct size of collet is a satisfactory substitute. An electrosurgical unit with cutting current capabilities can be used as back-up for CO_2 laser.

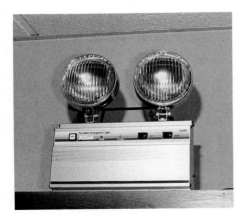

Figure 15 An alternate light source should be available in case of power failures. This light charges continuously when plugged into a standard outlet. It turns on automatically if the power is interrupted.

Individual Protective Equipment

Because of increasing concerns about physician and employee exposure to contagious diseases, such as human immunodeficiency virus and the hepatitis viruses, special attention needs to be directed at protecting the medical care worker. Surgical gloves should be worn for virtually all procedures, including injections. Employees should also wear gloves when handling and sorting used instruments. Strong consideration should be given to the use of masks and eye protection for nearly all surgical procedures. There is now evidence that the smoke generated by lasers and electrosurgery has a potential for carrying viable viruses. We need to reevaluate the protective value of surgical masks, and more sophisticated masks may be the standard in the future. The ordinary surgical masks used today do more to protect the patient from droplet exposure generated by the medical personnel than to protect the mask user. These masks are only marginal filters for small contaminated particles.

All offices should be equipped with devices that permit medical personnel to provide mouth-to-mouth resuscitation without risk of contamination. Such masks equipped with one-way valves should be available to all of the treatment areas.

Accreditation

Considering the procedures performed by dermatologic surgeons, it seems feasible at the present time to design an operating room for office use without compliance with regulatory criteria necessary for a licensed operating room. Many of the strict license requirements apply to major ambulatory surgical procedures. These are defined as operative procedures performed on nonhospitalized patients under any form of anesthesia that requires a period of postoperative recovery or observation. Minor ambulatory surgical procedures are those performed under local anesthesia with immediate discharge of the patient. This latter category applies to most cutaneous surgery. However, the licensing requirements cover the broad category of ambulatory surgery.

Accreditation is obtained through the Accreditation Association for Ambulatory Health Care, which is a byproduct of the Joint Commission of Accreditation of Hospitals. The laws for state licensing vary and may be different from requirements of the national agencies.

BIBLIOGRAPHY
Surgical Preparation of the Skin

Aly R, Maibach HI. *Clinical Skin Microbiology*. Springfield, IL, Charles C Thomas, 1978, pp. 30–35.

Atkinson LJ, Kohn ML. *Berry and Kohn's Introduction to Operating Room Technique*. New York, McGraw-Hill, 1986.

Butcher HR, Ballinger WF, Gravens DL, et al. Hexachlorophene concentrations in the blood of operating room personnel. *Arch Surg* 1973;107:70–74.

Chlorhexidine and other antiseptics. *Med Lett Drugs Ther* 1976;18:21,85–86.

Contaminated povidone-iodine solution. Northeastern United States. *MMWR* 1980;29:553–555.

Cruse PJE, Foord R. The epidemiology of wound infection. A ten year prospective study of 62,939 wounds. *Surg Clin North Am* 1980;60:27–40.

Dixon RE, Kaslow RA, Mackel DC, et al. Aqueous quarternary ammonium antiseptics and disinfectants: use and misuse. *JAMA* 1976;236:2415–2417.

Elliott RA, Hoehn JG. The office surgery suite. *Clin Plast Surg* 1983;10:225–246.

Engley FB. Evaluation of mercurial compounds as antiseptics. *Ann NY Acad Sci* 1950;53:197–206.

Evans CA, Smith WM, Johnston EA, Giblett ER. Bacterial flora of the normal human skin. *J Invest Dermatol* 1950;15:305–324.

Gradinger GP. Advantages and disadvantages of office surgery. *Clin Plast Surg* 1983;10:309–32.

Harvey SC. Antiseptics and disinfectants: Fungicides; ectoparasiticides. In *Goodman and Gilman's The Pharmacological Basis of Therapeutics*. AG Gilman, LS Goodman, A Gilman, TW Rall, F Murad, eds. New York, Macmillan, 1985, pp. 959–979.

Kaul AF, Jewett F. Agents and techniques for disinfection of the skin. *Surg Gynecol Obstet* 1981;152:677–685.

Kimbrough RD. Review of recent evidence of toxic effects of hexachlorophene. *Pediatrics* 1973;51:391–394.

Lockhart JD. How toxic is hexachlorophene? *Pediatrics* 1972;50:229–235.

Rodeheaver G, Bellamy W, Kody M, et al. Bactericidal activity and toxicity of iodine-containing solutions in wounds. *Arch Surg* 1982;117:181–186.

Rosenberg A, Alatary SD, Peterson AF. Safety and efficacy of the antiseptic chlorhexidine gluconate. *Surg Gynecol Obstet* 1976;143:789–792.

Sebben JE. Avoiding infection in office surgery. *J Dermatol Surg Oncol* 1982;8:455–458.

Selwyn S, Ellis H. Skin bacteria and skin disinfection reconsidered. *Br Med J* 1972;1:136–140.

Seropian R, Reynolds BM. Wound infections after preoperative depilatory versus razor preparation. *Am J Surg* 1971;121:251–254.

Simmons BP. Guidelines for hospital environmental control. *Infect Control* 1982;2:131–137.

Simmons BP. Guidelines for prevention of surgical wound infections. *Infect Control* 1982;3:187–196.

Steere AC, Mallison GF. Handwashing practices for the prevention of nosocomial infections. *Ann Intern Med* 1975;83:683–690.

Strachan C. Antibiotic prophylaxis in "clean" surgical procedures. *World J Surg* 1982;6:273–280.

Ulrich JA. Techniques of skin sampling for microbial contaminants. *Hosp Topic* 1965;43:121–123.

White JJ, Wallace CK, Burnett LS. Skin disinfection. *Johns Hopkins Med J* 1970;126:169–176.

Preparation and Sterilization of Surgical Instruments

Altemeier WA, Burke JF, Pruitt BA, Sandusky WR. *American College of Surgeons Manual on Control of Infection in Surgical Patients*. Philadelphia, J.B. Lippincott, 1976.

Association for Advancement of Medical Instrumentation Sterilization Committee. *Good Hosptial Practice: Ethylene Oxide Gas-Ventilation Recommendations and Safe Use*. AAMI, 1981.

Bond WW, Favero MS, Petersen NJ, et al. Inactivation of hepatitis B virus by intermediate-to-high level disinfectant chemicals. *J Clin Microbiol* 1982;18:535–538.

Caputo RA, Odlaug TE. Sterilization with ethylene oxide and other gases. In *Disinfection, Sterilization, and Preservation*. CA Lawrence, SS Block, eds. Philadelphia, Lea & Febiger, 1983, pp. 47–64.

Ernst RR. Sterilization by heat. In *Disinfection, Sterilization, and Preservation*. SS Block, ed. Philadelphia, Lea & Febiger, 1977, pp. 481–521.

Gorman SP, Scott EM, Russell AD. A review: Antimicrobial activity, uses and mechanism of action of glutaraldehyde. *J Appl Bacteriol* 1980;48:161–190.

Kuhn R. Care and handling of surgical instruments. Part II. *Med Product Sales* 1982;13:84–86.

Mallison GF, Standard PG. Safe storage times for sterile packs. *Hospitals* 1974;48:77–80.

Pepper RE. Comparison of the activities and stabilities of alkaline glutaraldehyde sterilizing solutions. *Infect Control* 1980;1:90–92.

Perkins JJ. *Principles and Methods of Sterilization in Health Sciences*. Springfield, IL, Charles C Thomas, 1980, pp. 154–167, 286–311.

Sebben JE. Sterilization and care of surgical instruments and supplies. *J Am Acad Dermatol* 1984;11:381–392.

Simmons BP. Guidelines for hospital environmental control. *Infect Control* 1981;2:133–146.

Spaulding EH, Cundy KR, Turner FJ. Chemical disinfection of medical and surgical materials. In *Disinfection, Sterilization, and Preservation*. CA Lawrence, SS Block, eds. Philadelphia, Lea & Febiger, 1977, pp. 654–684.

Surgical Facility

Accreditation Handbook for Ambulatory Health Care. Skokie, IL, Accreditation Association for Ambulatory Health Care, Inc., 1985.

American National Standard for the Safe Use of Lasers: ANSI Z126.1, New York, American National Standards Institute, Inc., 1980.

Elliott RA. Organization and efficient function of office surgery. In *Outpatient Surgery*. RC Schultz, ed. Philadelphia, Lea & Febiger, 1979, pp. 52–75.

Elliott RA. The design and management of an aesthetic surgeon's office and surgery suite. In *Aesthetic Plastic Surgery: Principles and Techniques*. P Regnault, R Daniel, eds. Boston, Little, Brown, 1984.

Mallison GFL. The inanimate environment. In *Hospital Infections*. JV Bennett, PS Brachman, eds. Boston, Little, Brown, 1979, pp. 81–92.

Sebben JE. Fire hazards and electrosurgery. *J. Dermatol Surg Oncol* 1990;16:421–424.

Tobin HA. Designing the facility. In *Ambulatory Surgery and Office Procedures in Head and Neck Surgery*. KJ Lee, C Stewart, eds. Orlando, FL. Grune & Stratton, 1986, pp. 303–314.

Tomita Y, Mihashi S, Nagata K, et al. Mutagenicity of smoke condensates induced by CO_2-laser irradiation and electrocauterization. *Mutat Res* 1981;89:145–149.

Trier WC. Plastic and reconstructive surgery. In *Major Ambulatory Surgery*. JE Davis, ed. Baltimore, Williams & Wilkins, 1986, pp. 333–366.

Watson AB, Loughman J. The surgical diathermy: Principles of operation and safe use. *Anesth Intensive Care* 1978;6:310–321.

2

Informed Consent*

Abel Torres
Loma Linda University School of Medicine, Loma Linda, California

Richard F. Wagner
The University of Texas Medical Branch, Galveston, Texas

Steven Proper
The University of Florida School of Medicine, Tampa, Florida

Physicians practicing medicine in the United States are not usually free to render treatment until the patient's consent is obtained. Consent consists of the right to agree (consent) to treatment, which is based on the law of battery and its underlying concept that all individuals should be free from harmful or offensive touchings of their person. Consent also requires that the individual (patient) agreeing to treatment is competent to agree and receives sufficient information to make the agreement meaningful (informed consent). The latter concept is based on an individual's (patient) right to self-determination and on the law of negligence.

SIMPLE CONSENT

The right to consent is best exemplified by the *Schoendorff v. New York Hospital* case. In that case, the court found that "every human being of adult years and sound mind has a right to determine what shall be done with his own body: and a surgeon who performs an operation without his patient's consent commits an assault, for which he is liable in damages." This unauthorized surgery or procedure can constitute a battery since the latter is defined as the use of force upon or intentional touching of another person without the person's consent. A battery may also occur when the physician exceeds the scope of the patient's consent such as when the wrong procedure is performed or a procedure is performed by a different physician without giving prior notice to the patient. If a battery is alleged by a patient, he or she can seek ordinary and/or punitive damages whether or not the procedure was properly performed. Such damages, if awarded, may not be covered by malpractice insurance.

Consent can be implied or express. Implied consent occurs when the conduct of the patient indicates awareness of the planned treatment. The patient must have some understanding of the nature and risks of the treatment and have an opportunity to withdraw from the proposed treat-

*Disclaimer: The information presented is intended as a general academic presentation about medicolegal issues. Specific legal advice should be sought from a licensed attorney in the involved jurisdiction.

ment. Unless consent is implied by statute, the burden will generally rest on the physician to prove that the patient's conduct implied consent, and thus relying on implied consent is risky. Express consent requires oral or written authorization by the patient. Oral consent poses the problem that the witnesses to the consent may no longer be available if needed in the future. Written consent provides better evidence of consent but, as will be discussed below, may not necessarily establish informed consent. If a physician obtains consent for treatment of a condition rather than a specific procedure, this may help avoid a scope of consent issue.

Consent must be obtained from a competent adult or, in the case of minors or incompetent adults, from authorized decision makers. It is incumbent upon practicing physicians to be familiar with the laws of their state, which define a competent adult and authorized decision makers for minors or incompetent adults.

INFORMED CONSENT/REFUSAL

The premise underlying the informed consent/informed refusal doctrine in many states is that patients should receive enough information about their condition to permit them to choose among potential interventions, including the option of no further treatment. In the extreme, a competent patient's autonomy permits him or her to refuse treatment for a potentially deadly but curable disease, even if the cure is minimally intrusive and well accepted by the medical community.

Informed consent constitutes an affirmative decision by a competent adult, which permits the physician to treat the patient in an agreed manner. Although selecting one treatment often precludes the use of another intervention, informed consent encompasses both concepts. In contrast, an informed refusal situation is usually encountered when a competent adult decides to forego a recommended test or treatment. Conflict around informed consent and informed refusal can arise when well-meaning physician interventions deprive a patient of his or her autonomy, especially when damages (harm) ensue. In the context of posttreatment injury, the patient is likely to learn of previously undisclosed alternative treatment options or risks. Under such circumstances the patient may conclude that had these relevant facts been explained, he or she would have selected a different treatment and the complication might have been avoided. To educate patients and protect patient autonomy in medical decision making, some states require physicians to distribute a written list of treatment options to patients who have or are suspected of having a certain disease.

The best way for physicians to avoid problems with informed consent and informed refusal issues is to fully communicate to patients the diagnosis or potential diagnosis, its natural course if untreated, the recommended treatment along with its potential benefits and risks, and the alternative treatments including their potential benefits and risks. Specialists often are held to a special responsibility for detailing available treatment options before undertaking treatment. Physician failure to obtain informed consent or informed refusal could potentially result in legal allegations of an intentional tort (assault, battery), breach of contract, or negligence. Negligence appears to be the most frequently employed allegation in instances where informed consent or informed refusal was not obtained or was defective. Two key legal components required to prove that a physician was negligent in rendering medical care are first to establish that the physician owed a particular duty to the patient and then to show that the physician breached that duty through an omission or commission. When a physician is accused of failing to obtain informed consent or informed refusal, it amounts to a claim that the physician had a legal duty to disclose more information to the patient but failed to do so.

The legal literature is full of reports where rare but serious potential complications were not disclosed to patients during the informed consent process. Although physicians are not held to the standard of disclosing every possible complication of a treatment, dermatology practitioners should remember that the risk of life-threatening or potentially disabling or disfiguring outcomes should be disclosed to and understood by the patient prior to treatment. Likewise, treatments involving medicines as well as medical and surgical procedures are subject to informed consent requirements.

Exceptions to informed consent and the informed refusal doctrine exist. Medical and surgical emergencies, especially when the patient is unconscious or incompetent to make medical decisions and no authorized person with decisional capacity is available, tends to diminish or negate simple consent or informed consent requirements. However, such situations are rare in dermatology practice. Medical information that is generally known by the public is also often exempted from informed consent requirements. However, physician reliance on this exception will be retroactively scrutinized in the event of a lawsuit. It is usually better for the physician to assume the outlook of some courts and presume that the patient has no knowledge about his or her condition and what risks the treatment will entail. This approach places responsibility on the physician to explain more information to the patient, so that the patient can make an informed choice about his or her health care.

Many in the field of risk management prefer some form of written informed consent or informed refusal that is signed by the patient before treatment is given or withheld. A writing of this nature in the medical record documents that informed consent or informed refusal was obtained from the patient. Also, signing a standardized informed consent or informed refusal form may diminish a patient's perception of his or her chances for successful litigation. In some states, such as California, written documentation of informed consent is required for procedures such as blood transfusions, sterilizations, and breast biopsies. However, since informed consent and informed refusal is really a process, defects in the process can serve to invalidate signed documents. A defect in the process that can serve to invalidate informed consent centers around the issue of who is responsible for obtaining informed consent. Although nurses and other non-physicians can help inform the patient, the courts have generally placed the responsibility for obtaining informed consent on the physician.

Some institutions prefer to use a note in the patient's medical record by the physician detailing the informed consent or refusal in place of having the patient sign a document. Others advocate that the patient sign or initial that note to acknowledge the informed consent process. Still others advocate the note and a signed consent document. In any case, all of these approaches have the merit of asking the physician to actively participate and document his or her role in the process.

Various approaches to the doctor–patient relationship may affect the informed consent and informed refusal processes. In an effort to determine the ideal relationship between patients and physicians, Emanuel and Emanuel (1992) delineated four theoretical models of interaction between the physician and patient: paternalistic, informative, interpretive, and deliberative. The paternalistic model is problematic for both informed consent and informed refusal processes because paternalism or beneficence is based upon the physician's perceptions about what is best for the patient. The currently dominant informative model views the physician as a competent technician who provides essential information to the patient and then implements the patient's decision. In the interpretive model, the physician serves as a counselor to the patient, helping to clarify values and desires and then aiding the patient in the selection of treatment that is consistent with his or her outlook. Some authors conclude that the deliberative model, where the physician acts as a friend or teacher, is preferable because conversation between the patient and physician may help the patient to select the best treatment. Adoption of the deliberative model could potentially improve the informed consent process, but care must be taken by the physician to avoid imposing an undesired intervention upon the patient.

TRANSLATION AND INFORMED CONSENT

The United States continues to become more multicultural. Encountering patients who do not speak or understand English is increasingly common. When it is necessary to employ a translator in order to communicate with a patient, it is usually a better medical practice to use a bilingual employee or translation service than to use a patient's friend, employee, or family member. In a recent lawsuit, a plastic surgeon amputated the toe of a non–English-speaking patient for the purpose of replacing a thumb lost to traumatic amputation. The patient did not speak English, so the patient's friend translated and the surgeon was satisfied that he had obtained adequate consent. However, the patient later claimed that he had agreed to skin grafting and not to amputation of his toe. A jury awarded this patient $413,000 in damages in addition to interest.

ALTERNATIVE TREATMENTS

A patient can allege that failure by a physician to disclose alternative treatment options is a defect that invalidated his or her consent to treatment and deprived the patient of the right to select another treatment. Many courts require an objective standard to these types of complaints, and rather than accepting the harmed patient's testimony that "I would have never agreed had I known of less risky alternatives," focus instead on what information a hypothetical reasonable person would have needed before rendering a valid informed consent.

In general, courts recognize no liability where there is more than one recognized and acceptable method of diagnosis or therapy, and the physician was not considered to have been negligent if, while exercising best judgment, he or she selected a method that later turned out to have been wrong. However, the other question that can still be raised is whether a physician is expected to inform the patient of procedures (alternatives) that are not recommended. Generally, appellate courts have rejected a general duty of disclosure concerning a treatment or procedure that a physician does not recommend since the landmark court case of *Cobbs v. Grant* stated that informed disclosure and consent laws "do not require a minicourse in medical science." This type of reasoning has been recently validated in an appeals court case from California (*Parris v. Sands*), which held that the doctor was not obligated to inform the patient of a treatment he did not recommend. Thus, failure by the physician to discuss all possible medical treatment options may not constitute a lack of informed consent. However, as articulated in the Connecticut Supreme Court case of *Logan v. Greenwich Hospital Association*, a patient might be found to reasonably rely upon a specialist to provide such information. This is somewhat supported by the California *Parris v. Sands* court case cited above, which implied that a case involving surgery, cancer diagnosis, cancer treatment, or other life-threatening procedures might bring a different conclusion to the scope of discussion of alternative treatments. With this in mind, specialists such as dermatologic surgeons should be careful when choosing not to discuss alternative treatments they do not recommend. In addition, if the physician is unaware of possible medical treatment options because he or she has not kept reasonably abreast of medical advances, then there may arise a standard of care issue (medical negligence).

Identifying potential conflicts of interest between a physician and patient may permit greater appreciation of why problems with informed consent may arise. Trust is required for a successful physician–patient relationship, and undisclosed conflicts of interest tend to undermine trust. Through the identification and disclosure of potential conflicts of interest with a patient during the informed consent process, the physician is likely to gain patient respect and trust appropriately and, at the same time, improve the chances that a valid informed consent will be obtained.

INFORMED REFUSAL

Legal concepts about informed consent and informed refusal continue to expand and evolve. In an important case from California, a family physician who failed to warn a young woman about the life-threatening danger involved in refusing a pap smear was held liable when the patient later died of cervical carcinoma. Just as informed consent is required before the physician performs a procedure on a patient, obtaining a patient's informed refusal is necessary if the patient refuses a potentially beneficial examination or procedure. The major policy concept behind informed refusal is that by warning a competent person about the potential negative outcomes of refusing an examination or treatment, a reasonable person would reconsider and agree. Without knowing about the risks of refusing, a patient is deprived of his or her autonomy to make health care decisions in much the same manner as would occur if a nonemergency procedure were performed upon a competent adult who did not have other treatment options explained.

An area where the issue of informed refusal may arise for dermatologists concerns "the complete skin examination" for new patients. A great potential benefit of a complete skin examination is that a previously undetected melanoma may be diagnosed and treated while it is still a curable tumor. Some dermatologists offer a complete skin examination routinely. Yet it is not uncommon for patients to reject a complete skin examination. Initial patient objections to complete skin examination, such as inconvenience, modesty or privacy concerns, and increased time requirement, are likely to abate once the potential life-saving purpose of the examination is disclosed. However, if the patient refuses the complete skin examination, it would be prudent for the physician to document the informed refusal by the patient. If the physician does not routinely offer a complete skin examination on all new patients, then informed refusal may not be an issue, although depending on the reasons and circumstances there may be a standard of care issue.

BIBLIOGRAPHY

Ashcraft v. King, 228 Cal. App. 3d 604 (1991).
Bommareddy v. Superior Court, 222 Cal. App. 3d 1017 (1990).
California Health and Safety Code, section 1704.5.
Cobbs v. Grant, 8 Cal.3d 229 (1972).
Emanuel EJ, Emanuel LL. Four models of the physician-patient relationship. *JAMA* 1992;267:2221–2226.10.
Frank, Flannery, et al. *Consent to Treatment, Legal Medicine: Legal Dynamics of Medical Encounters.* St. Louis, C.V. Mosby, 1988.
Leffell DJ, Berwick M, Bolognia J. The effect of preeducation on patient compliance with full-body examination in a public skin cancer screening. *J Dermatol Surg Oncol* 1993;19:660–663.
Logan v. Greenwich Hosp. Ass'n, 191 Conn. 282 (1983).
Parris v. Sands, 93 Daily Journal DAR 16233.
Sard v. Hardy, 281 Md. 432 (1977).
Schoendorff v. New York Hospital, 211 N.Y. 215 (1914).
Truman v. Thomas, 27 Cal. 3d 285 (1980).
UT System Closed Claim Study. *UT System Health Law Bulletin* 1993; (Oct.):7.

3

Anesthesia

J. Corwin Vance
University of Minnesota and Hennipen County Medical Center,
Minneapolis, Minnesota

The proper use of local anesthesia is a critical factor in the practice of dermatologic surgery. When good technique and the appropriate agents are used, pain can be minimized, which in turn dramatically affects how the patient reacts to the procedure and how the outcome is perceived. Attention to the details of local anesthesia can therefore be just as important as the procedure.

LOCAL ANESTHETICS

Ideally, local anesthetics should have a rapid onset of action, and the duration of anesthesia should be long enough to allow completion of the procedure. It is important to be familiar with the chemical structures of common anesthetic agents and how minor modifications affect their clinical efficacy. The chemical structures of most local anesthetics have many general properties in common. There are two chemical domains: a hydrophilic end that usually consists of a secondary or tertiary amine and a hydrophobic end that consists of an aromatic residue. They are linked by either an ester or an amide group. This linkage is important, affecting the functional properties of the anesthetic (Table 1). Ester linkages are readily degraded in the plasma by esterases, and thus are rapidly inactivated, resulting in a shorter duration of action. Amide linkages are less readily hydrolized in tissue, so they remain intact longer and are more likely to be excreted without enzymatic alteration and inactivation.

Ester-linked local anesthetics are exemplified by procaine, which has the following chemical structure:

$$H_2N-\langle\bigcirc\rangle--\overset{O}{\underset{}{C}}-\overset{}{\underset{}{O}}-CH_2-CH_2-N\overset{C_2H_5}{\underset{C_2H_5}{}}\ ----\ HCl$$

Table 1 Classes of Local Anesthetics

Ester	Amide
Procaine	Lidocaine
Tetracaine	Mepivacaine
Benzocaine	Dibucaine
Cocaine	Bupivacaine
	Etidocaine

Amide-linked local anesthetics are exemplified by lidocaine, which has this structure:

The salt form of the anesthetic is soluble in water and stable, so most commercial preparations are bonded with hydrochlorides. The active molecules diffuse through tissue to the nerves. At the nerve cell membrane, as the lipid-soluble base, it dissociates to the active cation form that is responsible for causing the nerve conduction carbon atoms joining the linkage group to the amine (hydrophilic) tail to increase fat and decrease water solubility. Both potency and toxicity increase. But precipitation goes up. Thus, a balance between one and three carbon atoms seems to be ideal.

The pH of the ambient solution and tissue is important in determining anesthetic action. Alkalinization of the solution in which the anesthetic is dissolved speeds the onset of action but also can result in precipitation of the base. Commercial local anesthetics are thus usually buffered. The inflammatory response surrounding an infected site acidifies the tissue, which in turn impairs the clinical effectiveness of anesthetics. This explains the clinical phenomenon of reduced benefit of local anesthesia when injected into infected tissue, such as when one is draining an abscess. In addition, because of the important role of pH, it is imperative that caution be used when mixing other solutions with local anesthetics. The anesthetic action may be impaired by injudicious use of a mixed solution in which the pH is altered by the additive.

Local anesthetics diffuse through the tissue to the nerves and then pass through the nerve cell membrane to block electrical conduction. Smaller nerves, such as C-fibers that carry pain, are more easily anesthetized than the larger A-fibers that carry touch and deep pressure. Cold and warmth are transmitted by intermediate-sized fibers. A resting nerve is less susceptible to the action of local anesthetics, since electrical conduction enhances the penetration of the molecule to the active site. Light stimulation of the site just before injection of the anesthetic may speed the effectiveness of the injection and can be used to distract the patient when inserting the needle.

The duration of action of the local anesthetic can be prolonged by the addition of a vasoconstrictor, which slows capillary circulation at the site and prevents the outward diffusion of anesthetic. In addition to prolonged action, the systemic toxicity is reduced. The slower absorption allows the amount in circulation to be kept low by continued inactivation. Epinephrine is generally used and should be diluted to the minimally effective level. This avoids the systemic and local toxicity associated with this class of drugs. Restlessness, tachycardia, palpitations, and chest pain are the systemic effects that can result from excessive use of vasoconstrictors. The relative hypoxia that results locally can delay wound healing. This is a particular problem when dealing with areas that have limited collateral circulation such as the fingers and toes. Most local anesthetics have vasodilating activity that can be balanced by the vasoconstrictive agent added to the anesthetic. Cocaine is an exception, having intrinsic vasoconstrictive action.

Types

There are four clinically distinct methods by which local anesthesia can be given: local tissue infiltration, nerve block, intravenous regional block (Bier), and topical application.

Local Tissue Infiltration

This is the primary technique used by dermatologic surgeons, and lidocaine is the agent most commonly used. Lidocaine is available in concentrations of 0.5–2% and is supplied with or without epinephrine. Its onset of action is very rapid, and it has an intermediate duration of anesthesia, ranging from 1 to 2 hr depending upon the vascularity of the site, the presence of a vasoconstricting agent, and other local factors. Metabolism by the liver is rapid, and the unchanged drug and its metabolites are excreted by the kidneys. The half-life of lidocaine in plasma is 1½–2 hr, but that is prolonged twofold or more in the presence of liver dysfunction. Thus, liver disease in the patient may necessitate dosage adjustment. Renal dysfunction, on the other hand, has less effect on lidocaine's metabolism.

The longer-acting local anesthetics such as bupivacaine and etidocaine are particularly useful if a prolonged or repetitive procedure is contemplated. Fewer injections result in less tissue trauma and pain. If the hemostatic effect of the vasoconstrictive agent is required, a shorter-acting agent such as lidocaine is used because of the limited duration of vasoconstriction. The onset of vasoconstriction from epinephrine is slower (15–20 min) than the onset of the anesthetic action of the lidocaine. Thus, some delay may be necessary for the full action of the epinephrine to be present before the surgery can begin.

Two types of pain are caused by giving local anesthetics: the "sharp" entry of the needle into the skin and the "burning" caused by distention of the tissue by the anesthetic. Both can be reduced by careful technique. First, and most important, a small (30-gauge) needle should be used. A slow insertion has been recommended, but a rapid needle penetration into tensed skin area along with distractive stimulation is most effective. The patient should be prepared for the needle, but confident distraction, such as conversation, is helpful as well.

The injection of the anesthetic, however, should be as slow as is practical; one should slowly advance and withdraw the needle. A dermal wheal gives immediate anesthesia, whereas subcutaneous injection requires some time for diffusion of the lidocaine to take place. Individual carpules of lidocaine are available, which can be heated to body temperature to reduce the pain of injection. Needle pricks to test the effectiveness of the anesthesia should be used sparingly since skin trauma results, which can be painful postoperatively. When advancing the needle, avoid intramuscular injection since toxicity may result. If an injection about the face is given intravascularly, it may be forced retrograde into the central nervous system and result in an immediate seizure. Aspiration to test for intravascular location of the needle is not as reliable with a 30-gauge needle as with a 27- or 25-gauge needle. Thus, if a perivascular injection is being given, it may be best to initiate local anesthesia with the smallest needle to reduce pain and then change to a larger one to avoid intravascular injections.

Nerve Block Anesthesia

Large areas of skin can be safely anesthetized using a small amount of anesthetic agent when one considers the anatomic distribution of sensory nerves and uses a nerve block (Fig. 1). There is less danger of anesthetic overdose, and such blocks often provide longer anesthesia and cause less tissue disturbance, allowing for better evaluation of cutaneous landmarks. The most com-

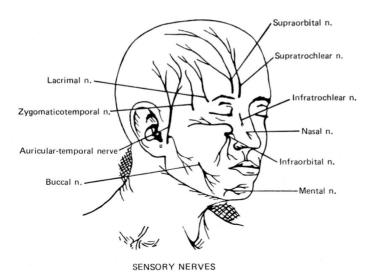

SENSORY NERVES

Figure 1   Distribution of facial sensory nerves amenable to nerve block anesthesia. (Courtesy of Ronald G. Wheeland, M.D.)

mon agents used are lidocaine, mepivacaine, bupivacaine, etidocaine, procaine, and chlorprocaine (Table 2). Higher concentrations of the agent are often used since a smaller volume is injected than in infiltration anesthesia. Epinephrine is used to prolong the anesthetic effect and slow absorption from the injected sites. Digital blocks, however, are usually used without epinephrine since there is some danger of anesthetic-induced vasospasm.

The method of injection differs somewhat from local infiltration. A small-diameter needle (30-gauge) should be selected and a small dermal wheal raised to initiate the block. Then a larger-diameter needle (25–27 gauge) is used to complete the block. The larger needle is used to avoid intravascular injection more accurately, since sensory nerves are usually accompanied by vessels. Systemic toxic reactions can occur from accidental intravascular injection. Hematomas can occur following nerve blocks and have caused permanent nerve damage. The needle is advanced to the desired site and depth, and 5–20 ml of anesthetic is infiltrated slowly while the needle is withdrawn. Five to 10 min are usually necessary for the block to become effective since diffusion into the nerve is required.

One should not attempt to inject directly into a foramen or the nerve trunk itself, since nerve damage can result with persistent radiating pain in the innervated areas. A shallow bevel-type needle is preferred over the long bevel type, since there is less likelihood of trauma to the nerve. If the needle touches the nerve, paresthesia will occur in the peripheral distribution of the nerve, and that can be used as an indication of needle position. It is uncomfortable, however, and should be relied upon only in relatively calm, stoic patients. The dermatologic surgeon should be familiar with the anatomy of the major sensory innervation of the facial skin. The nerves that can be safely and easily blocked are listed in Table 3 and Figure 1. Ankle and digital blocks are also useful.

Intravenous Regional Anesthesia (Bier Block)

This technique is useful for procedures on the hand or foot. It gives regional anesthesia while providing hemostasis with a low incidence of complications. An intravenous line is placed into

Table 2 Clinical Characteristics of Local Anesthetics

Anesthetic	Type	Uses	Concentration (%)	Onset	Duration	Max. single dose
Lidocaine (Xylocaine)	Amide	Infiltration	0.5, 1.2	Rapid	1–1½ hr	2 mg/lb
		Nerve block	1, 2			3 mg/lb with epi
		Topical ointment	5			
		Viscous	2			
Mepivacaine (Carbocaine)	Amide	Infiltration	1	3–20 min	2–2½ hr	400 mg[a] or 5–6 mg/kg
		Nerve block	1, 1.5, 2			
Dibucaine (Nupercaine)	Amide	Topical cream	0.5			1 oz/24 hr
		Topical ointment	1			
Bupivacaine (Marcaine)	Amide	Infiltration	0.025	2–10 min	Up to 7 hr	175 mg
		Nerve block[b]				225 mg with epi
						400 mg/24 hr
Etidocaine (Duranest)	Amide	Infiltration	1, 1.5	3–5 min	5–10 hr	400 mg or 8 mg/kg with epi or 300 mg or 6 mg after epi
Procaine (Novocain)	Ester	Infiltration	1, 2	Slow	30–45 min	500 mg
						600 mg with epi
Tetracaine (Cetacaine)	Ester	Topical spray	2	Rapid (30 sec)	Short	20 mg
						2-sec spray
(Pontocaine)		Spinal anesthesia	1	Rapid	2–3 hr	15 mg
Benzocaine (Anbesol)	Ester	Topical gel	6.3	Rapid	Short	
		Topical liquid				
(Chloraseptic)		Lozenges	5 mg	Rapid	Short	1/hr, 12/day
(Hurricaine)		Topical aerosol	20	Rapid	Short	
Cocaine	Ester	Topical solution	4, 10	2–10 min	10–30 min	150 mg
Chlorprocaine	Ester	Infiltration	1, 2	Rapid	1–2 hr	600 mg
		Nerve block	1, 2	Rapid		750 mg with epi

[a]Healthy, unsedated normal-sized adult.
[b]Not recommended for intravenous regional anesthesia (Bier block).

Table 3 Minor Nerve Blocks Useful in Cutaneous Surgery

Nerve	Site of block	Site of sensory innervation
Supraorbital	Above eyebrow in line with pupil (suborbital notch)	Forehead and scalp to the vertex
Supratrochlear	Above eyebrow approx. 2 cm medial to suborbital nerve	Midline forehead and scalp to the vertex
Infraorbital	4–6 mm below the midpoint of lower orbital margin, in line with the pupil (infraorbital foramen)	Lower eyelid, medial cheek and lateral nose to the upper lip; also maxillary gingiva, mucosa, cuspids, bicuspids, and maxillary incisor teeth
Mental	Midmandible, in line with pupil, between the bicuspid teeth just below their root apices (mental foramen)	Chin and lower lip including the mucous membrane and mandibular incisor teeth
Infratrochlear	Medial orbit, bridge of nose, 1 cm above medial canthus over nasal bone	Inner canthus, medial bulbar conjunctiva, and lacrimal sac
Nasalis	Junction of nasal bones and upper lateral cartilages	Nasal tip and supratip
Greater auricular, anterior cervical, lesser occipital	Posterior margin of sternocleidomastoid muscle	Neck and inferior ear
Auricular-temporal	Anterior to the tragus	Temporal scalp and superior ear

the distal part of the extremity to be blocked, and an extension line is attached. A pneumatic tourniquet is placed on the extremity. The extremity is raised to enhance venous drainage, and a firm elastic bandage is wrapped around the extremity from distal to proximal to evacuate the venous system. The proximal tourniquet is then inflated to approximately 50 cm above systolic blood pressure to prevent vascular refilling and the elastic bandage is removed. Local anesthetic is then injected via the intravenous catheter to fill the vascular system using a low concentration (0.5% lidocaine), giving 50–100 ml. Care must be taken when calculating the volume to avoid systemic toxicity when the tourniquet is released. The onset of anesthesia is rapid, occurring within 5–10 min.

The tourniquet can cause discomfort, so after anesthesia is obtained, a distal tourniquet may be inflated. It will be over an area of anesthesia and will not be felt. The proximal tourniquet can then be released.

The duration of anesthesia is approximately 1 hr. To end the block, the tourniquet is simply released. If a large volume has been used, the tourniquet can be briefly released and then reinflated to slow systemic absorption of the entire load of anesthetic agent. Systemic toxicity is rare if caution is used. Bradycardia can sometimes be detected, as well as transient asystole.

Topical Anesthesia

Pain from local injections may be reduced, and you may gain the confidence of anxious patients with the use of topical anesthetic. It is applied only to mucous membranes since topical anesthetics are not absorbed through an intact stratum corneum. Newer topical anesthetics (i.e., EMLA) are being developed in other countries and may soon be available for minor dermatologic surgical procedures. The five agents most widely used include lidocaine, dibucaine, tetracaine, benzocaine, and cocaine. They come in a variety of forms including solutions, creams, ointments, jellies, aerosols, and suppositories. In addition, proparacaine and tetracaine are used on the eyes to provide topical anesthesia to the mucous membranes of the sclera and conjunctiva. The onset of action of 0.5% proparacaine (Opthane) is rapid and has a duration of up to 30 min. This is particularly useful when treating eyelid lesions. Caution should be used since the anesthetized cornea is subject to trauma, and so the eye should be patched to prevent the patient from inadvertently rubbing it while it remains anesthetized.

For minor procedures such as snipping off small skin tags or curetting small seborrheic keratoses, anesthesia may not be necessary, provided that the instruments are sharp and the surgery done quickly. Skin refrigerants are useful to obtain temporary anesthesia while also causing the skin to become very firm, allowing for better curettage. Several types are available, including ethyl chloride, trichlorofluoromethane, dichlorodifluoromethane, and dichlorotetrafluoroethane.

The spray is directed toward the lesion on the skin from a distance of 4–12 inches and continued until the area turns white. The anesthesia is brief, lasting only a minute or so, and therefore it is useful to have an assistant apply the spray. This is particularly useful for minor procedures such as incising and draining furuncles and removing small growths. This anesthesia is also used for dermabrasion. There is some discomfort while thawing and, if excessively used, there may be cryonecrosis with delayed healing. Ethyl chloride is highly flammable and therefore should never be used when ignition is possible. Inhalation of the vapor should be minimized; ethyl chloride is a general anesthetic.

An ice cube held against the skin for several minutes will provide temporary reduction of painful stimuli and can be used to reduce the pain of local infiltration. Crushed ice in a plastic bag has the same effect and can be used over a wider area. It is particularly useful to reduce pain associated with argon laser treatment of hemangiomas, and no further anesthetic is required.

Toxicity

Most local anesthetics currently in use combine low tissue toxicity and negligible nerve damage with a low systemic toxicity. The possibility of systemic toxicity must be kept in mind, however, since all local anesthetics are eventually absorbed into the circulation from their site of local injection or application. This is important when large amounts are used or a particularly vascular area is treated, such as ring block for scalp reduction.

Certain toxic or allergic reactions are possible, however. They range from toxic cardiovascular or central nervous system reactions due to excessive systemic absorption of the medication to allergic skin reactions, ranging from contact dermatitis or hives resulting from allergic sensitivity to the agents, preservatives, or vasoconstrictors added to the solutions.

Systemic reactions are generally due to high plasma levels of the anesthetic agent. High levels may be due to any one of several causes, such as giving an excessive dose, rapid drug absorption, intravascular injection, or slowed detoxification and excretion secondary to liver disease.

Central Nervous System

Central nervous system reactions begin as excitatory phenomena and then become depressant. Excitatory signs may be minimal, and drowsiness is often an early indication of high plasma levels. Lightheadedness and nervousness may progress to confusion and dizziness, and even convulsions, unconsciousness, and respiratory depression. Respiratory depression requires prompt oxygen administration and assisted ventilation, if necessary. Acidosis and hypercarbia both decrease the threshold for induction of seizures by local anesthetic agents. If seizures occur and persist, they should be treated with intravenous benzodiazepam (Valium).

Cardiovascular

Cardiovascular side effects of high plasma levels begin with bradycardia and hypotension, which can progress to cardiovascular collapse and cardiac arrest. Hypoxia, acidosis, and hypercarbia all increase the depressant effect of local anesthetics. Support of the cardiovascular system includes intravenous fluids and vasopressors such as epinephrine or ephedrine. Cardiopulmonary resuscitation (CPR) should begin if cardiac or pulmonary arrest occurs. Dialysis, aimed at removing the excessive drug, is of negligible value. The more potent agents such as bupivacaine and etidocaine exhibit a higher degree of cardiovascular toxicity, and must be used with more caution.

Allergic Reactions

Systemic allergic reactions range from morbilliform rashes to itching, urticaria, wheezing, and, rarely, anaphylactic reactions. While local anesthetic agents are known to cause allergic reactions, preservatives in the multiple-dose vials such as methyl or prophylparaben can be the cause. In addition, lidocaine solutions with epinephrine may contain sodium metabisulfite, which may cause an anaphylactic reaction.

Vasovagal Reaction

The most commonly encountered systemic side effect is the vasovagal reaction. The patient becomes pale and diaphoretic, complains of lightheadedness, and may lose consciousness. The episode is brief, but must be quickly differentiated from a toxic or allergic reaction to the anesthetic agent, or myocardial infarction. It is most important that the vital signs be monitored. The pulse remains slow and regular, while the blood pressure is normal. Respirations remain unobstructed with no wheezing, as might be encountered in an allergic reaction. There is no loss of urinary or fecal continence or tonic-clonic movements as would be seen in a seizure. The treatment for these reactions consists of keeping the patient supine or in the Trendelenburg position, preventing a fall in which serious injury might result, and giving reassurance as the patient is gradually allowed to sit up.

INHALATION ANALGESIA

The administration of a general anesthetic requires special training and competence and will not be discussed here. However, analgesia and sedation can be obtained by administering subanesthetic concentrations of the anesthetic gases. The inhalation route of administration has the distinct advantage that the effects can be rapidly reversed and the dose titrated to the desired level of analgesia. It is particularly useful in anxious patients, especially children or those whose site of surgery is difficult to block locally.

Nitrous oxide is a particularly useful agent, being powerful but noninflammable and nontoxic. Many patients have become familiar with it, having received it to undergo dental work. It produces sedation and relaxation as well as elevation of the pain threshold and higher pain tolerance. Breathing 20% nitrous oxide produces analgesia equivalent to giving a narcotic, and at 80% most patients will become unconscious. If given alone in high concentrations, there is a danger of hypoxia. Concentrations between 10 and 60% mixed with oxygen can be safely administered by a variety of methods. Pregnant women and patients with obstructive pulmonary disease should not be given this form of analgesia.

The route of administration determines the efficiency of the system in delivering the gas to the patient. Nasal prongs deliver only 19% of the present concentration, a rebreathing mask deliver 34%, and a nonrebreathing mask delivers 95%. A patient-controlled method for self-administration has been developed so that when the patient becomes too sedated, he or she will be unable to continue taking the anesthetic and thus limit the amount received.

There must be a trained assistant present to monitor the patient and to observe for side effects. Minor side effects are common, occurring in as many as 20% of patients. They include nausea or vomiting, dizziness or lightheadedness, and excitement. Patients who are to receive nitrous oxide should be screened for possible vitamin B_{12} deficiency, since there may be an interaction resulting in the precipitation of neurologic disease. Avoid overtreatment with nitrous oxide, since loss of the gag reflux may result in aspiration.

The onset of action of nitrous oxide is rapid, and its effects are likewise rapidly terminated after administration is discontinued. Thus, there is little danger as long as the patient is closely observed. Some postanesthesia recovery observation is required after nitrous oxide is given to be sure that its effects have cleared before the patient is dismissed from the surgery area.

BIBLIOGRAPHY

Local Anesthesia

Allen ED, Elkington AR. Local anesthesia and the eye. *Br J Anaesth* 1980;52:689–694.

Bernstein G. Surface landmarks for the identification of key anatomic structures of the face and neck. *J Dermatol Surg Oncol* 1986;12(7):722–726.

Boberg-Ans J, Barner SS. Neural blockade for ophthalmologic surgery. In *Neural Blockade*. MJ Cousins, PC Bridenbaugh, eds. Philadelphia, JB Lippincott, 1980, pp. 443–462.

Garber JG. Neural blockade for dental, oral and adjoining areas. In *Neural Blockade*. MJ Cousins, PC Bridenbaugh, eds. Philadelphia, JB Lippincott, 1980, pp. 426–442.

Hanke CW, O'Brian JJ, Solow EB. Laboratory evaluation of skin refrigerants used in dermabrasion. *J Dermatol Surg Oncol* 1985;11:45–49.

Kennedy BR, Duthie AM, Parbrook GD, et al. Intravenous regional analgesia: An appraisal. *Br Med J* 1965;1:954–957.

Kew MC, Lowe JP. The cardiovascular complications of intravenous regional anesthesia. *Br J Surg* 1971;58:179.

Moore DC. *Regional Block*, 4th ed. Springfield, IL, Charles C Thomas, 1965.

Panje WR. Local anesthesia of the face. *J Dermatol Surg Oncol* 1979;5(4):311–315.

Schurman DJ. Ankle block anesthesia for foot surgery. *Anesthesiology* 1976;44:348.

Selander D, Dhuner KG, Lundborg G. Peripheral nerve injury due to injection needles used for regional anesthesia. *Acta Anesthesiol Scand* 1977;21:182.

Selander D, Edshage S, Wolff T. Paresthesia or no paresthesia? Nerve lesions after axillary blocks. *Acta Anaesthesiol Scand* 1979;23:27.

Thorn-Alquist AM. Intravenous regional anesthesia. A seven year survey. *Acta Anaesthesiol Scand* 1971; 15:23.

Tucker GT, Boas RA. Pharmacokinetic aspects of intravenous regional anesthesia. *Anesthesiology* 1971; 34:538.

Wooley EJ, Vandam LD. Neurological sequelae of brachial plexus nerve block. *Ann Surg* 1959;149:53.

Inhalation Analgesia

Dworkin SF, Schubert MM, Chen ACN, et al. Analgesic effects of nitrous oxide with controlled painful stimulae. *J Am Dent Assoc* 1983;107:581–585.

Lichtenthal P, Philip J, Sloss LJ, et al. Administration of nitrous oxide in normal subjects. *Chest* 1977; 72:316–322.

Philip BK, Covino BG. Local and regional anesthesia. In *Anesthesia for Ambulatory Surgery*. BV Wetchler, ed. Philadelphia, JB Lippincott, 1985, pp. 225–274.

Rubin J, Brock-Utne JG, Greenberg M, et al. Laryngeal incompetence during experimental "relative analgesia" using 50% nitrous oxide in oxygen. *Br J Anaesth* 1977;49:1005–1007.

Schilling RF. Is nitrous oxide a dangerous anesthetic for vitamin B_{12} deficient subjects? *JAMA* 1986; 255 (12):1605–1606.

Stewart RD, Paris PM, Stoy WA, et al. Patient-controlled inhalational analgesia in prehospital care: A study of the side-effects and feasibility. *Crit Care Med* 1983;11:851–855.

4

Tumescent Anesthesia

Patrick J. Lillis
University of Colorado Health Sciences Center, Denver, Colorado

INTRODUCTION

The intelligent and efficient use of local anesthesia for soft tissue surgery has been greatly influenced by dermatologists since dermatologic surgery became an integral part of our specialty. Dermatologic surgeons have been at the forefront in pioneering office-based local anesthesia for procedures previously performed in hospital operating rooms under general anesthesia.

During the 1970s and early 1980s there was little incentive for hospital-based surgeons to perform office surgery. Cost containment was not an important issue, and physicians predictably practiced in the manner in which they were trained.

In the early 1970s dermatologic surgery began to play a more prominent role in the specialty of dermatology. Sophisticated surgical training became available in many dermatology residencies and at various dermatology meetings. The dermatologist's anatomical, clinical, and histologic knowledge of the skin placed him or her in a uniquely advantageous position to render appropriate surgical treatment of skin problems.

Dermatologists treat the vast majority of skin cancers in an in-office outpatient setting. Even dermatologists who have acquired hospital surgical privileges rarely treat cases in the hospital. Efficiency, convenience for both doctor and patient, and a lower infection rate are noted as primary reasons to provide office-based surgery. Dermatologic surgeons have now been routinely performing in-office, sophisticated surgical procedures under local anesthesia for more than two decades.

Full-face dermabrasion, for example, has traditionally been considered a general anesthesia procedure when performed by nondermatologists. Dermatologic surgeons, however, have traditionally used a combination of methods (ice-packs, refrigerant sprays, nerve blocks, EMLA, and, now, tumescent anesthesia) to make this an office-based local anesthetic procedure.

In 1986 the most exciting development in the use of local anesthesia for soft tissue surgery was introduced in Philadelphia at the 2nd World Conference for Liposuction Surgery. The tumescent technique allowed liposuction to be performed in an office setting under local anesthesia. Other areas in which tumescent anesthesia is useful will be discussed.

HISTORY OF THE DEVELOPMENT OF THE TUMESCENT TECHNIQUE

The development of the tumescent technique has been the most significant contribution to liposuction surgery since the development of liposuction in Europe in the late 1970s. Dr. Jeffrey Klein is the originator of the tumescent technique. I was influenced by Dr. Klein in the "early days" of the development of the tumescent technique and have been in a position to contribute to the profound implications of Dr. Klein's work. I will convey from my perspective the history of the tumescent technique.

The 2nd World Congress of Liposuction was held in June 1986 in Philadelphia, Pennsylvania. At this meeting Dr. Klein presented the tumescent technique for liposuction surgery. Dr. Klein described a modification of the "wet technique" in which a very large volume of extremely dilute lidocaine/epinephrine solution was injected into subcutaneous tissue to the extent that swelling and firmness occurred.

At this meeting Dr. Klein also unveiled a specially designed device to efficiently infiltrate large quantities of the tumescent solution into the subcutaneous tissue. The "Klein needle," a blunt-tipped, 30-cm-long, 4.7-mm-diameter cannula contains a port into which a 60-cc syringe is inserted. One liter of dilute lidocaine/epinephrine solution is connected to the syringe by an intravenous line. The "needle" is inserted into the same incision site used for introduction of the suction cannula. The lidocaine/epinephrine solution is injected along a pathway in which the suction cannula will follow.

Klein reported that, by injecting a solution of 0.1% lidocaine with 1:1,000,000 epinephrine into 26 patients, he was able to infiltrate a mean lidocaine dose of 1250 mg (18.4 mg/kg), which was more than twice the recommended maximal dose of lidocaine (5–7 mg/kg). Blood lidocaine measurements at 1 hr postinfiltration yielded a mean serum lidocaine level of 0.36 μg/ml (toxicity range begins at approximately 5.0 μg/ml). The highest serum lidocaine level recorded in his patients was 0.614 μg/ml. In Klein's study the mean volume of fat extracted was 915 ml. There was no apparent change in hematocrits measured 48–72 hr postsurgery, indicating a significant decrease in expected blood loss.

Surprisingly, Klein's presentation generated little interest or discussion at this meeting. In retrospect, the lack of interest is understandable. The majority of those attending this conference were hospital-based surgeons trained in performing most procedures under general anesthesia.

Prior to the conference, I performed most of my liposuction surgery under general anesthesia in a hospital setting. Smaller cases were performed in my office with local anesthesia. These cases required a considerable amount of time to obtain adequate local anesthesia with a standard syringe and 25-gauge needle. I immediately realized the potential of the Klein needle for efficient delivery of local anesthetic. Klein's data on low serum lidocaine levels after subcutaneous injection of high doses of lidocaine were both promising and intriguing.

Over the ensuing 14 months I began performing larger-volume liposuction cases in my office using progressively larger doses of lidocaine and periodically checking 30- and 60-min postinfiltration serum lidocaine levels. Results were consistently found to be less than 1 μg/ml, even after greatly exceeding the recommended upper limit of 5–7 mg/kg.

High-volume liposuction cases were still performed under general anesthesia in a hospital operating room, but I now treated moderate-sized cases in my office with a combination of epidural anesthesia supplemented by tumescent anesthesia (for areas superior to those anesthetized by the epidural block). Smaller-volume cases were performed totally by the tumescent technique.

In cases using both epidural block and tumescent anesthesia, there was a striking difference between areas suctioned. The epidural block areas yielded grossly bloody aspirate, while the tumescent areas yielded bright yellow bloodless fat. Realizing the potential for decreased blood loss, I began injecting tumescent solution into areas suctioned in cases performed under general anesthesia. During my first case using tumescent anesthesia with general anesthesia, the anesthesiologist immediately commented on the noticeable absence of blood in the aspirate.

In March 1988, I initiated a study of 20 consecutive patients in which a minimum of 1500 cc of fat was removed to determine serum lidocaine levels and blood loss with the tumescent technique. The results of the study not only confirmed Dr. Klein's work, but showed that much larger doses of lidocaine could be safely administered allowing a larger volume of fat removal.

The average volume of fat removed in this study was approximately 2800 cc. The average amount of lidocaine administered was 66 mg/kg. The average preoperative hematocrit was 40.3 followed by an average one-week postoperative hematocrit of 40.0.

Prior to this study the most complete work on blood loss in liposuction surgery indicated that the average total blood loss (blood in the aspirate plus 3rd space blood loss) in females would decrease the one-week postoperative hematocrit by 0.5 for every 100 cc of aspirate. The predicted decrease in hematocrit in my study, with an average aspirate of 2800 cc, therefore would have been 14. Subsequent clinical experience has confirmed this virtual absence of significant blood loss with liposuction by the tumescent technique.

My study and Klein's "Anesthesia for Liposuction and Dermatologic Surgery" were published in October 1988. At the time of publication we believed the reason we were able to use such large doses of lidocaine was a combination of decreased concentration of lidocaine, vasoconstriction induced by epinephrine, and the relative avascularity of the adipose tissue prevented lidocaine from rapidly entering the bloodstream. We then assumed that we were removing most of the lidocaine during the liposuction process.

At the 1988 International Society of Dermatologic Surgery meeting, a presentation was given by Dr. John Skouge of Johns Hopkins University, who had measured the amount of lidocaine in liposuction aspirate. Skouge noted that only 5% of injected lidocaine was removed with the aspirate. These findings were subsequently confirmed by Bridenstine.

Klein subsequently performed a study in which a small number of patients were infiltrated with tumescent solution and liposuction was not performed. The same patients were later injected with an identical amount of the same solution and liposuction was performed. Blood lidocaine levels were obtained at regular intervals for 24 hr in both situations. Klein felt that the rate of absorption and peak lidocaine levels were a function of concentration of lidocaine and the rate of injection. Lower lidocaine concentration and slower injection would produce delayed and lower peak concentration. His study indicated that blood lidocaine levels peaked at approximately 12 hr, returning to zero by 24 hr. Peak levels were nearly equal whether or not liposuction was performed. These conclusions are consistent with studies showing that only a small amount of injected lidocaine is removed with the aspirate. It also explains why patients are virtually pain-free for the remainder of the postoperative day.

It also became apparent that when large volumes of fluid were injected into the fat 3rd spacing of vascular fluid into the treated areas was prevented. The injected fluid not only prevented 3rd spacing but also was absorbed into the vascular space if needed for fluid replacement. The need for estimating and providing intravenous fluid replacement was therefore eliminated.

An additional unexpected finding was the prolonged anesthesia that resulted with the tumescent technique. Prior to the tumescent technique, liposuction performed under general anesthesia would routinely cause patients to awaken in the recovery room in severe pain, usually with shaking chills.

When I initially used the tumescent technique I did not appreciate the prolonged anesthesia that resulted and would routinely place patients on postoperative narcotic analgesics. Postoperative nausea and vomiting was not uncommon. It was not clear to me whether this was due to rising blood levels of lidocaine or to the narcotic analgesics. Once the 12- to 18-hr duration of local anesthesia was appreciated and postoperative narcotics were no longer given, problems with postoperative nausea were virtually eliminated.

Prior to the development of the tumescent technique, Fournier and others advocated chilling the local anesthetic before injection to induce vasoconstriction, thereby decreasing blood loss. This practice would significantly lower body core temperature, producing shaking chills.

The development of the tumescent technique solved the problem of blood loss. It was noted, however, that even injecting large volumes of fluid at room temperature would frequently produce shaking chills. Heating the tumescent solution to body temperature, however, eliminated this problem.

The discovery that the addition of bicarbonate to local anesthetic significantly decreased the pain of injection by neutralizing the pH of lidocaine found immediate application in liposuction surgery. The decrease in discomfort when injecting buffered versus nonbuffered lidocaine was dramatic. Although the rate of infection with liposuction surgery was always quite low, the discovery that buffering lidocaine greatly enhanced its antibacterial properties is probably responsible for the virtual absence of infection with the tumescent technique.

A final serendipitous finding with the tumescent technique was the discovery that by magnifying the subcutaneous compartment by installation of copious amounts of fluid, fat extraction was not only physically easier to perform, but was more accurate and uniform. Ridges and irregularities, which were commonly seen prior to the tumescent technique due to locally excessive fat extraction, were uncommon with the tumescent technique. The ease of fat extraction led to the development of significantly smaller cannulas, further reducing the incidence of these irregularities.

During 1989 and 1990 many dermatologists attempted liposuction by the tumescent technique. My colleagues related in many instances the inability to obtain adequate anesthesia. The magnitude of tumescent solution required for this technique was difficult to comprehend. Once the concept was fully understood and mastered, this method proved a vast improvement over any previous attempts at local anesthesia. It is apparent that liposuction by tumescent technique is a procedure ideally suited to our specialty.

Tumescent technique liposuction became "state of the art" for dermatologic surgeons by 1990. In spite of this, other specialties were basically unaware of the existence or advantages of this approach.

At a 1990 workshop in Houston, Texas, conducted by Dr. Gary Fenno, I performed liposuction by tumescent technique under local anesthesia, extracting more than 6000 cc of nearly bloodless fat. Dr. Howard Tobin and Dr. Richard Dolsky, two prominent leaders in cosmetic surgery, were present. After observing this case, Drs. Tobin, Dolsky, and Fenno adopted the tumescent technique in conjunction with general anesthesia. They were instrumental in spreading the word to other cosmetic surgeons about the advantages of using the tumescent technique whether liposuction was performed by local, epidural, or general anesthesia.

The specialty of plastic surgery remained basically unaware of the tumescent technique until the publication of Pitman's textbook and Replogle's paper. As late as June 1992, Courtiss published "Large Volume Lipectomy—A Retrospective Analysis of 108 Patients." This article was a review of Courtiss's "high-volume" liposuction. "High volume" consisted of more than 1500 ml of aspirate. Courtiss's average volume removed was approximately 2700 cc. My paper, published 4 years earlier, also included patients with extracted fat volume greater than 1500 cc. My average extracted volume was coincidentally also approximately 2700 cc.

All of Courtiss's cases were performed in a hospital setting. Forty-four percent of his patients were admitted for at least one night postoperatively. Two hundred and twenty-seven units of autologous and two units of homologous blood were transfused. His average patient lost 2 L of blood, which accounted for an average of 40% of the total patient blood volume. The percentages of blood aspirate by body area consisted of thighs—30%, hips—35%, abdomen—45%, and flanks—46%. In spite of this significant blood loss, Courtiss concluded that high-volume liposuction was a "safe procedure." Our studies demonstrated total blood loss by tumescent technique to be less than 1%.

In November 1993 Klein published "Tumescent Technique for Local Anesthesia Improved Safety in Large Volume Liposuction." Pitman, in an editorial comment immediately following Klein's paper, acknowledged the distinct advantages of the tumescent technique but questioned the suitability of local anesthesia for most patients. He also stressed that this approach was very "technique-dependent." Recent publications in the plastic surgery literature have described approaches identical to the tumescent technique but have used terms such as "the distention technique" and "the pressure infusion technique."

The principles of tumescent anesthesia developed for liposuction have been proven to enhance hemostasis and prolong anesthesia. These principles can be applied to many other types of soft tissue surgery.

LOCAL ANESTHESIA

Anesthesia for cutaneous surgery may be local, regional, or general. Ideally, the safest method of anesthesia should be selected. General anesthesia carries a greater risk of morbidity and mortality than local anesthesia. Many procedures that were previously carried out under general anesthesia are now performed with regional or local anesthesia. The incidence of mortality caused by general anesthesia has been estimated to be approximately one in every 10,000 operations.

Use of local anesthesia on high-risk cardiac patients substantially reduces the risk of infarction when compared to general anesthesia. When using local anesthesia, the cardiovascular and respiratory systems are not compromised. Ideally, local anesthesia should be used whenever possible. In this regard, the development of tumescent anesthesia has eliminated the need for general and regional anesthesia in many procedures in which large amounts of local anesthetic are necessary.

Lidocaine was first synthesized in Sweden in 1943 under the trade name Xylocaine. It is almost entirely metabolized in the liver by microsomal oxidases by dealkylation. The metabolites monoethylglycinexylidide (MEGX) and glycinexylidide (GX) are then excreted by the kidneys. The plasma half-life for lidocaine is 1.5 hr.

The vasoconstrictor epinephrine shortens the time of onset, increases the depth of anesthesia, and prolongs the duration of anesthesia by increasing the intraneural concentration of the local anesthetic. Decreased blood flow induced by vasoconstrictors slows metabolism of the local anesthetic and decreases bleeding.

It was assumed that the minimum effective concentration of epinephrine was 1:200,000. With tumescent anesthesia, one observes profound prolonged vasoconstriction with concentrations of epinephrine of 1:2,000,000.

The duration of anesthesia is determined by the degree of protein binding of anesthetic to the nerve. The location of injection is important in determining the duration of anesthesia. Vascular areas such as the nose and scalp lead to increased absorption and decreased duration of action. Poorly vascularized areas such as fat are affected much longer by anesthesia.

The two major types of local anesthetic are amides and esters. Esters (e.g., procaine) have a lower toxicity potential than the amides (e.g., lidocaine). Esters have a much higher allergenic potential. The esters are hydrolyzed in the plasma by pseudocholinesterase, and the amides are degraded in the liver. All studies to date with tumescent anesthesia involve only lidocaine. Properties of other local anesthetic agents will not be discussed.

Rapid absorption of epinephrine may lead to increased heart rate, palpitations, and restlessness. Frequently, patients misinterpret the symptoms as an allergic reaction to local anesthetic. These symptoms are more often seen in situations in which concentrated solutions of epinephrine are injected into vascular areas. Although much larger quantities of epinephrine are used in tumescent anesthesia, the combination of dilute concentration and relatively avascular injection sites does not produce such adverse effects.

Cyanosis, sometimes seen after injection of epinephrine with local anesthesia, is exaggerated with tumescent anesthesia. Cyanosis is caused by blood pooling and the high content of deoxygenated hemoglobin. In tumescent anesthesia cyanosis may be so profound as to appear as bruising, particularly in the abdominal area.

Subjective symptoms of lidocaine toxicity may appear at plasma concentrations of 3–5 ng/ml. More serious symptoms may appear with concentrations of 6–10 ng/ml. Levels of 3 ng/ml of lidocaine are sometimes reached with tumescent anesthesia for liposuction surgery. These levels usually occur about 8–14 hr after injection and occasionally cause minor central nervous system subjective symptoms. Studies by Gotti et al. suggest that ingestion of diazepam prior to this "peak period" may decrease the degree of subjective symptoms.

Many factors are involved in determining blood levels of lidocaine. These include the concentration of lidocaine, site of injection, vascularity of the injection site, the presence of epinephrine, and the total dose of lidocaine injected. Theoretically, drugs such as phenytoin, which is metabolized by the liver, may increase the plasma concentration of lidocaine. In reality, the most common reasons for lidocaine toxicity is inadvertent intravascular injection.

The mechanism by which tumescent anesthesia works is not fully understood. It is assumed that the slower rate of absorption of lidocaine is due to four factors: lowered concentration of lidocaine, slower rate of injection, addition of epinephrine, and infiltration of lidocaine into relatively avascular subcutaneous tissue.

The sheer volume of local anesthetic exposes additional lengths of nerves to the local anesthetic, permeating the smallest nerve endings and producing more profound and prolonged anesthesia. There may also be a mechanical effect from the pressure generated by the large volume of fluid expanding the subcutaneous compartment.

A large volume of fluid also permeates the capillaries in much the same way, producing maximal and prolonged vasoconstriction. Many very small vessels and capillaries may be ruptured during liposuction, but maximal vasoconstriction prevents them from leaking red blood cells. Blanching of the treated areas is present even many hours postoperatively. This prolonged vasoconstriction not only prevents capillary oozing for many hours postoperatively, but also is likely to be responsible for sealing off the vessels so that oozing does not occur when vasoconstriction is no longer present.

Although in "blind" liposuction this total lack of capillary oozing is not visually present, it is readily apparent when using tumescent anesthesia for excision of large lesions on the trunk or extremities. The bright yellow fat appears wet and shiny, and the virtual absence of blood is impressive (Figs. 1, 2).

DELIVERY OF TUMESCENT ANESTHESIA

Prior to development of the Klein needle, the infiltration of local anesthetic for liposuction was primarily by laborious injection with multiple needlesticks. Only small cases of liposuction could be done in this manner. Total anesthesia was difficult to achieve. Anesthetizing a small lower

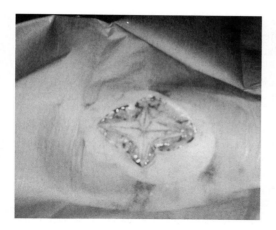

Figure 1   Incisions made for excision of skin prior to liposuction.

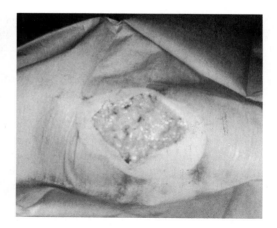

Figure 2   Skin removed. Fat exposed. Note how little blood is present.

abdominal case often required 30–60 min. The introduction of the Klein needle paved the way for efficient delivery of local anesthesia.

An advantage of the Klein needle (Fig. 3) is its ability to precisely inject local anesthetic into designated areas. Fibrous areas such as periumbilical fat or areas of fat that are fibrotic from previous liposuction are somewhat resistant to the passive diffusion of lidocaine. The tapered tip of the Klein needle is useful for "spearing" these fibrous areas and delivering local anesthetic to the exact area in which it is needed.

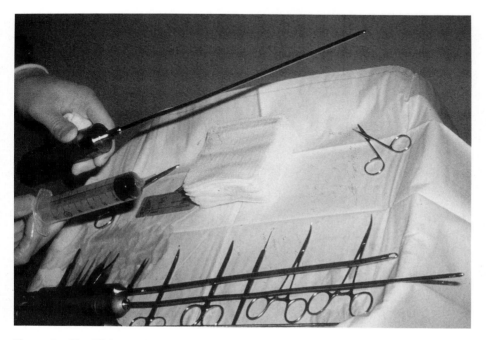

Figure 3   The Klein needle.

The needle is also useful for quickly testing areas for complete anesthesia after the subcutaneous tissue has been anesthetized by other, more efficient devices. When "hot spots" are encountered at this time or later during the procedure, the needle is a very efficient way to completely anesthetize a problem area.

The primary disadvantage of the Klein needle is the need to repeatedly pull back on the 60-cc syringe attached to the port. At least moderate strength and stamina are required to perform this task repeatedly.

Another disadvantage is the size of the injection cannula. Though the tip of the cannula is blunt and tapered, the 4.7-mm outside diameter may cause moderate to significant discomfort when advanced through nonanesthetized subcutaneous tissue. Injecting a small amount of local anesthetic prior to advancing the needle lessens the discomfort. In sensitive areas where fibrous fat is present (i.e., flanks, waist, upper abdomen, medial knees, and in younger leaner patients), the discomfort may be significant.

The cumbersome nature of the Klein needle led to the development of a simpler approach using intravenous tubing directly connected to a small injection cannula. A blood pump is placed around an intravenous bag and pumped up to create adequate pressure for injection (Fig. 4). This system rapidly injects fluid into the tissue. A drawback is the need for two people to operate the system efficiently: one to control the blood pump and another to inject the anesthesia. The rate of injection is also difficult to control. Rapid injection often causes unwanted discomfort in sensitive areas where a slower rate of injection is better tolerated. The system, however, is simple and inexpensive. It is useful for those just beginning to perform liposuction or for those performing liposuction on a limited basis.

A recent innovation has made the blood pump more efficient and easier to use. The Hunstad Handle incorporates a universal luer lock fitting for connection to an intravenous extension. The

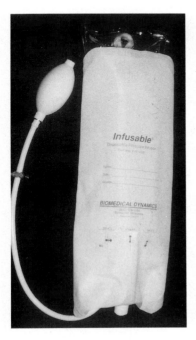

Figure 4   Modified injection system for tumescent anesthesia.

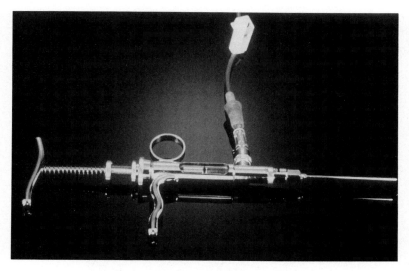

Figure 5   The Percutaneous Stik—a self-refilling system.

front of the handle accepts any luer lock needle. Solution flow is controlled by a simple depression of a button on the handle. Releasing the button stops the solution flow.

Glogau uses the McGhan disposable injection syringe developed to fill tissue expanders. A nondisposable similar self-refilling syringe, the Percutaneous Stik (Fig. 5), remains useful for anesthetizing small areas such as necks and medial knees. It also works well in anesthetizing fibrotic areas.

The "workhorse" injection system for many dermatologic surgeons performing a significant number of liposuction cases is the peristaltic pump. This pump incorporates a closed sterile system where local anesthetic can be injected at a variable rate through injection cannulas of different designs and diameters. The most commonly used peristaltic pump is the Klein Pump (Fig. 6). The Lamis Pump operates in a similar manner.

The use of the peristaltic pump greatly simplifies and speeds the delivery of local anesthesia, allowing the physician to treat larger cases more efficiently. The pump also simplifies training of assistants in administering the local anesthetic.

OTHER USES OF TUMESCENT ANESTHESIA

The beneficial features of tumescent anesthesia for other soft tissue surgery are apparent. Large doses of local anesthesia can be safely administered, achieving profound hemostasis and prolonged postoperative analgesia.

Tumescent anesthesia changed liposuction from a general anesthetic procedure with significant blood loss to a walk-in/walk-out local anesthetic procedure where blood loss is not a concern. The use of tumescent anesthesia to perform other soft tissue surgical procedures can include facial flap surgery, scalp surgery, facelifts, rhinophyma, hair transplantation, dermabrasion, treatment of axillary hyperhidrosis, ambulatory phlebectomy for large varicose veins, and surgical excision of lipomas or any other soft tissue mass. Although studies have not been done on lidocaine absorption rate when using tumescent anesthesia on the head and neck areas, the total amount of lidocaine used in these locations is typically well below 5–7 mg/kg.

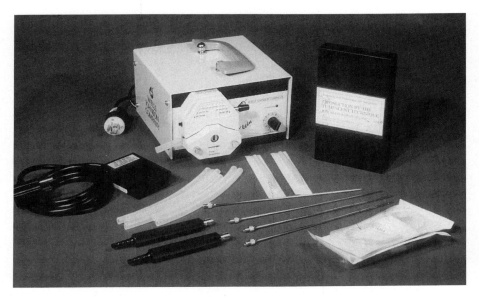

Figure 6 The Klein pump—a peristaltic pump.

In applying the principles of tumescent anesthesia to scalp surgery (scalp flaps, scalp reduction, hair transplantation), the profound hemostasis achieved is of significant benefit. Hydrodissection of the galea from the periosteum facilitates subgaleal undermining in scalp reduction and scalp flaps.

In hair transplantation using plugs, the "tumescence" of donor tissue mimics the common practice of instilling saline into the donor areas prior to harvesting. This creates a more cylindrical plug. The excellent hemostasis improves the surgical field of vision and decreases blood splatter if a power punch is used. In the recipient area, the "tumescence" of tissue provides a more efficient removal of discarded bald plugs. Total anesthesia lasts hours longer than traditional local anesthesia. Coleman elicited feedback from 10 consecutive hair transplant patients. All had previously undergone hair transplantation with traditional local anesthesia. All preferred tumescent anesthesia.

Tumescent anesthesia provides many advantages when used in facial dermabrasion. The firmness provided by "tumescing" the tissues eliminates the need for cryogens. Cryosurgical preparation of the skin prior to dermabrasion may increase the risk of scarring (especially over the bony prominences), pigmentary disturbances, and profound postoperative swelling and edema.

When tumescent anesthesia is used in rhinophyma or postsurgical dermabrasion of nasal scars and sebaceous skin, dermabrasion is facilitated. The significant hemostasis allows one to effectively dermabrade thick sebaceous skin, eliminating the considerable risk of scarring encountered in electrosurgery. Dermabrasion for acne scarring, wrinkles, actinic damage, and appendageal tumors such as neurofibromas and angiofibromas may also be performed with tumescent anesthesia.

The amount of local anesthetic needed for a facelift and other facial reconstructive procedures is reduced by the use of tumescent anesthesia. Profound hemostasis and prolonged anesthesia allow for a more uneventful and comfortable postoperative course. Risk of hematoma formation is decreased, and there is definite reduction in bruising.

Tumescent anesthesia has revolutionized the treatment of severe axillary hyperhidrosis. Prior to the development of the tumescent technique, severe recalcitrant axillary hyperhidrosis was routinely treated by axillary excision. Postoperative infections were frequent, and hematomas and wound dehiscence were not uncommon. Scar contractures would often limit range of motion at least to a minor degree. Unattractive scars were often a cosmetic problem, especially in female patients.

Liposuction of the axilla after tumescent anesthesia is an efficient simple procedure with a nearly 100% success rate when executed properly. Scars are two to three in number, 1/4 inch or less in diameter, and are well hidden. Infections are almost never encountered, probably due to the bactericidal properties of buffered lidocaine. Recovery is rapid, and scar contracture does not occur. Profound hemostasis virtually eliminates the risk of hematoma formation. Prolonged anesthesia provides for a comfortable postoperative recovery.

Tumescent anesthesia may also be useful in Mohs surgery, especially in large lesions when the amount of local anesthetic that is to be repeatedly injected surpasses the recommended maximum dose of 5–7 mg/kg. Tumescent anesthesia is also useful for raising perichondrium off of the cartilage. Anesthesia ia prolonged, and capillary oozing is lessened.

The use of tumescent anesthesia for ambulatory phlebectomy has recently been described by Seiger et al. Regional or general anesthesia is unnecessary when performing this procedure in this manner. Seiger et al. injected 0.05% lidocaine "through IV tubing into the Lamis TM injection syringe and pumped into the subcutaneous tissue as the blunt-tipped probe is passed directly below the vein and slowly advanced along the length of the vein until the skin surface becomes firm or tumescent." It is likely that tumescent anesthesia will make ambulatory phlebectomy a procedure ideally suited to an office-based dermatologic surgical practice.

Tumescent anesthesia is ideal for removal of any large soft tissue lesion (large congenital nevi, wide excision of melanomas, tattoo removal, etc.). Plastic surgery procedures presently performed under general anesthesia such as abdominal dermolipectomies and breast reduction could be performed under tumescent anesthesia.

It is not entirely clear why tumescent anesthesia works as it does. Dermatologic training provides a unique perspective from which to view cutaneous surgery. It is this unique training that has provided the setting for the development of tumescent anesthesia.

BIBLIOGRAPHY

Albright GA. Cardiac arrest following regional anesthesia with etidocaine or bupivacaine. *Anesthesiol* 1979; 51:285

Allen GD. Nitrous oxide-oxygen sedation machines and devices. *J Am Dent Assoc* 1974; 88:611

Bieter RN. Applied pharmacology of local anesthetics. *Am J Surg* 1936; 34:500

Bridenstein J. Letter to the editor. *J Dermatol Surg Oncol* 1989; 15(7):775–776.

Coleman WP III, Klein JA. Use of tumescent technique for scalp surgery, dermabrasion and soft tissue reconstruction. *J Dermatol Surg Oncol* 1992; 18:130–135

Courtiss EH, Choucair RJ, Donelan MB. Large volume suction lipectomy: An analysis of 108 patients. *Plast Reconstr Surg* 1992; 89:1080–1082

Dolsky R, Fetzek J, Anderson R. Evaluation of blood loss during liposuction surgery. *Am J Cosm Surgery* 1987;4:257–261.

Gotta AW, et al. Diazepam versus midazolam in the prevention of lidocaine toxicity in rats. *Anesth Analg* 1989; 68:S1–S321

Karlsson E, Collste R, Rawlins MD. Plasma levels of lidocaine during combined treatment with phenytoin and procainamide. *Eur J Clin Pharmacol* 1974; 7:455

Klein JA. Anesthesia for liposuction and dermatologic surgery. *J Dermatol Surg Oncol* 1988;14:1124–1132.

Klein J. Tumescent technique. *Am J Cosm Surg* 1987;4:263–267.

Klein JA. Tumescent technique for local anesthesia: Improved safety in large volume liposuction. *J Plas Reconstr Surg* 1993; 92:1085–1098

Klein JA. Tumescent technique for regional anesthesia permits lidocaine doses of 35 mg/kg for liposuction. *J Dermatol Surg Oncol* 1990;16:248–263.

Klingenstrom P, Westermark L. Local effects of adrenalin and phenylalanyl-lysyl-vasopressin in local anesthesia. *Acta Anesthesiol Scand* 1963; 7:131

Lillis PJ, Coleman WP III. Liposuction for treatment of axillary hyperhidrosis. In: Lillis PJ, Coleman WP III, eds. *Dermatologic Clinics: Liposuction* Philadelphia: Saunders, 1990; 8 (3):479–482

Lillis PJ. Liposuction surgery under local anesthesia: Limited blood loss and minimal lidocaine absorption. *J Dermatol Surg Oncol* 1988;14:1145–1148.

Lillis PJ. The tumescent technique for liposuction surgery. In *Dermatologic Clinics: Liposuction.* Philadelphia, Saunders, 1990; 8 (3):439–450

Lunn JN, Mushin WW. Mortality associated with anesthesia. *Anesthesiology* 1982; 37:856

McKay W, Morris R, Mushlin P. Sodium bicarbonate attenuates pain on skin infiltration with lidocaine with or without epinephrine. *Anesth Analg* 1987; 66:572

Metz H III, Gilliland M, Patronella C. Abdominal etching: Differential liposuction to detail abdominal musculature. *Anesth Plas Surg* 1993; 17:287–290

Physician's Desk Reference. Oradell, N.J., Medical Economics Co, Inc., 1989, p. 640.

Pitman G. Editorial comment. *J Plas Reconstr Surg* 1993; 92:1099

Pitman G. Liposuction and Aesthetic Surgery. Textbook Quality Medical Publishing Co., 1993

Promotional material for Dr. Gerald Pitman's videotape. Liposuction and Aesthetic Surgery

Replogle S. Experience with tumescent technique in lipoplasty *Anesth Plas Surg* 1993; 17:205–209

Seiger E, Goldman S, Cohn M. Ambulatory phlebectomy using the tumescent technique for local anesthesia. *J Dermatol Surg* 1995 (April).

Steen PA, Tinker JH, Tarhan S. Myocardial reinfarction after anesthesia and surgery. *JAMA* 1978; 239:25–66

Sung CY, Truant AP. The physiological disposition of lidocaine and its comparison in some respects with procaine. *J Pharmacol Exp Ther* 1954; 112:432

Thompson K, Welykyj S, Massa M. Antibacterial activity of lidocaine in combination with a bicarbonate buffer. *J Dermatol Surg Oncol* 1993; 19:216–220

5

Medical Evaluation and Universal Precautions

Mark R. Balle and Edward A. Krull
Henry Ford Hospital, Detroit, Michigan

Many dermatologic surgical procedures are so uncomplicated that extensive patient evaluation is unnecessary. But physicians should not be lulled into complacency because of the apparent simplicity of the surgery. These procedures include limited cryosurgery, curettage, electrosurgery, punch and saucerization biopsies, and simple excisions. There is a greater need for patient evaluation with more complex procedures such as dermabrasion, hair transplantation, flaps, and grafts. Patient evaluation, appropriate to the surgery, is a necessity to reduce the possibility of surgical complications. This includes laboratory workup when indicated (Table 1). Patient evaluation can be viewed in terms of general considerations, as well as those more relevant to the surgery being contemplated. During the evaluation of the patient, it is also an ideal time to establish a rapport and to discuss possible complications and expectations pertinent to the anticipated surgery. Possible side effects should be documented and be a part of the patient consent form.

GENERAL CONSIDERATIONS: AN EMERGENCY PLAN

Emergencies can occur in physicians' offices at the time of surgery, either completely unrelated to or directly related to some aspect of surgery. Physicians and nurses must be prepared for such problems, first by being trained in cardiopulmonary resuscitation. Basic equipment and supplies such as oxygen, intravenous fluids, and basic drugs for cardiopulmonary resuscitation should be available. Bag-valve devices for respiration avoid the risk of infection due to mouth-to-mouth resuscitation. The physician should be versed in the use of all drugs in the emergency kit. The availability of an emergency service should be known to all of the staff and emergency service phone numbers prominently displayed at the telephone. If the physician is in a multispecialty building, then an emergency plan for the building should be developed utilizing the skills of other practitioners in the office building.

Table 1 Laboratory Evaluation Prior to Dermatologic Surgery

Commonly indicated laboratory tests
  Complete blood count with platelets
  Serum chemistry screen
  Prothrombin time
  Partial thromboplastin time
  Bleeding time
  Electrocardiogram
Laboratory tests indicated in special situations
  Platelet function (aggregation)
  RPR (syphilis)
  HIV (HTLV-III; AIDS)
  Hepatitis B screen (surface Ag, core Ab)
  Zinc levels
  Vitamin A levels
  Vitamin C levels
  Peripheral vascular studies (i.e., Doppler flow, oximetry)
  Soft tissue x-ray
  Cryoglobulins
  Cryofibrinogen

PREVENTION OF EMERGENCIES AND COMPLICATIONS THROUGH PATIENT EVALUATION

In some instances, emergencies can be prevented, or their likelihood greatly reduced, with appropriate evaluation and preparation. Myocardial infarctions and strokes can occur in many situations unrelated to dermatologic surgical procedures. Anaphylaxis and less severe allergic reactions may occur without a previous history of allergy to a medication being administered. However, it is important to undertake whatever steps are possible to reduce the chance of such occurrences.

For even the simplest procedures, it is advisable to establish the general health of the patient, current medications, allergies (especially to medication planned for the procedure), and bleeding tendencies. General questions about allergies, specifically those related to medication that will be used, are a discipline that must be maintained by anyone prescribing or administering medication. No injection should be given without asking such questions. The same discipline should be repeated each time a medication is administered, because patients sometimes forget minor reactions resulting from the last administration of the medication. Allergies should be clearly noted on the patient's chart.

Elicit a history of current medical problems and a list of medications. This may provide significant information about the patient's general health. In fact, this may be more helpful than casually asking about the patient's health. Knowing the medications a patient takes gives insight into his or her general health and also reveals the potential for drug interactions with anesthetics or other agents used during surgery.

Although a history of bleeding diatheses should be elicited for even minor surgical procedures, some coagulopathies will not affect operations in which electrosurgery is used. Aspirin should be avoided for at least 1 week prior to significant surgical operations, and anticoagulants may have to be discontinued for 2 or more days prior to more extensive skin surgery. The bleeding diathesis in some of these circumstances may be controlled by coagulation with electrosurgery or laser surgery.

For even minor surgery, know whether the patient has cardiac valvular disease, prosthetic heart valves, or joint prostheses because of the risk of transient bacteremia, which can result in more serious problems for the patient. For more extensive specialized dermatologic surgery, a more complete patient history, detailed questions relevant to the contemplated procedure, and laboratory assessment may be required. Not only is this preoperative evaluation important to minimize complications, but it helps establish the medical background to help interpret difficulties the patient may have, related or unrelated to the surgery. For complex dermatologic surgery, both a general history and a more procedure-oriented evaluation of the patient is needed.

GENERAL HISTORY

It is unlikely that any medical history evaluation or questionnaire will satisfy every dermatologic surgeon, but all such inquiries should explore elements of general health, allergies, current medications, bleeding tendencies, and wound healing. Gross developed an acronym, HAMM, to serve as a framework for preoperative history-taking. H represents general health, A stands for allergies, the first M for medications, and the second M for miscellany (see Table 2). Gen-

Table 2   Preoperative History

I. Health	II. Allergies
A. Cardiovascular system	A. Atopy
1. Hypertension	1. Atopic dermatitis
2. Angina	2. Seasonal rhinitis
3. Pacemaker	3. Asthma
B. Hematological system	B. Acquired sensitivities
1. Anemia	1. Common drugs by mouth or injection
2. Nosebleed; easy bruising	a. Salicylates
3. Excessive menstrual bleeding	b. Laxatives
C. Respiratory system	c. Antibiotics
1. Bronchial asthma	d. Anesthetics
2. Emphysema	2. Common agents topically applied
3. Chronic cough	a. Mercurials
D. Hepatic system	b. Antibiotics
1. Hepatitis	c. Anesthetics
2. Gallbladder disease	III. Medicines
3. Cirrhosis	A. Drugs taken concurrently
E. Renal system	1. Analgesics
1. Glomerulonephritis	2. Tranquilizers
2. Calculi	3. Antihypertensives
3. Pyelonephritis	4. Anticoagulants
F. Endocrine system	5. Antibiotics
1. Diabetes mellitus	IV. Miscellany
2. Hyperthyroidism	A. Pregnant currently
3. Hypothyroidism	B. Previous surgery
G. Infections	C. Healing and scarring problems
1. Syphilis	D. Psychological problems
2. Impetigo	E. Domestic problems
3. Furunculosis	F. Occupation
4. Herpes simplex	G. Location of residence
5. Hepatitis	H. Financial problems

Source: Gross, 1981.

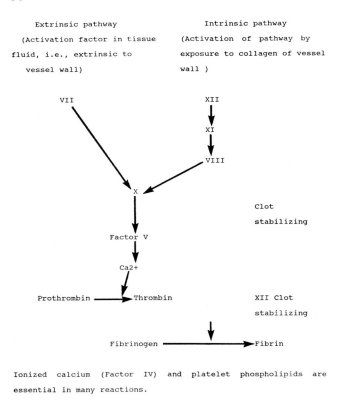

Ionized calcium (Factor IV) and platelet phospholipids are essential in many reactions.

Figure 1 Simplified illustration of the coagulation system.

infection to the risk of complications from antibiotic therapy leads many to use prophylactic antibiotics for dental conditions in only special circumstances such as acute dental infections, chronic bacteremia, predisposing conditions, or evidence of prior infection in the joint. The incidence of delayed infection in orthopedic implants (i.e., arising at least 3 months or more after the operations) is reported at 0.5–5%. According to Jacobson and Matthews, the incidence of delayed infection of a total hip replacement is about 1%, and possibly 0.04% are related to bacteremia from dental procedures. Gram-positive organisms accounted for 72% of the organism cultures, with *Staphylococcus epidermidis* being twice as common as *Staphylococcus aureus*. The remaining cultures grew gram-negative organisms, an increasing percentage over the 10 years of study. Aminoglycosides (gentamicin) were considered most effective for the gram-negative organisms; cephalosporins were next most effective, but one half of the gram-negative organisms were resistant. If prophylaxis for dental procedures for patients with joint replacements is indicated, cephalosporins are the agent of choice because they are effective against all but one gram-positive organism and about 50% of the gram-negative organisms. The increasing number of late gram-negative infections in joint replacements may require reconsideration of combination therapy for both gram-positive and gram-negative organisms.

Patients with valvular heart disease, prosthetic heart valves, and synthetic devices in the arterial circulation, as in vascular bypass, are at risk from hematogenous seeding of bacteria. The recommendation for prevention of bacterial endocarditis is clearly antibiotic prophylaxis for dental, genitourinary, and gastrointestinal procedures. The use of antibiotic prophylaxis for patients with mitral valve prolapse is less clear than for other valvular disease and may be advised only for those having an associated murmur. Institution of antibiotic prophylaxis in mitral valve prolapse, where the risks are less certain, is more inconsistent. The opinion of local experts is important when deciding whether to use antibiotic prophylaxis for mitral valve prolapse.

The use of antibiotic prophylaxis in skin surgery for prevention of bacterial endocarditis or prosthetic joint infection is less clear. About one third of patients develop transient bacteremia following a 10-min massage of staphylococcal furuncles. Sabetta and Zitelli found a maximum 8.4% incidence of bacteremia at a 95% level of statistical significance during surgery of non-infected but ulcerated tumors of the skin; no bacteremia was observed in skin surgery of tumors with intact skin surfaces. They recommended antibiotic prophylaxis for patients in whom skin surgery was contemplated on eroded but not infected skin lesions for only those patients with an unusually high risk of endocarditis, such as those with prosthetic heart valves or a systemic-pulmonary shunt. Prophylactic therapy should be directed toward staphylococci and streptococci with cephalosporin or dicloxicillin (1–2 g 1 hr preoperatively and 500 mg every 6 hr for one to two doses). In patients with heart valve replacement of less than 60 days' duration, vancomycin is suggested because of the increased incidence of diphtheroid infections. Since the incidence of transient bacteremia may be higher for infected skin than noninfected ulcerated skin, it might be preferable to use the same guidelines in skin surgery as for oral surgical prophylaxis. In fact, the American Heart Association Committee report recommended chemoprophylaxis to prevent endocarditis for surgery on any infected or contaminated tissue. Antibiotic prophylaxis for skin surgery in patients with joint replacement has not been established; but orthopedists often recommend antibiotic prophylaxis in those patients, especially when working on infected skin.

WOUND HEALING

Examination and history of excessive scar formation from trauma and surgery should be assessed. Keloids are more common in blacks and dark-skinned persons and may be familial, both autosomal recessive and dominant, especially when severe or when more than one are present.

Wound healing may be adversely affected by corticosteroids and deficiencies of zinc and vitamins A and C. A clinical effect on wound healing is usually not noted with corticosteroids unless given in repeated dosages at a level of 40 mg of prednisone or more and started prior to the surgery. Prednisone at 30 mg per day has a minor effect on the tensile strength of wounds, and 10 mg or less probably has no effect.

Antineoplastic and immunosuppressive agents have variable effects on wound healing. Actinomycin, bleomycin, or BCNU cause greater impairment than does vincristine, methotrexate, 5-fluorouracil, or cyclophosphamide. Most of these drugs have little significant effect on minor dermatologic surgical procedures.

Penicillamine at clinical dosages decreases wound tensile strength. Colchicine may have antifibroblastic properties. Diphenylhydantoin may stimulate healing wounds, as may zinc and vitamins A and C.

A number of skin and internal medical conditions are associated with decreased wound healing or with difficulty in handling tissue during the operation. These include chronic illnesses (liver, kidney, hematopoietic, cardiovascular, autoimmune diseases, and malignancy), endocrine disorders (diabetes mellitus and Cushing's syndrome), systemic vascular diseases (vasculitis), and connective tissue disease (Ehlers-Danlos syndrome).

Smoking can impair wound healing. It can be an important cause of flap necrosis, especially where there is extensive undermining. Patients should be encouraged to stop smoking several days prior to surgery and for 3 weeks after when flap surgery is anticipated. Admittedly, this may be a difficult task.

SPECIAL PROCEDURES AND CONSIDERATIONS

The degree of general patient evaluation is to some extent dependent on the complexity of surgery. For example, a small saucerization biopsy probably requires little more than a few questions about current health, allergies with special attention addressed to the anesthetic planned, bleeding diatheses, current medication, and nature of scar formation.

However, more extensive procedures such as dermabrasion, hair transplantation, flaps, and nail surgery may require more comprehensive evaluation. In addition to the general medical history, inquiry should be specifically directed to special aspects of the procedure and the site of surgery (i.e., dermabrasion, hair transplants, toenail surgery).

DERMABRASION

Herpes simplex may disseminate on the denuded skin of a dermabraded site during the healing phase. Acyclovir has been used as treatment and also to prevent this occurrence in patients with a history of recurrent herpes simplex. Acyclovir is given 1–2 days prior to dermabrasion and continued during the time of healing.

Skin refrigerants are used in dermabrasion for anesthesia, hemostasis, and to establish a firm surface. Cryopathies and diseases associated with cryopathy should be investigated in the medical history. The author tests for cryoglobulin and cryofibrinogen levels prior to dermabrasion. In addition, some of the refrigerants have been associated with increased scarring. This may be due to the loss of natural depth landmarks and also because the surgeon freezes or dermabrades too deep. The margin of safety of a new agent, Cryoesthesia (–30 to –60; containing Freon 11 and 12), is considered small and felt to present a hazard to dermabrasion. Skin refrigerants with pure Freon 12 (dichlorodifluoromethane) or in high percentages in mixtures with Freon 11 (trichlorofluoromethane) are colder and increase the risk of scarring with dermabrasion due to cryonecrosis. Products that are less cold (dichlorotetrafluoroethane [Freon 114, Frigiderm] or mixtures of Freon 114 with ethylchloride [Fluoro Ethyl]) are less likely to cause this complication.

Isotretinoin has been associated with unusual postoperative scarring after dermabrasion, despite intervals as long as 6–14 months between discontinuation of the isotretinoin and dermabrasion. The statistical incidence and significance of this relationship has not been established, and the mechanism is not known. These early reports, however, caution against performing dermabrasion on patients who have been previously treated with isotretinoin.

A personal and family history of a bleeding diathesis or of drugs affecting hemostasis should be identified. Patients with altered wound healing in terms of excessive or inadequate scar formation present hazards for dermabrasion.

HAIR TRANSPLANTATION

The main concern for preoperative evaluation of patients to undergo hair transplantation is bleeding problems. Some become manifest only when stressed with hair transplantation of the scalp, a highly vascular field, in which the donor sites are frequently not sutured. Therefore, a careful personal and family history of bleeding diatheses should be elicited as well as evaluating drugs that affect hemostasis, such as aspirin. Since bleeding disorders have been unmasked by hair transplantation, especially platelet dysfunction and von Willebrand's disease, the authors feel it is preferable to perform the following tests prior to hair transplant surgery: (1) platelet count or estimation, (2) activated partial thromboplastin time, (3) prothrombin time, and (4) bleeding time. A trial hair transplant, with a few plugs, may also identify a bleeding problem.

CRYOSURGERY

For extensive cryosurgery, such as cryoabrasion, evaluate for cryopathies and diseases in which cryopathy more frequently occurs. Measuring cryoglobulins and cryofibrinogens may be valuable, because at times the most serious adverse reactions to cold are in those patients with minimal symptomatology. If cryosurgery is used in acral areas, then Raynaud's phenomenon and other vasospastic or peripheral vascular disease should be assessed.

ELECTROSURGERY

The electromagnetic emission from electrosurgery may interfere with cardiac pacemakers. A false signal generated by electrosurgery may be interpreted as a QRS by a ventricular-inhibited pacemaker. In these circumstances, the pacemaker could remain in the standby mode in the face of cardiac standstill. If the electrosurgical unit is used for 3 sec followed by a pause of 10 sec, probably no more than three ventricular contractions would be missed, while cardiac function and peripheral blood flow would be reinstated while electrosurgery is discontinued. Some have recommended short bursts for 5 sec, with appropriate grounding, monitoring (pulse check), and avoiding work near the heart or pacemaker. The use of a biterminal electrode can more safely direct current flow away from the heart. Some suggest the use of laser surgery for patients with cardiac pacemakers. Today's modern pacemakers are better filtered and shielded. Electrosurgical interference, therefore, is much less of a potential problem than it has been in the past.

TOENAIL SURGERY

The most specific evaluation related to toenail surgery is the adequacy of the peripheral vascular system. Investigation should be directed at assessing peripheral vascular disease such as intermittent claudication or evidence of arteriosclerotic disease in other sites such as the heart or the brain. Peripheral pulses should be palpated before toenail surgery. Cutaneous signs of vascular insufficiency include thin shiny skin, thickened ridged nails, absence of dorsal digital hair, and dependent rubor followed by a pallor with elevation. Appropriate consultation and vascular flow studies may be indicated.

SURGERY IN ANATOMIC DANGER ZONES

Four anatomic areas are commonly referred to as danger zones because the motor nerves in these areas run superficially. These are the superficial temporal, zygomatic, and marginal mandibular branches of the facial nerve, and the spinal accessory nerve as it courses through the posterior triangle of the neck. Damage to these nerves can result in significant motor deficits. Extreme caution should be exercised when considering surgery in these areas. Unnecessary surgery should be avoided. If surgery is necessary, blunt dissection and minimization of incisions is important. Prior to undergoing any surgery, the patient must be made fully aware of the risks and consequences should damage to these nerves occur.

SURGERY NEAR THE EYE

Possible complications that can result when doing surgery near the eye range from ectropion, corneal abrasion, and lacrimal system injury to retrobulbar hemorrhage when performing a blepharoplasty. When doing extensive surgery near the eye, it is wise to have the patient obtain a presurgical eye examination to document visual acuity. If the patient claims to have any change in acuity resulting from the surgery, a comparison between pre- and postsurgical acuity can be helpful. It is also helpful when doing extensive work to have an oculoplastic surgeon readily available should an emergency arise.

UNIVERSAL PRECAUTIONS

Some infected patients may present a risk for the dermatologic surgeon. Berberian and Burnett reported that blood was found spattered from 1 to 29 cm (average 11–15 cm) away from the operating site of electrosurgery, regardless of whether epinephrine was used in the anesthesia. Sheretz et al. found that the active electrode tip retains hepatitis B surface antigen after the tip has been used for electrosurgery. This is not surprising, since the active tip used for high-frequency electrosurgery is not hot, but only a point source of electromagnetic emission. It has not been established whether the hepatitis B surface antigen is transmitted to tissue that has been electrosurgically treated.

The dermatologic surgeon and his or her staff must assume that all patients potentially have hepatitis B or AIDS or other transmissible infection. A series of guidelines that are collectively referred to as universal precautions must be followed whenever there is the potential for contact with blood or other body fluids. Hand washing is the single most effective means of preventing transmission of infection. Gloves should be worn and changed if torn or punctured. Masks and protective eyewear or face shield should be worn if splatter with blood or body fluids is anticipated. Gowns or impermeable aprons should be worn during all procedures likely to cause splashing or soiling from blood or body fluids.

In addition to hand washing and the wearing of gloves, masks, protective eyewear, and gowns, measures must be taken to prevent injury from needles and other sharp objects. All used sharps are considered to be contaminated and therefore must not be bent, broken, or manipulated by hand after use. The recapping of contaminated needles should be avoided. All sharp objects should be placed in a sharps disposal box. No attempt should be made to remove anything from the box.

Emergency equipment that minimizes direct mucous membrane contact should be readily available. Resuscitation devices such as ambu-bags and other ventilation devices should be used instead of mouth-to-mouth resuscitation whenever possible.

All laboratory specimens should be handled with care. When transporting specimens, personnel should wear gloves and wash hands after handling accordingly. Specimens should be transported in proper containers. Waste should be properly disposed in containers and materials appropriately designated for them.

Finally, all new staff employees should receive a formal orientation to universal precautions. Annual educational updates are essential. These guidelines should be modified as necessary to correlate with changing government regulations. Each office should tailor the general guidelines to their own specific setting. Adherence to universal precautions is the only insurance the surgeon and his staff have of minimizing the likelihood of exposure to transmissible infection.

BIBLIOGRAPHY

Amrein PC, Ellman L, Harris WH. Aspirin-induced prolongation of bleeding time and perioperative blood loss. *JAMA* 1981;245:1825–1828.
Berberian BJ, Burnett JW. The potential role of common dermatologic practice technics in transmitting disease. *J Am Acad Dermatol* 1986;15:1057–1058.
Cruess RL, Bickel WS, von Kessler KL. Infections in total hips secondary to a primary source elsewhere. *Clin Orthop* 1975;106:99–101.

Czapek EE, Deykin D, Salzman E, et al. Intermediate syndrome of platelet dysfunction. *Blood* 1978;52:103–113.

Downs JR. Joint replacement and prophylaxis. *J Am Dent Assoc* 1977;94:429.

Dzubow LM. Blood pressure as a parameter in dermatologic surgery. *Arch Dermatol* 1986;122:1406–1407.

Dzubow LM. Histologic and temperature alterations induced by skin refrigerants. *J Am Acad Dermatol* 1985;12;796–810.

Ferraris VA, Swanson E. Aspirin usage and perioperative blood loss in patients undergoing unexpected operations. *Surg Gynecol Obstet* 1983;156:439–442.

Fisher HW. Surgery on patients receiving anticoagulants. *J Dermatol Surg Oncol* 1977;3:210–212.

Goldsmith SM, Leshin B, Owen J. Management of patients taking anticoagulants and platelet inhibitors prior to dermatologic surgery. *J Dermatol Surg Oncol* 1993;19:578–581.

Gross D. On history-taking before surgery. *J Dermatol Surg Oncol* 1981;7:71–72.

Hanke CW, O'Brian JJ, Solow EB. Laboratory evaluation of skin refrigerants used in dermabrasion. *J Dermatol Surg Oncol* 1985;11:45–49.

Hanke CW, Pinski JB, Roenigk HH Jr, Alt TH. Caution: New skin refrigerants. *J Dermatol Surg Oncol* 1984;10:167.

Hanke CW, Roenigk HH Jr, Pinski JB. Complications of dermabrasion resulting from excessively cold skin refrigeration. *J Dermatol Surg Oncol* 1985;11:896–900.

Hickey AJ, MacMahon SW, Wilcken DEL. Mitral valve prolapse and bacterial endocarditis: When is antibiotic prophylaxis necessary? *Am Heart J* 1985;109:431–435.

Hicks PD Jr, Stromberg BV. Hemostasis in plastic surgical patients. *Clin Plast Surg* 1985;12:17–23.

Hull R, Hirsh J, Jay R, Carter C, et al. Different intensities of oral anticoagulant therapy in the treatment of proximal vein thrombosis. *N Engl J Med* 1982;307:1676–1681.

Irvin TT. *Wound Healing: Principles and Practice*. London, Chapman and Hall, 1981, p. 34.

Jacobson JJ, Matthews LS. Bacteria isolated from late prosthetic joint infections: Dental treatment and chemoprophylaxis. *Oral Surg* 1987;63:122–126.

Jacobson JJ, Millard HD, Plezia R, Blankenship JR. Dental treatment and late prosthetic joint infections. *Oral Surg Oral Med Oral Pathol* 1986;61:413–417.

Ketchum LD, Cohen IK, Masters FW. Hypertrophic scars and keloids: A collective review. *Plast Reconstr Surg* 1974;53:140–154.

Koranda FC, Grande DJ, Whitaker DC, Lee RD. Laser surgery in the medically compromised patient. *J Dermatol Surg Oncol* 1982;8:471–474.

Krull EA, Anbe DT. Diagnosis and treatment of surgical emergencies. In *Skin Surgery*, 5th ed. E Epstein, E Epstein Jr, eds. Philadelphia, W. B. Saunders, 1982, pp. 114–132.

Krull EA, Pickard SD, Hall JC. Effects of electrosurgery on cardiac pacemakers. *J Dermatol Surg Oncol* 1975;1:43–45.

McGowan DA, Hendrey ML. Is antibiotic prophylaxis required for dental patients with joint replacements? *Br Dent J* 1985;336–338.

Mulligan R. Late infections in patients with prostheses for total replacement of joints: Implications for the dental practitioner. *J Am Dent Assoc* 1980;101:44–46.

Murray JC, Pollack SV, Pinnell SR. Keloids: A review. *J Am Acad Dermatol* 1981;4:461–470.

Pollach A. *Surgical Infections*. Baltimore, Williams & Wilkins, 1987, pp. 225–233.

Pollack SV. Wound healing; A review part IV. Systemic medications affecting wound healing. *J Dermatol Surg Oncol* 1982;8:667–672.

Rees TD, Liverett DM, Guy GL. The effect of cigarette smoking on skin-flap survival in the face lift patient. *Plast Reconstr Surg* 1984;73:911–915

Retchin SM, Fletcher RH, Buescher PC, et al. The application of official policy. Prophylaxis recommendations for patients with mitral valve prolapse. *Med Care* 1985;23:1156–1162.

Richards JH. Bacteremia following irritation of foci of infection. *JAMA* 1932;99:1496–1497.

Rubenstein R, Roenigk HH Jr, Stegman SJ, Hanke CW. Atypical keloids after dermabrasion of patients taking isotretinoin. *J Am Acad Dermatol* 1986;15:280–285.

Sabetta JB, Zitelli JA. The incidence of bacteremia during skin surgery. *Arch Dermatol* 1987;123:213–215.

Salasche SJ. Acute surgical complications: Cause, prevention, and treatment. *J Am Acad Dermatol* 1986;15:1163–1185.

Salasche SJ, Bernstein G, Sentarik M. *Surgical Anatomy of the Skin*. Appleton and Lange, 1988.

Salzman EW. Hemostatic problems in surgical patients. In *Hemostasis and Thrombosis: Basic Principles and Clinical Practice*, 2nd ed. Philadelphia, Lippincott, 1987, pp. 920–925.

Sebben JE. Electrosurgery and cardiac pacemakers. *J Am Acad Dermatol* 1983;9:457–463.

Sebben JE. *Cutaneous Electrosurgery*. Chicago, Year Book Medical Publishers, 1989, p. 106.

Sharkey I, Brughera-Jones A. Evaluation of potential bleeding problems in dermatologic surgery. *J Dermatol Surg* 1975;1:41–44.

Sheretz EF, Davis GL, Rice RW, et al. Transfer of hepatitis B virus by contaminated reusable needle electrodes after electrodesiccation in simulated use. *J Am Acad Dermatol* 1986;15:1242–1246.

Shulman ST, Amren DP, Bisno AL, et al. Prevention of bacterial endocarditis. A statement for health professionals by the Committee on Rheumatic Fever and Infective Endocarditis of the Council on Cardiovascular Disease in the Young. *Circulation* 1984;70:1118A–1122A.

Silverman AK, Laing KF, Swanson NA, Schaberg DR. Activation of herpes simplex following dermabrasion. Report of a patient successfully treated with intravenous acyclovir and a brief review of the literature. *J Am Acad Dermatol* 1985;13:103–108.

Smith JG Jr, Chalker DK. Should dermatologists be immunized against hepatitis B? *J Am Acad Dermatol* 1983;8:252–254.

Stewart RH, Graham GF. Cryo corner: A complication of cryosurgery in a patient with cryofibrinogenemia. *J Dermatol Surg Oncol* 1978;4:743–744.

Stinchfield FE, Bigliani LU, Neu HC, et al. Later hematogenous infection of total joint replacemtn. *J Bone Joint Surg (Am)* 1980;62:1345–1350.

Storm O, Hansen AT. Mitral commissurotomy performed during anticoagulant prophylaxis with dicumarol. *Circulation* 1955;12:981.

Stuart MJ, Miller ML, Davery FR, Wolk JA. The post-aspirin bleeding time: A screening test for evaluating haemostatic disorders. *Br J Haemotol* 1979;43:649–659.

Update: Human immunodeficiency virus infections in health-care workers exposed to blood of infected patients. *MMWR* 1987;36.

Update: Universal precautions for prevention of transmission of human immunodeficiency virus, hepatitis B virus, and other bloodborne pathogens in health care settings. *MMWR* 1988;37.

Yarborough JM. Preoperative evaluation of the patient for dermabrasion. *J Dermatol Surg Oncol* 1987;13:652–653.

6

Preoperative Psychological Evaluation

Hugh M. Gloster, Jr.
University of Cincinnati, Cincinnati, Ohio

Randall K. Roenigk
*Mayo Clinic/Foundation and Mayo Medical School,
Rochester, Minnesota*

The preoperative evaluation of candidates for dermatologic surgery is often as important as the surgery itself. Fortunately, the risks and complications of minor skin surgery occur infrequently. Cosmetic surgery, however, requires a minimum risk of complications since patients' expectations are so high. Most dermatologic surgery can be performed under local anesthesia in an office or outpatient surgical suite without the need for general anesthesia or sedation. Therefore, even patients who have significant medical problems or are elderly can undergo these procedures safely. More time should be spent explaining a procedure and possible risks, because an anxious patient usually lacks understanding about what is going to happen. Patients are more cooperative and relaxed once they understand the procedure and its expected results.

The preoperative psychological management of patients undergoing skin surgery should be classified into three treatment groups: minor dermatologic surgery, oncologic dermatologic surgery, and cosmetic dermatologic surgery. Patients with skin cancer are highly motivated to undergo treatment as soon as possible. The final cosmetic result is usually secondary and not the main concern. Cosmetic dermatologic surgery patients may not have objective disease but are motivated to have surgery for a variety of reasons. Some patients want specific problems corrected, while others think they need "new skin." These patients may have unique personalities, and although all dermatologic surgeons may not find themselves qualified to evaluate them, time and experience are required to prepare patients for cosmetic surgery, lest one perform procedures on inappropriate patients.

The preoperative psychological evaluation of dermatologic surgery patients is difficult to teach and is learned through experience. Some surgeons never master this art of medicine and have difficulty communicating with patients. Patient satisfaction is determined not only by the technical quality of the surgery performed, but also by a good physician–patient relationship.

THE NONCOSMETIC CONSULTATION

Minor dermatologic surgery involves the removal of such benign neoplasms as nevi, cysts, and cherry angiomas. Removal of these lesions is done for both medical and cosmetic reasons but seldom involves stress on the part of the patient. Usually, patients understand the risks to be minimal and generally are not anxious about the results but do expect little or no resulting scar. Most malignant oncologic dermatologic surgery involves the treatment of basal cell carcinoma and squamous cell carcinoma. Simple outpatient therapy such as electrodesiccation and curettage seldom evokes emotional stress in patients, especially when a patient has been adequately instructed on the risk of these tumors. Finally, malignant melanoma is potentially life-threatening and requires more emotional support and discussion. Most dermatologists do not treat clinical stage II and III metastatic disease and therefore are not encumbered with handling the more emotional end stages and deaths in these patients. This is best left to the oncologist and others who deal with these problems routinely.

Once a diagnosis of basal cell carcinoma or squamous cell carcinoma has been made, it is important to explain the likely morbidity. The best approach is to be honest and give factual medical advice in a simplified fashion so that the patient understands completely. Of course, the patient may forget much of this information, and written material is always helpful. Aside from exceptional cases that require extensive surgery and reconstruction, reassurance about the outcome of basal cell carcinoma treatment is the best approach. The cosmetic result from reconstruction is secondary but important. The same can be said for most squamous cell carcinomas, since the risks for metastatic disease are minimal in most cases.

The treatment of nonmelanoma skin cancer can be thought of as a two-staged procedure. The first stage is treatment of the disease, and the second is reconstruction. Many patients are only concerned with the first stage and not with the cosmetic result when the diagnosis is first made. Most standard treatments for nonmelanoma skin cancer combine both stages. Electrodesiccation and curettage, fusiform excision, and cryosurgery often result in an excellent cosmetic scar that needs no further revision. Mohs micrographic surgery is generally reserved for more difficult tumors. The tumor-free margins obtained with Mohs micrographic surgery result in a defect that must be closed or allowed to heal by second intention. Reconstruction may involve the use of more advanced flaps or grafting procedures, and therefore a more complete discussion with the patient is required.

Patients with malignant melanoma have what might be a life-threatening tumor. The approach to these patients depends greatly on the clinical stage and histologic depth of the tumor. Most patients with thin melanomas (Breslow level less than 0.85 mm) classified as clinical stage I can be treated by simple excision with adequate margins and can expect very high cure rates. Despite the fact that we can reassure these patients, it is important to detail factual information about the long-term risks of this disease. Patients appreciate getting factual medical advice and simple, complete answers to their questions. In studies comparing patients with malignant melanoma and those with other dermatologic disorders, it has been shown that those with melanoma scored approximately equal to the general public and strikingly superior to other dermatologic patients in tests for emotional well-being. While patients with chronic dermatologic disease may have low self-esteem and self-image, patients with melanoma or other life-threatening cancer have the ability to "respond to the challenge" and emotionally "attack" the disease. Many cancer patients exhibit hopeful and goal-oriented thinking with a positive attitude.

In general, patients with skin cancer are anxious to be cured and require little discussion about whether surgery should be performed. Secondarily, they would like the final result to be cosmetically acceptable. When the cosmetic result takes precedence, there should be concern that the patient does not have a clear understanding about the tumor.

THE COSMETIC CONSULTATION

The preoperative consultation for patients undergoing cosmetic dermatologic surgery includes some basic determinations (Table 1). The first is the patient request, during which the patient describes the problem to be corrected. Second is the physical examination: the surgeon evaluates the patient based on his or her request and plans treatment. The third is a medical evaluation to determine if there are contraindications to the procedure. The final evaluation is the psychological assessment, which begins at the first meeting and continues through surgery and during all follow-up visits.

During the patient request, let the patient do all the talking. Give him or her a mirror and a pointer to show you the specific problems. The surgeon should listen to the patient's requests and not intercede with suggestions.

The physical examination is done to evaluate the patient and to determine if his or her request is reasonable. The surgeon can then point out additional problems that can be treated. The surgeon then plans his or her approach and tells the patient what can be done and what results can be expected. At this stage you must assess whether the patient has a reasonable understanding of what can be corrected based on the planned procedure. The patient must also demonstrate an understanding of the wound-healing process and the possible need for subsequent procedures. If a procedure can be performed, a determination of the patient's medical ability to undergo the operation is completed next (see Chap. 5).

The preoperative psychological assessment includes an evaluation of the patient's expectations and motivations for surgery. At this time, the surgeon must develop insight into the patient's own body perception for a successful surgical outcome. Important aspects of the preoperative psychological assessment of the cosmetic patient are listed in Table 2. It is necessary to determine the patient's motivations for surgery. A personal wish to change is essential to prevent later resentment. Patients who seek cosmetic surgery affecting body image for internal reasons are more likely to be pleased with their operation than those with externally directed motives. Internal motivations to undergo aesthetic surgery include a patient's desire to change his or her appearance in order to improve self-image or to meet a personal standard of physical attractiveness. Externally motivated patients, however, either respond to pressure from others (e.g., spouse, friend, or relative) to change their appearance or are driven to achieve some change external to themselves by undergoing surgery (e.g., to guarantee success in love and marriage). In other words, the disfigurement has become a focus for other psychological problems. The surgeon is usually unable to satisfy such patients. Preoperative assessment can provide the surgeon with information that allows the classification of patient motivations as internal or external. A direct way to evaluate patient motivations is to simply ask how and why they chose this time to undergo cosmetic surgery.

There is a developing consensus in the professional literature that the most important factor in the process of preoperative evaluation is the assessment of patient expectations regarding the outcome of aesthetic surgery. Expectations, which critically influence the patient's perception of surgical outcome, should be realistic, and the patient should not believe that surgery will improve

Table 1   The Cosmetic Consultation

Patient request
Physical examination
Medical evaluation
Psychological assessment

Table 2 Important Aspects of the Preoperative
Psychological Assessment of the Cosmetic Patient

Motivation for surgery
Expectations of surgery
Understanding of the risks and implications of surgery
Anxiety level
Ego strength

occupational problems, solve financial difficulties, resolve personal conflicts, or render physical perfection. From a medical-legal standpoint, it is important that the patient understand what results can be expected, good or bad. The use of before and after photos and written material on a procedure may help to explain a cosmetic procedure. Adequate physician–patient communication cannot be stressed enough.

The patient must understand the risks and implications of surgery in order to be sufficiently well informed to make an intelligent decision about whether or not to proceed with the operation. It is often helpful to delay the patient's decision about whether to have surgery. After the consultation, the patient may not fully understand all of the risks, benefits, and alternatives and may think of other questions later. The patient needs to understand the procedure completely as well as the follow-up care expected. Patients should also understand that the surgeon cannot predict the final outcome precisely. It is therefore important to document the nature and purpose of the procedure and alternatives; the risks involved need to be discussed and documented in the chart. Well-written and specific informed consent is essential.

The patient's anxiety level should be assessed. No anxiety indicates denial and a possible failure of the patient to fully comprehend the risks of surgery. Unwarranted, excessive anxiety may result in a decision to cancel surgery unnecessarily.

Finally, the surgeon must determine the patient's ego strength. An individual with normal ego strength is stable, capable of tolerating the stress of surgery, and will not be governed by irrational fears or fantasies.

To do an adequate consultation, it is not reasonable to see patients briefly. Cosmetic surgery consultations should be scheduled and uninterrupted (30–45 min). The consultation should not be hurried. If there is not enough time, the cosmetic surgery consultation should be rescheduled. During an extended discussion, the patient reveals more to the physician. If there are psychosocial motivations for surgery, these can be discussed. If the patient does not understand what can be expected, the procedure can be delayed. In addition, if complications occur later, the patient knows the surgeon better and recognizes that the surgeon wants to help him or her through the problem.

Dermatologic surgeons are not trained in psychology but deal with these issues routinely. A psychiatrist or psychologist can evaluate the patient in special situations, but generally this is not necessary if the surgeon pays particular attention to this part of the evaluation. If the patient is already under the care of a psychologist or psychiatrist, he or she should be contacted before the surgeon agrees to proceed with cosmetic surgery.

GOOD CANDIDATES FOR COSMETIC SURGERY

Good candidates for cosmetic surgery can be grouped as having either major or minor disfigurements (Table 3). Examples of patients with major disfigurements include those with severe acne scarring, neurofibromatosis, multiple cylindromas, and scarring alopecia. These patients have

Table 3 Good Candidates for Cosmetic Surgery

Major disfigurement	Minor disfigurement
Most accepting	Public appearance occupation (solid motive)
Greatest need	Do not like aging appearance
Best chance for improvement	The information seeker
Psychiatric issues relate to the disease, not surgery	

a physical deformity, and surgery may be considered reconstructive in most cases. They have the greatest need for help and have the best chance for physical improvement. Psychiatric issues regarding the surgery are minimal since the disfigurement has already created a problem that may be improved by the operation.

Patients with minor disfigurements can also be good candidates for cosmetic surgery. Examples are patients with small nevi, Norwood's type I-III male pattern alopecia, or superficial rhytids that require soft tissue augmentation. Correction of a specific problem can be very satisfying. Inquire why the patient wants surgery performed. Patients who work in public contact occupations are good candidates, because they have strong motivation. Older patients who simply do not like their aging appearance are appropriately motivated: they see specific changes over the years that can be corrected. Another good candidate is the information seeker. These patients consider surgery for many years, read all they can, and seek the consultation of several surgeons. Once the information seeker decides to undergo surgery, he or she already has a good understanding of what can be expected.

It is difficult to be certain who will be the best candidate for cosmetic surgery. The close relationship between cosmetic surgery and psychological factors has long been recognized. Early investigators felt that the desire to change the appearance of the body may reflect failure to resolve underlying psychological conflicts. Requests for cosmetic surgery were thus interpreted as a symptom of neurosis. Several studies performed 25 to 30 years ago investigated the mental status of patients seeking aesthetic surgery. Forty to 72% of patients were classified as either psychotic, neurotic, or having a personality trait disorder. Nevertheless, it has been determined that despite the high incidence of psychopathology preoperatively, most cosmetic patients are satisfied with their operation. As a result, cosmetic surgery often promotes positive changes in many aspects of psychosocial functioning, such as self-confidence and self-esteem. Patients usually become more socially outgoing and have an increased sense of well-being after aesthetic surgery. Thus, a history of psychiatric disease should not be an absolute contraindication to cosmetic surgery since well-chosen cases may have positive benefits on the overall adjustment of the individual.

A more recent evaluation of patients seeking cosmetic surgery showed that approximately 25% had psychological abnormalities as measured by the Minnesota Multiphasic Personality Inventory. This decline in the number of patients with an "abnormal" psychological profile seeking cosmetic surgery reflects current social changes such as the high value placed on physical attributes, the emphasis on youthfulness as being synonymous with capability at the workplace, the greater exposure of the body in modern clothing and sport trends, and increasing public awareness that cosmetic surgery procedures are readily available. In fact, there has been an astounding increase in the demand for such surgery over the past 20 years.

Based on a questionnaire and interview study of more than 60 consecutive cosmetic surgery patients, one author (RKR) found that the average patient who had cosmetic surgery performed would be approximately 40 years old, female, and having attained only a high school education.

These patients are likely to be in public contact occupations. They feel average or normally attractive and are slightly concerned about their appearance. These patients have considered surgery for 3–4 years before one or two consultations are obtained. The patient expects some improvement in physical appearance but still expects to be basically the same person after surgery. An improved sense of self-esteem is expected by the patient, but this is subjective. These patients do not expect that cosmetic surgery will improve their occupation but often consider this possibility. The primary reason for undergoing the surgery is that the patient alone will notice the improved appearance and feel better about himself or herself, thus enhancing the quality of life.

POOR CANDIDATES FOR COSMETIC SURGERY

Though most patients do benefit from cosmetic surgery, a small number of individuals will not be satisfied with the outcome of well-executed surgical procedures. An even smaller minority may be psychologically harmed by aesthetic surgery. The profiles of poor candidates for cosmetic surgery are listed in Table 4. Patients with recurrent psychiatric illness, especially those requiring hospitalization, should be carefully evaluated. Psychiatric disease is not an absolute contraindication to cosmetic surgery, and a pleasing outcome can result. Neurotic patients may be anxious and worry. Somatic complaints are a defense against this stress. With adequate counseling, treatment with surgical intervention of a monosymptomatic neurosis directed at a cosmetic problem may result in improvement.

Psychotic patients have escaped into their own psychological island without stress, conflict, or reality checks. Psychiatric consultation for these patients is important. Some people feel that the danger of operating on psychotics is exaggerated, and sometimes psychological improvement is realized postoperatively. However, schizophrenics are characterized by disorganized thought, and paranoid schizophrenics can be dangerous. Surgery is best avoided in these patients. In general, surgery for psychotic patients should be limited to severe deformities that are not involved in the patient's delusions or hallucinations. Close liaison between the surgeon and the psychiatrist is necessary to manage such patients.

Patients with personality disorders, including those with maladaptive behavior or who are sociopathic, can easily disguise their problem and persuade a surgeon to operate. The surgery will not affect their behavior, and these patients are prone to sue for medical malpractice. Under no circumstances should the surgeon operate with the intent to treat a patient's personality problem. Other patients with personality disorders to be aware of include the obsessive-compulsive or hysterical patient. These patients may be flighty, reactive, and compulsive with excessive anxiety. They may have a positive response to surgery, but the course can be rocky and emotional. It is also important to be familiar with the polysurgical syndrome (Munchausen's syndrome) or the surgical addict. These patients give a history of surgical failures and a futile outlook. Surgery is fantasy for them, and it is important to resist their pleas for further procedures.

Table 4 Poor Candidates for Cosmetic Surgery

Recurrent psychiatric illness/hospitalization
The minimal defect patient
Surgeon shopping: seeing more than three surgeons reflects patient indecision
The sudden whim
Unreasonable motive: "My husband will stop cheating on me . . . "
The solution to all problems

Certain patients seeking cosmetic surgery present to the surgeon with a conviction of having a physical defect, although their appearance is normal or very close to normal. These patients focus on one aspect of their body, which they find distasteful. This delusional preoccupation with some imagined defect in a normal-appearing person is called "dysmorphophobia," and most of these patients have a severe personality disorder or frank schizophrenia. Invariably, such patients are not pleased with surgery.

Besides the patient with specific psychopathology, another poor candidate for cosmetic surgery is the patient who gives a history of repeated surgery resulting in dissatisfaction and makes comments such as "the last doctor did it wrong" or "just a little change is needed here." The patient may be correct in believing that the last doctor did it wrong or that some modification may be required, but this should arouse suspicion that you, too, may not be able to meet the patient's expectations. In general, these patients have a severe disturbance in their object relations and carry a diagnosis of personality disorder with sadomasochistic, borderline, narcissistic, or antisocial traits.

The surgeon shopper is another patient to avoid. This is the patient who cannot make up his or her mind to have the procedure performed but seeks a number of consultations. After seeing two or three surgeons, most patients should be able to come to a decision. Indecision on the part of the patient may result in regret after the surgery has been performed. This decision is important, and if the patient is uncertain, a delay is warranted. Conversely, patients with the sudden whim to have cosmetic surgery should be considered poor candidates. An advertisement the patient saw in last week's Sunday sports section is unlikely to provoke serious thought about the consequences of his or her decision.

Some patients have unreasonable motives for having cosmetic surgery performed: "My husband will stop cheating on me if only I get this fixed." No cosmetic surgical procedure can be the solution to psychosocial or economic problems. It is unlikely that the surgeon will be able to meet such expectations.

Males requesting aesthetic surgery have traditionally been viewed suspiciously. Malignantly dissatisfied patients who tend to have aberrant reactions to cosmetic surgery are more likely to be men. Also, male cosmetic surgery patients appear to be more emotionally unstable than female patients. Changing sociocultural trends have lessened these concerns about the male psyche since it is currently more acceptable for men to want to alter their physical appearance. Hair replacement surgery is among the most commonly performed procedures today.

If, after the preoperative assessment, the surgeon is concerned about the presence of psychopathology in a patient, it is worthwhile to seek psychiatric consultation. A thorough preoperative evaluation by a psychiatrist is better patient care, and high-risk patients can be screened. The psychiatrist is better qualified to clarify the patient's mental health, motivations, expectations, personality make-up, anxiety level, ego strength, and ability to understand the risks and implications of surgery. After the preoperative assessment, the surgeon and/or the psychiatrist may feel that the patient is not an ideal candidate for cosmetic surgery. In such cases, the following courses of action may be taken, each requiring the participation of the surgeon and psychiatrist:

1. A decision against surgery based on the patient's impaired psychological functioning along with a recommendation that the patient seek further psychiatric treatment. This course is most commonly chosen when the patient is externally motivated, unable to understand the procedure, or when the body image goal is surgically unfeasible and linked with other psychopathology.
2. Deferring surgery for several months and, in the meantime, offering psychotherapy to clarify expectations and motivations for surgery.
3. Deciding not to perform surgery unless the patient agrees to psychiatric follow-up postoperatively.

4. Deciding not to perform surgery on the basis of the surgeon's belief that the operation would be of no benefit (e.g., the "minimal defect" patient).
5. Recommending preoperative supportive treatment.
6. Referral to another surgeon. This is done when the patient is a good candidate but has a poor personality fit with the first surgeon. The patient's willingness to accept consultation has been positively correlated with the ability to accept surgical results.

THE DAY OF SURGERY

Although the psychological evaluation should be complete by the time surgery is performed, a relationship between the surgeon and patient continues. The patient has placed his or her confidence in the surgeon and expects technical perfection. Patients have few ways of evaluating surgical expertise and rely heavily on how the surgeon appears or whether they like the surgeon. On the day of surgery, the surgeon should appear happy, efficient, and organized. The surgeon should greet the patient and establish that the surgery is a happy event. The surgeon's perspective about the operative outcome can strongly influence the patient's reactions to the operative results. Patient anxiety is normal and should be expected. Most patients want to know that everything is going as it should on a routine basis. Since most dermatologic surgery is performed with local anesthesia, the patient is acutely aware of all that is said during the procedure. It is important that intraoperative problems be dealt with quietly and efficiently. Patients are unsettled by complications and would rather be assured that everything is proceeding routinely (never say "oops" during the procedure).

FOLLOW-UP

Follow-up care is just as important as the preoperative consultation. Wound care is dealt with elsewhere in this book, but in addition to medical treatment, the patient must also be given psychological support. If there is a problem and the patient is dissatisfied, listen to the patient's complaint and do not try to argue. Although the patient may be disappointed, he or she still wants your help through the follow-up care. Most dissatisfied patients are not litigious and simply want the doctor to stand by and be attentive to their feelings of disappointment. Recent research has shown that the majority of patients are in the physician's corner and not "out to get them." If the patient becomes troublesome, resist the temptation not to schedule follow-up appointments. It would be more prudent to schedule more frequent visits and give the patient more time. If the surgeon is dissatisfied with the results, his or her feelings should be dealt with away from the patient. Once the surgeon is relaxed, he or she can then better deal with the patient's problem. Never completely dismiss a post–cosmetic surgery patient. Always leave the door open for later consultation and reevaluation.

The three main causes of patient dissatisfaction with the outcome of cosmetic surgery are listed in Table 5. Physical complications must be discussed in a straightforward manner with the patient. The surgeon should not deny the existence of a complication, as this implies guilt and projects blame to the patient. The surgeon must reestablish the patient's confidence so the patient will be receptive to a secondary, corrective procedure.

Table 5   Reasons for Patient Dissatisfaction with Surgery

Physical complication or disappointment in anatomic change
Unrealistic psychological expectations
Lack of rapport between the physician and the patient

Postoperatively, it is difficult to deal with the patient who is dissatisfied as a result of unrealistic expectations. It is easier to screen such patients during the preoperative assessment. After carefully listening to the patient's complaints, the surgeon should simply state what he or she is capable of doing without dwelling on the patient's unreasonable arguments.

Because lack of rapport between the patient and physician has been documented as the major cause of medical malpractice suits, it is critical that the surgeon establish a good relationship with the patient. This can be done by listening to the patient and responding to complaints and concerns in an understanding rather than defensive manner.

The occasional patient may become malignantly dissatisfied with cosmetic surgery. Such patients tend to be male and may react psychopathologically to surgery with suicide attempts, delusional fixation upon the "damaged" organ, pursuit of further operations, or paranoid attitudes toward successive physicians. The occasional murder of physicians by such patients should provide ample incentive for surgeons performing cosmetic procedures to be adept at recognizing this potentially dangerous personality trait.

Cosmetic surgery may result in a significant change in body image, which requires psychological readjustment and adaptation to a new appearance. Therefore, most patients experience a transient, brief psychiatric disturbance in the immediate postoperative period, which may be manifested by irritability, emotional liability, and interpersonal conflict. Patients who are forewarned about these kinds of emotional fluctuations are more likely to have an easier time adjusting to them if they occur. These preoperative presence of psychosis or neurosis may intensify emotional disturbances during the postoperative period. Alternatively, hidden psychiatric disease may be unmasked following an operation.

Postoperative depression is a common phenomenon. In one study, varying degrees of depression occurred at a rate of 57%. In that study, 19% of patients required hospitalization for psychiatric observation. Transient postoperative depression usually occurs at rates of 12–16% 5–14 days (rarely longer) after surgery. Surgeons should be aware than when a patient is depressed preoperatively, the depression will likely intensify postoperatively. Some dermatologic surgical procedures such as dermabrasion and deep chemical peel result in erythema that persists for 2–3 months. Although many patients understand this preoperatively, it is reasonable to expect them to feel disappointed at some point that the wound healing is not more expeditious.

Patient satisfaction with cosmetic surgery sometimes fails to correlate with the technical quality of the surgery performed. This paradox is perplexing. The use of good preoperative and postoperative photos is valuable as documentation of what has been achieved, good or bad. Generally, when a patient is well informed and the procedure is performed satisfactorily, the surgeon and patient are happy with the results. Predictably, when problems arise, the patient may be disappointed, but when treated appropriately he or she may still be pleased with the outcome. It is surprising that surgery performed poorly with substandard results may be acceptable to some patients. The problem occurs when patients are never pleased despite flawless technique and excellent results. It is therefore imperative that some assessment of patients' expectations and psyche be made during the preoperative consultation to determine whether or not the surgeon is capable of improving the perceived problem. Judging patients' psyches is an inexact science at best. This problem is more profound for the cosmetic surgery patient than the oncologic patient. However, understanding patients' expectations helps surgeons to prevent dissatisfaction postoperatively.

BIBLIOGRAPHY

1. Adams GR. The effects of physical attractiveness on socialization process. In *Psychological Aspects of Facial Form*. GW Lucker, KA Ribbens, JA McNamara Jr., eds. Ann Arbor, MI, Center for Human Growth and Development, 1981.

2. Hazards of cosmetic surgery. Editorial. *Brit Med J* 1967;1:381.

3. Arndt EM, Travis F, Lefebvre A., et al. Beauty and the eye of the beholder: Social consequences and personal adjustments for facial patients. *Br J Plast Surg* 1984;37:313–318.

4. Baker JT. Patient selection and psychological evaluation. In *Clinics in Plastic Surgery: The Aging Face.* R. Webster, ed. Philadelphia, Saunders, 1978, pp. 3–15.

5. Belfer ML, Mulliken JB, Cochran, TC. Cosmetic surgery as an antecedent of life change. *Am J Psychiatry* 1979;136:199–201.

6. Berscheid E, Gangestad S. The social psychological implications of facial physical attractiveness. *Clin Plast Surg* 1982;9(3):289–296.

7. Cassileth BR, Lusk EJ, Tenaglia AN. A psychological comparison of patients with malignant melanoma and other dermatologic disorders. *J Am Acad Dermatol* 1982;7:742–746.

8. Cassileth BR, Zupkis RV, Sutton-Smith K, et al. Information and participation preferences among cancer patients. *Ann Intern Med* 1980;92:832–836.

9. Cone JCP, Hueson JT. Psychological aspects of hand surgery. *Med J Aust* 1974;1:104–108.

10. Connolly FH, Gipson M. Dysmorphophobia-a long-term study. *Br J Psych* 1978;132:568–570.

11. Deaton AV, Langman MI. The contribution of psychologists to the treatment of plastic surgery patients. *Prof Psychol: Res Pract* 1986;17(3):179–184.

12. Edgerton MT, Jacobson WE, Meyer E: Surgical-psychiatric sutdy of patients seeking plastic (cosmetic) surgery: Ninety-eight consecutive patients with minimal deformity. *Br J Plast Surg* 1961;13:136–145.

13. Edgerton MT, Knorr NJ. Motivational patterns of patients seeking cosmetic (aesthetic) surgery. *Plast Reconstr Surg* 1971;48:551–557.

14. Gifford S. Cosmetic surgery and personality change: A review and some clinical observations. In *The Unfavourable Result in Plastic Surgery.* R. M. Goldwyn, ed. Boston: Little, Brown and Company, 1972, pp. 11–35.

15. Goin JM, Goin MK. *Changing the Body, Psychological Aspects of Plastic Surgery.* Baltimore, Williams and Wilkins, 1981.

16. Goin MK, Burgoyne RK, Goin JM. Face-lift operations: The patient's secret motivations and reactions to informed consent. *Plast Reconstr Surg* 1976;58:273–279.

17. Goin MK, Burgoyne RW, Goin JM, Staples FR. A prospective psychological study of 50 female face-lift patients. *Plast Reconstr Surg* 1980;65:436–442.

18. Goldwyn RM. The consultant and the unfavorable result. In *The Unfavorable Result in Plastic Surgery.* RM Goldwyn, ed. Boston, Little, Brown and Company, 1972, pp. 1–4.

19. Hay GG. Psychiatric aspects of cosmetic nasal operations. *Br J Psychiat* 1970;116:85–97.

20. Hay GG, Heather BB. Changes in psychometric test results following cosmetic nasal operations. *Br J Psychiatr* 1973;122:89–90.

21. Hill G, Silver AG. Psychodynamic and esthetic motivations for plastic surgery. *Psychosom Med* 1950;12:345–355.

22. Hueston J, Dennerstein L, Gotts G. Psychological aspects of cosmetic surgery. *J Psych ObGyn* 1985; 4:335–346.

23. Jacobson WE, Edgerton MT, Meyer E, et al. Psychiatric evaluation of male patients seeking cosmetic surgery. *Plast Reconstr Surg* 1960;26:356–372.

24. Knorr NJ, Edgerton MT, Hoopes JE. The "insatiable" cosmetic surgery patient. *Plast Reconstr Surg* 1967;40:285–289.

25. Marcus P. Psychological aspects of cosmetic rhinoplasty. *Br J Plast Surg* 1984;37:313–318.

26. Merloo JAM. The fate of one's face with some remarks on the implications of plastic surgery. *Psychiatr Q* 1956;30:31–43.

27. Mohl PC. Psychiatric consultation in plastic surgery: The psychiatrist's perspective. *Psychosomatics* 1984;25(6):471–476.

28. Pruzinsky T. Psychological factors in cosmetic plastic surgery: Recent developments in patient care. *Plast Surg Nurs* 1993;13(2):64–72.

29. Pruzinsky T, Persing JR. Psychological perspectives on aesthetic applications of reconstructive surgery techniques. In *Aesthetic Applications of Craniofacial Techniques.* DK Ousterhout, ed. Boston, Little, Brown and Company, 1991, pp. 43–56.

30. Reich J. Aesthetic plastic surgery development and place in medical practice. *Med J Aust* 1972; 1: 1152–1156.
31. Reich J. The surgery of appearance: psychological and related aspects. *Med J Aust* 1969;2:5–13.
32. Rosenthal GK. Preventing malpractice claims. *Washington University Magazine* 1977;47:7–13.
33. Schneitzer I. The psychiatric assessment of the patient requesting facial surgery. *Aust NZ J Psychiatry* 1989;23:249–254.
34. Schneitzer I, Hirschfeld JJ. Post-rhytidectomy psychosis: A rare complication. *Plast Reconstr Surg* 1984;74:419–422.
35. Sihm F, Jagd M, Pers M. Psychological assessment before and after augmentation mammoplasty. *Scand J Plast Reconstr Surg* 1978;12:295–298.
36. Shulman BH. Psychiatric assessment of the candidate for cosmetic surgery. *Otolaryngol Clin North Am* 1980;12(2):383–389.
37. Wright MR. How to recognize and control the problem patient. *J Dermatol Surg Oncol* 1984; 10(5): 389–395.
38. Wright MR. Management of patient dissatisfaction with results of cosmetic procedures. *Arch Otolaryngol* 1980;106:446–471.
39. Wright MR, Wright WK. A psychological study of patients undergoing cosmetic surgery. *Arch Otolaryngol* 1975;101:145–151.
40. Young JK. Lay-professional conflict in a Canadian community health center. *Med Care* 1975; 13: 897–904.

7

Emergencies in Skin Surgery

Rufus M. Thomas
Private Practice, Waynesville, North Carolina

Rex A. Amonette
University of Tennessee, Memphis, Tennessee

Emergencies in dermatologic office surgery fortunately are rare. Dermatologists have long been the leaders in performing office surgical procedures and today are doing even more complex procedures in the office setting. This, coupled with an increasingly older patient population, makes the risk of an emergency occurring much more likely. Therefore, it is essential for the dermatologist to become thoroughly familiar with the recognition and proper management of surgical emergencies. Training, planning, and availability of basic equipment and medication are the keys to the successful management of an emergency.

Excellent training in the management of cardiovascular emergencies such as myocardial infarction, cardiac arrhythmias, or cardiac arrest can be obtained by completing the Basic Life Support (BLS) course and the Advanced Cardiac Life Support (ACLS) course, which are offered through the Red Cross or American Heart Association in most communities. It is strongly recommended that all physicians and nursing personnel in an office receive training in one or both of these courses as well as annual refresher courses. A cardiopulmonary resuscitation (CPR) instructor can give the annual refresher course in the familiarity of the office to the entire office staff using the "Annie" mannequin. Additional training in the recognition and handling of other types of emergencies such as hemorrhage, allergic reactions, or convulsions may be obtained through many hospitals, medical schools, or medical societies.

Planning for an emergency begins with a written plan stating each staff member's role in an emergency situation. These roles include (1) someone to activate the emergency medical system, (2) someone to record accurately the time of events, vital signs, medications, (3) someone to perform basic CPR, and (4) someone to start intravenous infusions. Drills performed on a regular basis sharpen the skills, confidence, and response time of the office staff. The goal of managing an office emergency is to stabilize and transport the patient to an emergency care facility as quickly as possible. The telephone number for the local response team (emergency medical system or "code blue" team if you are adjacent to a hospital) should be placed near all office telephones.

Arrangements should be made in advance with internist or cardiologist colleagues within the building or local area to assist in the care of emergency patients.

Equally as important as training and planning is having available basic equipment and medications for emergencies. Oxygen that can be given by mask is an essential part of the basic emergency equipment. The oxygen tank and delivery system should be checked on a regular basis for adequacy and volume. Surgical tables that can be either manually or automatically placed into the Trendelenburg position are desirable. If the surgical table is firm, a cardiac board is probably not needed. Various intravenous fluids, tubing, and intravenous catheters as well as a suction device are necessary. A cardiac monitor and defibrillation unit, laryngoscope, and endostracheal tubes are optional equipment that should be restricted to medical personnel who are highly trained in their use (Fig. 1). Essential pharmaceuticals along with other equipment can be conveniently kept in an emergency tray or rolling cart (Fig. 2). Contents, expiration dates, and proper labels on all drugs should be reviewed on a regular basis. Appropriate adult and pediatric dosages listed in table form and kept in the emergency kit may be very helpful in an emergency.

TREATMENT OF SPECIFIC EMERGENCIES

Syncope

Syncope is probably the most frequent emergency in dermatologic surgery. It is caused by the loss of peripheral vasomotor tone with secondary visceral blood pooling and inadequate return to the heart. Patients frequently have a past history of syncopal episodes associated with vaccinations, venipuncture, or seeing trauma or blood. A family history of similar episodes is not uncommon. In the dermatologic setting, patients may experience syncope following the most minor procedure such as a shave biopsy. Certain measures can effectively prevent syncopal episodes. This includes explaining to the patient what to expect from a procedure in regard to discomfort. Speaking in a calm, reassuring tone is important. Allowing the patient to view a procedure or a specimen taken in a procedure should be avoided. The family member or friend who may accompany the patient should also be restricted from viewing the procedure, since they may also experience syncope. After the procedure is completed, the patient should slowly be assisted into a sitting position and observed for signs and symptoms of syncope before standing is allowed.

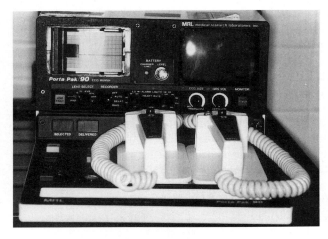

Figure 1   Portable monitor-defibrillator unit.

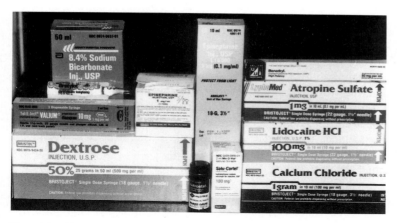

Figure 2 Essential pharmaceutical agents.

Signs of syncope include diaphoresis, pallor, and loss of consciousness. These signs help the physician distinguish syncope from other causes of unconsciousness. Treatment includes immediately placing the patient in the Trendelenburg position, applying cool compresses to the face, loosening the clothing, and administering oxygen. Spirits of ammonia may be used to stimulate the patient. Vital signs should be taken and recorded. Full restoration of mental status and cardiopulmonary function should occur quickly—within seconds to minutes. Atropine, 0.5 mg IV, should be considered if the syncopal episode is severe or prolonged and associated with bradycardia. If the patient does not promptly return to full mental and cardiopulmonary status, other more serious causes of syncope must be considered. These include stroke, seizure, cardiac arrythmias, myocardial infarction, and hypoglycemia.

Convulsions

Convulsions may occur as a result of a variety of disorders including drug reactions, insulin shock, cerebrovascular accidents, syncope, and convulsive disorders. The signs and symptoms include auras, excessive salivation, convulsive movements of the extremities, and loss of consciousness. Therapy is primarily aimed at protecting the patient from personal damage. Patients should be placed in a position in which they cannot hurt themselves by knocking against hard objects. If possible, they should be kept in a side-lying position, so that mucus and saliva will flow freely and not block the airway. Tight clothing, especially around the neck, should be removed. A padded tongue blade or a plastic airway should be inserted between the teeth to prevent trauma to the tongue and cheeks. Status epilepticus constitutes a medical emergency and refers to a stage of recurrent major motor seizures between which the patient does not completely regain consciousness.

Less than one half of status epilepticus occurs in confirmed epileptics; therefore, it is essential to search for and correct metabolic disturbances such as hypoglycemia, hyponatremia, hypomagnesemia, and hypocalcemia. Before administering anticonvulsive therapy, 50 ml of 50% dextrose in water should be given IV. Prior to this, a blood sample should be drawn to measure for levels of glucose, various chemicals, and anticonvulsive drug levels. Diazepam very effectively controls status epilepticus and should be given IV at a rate no greater than 5 mg/min in adults. If the seizure has not stopped within 10 min, another 5–10 mg is given. Blood pressure and respirations must be closely monitored. If status it not terminated, the administration of phenobarbital and/or phenytoin must be considered.

Allergic Reactions and Anaphylaxis

Type I allergic reactions follow antigen exposure in a sensitized person. These are mediated by IgE and involve the release of chemical mediators from mast cells and basophils. Exposure to substances such as pollens, drugs, foreign serum, insect stings, vaccines, local anesthetics, and food products may induce allergic reactions in susceptible individuals. In the dermatologist's office, the most common cause of allergic reactions is the injection of medications or local anesthetics. There is a broad spectrum of the clinical manifestations of allergic reactions. Minor reactions can be limited to the skin and include severe pruritus or urticaria. Angioneurotic edema with swelling of the lips, eyelids, cheeks, pharynx, and larynx may occur. Signs of progression to anaphylactic reaction include laryngospasm, bronchospasm, hypotension, and circulatory collapse. In severe anaphylaxis, death may occur within minutes.

True allergic reactions to the newer local anesthetics appear to be rare. Older local anesthetic agents such as the ester linkage group, which includes procaine, chloroprocaine, and tetracaine are associated with allergic reactions at a rate of 1%. The larger amide linkage group of local anesthetics are used almost exclusively today. This group includes lidocaine, bupivacaine, carbocaine, etidocaine, and prilocaine. Neither cross-reactivity nor cross-sensitivity has been shown between the ester and amide anesthestics, which are chemically dissimilar. Nor is there cross-reactivity between the various amide-type anesthetics. Most allergic reactions to the amide group reported in the literature are of the delayed response type, with very few cases of anaphylaxis reported.

Allergic reactions to methylparaben, a preservative used in multidose vials, may account for the few cases that occur with the amide linkage anesthetics. Cardiac lidocaine or single-dose vials do not contain parabens. In the case of a documented allergic reaction to an amide anesthetic, normal saline or diphenhydramine may be used and is very effective for smaller procedures such as a shave or punch biopsy.

Epinephrine is the drug of choice for the initial treatment of allergic reactions. In the adult 0.3–0.5 ml of a 1:1000 solution should be given subcutaneously every 20–30 min as needed, for up to three doses. In the child 0.01 ml/kg of a 1:1000 solution should be administered. For life-threatening anaphylactic reactions, 5 ml of a 1:10,000 solution should be given IV and repeated every 5–10 min as needed. Sublingual or endotracheal administration may be used if an IV cannot be established. Maintenance of a patent airway along with the administration of oxygen is critical. With signs of upper airway compromise, endotracheal intubation should be performed. In cases of severe laryngeal edema, cricothyrotomy or tracheostomy may be necessary. Initially, bronchospasm may be treated with inhaled bronchodilators such as metaproterenol or albuterol. Secondary treatment of bronchospasm would include aminophylline 6 mg/kg infused IV over 20–30 min. Volume expansion with normal saline or Ringer's lactate solution may be needed as large losses of fluid from the intravascular compartment commonly occur.

A dopamine hydrochloride infusion of 2–50 µg/kg min is the vasopressor agent of choice to manage hypotension that is unresponsive to volume expansion. Antihistamines, although of little value in treating the acute episode, by blocking further histamine binding to target tissues may shorten the duration of reaction and prevent relapses. Diphenhydramine hydrochloride, 25–50 mg, may be given IV over several minutes. Intramuscular or oral routes may also be used. Corticosteroids are not rapidly efficacious but may be useful in protracted anaphylaxis. Their major role is in preventing recurrence of the allergic reaction. Hydrocortisone sodium succinate, 500 mg, or its equivalent, should be administered IV.

A venous tourniquet proximal to an injection site may be used to delay absorption of an injected antigen, and epinephrine, 0.3 ml of a 1:1000 solution, may be injected subcutaneously into the site. All patients experiencing anaphylaxis should be admitted to a hospital for careful monitoring and observation.

Drug Toxicity

Toxic reactions related to local anesthetics are either local or general. Local toxicity involves the tissue at the site of injection and includes cellulitis, ulceration, abscess formation, and tissue slough. These manifestations may be due to contamination of the anesthetic agent, traumatic administration, or reactions to the anesthetic itself, preservatives, or vasoconstrictors. General toxicity is characterized by systemic reactions due to excessive dosage, rapid absorption, inadequate metabolism, and redistribution or unintentional intravascular injection. Systemic toxic reactions to local anesthetics are due to overdosage most of the time and can be prevented by always aspirating, injecting slowly, and keeping the dosage compatible with the patient's body weight. The physician should be thoroughly familiar with the toxic dosage of the anesthetic used. For example, the toxic dosage of 1% lidocaine, the most commonly used anesthetic, is 300 mg when used without epinephrine and 500 mg when used with epinephrine in a healthy adult patient.

Early symptoms of systemic toxicity to local anesthetics may include yawning, drowsiness, coughing, twitching, restlessness, or numbness of the tongue and perioral tissues. The central nervous system is the primary target of toxic levels of anesthetics with biphasic excitatory and depressant stages. The excitatory stage is characterized by lightheadedness, nervousness, apprehension, euphoria, confusion, dizziness, tinnitus, diplopia, vomiting, tremors, and convulsions. The excitatory stage may be brief or may not occur at all, in which case the first manifestation of toxicity may be the depressant state characterized by extreme drowsiness merging into unconsciousness, respiratory depression, and arrest. Respiratory arrest is the most common cause of death directly attributable to reactions to local anesthetics. Cardiovascular manifestations are usually depressant and include myocardial depression, with concurrent peripheral vasodilation, hypotension, bradycardia, and cardiovascular collapse that may lead to cardiac arrest.

Management of local anesthetic emergencies begins first with careful monitoring of cardiovascular and respiratory vital signs and the patient's state of consciousness after each injection of local anesthetic. At the first sign of change in any of these areas, immediate attention should be given to the maintenance of a patent airway, administration of oxygen, and institution of an intravenous infusion. Convulsions that persist despite adequate respiratory support should be treated with small increments of an ultra-short-acting barbiturate (thiopental 1–2 mg/kg) or diazepam (2.5–5.0 mg) given IV. Since these medications inhibit respirations, close attention should be given to the patient's respiratory rate. Supportive treatment of circulatory depression may require administration of IV fluids and a vasopressor as directed by the clinical situation. Standard cardiopulmonary resuscitative measures should be instituted in severe toxic reactions leading to respiratory or cardiac arrest.

Vasoconstrictive agents, most commonly epinephrine, are frequently given with local anesthesics. The vasoconstriction prolongs the duration of local anesthesia, lessens bleeding at the surgical site, and inhibits absorption of both itself and the local anesthetic, thereby minimizing the possibility of systemic toxicity. Toxic reactions can occur with epinephrine when a high dosage is used or with intravascular injection. Manifestations may include palpitations, throbbing headache, tremor, tachycardia, tachypnea, and cardiac arrhythmias. Fortunately, the half-life of epinephrine in serum is short and specific therapy is usually not needed.

Absolute contraindications to the use of epinephrine are hyperthyroidism and pheochromocytoma. It should be used with caution in patients with heart disease. Recently, a possible interaction with epinephrine-containing local anesthetics given to patients receiving propanolol was described. This interaction is most likely associated with higher doses of epinephrine and may lead to malignant hypertension, stroke, and cardiac arrest. The proposed mechanism of the interaction is thought to be propanolol-induced blockade of the beta-2 vascular bed receptors, with resultant unopposed alpha pressor effect. In all cases, the lowest dosage and concentration of epinephrine should be used. Concentrations of 1:200,000 or less should be used since higher concentrations add little to the degree of vasoconstriction.

Hemorrhage

Significant hemorrhage occurring intraoperatively or postoperatively is an emergency situation caused either by a preexisting bleeding disorder or by inadequate intraoperative hemostasis. Adequate history and physical examination should reveal a preexisting bleeding disorder prior to surgery. Inquiry should be made into a family history of bleeding problems as well as personal history of prolonged bleeding after trauma, unprovoked nosebleeds, or bleeding from the gums. Most importantly, a complete list of medications that the patient takes, including all over-the-counter products, should be made. Many patients take aspirin-containing over-the-counter products and are unaware that these products contain aspirin. Petechiae and ecchymoses found on physical examination would confirm a significant bleeding diathesis.

Screening laboratory tests should also be used to evaluate hereditary or acquired coagulopathy. These tests include a complete blood count, platelet count, peripheral smear for platelet morphology, prothrombin time, partial thromboplastin time, and bleeding time. The prothrombin time measures the extrinsic system of the coagulation cascade, while the partial thromboplastin time measures the intrinsic system.

Drug-induced coagulopathy may be caused by aspirin, nonsteroidal anti-inflammatory drugs, and anticoagulants. Patients who are undergoing parenteral anticoagulation with heparin are not candidates for elective dermatologic surgery. However, many patients require chronic anticoagulation with a coumarin-type drug, and dermatologic surgical procedures can be undertaken in these patients with caution. In consultation with the patient's internist, the drug may be stopped 4 days prior to the surgical procedure and reinstituted 1 week after surgery. If the patient's medical condition does not warrant discontinuation of anticoagulation, the procedure may be performed but with meticulous attention given to intraoperative hemostasis and the application of a pressure dressing. Use of the carbon dioxide laser, focused as a cutting instrument, may be an option since small-gauge capillary vessels are sealed immediately, often resulting in a bloodless incision. Oral or parenteral vitamin K can be administered to control persistent bleeding.

Aspirin and nonsteroidal anti-inflammatory drugs such as ibuprofen, acetylate platelet cyclo-oxygenase, block the pathway from arachidonic acid to cyclic endoperoxides and subsequently to thromboxane A_2. Patients should avoid these drugs for 7–14 days before surgery and 1 week after to diminish problems with hemorrhage. Alcohol is another drug that should be avoided during the perioperative period because it is a potent vasodilator.

Hemorrhage secondary to inadequate intraoperative hemostasis is a preventable problem. Careful and thorough cautery or ligation of all bleeding points should be accomplished prior to closure. Adequate closure of all dead space should be performed using subcutaneous, dermal, and skin sutures as needed.

Special attention should be given to the application of an effective pressure dressing during the first 24 hr postoperatively. Postoperative hemorrhage requiring a return visit to the physician necessitates a complete examination of the surgical wound, which may include evacuation of a hematoma and ligation of any bleeding points. Antibiotic therapy would be indicated at this juncture if it had not already been started.

Myocardial Infarction

Myocardial infarction is an emergency requiring careful management during the acute phase because most deaths occur during the first few hours and are due to ventricular fibrillation. The classic signs and symptoms of acute myocardial infarction include severe crushing substernal chest pain, diaphoresis, cyanosis or pallor, and nausea or vomiting. The pain is more severe than that of angina and is generally unrelieved by nitroglycerin tablets.

The following measures are recommended for any patient strongly suspected of having acute myocardial infarction. Surgery should be terminated and the emergency medical system activated. Because of the high incidence of ventricular fibrillation and other serious arrhythmias during the early hours of infarction, electrocardiographic (ECG) monitoring should be initiated immediately, if available. Oxygen should be administered by mask or nasal cannula at a flow rate of 4–6 liters/min. Routine administration of oxygen may minimize the extent of myocardial damage. An intravenous line should be established promptly.

Vital signs should be measured frequently and recorded by one member of the office team. Relief of pain should have a high priority, with a trial of nitroglycerin 0.4 mg given sublingually if the patient is normotensive or hypertensive. If this is unsuccessful or if pain is severe, morphine sulfate should slowly be given IV at doses of 1–5 mg as often as every 5 min.

Ventricular fibrillation occurs in the first hours of acute myocardial infarction. It may occur suddenly without preceding arrhythmia. Early prophylactic administration of lidocaine can substantially reduce the incidence of primary ventricular fibrillation. Therefore, in patients highly suspected of having myocardial infarction even in the absence of ventricular ectopy, prophylactic therapy with lidocaine should be started at the earliest possible time. A bolus of 1 mg/kg 1% lidocaine should be given initially. A continuous infusion should then be initiated at 2 mg/min. The dosage should be reduced in the presence of decreased cardiac output, in patients older than 70 years, and in those with hepatic dysfunction. These patients should be given one-half the normal bolus dosage and observed closely for signs of drug efficacy and toxicity.

Cardiac Arrest

The most feared emergency in dermatologic office surgery is cardiac arrest, which may occur as the unexpected result of a medication administered or secondary to a toxic dose of local anesthetic. Most commonly, however, patients who suffer cardiac arrest have preexisting coronary artery disease. The survival rate from cardiac arrest is dramatically increased whenever early CPR is coupled with an efficient emergency medical system (EMS) and advanced cardiac life support capability.

Extensive training in the recognition and management of cardiac arrest is mandatory. A textbook chapter cannot substitute for hands-on training given in the BLS and ACLS courses. Recent significant changes in both the BLS and ACLS courses were made by the 1985 National Conference on Standards and Guidelines for Cardiopulmonary Resuscitation and Emergency Cardiac Care.

The sequence of BLS—opening the airway, rescue breathing, and external chest compression, also known as the ABCs of CPR—is unchanged. Each of the ABCs begins with an assessment phase: "determine unresponsiveness," "determine breathlessness," and "determine pulselessness,"respectively. Determining unresponsiveness is important to prevent injury from attempted resuscitation of a patient who is not truly unconscious. This can be accomplished by gently tapping or shaking the patient and shouting, "Are you O.K.?" If the patient is unresponsive, summon someone to help activate the EMS system.

The airway should be opened immediately. The head-tilt/chin-lift maneuver (Fig. 3) is recommended to open the airway rather than the previously recommended head-tilt/neck-lift. The former more effectively opens the airway. The assessment for breathlessness should take no more than 5 sec and should include (1) looking for the rise and fall of the patient's chest, (2) listening for the air escaping during exhalation, (3) feeling for the flow of air from the patient's nose or mouth. This should be done while the opened airway is maintained. If the patient shows no signs of spontaneous respiration, mouth-to-mouth rescue breathing should be initiated while keep-

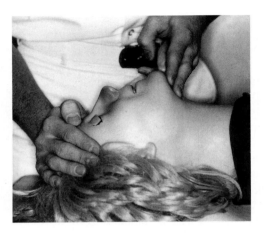

Figure 3 Head-tilt/chin-lift maneuver for opening the airway.

ing the airway open with the head-tilt/chin-lift maneuver and gently pinching the nose closed using the thumb and index finger of the hand on the forehead. After taking a deep breath and creating an airtight seal around the patient's mouth, two breaths of 1–1½ sec each should be given, rather than the four "quick" initial ventilations formerly recommended.

An assessment of pulselessness should be done carefully by checking the carotid pulse for 5–10 sec. If a pulse is present but there is no breathing, rescue breathing should be done at a rate of 12 times/min (once every 5 sec) after the first two breaths. The diagnosis of cardiac arrest is confirmed if no pulse is palpable. If this has not been done earlier, the EMS system should be activated and external chest compression begun.

The hand positioning and compression technique is unchanged. The heel of the hand nearest the patient's head is placed over the lower half of the sternum and the other hand placed on top of the hand on the sternum. The elbows are locked and the shoulders positioned directly over the hands so that each chest compression is directed down on the sternum. The sternum must be depressed 1½–2 inches for a normal-sized adult. External chest compression must be released completely and the chest allowed to return to its normal position after each compression.

A compression rate of 80–100/min for single and two-rescuer CPR is now recommended. The single rescuer should perform 15 external chest compressions at the 80–100/min rate. The mnemonic "one and, two and, three and, four and, five" helps to establish the proper compression rate. The airway should be opened again and two rescue breaths delivered, each lasting 1½ sec. Four cycles of 15 compressions and 2 ventilations should be performed before the carotid pulse is checked. If CPR is continued, the pulse and breathing can be checked every few minutes without interrupting CPR for more than 7 sec.

Two-rescuer CPR is now recommended only for professionals, and mouth-to-mask ventilation (Fig. 4) is an acceptable alternative for rescue breathing. A properly fitted mask equipped with a one-way valve diverts the patient's exhaled gas away from the rescuer and is an effective, simple method of providing ventilation. The mask is easier to use and provides larger tidal volumes than the bag-valve-mask technique. Mouth-to-mask ventilation with supplemental oxygen is preferred over bag-valve-mask devices until an endotracheal or esophageal airway is in place. The compression-ventilation rate for two rescuers is 5:1, with a pause for ventilation of 1–1½ sec. If an esophageal obturator or endotracheal tube is placed, ventilations may be given at a rate of 12–15/min.

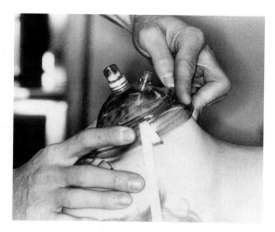

Figure 4 Mouth-to-mask ventilation with supplemental oxygen is a simple, effective method of artificial ventilation until an endotracheal or esophageal airway is in place.

The placement of any type of airway (oropharyngeal, nasopharyngeal, esophageal obturator, endotracheal) ensures the delivery of a high concentration of oxygen to the lungs. However, because of the delays and complications that can arise from the placement of these airways, their use should be restricted to medical personnel who are highly trained and who either use them frequently or are retrained frequently. The maximum period of interruption of ventilation when placing an airway should not exceed 30 sec. Suction may be required to remove oral and gastric secretions in order to place an endotracheal tube properly. Once an airway is in place, ventilation need not be synchronized with chest compression but should be performed at a rate of 12–15/min.

Cardiac arrest frequently results from several types of arrhythmias that may respond to electrical therapy. The electrocardiographic patterns of cardiac arrest most frequently encountered include ventricular fibrillation, pulseless ventricular tachycardia, asystole, and electromechanical dissociation. The success of resuscitation of patients with ventricular fibrillation and pulseless ventricular tachycardia is directly related to the rapidity of defibrillation. A monitor defibrillator unit is generally necessary to determine which cardiac arrest pattern is present. However, many emergency personnel today are using automated external defibrillators. These are highly sophisticated devices, which, when attached to the patient to record the rhythm, analyze the rhythm and, if ventricular fibrillation is present, deliver the appropriate shock.

After appropriate rhythm diagnosis using a cardiac monitor with quick-look paddles and prompt defibrillation as indicated, the next priority should be establishing a reliable intravenous line to administer medications. Antecubital veins should be the first choice to establish venous access since cannulation of either the jugular or subclavian veins not only interrupts CPR but is also associated with significant complications if improperly performed. Five percent dextrose in water is generally used to keep the IV line open. The three drugs of most value in the acute management of cardiac arrest are epinephrine 1:10,000, lidocaine 1% or 2%, and atropine (see Table 1). These three medications have a distinct advantage in that they can be administered via an endotracheal tube if difficulty has been encountered in establishing an IV line. All cardiac medications should be purchased in premixed, ready-to-inject syringes. Calcium chloride and sodium bicarbonate, which had previously been used routinely in the treatment of cardiac arrest, are now used infrequently or in very specific settings. Calcium chloride is indicated only in

Table 1 Basic Cardiopulmonary Resuscitation Drugs

Drug	Dosage	How Supplied	Remarks
Epinephrine	5–10 ml	1:10,000 (0.1 mg/ml)	IV or endotracheal administration is preferable to intracardiac. Give every 5 min during resuscitation attempt
Lidocaine	1 mg/kg	10 mg/ml (1%) 20 mg/ml (2%)	Only bolus therapy should be used in cardiac arrest setting. Repeat at 0.5 mg/kg every 8–10 min as needed to a total of 3 mg/kg
Bretylium	5 mg/kg	500 mg/10ml	IV bolus for refractory ventricular fibrillation, followed by 10 mg/kg in 15 min if needed. Repeat at 15–30 min intervals to a total of 30 mg/kg
Atropine	0.5–1.0 mg	0.1 mg/ml	1.0 mg IV for asystole. Repeat at 5 min if asystole persists
Sodium bicarbonate	1 mEq/kg	1 mEq/ml	Not recommended for routine cardiac arrest sequence. If used, half the initial dose may be repeated every 10 min
Calcium chloride	2–4 mg/kg	100 mg/ml	Use only in cases of hyperkalemia, hypocalcemia, or calcium channel block toxicity

specific situations such as cardiac arrest related to hyperkalemia, profound hypocalcemia, or calcium channel blocker toxicity. Sodium bicarbonate should only be used after defibrillation, chest compressions, ventilatory support, including intubation, epinephrine, and antiarrhythmics have been used, and then only when blood gases are available and indicate a profound acidosis.

The great majority of outpatient cardiac arrests are due to ventricular fibrillation. Treatment of this rhythm disturbance begins with CPR and activation of the emergency medical system (Table 2). If a defibrillator is available, immediate defibrillation is critical and is carried out initially with 200 J. If defibrillation is persistent, a second shock should be administered at a strength of 200–300 J. If the first two shocks are ineffective in establishing a life-sustaining rhythm, a third shock not exceeding 360 J should be delivered immediately. Proper paddle electrode positioning is important. One electrode should be placed to the right of the upper sternum and below the clavicle; the other should be placed to the left of the nipple with the electrode in the center of the midaxillary line. Approximately 25 lb of pressure should be applied to each paddle. In patients with permanent pacemakers, the electrodes should not be closer than 5 inches from the pacemaker generator.

If initial defibrillation is unsuccessful, epinephrine should be administered immediately after establishing an IV line. Epinephrine is administered in a dose of 5–10 ml of a 1:10,000 solution every 5–10 min during resuscitation. Intracardiac administration of epinephrine should be avoided unless both IV and endotracheal routes are not readily available because of the risk of coronary artery laceration, cardiac tamponade, or pneumothorax. When epinephrine is administered in an intracardiac fashion, there is also an interruption of external compressions and ventilation. Epinephrine with its potent alpha-adrenergic receptor-stimulating properties increases myocardial and CNS blood flow during ventilation and chest compression.

Table 2 Ventricular Fibrillation (VF) and Pulseless Ventricular Tachycardia (VT)

Begin CPR until a defibrillator is available.
If monitor confirms VF (pulseless VT treated identically), defibrillate with 200 J. Repeat a second time with 200–300 J and a third time with up to 360 J if VF persists.
Continue CPR if no pulse and give epinephrine, 1:10,000, 5–10 ml IV push. Epinephrine should be repeated every 5 min as needed.
Intubate if possible. Do not interrupt CPR for more than 30 sec.
Defibrillate again with up to 360 J.
If unsuccessful, give lidocaine 1 mg/kg IV push and defibrillate again with up to 360 J.
If unsuccessful, give bretylium 5 mg/kg IV push, and defibrillate again with up to 360 J.
Consider the use of bicarbonate at this time.
If unsuccessful, give bretylium 10 mg/kg IV push, and defibrillate again with up to 360 J.
Boluses of lidocaine or bretylium may be repeated at the recommended intervals to the maximum limit.
Each bolus should be followed by defibrillation of up to 360 J.

The drug of choice for ventricular ectopy including ventricular tachycardia and ventricular fibrillation is lidocaine. Lidocaine is recommended when these arrhythmias are resistant to defibrillation since it may improve the response to electrical therapy. When ventricular fibrillation is present, an initial dosage of 1 mg/kg of lidocaine is given IV push. After this dose, additional boluses (0.5 mg/kg) can be given every 8–10 min if necessary up to 3 mg/kg. In the cardiac arrest setting only bolus therapy should be utilized. A continuous infusion of 2–4 mg/min should be started after successful resuscitation. The dosage should be reduced to half the normal bolus dose in the presence of decreased cardiac output, in patients older than 70 years, or in patients with hepatic dysfunction. If signs of lidocaine toxicity (slurred speech, altered consciousness, muscle twitching, seizures) are observed, the drug dosage should be reduced immediately.

In ventricular fibrillation refractory to defibrillation and lidocaine, bretylium is given as an IV bolus (5 mg/kg). This is followed by a single electrical defibrillation up to 360 J. The dosage of bretylium can be increased to 10 mg/kg and given at 15- to 30-min intervals until a maximum dosage of 30 mg/kg has been given for persistent ventricular fibrillation. Both lidocaine and bretylium may take up to 2 min to reach the cardiac circulation.

Atropine may be efficacious in the treatment of cardiac arrest due to ventricular asystole. Its parasympatholytic actions include decreasing cardiac vagal tone, increasing the rate of discharge of the sinus node, and enhancing atrioventricular (AV) conduction. The recommended dosage of atropine for asystole is 1.0 mg given IV. This is repeated in 5 min if asystole persists. Full vagal blockage results after a total dosage of 2.0 mg. Epinephrine should be administered prior to atropine and repeated every 5 min in ventricular asystole (Tables 3 and 4).

Table 3 Treatment of Asystole

If the rhythm is unclear, and possible VF, defibrillate as for VF.
Once diagnosis of asystole is confirmed, establish IV and give epinephrine 1:10,000, 5–10 ml IV push, while continuing CPR. Repeat epinephrine every 5 min as needed.
Intubate if possible. Do not interrupt CPR for more than 30 sec.
Give atropine 1.0 mg IV push. Repeat in 5 min if asystole persists.
Consider the use of bicarbonate at this time.
If there is no response, insertion of a pacemaker should be considered.

8

Suture Materials

Clifford Warren Lober and Neil A. Fenske
University of South Florida College of Medicine, Tampa, Florida

For thousands of years we have been searching for an ideal suture material. Naturally occurring materials such as cotton, bark fiber, horse tails, and the mouth parts of pitcher ants have been used to close wounds. Innovative physicians tried violin strings, wooden sticks, and other devices for the same purpose. When synthetic materials such as nylon were developed for other purposes, surgeons adapted them to wound closure. It was not until the 1970s that synthetic polymers were developed specifically for use as suture materials on the basis of their physical, chemical, and biologic properties.

Suture materials may be made of naturally occurring substances or synthetic polymers, monofilament or multifilament, dyed or undyed, and can be coated or uncoated. The chemical composition of a suture material may be either well determined (e.g., synthetic chemical polymers) or less specifically defined (e.g., catgut). Both the chemical composition and the physical construction of the suture determine the final properties of the suture material.

Several parameters are used to describe the physical characteristics of sutures. Tensile strength is calculated by dividing the maximum load by the original cross-sectional area of suture material. Breaking strength is that load required to cause the suture material to rupture. Elasticity is the ability of a substance to undergo nonpermanent deformation, and plasticity refers to the ability of the material to stretch nonelastically without rupturing or the ability of a substance to be permanently deformed without fracturing. Materials stretch elastically prior to undergoing plastic deformation. Memory is the ability of a substance to return to its original physical configuration following deformation.

Capillarity refers to the ability of suture material to conduct fluids. Multifilament and uncoated sutures tend to have a greater capillarity than monofilament and coated sutures. It has been clearly shown that multifilament and uncoated sutures tend to permit greater passage of bacteria into wounds and promote infection.

Sutures should elicit a minimal degree of tissue reactivity. Naturally occurring materials such as catgut and silk, which are absorbed by phagocytosis and enzymatic degradation, tend to induce a greater degree of inflammatory response than synthetic polymers such as polyglycolic acid or polyglycan 910, which are degraded primarily by hydrolysis.

In addition to evaluating sutures on the basis of measurable physical characteristics, surgeons compare sutures on the basis of "performance characteristics." These subjectively evaluated parameters include pliability, ease of handling, visibility, and knot security. The latter is the ability of a knot to hold without breaking or stretching and reflects the material's elasticity, plasticity, tensile strength, and memory.

Suture materials are available in different sizes. The number of zeros indicated on a suture package reflects the size of the enclosed suture material. As the number of zeros increases, the size of the suture material decreases. A 6–0 nylon suture, for example, is smaller than a 4–0 strand of nylon suture. The designation in terms of zeros, however, does not correspond to an exact physical size but to a range of sizes allowed by the United States Pharmacopoeia to attain a given tensile strength. For this reason a strand of 4–0 polyglycan 910, for example, is not necessarily of the same diameter as a 4–0 strand of catgut.

Suture materials have been arbitrarily designated by the United States Pharmacopoeia as either absorbable or nonabsorbable. A nonabsorbable suture is defined as one that persists in tissue for more than 60 days. An absorbable material, conversely, is a substance that is not present in the tissue 60 days following implantation. Many of the so-called nonabsorbable sutures are, in fact, physiologically absorbable. Cotton, for example, which is a nonabsorbable suture according to the United States Pharmacopoeia definition, loses 50% of its tensile strength in 6 months.

In order to understand what we can expect of sutures, we must have a basic understanding of the physiology of wound healing. During the first 4–6 days following wounding there is a minimal gain in wound strength and the surgical site is virtually totally dependent upon sutures to maintain closure. During the burst of fibroplasia and collagen production that begins between the fifth and sixth day, there is a rapid gain in wound strength. This gain in strength continues as remodeling of the wounded dermis progresses and plateaus after approximately 70 days. The maturation phase of wound healing continues for at least 1 year.

A surgical wound never attains the same cutaneous tensile strength of normal uncut skin. Two weeks after sutures are implanted, at a time when many surgeons elect to remove them, surgical wounds have achieved only 3–5% of the original skin strength or approximately 7% of the ultimate tensile strength the repaired wound will achieve. By the end of the third week 20% of final tensile strength is achieved, and by 1 month only 50% of ultimate wound strength (or 35% of the original strength) is attained. Wounds never gain more than 80% of the strength of intact unwounded skin.

All sutures are foreign bodies and produce an inflammatory response in the host dermis that peaks between the second and seventh day following implantation. Between the second and seventh day there is an abundance of polymorphonuclear leukocytes, lymphocytes, and large monocytes. By the fourth day, there is an increasing number of mononuclear cells, macrophages, and fibroblasts. Between the third and eighth day the epithelial cells deeply invade suture tracts and do not cease their migration until cells migrating from the needle entrance site meet cells advancing from the needle exit site (contact inhibition). In the case of absorbable sutures the inflammatory cell reaction is noted to increase when absorption begins and persists until all of the foreign material is eliminated. In the case of nonabsorbable sutures, a comparatively acellular reaction persists, in which a fibrous capsule is laid down around the sutures at 10–16 days. In general, monofilament sutures produce less inflammatory response than multifilament sutures.

ABSORBABLE SUTURES

Absorbable sutures are placed into the subcutaneous tissue to minimize tissue tension during wound healing. It is important to remember that absorbable sutures must be placed well into the dermis to facilitate their subsequent absorption by inflammation or hydrolysis. If absorbable sutures are placed superficially, they may persist for a prolonged period of time and may have an increased tendency to be eliminated ("spit") from the wound. One must also remember that absorbable sutures are not intended to be used to close the skin surface, because their delayed absorption may permit the epithelialization of the suture tunnels and leave permanent suture tracts on the patient.

Catgut

The first reference to catgut as an absorbable suture is by Galen of Pergamon, circa 175 A.D. Although the origin of the name catgut is obscure, it has nothing to do with cats. It has been suggested that it was derived from the word "kitgut," from "kit," an Arabian dancing master's fiddle that had strings made from sheep intestine.

Catgut sutures are derived from the submucosal layer of the small intestine of sheep and the serosal layer of the small intestine of cattle. Since they are derived from organic sources, there is no assurance of chemical uniformity among catgut sutures. Manufacturing procedures may produce weak spots and tear fibrils. This may cause uneven absorption and premature rupture of the sutures. Similarly, the physical parameters (e.g., width) of a given strand of catgut may vary.

In comparison to other absorbable suture materials presently available, catgut sutures tend to lose their strength rapidly. Although markedly variable for the above-cited reasons, approximately 60% of the tensile strength of catgut is lost 1 week following implantation into a wound, and, effectively, no tensile strength remains in 2 weeks. Catgut is a foreign organic substance in recipient tissue and elicits a markedly inflammatory response. Through this inflammatory response catgut is broken down and absorbed. Histologic examination of tissues sutured with catgut reveals a striking inflammatory response within 4 days, peaking at day 9.

In an attempt to retard the absorption of catgut sutures, they have been coated with chromic salts. Although physical absorption is delayed, the actual retention of tensile strength beyond 14 days is negligible. Chromic catgut sutures may persist beyond 2 weeks in the dermis and a continuous inflammatory reaction persists until they are absorbed.

Although the use of catgut sutures has decreased during the last decade, there is one form in which catgut is still widely used. In procedures such as blepharoplasty, surgeons frequently wish to have sutures in place for only a few days. Under these conditions, the use of "mild ophthalamic chromic gut" or "fast-absorbing surgical gut" may be advantageous. The sutures are removed when the dressing is taken off in 2 days.

Polyglycolic Acid

Polyglycolic acid (Dexon, Davis & Geck) became commercially available in 1971. This synthetic homopolymer of glycolic acid (hydroacetic acid) provided for the first time a suture of uniform chemical composition. Glycolic acid is initially reacted with itself to form the cyclic ester glycolide, which is subsequently converted to a high molecular weight linear chain polymer. This polymer is made into sutures when, in either its dyed or undyed form, it is crushed into small granules, melt-extruded through a dye to form fibers, heat-stretched, braided, restretched, and heat-treated again to make the braiding tight and more uniform. A needle is attached and the suture is wound onto a paper holder that is subsequently wrapped prior to sterilization with ethylene oxide.

Since polyglycolic acid is not a naturally occurring organic substance, it elicits far less inflammatory response than catgut. It is absorbed primarily by hydrolysis rather than by a host inflammatory response. Polyglycolic acid possesses good tensile strength and excellent knot security. According to the product description prepared by the manufacturer, 2 weeks after implantation into a wound approximately 55% of the initial tensile strength of polyglycolic acid sutures remains and at 3 weeks approximately 20% of the original tensile strength remains.

Many surgeons report noticeable tissue resistance to the passage of polyglycolic acid sutures. To improve the handling characteristics of this material, a newer polyglycolic acid suture was introduced in 1978. It has smaller multifilament strands and a tighter weave. Additionally, a coating of polyoxamer 188 has been used to minimize tissue drag and facilitate handling.

Polyglycan 910

With the appearance of polyglycan sutures (Vicryl, Ethicon) in 1974, surgeons were able to use a synthetic heteropolymer consisting of 90% glycolide and 10% lactide. Glycolide and lactide are cyclic intermediates of lactide and glycolic acid that are more easily converted into fiber-forming polymers than are their parent free acids. The addition of lactic to the glycolic acid reduces crystalinity and increases pliability. In the manufacturing of polyglycan 910 sutures the heteropolymer is melted in the presence of a catalyst, extruded into fibers, braided, heat-stretched to make the braiding tighter and more uniform, and sterilized using ethylene oxide. Polyglycan 910 is a light tan or gold suture, but it may be colored to enhance visibility by the addition of Drug and Cosmetic Violet No. 2 dye during polymerization. The dye is thus uniformly distributed throughout each fiber. This synthetic polymer is degraded by hydrolysis to water and carbon dioxide. It thus induces less tissue reactivity than does catgut. An absorbable coating composed of a mixture of calcium stearate and a copolymer derived from 65% lactide and 35% glycolide may be applied to polyglycan 910 to improve the overall handling properties of this multifilament braided suture.

It is important that our absorbable suture material retain significant functional tensile strength for several weeks following implantation into a wound. The residual tensile strength of a 4–0 suture of polyglycan 910 is consistently greater than that of polyglycolic acid when measured weekly. The difference in tensile strength between these two materials, however, should be of minimal clinical significance if we close wounds of the skin and subcutaneous tissues using appropriate surgical techniques that minimize skin tension of our wounds.

We would like our absorbable suture material to disappear as rapidly and completely as possible following its loss of functional tensile strength. Polyglycan 910 is absorbed more rapidly than is polyglycolic acid. In one study the absorption of polyglycan 910 began at approximately 40 days following its implantation into rabbits and was nearly complete by day 70. At 90 days, no polymer remained in the tissue. Although the absorption of polyglycolic acid was also noted to begin 40 days following its implantation, approximately half of the material remained in the tissue at 90 days and "significant quantities" were present when the study was terminated at 120 days.

Polydioxanone

In 1982 the synthetic homopolymer polydioxanone (PDS, Ethicon) became available commercially. It is prepared by polymerizing the monomer paradioxanone to a high molecular weight compound that can be melt excluded into a monofilament. The suture may be dyed using Drug and Cosmetic Violet No. 2 dye and thus be highly visible. Monofilament polydioxanone is particularly valuable when potential wound infection is a concern, because its monofilament construction prevents organisms from being entrapped by or traveling along the interstices of suture strands.

Polydioxanone is similar to polyglycolic acid and polyglycan 910 in that it is degraded by hydrolysis rather than by phagocytosis and inflammation. Compared to polyglycan 910, a far less severe host inflammatory response in induced by polydioxanone.

A major advantage of polydioxanone suture is that it retains significant tensile strength for over a month. Two weeks following implantation, approximately 70% of its original tensile strength remains. At 4 weeks polydioxanone still retains 50% of its tensile strength, and approximately 25% of its tensile strength remains at 6 weeks. One study revealed that 14% of initial tensile strength was still present 8 weeks following implantation. Since we are aware that surgical wounds attain only 3–5% of the original skin strength 2 weeks following the placement of sutures, this added tensile strength may be clinically significant in those wounds closed under some degree of tension. Polydioxanone is rapidly absorbed between 140 days following its implantation, at which time approximately 80% of the polymer remains, and 180 days, at which time no significant material is present in the host tissue.

NONABSORBABLE SUTURES

Nonabsorbable sutures may be used subcutaneously ("buried") to provide prolonged mechanical support for a healing wound or to approximate the skin surface. The use of nonabsorbable sutures in the subcutaneous tissues should not be viewed as an alternative to proper surgical techniques (e.g., proper planning of wound configuration, undermining, etc.) that minimize wound tension. When used to oppose the skin surface, the sutures should be just tight enough to approximate, not strangulate, tissues. The wound edema that develops postoperatively increases the tension on the sutures and may cause them to "cut in" if they are firmly placed at the time of surgery.

Silk

Silk has been used for centuries to close wounds. For the first half of this century absorbable catgut and nonabsorbable silk were the standards for virtually all wound closures. Silk is a naturally occurring organic substance and induces a striking host inflammatory response. It is degraded by phagocytosis and the actions of enzymes. Like catgut and other organic materials, silk may vary in its exact chemical composition and the diameter of each strand may be somewhat nonuniform.

An outstanding quality of silk is its ease of handling. Despite the development of numerous synthetic polymers, silk remains the standard by which all suture materials are judged with regard to ease of handling. Its ease of passage through tissue and pliability remain unsurpassed by any other material presently available.

Although silk is classified as a nonabsorbable suture according to the arbitrary United States Pharmacopoeia definition, it is in fact gradually absorbed. Postlethwait reported that 8 months after implantation silk lost 38% of its initial strength. It loses approximately 50% of its strength in 1 year and has no significant tensile strength 2 years after implantation.

Nylon

In the 1930s and 1940s numerous synthetic materials were developed for the clothing industry, the rubber industry, and other commercial ventures. Surgeons were quick to adapt these synthetic polymers as suture materials. Nylon, polyester, rayon, and other materials were tried. These synthetic polymers were uniform in composition and, as nonorganic materials, generally elicited less tissue reactivity than organic materials. They are available in either mono- or multifilament forms. Monofilament nylon has a great deal of memory, and its proclivity to permit knot slippage is well recognized.

Like silk, some synthetic polymers are gradually absorbed by host tissues. Nylon, for example, loses 25% of its tensile strength over a 2-year period.

Polypropyline

In 1970 polypropyline was introduced as the first synthetic nonabsorbable material specifically developed for use as sutures. It is an isotactic crystalline stereoisomer of a linear homopolymer containing few or no unsaturated bonds. This material has tensile strength exceeding that of nylon, passes easily through tissue, and induces a minimal host inflammatory response. It is not absorbed to any significant degree over a period of at least 1 year. It is highly visible when dyed blue and has slightly more memory than nylon.

Polybutester

In 1984 polybutester (Novafil, Davis & Geck) was introduced as a synthetic monofilament heteropolymer of polytetramethylene ether glycol terephthalate (16%) and polybutylene terephthalate (84%). Polybutester suture passes easily through tissue and induces a minimal host inflammatory response. Its functional tensile strength is similar to that of nylon.

Polybutester has a marked degree of plasticity and memory. It feels like a rubber band. This enables the suture material to expand as the wound undergoes its edematous healing phase and subsequently to contract as the edematous phase resolves.

Staples

Surgical staples are used because they permit rapid wound closure, reduce tissue trauma, elicit minimal inflammatory response, and are cost-effective. The stapling guns presently available tend to evert wound edges and thus facilitate the healing wounds. Surgical staples may be particularly useful in hair-bearing areas such as in closing scalp reductions or closing donor sites following hair transplantation.

On nonfacial skin the results obtainable by staples are comparable to those one might expect using other nonabsorbable sutures. On facial areas, however, many believe that a more exact approximation of tissue and thus a better cosmetic result may be obtainable using sutures other than staples.

Skin staples and steel ligatures are available from several manufacturers in disposable stapling units. Several units have rotatable heads that make them easier to use in hard-to-reach locations. In 1987 Ethicon Corporation released the Quantum skin stapler (Fig. 1). This stapler has a rotatable head and dispenses Teflon-coated staples. This coating makes removal of the staples easier postoperatively. The Quantum stapler may be precocked into a position of partial staple closure and thus facilitates the placement of grafts by "hooking into" the graft tissue and opposing wound edges.

SUTURE REMOVAL

The size of the suture and needle used to insert it are relatively unimportant in terms of final cosmetic result. Sutures removed within 7 days generally leave no skin marks, while those left in place over 2 weeks produce persistent marks. This is understandable in view of the time course of wound healing and the host inflammatory response to sutures as previously detailed.

It has been suggested that all sutures on the face be removed by the fifth day, with alternating sutures having been removed on the second to third day following placement. The same author suggests that sutures in the eyelids be completely removed by the second to third day, those in the extremities and anterior trunk at the sixth or seventh day, and those on the sole of the foot and back at 7–10 days. Others have suggested that sutures on the back and those placed in areas affected by a great deal of motion be left in place for 2 weeks or longer. These gener-

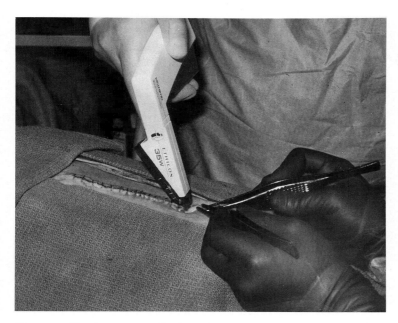

Figure 1 The Quantum stapler features a rotatable head and dispenses Teflon-coated staples. (Photograph courtesy of Ethicon Corporation.)

alizations can only be used as guidelines. The proper time to remove sutures is determined by balancing cosmetic considerations, which dictate removal of sutures as rapidly as possible to avoid suture marks, and functional considerations such as ensuring that the wound does not dehisce. These considerations will reflect the anatomy of the site involved, the degree of tension on the wound, the use of subcutaneous sutures, and the amount and direction of tension exerted by underlying muscles.

SURGICAL NEEDLES

Virtually all sutures in use today are directly attached to the needles (swaged or swedged) rather than being threaded through a hole in the needle. This permits use of a smaller-diameter needle and thus less tissue trauma when sutures are placed.

The majority of needles used by dermatologic surgeons have an arc of 135 degrees. The terminology used to describe needles has developed in a totally haphazard fashion. One must determine which needles one prefers and learn the terminology of that particular manufacturer. Since Ethicon Corporation presently manufactures 80–85% of all surgical sutures and needles in North America, a few words about their terminology are in order.

The conventional cutting needle has a triangular point and body. The flat base of the triangle faces away from the wound and the apex of the triangle faces toward the wound. This permits the suture to "ride" in the needle tract; if there is any tension on the wound the suture will tend to "cut in" towards the wound edges. To avoid this difficulty, the reverse cutting needle was developed. Like the conventional needle, the reverse cutting needle has a triangular configuration but the apex of the triangle points away from the wound incision rather than toward it. This needle is particularly good for tough and difficult-to-penetrate tissues.

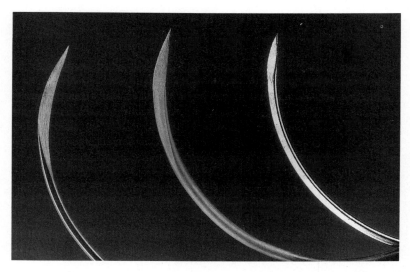

Figure 2   The PC needle (left) is honed to a finer point than either the PS needle (center) or the FS needle (right). The latter two needles are reverse cutting needles. (Photograph courtesy of Ethicon Corporation.)

In addition to differences in the geometric shape of the needle, needles may also differ in the type of surgical steel from which they are manufactured and their degree of sharpness. The FS ("for skin") series of needles is the least expensive needle and is used primarily for noncosmetic surgery. The P ("plastic") or PS ("plastic skin") and PC ("precision cosmetic") series of needles are made of a higher-quality steel and are honed to a greater degree (Fig. 2). The P or PS series, for example, is honed 24 times more than the FS series. These needles pass more easily through tissue and are useful when cosmetic considerations are important. The PC needles are made of stronger stainless steel alloy and have a modified, flattened, conventional cutting point.

BIBLIOGRAPHY

Albom MJ. Cutaneous surgery, including Mohs surgery. In *Dermatology*. Moschella SL, Hurley HJ, eds. Philadelphia, W.B. Saunders Company, 1992, pp. 2314–2402.

Albom MJ. Dermatologic surgery. In *Clinical Dermatology*. Demis DJ, ed. Philadelphia, J.B. Lippincott Company, 1991, pp. 1–81.

Artandi C. A revolution in sutures. *Surg Gynecol Obstet* 1980;150:235–236.

Aston SJ. The choice of suture material for skin closure. *J Dermatol Surg* 1976;2:57–61.

Becker H, Davidoff MR. The physical properties of suture materials as related to knot holding. *S Afr J Surg* 1977;15:105–113.

Blomstedt B, Jacobsson S. Experiences with polyglactin 910 (Vicryl®) in general surgery. *Acta Chir Scand* 1977;143:259–263.

Blomstedt B, Osterberg B. Suture materials and wound infection. *Acta Chir Scand* 1978;144:269–274.

Chu CC. Mechanical properties of suture materials, an important characterization. *Ann Surg* 1981; 193:365–371.

Chusak RB, Dibbell DG. Clinical experience with polydioxanone monofilament absorbable sutures in plastic surgery. *Plast Reconstr Surg* 1983;72:217–221.

Conn J Jr, Beal JM. Coated Vicryl synthetic absorbable sutures. *Surg Gynecol Obstet* 1980;150:843–844.

Craig PH, Williams JA, Davis KW, Magoun AD, Levy AJ, Bogdansky S, Jones JP Jr. A biologic comparison of polyglactin 910 and polyglycolic acid synthetic absorbable sutures. *Surg Gynecol Obstet* 1975; 141:1–10.

Crikelair GF. Skin suture marks. *Am J Surg* 1958;96:631–639.

Deutsch HL. Observations on a new absorbable suture material. *J Dermatol Surg* 1975;1:49–51.

Edstrom LE. Clinical experience with polydioxanone monofilament absorbable sutures in plastic surgery. *Plast Reconstr Surg* 1983;72:221.

Ethicon Inc. *Wound Closure Manual, Use and Handling of Sutures, Needles and Mechanical Wound Closure Devices*. Ethicon, 1985.

Garrett AB. Wound closure materials. In *Cutaneous Surgery*. Wheeland RG, ed. Philadelphia, W.B. Saunders Company, 1994, pp. 199–205.

Georgiade G, Riefkohl R, Serafin D, Georgiade N. Use of skin staples in plastic surgery. *Ann Plast Surg* 1980;5:324–325.

Guyuron B, Vaughn C. A comparison of absorbable and nonabsorbable suture material for skin repair. *Plast Reconstr Surg* 1992;89:234–236.

Harris DR. Healing of the surgical wound, I. Basic considerations. *J Am Acad Dermatol* 1979;1:197–207.

Harris DR. Healing of the surgical wound, II. Factors influencing repair and regeneration. *J Am Acad Dermatol* 1979;1:208–215.

Herrmann JB. Changes in tensile strength and knot security of surgical sutures in vivo. *Arch Surg* 1973; 106:707–710.

Herrmann JB, Kelly RJ, Higgins GA. Polyglycolic acid sutures, laboratory and clinical evaluation of a new absorbable suture material. *Arch Surg* 1970;100:486–490.

Holt GR, Holt JE. Suture materials and techniques. *Ear Nose Throat J* 1981;60:12–18.

Horton CE, Adamson JE, Mladick RA, Carraway JH. Vicryl synthetic absorbable sutures. *Am Surg* 1974; 40:729–731.

Howes EL. Effects of suture material on the tensile strength of wound repair. *Ann Surg* 1933;98:153–155.

Howes EL. Strength studies of polyglycolic acid versus catgut sutures of the same size. *Surg Gynecol Obstet* 1973;137:15–20.

Howes EL. The immediate strength of the sutured wound. *Surgery* 1940;7:24–31.

Howes EL. The strengh of wounds sutured with catgut and silk. *Surg Gynecol Obstet* 1933;57:309–311.

Howes EL, Harvey SC. The strength of the healing wound in relation to the holding strength of the catgut suture. *N Engl J Med* 1929;200:1285–1291.

Jenkins HP, Hrdina LS, Owens FM, Jr. Swisher FM. Absorption of surgical gut (catgut). *Arch Surg* 1942; 45;74–102.

Katz AR, Turner RJ. Evaluation of tensile and absorption properties of polyglycolic acid sutures. *Surg Gynecol Obstet* 1970;131:701–716.

Laufer N, Merino M, Trietsch HG, DeCherney AH. Macroscopic and histologic tissue reaction to polydioxanone , a new, synthetic, monofilament microsuture. *J Reprod Med* 1984;29:307–310.

Lerwick E. Studies on the efficacy and safety of polydioxanone monofilament absorbable suture. *Surg Gynecol Obstet* 1983;156:51–55.

Lober CW, Fenske NA. Suture materials for closing the skin and subcutaneous tissues. *Aesthetic Plast Surg* 1986;10:245–247.

Lynch WS. Wound healing. In *Skin Surgery*. E Epstein, E Epstein, Jr, eds. Philadelphia, WB Saunders, 1987, pp. 56–70.

Mackenzie D. The history of sutures. *Med Hist* 1973;17:158–168.

MacKinnon AE, Brown S. Skin closure with polyglycolic acid (Dexon). *Postgrad Med J* 1978;54:384–385.

Madsen ET. An experimental and clinical evaluation of surgical suture materials. *Surg Gynecol Obstet* 1953;97:73–80.

Nilsson T. Mechanical properties of Prolene® and Ethilon® sutures after three weeks in vivo. *Scand J Plast Reconstr Surg* 1982;16:11–15.

Novafil Polybutester Suture. Proceedings of a symposium. American Cyanamid, Wayne, NJ, 1984

Osterburg B, Blomstedt B. Effect of suture materials on bacterial survival in infected wounds. *Acta Chir Scand* 1979;145:431–434.

Postlethwait RW. Long-term comparative study of nonabsorbable sutures. *Ann Surg* 1970;171:892–898.

Postlethwait RW. Polyglycolic acid surgical suture. *Arch Surg* 1970;101:489–494.

Postlethwait RW, Smith BM. A new synthetic absorbable suture. *Surg Gynecol Obstet* 1975;140:377–380.

Postlethwait RW, Willigan DA, Ulin AW. Human tissue reaction to sutures. *Ann Surg* 1975;181:144–150.

Ray JA, Doddi N, Regula D, Williams JA, Melveger A. Polydioxanone (PDS), a novel monofilament synthetic absorbable suture. *Surg Gynecol Obstet* 1981;153:497–507.

Rodeheaver GT, Kurtz LD, Bellamy WT, Smith SL, Farris H, Edlich RF. Biocidal braided sutures. *Arch Surg* 1983;118:322–327.

Salthouse TN. Biologic response to sutures. *Otolaryngol Head Neck Surg* 1980;88:658–664.

Sato RM, Tebbetts JB, Suarez AJ, Hunt JL, Baxter CR. Staples: Their use in achieving biological coverage of burn patients. *Burns* 1979;6:261–263.

Stegman SJ, Tromovitch TA, Glogau RG. Suture material. In *Basics of Dermatologic Surgery,* SJ Stegman, TA Tromovitch, RG Glogau, eds. Chicago, Year Book Medical Publishers, 1982, pp. 36–40.

Stroumtsos O. *Perspectives on Sutures.* Davis & Geck, American Cyanamid Company, 1978.

Swanson NA, Tromovitch TA. Suture materials, 1980s: Properties, uses, and abuses. *Int J Dermatol* 1982; 21:373–378.

VanVlack LH. *Elements of Materials Science*, Reading MA, Addison-Wesley, 1964, p. 139.

VanVlack LH. Engineering requirements of materials. In *Elements of Materials Science*. Reading, MA, Addison-Wesley, 1964, pp. 1–7.

Van Winkle W Jr, Hastings JC. Considerations in the choice of suture material for various tissues. *Surg Gynecol Obstet* 1972;135:113–126.

Varma S, Ferguson HL, Breen H, Lumb WV. Comparison of seven suture materials in infected wounds—an experimental study. *J Surg Res* 1974;17:165–170.

Watts GT. Sutures for skin closure. *Lancet* 1975;1:581.

Yu GV, Cavaliere R. Suture materials, properties and uses. *J Am Podiatry Assoc* 1983;73:57–64.

9

Wound Healing by First and Second Intention

John A. Zitelli

Shadyside Medical Center, Pittsburgh, Pennsylvania

People have always searched for ways to improve wound healing, particularly to decrease pain and speed the time needed for complete healing. In ancient mythology, Aesculapius, the Greek god of healing, Ningishzida, a Babylonian god of healing, and Hermes, the Roman Mercury, were symbolized with a staff entwined with one or two snakes. The significance of the snake was its ability to repeatedly shed and regenerate its skin, a capability envied by physicians of the day.

The quest for a better understanding of wound healing has continued slowly. Some ancient methods of wound management such as wet linen wraps are similar to more modern methods of occlusive or semiocclusive dressings. Although Hippocrates advocated that wounds be kept dry, most wounds were covered with fat- or oil-based ointment after being washed in wine or vinegar. Wound management took a step backward during medieval times when it was common to treat open wounds with hot coals and caustic substances that we now recognize delay wound healing. The concept of asepsis resulted in more control of wound healing than any other approach, and as a science, wound healing became the primary interest of surgeons. However, in the last few decades, clinical and basic science research in dermatology has significantly contributed to our understanding of cutaneous wound healing so that we can better enhance this process.

NORMAL EVENTS OF WOUND HEALING

Normal wound healing is a complex series of events occurring simultaneously in the epidermis, dermis, and subcutaneous tissue. It is easy to differentiate epidermal healing from dermal healing, although it is important to remember that the events occur at the same time (Fig. 1).

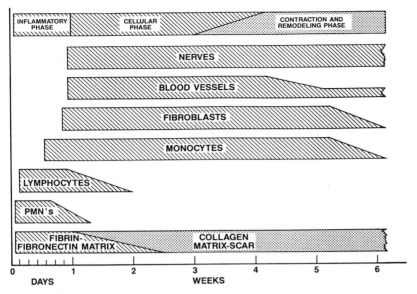

Figure 1 Normal events of dermal wound healing.

Dermal Wound Healing

Wound healing begins when an injury to the skin causes bleeding. Extravasated blood clots rapidly and forms an insoluble, water-holding gel matrix of fibrin, fibronectin, and platelets as well as blood cells. Exposure of collagen to Hageman factor XII activates the coagulation pathway; fibrinogen is activated to form fibrin, and platelets are activated releasing platelet-derived growth factors and chemoattractants for connective tissue cells. For wounds created without bleeding (burns, cryosurgery), other mechanisms such as activation of complement and stimulation of the cellular immune response may participate in the first phase of wound healing.

Serum factors such as fibronectin, laminin, and vasoactive amines (i.e., kinin) are also important in attracting polymorphonuclear leukocytes (PMNs) and maintaining increased vascular permeability. Fibrin and fibronectin are very important proteins in healing wounds. As vascular permeability increases, serum proteins, including fibrin and fibronectin, enter the extravascular space. Together fibrin and fibronectin form the initial wound matrix. Fibrin in the matrix is covalently cross-linked to provide strong tensile strength. Later, as normal vascular permeability is restored, fibroblasts appear and begin synthesizing fibrin and fibronectin to maintain the integrity of the matrix while monocytes, endothelial cells, and epidermal cells migrate into the wound.

Inflammatory Phase

The inflammatory phase of wound healing is defined as the period where the effects of chemical mediators and inflammatory cells predominate. The inflammatory phase in a sutured wound may go unrecognized, lasting only 4–5 days with mild redness and swelling. In a clean open wound, the inflammatory phase is characterized by a copious exudate lasting 7–10 days, or longer in wounds complicated by the presence of denatured protein or necrotic tissue caused by infection, laser, electrosurgery, cryosurgery, topical acids, or caustics. Clinically, this is the period when an open wound is best managed with adsorbent dressings or more frequent dressing changes than those required during later stages of wound healing.

The inflammatory phase of wound healing begins when vasoactive substances are released from platelets or mononuclear cells, or when complement is activated in the initial events of healing. These signals increase vascular permeability, and with specific leukocyte chemotactic factors stimulate polymorphonuclear cell migration into the wound. Within hours, PMNs are the predominant inflammatory cell around the wound, although their function is not clear. They may play a role in preventing infection as well as debriding the wound of necrotic tissue by enzymatic digestion and phagocytosis of debris. However, it is known that wounds in neutropenic animals heal in a normal fashion and, therefore, PMNs may only be useful in complicated wounds.

Lymphocytes are also a prominent cell in the inflammatory infiltrate of wounds, first appearing after 6–12 hr. Although activated T cells release factors chemotactic for fibroblasts, their role is poorly understood. Wounds in lymphopenic animals heal well also.

The most important cell orchestrating the events of wound healing is the monocyte. Unlike neutropenic or lymphopenic animals, animals depleted of monocytes do not heal normally. The monocyte comes from the blood and migrates into the wound after 4–5 days. The stimulus for monocyte migration includes platelet factors, cell-derived chemotactins, and fibrin. The monocyte continues many of the functions of the neutrophil including phagocytosis and debridement, but, more importantly, it releases factors (monokines) that control subsequent events in healing. Monokines attract more monocytes and fibroblasts, stimulate fibroblast replication and collagen synthesis, and stimulate angiogenesis. Under altered conditions in vitro, the monocyte can also inhibit fibroblast collagen synthesis, which suggests that monocytes may control the signal that halts wound healing as well. Clinically, any drug or condition that alters monocyte function may affect wound healing.

Cellular Phase

Transition from the inflammatory phase to the cellular phase of wound healing is characterized in a clean, open, second intention wound by a decrease in exudate as the vascular permeability returns to normal. Healthy granulation tissue appears composed of monocytes, fibroblasts, and numerous capillaries. This usually occurs after 7–10 days. In a sutured wound this phase may also go unnoticed.

The fibroblasts, which first appear on day 5, begin to replicate under the continued stimulation of monokines. New fibroblasts continue to migrate into the wound under the stimulus of fibrin and fibronectin. Ground substance is produced and collagen synthesis occurs, peaking at 6–7 days and continuing for 2–4 weeks. The collagen is synthesized intracellularly and is secreted extracellularly as fibrils in a random and haphazard fashion. As new collagen is formed, it is deposited on preexisting fibrin. The initial fibrin-fibronectin gel matrix is replaced and eventually transformed into a dense collagen matrix: scar tissue. As extracellular collagen cross-linking occurs, wound tensile strength slowly increases.

Monocytes also stimulate proliferation of endothelial cells, and vessel growth is stimulated by low oxygen tension and high lactate concentrations derived from cellular metabolism in the wound. This new vessel growth occurs simultaneously with fibroblast proliferation and synthesis of collagen and ground substance and allows the delivery of oxygen and nutrients as well as disposal of toxic by-products of wound metabolism.

The cellular phase, therefore, begins as monocytes and fibroblasts, and new vessels predominate with the appearance of granulation tissue and a decrease in wound exudate. Granulation tissue expands to fill the wound. Later this is replaced with new collagen covered with epidermis, which essentially regenerates the lost skin.

Wound Contraction

Wound contraction is a phase of wound healing that overlaps the cellular phase. A decrease in the size of the wound begins after 7 days but is usually not noticed clinically until 14 days. The most important cell responsible for wound contraction is the myofibroblast, a fibroblast containing large amounts of actin and myosin filaments. Granulation tissue is rich in myofibroblasts and contains as much actinomyosin per gram of tissue as the uterus from a pregnant rat. After 2 weeks these myofibroblasts line up end to end, exerting tension on the margins, pulling towards the center. This results in a decrease in the size of the wound and teleologically minimizes the area to be repaired and the time to complete wound healing.

In wounds closed primarily, ordinary synthetic fibroblasts predominate and myofibroblasts are rare. No specific biochemical or cellular stimulus has been found to account for the transformation of ordinary fibroblasts to myofibroblasts. However, some findings have pointed to inflammatory cells or by-products of inflammatory cells as the stimuli to induction of myofibroblasts. This evidence includes the parallel, temporal relationship of inflammatory cells to myofibroblasts in the sequence of events of healing, and the finding of most myofibroblasts near to inflammatory foci of wounds. However, the stimulus to form myofibroblasts has yet to be elucidated.

The control of wound contraction is difficult. In vitro studies of collagen lattices populated with fibroblasts in Petri dishes have shown that the collagen lattices contract when fibroblasts differentiate toward myofibroblasts. This contraction may be inhibited by drugs such as dilantin, cytochalasin B, and steroids. Other drugs have also been shown to influence wound contraction, such as colchicine, smooth muscle antagonists (thiphenamil), and vinblastine. In theory, contraction might be inhibited without affecting wound healing by using a combination of steroids and vitamin A. Steroids inhibit contraction and epithelialization, while vitamin A reverses the adverse effects of epithelialization but does not reverse steroidal inhibition of contraction. However, the clinical effect of these drugs has been poor, and, other than delaying wound contraction, they seem to have no significant clinical usefulness.

Indirect methods have been used to control wound contraction. These include skin flaps and grafts, since contraction of wounds repaired in this fashion is minimal. It appears that the presence of reticular dermis is important to inhibit contraction. While wounds repaired with full-thickness skin grafts contract very little, split-thickness skin grafts with very little reticular dermis will contract approximately 40%. Superficial wounds, into papillary dermis alone, that heal by second intention contract very little, while full-thickness wounds devoid of reticular dermis contract significantly. This may be explained by the finding of myofibroblasts in reticular dermis but not in the superficial papillary dermis.

Guiding sutures may affect this process by allowing the surgeon to control the direction of wound contraction. Sutures pulled across the wound edges in one direction will create laxity in the direction perpendicular to the sutures and will, therefore, minimize any deformity caused by contraction in that direction. Thus, guiding sutures are useful to prevent ectropion, distortion of the brow, lip, or ala nasi (Fig. 2).

During the cellular phase of wound healing, nerve regeneration also takes place. For superficial wounds, reinnervation starts in 3 days from the edge and the base of the wound. After 2 weeks, some hyperinnervation is present, and by 4–5 weeks sensation is normal. In full-thickness wounds healed by second intention, return of sensory function is slow and often incomplete, particularly in large wounds.

Wound Remodeling

Wound contraction continues through the cellular phase into the remodeling phase. Even after the wound is covered with epidermis, contraction continues. Later wound remodeling may cor-

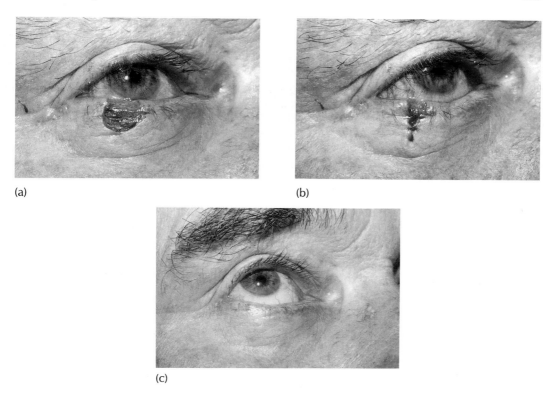

(a)

(b)

(c)

Figure 2 Guiding sutures to control wound contraction. (a) A full-thickness wound on the eyelid and lid margin. (b) Guiding absorbable sutures placed across the wound increase the laxity in the vertical direction. (c) Final result. An ectropion may have occurred with uncontrolled wound contraction.

rect some deformities caused by wound contraction such as ectropion, mild contractures, and distortion of adjacent structures.

Once an open wound is covered, the scar is still red from the dense network of capillaries. During the remodeling phase, these capillaries regress and the red color and mild persistent edema associated with the early scar formation diminish. Fibroblast proliferation slows and gradually the scar becomes relatively acellular. Remodeling of collagen continues for many months. Cross-linking continues, and as the original collagen is digested and replaced, bundle orientation occurs in an organized fashion, aligned parallel to the vector of stress in the skin. Thus, both cross-linking and bundle reorientation add to the slow increase in tensile strength noted over the first 6 months. Collagen remodeling is also responsible for some relaxation of wound contraction. When wound contraction has caused distortion of an adjacent structure, remodeling may allow partial or complete return of that structure to a normal position. This is desirable in some locations such as the ala nasi or lip. In other situations this is undesirable, such as when continued pull across a wound causes a narrow scar to widen.

Epidermal Healing

Reepithelialization begins rapidly after wounding. Within 12 hr of epidermal injury, changes in epidermal cell morphology and function occur. Cells at the wound margin cease to form keratin and prepare for cell migration and proliferation. The earliest cells that begin to cover the wound are not newly divided cells but suprabasal cells that move over into the position of a basal cell. This migration of suprabasal to basal cell position occurs before mitosis and cell division. These migrating basal cells begin to proliferate and form new suprabasal cells that again migrate toward the center of the wound. No single cell travels across the entire wound; instead, the process of migration and mitosis allows for epidermal healing.

In full-thickness wounds, the epidermal parent cells are located only at the margin, and this leap-frog migration and mitosis must occur over the entire surface. In partial-thickness wounds, parent epidermal cells are found in transected appendages such as hair follicles and sebaceous and eccrine ducts. Thus, in partial-thickness wounds, reepithelialization begins not only at the wound margin but also at the transected pores of these appendages within the wound. This reduces the distance that epidermal cells must migrate and allows for more rapid reepithelialization.

The factors that initiate, maintain, and halt reepithelialization are complex and poorly understood. Epithelial migration may be stimulated by serum factors such as epibolin (serum spreading factor), epidermal growth factor, and platelet-derived growth factor. In addition, it has been suggested that the epidermis is normally controlled by epidermally derived chalones, or factors that inhibit proliferation and migration. Wounding the epidermis may inhibit chalone production and release the epidermis from the inhibition. Once reepithelialization is complete, chalone synthesis resumes and proliferation is once again inhibited. Other theories suggest that epidermal injury allows circulating stratum corneum antibodies to bind to exposed stratum corneum, activate complement, and signal the beginning of epidermal repair.

An important factor in epidermal healing is substrate. Epidermis will only migrate over substrates of type I collagen, fibronectin, or basement membrane components such as laminin or type IV and V collagen. Epidermal cells will not migrate over a dry crust, desiccated collagen, neutrophils, and wound debris. The most important concept in epidermal wound healing is providing the proper substrate for epidermal migration. This includes a clean wound without denatured protein or necrotic debris, and a moist environment to maintain a viable substrate. An air-dried wound or a wound treated with topical alcohol, many hemostatics, caustics, lasers, electrosurgery, or cryosurgery will result in nonviable eschar. The new epidermal cells must slowly digest the eschar, wasting both energy and time required for reepithelialization.

Just as dermal wound healing continues after reepithelialization is complete, epidermal healing also continues after reepithelialization is complete. The process of contact inhibition may end epidermal migration, but epidermal maturation continues. The new epidermis is capable of rapidly forming stratum corneum, and thus the important barrier function is retained. However, new epidermis has few rete ridges and the attachment of the dermis is weak. Clinically, this is characterized by epidermal fragility, easy bruising, and blister formation. In addition, melanocyte repopulation and function is often incomplete. Partial-thickness wounds repopulate with functional melanocytes more quickly than full-thickness wounds. However, appropriate melanocyte function often lags behind repopulation. Clinically, this is seen as hypo- or hyperpigmentation, especially when the newly populated and immature melanocytes are stimulated by ultraviolet light, chemicals, or hormones (i.e., diazepam or estrogen). Full-thickness wounds do not quickly repopulate with melanocytes and, therefore, are usually hypopigmented for months, or permanently. In some patients, even large full-thickness wounds eventually repigment from the margins, but in most patients the ability of pigment to reappear is limited.

Final Result

The final result of any wound is a scar. A well-planned incision and closure should result in a fine line scar level with the skin and camouflaged by normal skin lines. If the wound is superficial (epidermis and papillary dermis only) true regeneration occurs so that clinically and histologically there is little or no evidence of scarring. The epidermis reforms its rete pegs and is quickly repopulated by melanocytes. Skin texture, color, and function all return to normal.

Deeper dermal or full-thickness second intention wounds leave a more noticeable scar with abnormal function compared to normal skin. The new dermis has disordered collagen bundles and a sparse vascular network with few or no melanocytes in the new epidermis, so that the scar appears white. The altered vascular network often results in widely dilated superficial vessels appearing as prominent telangiectasias. Finally, the scar lacks the elastic properties and tensile strength of normal dermis. Langerhans cell function may be altered in large scars, resulting in a local immune surveillance defect that may be responsible for the higher incidence of skin cancer in old scar tissue.

Therefore, only epidermal healing is truly regenerative. Deeper dermal wounds result in new skin that has both an altered appearance and function compared with normal skin (Fig. 3).

Kinetics

Understanding the kinetics of wound healing has important clinical implications. The kinetics of sutured wounds healing by primary intention differs from open clean wounds healing by second intention. Each type of wound will be considered separately here.

Primary Intention Healing

The most important aspect of primary intention healing is tensile strength. Reepithelialization occurs rapidly and has little clinical significance except that sutures should be removed to prevent epithelial-lined sinus tracts migrating into the dermis except around the suture.

The tensile strength of a wound develops slowly. At 4–5 days, when sutures are removed, collagen synthesis has not peaked and the wound edges are held together by fibrin. The tensile strength is less than 5% of normal skin. Sutures are removed at this time to prevent permanent suture marks, but there is enough strength to keep the skin edges together and everted without sutures if the wound is supported with adhesive strips and excess stress is avoided. Tensile strength is related more to collagen cross-linking than collagen synthesis. By 3 weeks (or longer in acral areas) 20% of normal tensile strength is present, usually enough to prevent dehiscence. In acral areas or when there is excess stress on the wound, special sutures or splinting techniques (i.e., running buried subcutaneous sutures) may be required to avoid complications. These wounds never have more than 80% of the tensile strength of normal skin, although the reduced strength of a scar is rarely a problem (Fig. 4).

Second Intention Healing

The kinetics of second intention healing are often misunderstood but are clinically important. The healing of partial-thickness wounds is related only to reepithelialization. In these superficial wounds there are many reservoirs of epidermis in the transected adnexal structures. After an initial lag period, the rate of epidermal movement is constant as the epidermis moves from one adnexal structure to the next. Therefore, healing time is not proportional to the size of the wound, but to the density of adnexal structures. For example, large and small superficial wounds heal more quickly on the face where adnexae are close together than on the trunk or extremities where the adnexae are sparse.

For full-thickness wounds, however, a number of factors influence the healing time. During the first week of healing, there is no change in the size of the wounds. Sometimes local swelling and elastic recoil of surrounding skin actually result in the wounds enlarging. This is called the *lag period* and correlates with the inflammatory, exudative phase of wound healing. Later, healing occurs at a constant rate: the *exponential phase*.

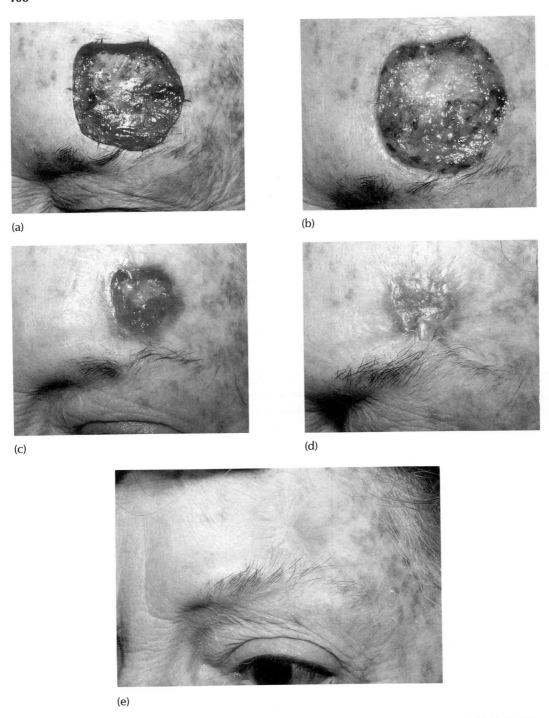

(a)

(b)

(c)

(d)

(e)

Figure 3 Clinical phases of wound healing. (a) Fresh full-thickness wound of the forehead. (b) Full-thickness wound 1 week later. The exudate has diminished and granulation tissue begins to form. (c) Wound healing at 3 weeks. Wound contraction is beginning, and reepithelialization has begun from the wound edge. (d) The wound at 9 weeks. Wound contraction and epithelialization are complete and collagen synthesis and degradation are in delicate balance. (e) The wound 6 months later.

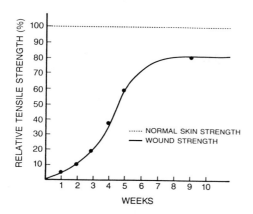

Figure 4 Wound tensile strength increases slowly after wounding, with less than 10% of normal strength present at the time of suture removal and a maximum of only 80% of the strength of normal skin. (Reproduced with permission from Zitelli, Yearbook Medical Publishers Inc., 1987.)

Effect of Wound Size.   One misconception is that the healing time for full-thickness wounds is directly proportional to the size of the wound. One might imagine that a 16-cm wound would take 16 times longer to heal than a 1-cm wound. However, weekly plots of wound area in full-thickness wounds document that healing time instead is related to the *logarithm* of the wound area; thus larger wounds take only slightly longer to heal than smaller wounds (Fig. 5). More realistically, if a 10-cm wound (10 to the first power) takes 5 weeks to heal, a 100-cm wound (10 to the second power) will take only twice as long—10 weeks (the log of the larger wound

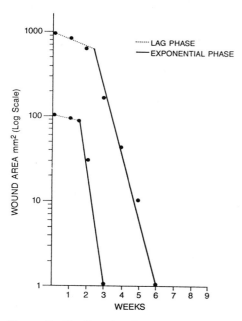

Figure 5 Healing time is proportional to the log of area, and thus large wounds often heal faster than expected. Wound size changes slowly during the first 1 or 2 weeks (lag phase) until entering the exponential phase. (Reproduced with permission from Zitelli, Yearbook Medical Publishers, Inc., 1987.)

is twice that of the smaller wound). More simply put, since the healing time is proportional to the logarithm of the area and the area is a function of the log of the radius, the best predictor of healing time is the width of the wound. Clinically, it makes little sense to treat a 6-cm lesion in four sessions, each time destroying a 3 × 3 cm quadrant, when total wound healing time would be half as long if one treated the entire lesion at once.

Effect of Wound Shape. Other variables are important, including wound location, shape, method of wounding, and skin temperature. The effect of wound shape is often misunderstood. Hippocrates taught that circular wounds were difficult or impossible to heal. Some surgeons purposely transformed circular wounds into stellate-shaped wounds to quicken the healing time. However, their perceptions were inaccurate since the *rate* of wound closure is independent of wound shape. A long, thin elliptical wound will heal in less time than a circular wound of the same area only because the wound edges are closer together. Thus, although the rate of wound edge migration is the same in both shapes, the relationship of *healing time* to shape is best described as being dependent on the diameter of the largest circle that can be contained within the wound margins (Fig. 6). Enlarging the wound by altering its shape will not expedite healing time.

The Effect of Wound Location. Location is a variable that will significantly affect healing time. Wounds of identical size, depth, and shape made on the face and leg will heal in different times. Generally, wounds in acral locations take longer to heal than more centrally located wounds, and wounds on the face heal most quickly. Although the reasons for this are unknown, it has been observed that the lag period before the exponential phase of healing is longer in acral areas (Fig. 7).

FACTORS AFFECTING WOUND HEALING

The search for better methods of managing wounds created by war or accident has led to our understanding of the importance of asepsis and improved surgical techniques. More recently, the search has continued in sophisticated laboratories for chemical factors or natural hormones that might enhance healing. While we still have no true method of enhancing wound healing, many factors, if uncontrolled, might slow wound healing.

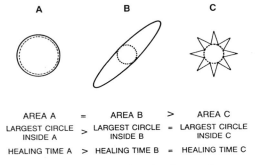

AREA A	=	AREA B	>	AREA C
LARGEST CIRCLE INSIDE A	>	LARGEST CIRCLE INSIDE B	=	LARGEST CIRCLE INSIDE C
HEALING TIME A	>	HEALING TIME B	=	HEALING TIME C

Figure 6 Healing time is related not only to wound area but also to wound shape. Healing time is best related to the diameter of the largest circle that can fit inside the wound margins. Although the area of A and B are equal, the largest circle fitting within wound A (dotted line) is greater than the largest circle within wound B and corresponds to the greater healing time for wound A. Similarly, although the area of wound B is larger than wound C, the diameter of the largest circle within each wound is the same, and the healing times will be similar. (Reproduced with permission from Zitelli, Yearbook Medical Publishers Inc., 1987.)

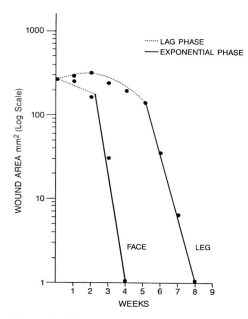

Figure 7 Wounds on acral locations often heal more slowly than wounds on the face. Once in the exponential phase, healing occurs at the same rapid rate. (Reproduced with permission from Zitelli, Yearbook Medical Publishers, Inc., 1987.)

Method of Healing

One important variable that can be controlled is the method of wounding. The most rapid healing occurs in a wound devoid of denatured proteins, necrotic debris, or infection. Wound healing is delayed if the lag phase is prolonged while necrotic debris is digested or while epidermis migrates under a dry, denatured collagen crust. Thus, slower healing times for wounds of identical size and location will occur if the wound was created by cryosurgery, electrosurgery, laser surgery, hot cautery (Shaw scalpel), or acids. Slower healing will also occur if the wound is further damaged by caustics, some antiseptics such as gentian violet, and many commonly used hemostatic agents. X-irradiation of the skin 24 hr before or after wounding significantly inhibits healing, although radiation of a healing wound after 2 weeks does not seem to retard healing.

Wound Temperature

Lower than normal temperature slows wound healing. Wounds in rabbits subjected to hypothermia or cold environments take longer to achieve expected wound tensile strength. Patients should be instructed to avoid low temperatures during the postoperative period while wound tensile strength increases.

Infection

Infection will delay healing time for an open wound and will delay the development of tensile strength in a sutured wound. Since treatment of wound infection is important, recognition of infection is also important. However, signs of infection are often confused with normal signs of healing.

Bacterial wound infection is defined as the presence of greater than 10,000 organisms/g tissue in a wound with clinical signs of infection. Organisms present at lower concentrations may represent only surface contaminants and not affect wound healing. The clinical signs of wound infection include redness more than 3–5 mm from the sutured wound margin, swelling, purulent discharge, pain, fever, or other systemic symptoms. Healing does not occur without inflammation, so all surgical wounds are tender. In open wounds, early signs of infection may be difficult to detect, especially if a dry crust or necrotic debris is present. When a swollen wound becomes painful and exudate and redness are excessive, a diagnosis of infection is made. Quantitative bacteriologic study to determine if more than 10,000 organisms are present in a gram of tissue is impractical. Cultures are important only to determine the type of bacteria and antibiotic sensitivity, once the clinical diagnosis is made.

Colonization of wounds by resident flora does not interfere with wound healing. Colonization by *Staphylococcus aureus* does not adversely affect healing unless the organism is present at high levels, when a yellowish exudate is often seen. Herpes simplex infection is recognized as a complication of dermabrasion wounds. Yeasts, especially *Candida*, are often overlooked as wound pathogens and should also be considered pathogenic. Their presence should be considered in a tender, open wound that is not healing after 3–5 weeks with topical antibiotic ointments and semiocclusive dressings. The diagnosis can often be made by microscopic examination of the wound surface exudate, which demonstrates pseudophyphae and budding yeasts, and can be confirmed by culture. Topical antimycotic creams will allow the wound to resume normal healing.

Drugs

Steroids are probably the most potent and commonly used drugs that affect wound healing. Steroids inhibit wound healing and delay the development of tensile strength if given before or during the first 3 days after wounding. This is due to inhibition of migration of the important monocyte. After 3 days, high-dosage steroids (40 mg/day prednisone) are necessary to effect fibroplasia and collagen remodeling. Topical steroids also inhibit wound healing. Fluorinated compounds are most potent, while 1% hydrocortisone has little or no effect.

The inhibition of healing by steroids may be reversed by the systemic administration of vitamin A (25,000 IU/day), although the therapeutic effects of the steroid may then be affected. To reverse steroid inhibition locally, investigators have recommended the topical application of vitamin A or retinoic acid. It is curious that vitamin A administration will not reverse steroid inhibition of wound contraction, suggesting that a combination of the two drugs may be a way to control wound contraction.

One might also suspect that immunosuppressive and antineoplastic drugs would interfere with wound healing because of their role in inhibiting inflammatory cell function. Some laboratory evidence suggests that drugs such as actinomycin D, bleomycin, or BCNU are more likely to impair healing than methotrexate, 5-fluorouracil, or cyclophosphamide. However, clinical studies have shown no impairment in wound healing when resections of internal malignancies were accompanied by adjuvant chemotherapy using combinations of thiotepa, nitrogen mustard, cyclophosphamide, 5-fluorouracil, actinomycin D, or chlorambucil. The benefits of these drugs are likely to outweigh the theoretical risk of impairing wound healing.

Other drugs have been reported to have adverse effects on cell function or biochemical pathways of cells important in wound healing. Nonsteroid anti-inflammatory drugs such as aspirin and phenylbutazone decrease tensile strength of wounds in animals, but extrapolation of these findings to humans has not been documented. It is important for patients to avoid these drugs because of their effect on platelet function, causing an increased risk of bleeding or hematoma formation.

Vitamins A, C, E, and minerals (zinc, copper, iron, and manganese) all have important functions in wound healing. Deficiencies in these substances affect collagen synthesis, collagen cross-linking, and the ability to generate superoxides to kill bacteria. Wound healing in patients who are deficient in these vitamins and minerals will be enhanced by supplementation. This is important to remember in older patients with prolonged illness. Otherwise, vitamin-mineral supplementation of otherwise healthy patients will not improve wound healing.

COMPLICATIONS

Occasionally, wound healing is complicated or influenced by systemic or external factors. If we can appropriately manage or avoid these problems, wound healing may continue a normal course.

Seborrheic Dermatitis

The most common cause of widespread erythema and even superficial erosions surrounding the wound is acute seborrheic dermatitis. The clinical picture is similar to acute contact dermatitis since it often occurs under the dressing. Patch testing is negative, and it occurs in patients with preexisting seborrheic dermatitis. This usually occurs in locations characteristic for seborrheic dermatitis (midface, periauricular, scalp, and upper trunk). It can also be confused with infection, but the eruption is not painful and responds quickly to topical steroids. Later, after the scar matures, seborrheic dermatitis may be localized to the scar surface itself (Fig. 8).

Excess Granulation

The formation of granulation tissue in an open wound is necessary before reepithelialization takes place. Occasionally, however, granulation tissue continues to form unchecked until a large nodule or even a pedunculated mass accumulates on the wound bed. This is more common in wounds managed by total occlusion or stimulated by embedded hair or other foreign bodies, but often occurs for no apparent reason. Management of this complication should first be directed at removing any external stimulus such as plucking or shaving hairs and removing unnecessary suture material or other foreign bodies.

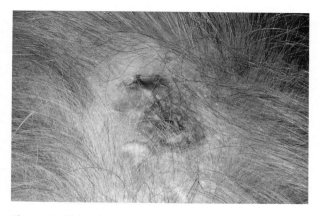

Figure 8 Seborrheic dermatitis in a scar.

It is a common practice to remove excess granulation tissue by curettage or application of caustics such as silver nitrate, even though there is no evidence that this procedure is effective. To ascertain the value of this practice, excess granulation tissue was removed from one-half of each of five wounds. In two cases, the granulation tissue was pedunculated and hung over the healing wound edge. In both of these cases, the area healed rapidly where granulation tissue was excised. In the remaining three cases, wound granulation extended above the level of the skin, but did not overhang the skin edge. In these cases, removal of half the granulation tissue did not improve the wound healing rate (Fig. 9). If removal of granulation tissue is done, it is most reasonable to use a curet or scalpel. The capillary oozing stops rapidly with pressure. Other techniques, such as silver nitrate, rewound the site and produce an eschar of denatured material that must be digested and, therefore, delays wound healing.

Hypertrophic Scars and Keloids

Hypertrophic scars and keloids are uncommon complications of superficial wounds but are not uncommon in full-thickness wounds, particularly in certain locations. The event that signals an end to wound healing is unknown, although some evidence suggests that monocytes may be involved. In any case, the cell responsible for hypertrophic and keloidal scars appears to be the myofibroblast. In sutured wounds or wounds covered with full-thickness and even split-thickness grafts, the proliferation of myofibroblasts is inhibited. In open wounds, the myofibroblast appears shortly after the fibroblasts, 5 days after wounding. Normally, some balance exists between fibroblasts, myofibroblasts, collagen synthesis, and collagen degradation. When this balance is altered, a keloid or hypertrophic scar may result from a more cellular, metabolically active scar. Fibroblasts cultured from keloids are similar to fibroblasts from normal skin. No conclusive difference in the characteristics of collagen have been found. Keloids have a higher density of mast cells, which may be important since histamine stimulates cell growth. It also explains the pruritus often noted in keloids and early hypertrophic scars.

Prevention and control of keloids and hypertrophic scars are difficult. Wound location is an important factor in predicting the likelihood of keloids and hypertrophic scar formation. On the face, hypertrophic scars are most likely to occur on convex surfaces such as the cheek, chin, upper lip, or side of the nose. Keloids are most common on the earlobes, upper trunk, and deltoid areas. With this in mind, surgery in these areas should be done using techniques known to inhibit myofibroblasts such as primary closure, skin flaps, and grafts. Gentle surgical manipulation minimizes skin necrosis and inflammation. Healing by second intention encourages myofibroblast growth and should be avoided in these areas.

Controlling these complications in open wounds after myofibroblasts have appeared is more difficult. Intralesional steroids are the most effective approach. Occlusive topical dressings such as silashe sheets over prolonged periods (months) will help to resolve hypertrophic scars. Other techniques such as laser surgery have theoretical advantages but have been of little practical help. Drugs affecting fibroblast growth and collagen metabolism such as colchicine and beta-amino proprionitrile (BAPN) are being studied.

Wound Fragility (Blisters, Erosions, and Delayed Bleeding)

As the epidermis migrates over newly formed dermis in second intention healing, the cohesive bonds are not mature and the epidermal attachment is easily broken, resulting in blisters after epithelialization is complete or nearly complete; this may also happen in the first few months after the wound has healed. It is more likely to occur in locations where the skin is least mobile such as the forehead or scalp and is very common in the center of scars greater than 10 cm. It may be caused by very minor trauma, particularly shearing forces, or by injury from remov-

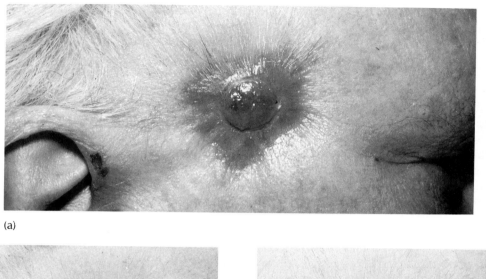

(a)

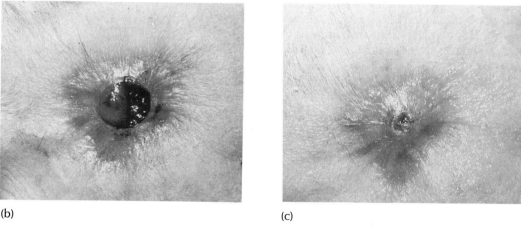

(b)   (c)

Figure 9 Excision of excess granulation tissue. (a) Excess granulation tissue during healing of a full-thickness wound. (b) Excision of the medial half with a scalpel. (c) Appearance 1 week later: no apparent effect from excision of granulation tissue. (Reproduced with permission from Zitelli, JB Lippincott, 1984.)

ing adhesive-backed wound dressings that adhere more strongly to the epidermis than the epidermis adheres to the dermis. It also can occur with the use of hydrogen peroxide, which releases oxygen under enough pressure to lift the epidermis. The cause of the epidermal fragility is unclear, but some evidence suggests that it may be due to the lack of anchoring fibrils and epidermal rete peg architecture. It is important to recognize this potential complication and warn patients to avoid trauma. This avoids confusion over the cause of erosions, which may easily be considered as infection or recurrence of tumor following tumor surgery.

Delayed bleeding is also related to wound fragility. Although most postoperative bleeding occurs within the first 24 hr, spontaneous bleeding may occur in sutured wounds up to 1 week later and is related to clot lysis in larger vessels before collagen synthesis and cross-linking seals them adequately. In open wounds, delayed bleeding may occur after the wound is epithelialized, presenting as subepidermal ecchymoses. It may also be due to fragile, immature capillaries and small vessels that rupture with minor trauma. Recognition of these complications allows the physician to reassure the patient that no significant problem exists.

The Nonhealing Wound

The nonhealing wound is a significant problem in some patients. The mechanisms of wound healing discussed so far pertain to normal healthy tissues, but occasionally pathologic processes, either systemic or local, affect these mechanisms and cause an interruption in normal healing.

An approach to the nonhealing wound should first include a search for correctable causes. This includes evaluation and treatment of infection, including organisms often overlooked and not detected by normal bacterial culture techniques such as anaerobic bacterial infection, *Mycobacteria*, spirochetes, viruses, yeasts, fungi, and protozoa. A skin biopsy with additional studies such as immunofluorescence if indicated is an important tool. Allergic contact dermatitis to many topically applied wound remedies is not uncommon. The patient may also be applying agents other than those prescribed by the doctor. A careful history may reveal these home remedies. Nutritional factors in malnourished or chronically ill patients require protein and vitamin-mineral supplementation. Drugs such as glucocorticoids and penicillamine may delay wound healing, but they rarely prevent wounds from healing. Malignant and large benign tumors may ulcerate and masquerade as a nonhealing wound until skin biopsy confirms the correct diagnosis. Other diseases may produce chronic ulcers or erosions; these include pyoderma gangrenosum, Behçet's disease, and some blistering disorders. Arterial vascular occlusion may produce peripheral ulcers alone or in combination with other disorders such as scleroderma, Raynaud's disease, Buerger's disease, embolic disease, or severe vasculitis.

Two of the most common and frustrating causes of nonhealing wounds include decubitus ulcers and venous hypertension ulcers of the leg. The goal in treating decubitus ulcers is to remove the prolonged pressure on the skin that results in necrosis. Management is complex and involves treating complications such as secondary infection, nutritional deficiencies, and good wound care, which often requires tissue replacement with local flaps. Chronic leg ulcers from venous hypertension are also a frustrating problem. The mechanism of ulcer formation is unclear, but fibrin deposits around capillaries and venules that block the perfusion of oxygen and nutrients are thought to be important in the pathogenesis of these ulcers. Again, treatment is complex and requires good wound management and an attempt to reverse or prevent additional accumulation of fibrin around the vessels.

There are numerous uncorrectable disorders in which abnormal healing may occur. Atrophy and ulceration may occur in tissue deprived of pain, temperature, and light touch. This is common after transection of the trigeminal nerve but may occur after transection of other sensory nerves. In addition, inherited disorders of connective tissue may present with abnormal wound healing. However, when no apparent reason for a nonhealing wound can be found, factitial ulcers should be considered.

CLINICAL CORRELATIONS: WOUND MANAGEMENT

Applying the basics of wound healing to clinical practice minimizes complications and provides better control over wound healing. This can be translated into a number of useful guidelines for wound management in dermatologic surgery. For convenience, these guidelines are classified into primary and second intention healing even though the events of healing are similar for both types of wound management.

First Intention Healing

Wounds to be sutured are usually clean, without necrotic debris. Aseptic surgical technique reduces the chance of wound infection, which would delay healing and increase the likelihood of wound dehiscence and scar spreading. Chlorhexidine is a favorite presurgical scrub because its antiseptic action persists for days and it is active in the presence of serum or blood.

Intraoperatively, attention should be paid to careful hemostasis. Hemostasis induced by electro-surgery, cautery, or suture ligature always produces tissue necrosis. Wound healing can occur normally with small amounts of necrosis. However, if there is extensive necrosis, healing is delayed while inflammatory cells digest the necrotic tissue and replace it with granulation tissue, collagen, and scar. For dermatologic surgery, a fine-tipped needle is best, especially when applied to a dry field. Larger vessels require suture ligation rather than deep, extensive electro-coagulation. Hemostasis is also achieved with a pressure dressing applied for 24 hr. This will help to eliminate dead space until fibrin glues the tissue together. Since fibrin has little tensile strength and collagen synthesis does not peak for 5 days, physical activity should be restricted until the wound has stabilized by collagen cross-linking and achieved adequate tensile strength. This may take 2 weeks for facial wounds closed without tension, or 5–6 weeks on extremities, especially if the wound edge was closed with tension.

Good suturing technique is important to minimize complications and enhance both healing and the final cosmetic result. Multilayered suture techniques are more effective than a single layer of skin sutures. Buried intradermal sutures have a number of important functions. They effectively minimize dead space that leads to hematoma and seroma, and they provide prolonged wound support. Since sutures are removed 5–7 days after surgery to prevent cross-hatching when the wound has only 3% of eventual tensile strength, the additional support provided by the buried sutures is important to prevent scar spread. Buried sutures also help to evert wound edges. As wound remodeling and contraction occurs, an everted wound will contract and result in flat, unnoticeable scar. Without wound edge eversion, the scar contracts below the level of surrounding skin, creating shadows and a more noticeable scar.

Knowledge of the events of healing is important when choosing suture material as well as timing suture removal. Wounds closed under considerable tension, or when prolonged support is needed (acral areas), or in patients taking systemic steroids, should be closed with buried sutures that are nonabsorbable (nylon, Prolene) or have prolonged tensile strength (Vicryl, Dexon, PDS). In addition, skin sutures may be left in place longer than normal. A running subcuticular suture technique can be used to minimize the chance of permanent suture marks when sutures need to be left in place for longer than 1 week.

After suture removal, external splinting with tape provides additional support until tensile strength increases. During this time, exercise that stretches the skin should be avoided to minimize scar spreading. Patients are usually more tolerant of red suture lines or minor distortion if they are informed that the redness will fade and slight tissue protrusions or displacements will resolve as remodeling occurs over 3–6 months.

Second Intention Healing

Dermatologic surgery is unique because of the various surgical techniques used to treat skin lesions. These techniques often result in wounds managed by second intention healing and include chemical destruction, cryosurgery, electrosurgery, laser surgery, punch biopsy, curettage, and tangential scalpel excision. Dermatologists also manage many nonsurgical erosive or ulcerative skin lesions for which guidelines for wound management are useful.

Today, wound management is best summarized by "wet is best." Semiocclusive dressings provide the best environment for wound healing. Even in a wound that has been allowed to air dry, a crust eventually forms, and wound healing occurs at the top of the moist portion of the wound under the crust. Of course, this slows wound healing and occurs at the expense of deepening the wound by the desiccated, denatured collagen lost when the crust is formed. Despite voluminous literature on the advantages of occlusive wound management, many physicians still recommend antiseptic tinctures, alcohol washes, and air exposure. These methods have at least three major problems: (1) enhanced tissue necrosis and deepening of the wound because of alcohol fixation and air desiccation of tissue, (2) slow healing because the epidermis is forced to migrate under the crust, and (3) increased pain.

Topical Agents

Topical agents are frequently applied to wounds for hemostasis, antisepsis, and to promote healing. However, many agents used for topical hemostasis delay wound healing. Ferric subsulfate (Monsel's solution) and aluminum chloride 30% both cause delays in healing and slightly larger, less cosmetically acceptable scars. Topical silver nitrate, trichloracetic acid, and oxidized cellulose likewise cause additional tissue damage and delay wound healing.

Topical gelatin and collagen cause little or no damage to the wound and only interfere with healing if large amounts are placed in superficial wounds. Collagen sponge matrices may enhance the healing of full-thickness wounds. A safe topical hemostatic is thrombin, but the safest is simple temporary pressure until natural hemostatic mechanisms stop bleeding.

Many popular antiseptic agents are also toxic. Chlorhexidine (0.5%), 1% povidone-iodine (Betadine), 0.5% sodium hypochlorite (Daiken solution), 0.2% acetic acid, and 3% hydrogen peroxide are highly toxic to granulation tissue or cultured fibroblasts. More dilute solutions seriously affect the chemicals' antimicrobial activity, although povidone-iodine at dilutions of 0.001% and sodium hypochlorite 0.005% remain bactericidal while no longer damaging fibroblasts. These in vitro studies suggest that many topical antiseptics may interfere with healing, although in vitro studies have shown that hydrogen peroxide does not inhibit the growth of granulation tissue the way other toxic substances do.

Topical steroids and antibiotic ointments are also commonly applied to wounds. Potent fluorinated steroids retard epidermal resurfacing and reduce collagen biosynthesis. One percent hydrocortisone has been shown to exert little or no inhibition of wound healing. Topical nitrofurazone and a liquid detergent inhibited wound healing in pigs. Wounds treated with 70% ethanol heal as fast as air-exposed wounds. Oil and water cream, Neosporin ointment, Silvadene cream, and benzoyl peroxide lotion (10% and 20%) enhance epidermal wound healing. Topical retinoic acid, which stimulates mitoses, may enhance reepithelialization after dermabrasion if applied to intact skin 10 days before wounding but may inhibit reepithelialization if applied to superficial wounds.

Using this information to avoid the toxic effects and minimize any inhibition of wound healing, topical antibiotic ointments may be helpful, especially if common sensitizers can be avoided (neomycin). If an anti-inflammatory topical is needed around a chronic ulcer or on damaged skin, hydrocortisone is least likely to interfere with healing.

Wound Dressings

The ideal wound dressing should enhance healing, reduce pain, absorb wound exudate, and be easy to apply and replace without causing irritation. It should protect the wound from trauma, toxins, and bacteria and not induce allergic contact dermatitis.

Many modern wound dressings available today fulfill most of these requirements. Occlusive and semiocclusive dressings provide a moist environment for the wound, preventing desiccation and, most importantly, enhancing both reepithelialization (30–45%) and collagen synthesis compared to air-exposed wound controls. This enhanced healing is seen in acute partial-thickness and full-thickness wounds as well as some chronic wounds such as leg ulcers.

Occlusive dressings also reduce the pain of surgical wounds, leg ulcers, skin graft donor sites, and dermabrasion. The moist wound bed created by these dressings is flexible. There is less inflammation in contrast to the air-dried wound with its immobile hard crust that adheres tightly to the wound and pulls with any movement. Some investigators report better cosmetic results with occlusive dressings used both on sutured wounds and wounds allowed to heal by second intention.

In the past decade, the popularity and usefulness of occlusive dressings have led to the marketing of many types. The most commonly used dressings can be classified into four main groups: (1) perforated plastic films with absorptive pad backing (band-aid, Telfa), (2) hydrogel dressings (Vigilon, Second Skin), (3) hydrocolloid dressings (Duoderm), and (4) adhesive polyurethane dressings (Op-Site, Tegaderm) (Table 1).

The most commonly used commercial dressing, and the closest to an ideal dressing, is the perforated plastic film with an absorptive pad backing. These are commercially available in many sizes, inexpensive, and easy to apply and change, and they absorb the wound exudate. Thus they are convenient for patients and have all the advantages of occlusive dressings. For small wounds, Band-Aids suffice as the dressing, but for larger wounds pads must be used and cut to overlap the wound margins, and are then held in place with tape.

The hydrogel dressings are polymers of polyethylene oxide holding 96% sterile water in the form of a gelatinous sheet. This gelatinlike sheet is packaged between two thin plastic sheets. The bottom layer is usually removed before the dressing is applied so that the gelatinous layer is in direct contact with the wound and the outer plastic film prevents evaporation of the water from the gel. This dressing may also be cut to overlap the wound edges and must be held in place with tape since it is nonadhesive. This dressing feels soothing and is best for superficial, rapidly healing wounds such as dermabrasion. This dressing has been shown to selectively permit the growth of gram-negative organisms in wounds of animals and humans, resulting in an increased incidence of wound infection. A more recent improvement of this type of dressing has been the impregnation of povidone-iodine into the hydrogel to provide an antimicrobial dressing.

Some dressings have adhesive that obviates the need for additional tape. Ideally, they stick to the normal skin surrounding the wound but not the moist wound bed. Unfortunately, these adhesive dressings also stick to the newly migrated epidermis and can cause rewounding during dressing changes. For this reason, when using these dressings it can be helpful to apply a thin coat of petrolatum or antibiotic ointment over the new epidermis to prevent adherence and to change the dressing infrequently to minimize trauma. One advantage of the adhesive dressings is that they protect the wound from environmental bacterial contamination.

The hydrocolloid dressing is composed of gelatin and pectin hydrocolloid particles in a polymer. This is a thicker, more protective dressing and is easy to cut and apply to the wound. It appears to be very effective for stimulating granulation tissue, possibly because of the low oxygen permeability. It is useful in chronic leg ulcers and decubitus ulcers. Patients should be warned that the dressing dissolves on contact with wound exudate, and the yellow mixture under the dressing often has a foul odor that should not be confused with pus or sign of infection.

Adhesive-backed polyurethane films are transparent and do not require tape, and thus are quite useful on small facial wounds where an inconspicuous dressing is desired. They are also useful for wounds after the exudative phase of healing (lag phase) since they have no absorptive capacity. In acute wounds, the exudate accumulates under the dressing, requiring frequent changes,

Table 1 Occlusive Wound Dressings

Types	Enhances healing	Reduces pain
Perforated plastic with absorbent pad	+	+
Hydrogel	+	+
Hydrocolloid	+	+
Polyurethane	+	+

or unpredictable leakage of the accumulated contents under the film may occur. This type of dressing is often difficult to apply since it easily folds and adheres to itself. Improvements in packaging have helped somewhat.

The choice of wound dressing may depend on a number of variables. One important feature is the ability to absorb exudate. During the exudative phase of healing, an absorptive occlusive dressing such as the perforated plastic films with a pad backing is most desirable to handle the copious exudate. If protection of the wound from environmental bacterial contamination is important, one of the adhesive-backed dressings, polyurethane films, or hydrocolloid dressings may be helpful. When these dressings are used during the exudative phase, daily dressing changes are needed to clean the exudate. Later, they only need to be changed every 4–5 days. In chronic wounds, the hydrocolloid dressings seem to be effective in helping to debride the wound and promote the growth of granulation tissue.

Concerns about the use of occlusive dressings include oxygen permeability and the chance of infection. While some dressings are oxygen permeable (polyurethane films) and others are impermeable (hydrocolloid dressings), the rate of wound healing is similar. Thus the theoretical concern about oxygen tension under the wound dressing has little clinical application. However, bacteria do proliferate under occlusive dressings, but clinical infection is rare. The advantages of occlusive dressings outweigh the theoretical increased risk of infection. A number of factors may account for the low infection rate. Neutrophils in the exudate under occlusive dressings are active for 24 hr, actively phagocytizing and killing bacteria. The adhesive of some polyurethane films or the acid pH of the dissolved hydrocolloid dressings inhibits bacterial growth. Finally, many dressings are used in combination with antibiotic ointments.

When infection does occur, it may present differently from normal. There may be less inflammation or pain. A delay in wound healing may be the most important sign of infection to

Absorbent	Adhesive	Ease of application
+	–	+
+/–	–	+
–	+	+
–	+	–

monitor. In addition, the organisms more likely to be involved include gram-negative bacteria and yeasts as well as *Staphylococcus* (Fig. 10).

Wound Management

The goal of wound management is to minimize bacterial colonization, prevent desiccation of the wound, and provide a moist wound environment, all at low cost and convenience for the patient. The surgical procedure chosen should be the most effective technique that causes the least amount of necrotic tissue. If hemostasis is necessary, powdered gelatin, collagen, or topical thrombin with or without pinpoint electrocoagulation is best. Most other hemostatic agents are toxic and delay healing (i.e., Monsel's solution, aluminum chloride, silver nitrate, oxidized cellulose) and should be used only when necessary to ensure hemostasis. An occlusive dressing should be applied (i.e., perforated plastic film with an absorbent pad) and a pressure dressing if necessary. After 24 hr, patients may remove the dressing and compress the wound with tap water or 1–3% hydrogen peroxide. Hydrogen peroxide is used because it produces effervescence and mechanically softens and removes any crusts or blood clots. If no crusts are present, tap water cleansing is recommended to prevent epidermal blisters caused by hydrogen peroxide during the later stages of healing. A nonsensitizing antibiotic ointment is applied to the wound surface before a clean occlusive dressing is reapplied. This procedure is repeated daily until the wound is covered with epidermis.

Managing Complex Wounds

Most wounds created by dermatologic surgeons involve skin and subcutaneous tissue. The treatment plan outlined above is also effective in areas of exposed fat, muscle, and fascia. However,

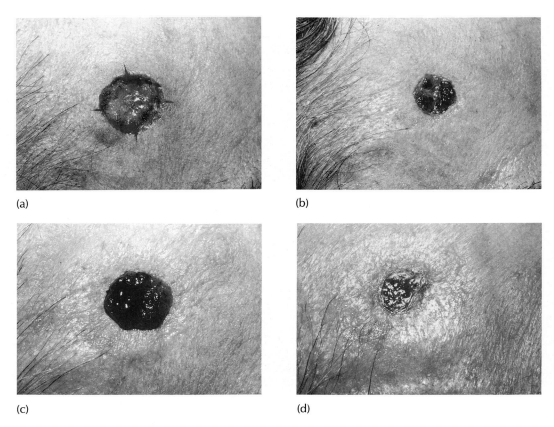

(a)   (b)

(c)   (d)

Figure 10   Effect of infection on wound healing. (a) Full-thickness wound on the temple managed using occlusive therapy. (b) Appearance 2 weeks later shows progress as expected. (c) Wound 6 weeks after wounding shows no further healing. Culture documents infection with *Serratia marcescens*, but wound shows little surrounding redness, although it is painful. (d) Rapid healing 1 week later, after topical antibiotic is applied with occlusive dressing.

wounds that expose cartilage, bone, or contain necrotic tissue from disease or infection will not support epidermal migration. In these cases, additional care is needed to stimulate granulation tissue that will support epidermal migration. If small areas of bone or cartilage (less than 1 cm) are exposed, the only alteration from routine treatment is the more frequent and liberal use of antibiotic ointments to ensure an occlusive environment to prevent desiccation necrosis. Areas of exposed cartilage larger than 1 cm can be excised if they are located in concave areas, exposing the perichondrium from the opposite surface. This provides a good blood supply for granulation tissue and later reepithelialization. On convex surfaces (helix, antihelix, and nasal cartilages), the structural support of the cartilage must be preserved to prevent significant deformities. This may be done by removing small discs of cartilage with a 3-mm dermal punch, exposing islands of perichondrium to support granulation tissue growth over the lattice of remaining cartilage (Fig. 11).

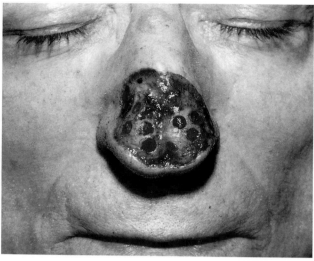

(a)

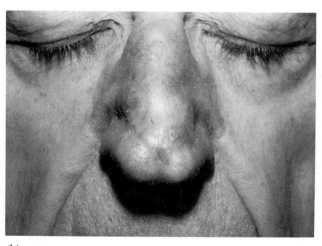

(b)

Figure 11 Excision of cartilage to promote healing. (a) A full-thickness wound on the nose, exposing the cartilage. Discs of cartilage (3 mm) have been removed to maintain cartilage support and promote granulation tissue growth. (b) Healed wound 6 months later. (Reproduced with permission from Zitelli, CV Mosby Co., 1983.)

When large areas of bone are exposed, a blood supply must be obtained from the medullary portion of bone by removing a portion of the outer cortex. This may be done with a bone chisel, high-speed dental burr or drill, or carbon dioxide laser. If the need to remove bone or cartilage is in question, the decision may be delayed for 3 weeks to wait for the spontaneous appearance of granulation tissue from small perforating vessels. Although exposed cartilage and bone require special care, these procedures can be done quickly and painlessly on an outpatient basis; the

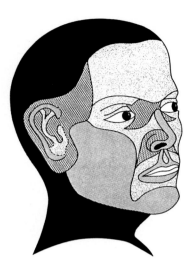

Figure 12 The effect of location on the cosmetic result of wounds managed by second intention healing. Wounds in concave areas heal well. Wounds on flat surfaces usually heal satisfactorily. Wounds on convex surfaces heal with variable cosmetic results, and deep wounds often look best if repaired surgically. (Reproduced with permission from Zitelli, Yearbook Medical Publishers Inc., 1987.)

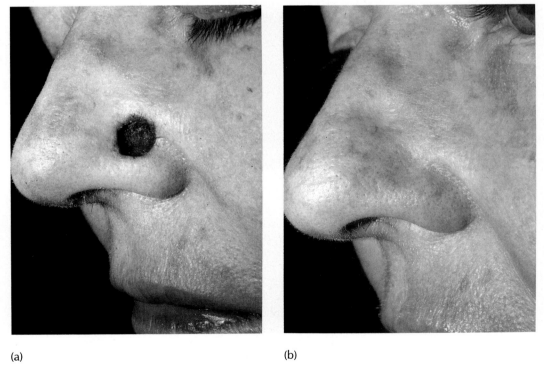

(a)   (b)

Figure 13 (a) A full-thickness wound on the crease of the nasal ala. (b) Cosmetic result 6 months after healing by second intention. (Reproduced with permission from Zitelli, Yearbook Medical Publishers Inc., 1987.)

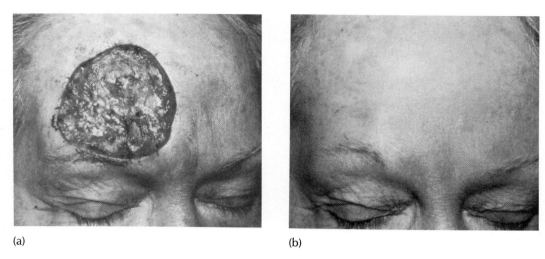

(a)   (b)

Figure 14 (a) A large full-thickness wound that might be managed with a skin graft. Local flaps would be likely to distort nearby landmarks. (b) Cosmetic result 1 year later after healing by second intention with guiding sutures.

options for wound management can be increased by adding grafts and second intention healing in addition to local flap coverage.

In wounds complicated by necrosis, control of the disease process and debridement are essential. Superficial debridement can be done with an occlusive hydrocolloid dressing or more rapidly by gentle curettage until healthy bleeding tissue is exposed. Otherwise, more aggressive debridement with a scalpel is required to remove necrotic tissue and enhance healing.

Predicting the Cosmetic Result

Dermatologic surgeons have a variety of surgical techniques at their disposal for the treatment of skin lesions. It is helpful to be able to predict the cosmetic result when choosing between surgical repair and a method requiring healing by second intention. Although many factors influence the cosmetic result, the location of the wound is the most important factor that predicts the result after second intention healing. Wounds located in concave areas heal with excellent cosmetic results. Wounds on flat surfaces usually heal with satisfactory results, and wounds on convex surfaces often heal with a noticeable scar (Fig. 12).

Wounds in the inner canthus, crease of the nasal ala, nasolabial fold, temple, and concave areas of the ear usually heal with a cosmetic result equal or superior to the result from surgical repair (Fig. 13). Wounds on flat surfaces such as the forehead, sides of the nose, and periorbital areas may look best if a surgical repair can be designed to maintain normal tension lines and cause no distortion of important structures; otherwise they may look best if allowed to heal by second intention (Fig. 14). Wounds on the convex surface on the malar cheeks, tip of the nose, or vermilion border usually look best if a surgical repair is done (Fig. 15). Often wounds on the trunk or extremities look best when allowed to heal by second intention especially if wound closure is complicated or requires considerable tension.

Other factors that influence the cosmetic result include wound depth, skin color, and wound size. Skin color is an important factor to consider. Since scars from all but the most superficial

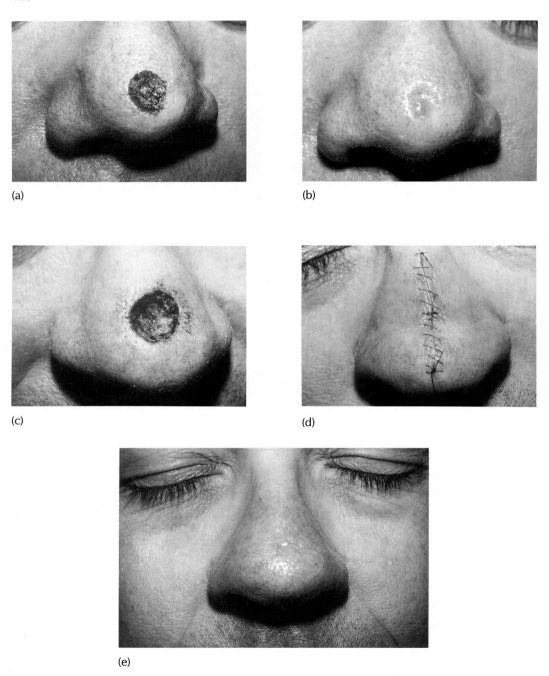

Figure 15 (a) Full-thickness wound on the tip of the nose. (b) Cosmetic result 6 months later with depressed scar from second intention healing. (c) Full-thickness wound on the tip of the nose (similar to a). (d) Primary closure without distortion of the nose. (e) Cosmetic result 6 months later. (a and b reproduced with permission from Zitelli, Yearbook Medical Publishers Inc., 1987.)

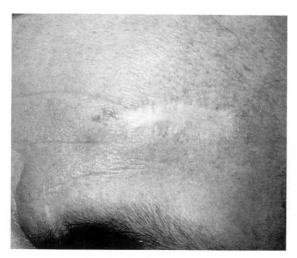

Figure 16 Hypopigmented avascular scar.

wounds are hypopigmented and avascular, the healed wound will be less noticeable in light-colored skin than in darkly pigmented or telangiectatic skin (Fig. 16). Small wounds heal with better cosmetic results than large wounds, especially in older patients in whom other skin changes such as lentigines, keratoses, and wrinkles help to camouflage the scar.

BIBLIOGRAPHY

Forrest RD. Early history of wound treatment. *J R Soc Med* 1982;75:198–205.

Johnston LC. Yet more, yet older, snakes (letter). *JAMA* 1986;255:2445.

Dermal Wound Healing

Albright SD. Surgical gem: Placement of "guiding sutures"to counteract undesirable retraction of tissues in and around functionally and cosmetically important structures. *J Dematol Surg Oncol* 1981;7:446–449.

Aldskogius H, Hermanson A, Jonsson E. Re-innervation of experimental superficial wounds in rats. *Plast Reconstr Surg* 1987;79:595–599.

Clark RAF, Winn HJ, Dvorak HG, Colvin RB. Fibronectin beneath reepithelializing epidermis in vivo: Sources and significance. *J Invest Dermatol* 1983;80:026s–30s.

Clark YK, Stone RD, Leung D, et al. Role of macrophages in wound healing. *Surg Forum* 1976;27:16.

Corps BVM. The effect of graft thickness, donor site, and graft bed on graft shrinkage in the hooded rat. *Br J Plast Surg* 1969;22:125.

Eaglstein WH. The genesis of wound repair. In *The Pathogenesis of Skin Disease*. B Theirs, R Dobson, eds. New York, Churchill Livingstone, 1986, pp.617–623.

Ehrlich HP, Buttle DJ, Trelstad R, Hayashi K. Epidermolysis bullosa dystrophica recessive fibroblasts altered behaviour in a collagen matrix. *J Invest Dermatol* 1983;80:56.

Ehrlich HP, Hunt TK. Effects of cortisone and vitamin A on wound healing. *Ann Surg* 1968;167:324–328.

Leibovich SJ, Ross R. The role of the macrophage in wound repair: A study with hydrocortisone and anti-macrophage serum. *Am J Pathol* 1975;78:71.

Majno G. The story of the myofibroblasts. *Am J Surg Pathol* 1979;3:535.

Majno G, Gabbiani G, Hirschel BJ, et al. Contraction of granulation tissue in vitro: Similarity to smooth muscle. *Science* 1971;173:548–550.

McGrath MH. Healing of the open wound. In *Problems in Aesthetic Surgery*. R Rudolph, ed. St. Louis, CV Mosby, 1986, pp. 13–48.

McGrath MH, Hundahl SA. The spatial and temporal quantification of myofibroblasts. *Plast Reconstr Surg* 1982;69:975.

Postlethwaite AG, Snyderman R, Kang AH. Chemotactic attraction of human fibroblasts to a lymphocyte-derived factor. *J Exp Med* 1976;144:1188.

Rudolph R. Inhibition of myofibroblasts by skin grafts. *Plast Reconstr Surg* 1979;63:473.

Simpson DM, Ross R The neutrophilic leukocyte in wound repair. A study with antineutrophil serum. *J Clin Invest* 1972;51:2009–2023.

Weiss RE, Reddi AH. Role of fibronectin in collagenous matrix-induced mesenchymal cell proliferation and differentiation in vivo. *Exp Cell Res* 1981;133:247–254.

Woodley DT, O'Keefe EJ, Prunieras M. Cutaneous wound healing: A model for cell-matrix interactions. *J Am Acad Dermatol* 1985;12:420–433.

Zitelli JA. Secondary intention healing—an alternative to surgical repair. *Clin Dermatol* 1984;2:92–106.

Epidermal Healing

Beutner EH, Binder WL, Jablonska S, et al. Nature of stratum corneum autoantibodies, antigens, and antigen conversion and their role in healing and psoriasis. In *The Epidermis in Disease*. R Marks, E Christophers, eds. Philadelphia, JB Lippincott, 1981, p. 333.

Cohen S. Isolation of a mouse submaxillary gland protein accelerating incisor eruption and eyelid opening in the new-born animal. *J Biol Chem* 1962;237:1555–1562.

Dillman T, Penn J. Studies on repair of cutaneous wounds II. The healing of wounds involving loss of superficial portions of the skin. *Med Proc* 2:150,156,

Ferreira JA. Dermabrasion of the skin: Prevention and/or treatment of hyperpigmentation. *Aesthet Plast Surg* 1978;1:381.

Ferreira JA. The role of diazepam in skin hyperpigmentation. *Aesthet Plast Surg* 1980;4:343.

Hebda PA, Alstadt SP, Hileman WT, Eaglstein WH. Support and stimulation of epidermal cell outgrowth from porcine skin explants by platelet factors. *Br J Dermatol* 1986;115:529–541.

Krawczyk W. Pattern of epidermal cell migration during wound healing. *J Cell Biol* 1971;49:247–263.

Stenn KS. Epibolin: A protein in human plasma that supports epithelial cell movement. *Proc Natl Acad Sci USA* 1981;78:6907.

Winter GD. Epidermal regeneration studied in the domestic pig. In *Epidermal Wound Healing*. HI Maibach, DT Rovee, eds. Chicago, Yearbook Medical Publishers, 1972.

Kinetics of Wound Healing

Levenson SM, Geever EF, Crowley LV, et al. The healing of rat skin wounds. *Ann Surg* 1965;161:293–308.

Majno G. *The Latros in the Healing Hand: Man and Wound in the Ancient World*. Cambridge, MA, Harvard University Press, 1977, pp. 154–156.

McGrath MH, Simon RH. Wound geometry and the kinetics of wound contraction. *Plast Reconstr Surg* 1983;72:66.

Peacock EE, Madden JW. Some studies on the effect of β-aminopropionitrile on collagen in healing wounds. *Surgery* 1966;60:7–12.

Robins P, Day CL, Lew RA. A multivariate analysis of factors affecting wound healing time. *J Dermatol Surg Oncol* 1984;10:219–221.

Zitelli J. Wound healing for the clinician. *Adv Dermatol* 1987;2:243–267.

Factors Affecting Wound Healing

Epstein E. Effects of tissue-destructive technics on wound healing (letter). *J Am Acad Dermatol* 1986; 14:1098–1099.

Grillo HC, Potsaid MS. Studies in wound healing. IV. Retardation of contraction by local x-irradiation: Observations relating to the origin of fibroblasts in repair. *Ann Surg* 1958;148:145.

Hell E, Lawrence JC. The initiation of epidermal wound healing in cuts and burns. *Br J Exp Pathol* 1979; 60:171–179.

Hunt TK. Vitamin A and wound healing. *J Am Acad Dermatol* 1986;15:817–821.

Klausner JM, Lulcuk S, Inbar M, et al. The effects of perioperative fluorouracil administration on convalescence and wound healing. *Arch Surg* 1986;121:239–242.

Krizek TJ, Robson MC. Evolution of quantitative bacteriology in wound management. *Am J Surg* 1975; 130:579–581.

Leyden JJ. Effect of bacteria on healing of superficial wounds. *Clin Dermatol* 1984;2:81–85.

Lundgren C, Muren A, Zederfeldt B. Effect of cold vasoconstriction on wound healing in the rabbit. *Acta Chir Scand* 1959;118:1–4.

Marks JG, Cano C, Leitzel K, et al. Inhibition of wound healing by topical steroids. *J Dermatol Surg Oncol* 1983;9:819–821.

Mertz PM, Eaglstein WH. The effect of a semiocclusive dressing on the microbial population in superficial wounds. *Arch Surg* 1984;119:287–289.

Mobacken H. Gentian violet and wound repair (letter). *J Am Acad Dermatol* 1986;15:1303.

Moreno RA, Hebda PA, Zitelli JA, et al. Epidermal cell outgrowth from CO_2 laser- and scalpel-cut explants: Implications for wound healing. *J Dermatol Surg Oncol* 1984;10:863–868.

Pollack SV. Wound healing. A review III: Nutritional factors affecting wound healing. *J Dermatol Surg Oncol* 1979;5:615–619.

Pollack SV. Wound healing. A review IV: Systemic medications affecting wound healing. *J Dermatol Surg Oncol* 1982;8:667–672.

Robson MC, Heggers JP. Delayed wound closures based on bacterial counts. *J Surg Oncol* 1970;2:379–383.

Sawchuk WS, Friedman KJ, Manning T, Pinnell SR. Delayed healing in full-thickness wounds treated with aluminun chloride solution. *J Am Acad Dermatol* 1986;15:982–994.

Selden ST. Candida; A common culprit. *J Dermatol Surg Oncol* 1985;11:958.

Siegle RJ, Chiaramonti A, Knox DW, Pollack SV. Cutaneous candidosis as a complication of facial dermabrasion. *J Dermatol Surg Oncol* 1984;10:891–895.

Sowa DE, Masterson BJ, Nealon N, von Fraunhofer JA. Effects of thermal knives on wound healing. *Obstet Gynecol* 1985;66:436–439.

Spebar MJ, Pruitt BA. Candidiasis in the burned patient. *J Trauma* 1981;21:237–239.

Zanini V, Viviani MA, Cava L, et al. Candida infections in the burn patients. *Pan Minerva Med* 1983; 25:163–166.

Complications

Gruber RP, Vistnes L, Pardoe R. The effect of commonly used antiseptics on wound healing. *Plast Reconstr Surg* 1975;55:472–476.

Howell JB. Neurotrophic changes in the trigeminal territory. *Arch Dermatol* 1962;86:442–448.

Krull EA. Chronic cutaneous ulcerations and impaired healing in human skin. *J Am Acad Dermatol* 1985; 12:394–401.

Murray JC, Pollack SV, Pinnell SR. Keloids and hypertrophic scars. *Clin Dermatol* 1984;2:121–133.

Peacock EE. Pharmacologic control of surface scarring in human beings. *Ann Surg* 1981;193:592–597.

Sproat JE, Dalcin A, Weitaver N, Robert RS. Hypertrophic sternal scars: Silicone gel sheet versus Kenalog injection treatment. *Plast Reconstr Surg* 1992;90:988–992.

Second Intention Healing and Special Dressings

Albom MJ. Surgical gems. *J Dermatol Surg Oncol* 1975;1:60.

Alper JC, Welch EA, Ginsberg M, et al. Moist wound healing under a vapor permeable membrane. *J Am Acad Dermatol* 1983;8:347–353.

Alvarez OM, Mertz PM, Eaglstein WH. The effect of occlusive dressings on collagen synthesis and re-epithelialization in superficial wounds. *J Surg Res* 1983;35:142–148.

Ariyan S, Krizek TJ. In defense of the open wound. *Arch Surg* 1976;111:293–296.

Eaglstein WH, Mertz P, Alvarez OM. Effect of topically applied agents on healing wounds. *Clin Dermatol* 1984;2(3):112–115.

Eaton AC. A controlled trial to evaluate and compare a sutureless skin closure technique (Op-Site skin closure) with conventional skin suturing and clipping in abdominal surgery. *Br J Surg* 1980;67:857–860.

Field LM. Letter to the editor. *J Dermatol Surg Oncol* 1981;7:597.

Fox SA, Beard C. Spontaneous lid repair. *Am J Ophthamol* 1964;58:947–952.

Geronemus RG, Robins P. The effects of two new dressings on epidermal wound healing. *J Dermatol Surg Oncol* 1982;8:850–852.

Goldwyn RM. Value of healing by secondary intention seconded (letter). *Ann Plast Surg* 1980;4:435.

Holland KT, Davis W, Ingham E, Gowland G. A comparison of the in-vitro antibacterial and complement activating effect of "Op-Site" and "Tegaderm" dressings. *J Hosp Infect* 1984;5:323–328.

James JH, Watson CH. The use of Op-Site, a vapor permeable dressing, on skin graft donor sites. *Br J Plast Surg* 1975;28:107–110.

Katz S, McGinley K, Leyden JJ. Semipermeable occlusive dressings. *Arch Dermatol* 1986;122:58–62.

Lineaweaver W, McMorris S, Soucy D, Howard R. Cellular and bacterial toxicities of topical antimicrobials. *Plast Reconstr Surg* 1985;75:394–396.

Linsky CB, Rovee DT, Dow T. Effect of dressing on wound inflammation and scar tissue. In *The Surgical Wound*. P Dineen, G Hildick-Smith, eds. Philadelphia: Lea & Febiger, 1981, pp. 191–205.

Mandy SH. A new primary wound dressing made of polyethylene oxide gel. *J Dermatol Surg Oncol* 1983; 9:153–155.

Mandy SH. Tretinoin in the preoperative and postoperative management of dermabrasion. *J Am Acad Dermatol* 1986;15:878–879.

Mehta HK. Surgical management of carcinoma of eyelids and periorbital skin. *Br J Ophthalmol* 1979; 63:578–585.

Mertz PM, Marshall DA, Eaglstein WH. Occlusive wound dressings to prevent bacterial invasion and wound infection. *J Am Acad Dermatol* 1985;12:662–668.

Mertz PM, Marshall DA, Kuglar MA. Povidone-iodine in polyethylene oxide hydrogel dressing. *Arch Dermatol* 1986;122:1133–1138.

Mohs FE, Zitelli JA. Microscopically controlled surgery in the treatment of carcinoma of the scalp. *Arch Dermatol* 1981;117:764–769.

Niedner R, Schöpf E. Inhibition of wound healing by antiseptics. *Br J Dermatol* 1986;115(Suppl 31):41–44.

Silverberg B, Smoot CE, Landa SJF, Parsons RW. Hidradenitis suppurativa: Patient satisfaction with wound healing by secondary intention. *Plast Reconstr Surg* 1987;79:555–559.

Vanderveen EG, Stoner JG, Swanson NA. Chiseling of exposed bone to stimulate granulation tissue after Mohs surgery. *J Dermatol Surg Oncol* 1983;9:925–928.

Varghese MC, Balin AK, Carter M, Caldwell D. Local environment of chronic wounds under synthetic dressings. *Arch Dermatol* 1986;122:52–57.

Winter GD. Formation of scab and the rate of epithelization of superficial wounds in the skin of the young domestic pig. *Nature* (London) 1962;193:293–294.

Zitelli JA. Delayed wound healing with adhesive wound dressings. *J Dermatol Surg Oncol* 1984;10:709–710.

Zitelli JA. Wound healing by secondary intention, a cosmetic appraisal. *J Am Acad Dermatol* 1983; 9: 407–415.

10

Wound Dressings

Bari B. Cunningham, Leonard Bernstein, and David T. Woodley
Northwestern University School of Medicine, Chicago, Illinois

WOUND DRESSINGS

A wound dressing may vary from a clean, simple cloth to a sheet of cultured keratinocytes. Within the latter paradigm is the notion that a wound dressing can act as a delivery system for biological mediators in addition to providing a protective environment for a wound. Ideally, a dressing should serve as a barrier between the wound and the outside environment, absorb wound exudate, assert pressure to provide hemostasis, enhance the reepithelization process, splint the surrounding wound edges without restricting patient mobility, be easily applied and removed without disturbing the newly epithelized surface, and be inexpensive (Table 1). That any one dressing possesses all these traits is unlikely. However, throughout the healing process of a wound, the dressings one chooses should possess the qualities that are most applicable at that time.

In general, the dressing serves as a barrier between the wound bed and the external environment, including both physical and bacterial contamination. It temporarily replaces some of the functions of normal skin. Occasionally, however, wound dressings, whether through exhaustion of an ability to function or fundamental design, may act as an entry site for bacteria.

Studies have shown that reepithelization occurs more quickly in a moist environment than in an open, air-dried wound. This principle has led to the development of wound dressings that provide a moist environment for the healing wound bed by preventing evaporative water loss. The ability of a dressing to prevent water vapor loss, or its occlusivity, is based on several variables, the most important of which is the permeability of the outer layer of the dressing. One can categorize dressings in the following manner: impermeable to the passage of both fluid and water vapor, impermeable to fluid but permeable to water vapor, and permeable to both fluid and water vapor. This function is directly proportional to the porosity of the material in the outer layer of the dressing. The degree to which it can maintain a tight impermeable border depends on the dressing's flexibility and its adherence to the surrounding skin.

Table 1   Ideal Functions
of a Wound Dressing

Protective barrier
Absorb exudate
Promote hemostasis
Enhance reepithelization
Provide support
Easily applied and removed
Inexpensive

The need for the absorption of exudate varies in different wounds. The amount of wound fluid drainage may be minimal or extensive. Similarly, the absorption capacity of available wound dressings may vary from a minimal amount to many times its own volume. A dressing absorbs exudate via the principle of capillary flow—in essence, wicking the fluid away from the wound bed.

The ability of a dressing to repel or exert pressure varies according to its structure. It may absorb physical pressure and prevent its transference to the fragile neoepithelium by acting as a cushion against mechanical forces and an anchor for sheering forces. In addition, a firmly placed wound dressing will promote hemostasis and minimize hematoma formation, thereby minimizing endogenous mechanical forces.

The adherence of a dressing can be inherent to the dressing or be a part of a complex dressing. Many of the synthetic occlusive dressings contain adhesive compounds that maintain a tight seal at the periphery. Others may contain an adhesive across the entire surface of the dressing (Op-Site). A complex dressing may include several nonadherent layers secured with adhesive tape on the external surface.

DRESSING LAYERS

A wound dressing can be broken down into several functional components: ointment layer, contact layer, absorbing layer, contouring layer, and securing layer (Table 2). A given dressing may not have all of these characteristics. Complex dressings utilize different elements to accomplish several of these functions.

The ointment layer provides a moist and often antibacterial environment. The moisture promotes epithelialization and prevents the dressing from adhering to the underlying tissue. This layer is often provided by the use of one of the many antibiotic ointment preparations applied to a wound base. Should the patient have a sensitivity to these ointments, plain petrolatum can be substituted.

The contact layer is the part of the dressing that comes into contact with the wound base. It has three important roles. First, it must form a firm contact between the surface of the dressing and the wound to avoid fluid accumulation and to allow the absorbing layer to function. Second, it should be fluid permeable to allow the absorbing layer to absorb the exudate via capillary flow. Third, it should be nonadherent to avoid trauma to the fragile underlying epithelium when it is removed. Examples of common dressings addressing this concept are Telfa pads, Vaseline Petrolatum Gauze, and N-terface (a plastic over a monofilament membrane).

The absorbing layer, as mentioned above, is designed to remove the exudate from the wound surface. By removing the wound exudate, a good culture medium for bacteria, the wound base will be less likely colonized by large numbers of bacteria. Also, the wound will be less macerated. An example of this type of dressing is a cotton gauze dressing.

Table 2 Layers of a Wound Dressing

Layer	Function
Ointment layer	Provides moist environment Prevents adherence of dressing
Absorbing layer	Absorbs exudate
Contact layer	Provides close contact between wound and other layers
Contouring layer	Supports adjacent structures
Securing layer	Fastens dressing to bordering skin

The contouring layer may be used to support protruding structures, such as the ears, to avoid injury from the folding effect of the bandage or tape. It is also used to fill in anatomic depressions or sulci so that the dressing will be more securely placed. Common examples include cotton dental rolls or fluffed cotton gauze.

The securing layer fastens the underlying dressing to the wound surface and bordering skin. Examples include adhesive tape, Mastisol, and tincture of benzoin. Often dressings are manufactured with an adhesive surface combined to an absorptive surface. An example of the latter includes Band-Aids. In certain instances, a roll-type, self-adhesive dressing may be used to add pressure and support to the wound. Elastoplast or Coban wrap are examples of compressive dressings used to add pressure to the lower extremities in the treatment of venous stasis dermatitis or postsclerotherapy for varicose veins.

CLASSIFICATION OF DRESSINGS

Dressings can be classified in two manners. First, they may be categorized based on their synthetic components: natural, semisynthetic, and synthetic. Second, they can be categorized based on their permeability to fluids and vapor, as noted above. The latter of these two classifications is used here (Table 3).

Fluid- and Vapor-Permeable Dressings

Cotton Gauze

Cotton has been a longstanding constituent of wound dressings. It is used in many forms, including cotton balls, gauze, pads, and combination dressings, in which an absorbtion layer of cotton is placed between two layers of plastic (Telfa pads). The cotton is bleached prior to processing to remove the oils that inhibit its absorptive ability, a primary function of this type of dressing.

In the treatment of surgical wounds, the use of cotton gauze as the primary dressing is useful during the early postoperative period to absorb exudate. It is important to change the dressing frequently to prevent it from becoming a breeding ground for bacteria and promoting wound infection. Also, frequent changes prevent the incorporation of the dressing into the granulation tissue, which may damage the fragile reepithelized wound bed upon removal.

In some instances this possible disadvantage becomes an advantage. Gauze dressings are used to debride wounds. To accomplish debridement, the gauze is applied in two layers. The moist gauze layer lies directly over the wound bed covered by a layer of dry gauze. As the lower layer of gauze dries due to evaporation, the gauze becomes incorporated into the exudate and fibrin-

Table 3 Classification and Manufacturer Listing of Common Wound Dressings

Permeability	Category	Active component(s)
I. Fluid and water vapor permeable	1 Cotton (Plain)	Cloth Balls Rolls Gauze
	2 Cotton/Cellulose (Coated)	Pads Hydrophilic petrolatum Petrolatum Povidone-iodine o-tolylazo-o-tolyazo-beta-naphthol Bismuth tribromophenate Zinc oxide, calamine
	3 Polymers	Cadexomer iodine (beads) Dextranomer (beads) Plastic monofilament Polyester/Rayon Polyester/Rayon/Iodoform Polyester/Cellulose
	4 Alginates	Alginates (seaweed extracts)
II. Fluid impermeable, water vapor permeable	1 Polyurethane	Film Foam
	2 Hydrogels	Polyethylene oxide Agar/acrylamide Starch polymer
III. Fluid and water vapor impermeable	Hydrocolloids	Carboxymethylcellulose sodium
IV. Miscellaneous	Adhesive Wraps	

Group/Name	Manufacturer
	Johnson & Johnson
	Johnson & Johnson
Kling	Johnson & Johnson
Kerlix	Kendall Co
Gauze Sponges	Johnson & Johnson
Curity Gauze Sponges	Kendall Co
Steri-Pad	Johnson & Johnson
Aquaphor Gauze	Beiersdorf
Vaseline Petrolatum Gauze	Sherwood
Adaptic Non-Adherent Dressing	Johnson & Johnson
Betadine Gauze	Purdue
Scarlet Red Ointment Dressing	Sherwood
Xeroform Petrolatum Dressing	Sherwood
Dome-Paste	Miles
Gelocast	Beiersdorf
Medico-Paste	Graham-Field
Iodosorb	Perstorp AB
	Stuart Pharmaceuticals
Debrisan	Johnson & Johnson
N-Terface	Winfield Laboratories
Nu Gauze	Johnson & Johnson
Nova Gauze	Johnson & Johnson
Nu Gauze with Iodoform	Johnson & Johnson
Telfa	Kendallm Co
Sorbsan	Hickam
Kaltostat	Calgon/Vestal
Op-site	Smith & Nephew
Tegaderm	3M, Medical-Surgical
Acu-Derm	Acme United
Bioclusive	Johnson & Johnson
Uniflex	Pfizer
Synthaderm	Derma-Lock Medical Corp
Epi-Lock	Calgon/Vestal
	Derma-Lock Medical Corp
Vigilon	Bard Home Health
Zenoderm	Zenith Tech Group
Bio-Film	BF Goodrich
Gelliperm	Geistlich Pharmaceuticals
Bard	Bard Home Health
DuoDerm	Squibb (Convatec)
Coban	3M
Elastoplast	Beiersdorf

ous debris on the wound surface. Upon removal of the dressing, the wound bed is debrided with the removal of the dried serum coagulum, necrotic tissue, and fibrin.

Often gauze is applied to a wound, in a wet-to-dry manner, with an antibacterial solution soaked into its network. In addition to debriding the wound base, the dressing serves to decrease the population of bacteria at the surface of the wound. Sodium hypochlorite (Dakin's solution) is commonly used for this purpose.

Medicated Gauze

Cotton gauze can be combined or coated with ointments and medications. The combination of petrolatum with cotton gauze allows for an effective ointment layer to be formed, however, the absorbtive capacity is decreased due to its hydrophobicity. The substitution of hydrophilic ointment, which can absorb many times its own volume of water, eliminates this problem. This combination provides a moist environment for wound healing, inhibition of dressing incorporation into the healing wound bed, and greater absorption of exudate.

Infection is known to slow wound healing. Antibacterial agents, such as povidone-iodine and silver sulfadiazine, have been combined in cotton gauze dressings in an effort to decrease bacterial colonization. Iodoform gauze strips are useful for packing cavitary lesions to allow for absorption and drainage of exudate while decreasing bacterial counts. However, iodine is cytotoxic to fibroblasts at all but very low concentrations. Therefore, the use of iodine in wound dressings may actually slow wound healing.

Polymers

Starch Polymers (Iodosorb, Debrisan)

Cadexomer iodine (Iodosorb) is a highly hydrophilic network of a starch polymer in the form of beads with iodine immobilized within its matrix. Upon absorption of water, the porosity of the beads increases, releasing the iodine into the wound in a timely fashion. This dressing is very effective in absorbing exudate and at the same time introduces a bacteriostatic agent to the surface of a wound. A decrease in bacterial counts on the wound surface has been demonstrated in animal models. The slow release of iodine as the porosity increases maintains a very low iodine concentration at the wound surface. This low concentration may have significant antimicrobial activity with little to no cytotoxic effects to the fibroblasts.

The dextranomer (Debrisan) dressing is a 90% dextranomer with polyethylene glycol and water combination in the form of beads. It has moderate absorptive capacity. The beads absorb low molecular weight particles, and the larger molecules move between the beads via capillary action, resulting in the lifting away of necrotic tissue from the wound surface. It is less absorptive than cadexomer iodine and lacks antibacterial properties. Both dressings in this category require an outer layer to absorb excess exudate and to secure the dressing to the wound.

Polymer Blend (N-Terface)

This dressing is a synthetic, high-density plastic polymer in a monofilament woven, nonadherent dressing. It allows fluid to flow though its network into an absorbant overlying dressing while preventing adherence to the new epithelial surface. This dressing is commonly used on fresh surgical wounds.

Although this is considered a nonadherent dressing, Weber described the possibility of extention of granulation tissue into the woven matrix of the dressing. Because this would lead to trauma to the wound bed upon removal of this dressing, it is recommended that this dressing be changed weekly.

Alginates (Sorbsan, Kaltostat)

Alginates are natural polysaccharides extracted from seaweed. Sorbsan is a calcium salt of alginic acid prepared in a woven fiber for wound dressings. It has a high absorptive capacity and forms a gel that conforms well to the dimensions of the wound base. This dressing also requires an overlying dressing to absorb excess fluid and secure this gel dressing to the wound.

Water-Impermeable and Vapor-Permeable Dressings

This category contains many of the semisynthetic and synthetic dressings. The water impermeable membranes produce a moist environment for the wound bed and prevents external contamination by bacteria. The vapor permeable membrane allows for some air and water vapor to transfer between the wound and the environment. This category includes the polyurethane films/membranes and the hydrogels.

Polyurethane Films and Membranes (Op-site, TegaDerm, Acu-Derm, Bioclusive)

Polyurethane films are transluscent, self-adherent, water impermeable, and vapor permeable dressings. They lack an absorbing layer, so that exudate will accumulate under this dressing. To prevent the frequent changing of this dressing and to reduce the potential trauma to the fragile wound, a sterile needle can be used to puncture the surface and remove the collection of exudate. This hole can be resealed by applying a small piece of a new film over it. The translucent feature of this membrane allows for the monitoring of the wound bed for signs of infection without removing the dressing. This is one major advantage over the more occlusive dressings discussed below. In addition, these dressings are quite thin and flexible. This flexibility allows effective contouring of the dressing over concave and convex surfaces, and mobility when placed over joints.

These dressings are useful for holding pinch grafts in place in the treatment of leg ulcers. They allow visualization of the wound bed and hold the grafts in place until engraftment. They may be used in the treatment of early decubiti ulcers, split-thickness graft donor sites, and over sites of dermabrasion.

As mentioned above, the adherent nature of this dressing must be considered when using it for skin grafts. The removal of this dressing prematurely may traumatize grafted tissue. For this reason, it is recommended that the dressing be allowed to remain in place until it falls off on its own, usually after 1 or 2 weeks.

Hydrogels (Polyethylene Oxide—Vigilon and Bio-Film; Starch Polymer—Bard)

The hydrogel dressings are semiadherent, absorbant, water-impermeable, and vapor-permeable membranes. They are of two major types. First, the 4% polyethylene oxide/96% water hydrogel (Vigilon) is a gel sandwiched between two removable sheets of polyurethane. The permeability to water vapor is increased as each of the outer and inner membranes is removed. If both are removed, the dressing becomes permeable to fluid. The second type, the starch hydrogel (Bard), is a compound polymerized from cornstarch that is transformed into a gel with hydration at the time of its use.

Unlike the polyurethane dressings, the hydrogels have significant absorptive capacity—between 100 and 200% of their volume. These dressings are semiadhesive at the wound site by forming a gel that conforms to the edges of the wound. The polyethylene dressings are easily removed from the wound without trauma, while the starch polymer dressing requires water to be applied to the surface to aid in its removal. Frequently these dressings are secured in place with a gauze wrap. Geronemus and Robins showed an average 25–45% faster reepithelization rate in pig skin wound models using hydrogels compared to open wound controls. Vigilon dressings may be used on dermabrasion wounds, venous ulcers, and surgical wounds, healing by second intention.

Water- and Vapor-Impermeable Dressings

This class of dressings is impermeable to both fluid and water vapor. Such dressings provide a very moist environment for wound healing, reduce pain at the wound site, and need less frequent changes than permeable dressings.

Hydrocolloid Dressings (DuoDerm)

This is a self-adherent, opaque, fluid and water vapor–impermeable, gel-forming dressing composed of carboxymethylcellulose sodium, gelatin, and polyisobutylene, which is able to absorb approximately 100% of its volume in water. The contact layer forms a gel with hydration and readily conforms to the shape of the wound. The adhesive nature of this dressing often precludes the need for a securing dressing. The ability of this dressing to form an impermeable barrier allows the phagocytic cells and the active proteases from the exudate to accumulate in a very moist environment to assist in the debridement of a wound base.

The disadvantages of this dressing include a malodorous discharge upon removal, maceration of the surrounding normal tissue, leakage of excessive tissue exudate, and the potential formation of exuberant granulation tissue. These problems can be circumvented by the proper selection of a secondary dressing for a highly exudative wound and more frequent dressing changes.

Xakellis et al. performed a cost analysis of treating decubiti ulcers with hydrocolloid dressings vs. wet-to-dry saline gauze dressings in a nursing home. The cost of each hydrocolloid dressing was much greater than the cost of cotton gauze, and the healing times were very similar. Nevertheless, the real savings in cost was the amount of nursing time saved because the hydrocolloid dressings required significantly fewer dressing changes than a gauze dressing.

OCCLUSIVE VERSUS NONOCCLUSIVE DRESSINGS

In the early 1960s it was demonstrated that reepithelization was promoted by a moist wound environment when compared with a wound allowed to air-dry. The development of a semipermeable and impermeable synthetic dressings arose from this finding. Many theories have been postulated to explain why moist wounds heal better. These include increased partial oxygen tension of the wound environment, easier mobility of epithelial cells in a moist environment, elimination of eschar formation, and the concentration of growth factors in the wound.

Silver examined various occlusive dressings with regard to the oxygen tension at the wound site. He found that the rate of reepithelization was related to the oxygen permeability of the dressing. Another study, comparing vapor-impermeable and semipermeable dressings, demonstrated that the less permeable dressings (and by extension having less oxygen tension) had a faster rate of reepithelization.

Jonkman et al., using various vapor-permeable dressings, showed that an intermediate moist environment (provided by highly vapor-permeable dressings) created the best foundation for the formation of a fibrin and fibronectin matrix in the wound bed. This in turn provides a platform for reepithelization until there is reformation of the basement membrane.

The presence of an eschar, or scab, will slow the reepithelization process by forcing the epithelial cells to tunnel under an adherent dessicated structure in order to cover the wound base. The higher the degree of desiccation, the deeper into the dermis the scab will form and the slower the reepithelization rate. The occlusive nature of synthetic dressings prevents scab formation in two ways. First, it maintains a moist environment, preventing desiccation. Second, a collection of enzymatically active cells is maintained at the wound surface to degrade necrotic tissue and prevent scab formation.

Another concern in the early use of occlusive dressings are that of bacterial infections. Wound exudate is known to be a good culture medium for bacterial growth. The bacterial concentration in a wound has been shown to increase with the use of occlusive dressings compared with open wounds. This increase may be due, in part, to changes in the pH, oxygen concentration, and moisture content. Nevertheless, many studies comparing the rate of bacterial infection of wounds using occlusive and nonocclusive dressings have shown no significant difference. In fact, the growth of bacterial organisms, which normally colonize most wounds, may have a protective role in occlusive situations by preventing pathogenic organisms from invading the tissue. Also, it has been shown that occlusive dressings have a strong barrier function, which prevents the penetrance of bacteria from the outside environment.

CULTURED EPIDERMAL GRAFTS

Human epidermal keratinocytes can now be grown reliably in vitro to form large sheets of epithelium, which can be grafted unto cutaneous ulcers or surgical defects. The procedure can be performed using autografts (skin biopsy from patient) or allografts (biopsy from donor). Cultured keratinocyte grafts can be cultivated by digesting whole skin with trypsin followed by growing the digest on irradiated 3T3 mouse fibroblasts, which support rapid keratinocyte proliferation. Within several weeks, a 1 cm^2 skin sample can be expanded to generate a cultured epithelium large enough to cover an entire body surface.

Autografts

This technique was first used successfully in 1981 in two men with third degree burns using cultured keratinocyte autograft. Subsequently, cultured keratinocyte autografts have gained moderate acceptance by centers in Europe and the United States with varying success rates. The graft "take" rate varies from 30 to 80% depending on host factors, postoperative care, depth of cutaneous defect, etc. The graft's acceptance into mainstream wound care has been limited by several factors, including the vulnerability of these grafts in the postoperative period. The patient must remain immobilized for several days postoperatively in order to facilitate graft "take." Grafts that survive beyond 6 months have long-term durability and texture that is equivalent to split-thickness skin grafts.

There are few studies of histologic changes within these grafts after transplantation. There is evidence that the epidermis differentiates into basal, spinous, granular, and cornified layers. Rete ridges may not form for many years after grafting. Within 3 weeks of transplant, grafts develop basal lamina, hemidesmosomes, and anchoring fibrils. However, the anchoring fibrils are immature ultrastructurally and sparse when compared with normal skin. In addition to their fragility after transplant, autologous cultured keratinocyte grafts are exquisitely vulnerable in the laboratory. The major disadvantages of autologous keratinocyte grafts are the time required for the production (approximately 3 weeks), intensive postoperative care, and expense.

Allografts

More recently the technique of cultured keratinocytes has been applied to cultured epithelium delivered from an unrelated donor, a cultured allograft. Leigh et al. using skin obtained during mammoplasty as a source of donor keratinocytes, grafted chronic ulcers. Twenty-nine percent of the ulcers healed completely, with improvement shown in an additional 44%.

This procedure is limited by the fact that keratinocytes of older donors grow more slowly and are more senescent. With this knowledge, Phillips et al. treated 36 chronic ulcers with cultured epidermal sheets derived from neonatal foreskin. In 73% of ulcers there was complete healing within 8 weeks In the remaining ulcers there were marked reductions in size within 8 weeks. Pain was relieved within 24 hr after grafting. Unfortunately, this study, which looked at ulcers resulting from scleroderma, venous stasis disease, trauma, paraplegia, and rheumatoid arthritis, was uncontrolled and unblinded.

Although initially believed to survive permanently, cultured keratinocyte allografts are now believed not to "take" because they are rapidly rejected by the host. Using monoclonal antibodies against MHC specificities, which differ between host and donor keratinocytes, replacement of grafted keratinocytes by host cells is observed within 2 weeks following cultured allografting. Nevertheless, allografts improve healing of cutaneous wounds, perhaps by the production of growth factors. Keratinocytes in culture are known to elaborate soluble mediators that enhance cell proliferation and differentiation. The cytokines potentially relevant to wound healing after autologous grafts include interleukins 1 and 3, fibronectin, and transforming growth factor alpha (TGF-α).

Allografting is more convenient than autografts because it obviates that need for biopsy and cultivation 3 weeks prior to the grafting procedure. Additionally, these grafts could be harvested and stored for future use. Whether cultured keratinocyte grafts will ultimately be a routine part of the dermatologist's armamentarium will depend on well-controlled multicentered trials, which have not yet been performed.

VITAL DYES/ANTISEPTICS

Topical antimicrobial agents have long been promoted as important components of wound care. It is well documented that infection delays wound healing. This has led to the belief that reducing bacterial colonization will promote wound healing. This is accomplished by adding topical antibiotics and antiseptics to cutaneous wounds. This often occurs without regard to potential inhibition of normal wound healing. Furthermore, there are few studies to support the use of prophylactic antiseptics in wound healing. In fact, the presence of bacteria is not tantamount to skin infection. Bolton et al. showed that occluded wounds contaminated with 10^5 bacteria/0.01 ml did not heal slower than wounds with lower bacterial counts as measured by wound contraction. Studies must correlate the in vitro efficacy of antimicrobial agents with the clinical efficacy. Additionally, wounds treated with topical antibiotics may lead to the emergence of resistant bacteria.

The prolonged use of prophylactic topical antimicrobial agents during wound care is not recommended.

Povidone-Iodine

Povidone-iodine is one of the most commonly used antiseptics and is widely available in 10% solution, 2% detergent, and 2% ointment or wash. It is active against gram-positive and gram-negative organisms and spores. Despite its "broad-spectrum" characteristics, it is cytotoxic at certain concentrations. Rodeheaver et al. looked at varying concentrations and formulations of iodine products and their effects on wound infection in a guinea pig model. Povidone-iodine surgical scrub solution had the lowest degree of activity; in fact, it was incapable of sterilizing a single challenge of 10^{10} *E. coli* in a test tube. The povidone-iodine scrub solution significantly decreased the wound's ability to fight infection. Rodeheaver et al. postulate that the damaging effects of this solution may be related to its detergent characteristics, which are highly cytotoxic. Additionally, because iodine is insoluble in water, it may not be able to reach and kill the bacteria present in tissue. In the same study, bacteria present in 1.5-mm-thick tissue were unaffected by immersion in an iodine scrub solution. Lineaweaver et al. specifically addressed the cytotoxicity and bactericidal activity of varying concentrations of povidone-iodine. At standard strengths (1%), the antiseptic was 100% cytotoxic to fibroblasts in culture. Adult rat wounds irrigated with 1% povidone-iodine retained only 21% the tensile strength compared with controls. On the other hand, *diluted* iodine at 0.001% resulted in 100% fibroblast survival and no bacterial survival. This argues for a balance between cytotoxicity and bacterial cytotoxicity obtainable by dilution. The concentration of a wound antiseptic should be as low as possible while maximizing the antimicrobial properties.

Acetic Acid

Acetic acid is effective against a variety of gram-positive and gram-negative organisms. When combined with gauze it has a dessicating effect on a wound, permitting evaporative water loss. Gruber et al. compared acetic acid 0.25% solution with povidone-iodine (Betadine) and 3% hydrogen peroxide applied to partial thickness wounds on rats. The acetic acid solution had no significant gross or microscopic effect on the wounds. When compared with a 0.5% sodium hypochlorite (Dakin's solution) and 1% povidone-iodine, 0.25% acetic acid solution was as toxic to fibroblasts but less bactericidal, decreasing only 20% bacterial survival. Dilution of acetic acid to 0.025% and 0.0025% allowed increased fibroblast survival, but was associated with unacceptable antibacterial activity. At present, the use of acetic acid as an antimicrobial agent in wound care is not recommended.

Hydrogen Peroxide

Despite its global acceptance and use as a wound cleanser, hydrogen peroxide is a poor antiseptic. Its benefits are likely a consequence of its effervescence and debridement rather than its antibacterial effect. Hydrogen peroxide is rapidly decomposed by catalase, an enzyme ubiquitous in living tissue, into oxygen and water. The released oxygen is thought to have little antibacterial effect. Furthermore, the use of hydrogen peroxide under pressure dressings in a closed lesion should be avoided due to a concern for the possibility of air emboli.

Most studies of topical antimicrobial toxicity have used various bacterial toxicity assays where different concentrations of hydrogen peroxide are suspended with aliquots of bacteria and plated for growth on agar. Because they do not take into account the in vivo phenomenon of catalase-driven degradation of hydrogen peroxide, many of these studies are flawed. Full-strength 3% hydrogen peroxide is completely cytotoxic to bacteria in a test tube, but its in vivo effect is unclear. Early studies in the plastic surgery literature tauted hydrogen peroxide as *shortening* the healing time of artificially created wounds in rats. At present, hydrogen peroxide is considered more innocuous than Betadine but has minimal in vivo antimicrobial activity.

Various Antimicrobials

At strengths generally used in wound care, sodium hypochlorite (0.05%) (Dakin's solution) is toxic to both fibroblasts and bacteria. At a dilution of 0.005%, however, Dakin's solution may afford a favorable balance as it allows for 97% fibroblast survival and no bacterial survival. Various other antiseptics including pyoctanin 0.5%, brillant green 0.5%, chlorhexidine 0.5%, chloramine-T 10%, and silver nitrate 1.0% inhibit granulation tissue formation. In fact, chlorhexidine, brillant green, and pyoctanin actually are more toxic to granulation tissue than silver nitrate, a compound that has been used therapeutically for its caustic antigranulation effects.

TOPICAL ANTIBIOTICS

Silver Sulfadiazine

Silver sulfadiazine (Silvadene) 1% cream is water soluble and water absorbant and is widely used for its antimicrobial properties in the treatment of burns. Geronemus et al. compared Silvadene cream, Pharmadine (povidone-iodine), Neosporin ointment (neomycin sulfate, polymyxin B sulfate, and bacitracin zinc), and Furacin (nitrofurazone). They demonstrated that topical antimicrobial agents affect the rate of reepithelization as monitored experimentally in pigs. Silvadene cream promoted healing at the fastest rate of the four agents examined, being 28% faster than controls.

The faster reepithelization, however, is not solely a result of antimicrobial activity because the vehicle alone significantly increased the reepithelization rate by 21%. Inert vehicles affect wound healing. In pig dermatome wounds, USP White Petrolatum retarded reepithelization by 17% compared to untreated wounds. An oil-in-water vanishing cream increased reepithelization by 24%, and a lotion of PEG-20, stearic acid, isopropyl palmitate, propylene glycol, and zinc soap increased reepithelization by 15%. McGrath showed that USP White Petrolatum increased tissue survival of skin flaps in rats.

Several cases of transient leukopenia have been reported in patients receiving topical silver sulfadiazine. The leukopenia is primarily a neutropenia with maximal white blood cell depression occurring within 2–4 days of therapy initiation. The recovery of leukocyte levels to normal occurs despite continuation of silver sulfadiazine therapy. A higher incidence of this transient leukopenia has been reported in patients using cimetidene concomitantly.

Nitrofurazone

Although Furacin has an antimicrobial spectrum similar to silver sulfadiazine, it significantly retards reepithelization. Furacin, which contains nitrofurazone in Solubase (a water-soluble base of propylene glycol), showed a 24% retardation of reepithelization compared wtih Solubase alone and controls. This retardation of reepithelization may be due to inhibition to ornithine decarboxylase and subsequent cell proliferation. The use of Furacin over large body surface areas may lead to significant absorption of propylene glycol. High serum levels of propylene glycol can cause renal failure in patients with baseline renal impairment.

Neomycin

This antibacterial is primarily effective against gram-positive organisms. A small number of patients may develop an allergic contact dermatitis to neomycin. Patients with a history of hypersensitivity to neomycin may cross-react to gentamicin. In an ointment base it has been shown to promote reepithelization.

Benzoyl Peroxide

Benzoyl peroxide is a potent oxidizer, which has been widely used in dermatologic therapy for its antimicrobial, keratolytic, and antifungal properties. It is converted in skin to benzoic acid. Its use has been limited by a 10% incidence of allergic contact dermatitis. Systemic toxicity has not been reported. Keratome wounds created in pigs were shown to reepithelize faster when treated with 20% benzoyl peroxide lotion. Coleman and Roenigk evaluated the clinical and histological effects of varying concentrations of benzoyl peroxide on the healing of pig wounds created by a dermatome. Twenty percent benzoyl peroxide lotion was associated with the most rapid reepithelization. Differences were attributed to antimicrobial and debriding properties of benzoyl peroxide. However, bacteriostatic activity has not been shown, in subsequent studies, to correlate with earlier reepithelization. Regardless of the mechanism of action, the concentration of benzoyl peroxide seems to be important for reepithelization because 10% benzoyl peroxide did not demonstrate any benefit on chronic leg ulcers. High benzoyl peroxide concentrations may be toxic to wounds. Fifty percent benzoyl peroxide lotion significantly retarded wound healing in pigs. The toxic effects of benzoyl peroxide may relate to its particle size. As the benzoyl peroxide concentration increases, the size of the particle also increases. Formulations with larger particles have a higher ocular irritation potential.

HEMOSTATIC AGENTS: MONSEL'S SOLUTION AND ALUMINUM CHLORIDE

Monsel's solution (ferric subsulfate) and aluminum chloride are commonly used hemostatic agents. They are convenient and rapid acting. For many years. Monsel's solution was the most popular agent for hemostasis. However, due to concern over tattoo formation in cosmetically important skin using Monsel's solution, aluminum chloride has been used with increasing frequency. More recently, these agents have been found to delay reepithelization and result in less cosmetically acceptable scars. Ferric subsulfate and aluminum chloride may inhibit wound healing by dessication of the wound bed with inhibition of fluid exudation. This interferes with the delivery of cellular and soluble substances to the wound surface, which are necessary for wound healing. Both hemostatic agents result in scars 0.5–2 mm larger than controls in miniature pigs. These data were confirmed by earlier work by Harris and Youkey.

GROWTH FACTORS

Transforming Growth Factor Beta

Locally applied growth factors may modify and enhance the wound-healing response; they may be attractive additions to wound care. Mustoe et al. analyzed the effects of transforming growth factor beta (TGF-β) on surgical incisions in rats. They found a dose-related direct stimulatory effect on tensile strength after a single application of TGF-β. The increase in wound strength was associated with marked increase in collagen deposition, increased influx of mononuclear cells, and fibroblasts. Their results show that TGF-β can accelerate wound healing in an in vivo model. However, they did not comment on the final appearance of the surgical scar after remodeling. Because TGF-β is known to stimulate collagen synthesis and inhibit collagenase, there may be the potential for excessive collagen synthesis, resulting in hypertrophic, keloidal, and/or sclerotic scars in humans. Whether TGF-β will be used therapeutically in wound dressings remains to be determined. Large multicenter controlled trials in humans have yet to be performed.

Epidermal Growth Factor

Brown et al. evaluated the effect of locally applied epidermal growth factor (EGF) and TGF-β confirming earlier work by Mustoe et al. The EGF, however, was ineffective after one application. When EGF was incorporated into multilamelar liposomes, prolonging the exposure of the wound bed to EGF, there was a 200% increase in tensile strength of the wound. This was associated with increased collagen production and fibroblast proliferation.

DRESSINGS FOR DIFFICULT ANATOMIC AREAS

Scalp

Because the scalp is usually covered with hair, securing a dressing is difficult. Therefore, dressings on the scalp are usually held in place by successive turban wrapping with Kerlix or Kling. Although easy to apply, this technique results in bothersome, cosmetically unappealing dressings. Robinson recommends the use of the elastic panty portion of pantyhose and a small coin to avoid bulky turbans. The wound is covered by small eye pads, and the elastic end of a pantyhose is pulled over the head (and wound). This dressing is secured in place by twisting the nylon over a small coin above the pinna of the ear. This dressing may then be concealed by a hat.

An alternative is a modified Russian technique, which is comfortable and cosmetically acceptable. Kerlix or other gauze approximately 4 inches wide and 9–10 yards long is needed. An anchoring piece of gauze is draped over the scalp and another piece is used to form a modified turban by interlocking with alternating arms of the anchoring piece. The free end is tied into a knot, while the anchoring piece is tied under the chin.

Turban head dressings are often unappealing to patients. For dressing small wounds on a scalp with moderate hair growth, one can utilize the hair in securing the dressing. Applying a coating of Mastisol (a gum mastic with styrax and methyl salicylate) to several hairs on each side of the dressing will create tacky anchored ties. Tying opposite ties over a dressing will secure it to the wound surface and eliminate the need for cosmetically unacceptable head wraps. Removal of the dressing requires the simple cutting of the few hairs used in the ties. Often this type of dressing can be hidden by hairstyling until removed.

Nose

Some nasal wounds can be dressed with Telfa, an eye pad, and tape without additional bulk. However, the materials must be taped in three directions. First, a horizontal piece of tape is used. Additional pieces of tape form an X at the glabella. The key is to use tape that is wide and long enough; ½-inch tape works well.

Sometimes a dressing on the nose will collapse the nostril. If this occurs, counterpressure can be applied by inserting a dental roll or the cut rubber finger from a surgical glove, filled with gauze and coated with ointment, into the nostril. Obviously, it is essential when inserting an object into a nostril to ensure that the patient can breathe adequately via the other nostril and mouth.

Because of the abundance of oil secretion from the sebaceous glands on the nose, the adhesive tends not to stick as well. Therefore, the dressing may require more frequent changes.

Ears

The most efficient way to dress a wound on the ear is to provide bulk. The ear is contoured with fluffed dry gauze both anteriorly and posteriorly. Tape may be applied directly to the gauze. If additional pressure is required, Kerlix can be wrapped around the scalp, leaving the contralateral ear uncovered by twisting the roll of gauze as it passes.

Axilla

The axilla is a problem area because tape is too rigid to provide for free range of motion of the ipsilateral arm. Winton suggests using Kerlix wrapped in a figure-8 conformation across the back and around the contralateral shoulder and axilla.

Hands, Feet, and Digits

Tubular gauze is commonly used to secure dressings on the fingers and toes. One must take care to avoid taping the gauze too tightly or circumferentially to avoid constriction of digital blood vessels. Bennett recommends gauze taped *obliquely*. Finger dressings may also be wound loosely around the finger and secured with gauze wrap tied at the wrist.

The use of a sling may reduce pain. However, the hand should not be elevated more than 90 degrees at the elbow to avoid diminishing blood flow. Specially designed shoes are available to facilitate ambulation postoperatively. The Reese boot and Zimmer boot are open-toed wood-soled shoes, which can be laced in front and accommodate dressings, edema, and pain.

SPECIAL SITUATIONS

Keloids

Keloids and hypertrophic scars have been treated with lasers, radiation, surgery, cryosurgery, topical steroids, and topical retinoids. More recently, the use of nonpressure dressings consisting of silicone gel have been described. Perkins et al. first described using these in 1982 for treating burn scars. This dressing is a nonadherent semi-occlusive, synthetic polymer of silicone (Silastic Gel) applied to keloids without pressure and secured with tape.

Gold recently showed the benefit of a silicone gel in a three-phase study evaluating treatment of hypertrophic scars with silicone alone, prevention of recurrence with silicone following destructive treatment with a CO_2 laser, and in treating thermal burns with silicone alone. He found that 57% (12/21) of the patients had moderate improvement of the hypertrophic scar with silicone gel alone. There was one recurrence out of eight patients using silicone after laser treatment, as opposed to three recurrences out of eight patients not using silicone after laser treatment. Minimal to moderate change was observed using silicone gel with thermal burns ($n = 5$).

The mechanism for the effectiveness of silicone is not known. There is no evidence that pressure plays a role, that silicone penetrates the skin, or that oxygen tension changes on the surface of the scar. It has been postulated by Sawanda and Sone that hydration of the skin under the dressing may play a role. However, it is difficult to imagine how simple hydration of the stratum corneum would affect fibroblastic activity in the underlying dermis.

Leg Ulcers

The etiology of the leg ulcer is important in determining which dressing is most suitable (see Chap. 39). In this section, treatment of leg ulcers related to venous insufficiency, which constitute the majority of ulcers due to circulatory problems seen in a dermatology office, is discussed.

To treat a venous ulcer effectively, an understanding of the fundamental pathophysiology is needed. Intrinsic causes of venous ulcerations include incompetent valves that allow backward flow of blood in the extremities and increase hydrostatic pressures. This increase in pressure causes dilation of the vessels with leakage of fluid through stretched pores in the vessel walls and the formation of a fibrin cuff around the dermal blood vessels.

Extrinsic causes may include thrombosis of a deep vessel secondary to prolonged compression. This will also cause a backup of blood flow and increase hydrostatic pressure. Whether the cause of venous failure is intrinsic to an individual or extrinsic is not as important as the fact that they can both produce the same fundamental problem, edema.

The ulceration process occurs when the edema increases the pressure on the tissue within the leg to such a degree that the skin surface becomes eczematous. At this point, only a small degree of trauma can induce tissue breakdown and ulcer formation.

The main goal in the treatment of venous insufficiency should be the prevention of ulcerations. Leg elevation and pressure stockings are useful, but both depend greatly on patient compliance. Compressive dressings, on the other hand, can often be applied in a physician's office and left on for a week. This obviates the need for compliance and provides for more physician control of the wound. Compression dressings have the disadvantages that they are frequently too warm to wear continuously in warm climates and need to be protected from getting wet.

Any successful approach to healing venous stasis leg ulcers will require addressing the main source of the problem, edema. Compression dressings may vary from fairly nonabsorbant, compressive adhesive wraps (Elastoplast, Coban) to the minimally absorbant, moderately compressive paste wrap. Unna utilized a gauze wrap, manually impregnated with zinc paste, now referred to as the Unna Boot, in treating venous ulcers. Prepackaged zinc paste wraps are now available, some combined with calamine for patient comfort (Unna Pak, MedicoPaste). Burton has combined the use of a hydrocolloid gel placed directly on the wound with a secondary zinc paste gauze wrap and a tertiary compressive layer (Coban). This three-phase dressing has been called the Duke Boot. This combination adds increased pressure to the lower extremities while wicking away a good deal of exudate.

BIBLIOGRAPHY

Alper JC, Welch EA, Ginsberg MP, et al. Moist wound healing under a vapor permeable membrane. *J Am Acad Dermatol* 1983;8:347–353.

Alvarez OM, Mertz P, Eaglstein WH. Benzoyl peroxide and epidermal wound healing. *Arch Dermatol* 1983;119:222–225.

Barrandon Y, Green H. Three clonal types of keratinocytes with different capacities for multiplication. *Proc Natl Acad Sci USA* 1987;84:2303–2306.

Bennett RG. Dressings and miscellaneous surgical materials. In *Fundamentals of Cutaneous Surgery*. St. Louis, CV Mosby Co, Inc., 1988.

Bolton L, Oleniacz W, Constantine G, et al. Repair and antibacterial effects of topical antiseptics in vivo. In *Animal Models in Dermatopharmacology and Dermatotoxicology*. Lowe NJ, Maibach HI, eds. Basel, S. Karger AG, 1984,

Brown GL, Curtsinger LJ, White M, Mitchell TO, Pietsch J, Nordquist R, vonFraunhoffer A, Schultz GS. Acceleration of tensile strength of incisions treated with EGF and TGFβ. *Ann Surg* 1988;208:788–794.

Bucknall TE. The effect of local infection upon wound healing; An experimental study. *Br J Surg* 1990; 67:851–855.

Burton CS. Treatment of leg ulcers. In *Current Therapy*. BH Thiers, ed. Philadelphia, W.B Saunders Co., 1993, pp. 315–323.

Coffey RJ, Derynk R, Wilcos JN, et al. Production and autoinduction of transforming growth factor alpha in human keratinocytes. *Nature* 1987;328:817–820.

Coleman GJ, Roenigk HH. The healing of wounds in the skin treated with benzoyl peroxide. *J Dermatol Surg Oncol* 1978;4:705–707.

Compton CG, Gill JM, Bradford DA, et al. Skin regenerated from cultured epithelial autografts on acute burn wounds: A light, electron microscopic and immunohistochemical study. *Lab Invest* 1989; 60: 600–612.

Davis RS, Surgical dressings and postoperative care. In *Outpatient Surgery of the Skin*. Coleman WP, Colon GA, Davis RS, eds. New Hyde Park, NY, Medical Examination Publishing, Co, Inc., 1983, p. 232.

deHaan BB, Ellis H, Wilks M. The role of infection on wound healing. *Surg Gyn Ob* 1974;138:693–700.

Eaglstein W, Mertz P. Inert vehicles do affect wound healing. *J Invest Dermatol* 1980;74:90–91.

Falanga V. Occlusive wound dressings. *Arch Dermatol* 1988;124:872–877.

Geronemus R, Mertz P, Eaglstein W. Wound healing: The effects of topical antimicrobial agents. *Arch Dermatol* 1979;115:1311–1314.

Geronemus RG, Robins P. The effect of two new dressings on epidermal wound healing. *J Dermatol Surg Oncol* 1982;8:850–852.

Gielen V, Faure M, Mauduit G et al. Progressive replacement of human cultured epithelial allografts as evidenced by HLA class I antigen expression *Dermatologica* 1987;175:166–170.

Gilchrest BA, Karassik RL, Wilkins, et al. Autocrine and paracrine growth stimulation of cells derived from human skin. *J Cell Physiol* 1983;117:235–240.

Gold M. Topical silicone gel sheeting in the treatment of hypertrophic scars and keloids, a dermatologic experience. *J Dermatol Surg Oncol* 1993;19:912–916.

Goodman LS, Gilman A, eds. *The Pharmacologic Basis of Therapeutics*. New York, Macmillan Publishing Co., Inc., 1990.

Gruber R, Vistnes L, Pardoe R. The effect of commonly used antiseptics on wound healing. *Plast Reconstr Surg* 1975;55:472–476.

Harris DR, Youkey IR. Evaluating the effects of hemostatic agents on the healing of superficial wounds. In *Epidermal Wound Healing*. Rovee DT, Maibach HI, eds. Chicago, Year Book Medical Publishers Inc., 1972, pp. 343–355.

Harvey SC. Antiseptics and disinfectants, fungicides, ectoparasiticides. In *The Pharmacologic Basis of Therapeutics*. Gilman AG, Goodman LS, Gilman A, eds. New York, Macmillan Publishing Co., Inc., 1980, pp. 964–987.

Hillstrom I. Iodosorb compared to standard treatment in chronic venous leg ulcers—a multicenter study. *Acta Chir Scand Suppl* 1988;544:53–56.

Hinman CD, Maibach H. Effect of air exposure and occlusion on experimental human skin wounds. *Nature* 1963;200:377–378.

Jonker M, Hoogeboom J, vanLeeuwen, et al. The influence of matching for HLA–DR antigens on skin graft survival. *Transplantation* 1979;27:91–94

Jonkman MF, Hoeksma EA, Nieuwenhuis: Accelerated epithelization under a highly vapor permeable wound dressing is associated with increased precipitation of fibrinogen and fibronectin. *J Invest Dermatol* 1990; 94:477–484.

Kupper TS, Ballard DW, Chua AO, et al. Human keratinocytes contain mRNA indistinguishable from monocyte interleukin 1 alpha and beta mRNA: Keratinocyte epidermal cell-derived thymocyte-activating factor is identical to interleukin 1. *J Exp Med* 1986;164L:2095–2100.

Kuroyanagi Y, Kim E, Shioya N. Evaluation of a synthetic wound dressing capable of releasing silver sulfadiazine. *J Burn Care Rehabil* 1991;12:106–115.

Lebovits PE, Dzubow LM. A pressure dressing on the scalp by a modified Russian technique. *J Dermatol Surg Oncol* 1980;6:259–263.

Leigh IM, Purkis PE, Navsaria H, et al. Treatment of chronic venous stasis ulcers with sheets of cultured allogeneic keratinocytes. *Br J Dermatol* 1987;117:591–597.

Lesiewicz J, Goldsmith CA. Inhibition of rat skin ornithine decarboxylase by nitrofurazone. *Arch Dermatol* 1980;116:1225.

Lineaweaver W, Howard R, Soucy D, McMorris S, Freeman J, Crain C, Robertson J, Rumley T. Topical antimicrobial toxicity. *Arch Surg* 1985;120:267–270.

Lookingbill DP, Miller SH, Knowles RC. Bacteriology of chronic leg ulcers. *Arch Dermatol* 1978;114:1765.

Lorenzetti OJ, Wernet T, McDonald T. Some comparisons of benzoyl peroxide formulations. *J Soc Cosmet Chem* 1977;28:533–549.

Luger TA, Wirth U, Kock A. Epidermal cells synthesize a cytokine with interleukin 3 like properties. *J Immunol* 1985;134:915–919.

McGrath MH. How topical dressings salvage questionable flaps: Experimental study. *Plast Reconstr Surg* 1981;67:653.

Marshall DA, Mertz PM, Eaglstein WH. Occlusive dressings—Does dressing type influence the growth of common bacterial pathogens. *Arch Surg* 1990;125:1136–1139.

Melski JW, Arndt KA. Topical therapy for acne. *NEJM* 1980;302:503–506.

Mertz PM, Eaglstein WH. The effect of a semiocclusive dressing on the microbial population in superficial wounds. *Arch Surg* 1984;119:287–289.

Mertz PM, Marshall DA, Eaglstein WH. Occlusive wound dressings to prevent bacterial invasion and wound infection. *J Am Acad Dermatol* 1985;12:662–668.

Mustoe TA, Pierce GF, Thomason A, Gramates P, Sporn MB. Devel TF. Accelerated healing of incisional wounds in rats induced by transforming growth factor beta. *Science* 1987;237:1333–1335.

Nieder R, Schopf E. Inhibition of wound healing by antiseptics. *Br J Dermatol* 1986;115:41–44.

O'Connor NE, Gallico GG, Kehinde O, et al. Grafting of burns with cultured epithelium prepared from autologous epidermal cells: II. Intermediate term results on three pediatric patients. In *Soft and hard Tissue Repair. Biological and Clinical Aspects*. Vol. 2 Hunt TK, Hepenstall HBS, Pines E, et al, eds. New York, Praeger Publishers, 1984, pp. 283–292.

O'Connor NE, Milliken JB, Banks-Schlegel E, et al. Grafting of burns with cultured epithelium prepared from autologous epidermal cells. *Lancet* 1981;1:75–78.

Perkins K, Davey RB, Wallis KA. Silicone gel: A new treatment for hypertrophic scars. *Burns* 1982; 9: 406–410.

Phillips TJ, Gilchrest BA. Cultured epidermal grafts in the treatment of leg ulcers. In *Adv Derm* Chicago, Year Book Medical Publishers Inc., 1990, pp. 33–40.

Phillips T, Kehinde O, Green H, Gilchrest B. Treatment of skin ulcers with cultured epidermal allografts. *J Am Acad Dermatol Physicians Desk Reference*, 47th ed. Montvale, Medical Economics Co., 1978.

Reed BR, Clark RA. Cutaneous tissue repair practical implications of current knowledge. II. *J Am Acad Dermatol* 1985;13:919–941.

Robinson JR. An effective pressure dressing on the scalp that is easily made and is cosmetically acceptable. *J Dermatol Surg Oncol* 1981;7:607.

Rodeheaver G, Bellamy W, Kody M, et al. Bactericidal activity and toxicity of iodine containing solutions in wounds. *Arch Surg* 1982;117:181–185.

Sawada Y, Sone K. Hydration and occlusion treatment for hypertrophic scars and keloids. *Br J Plastic Surg* 1992;45:599–603.

Sawchuk WS, Friedman KJ, Mannin T Pinnell SR. Delayed healing in full thickness wounds treated with aluminum chloride solution. *J Am Acad Dermatol* 1986;15:982–989.

Silver I. Oxygen tension and epithelization. In *Epidermal Wound Healing*. H Maibach, D Rovee, eds. Chicago, Year Book Medical, 1972, pp. 291–305.

Tan ST, Roberts RH, Sinclair SW. A comparison of Zenoderm with DuoDerm E in the treatment of split skin graft donor sites. *Br J Plastic Surg* 1993;46:82–84.

Topical PEG in burn ointments. *FDA Drug Bull* 1982;12:25.

Weber W. Use caution with mesh dressing. *J Dermatol Surg Oncol* 1986;12:911.

Wickner Ne, Persichitte KA, Baskin JB, et al. Transforming growth factor beta stimulates the expression of fibronectin by human keratinocytes. *J Invest Dermatol* 1988;91:207–212.

Winter GD. formation of the scab and the rate of epithelization of superficial wounds in the skin of the young domestic pig. *Nature* 1962;193:293–294.

Winter GD, Scales JT. Effect of air drying and dressings on the surface of a wound. *Nature* 1963;197:91–92.

Winton GB, Salasche SJ. Wound dressings for dermatologic surgery. *J Am Acad Dermatol* 1985; 13: 1026–1044.

Xakellis C, Chrischilles EA. Hydrocolloid versus saline-gauze dressings in treating pressure ulcers: A cost-effectiveness analysis. *Arch Phys Med Rehabil* 1992;73:463–469.

11

Complications of Cutaneous Procedures

Thomas Stasko
Vanderbilt University Medical Center, Nashville, Tennessee

The word "complicate" comes from the Latin word *complicare*, meaning to fold up, and is defined as a verb meaning to make or become complex or intricate. In medicine a complication is a secondary disease or condition aggravating a previous one. In cutaneous surgery, complications are the result of a deviation from the original planned outcome. At times a simple step may lead directly to a single change in outcome. More often a series of small events interrelates until the final result is reached at the end of a series of twists and turns. As a consequence, complications in cutaneous surgical procedures are rarely single isolated events. Instead, a complication, as the surgeon finally sees it, is the end result of a cascade of multiple events. Each event is enabled by a previous event and provides the proper conditions for the development of the next step in the sequence.

Some complications are the unavoidable results of factors beyond the control of the surgeon or of the patient. In spite of optimal planning and care, the diversity of human response to injury and disease yields an outcome different from that intended and provides additional problems, which must be dealt with. However, it must be stated from the outset that the best approach to complications is prevention. By avoiding even one or two of the small events that contribute to an adverse result, the cascade towards a complication can be averted. Attention to each individual, routine detail is probably the best means of preventing complications. The surgeon must also remember that each deviation from one's usual standards and routines may set the stage for the initiation of such a cascade. "Bending the rules" to accommodate a particular patient's needs or desires or changing the routine to fit unusual circumstances is a particularly insidious manner in which complications start. The surgeon can be flexible but must be aware of the possible consequences of these alterations to the routine.

Ultimately, complications are events that threaten the patient's life, efficient wound healing, cosmesis or litigation. The most serious of all complications are those that are life threatening. Although emergencies in cutaneous surgery are fortunately extremely rare, the surgeon must be prepared to deal with acute cardiac problems, seizures, reactions to anesthesia, and the like. The details of developing a plan to prevent most such emergencies and deal with those that do arise are covered in Chapter 7. Also of serious concern is the possible development of bacterial endocarditis or infection of prosthetic joints as a result of bacteremia from skin surgery. The prophylactic use of antibiotics in such situations is discussed in Chapter 5.

COMPLICATIONS THAT THREATEN EFFICIENT WOUND HEALING

Wound-Healing Basics

Wounding of the skin initiates a remarkable series of events at a molecular and cellular level, which lead to repair of the injury. The inflammatory phase follows the clotting cascade, which occurs initially after wounding. This phase then leads to the formation of granulation tissue, reepithelization, neovascularization, and fibroplasia. Finally, the extracellular matrix is rebuilt and remodeled. Although the details of our understanding of wound healing are covered in Chapter 9, on a more macroscopic level, it is intuitive that events that disrupt this orderly progression will inhibit wound healing and lead to complications.

An interrelated set of complications that can lead to adverse outcomes in cutaneous surgical procedures has been referred to as the "terrible tetrad." Bleeding, infection, necrosis, and dehiscence can singly or in combination lead to a failure of optimal wound healing. This terrible tetrad can disrupt the process of wound healing in a cascading-type effect (Fig. 1.)

Mechanisms of Hemostasis

When a vessel is disrupted by surgery or trauma, blood escapes. A tightly interwoven sequence of events begins to halt the blood loss and begin repair of the wounded site.

The initial response to the transection of a vessel is vasoconstriction. This reduces the area of transected vessel that must be filled with aggregated platelets and reduces blood loss prior to formation of the platelet plug. This vasoconstriction also slows the blood flow and prolongs the exposure of the blood to the subendothelial collagen and coagulation factors, which results in enhanced platelet adherence to the injury site. Most local anesthetics, with the exception of cocaine, produce vasodilatation as a result of the relaxation of the smooth muscle of the vessel wall. It is essential for the surgeon to remember this action when using local anesthesia without epinephrine. Epinephrine is often added to local anesthetic solution to counteract this action and indeed provide additional vasoconstriction. The use of epinephrine in a concentration as low

POSTOPERATIVE COMPLICATIONS

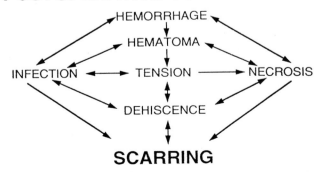

Figure 1 The tangled web of events that may interfere with wound healing.

as 1:500,000 can provide potent vasoconstriction and a much drier surgical field. The surgeon must be aware that this effect is very time-limited and fresh bleeding may occur when the vessel returns to its normal diameter as the effect of the epinephrine wears off. Such bleeding may occur during the final stages of a prolonged procedure or in the immediate postoperative period. Alcohol is also a potent vasodilator. The ingestion of alcohol during the postoperative period may result in fresh bleeding from dilated vessels. This effect plus the possible loss of protective inhibitions with alcohol consumption make it important to prohibit drinking during the postoperative period.

After vasoconstriction, primary hemostasis is obtained by the formation of a platelet plug. Platelets adhere to the subendothelial connective tissue collagen exposed by the injury. Von Willebrand's factor enhances this adherence by forming a cross-link between the exposed collagen and platelet receptor sites. The binding of collagen to the platelet receptor initiates the activation of platelet membrane lipases (phospholipase C and A$_2$) and begins the cascade. The ultimate result is platelet aggregation. The exposed endothelial collagen also initiates the intrinsic and extrinsic coagulation pathways. These pathways provide the fibrin to cross-link with the platelet plug to form the hemostatic plug or clot (Fig. 2).

Several common drugs interfere with hemostatic functions. The list of drugs that impair platelet function is lengthy, but only a limited number of commonly used drugs are usually of concern:

Aspirin.   The most common drug with significant inhibition of platelet function is aspirin. Aspirin irreversibly acetylates platelet cyclooxygenase. This action impairs platelet aggregation.

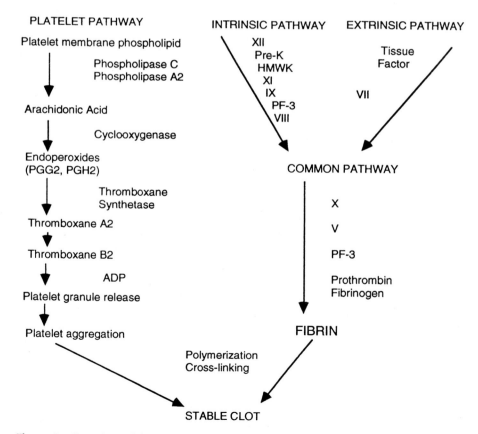

Figure 2   Overview of the clotting mechanism.

As the platelet cannot replace the defective enzyme, the effect persists as long as the platelet survives. A single dose of aspirin will impair platelet function for the entire 9.5-day platelet lifespan. The increased bleeding from aspirin can be difficult to control in the form of diffuse oozing at the time of surgery and can lead to postoperative bleeding and more extensive ecchymoses than are usual. Elective use of aspirin as an analgesic or antiinflammatory agent should be discontinued 2 weeks prior to surgery. Aspirin is now "prescribed" in many patients for its action in possibly preventing clot formation and the prophylaxis of myocardial infarction and stroke. Discontinuation of aspirin in such cases should be made in consultation with the prescribing physician. If the ingestion of aspirin cannot be discontinued, surgery can be performed, but consideration should be given to limiting the extent of the procedure and deferring elective cosmetic procedures. Aspirin ingestion postoperatively will not effect a well-established solid fibrin-platelet clot.

Nonsteroidal Antiinflammatory Drugs.   Most nonsteroidal antiinflammatory drugs act on platelets in a manner similar to that of aspirin. Their effect is usually much less severe and is reversible. The duration of the effect is related to the half-life of the drug and only continues if adequate blood levels are maintained.

Dipyridamole.   Dipyridamole interferes with ADP-induced platelet aggregation. Dipyridamole usually does not alter platelet function to such an extent that the effect is noticeable at the time of surgery, but may lead to postoperative bleeding.

Antibiotics.   Many antibiotics can interfere with platelet aggregation and platelet granule release. Any resulting dysfunction is usually minor. However, at therapeutic dosages, carbenicillin and other beta-lactam antibiotics may have sufficient effect to prolong bleeding times and produce an increased risk of bleeding.

Ethanol.   Ethanol also inhibits ADP-induced platelet aggregation and platelet granule release. By itself, this effect is minor, but ethanol does appear to accentuate the increase in bleeding time caused by aspirin.

Omega-3 Fatty Acids.   Ingestion of large amounts of certain fish oils may increase bleeding time by an interference with platelet function. This effect may also be additive with aspirin.

Drugs may also cause anticoagulation by interfering with the intrinsic and extrinsic pathways of coagulation.

Coumadin.   Coumadin is a structural analog of vitamin K, and its ingestion inhibits the functional forms of factors VII, IX, X and prothrombin. Anticoagulation with Coumadin can lead to significant intraoperative and postoperative bleeding. Although simple biopsies and excisions may be performed on such patients if care is taken to obtain good hemostasis during the procedure and the patient is closely observed during the postoperative period, more extensive procedures can be difficult and subject to considerable complications. Discontinuing Coumadin should be done only in coordination with the physician maintaining the patient's anticoagulation. Many patients can go without anticoagulation for short periods. In these cases the drug may be discontinued for 2 days prior to the procedure and the prothrombin time checked immediately prior to the procedure. If there is good intraoperative and postoperative hemostasis, the Coumadin may be restarted the evening or morning after surgery. If discontinuation of anticoagulation is not possible and another procedure cannot be substituted, consideration should be given to hospitalization for substitution of heparin for the Coumadin.

Heparin.   Heparin must be given parenterally. Heparin acts primarily as an antithrombin factor. The operative and postoperative bleeding problems caused by heparin can be significant. Fortunately, heparin has a short half-life (1 hr) and may be rapidly reversed by protamine sulfate. Heparin can be utilized for patients who require a procedure but can go without anticoagulation for very limited periods of time. The patient can be hospitalized and heparin substituted for Coumadin. The heparin may then be discontinued just hours before surgery (or reversed with protamine sulfate) and the procedure performed. The heparin can then be immediately restarted in the controlled, closely observed hospital setting.

The evaluation of a patient prior to surgery with regard to the risk for excessive bleeding should begin with a brief but thorough history. The use of prescription drugs is usually easy to elicit, but covering all of the over-the-counter medications that contain aspirin can take some time and patience. A large number of inherited and acquired medical problems may also result in coagulation defects. Obviously the patient should be asked whether he or she has any known defect of coagulation. The patient should also be questioned about previous surgical procedures, trauma, and the like. Was there excessive bleeding at the time of surgery or in the postoperative period? Has the patient had extensive bleeding with tooth extractions or other dental work? Does the patient have prolonged bleeding with minor cuts and scratches? Finally, does the patient develop large ecchymoses (greater than the size of a half-dollar) without known trauma? If the patient answers no to all of these questions and has had a history of sufficient hemostatic challenge, then no further preoperative workup is required. If the patient has a known defect of coagulation abilities, consultation with the patient's appropriate specialist is in order. If the history reveals only a general sense of "easy bleeding" without a contributing drug or medical history, some preoperative evaluation may be warranted. Screening the patient with a complete blood count including a platelet count can exclude chronic blood loss sufficient to cause anemia and provide a quantitative evaluation of platelets. A bleeding time can give an estimation of platelet function. Finally, a prothrombin time (PT) and partial thromboplastin time (PTT) can give an evaluation of the intrinsic, extrinsic, and common pathways of coagulation. If these screening tests are normal, the procedure can be undertaken with relative surety of the patient's ability to coagulate.

RESULTS OF EXCESSIVE BLEEDING

Exsanguination

Although it is possible for bleeding from cutaneous surgery to reach levels at which it presents with hemodynamic significance, this situation is extremely rare. The unusual cases in which such a situation might occur include Mohs procedures in which tumors might be traced to depths at which large major vessels could be encountered (e.g., the carotid artery, femoral artery, etc.) scalp procedures without suturing (e.g., hair transplants), and surgery in which bleeding into a large dead space is possible. This situation can always be aggravated by preexisting hematologic abnormalities and drug-induced coagulopathies.

Intraoperative Bleeding

Intraoperative bleeding can distress the surgeon and the patient. Even for experienced surgeons, bleeding raises the general anxiety level in the operating room, and flowing blood can be very distressing to the patient. Blood obscuring the operative site can interfere with the careful dissection desirable. By minimizing the potential causes of increased bleeding and using epinephrine, the surgeon can decrease the effects of this blood loss. The use of suction can help maintain good visualization in a bloody field. Immediate drying of the surgical field can sometimes be obtained by applying pressure to the periphery of the operative site. An assistant can provide traction across the wound surface with gloved hands or a ringed instrument, such as a scissors handle (Fig. 3). This can allow the completion of the immediate portion of the procedure. Intraoperative bleeding can then be controlled as soon as practical. Individual small vessels should be isolated and cauterized with electrocautery or hot-tipped cautery. Various types of instruments are available for this purpose, each with advantages and disadvantages (see Chap. 15). Such

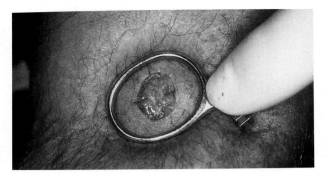

Figure 3   The use of ringed scissor handles to help dry the operative field.

cautery should be precise as possible to avoid excessive tissue destruction and leaving excessive char in the operative site as a cause of increased inflammation and a nidus for infection. Slightly larger vessels should be grasped with an appropriately sized hemostat and then cauterized (Fig. 4). This action tends to limit the extent of the destruction. Larger, muscular vessels should be ligated with ties of absorbable sutures. Cautery of such vessels may provide immediate hemostasis but may lead to delayed bleeding if the clot retracts into the large vessel lumen. The surgical field should be as dry as possible prior to closure. Particular attention should be paid to the apices of ellipses and flaps. In addition, cut muscle may have several small bleeding points.

   If bleeding has been particularly difficult to control during the initial portion of a procedure, the surgeon may wish to consider modifying the extent of the operation. Limiting undermining or choosing a linear closure rather than a flap or graft will limit the potential "dead space" in which blood may accumulate postoperatively. In addition, tightly suturing small wounds may tamponade small vessels to provide hemostasis. If bleeding has been difficult to control during the performance of a flap or a large multilayered closure, the placement of a drain may prevent hematoma formation. A simple drain may be created from a sterilized rubber band, a fenestrated penrose drain may be placed (Fig. 5.), or a more elaborate drain such a Jackson-Pratt drain may

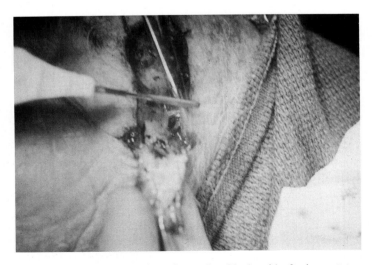

Figure 4   Electrocoagulation of vessels with the aid of a hemostat.

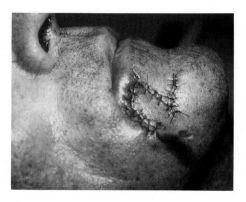

Figure 5 A Penrose drain placed.

be utilized. Such a drain can usually be removed 24–48 hr after the procedure when any bleeding has become minimal. Although placement of a drain may cause a small delay in healing and slightly increase the risk of infection, some surgeons choose to place drains after any extensive procedure to allow for small amounts of postoperative bleeding.

A layered pressure dressing can aid in hemostasis. This firmly applied series of bandages can also wick away small amounts of bleeding from the wound site. However, if the dressing becomes saturated with blood, it rapidly loses any compressive qualities and will not impede bleeding.

Dressings and/or splints may also be utilized to decrease wound site motion after a procedure. Movement of the site may dislodge clots or electrocoagulation char and precipitate new bleeding. The proper application of a dressing can protect the wound site from external trauma with its resulting risk of bleeding. The patient should be given strict, explicit instructions regarding activity after each procedure. These instructions may range from essentially only restrictions on wetting the area for simple shave procedures to modified bedrest for large, extensive flaps. The patient must be instructed in such circumstances to avoid putting the wound in dependent positions. The patient must be told in straightforward terms which activities are allowed and which are prohibited. Perioral wounds may require a soft diet and restrictions on talking; lower extremity wounds may require limitations on standing and walking. The patient needs to be told when and at what level normal activities can be resumed. Especially now that regular exercise is an important part of many patients' routines, a simple "take it easy" may be insufficient in many circumstances.

Postoperative Bleeding

In spite of careful preoperative evaluation and intraoperative hemostasis and careful limitation of patient activities, postoperative bleeding will occur in a small number of cases. The bleeding may be a continuation of a slow ooze that was present at the end of the procedure, or it may have begun fresh. The first few hours after the surgery present the greatest risk. As the patient returns home after surgery, the clots are still fragile and bleeding may be precipitated by sudden movements or changes in blood pressure. In addition, the loss of the epinephrine effect may yield small vessel bleeding. The patient should be instructed that a small amount of blood on the wound dressing is normal. If the bloodied area is increasing or blood is dripping from the dressing, the patient should be instructed to apply firm pressure directly to the wound site for 20 min. The patient must be instructed not to remove pressure to look at the site during this period. The time will always be underestimated if it is not measured by the clock. If the dressing was saturated with blood, the dressing should be removed prior to applying pressure and replaced with sterile dry dressing material. If the pressure is successful in stopping the bleeding, this dressing or the original one can be reinforced with additional gauze and tape.

If the bleeding persists, the surgeon should see the patient. A trial of direct pressure can again be initiated. If this fails, the wound must be opened and explored for the source of the bleeding. The infiltration of local anesthesia is usually necessary prior to such exploration. The use of epinephrine in the anesthesia mix will provide a drier field but may obscure the bleeding sites. Rarely, the bleeding may be from a single large vessel. In this event, the vessel should be isolated and cauterized or ligated as appropriate. The wound can then be resutured. In most cases, however, the bleeding is from multiple small vessels. These bleeding points should be isolated and cauterized. If a *very* dry surgical field is not obtainable, consideration should be given to the placement of a surgical drain.

Hematoma

Bleeding through a sutured wound is troublesome; however, blood collecting as a large clot in the dead space of a wound can cause even greater problems. The development of a hematoma may be accompanied by external bleeding, but most often it is not. The most frequent symptom of a large, expanding hematoma is the onset of a new, often throbbing, pain. If the hematoma is smaller, only pressure may be experienced. Removal of the dressing will reveal an ecchymotic, firm, yet fluctuant mass under all or part of the wound (Fig. 6). Early hematomas should be evacuated. The blood clot of the hematoma provides an excellent medium for the growth of bacteria. The presence of the hematoma prevents wound healing and can lead to dehiscence. Finally, the hematoma may cause increased tension on the wound edge or the flap pedicle and lead to necrosis. Pressure to the wound may express small amounts of blood, but the hematoma itself cannot usually be evacuated in that manner. The early hematoma consists of gelatinlike clots of blood. By removing several sutures and opening a tract to the dead space of the wound with scissors or a hemostat, large portions of the hematoma may be evacuated (Fig. 7). The hematoma, however, is often fragmented into numerous smaller clots, and the wound may need to be widely opened to remove the entire contents. The site should then be irrigated and inspected for bleeding sites. Local anesthesia is required. The surgeon should be aware that the walls of the dead space that abutted the hematoma will now appear dusky and ecchymotic, rather than exhibiting the pink, fresh appearance that was present at the initial surgery. Again, a single bleeding ves-

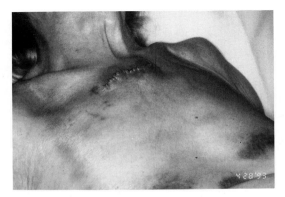

Figure 6 Hematoma under the suture line with marked ecchymosis remotely distal to the surgical site in dependent areas.

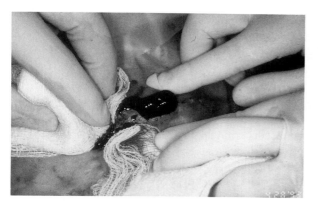

Figure 7 Gelatinlike clots of a hematoma being expressed.

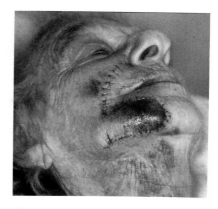

Figure 8 Organized hematoma at one week postoperative.

sel may be found, but most often there are multiple small bleeding points, which should be isolated and cauterized. The wound may then be reclosed. Strict attention should be paid to closing any dead space. If there is any difficulty obtaining a dry field, a drain should be placed. Because of the increased risk of wound infection, the empirical use of antibiotics is advocated by many surgeons.

If the hematoma is not recognized or treated early, within several days the clot becomes organized. It develops a thick fibrous texture and adheres to the surrounding tissue. Large or expanding hematomas are probably best still evacuated at this stage to decrease the risk of infection and limit the necrosis from increased wound tension. After the infiltration of local anesthesia, the area over the hematoma is opened and as much of the organized clot is removed as is possible. The original bleeding has most often stopped, but fresh bleeding may be caused by the removal of the adherent material. Most often the wound is not resutured but is allowed to heal by second intention. Because a dead space is created by the evacuation of the hematoma, such a wound often requires packing with daily changes of the packing material.

A small, stable hematoma may be observed, rather than evacuated. This hematoma will be quite firm with an ecchymotic appearance (Fig. 8). Gentle heat applied for 30- to 60-min intervals several times each day may speed the resolution of the hematoma.

With time the hematoma is liquefied by the action of the fibrinolytic system. With small hematomas, this liquefied material is reabsorbed by the body and no further action is necessary. Larger hematomas may develop a fluctuant mass that needs aspiration. This usually occurs between 1 and 2 weeks postoperatively. Aspiration can usually be accomplished with a large-bore needle (16–18 gauge) and may have to be repeated over several days.

Ecchymosis

Ecchymosis or bruising is caused by the leakage of small amounts of blood into the interstitial space. Ecchymoses often develop after surgical procedures, especially if there is loose, distensible tissues such as in the periorbital region or on the chest or forearms in elderly individuals. The trauma of skin surgery, beginning with the distention of the tissue with the injection of local anesthesia, can lead to ecchymoses in the surgical area. The area of bruising initially is black and blue from the reduced hemoglobin in the extravasated blood. As the hemoglobin is degraded to bilirubin, the colors change to green and yellow and finally resolve. Ecchymoses can extend widely from the surgical site, usually migrating to dependent areas under the influence of gravity (Fig. 6). In the periorbital area a unilateral black eye may result or bilateral "raccoon's eyes" may appear, even with relatively minor procedures (Fig. 9). Ecchymoses may be alarming to the patient but will resolve with time, usually with no sequelae.

Infection

The risk of infection in cutaneous surgery is generally very low. However, when it develops, infection can lead to severe problems in wound healing. As with most complications, the best treatment is prevention. Most extensive studies concerning wound infection have been done on populations of general surgery patients and head and neck surgery patients, and extrapolation to skin surgery is somewhat speculative. The risk of infection is directly proportional to the level of wound contamination and inversely proportional to the body's level of tissue defense. Few studies are available in the dermatologic surgical literature to help accurately predict infection rates, but those available and communications from individual dermatologic surgeons would indicate the rate of significant infections to be less than 5% and often 1–2%. These perceived rates often do not distinguish between patients who receive prophylactic antibiotics and those who do not. This low apparent rate of infection makes studies of the effectiveness of prophylactic antibiotics and other preventive measures difficult. It also brings into question the dermatologic surgeon's sense of having prevented infections by prescribing antibiotics.

It is generally accepted that systemic factors can lower the individual's resistance to the development of infection. Abnormalities that alter the immune system by the reduction in number or effectiveness of granulocytes or lymphocytes may lead to infection with common and unusual pathogens in both the surgical and nonsurgical setting. Patients with AIDS certainly have an increased risk of many infections; however, the risk of developing infections after cutaneous procedures has not been quantitated. Processes that alter the body's ability to produce effective immunoglobulins may also predispose the individual to infection. The presence of uncontrolled diabetes mellitus, liver failure, renal failure, or malnutrition may each contribute to an increased risk of infection. Immune defenses may also be compromised by systemic medications. Corticosteroids, immunosuppressants, and cytotoxic agents may also increase the risk of infection. Significant numbers of patients are now receiving long-term immunosuppression for organ transplantation, oncologic, rheumatologic, and dermatologic conditions.

A careful history must be taken to elucidate systemic factors that might predispose the patient to infection. As a significant number of patients will have one or more such factors, the der-

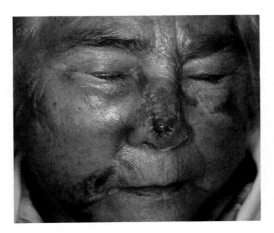

Figure 9 Extensive periorbital and facial ecchymoses after a procedure on the nose.

matologic surgeon must develop a rationale for approaching these situations. Patients with severe immunodeficiencies should be treated in consultation with the appropriate specialists to determine the proper antibiotic coverage to forestall infections. Patients with relative immunosuppression have a much smaller risk, and the dangers of adverse reactions to antibiotics must be weighed against this risk. If the patient is anticipated to have additional nonsystemic risk factors discussed below, prophylaxis should be considered. If no other risk factors are anticipated, such action is probably not warranted.

Local wound factors can also inhibit defenses against infection. As discussed above, hematoma can provide an area not well penetrated by the body's immune response and a good media for bacterial growth. Excessive wound tension from closure or an expanding hematoma may decrease the blood supply to a wound, providing devitalized tissue as a nidus for infection. Foreign bodies such as suture and char from electrocautery may incite an inflammatory response and also serve as a focus for infection.

Existing bacterial infection at the operative site such as an infected epidermoid cyst or a necrotic tumor or even an infection at another remote site can greatly increase the risk of wound infection. If possible, such infections should be completely treated prior to elective procedures. Consideration should be given to delaying closure in procedures classified as "dirty and infected." Procedures in certain anatomic sites such as the groin, mouth, and axilla may also carry an increased risk of wound infection.

The most critical time with regard to contamination of the surgical wound is the immediate preoperative period until the closure is complete. Techniques for preparation for surgery and maintenance of a clean operative field are discussed in Chapter 1 and should be adhered to. In the general surgical literature, wounds are classified according to Table 1. Most skin surgery wounds fall into Class I—Clean—or Class 2—Clean-Contaminated. Significant breaks in sterile technique resulting in gross contamination should be corrected and the institution of antibiotics considered. Prolonged procedures have a higher infection rate. In general surgery patients it has been established that infection rates are higher in procedures that extend beyond 3 hr. Many Mohs micrographic surgery procedures would have such a prolonged operating time. Shaving of the surgical site prior to surgery also increases the risk of wound infection. Hair should only be removed if it will grossly interfere with the surgical procedure. If possible, it should then be clipped with scissors or hair clippers or a depilatory employed just prior to the procedure.

Prophylactic antibiotics are most effective if administered just prior to the surgical wounding. The reduction in infection rates may be diminished if antibiotics are given earlier. Parenteral antibiotics are given within 30 min of the start of a procedure. By extrapolation, oral antibiotics should be administered approximately 1 hr before wounding. The duration of prophylactic antibiotic administration is less well documented but should probably be much shorter than is generally employed in current dermatologic practice. Some studies have suggested that the single preoperative dose is optimal, while other reports suggest that a second dose is helpful in prolonged procedures. There is no evidence to suggest that the extension of prophylactic antibiotic coverage beyond 24 hr is required. While it has long been recognized that having antibiotics in the surgical site prior to wounding is optimal, postoperative administration of prophylactic antibiotics, common in dermatologic surgery, may not provide the maximum reduction in wound infection but may still be able to reduce wound infection in a significant manner.

The choice of antibiotic for wound infection prophylaxis should be made on the basis of the most likely causal organism. This decision should be based on the organism most often found in wound infections in the anatomic site rather than the resident flora. At least in head and neck cancer surgery, most wound infections are polymicrobial and involve both aerobic and anaerobic organisms. The flora of the wound infection cannot be predicted on the basis of the preoperative flora. Attention should also be paid to less likely infectious organisms, which could

Table 1 Operative Wound Classification

Classification	Characteristics	Risk of infection (%)
Clean	No break in technique	1–4 %
	No inflammation	
	Respiratory, GI, GU tracts not entered	
Clean-contaminated	Minor break in technique	5–15
	Noninfected respiratory, GI, or GU tract entered without gross spillage	
Contaminated	Major break in technique	6–25
	Gross spillage from respiratory, GI, or GU tract	
Dirty and infected	Surgical wound includes acute bacterial infection with or without pus	>25 (?100)

lead to more significant consequences. Because the organisms likely to be encountered in wound infections are somewhat limited, a first-generation cephalosporin is often the drug of choice. These agents have broad-spectrum activity against the most common pathogenic gram-positive cocci (*S. aureus* and *Streptococcus viridans*) as well activity against *Escherichia coli, Klebsiella,* and *Proteus mirabilis*. A usual dosage would be Cephalexin 1 g p.o. 1 hr prior to the procedure followed by 500 mg 6 hr later. The use of a sterile cephalosporin powder sprinkled into the wound may also decrease the incidence of wound infection. In the hospital setting if methicillin-resistant *S. aureus* is a concern or if enterococcus is a concern with GI/GU procedures, vancomycin may be required, which must be administered IV. The usual dosage is 500 mg IV 30 min prior to the procedure followed by 250 mg IV 6 hr later if felt necessary. Vancomycin may also be utilized for cephalosporin-sensitive patients. If coverage for *P. aeruginosa* is desired, ciprofloxacin 500 mg 1 hr prior followed by 500 mg 12 hr later may be considered.

In deciding on the use of prophylactic antibiotics, the risk of infection and the consequence of such an infection must be weighed against the risk of the administration of the antibiotic and the cost of the administration. Fortunately, the medical risk of the administration of such antibiotics for short periods of time is quite low.

Topical antibiotic ointments and creams have been commonly utilized to prevent wound infection and promote wound healing. There is evidence that topical antibiotics can reduce bacterial counts in open wounds and around catheter sites, but there is no substantial evidence that wound infections are prevented. The increased efficacy of the administration of systemic antibiotics prior to wounding has been well established. Topical application of benzoyl peroxide for 7 days prior to surgery has been shown to reduce the rate of wound infection in surgical procedures to the centrofacial area.

The postoperative period is not commonly a time when wound infections develop. However, early contamination of wounds is possible if poor wound care practices are followed. The failure to remove blood-soaked dressing increases bacterial contamination. The site may also be contaminated by poor hand washing and dressing changes and excessive manipulation or exposure during the first 24–48 hr. After this time the wound is more resistant to contamination.

Although, in most cases, the infection truly begins at the time of surgery, most wound infections becomes evident 4–8 days postoperatively. The onset is usually an exaggeration of the inflammation that accompanies normal healing. There is an increase of erythema and edema, with the wound often becoming warm (Fig. 10). In most cases, pain and tenderness increase, reversing the normal postoperative course. The erythema may extend rapidly, with the red streaks of lymphangitis becoming evident and lymphadenopathy becoming present. The swelling at the

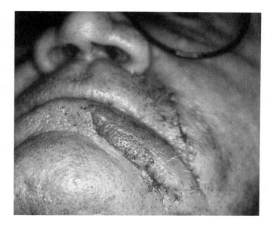

Figure 10   Wound infection one week post-op. The area is red, warm, and tender. Exudate can be expressed.

wound site may give way to a fluctuance, and purulent material may be discharged or expressed from the wound margins. Systemic symptoms including fever and chills may be symptoms of spreading infection.

The treatment of an established wound infection should follow the principles established in general surgery—drainage, heat, elevation, and rest. In a wound that is red, warm, and has prulent drainage, the precept of draining the infection should be followed. Any remaining sutures should be removed, and if an abscess is present, it should be opened and drained. In this situation deep absorbable sutures may also have to be removed as they too compromise the body's defenses. The wound should be left open to allow additional drainage, and if deep cavities are present the wound should be packed lightly with iodoform gauze to maintain drainage. Packing should be changed daily and the wound cleaned until the discharge ceases. Gentle heat to the area may aid in the resolution of the infection by increasing local blood flow. In addition, appropriate antibiotic measures should be initiated. If a discharge or other exudative material is present, a specimen for culture and sensitivity should be collected. The specimen should be Gram stained to aid with early therapy. Initial antibiotic therapy should be guided by the Gram stain as well as the likely organism based on the anatomic site, the patient's overall medical condition, and the surgeon's most recent experiences with wound infection. Although many wound infections are the result of the growth of multiple organisms, *S. aureus* is the most frequently cultured organism. If *S. aureus* is suspected, a penicillinase-resistant penicillin or a first-generation cephalosporin should be initiated. If gram-negative organisms are likely, a cephalosporin would be the initial choice. If *Pseudomonas* is suspected, an agent with action toward the organism such as ciprofloxacin would be required. Further antimicrobial therapy should be guided by the culture and sensitivity and the clinical response.

In a patient with a rapidly spreading infection, extensive lymphangitis, or systemic symptoms, hospital admission for parenteral antibiotics and aggressive wound care should be considered. Immunosuppression and poor general health should also be considered as factors that may predispose a patient to a severe infection and possible inadequate response to oral antibiotic therapy.

Early or mild infection should be treated aggressively. If the patient reports the onset of increased erythema, pain or discharge, the wound should be examined by the surgeon. In the face of spreading erythema, exudate, or induration, any remaining sutures should be removed, and if the wound opens it should be treated as above. If only mild erythema is present, sutures that can safely be removed should be. Antibiotic treatment should be initiated and the wound closely observed. If the infection is controlled by such measures, the remaining sutures can be removed at the usual time.

It is important to consider that conditions other than bacterial infections may also present with similar symptoms. If the skin surrounding the wound has vesicles, pustules, or scale in addition to the erythema, one must consider an infection with dermatophytes or *Candida*. A KOH examination and culture will aid in the evaluation in such circumstances. The occlusive dressings often used after surgery may provide the proper conditions for the growth of these organisms.

If the erythema closely follows only the area to which the antibiotic cream or ointment has been applied, contact dermatitis must be considered (Fig. 11). Again, the occluded environment provides an almost "patch test" situation. In a similar manner, if the erythema follows the contact areas of the tape of the dressing, a contact sensitivity or irritant reaction is likely. Scale and vesiculation may also be present if the reaction is vigorous. Pruritus often accompanies irritant and allergic reactions rather than increased pain. Contact and irritant reactions can be minimized by avoiding, when possible, commonly sensitizing agents. Neomycin, present in Neosporin and other triple antibiotic ointments, is probably the most common sensitizer, with up to 6–8% of patients reacting to it. Although bacitracin alone does not appear to be a potent sensitizer, many patients sensitive to neomycin are also sensitive to bacitracin. If contact sensitivity is suspected, the antibiotic ointment should be discontinued. If possible the wound should be left open and a mild- to medium-potency topical steroid may be applied to the area *surrounding* the wound.

An inflammatory reaction to suture material may also be mistaken for a wound infection. Erythema or an erythematous papule may develop at each suture site. At its extreme, small pustules may be observed. Such a reaction may be recognized by its localization to the site of the individual sutures (Fig. 12). The reaction is aborted by the removal of the sutures.

Necrosis

Necrosis is the death of previously viable tissue. Necrosis results from a loss of blood supply to the involved tissue. Any event that compromises blood flow can lead to necrosis. Necrosis may result directly from events initiated at the time of surgery, or it may arise as a consequence of other complications. The best treatment is prevention and many potential problems can be averted with good surgical planning.

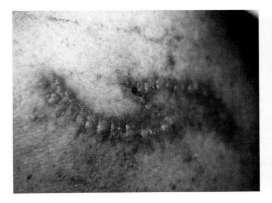

Figure 11 Contact dermatitis from the application of topical antibiotic. The redness is confined to the area of application.

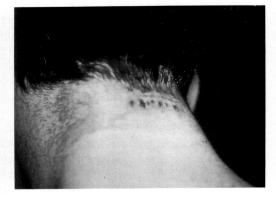

Figure 12 Brightly erythematous suture reaction.

It must be remembered that the blood supply to skin comes primarily from a subdermal arterial plexus, which in turn is supplied by small segmental arteries. These arteries may be musculocutaneous, supplying both skin and muscle or perforating vessels that directly supply the skin. The hair follicles and eccrine glands are supplied from the subdermal plexus, a horizontal dermal plexus, and plexuses in the area. Interruption of the segmental arteries may lead to areas of necrosis of several centimeters. However, the blood supply to most skin areas in the absence of other disease processes is quite rich with multiple anastamoses. As a result, the subdermal plexus continues to be supplied, albeit from a distance. A number of factors may decrease blood supply to the skin, thereby increasing the risk of necrosis (Table 2). The most controllable of these factors is cigarette smoking. Patients should be advised to quit smoking completely several days prior to surgery and extending through the postoperative period. If the patient is unable to do so, decreasing smoking to less than one pack of cigarettes a day may be helpful in decreasing the risk of necrosis.

Extensive undermining of wounds decreases the circulation to the distal wound margins. Superficial undermining may damage the subdermal plexus as well as the segmented arteries. Any situation that will further decrease blood flow may cause a sufficient loss of perfusion, resulting in necrosis. Wound swelling from edema or venous congestion may place external pressure on the arterioles and capillaries and diminish the blood flow. A hematoma may take this external pressure to the extreme. Even the tension on the wound edge created as the wound is pulled to closure will stretch the vessels and decrease flow. Small areas of blood flow may be completely obstructed by tight or improperly placed sutures. Orientation of the blood vessels in the dermis and the subdermis should be kept in mind as looping horizontally oriented sutures that have the potential to occlude portions of the plexuses should be avoided. As much tension as possible should be relieved from the skin edges by the placement of subcutaneous and deep dermal sutures. In addition, increased suture tension results from postoperative wound edema. The use of suture material that stretches slightly, such as monofilament polypropylene or nylon,

Table 2 Factors That Increase Risk of Necrosis

Systemic Factors
    Arteriosclerotic vascular disease
    Diabetes
    Collagen-vascular disease
    Systemic vasculitis
    Smoking
Local Factors
    Location: lower extremities, acral locations (fingers, toes, ears)
    Radiation dermatitis
    Lymphedema
    Stasis dermatitis
Wound Complications
    Hematoma
    Infection
    Edema
    Venous congestion
    Excessive wound tension
    Tight sutures
    Excessive undermining
    Inadequate random flap pedicle width
    Compromise of blood flow in arterial-based flap

can relieve some of this tension. Tension from postoperative edema can also be compensated for by employing the "loop stitch." A small 1- to 20-mm "loop" between the first and second throws of the knot allows room for expansion.

Flaps may also suffer from inadequate blood supply. Many flaps in dermatologic surgery are not based on a recognized blood vessel, but on a random blood supply to the subdermal plexus. In general, the width of the base of a flap should be at least one-third the length of the flap. If the width is not sufficient, distal necrosis may result (Fig. 13). In addition, rotation and transposition flap movement may create a standing cutaneous cone (dog-ear) at the base of the flap. Removal of this excess tissue must be taken in a manner such that the base is not decreased in width or the flap elongated to the point that the 1:3 ratio is exceeded. In many cases removal of this redundancy could be delayed until the distal flap has developed new collateral circulation. When flaps are based on an isolated blood vessel, extreme care must be exercised when handling the base that contains the vessel. Stretching or twisting the flap may compromise blood flow.

A full-thickness or split-thickness graft will necrose if it fails to establish a blood supply from the underlying wound bed. If a properly harvested and prepared graft fails, one or two events may have occurred. First, the underlying bed may have insufficient vasculature to support the graft. Grafts placed over areas with more than 1 cm^2 of exposed cartilage or bone will often partially necrose (Fig. 14). Full-thickness grafts placed on sites that have previously been exposed to therapeutic radiation also frequently fail. Second, blood or serous fluid may have prevented the graft from adhering to the bed and establishing a blood supply. Assuring a dry operative field prior to placement of the graft and use of basting sutures and tie-down bolsters can decrease the risk of necrosis due to this cause. Excessive physical activity by the patient can also interfere with adherence of the graft to the bed.

The earliest sign of vascular insufficiency may be pallor that fails to resolve after the epinephrine effect of the local anesthesia has worn off. More commonly, there is also venous insufficiency, which presents as cyanotic swelling of the wound edge or flap. At this early stage, intervention may aid in aborting necrosis. A hematoma, if present, should be evacuated. If wound tension or pressure can be relieved by judicious suture removal or replacement, it should be done. Gentle heat to the area may increase blood flow. Hyperbaric oxygen, if available, may also increase tissue survival.

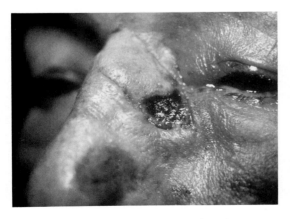

Figure 13 Necrosis of the distal portion of a transposition flap. Note also the hyperpigmentation from a full-thickness skin graft on the distal nose.

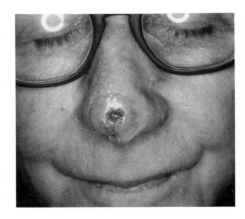

Figure 14 Necrosis of a full-thickness skin graft in an area placed over exposed cartilage.

After necrosis has begun, observation is usually the best course of action. The tissue loss may vary in depth from only slough of the epidermis to full-thickness loss of the skin and subcutaneous tissue. If infection does not intervene, an eschar will form. The area of necrosis should be cared for with only minimal cleaning and debridement. The extent of necrosis may be less than initially predicted, and vigorous debridement may extend the process. The eschar will ultimately separate from the wound bed as the base heals by second intention. Any infection present should be treated in the usual manner.

Dehiscence

Dehiscence is the separation of the surgical wound. When necrosis is present, the patient will often present with gapping of the surgical wound at the area of necrosis (Fig. 15). Likewise, when infection or hematoma are present, removal of the sutures to treat the underlying problem will often result in a separated surgical wound. In these circumstances, the problem has been caused by another complication and prevention of that complication might have prevented the dehiscence.

At other times, a wound may dehisce when the sutures are removed or shortly after suture removal. The most common cause of wound dehiscence is excessive wound tension. Unlike many other types of surgery, which result in a skin wound but no significant loss of cutaneous tissue, cutaneous surgery almost always involves the removal of a significant amount of skin tissue. Replacement of that tissue is most frequently accomplished by utilizing the "stretch" of surrounding tissue in the form of a primary closure or a local flap. This type of repair places tension on the skin edge. If the tension is significant, the wound may not be sufficiently healed at the time of suture removal to keep the wound edges apposed. There is a lag between wounding and the development of wound tensile strength (Table 3). As most skin sutures are removed between 5 and 14 days, it is not surprising that some wounds reopen. At this point, little fibroplasia has occurred and the wound surface is held only by the newly bridged epithelium, wound coagulum, and early neovascularization. Trauma or excessive wound movement may cause dehiscence. Excessive use of electrocoagulation or use of the CO_2 laser may also delay the development of tensile strength. Prolonged suture placement may decrease the risk of dehiscence but may also result in the formation of suture tracts. The practice of removing sutures in stages at intervals of several days can help minimize this problem while providing more prolonged support. Adhesive strips can provide some support after suture removal, but they will not provide prolonged protection in the face of significant wound tension. If there is wound tension, the proper place-

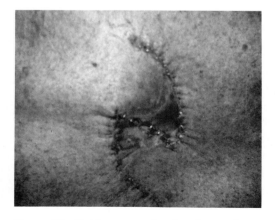

Figure 15 Dehiscence at the site of necrosis.

Table 3 Wound Tensile Strength

Time after wounding	Strength (%)
2 weeks	3–5
3 weeks	15
4 weeks	35
Final	80

ment of buried sutures may be essential to provide additional support to keep the wound edges approximated. Aside from wound tension, numerous factors can increase the risk of wound dehiscence. Cigarette smoking is a potentially controllable factor that can lead to impaired wound healing. Other systemic factors such as increased patient age (65 yr), systemic infection, hypoproteinemia, uremia, hypertension, pulmonary disease, and steroid use may also increase the risk of dehiscence.

The treatment of wound dehiscence varies with the cause of dehiscence. If the dehiscence is caused by infection or necrosis, the wound should be left open for drainage and to heal by second intention. A delayed closure or scar revision can be considered. If wound tension or trauma is the cause of dehiscence, immediate reapproximation of the wound edges can be considered if there is no evidence of infection. "Freshening" of the wound edges should be kept to a minimum, removing only nonviable tissue. Allowing the wound edges to remain "unfreshened" minimizes the lag period to fibroplasia and accelerates the development of tensile strength. The wound should be prepared in a sterile manner as for any closure, infiltrated with local anesthesia, and sutured closed with nylon or Prolene. Reclosure of dehisced wounds may greatly reduce healing times as opposed to allowing the area to heal by second intention.

Nerve Deficits

Sensory and motor nerves may be transected or injured during cutaneous surgery. Fortunately, most areas of the skin and the underlying muscles have diverse nerve innervation and unless a major nerve is injured, there is little permanent effect. The transection of cutaneous nerves happens with any skin incision. Patients may have relative anesthesia in the skin at primary closure sites and in the area of flaps. There will be hypoesthesia in any graft. Sensory nerves readily regenerate and reinnervate in areas of wounding. This action may take many months to complete, and the healing process may be accompanied by troublesome paresthesias, especially in the case of grafts. Normal sensation may never completely return to the operative state. In some locations larger sensory nerves may be injured leading to sensory deficits distal to the injury site. The most common sites for such injuries are on the forehead and anterior scalp, the posterior scalp, and the digits. The patient should be warned of the possibility of such nerve injuries prior to a procedure. In time, most of these deficits at least partially resolve.

Injury or transection of motor nerves can lead to paralysis of the innervated muscles. In general, the more proximal the nerve injury, the more severe the consequences. For example, injury to branches of the facial nerve medial to a line drawn from the lateral canthus to the angle of the mouth are unlikely to lead to severe consequences, while transection lateral to this area may lead to significant paralysis. Fortunately, most of the larger, more proximal branches are usually relatively deep and well protected. The most common area of injury to a major branch

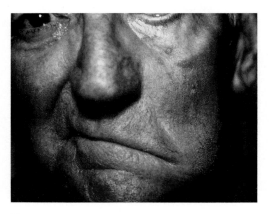

Figure 16 Loss of function of the main branch of the facial nerve due to local anesthesia.

of the facial nerve is to the temporal branch of the facial nerve as it crosses the zygomatic arch. The nerve is superficial and covered only by the superficial temporalis fascia. Transection will lead to paralysis of the frontalis muscle and loss of the ability to elevate the forehead on the affected side. Unless there is a preexisting brow ptosis, this loss is usually only of cosmetic consequence. Such a ptosis can be surgically corrected if necessary. The mandibular branch of the facial nerve may be encountered as it crosses the mandible, near the facial artery and vein. It is superficial at this point, being covered only by the skin and the platysma muscle. Loss of this nerve prevents use of the lip depressors and can give the face a distorted appearance when smiling and forming other facial expressions. There may be some interference with mouth function. Injuries to the buccal branch, zygomatic branch, or main trunk of the facial nerve are much rarer but can have significant sequelae. There may be loss of function of the muscles around the eye and the mouth with resulting inability to close the eye, drooling from loss of spincter control of the mouth, and a distorted facial appearance (Fig. 16). The spinal accessory nerve may be injured in the posterior triangle of the neck at Erb's point where it exits from behind the sternocleidomastoid muscle. Damage to the spinal accessory nerve can lead to a paralysis of the trapezius muscle with resulting winging of the scapula, difficulty abducting the arm, and possible chronic shoulder pain. A dilemma results when tumor involves the area of a major nerve. If isolation of the nerve from the tumor is possible, preservation of the nerve should be attempted. If it is not possible, either the nerve must be removed or alternative therapy for the residual tumor (such as radiation therapy) must be planned. There may be some regrowth and return of function when major branches are injured, however, when major branches are transected, consideration must be given to repair with reapproximation and/or nerve grafts. In addition while awaiting the return of function, muscle stimulation may be necessary to forestall muscle atrophy.

By design, local anesthesia will cause the temporary loss of function of sensory and motor nerves. If a major nerve is affected by the infiltration of local anesthesia or the nerve is injured but not severed by the procedure, it may not be possible at the conclusion of a procedure to fully assess the residual nerve function. The loss of function may be of varying duration (Table 4). While waiting to delineate the extent of any permanent deficit, care must be taken to provide for the necessary functions of the nerve. The eye may need to be patched closed if the ability to close the eye is lost. The patient must be warned to avoid hot liquids and chewing if sensation of the lips is compromised. In most circumstances, function will rapidly return.

Table 4 Duration of Nerve Deficits

Injury	Duration
Local anesthesia	~6 hr
Nerve block	~ 12 hr
Neuropraxia	Up to 6 months
Transection	May be permanent

PROBLEMS OF WOUND APPEARANCE

Suture Problems

Buried sutures can cause a variety of problems prior to their total absorption. Older sutures of gut or chromic gut are digested by neutrophils. As this digestion takes place, a sterile abscess may form. Pustules may be opened and the remaining suture gently removed. Newer synthetic absorbable sutures are absorbed without enzymatic action by hydrolysis. These sutures rarely result in pustules but may form firm papules in the suture line (Fig. 17). These suture reactions most commonly occur at 6 weeks with a range of 1–4 months. If the papule is deep, the skin cancer patient may be concerned that this thickening represents a return of the tumor. The papule usually resolves with time. The patient may "assist" in the resolution of the papule by applying gentle massage to the site. If the papule is near the skin surface, the suture may be extruded through the wound. Such a papule usually appears with little inflammation, and a small tuft of suture may protrude. It has been proposed that the spitting of absorbable sutures is the result of sutures placed too close to the surface of knots tied toward the surface rather than buried. Although these factors may account for some instances of suture extrusion, at times even properly placed deep sutures will split. If the suture is loose, it should be removed. If the loop is intact, the suture should be elevated with forceps and as much as possible should be clipped with the scissors, allowing the remaining suture to retract into the wound to be absorbed. The ultimate wound appearance is usually unaffected by this event.

The placement of skin sutures through the epithelium and the resulting presence of suture creates a tract for epithelial cell migration. Epithelization around the suture occurs between the

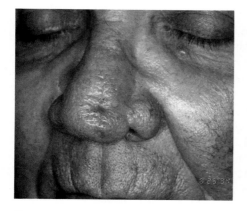

Figure 17 "Spitting" of Vicryl suture.

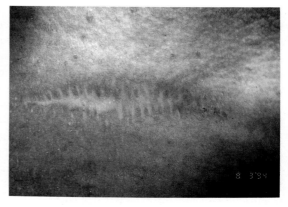

Figure 18 "Railroad tracking" at suture sites and early scar spreading.

third and eighth day. If the sutures are removed prior to complete epithelization, the tract regresses. If the tract completely epithelizes, several problems can develop. The keratinizing cells can incite an inflammatory response, which may persist after suture removal. This erythema may be confused with infection (Fig. 12). The inflammation may lead to scarring around the suture tracts with the development of pitted scars at the site. If the suture has also pressed tightly on the skin, it may create a linear scar linking the suture tract scars and yielding a "railroad track" appearance (Fig. 18). The longer sutures are in place, the more likely such marks are to develop. In addition, some anatomic sites are more prone to the development of suture reactions than others. The risk is greater on sebaceous areas of the face, the chest, back, and extremities and lower on the eyelids, palms, and soles of the feet. The best way to avoid cutaneous suture reactions is through early suture removal. This can be accomplished by minimizing wound edge tension through good surgical planning and the proper placement of buried sutures.

Hypertrophic Scars and Keloids

During the healing process, usually several weeks after the sutures have been removed, the wound site may become thickened, erythematous, or raised. Hypertrophic scars are frequently pruritic or painful. Unlike keloids, hypertrophic scars do not grow beyond the margins of the original wound. Hypertrophic scars are most frequent on the chest, including the breasts, back, and shoulders, but some degree of thickening can occur in any location, including the face. Although most hypertrophic scars will resolve given sufficient time, the larger and more firm a hypertrophic scar becomes, the more likely it is to result in a scar that is wide and has an irregular surface texture from dermal scarring and loss of adnexal structures (Fig. 19). Intervention at the early stages of hypertrophic scar formation may yield a more acceptable scar. High-potency topical glucocorticoids or intralesional glucocorticoid injections may decrease the thickness of the scar and relieve some of the symptoms. However, the use of steroids may lead to telangiectasias on the surface of the scar and possibly a widened scar. Smaller, less significant hypertrophic scars may respond to patient massage.

Keloids (see Chap. 36) are more extensive than hypertrophic scars and spread beyond the site of the original wound. Keloid formation tends to be hereditary. Although keloids are most prevalent in dark-skinned races, they occur in all racial and ethnic groups. A patient with a personal or family history of keloids is at risk of developing a keloid with any wounding injury. Keloids are more prevalent in some body locations such as the ear lobes, neck, and trunk. Keloid for-

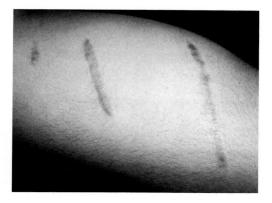

Figure 19 Hypertrophic scars from traumatic lacerations. Note the widened and stretched appearance of the scar as the hypertrophic elements regress (the longer scar).

Table 5 Treatment Modalities for Keloids

Surgical
  Cryosurgery
  Laser surgery
    CO_2
    Neodynium:YAG
  Replacement with flaps and/or grafts
Nonsurgical
  Radiation therapy
  Pressure garments
  Silicone gel sheeting
  Hydration and occlusion
  Steroids—topical or intralesional
  Intralesional steroids plus hyaluronidase
  Topical retinoic acid
  Intralesional interferon—gamma and alpha 2-b
Systemic Medications
  Colchicine
  Methotrexate
  Penicillamine

mation is rare on the face, but they have been reported to occur on the eyelids, cornea, and mucous membranes. The treatment of keloids is difficult, as additional trauma to the skin may only exacerbate the problem. Keloids are often not only very unsightly, but also tend to be pruritic and tender. A variety of treatments have been employed (Table 5) with varying degrees of success. Often combining various modalities yields the best results.

In predisposed individuals and on predisposed body sites, even small procedures such as shave or punch biopsies can lead to hypertrophic scars or keloids (Fig. 20). Patients must be informed of this possibility.

Spread Scars

Tension across a wound can lead to a spreading of the finely approximated wound initially present after surgery, especially on the shoulders, back, and chest, but wound spread can occur in any

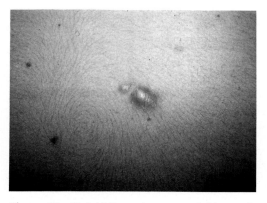

Figure 20 Keloid formation at punch biopsy site.

wound (Fig. 18). Scar spread seems to occur in skin with less elasticity (a thicker dermis) and fewer adnexal structures. Vigorous activity involving the area of wounding may also increase the rate of wound spread.

It is important to recognize the risk of widened scars in such locations and counsel the patient on the possible outcome prior to the procedure. With this knowledge, some cosmetic procedures in these locations may be deferred.

Most widening of the scar takes place during the first 6 months after surgery. Wide undermining to reduce wound tension may decrease spreading. Subcutaneous placement of longer-lasting absorbable sutures, such as Maxon or PDS, may also retard and decrease spread. Placement of nonabsorbable material such as clear nylon or Prolene as deep-buried sutures may also provide prolonged support to prevent wound spreading, as well as prolonged (6 month) placement of a running intradermal suture such as Prolene.

Reexcising a spread scar to achieve a narrower scar usually provides little improvement. A Z-plasty type excision to change the direction of closure and to remove significant wound tension may be successful.

Trap-Door Deformity

During the first few weeks after surgery, a "pincushion" appearance may develop, especially in transposition flap repairs. The central portion of the flap may elevate and recede towards the wound margins. The outer edges of the wound margins may also be raised (Fig. 21). Although the etiology of the trap-door deformity has not been convincingly demonstrated, it probably at least in part results from contraction of the wound bed upon which the flap has been transposed. Wide undermining of the skin edges of the defect to be filled by the flap or graft may distribute the contracture and minimize any trap-door effect. The more circular the wound edges, the more pronounced the deformity, if it develops.

Good flap planning and execution may prevent trap-door deformities in some circumstances. Some feel that rhombic flaps should be planned with their rhombic angles intact. After Mohs surgery it is often tempting to trim the flap to the round shape of the defect rather than remove more tissue to convert the wound to a rhombic shape. Maintaining the rhombic angles may cause the angles of contraction to be in various directions, rather than being directed in a radial fashion. This diffusion of the lines of contraction may minimize the amount of trap-dooring. Widely undermining around the defect margins will also spread the contraction over a larger area. Flaps should also be designed and cut so that they have to be stretched slightly to fit the defect in order

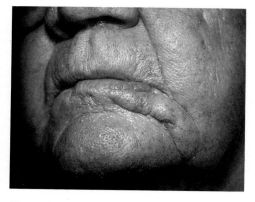

Figure 21   Trap-door deformity.

to reduce any redundant tissue. Trimming the underside of the flap of excess subcutaneous tissue also seems to inhibit trap-door formation.

If trap-dooring does occur, intervention may be helpful. Glucocorticoid injections of the wound margins and the central base help. Massage to the entire flap may also be useful. After the flap and the deformity have matured (6 months to 1 yr), a procedure to undermine, defat, and trim the flap may provide some improvement.

Pigmentary Alterations

Epidermal wounding may result in changes in pigment. As skin pigmentation is produced by epidermal melanocytes, the broader the epidermal wound site, the more likely the pigmentary alteration. Wounds closed primarily may produce a hypopigmented or hyperpigmented scar line, but rarely a more extensive deformity. Broader-based epidermal or full-thickness injuries such as those produced by electrosurgery, cryosurgery, CO_2 laser ablation, or dermabrasion may lead to more pronounced pigmentary alterations. The degree of melanocytic injury seems to play a role in whether hyperpigmentation or hypopigmentation results. Injury that destroys melanocytes such as deep cryosurgery leads to hypopigmentation. Partial injury, such as a superficial abrasion, often results in accelerated melanocytic activity in the recovery period and hyperpigmentation. Because wounds may often involve both melanocytic destruction and partial injury, many wounds develop mottled pigmentation. Hypopigmentation is obviously most noticeable in dark-skinned individuals. Because of the ability of the melanocytes in dark-skinned people to react so vigorously to stimulation, hyperpigmentation can also be very prominent.

Patients undergoing procedures likely to result in pigmentary changes should be advised to practice strict sun protection. UV exposure will accentuate pigmentary changes by augmenting hyperpigmentation and providing additional contrast to areas of hyperpigmentation. Patients should be advised to avoid intentional tanning and wear high-grade sun blocks for at least a year after the procedure. Consideration should be given to not performing elective procedures with a high risk of pigmentary alteration (such as dermabrasion) during the summer months. Full-thickness and split-thickness grafts are also prone to irregular pigmentation and should have strict photoprotection (Figs. 13 and 22).

Early or established hyperpigmentation may be treated with topical hydroquinones. Camouflage make-up may also be helpful.

Tattooing may also occur in surgical scars from chemical cauterants such as ferrous subsulfate (Monsel's solution) or silver nitrate. Such tattooing is usually permanent, unless treated by excision or laser.

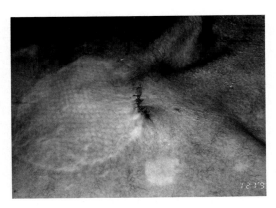

Figure 22 Hypopigmentation of a full-thickness graft on the chest.

Prominent Scar Lines

Scar lines may be raised and prominent rather than flat. At times there may appear to be an unevenness between the two sides of the scar. Such a situation may follow planned primary closures, flaps, grafts, or the closure of traumatic injuries. This type of scar also seems to be more common in younger individuals who exhibit more exuberant healing. Dermabrasion of the scar line 4–8 weeks after the original wounding appears to have a beneficial effect on the appearance of such scars. The beneficial effect may be diminished if the dermabrasion is delayed beyond 6–8 weeks.

Surgeon-Patient Complications

A surgical scar is the result of an interplay between the action of the surgeon, the patient, and nature. The patient's role must begin at the decision to proceed with surgery and continue through the postoperative period. Although informed consent has legal meaning and implications, it should mean that the surgeon shares with the patient what he or she knows, so that the patient can participate in his or her own care. The patient must be informed about the results to be reasonably expected and what might occur if complications arise. The patient may worry about how the procedure will affect his or her general health, appearance, or well-being. The surgeon must anticipate and address those concerns. The patient must also accept responsibility for his or her portion of preoperative preparation, cooperation with the surgical procedure, wound care, and having realistic long-term expectations. Since lifestyle habits such as smoking or drinking alcohol affect wound healing, the patient should be instructed to alter behaviors to improve the outcome, if necessary. The surgeon must provide detailed information, both oral and written, to help the patient with these responsibilities. If complications arise, the complication, its treatment, and the expected long-term result should be fully shared with the patient. Every surgeon experiences complications, and every patient presents the potential for complications. Good doctor-patient communication as well as involving the patient in his or her own care should, in most circumstances, prevent the additional complication of litigation.

BIBLIOGRAPHY

Becker G. Chemoprophylaxis for surgery of the head and neck. *Ann Otol Rhinol Laryngol* 1981;90:8–12.

Bencini PL, Galimberti M, Signorini M. Utility of topical benzoyl peroxide for prevention of surgical skin wound infection. *J Dermatol Surg Oncol* 1994;20:538–540.

Bencini PL, et al. Antibiotic prophylaxis of wound infections in skin surgery. *Arch Dermatol* 1991; 127: 1357–1360.

Bernstein G. The loop stitch. *J Dermatol Surg Oncol* 1984;10:587.

Bithell TC. Blood coagulation. In *Wintrobe's Clinical Hematology*. RG Lee et al., ed. Philadelphia, Lea & Febiger, 1993; pp. 566–615.

Bithell TC. Qualitative disorders of platelet disfunction. In *Wintrobe's Clinical Hematology*. RG Lee et al., ed. Philadelphia, Lea & Febiger, 1993; pp. 1397–1421.

Buell BR, E SD. Comparison of tensile strength of CO_2 laser and scapel skin incisions. *Arch Otolaryngol* 1983;109:465–487.

Burke JF. The effective period of preventive antibiotic action in experimental incision and dermal lesions. *Surgery* 1961;50:161–163.

Burke JF. Infection. In *Fundamentals of Wound Management*. TK Hunt and JE Dunphy, ed. New York, Appleton-Century-Crofts, 1979, pp. 170–240.

Clark RAF. Basics of cutaneous wound repair. *J Dermatol Surg Oncol* 1993;19:693–706.

Clark RAF. Cutaneous tissue repair: Basic biologic considerations. *J Am Acad Dermatol* 1985;13:701–725.

Classen DC, et al. The timing of prophylactic administration of antibiotics and the risk of surgical wound infection. *N Engl J Med* 1992;236(5):337–339.

Dellinger EP. Antibiotic prophylaxis of wound infections in skin surgery. Is 4 days too much? *Arch Dermatol* 1991;127:1394–1395.

Deykin D, Janson P, McMahon L. Ethanol potentiation of aspirin-induced prolongation of the bleeding time. *N Engl J Med* 1982;306:852.

Dodson MK, Magann EF, Meeks GR. A randomized comparison of secondary closure and secondary intention in patients with superficial wound dehiscence. *Obstet Gynecol* 1992;80:321–324.

Dzubow LM. *Facial Flaps: Biomechanics and Regional Application.* Norwalk, CT, Appleton & Lange, 1990.

Elliot D, Mahaffey PJ. The stretched scar: The benefit of prolonged dermal support. *Br J Plast Surg* 1989; 42:74–78.

Gette MT, Marks JG, Maloney ME. The frequency of postoperative allergic contact dermatitis to topical antibiotics. *Arch Dermatol* 1992;128:365–367.

Giandoni MB, Grabski WJ. Cutaneous candidiasis as a cause of delayed surgical wound healing. *J Am Acad Dermatol* 1994;30:

Goldminz D, Bennett RG. Cigarette smoking and flap and full-thickness graft necrosis. *Arch Dermatol* 1991;127:1012–1015.

Goth A. *Medical Pharmacology*, 7th ed. St. Louis, C.V. Mosby Co., 1974.

Grabb WC. A concentration of 1:500,000 epinephrine in a local anesthetic solution is sufficient to provide excellent hemostasis. *Plast Recconstr Surg* 1979;63:384.

Haas AF. Antibiotic prophylaxis. *Semin Dermatol* 1994;13:27–34.

Harris DR. Healing of the surgical wound. I. Basic considerations. *J Am Acad Dermatol* 1979;1:197–207.

Hirschmann JV. Topical antibiotics in dermatology. *Arch Dermatol* 1988;124:1691–1700.

Jones JK, Triplett RG. The relationship of cigarette smoking to impaired intraoral wound healing: A review of the evidence and implications for patient care. *J Oral Maxillofac Surg* 1992;50:237–239.

Kaiser AB. Antimicrobial prophylaxis in surgery. *N Engl J Med* 1986;315:1129–1138.

Katz BE, Oca MAGS. A controlled study of the effectiveness of spot dermabrasion ('scarabrasion') on the appearance of surgical scars. *J Am Acad Dermatol* 1991;24:462–466.

Maloney ME. Management of surgical complications and suboptimal results. In *Cutaneous Surgery*. RG Wheeland, ed. Philadelphia, W.B. Saunders Co., 1994; pp. 921–934.

Nanney LB. Biochemical and physiological aspects of wound healing. In *Cutaneous Surgery*. RG Wheeland, ed. Philadelphia, W.B. Saunders Co., 1994; pp. 113–121.

Nemeth AJ. Keloids and hypertrophic scars. *J Dermatol Surg Oncol* 1993;19:

Pellitteri PK, Kennedy TL, Youn BA. The influence of intensive hyperbaric oxygen therapy on skin flap survival in a swine model. *Arch Otolaryn* 1992;118:1050–1054.

Polk HC, et al. Guidelines for prevention of surgical wound infection. *Arch Surg* 1983;118:1213–1217.

Pollack SV. Management of keloids. In *Cutaneous Surgery*. RG Wheeland, ed. Philadelphia, W.B. Saunders Co., 1994, pp. 688–698.

Rappaport WD, et al. The effect of electrocautery on wound healing in midline laparotomy incisions. *Am J Surg* 1990;160:618–620.

Recommended Practices Coordinating Committee. Proposed Recommended Practices, Skin Preparation of Patients. *AORN J* 1992;55(2):555–561.

Riou JP, Cohen JR, Johnson H. Factors influencing wound dehiscence. *Am J Surg* 1992;163:324–330.

Salasche SJ. Acute surgical complications: Cause, prevention, and treatment. *J Am Acad Dermatol* 1986; 15:1163–1185.

Salasche SJ, Bernstein G, Senkarik M. *Surgical Anatomy of the Skin.* Norwalk, CT, Appleton and Lange, 1988.

Scherbenske JM, Winton GB, James WD. Acute pseudomomas infection of the external ear (malignant otitis externa). *J Dermatol Surg Oncol* 1988;14:165–169.

Sebben JE. Prophylactic antibiotics in cutaneous surgery. *J Dermatol Surg Oncol* 1985;11:901–906.

Sommerlad BC, Creasey JM. The stretched scar: A clinical and histologic study. *Br J Plast Surg* 1978; 31:34–45.

Stegman SJ, Tromovitch TA, Glogau RG. *Basics of Dermatologic Surgery.* Chicago, Year Book Medical Publishers, 1982.

Thorngren M, Shafi S, Born GV. Quantification of blood from skin bleeding time determinations: Effects of fish diet or acetylsalicylic acid. *Haemostasis* 1983;13:282.

Wilkin JK. Diseases of the blood vessels: Introduction. In *Clinical Dermatology*. DJ Demis, ed. Philadelphia, JB Lippincott Co., 1993; pp. 1–8.

Winton GB. Anesthesia for dermatologic surgery. *J Dermatol Surg Oncol* 1988;14:41–54.

Winton GB, Salasche SJ. Wound dressings for dermatologic surgery. *J Am Acad Dermatol* 1985; 13: 1026–1044.

Yarbrorough JM. Ablation of facial scars by programmed dermabrasion. *J Dermatol Surg Oncol* 1988; 14:292–294.

Zitelli JA. The naso-labial flap as a single state procedure. *Arch Dermatol* 1990;126:1445–1448.

12

Skin Biopsy

Bryan C. Schultz
Loyola University Stritch School of Medicine, Maywood, Illinois

Skin biopsy is a routine diagnostic tool used to evaluate the skin. Ease in sampling of skin has resulted in a large body of information correlating clinical with histopathologic data over more than a century. No other organ in the human body is so easily biopsied for diagnostic purposes. Advances in immunology, molecular biology, electron microscopy, and culturing techniques have contributed greatly to the breadth of knowledge obtained through skin biopsy. Techniques using immunohistochemistry, gene rearrangement, polymerase chain reaction (PCR), HPV typing, DNA flow cytometry, etc., are all rapidly evolving. There will be a greater demand for skin biopsy to aid in the diagnosis of both cutaneous and systemic disease.

The most common circumstances for biopsying the skin are (1) to rule out malignancy, (2) to evaluate diagnostically a benign tumor, and (3) to evaluate a dermatosis for histopathologic correlation with clinical data. It is extremely important that the physican consider all possible causes of the condition before performing a skin biopsy. If a nonspecialist who does not have an accurate differential diagnosis is doing the procedure, the dermatopathologist's ability to make the diagnosis is compromised. It is important that someone with a background in clinical skin disease and its pathologic correlations interpret the biopsy as it relates to the disease.

Surgical principles discussed elsewhere would apply to skin biopsy procedures. General procedures used for skin biopsy will be discussed, as well as considerations that must be taken into account with different diagnoses. Special concerns and preferable techniques in certain body locations are addressed.

GENERAL PROCEDURES AND TECHNIQUE

Skin Preparation

Prepare the skin with 70% isopropyl alcohol, including the area to be biopsied and approximately 5 cm surrounding. It is best to let the alcohol dry for a brief period after application. With this skin prep, less than 1 in 5000 infections occur, and infections have never been severe or clinically threatening in the author's experience. In fact, infection or significant pain after biopsy should be considered an unusual event. No skin prep can ever prevent infection entirely. Isopropyl alcohol does not discolor or distort clinical borders of the lesions. Povidone-iodine preparations are a favorite of many surgeons but may distort the clinical border of faintly colored or erythematous lesions. Some povidone-iodine solutions have had bacterial contaminants cultured from them. Chlorhexidine compounds are also an acceptable way of cleansing skin. Caution must be used with these agents, and they should not be used near the eye or ear canal because of reported problems with corneal clouding and ototoxicity. Both isopropyl alcohol and some chlorhexidine compounds are flammable. The skin should be thoroughly dried before any cautery is used. A rare patient may be allergic to isopropyl alcohol or povidone-iodine. In such cases, gentle mechanical cleansing with sterile saline or soap and water would be adequate for most skin biopsies.

For most small procedures such as punch skin biopsies a drape is unnecessary. Fenestrated drapes such as Steridrape with an adhesive backing and central circular fenestration can be useful. Allergies to this adhesive backing are rare. The adhesive backing also ensures that any blood from the biopsy site will run on the drape.

Anesthesia

For the vast majority of cases, either 0.5% or 1.0% plain lidocaine may be used. Epinephrine can be used in dilutions of 1:100,000, 1:200,000, or 1:500,000 for hemostasis. A 1:400,000 concentration can still give maximum vasoconstrictive effect, while minimizing the total amount of epinephrine used. Since most biopsies are performed in just a few minutes, it may not be necessary to use epinephrine for prolonged anesthesia. Side effects such as tachycardia and tachyarrhythmia may occur with epinephrine and should be avoided in patients with significant hypertension or vasoconstrictive cardiovascular disease. Severe bradycardia and hypertensive crises have resulted when using this agent in patients receiving a beta blocker such as propranolol (Inderal).

A 30-gauge needle is used for injecting the anesthestic into the skin. Larger-gauge needles cause significantly more pain during the injection. Thirty-gauge needles with a silicon coating will puncture skin smoothly and painlessly. A dental Cook-Waite type syringe with disposable carpules may be used. It is best to obtain the type that allows for aspiration. Carpules are easy to use and preferred by many dentists and physicians.

Allergy to most local anesthetics is uncommon. Frequently reactions are due to epinephrine used in the anesthetic. True allergic reactions are usually to the ester group of local anesthetics. The amide group, which includes lidocaine, rarely sensitizes an individual. When sensitization has occurred, it may be due to a preservative in a multiple-dose vial. In that circumstance, the physician may use a single-dose vial without a preservative. Another method of anesthetizing such allergic patients is to use a liquid nitrogen or carbon dioxide freeze of the area, and then quickly perform the biopsy. Others have used saline and diphenhydramine (Benadryl) infiltration for short anesthesia during biopsy. EMLA cream (eutectic mixture of local anesthetics), a combination of lidocaine and prilocaine, is quite helpful either alone (with occlusion for about 60 min) or to minimize the pain of local anesthetic injection.

Instrumentation

The standard instrument for skin biopsy is the dermal punch (Keyes' punch). High-quality sterilizable punches in sizes from 1.5 to 10 mm are available. Because the quality of these punches may be superior to some disposable punches, they remain the choice of some physicians. The convenience and safety of disposable punches make them appealing for small routine skin biopsies. The most important aspect is the sharpness of the punch. The operator should be able to penetrate the skin with one or two rotations of its axis. A good punch should penetrate the skin like a knife cutting butter. Adequate sharpness not only enables the operator to remove the tissue specimen easily but also minimizes trauma to the specimen and surrounding tissue. When obtaining subcutaneous tissue, a sharp punch is less likely to cause separation of the dermis from the subcutaneous tissue. Many disposable punches now provide superior cutting quality. They are not only equal to, but in many cases superior to, permanent punches.

PUNCH BIOPSY

Certainly the most common method of performing skin biopsies is the punch biopsy. The Keyes' punch is reminiscent of wood punches used by the carpenter. The instrument is ideal since many skin lesions grow in a radial fashion, resulting in a relatively circular configuration. Any lesion with such a configuration may be considered for punch biopsy. It is also an excellent instrument to obtain tissue for diagnosis of inflammatory processes.

If the punch biopsy is done for small lesions, it may also serve to excise. If the punch is used for total excision, accurate measurement of lesion diameter is important. If the lesion is slightly oval or irregular, the skin may be stretched at the time of biopsy to accommodate the smallest punch. Punches as small as 1.5 mm are available for dilated pores, while large sizes such as 9 and 10 mm are available for circular excision in nonfacial areas. When choosing a punch, the location of the lesion and the relative elasticity of the skin in that area will affect the size of circular excision that can be made to allow primary closure without dog ears. As a rule, do not use a punch greater than 5–6 mm on the face or 8–10 mm on the body. There are exceptions, and trimming of minute dog ears may be necessary in these circumstances.

It is helpful to outline the area to be biopsied prior to starting. Injection of local anesthetics, especially when epinephrine is used, will blanch the surrounding skin and make lesional borders less perceptible. This is especially important for lesions that do not have a sharp border or for faintly erythematous dermatoses that may blanch entirely upon injection.

The local anesthetic should be injected into the deep dermis. This provides almost immediate, complete anesthesia. A subcutaneous injection may be used in addition to this, but when used alone results in either delayed or often incomplete anesthesia.

The skin is stretched, with the fingers, perpendicular to skin tension lines so that the wound forms an oval (Fig. 1). In certain areas where tension lines are unclear, such as the nose, it may be preferable not to stretch the skin. This will give the physician a clue to the direction of closure of that defect. This technique will improve the appearance of the scar.

While holding or stretching the adjacent skin firmly with either the forefinger and thumb or the second and third fingers, gently rotate the punch, cutting to the appropriate depth for that lesion. If sharp punches are used, little pressure is needed to cut through to the subcutaneous tissue. In almost all circumstances, penetration should be at least to the superficial subcutaneous tissue, especially when closed with sutures. If dermis is left at the bottom of the wound and sutured, it will buckle the skin and cause a gap of the wound edges.

Removal of the biopsy tissue is done with a fine, single-toothed forceps. The tip is placed gently but firmly on dermal tissue, avoiding epidermis and subcutaneous fat. The tissue is gently lifted out until resistance is met, and iris scissors can be used to cut the tissue free at the subcutaneous level. The tissue may also be impaled with a 30-gauge needle used for anesthetics. The needle is lifted outward with the specimen and cut with either scissors or a #11 scalpel blade.

When penetrating subcutaneous tissue, knowledge of local anatomy, including blood vessel and nerve distribution, is important. Transecting nerves or vessels can be a difficult problem.

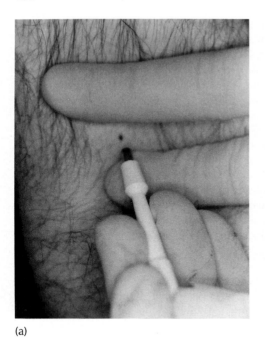
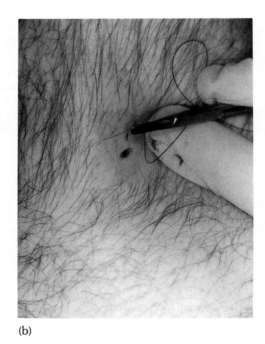

(a)   (b)

Figure 1   (a) Skin stretched perpendicular to skin tension lines before punch biopsy of small nevus. (b) Placing suture in resulting oval defect.

Examples of such structures would be the angular artery alongside the nose and the spinal accessory nerve beneath the subcutaneous fat of the posterior triangle of the neck.

Suture closure is preferred for many punch biopsies. This has the advantage of reestablishing a skin barrier to infection immediately. Superficial curet and shave biopsies are best left open to heal by second intention. Other methods to obtain hemostasis in an open-punch biopsy wound are Gelfoam, collagen matrix, and Monsel's solution. Styptic agents and cauterization should be avoided for hemostasis. Mild styptics such as 35% aluminum chloride in 50–70% isopropyl alcohol may be used for more superficial procedures when only epidermis and superficial dermis have been removed. They are applied for a few seconds with light pressure and the excess is dried with a small sponge. Any styptic (e.g., Monsel's, aluminum chloride) may delay wound healing, but this has been clinically imperceptible for small wounds in my experience.

Without a complete sterile surgical setup, the following technique may be used for sterile placement of two or three sutures (Fig. 2).

1. The wound is prepped with alcohol or povidone-iodine.
2. All instruments are taken from sterile wrappings. Touch only the handles, leaving the tips of the instruments sterile.
3. To sponge, pick up the ends of sterile gauze and use the center only to blot.
4. Suture packs are opened without touching the needle.
5. Grasp the sterile needle in the suture pack with the jaws of the needle holder.
6. The needle is gently pulled from the suture pack so that it may be passed through skin tissue.
7. After the first pass, the needle is grasped with the sterile needle holder as it exits the

skin. It is pulled through the wound until about 3 inches of suture material remain on the initial side.

8. Cut the suture material on the exit side leaving another 3 inches. The needle holder still holds a sterile needle.

9. To reposition the needle holder without touching the sterile needle or the jaws of the needle holder, the end of the remaining suture is grasped with the fingers and the needle is allowed to drop. The needle then may be repositioned on the needle holder. While holding the end of the suture material taut, pass the needle through the wound again.

10. After two or three sutures are placed, go back and tie all sutures that have been placed.

This procedure is best performed with clean, disposable examination gloves. This method enables one to place two or three sutures sterilely without a sterile field for both operator and assistant.

EXCISIONAL BIOPSY

The excisional biopsy may be done with either a punch for smaller lesions or a scalpel for larger lesions. For larger lesions, the excision is done with a scalpel forming elliptical or fusiform wound margins (see Chap. 13).The length of the excision traditionally is three times the width. A shorter length-to-width ratio can be closed in some areas where skin elasticity is greater.

The primary reason for excisional biopsy is to remove a lesion in toto. A common example would be biopsy of a suspected melanoma. If melanoma is suspected, complete excision of the lesion down to subcutaneous tissue is preferable. This is done to assess accurately the level of invasion; however, incisional or punch biopsy has not been shown to adversely affect the outcome of melanoma. Total excision may not be necessary for most linear pigmented uniform streaks seen in melanoma excisional scars, as these are probably benign. Punch biopsy for assurance may be an acceptable alternative to close observation for a concerned physician and patient.

Excisional biopsy may also be considered for Spitz nevi. Some have considered subtotal excision acceptable if the diagnosis is unequivocal, while others find the word "unequivocal" difficult to use with Spitz nevi. No definitive answer can be given for this dilemma, so evaluation of the clinal and histopathological evidence must still be weighed carefully in choosing treatment.

Excisional biopsy should be considered in larger lesions where a dog-ear effect may result from a punch biopsy. A gently curved fusiform excision will result in a linear scar and superior cosmetic results. Poorly defined tumors or infiltrative dermatoses may be excised to obtain a larger specimen for more accurate pathologic examination. Lesions with deeper pathology in subcutaneous tissue, such as erythema nodosum or panniculitis, are better biopsied using excision technique.

SCISSORS AND SHAVE BIOPSIES

When the pathologic condition is restricted entirely to epidermis or epidermis and superficial dermis (such as a benign pedunculated nevus or fibroepithelial polyp), either a scissors or scalpel shave biopsy may be considered. The lesion may be gently grasped with a small forceps and pulled to cause slight tenting of the epidermis and upper dermis. A curved iris scissors with fine points may be used to remove the lesion (Fig. 3). It is preferable to include the superficial dermis to examine for any extension into the dermis (Fig. 4). The base may be lightly electrodesiccated or a styptic applied. If the lesion is melanocytic (e.g., nevus), it is best to ask the

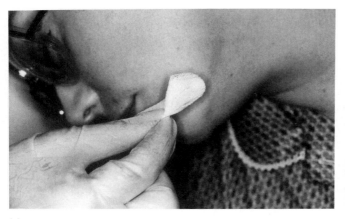

(a)

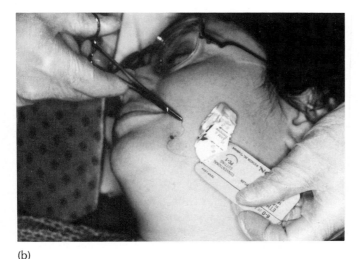

(b)

Figure 2   (a) Sponging with sterile center of sponges. (b) Needle holder grasping the needle as it emerges on the opposite side of the wound. (c) Cutting the suture while the needle holder is still grasping the needle. (d) Grasping the free-hanging needle with the sterile jaws of the needle holder while the unsterile hand holds the end of the suture. (e) Passing the needle through the skin for a second suture while holding the suture taut to prevent sagging onto surrounding undraped and unprepped skin. (From Schultz and McKinney, with permission.)

patient to look for any return of color. In experienced hands this will rarely happen, as both clinical assessment of proper depth before and immediately after a transected biopsy/excision can be judged with a significant degree accuracy. Any unusual pigment pattern or abnormal histopathology would necessitate a deeper excisional biopsy.

CURET BIOPSY

One of the most common skin biopsy techniques is the curet biopsy. A sharp, oval curet is best for most situations. It provides a wide, flat shearing force at the tip of the instrument. A circular curet is better for scooping out cavities or small pockets of tumor and for smaller lesions.

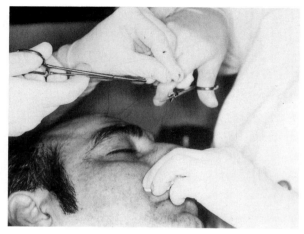

(c)

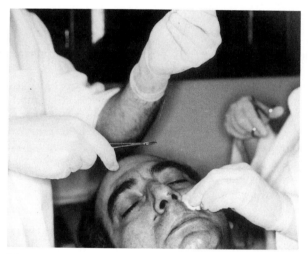

(d)

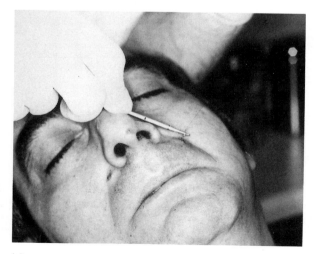

(e)

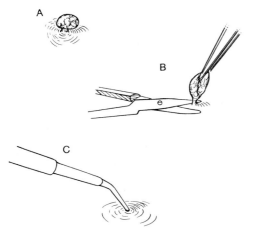

Figure 3 (A) Fibroepithelial polyp. (B) Polyp grasped with forceps and gently pulled outward. (C) Light electrocautery to base. (From Schultz and McKinney, with permission.)

Frequent use and autoclaving will necessitate either sharpening or purchase of new instruments on a regular basis. Disposable curets are available for one-time use.

The sharp shearing force of a curet easily removes epidermal and superficial dermal lesions. An example is a lesion on firm skin. This provides resistance to the shearing force of the curet. Seborrheic keratoses are ideal lesions for such removal (Fig. 5). The lesion can be removed with minimal scarring. If the skin is loose or thin, it may be more difficult to stabilize the skin and remove the lesion without tearing normal skin. Apply pressure to the surrounding tissue before curetting. An assistant may help apply pressure for larger lesions. Light electrodesiccation will facilitate curetting if material for histologic examination is not needed. The curet easily removes charred epidermal tissue at the epidermal-dermal junction, and scarring is minimal.

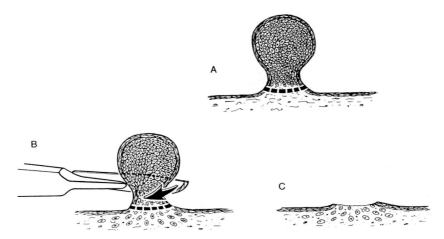

Figure 4 (A) Pedunculated nevus with nevus cells at or above the surrounding tissue. (B) Pedunculated nevus with some nevus cells penetrating lower into the dermis. (C) Shave biopsy may leave nevus cells behind, depending on the level of the shave and the location of the nevus cells. (From Schultz and McKinney, with permission.)

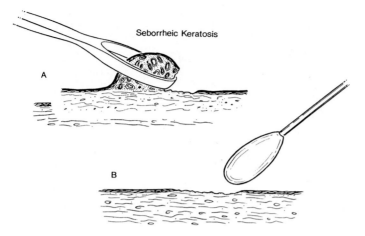

Figure 5 The curet easily removes a seborrheic keratosis with sharp shearing force. Aluminum chloride styptic is applied after removal of the keratosis. (From Schultz and McKinney, with permission.)

Superficial epidermal lesions that are amenable to curet biopsy include warts, cherry angiomas, and superficial epidermal cysts. Whenever malignancy is considered, the curet should penetrate the dermis to provide an adequate specimen for the pathologist. When curet biopsy of a cutaneous horn reveals squamous cell carcinoma, reexcision must be considered.

Curet biopsy may also be used for basal cell carcinoma. Biopsy of basal cell carcinoma should not penetrate to subcutaneous fat if curettage and electrodesiccation are the planned treatments (Fig. 6). Clinical tumor-free margins with this technique are best assessed by feeling healthy dermis with the curet. If the biopsy penetrates subcutaneous tissue, it is more difficult to determine the margins of the tumor during treatment with curettage and electrodesiccation. Basal cell carcinoma that clearly penetrates subcutaneous tissue may be best excised and submitted for pathologic confirmation of tumor-free margins.

Curettage may also be used to assess the margins of a basal cell carcinoma prior to excision. The curet is used to debulk or remove the tumor; the area that was curettaged is then excised. This results in an excision that is less likely to leave residual tumor. A delayed excision, after the wound from curettage and electrodesiccation has healed and contracted, may also be chosen. This is usually done to improve the cosmetic appearance of the scar.

SKIN BIOPSY IN SPECIAL LOCATIONS

Special considerations should be mentioned when doing skin biopsy in certain locations.

Eyes

A fine iris scissors is helpful for biopsy of epidermal or dermal lesions on the eyelid because of its fine point with a light curve at the tip. The operator can lay the scissors flat on the skin and remove tissue precisely. A fine gradle scissors with its tapered fine points is also ideal. To stabilize tissue, a small chalazion clamp is extremely helpful. Protective corneal shields are helpful for some but not mandatory for all eyelid work.

Hemostasis may be achieved with light cautery. Topical styptics can be used with extreme caution. A bottle of eyewash should be available. Styptic is applied with a moist (not wet) cot-

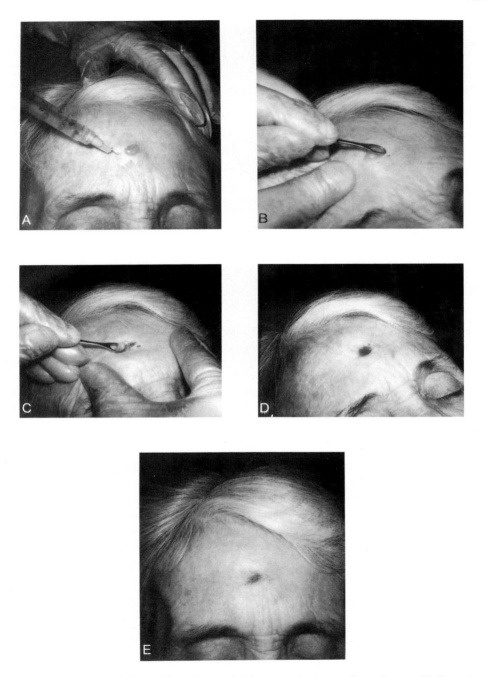

Figure 6   (A) Anesthetic is infiltrated in a circular fashion around a basal cell carcinoma. (B) Curet in place to begin curettage. (C) Curet removing the bulk of the tumor with the first pass. (D) Hemostasis is achieved after the first pass with aluminum chloride styptic alone. (E) Contraction of the wound immediately after electrodesiccation. (From Schultz and McKinney, with permission.)

ton-tipped applicator. Bottles of chemical styptic should not pass over the patient's eyes to avoid corneal burns from spillage.

Ears

When a biopsy is performed on the cartilaginous portion of the ear, care is taken to avoid trauma that may result in chondritis. When a large portion of cartilage is exposed, it may be necessary to punch small holes through it to allow granulation tissue to form from skin on the other side.

Forehead and Temples

Knowledge of the superficial anatomy is mandatory. Some vessels and nerves may be transected with punch biopsy. Hemostasis of a large-gauge vessel is more difficult through a small punch biopsy defect than larger wounds. On the forehead, the supraorbital and supratrochlear vessels run vertically from the medial third of the eyebrow. The superficial temporal arteries should be palpated laterally before biopsy is performed.

Nose

Before performing a punch biopsy of the nose, the elasticity of the nasal tissue should be evaluated, especially the alae and nasal tip. Curettage may be more acceptable, unless a deeper specimen is needed. Punch biopsies up to 4 mm can easily be closed with 6-0 nylon in these locations with good cosmetic results. Dog ears can be trimmed with a fine scissors.

A biopsy on the rim of the nose may result in notching. The columella presents no particular problem as long as width of the biopsy is slightly less than the columella. When using very sharp punches, one should be aware of the underlying cartilage and bone to avoid unwanted damage to the support structures. The operator can insert a gloved finger into the nasal airway to help orient the biopsy. Attention should be given to the angular artery as well.

Scalp

Be sure to angle the punch in the direction of the hair shafts and to include subcutaneous tissue to reveal follicular bulbs. The punch should be very sharp to do this properly.

When assessing various forms of alopecia, it may be helpful to request transverse sectioning of the specimen. Follicular density and diameters, as well as relative telogen counts, can be evaluated with this method of sectioning.

Large punch biopsies that are not sutured or deep curet biopsies occasionally form exuberant granulation tissue when healing on the anterior scalp and upper forehead. This tissue may be debulked surgically or with light chemical or electrocautery.

Fingers

Epinephrine is contraindicated as a vasoconstrictor agent in the local anesthetic when performing biopsies of the digit. Hemostasis may be obtained with a brief rubberband tourniquet at the base of the digit. Simple firm pressure with the operator's own finger is also adequate in many circumstances. Thorough knowledge of the anatomy including digital nerves and vessels is imperative (see Chap. 25), especially when performing deep or excisional biopsies.

Genital Area

Use of vasoconstrictors should be avoided on the penis. Suture closure is preferred if the biopsy is larger than 3-4 mm. For smaller superficial biopsies, cautery or light styptic may be used.

Mucous Membranes

Superficial biopsies of mucous membranes heal quite rapidly when a light styptic or chemical (e.g., silver nitrate) is used for hemostasis. Light cautery is also acceptable. For large or deep punch biopsies, closure with plain catgut is preferred. Other synthetic absorbables take too long to dissolve in mucosa. Nonabsorbables such as nylon may be used but may be removed in about 3 days since these areas heal so rapidly.

Nails

See Chapter 24.

TECHNICAL CONSIDERATIONS

Proper Locations

In many circumstances, different areas may be biopsied to obtain the pathologic diagnosis. It is most helpful to have a good idea of what pathologic changes you are looking for and where they are best found. For example, in dermatitis herpetiformis, a biopsy of perilesional skin is necessary to demonstrate characteristic histopathologic changes. To identify deposits of IgA by direct immunofluorescence, however, normal, intact skin is preferred. A generous portion of fat is required for the diagnosis of erythema nodosum, so biopsying a lesion not directly over the anterior tibial surface would be important. Amyloidosis may be diagnosed by biopsy of rectal mucosa and skin. Papulosquamous disorders should be biopsied in areas where disease is most characteristic and active, such as the volar surface of the lower forearm in lichen planus or thicker plaques on the buttocks for psoriasis.

Proper Depth and Width

Here again it is preferable to anticipate the diagnosis in order to perform the proper biopsy. Histologic diagnosis of lupus panniculitis or erythema nodosum requires a good portion of subcutaneous fat. If a generous amount of fat is present, a punch biopsy will frequently be adequate to see subcutaneous fat and the epidermal-dermal portion of the skin. If there is not a good deal of fat in the area that must be biopsied, an excisional biopsy may be preferable. To assess the follicular bulb in hair disorders, the biopsy must also penetrate to subcutaneous fat. For bullous disorders, an excision or a larger punch biopsy may be preferable to include the bulla and adjacent uninvolved tissue. The diagnosis of eosinophilic fasciitis requires examination of the superficial fascia and muscle to allow one to see the characteristic pathologic changes. It cannot be overstated that proper clinical diagnosis be used as a guide to obtain a proper specimen with characteristic pathologic appearance.

Multiple Biopsies

Several skin biopsies may be necessary for two reasons:

1. A widespread eruption presents with lesions distinctly different in clinical appearance in different locations. For a better possibility of obtaining the correct diagnosis, several lesions are biopsied (e.g., mycosis fungoides).
2. Some conditions change or develop over time so that nonspecific pathologic changes may later reveal more specific, characteristic changes.

Erythema multiforme may present in varying stages of development at the same time. Several biopsies over several months may be required before nonspecific precursor stages of mycosis fungoides demonstrate an infiltrate with Pautrier microabscesses. Conditions such as parapsoriasis and poikiloderma atrophicans vasculare may not shown pathologic changes consistent with mycosis fungoides for several months or years. Even in fully developed mycosis fungoides, some patches may not demonstrate all pathologic characteristics.

Handling and Processing of Biopsy Material

Most biopsies sent for routine processing are usually fixed in formalin and stained with hematoxylin and eosin. The amount of fixative in the biopsy container should be several times the volume of the biopsy itself. It is important, especially when it is mailed, that the specimen be completely immersed in fixative and that tight, leak-free caps are used. Usually specimens are fixed for 24 hr before processing. They are then embedded in paraffin wax and cut with a microtome. Hematoxylin and eosin are the most commonly used stains, but special stains, including immunohistochemistry, can also be performed from these blocks.

For a more rapid evaluation, frozen sections may be done. The specimen is transported either in liquid nitrogen or saline-moistened gauze. The specimen is frozen and cut in a cryostat. If therapy must be initiated quickly, as in some viral disorders and bullous disease, a frozen section biopsy may be very helpful. A second biopsy may be done for formalin-fixed, paraffin-embedded processing, since these slides are generally of better quality. Frozen sections are also helpful when checking the borders of a tumor at the time of excision (Mohs surgery).

When an infectious process is suspected, culturing and staining of biopsy material may be extremely helpful. A larger biopsy may be obtained and sectioned into segments for permanent processing and for tissue smears and culture. Material for culturing is usually placed in sterile gauze moistened with nonbacteriostatic saline or water in a sterile container. The tissue is homogenized and plated in the laboratory for appropriate cultures. The section for permanent processing may be placed in formalin as usual, and the lab can do special bacterial, acid-fast, or fungal stains.

Punch biopsies are done to obtain skin for direct immunofluorescent study. Specimens are transported in liquid nitrogen or dry ice, or an immunofluorescent transport media such as that described by Michel. Immunofluorescent staining techniques are done to identify immunoglobulins (IgG, IgM, IgA), fibrin, complement, and certain infectious antigens.

Electron microscopy is most commonly used for the study of bullous disorders, melanocytic disorders, the identification of abnormal lymphocytic cells such as in mycosis fungoides and Sézary syndrome, and in the identification of viral particles. Although it may be done on paraffin-embedded tissue, glutaraldehyde, kept cold to avoid polymerization, is a better fixative.

Fresh tissue may be preferred for some newer techniques such as gene rearrangement, PCR, HPV typing, and DNA flow cytometry. Techniques are changing rapidly and may vary from one laboratory to another. Some newer studies can still be done from fixed tissue, so it is best to check directly with the laboratory.

BIBLIOGRAPHY

Crabb WC. A concentration of 1:500,000 epinephrine in a local anesthetic solution is sufficient to provide excellent hemostasis. *Plast Reconstr Surg* 1979;63;834.

Davis TS, Graham WP, Miller SH. The circular excision. *Ann Plast Surg* 1980;4:21.

de Jong CA, Aston SJ. Propranolol-epinephrine interaction. A potential disaster. *Plast Reconstr Surg* 1983; 72:74–78.

Ho VC, Sober AJ. Pigmented streaks in melanoma scars. *J Dermatol Surg Oncol* 1990;16:663–666.

Kaye VN, Dehner LP. Spindle epithelioid cell nevus (Spitz nevus): Natural history following biopsy. *Arch Dermatol* 1990;126:1582–1583.

Lees VS, Briggs JC. Effect of initial biopsy procedure on prognosis in Stage I invasive cutaneous malignant melanoma: Review of 1086 patients. *Br J Surg* 1991;78:1108–1110.

Michel B, Milner Y, David K. Preservation of tissue-fixed immunoglobulins in skin biopsies of patients with lupus erythematosus and bullous diseases—preliminary report. *J Invest Dermatol* 1972;59:449–552.

Robinson JD. *Fundamentals of Skin Biopsy*. Chicago, Year Book Medical Publishers, 1986, pp. 21–22.

Schultz BC, McKinney P. *Office Practice of Skin Surgery*. Philadelphia, WB Saunders, 1985.

Torres A, Seeburger J, Robison D, Glogau R. The reliability of a second biopsy for determining residual tumor. *J Am Acad Dermatol* 1992;27:70–73.

Solomon AR. The transversely sectioned scalp biopsy specimen: The technique and an algorithm for its use in the diagnosis of alopecia. In *Advances in Dermatology*, Vol. 9. JP Callen, MV Dahl, LE Golitz, HT Greenway, LA Schachner, eds. St. Louis, Mosby, 1994.

13

Excision

Mark J. Zalla
*Mayo Clinic/Foundation and Mayo Medical School,
Scottsdale, Arizona*

Randall K. Roenigk
*Mayo Clinic/Foundation and Mayo Medical School,
Rochester, Minnesota*

INDICATIONS

The simple fusiform excision is the foundation of dermatologic surgery and is a tool for both diagnosis and definitive treatment. Although commonly called "elliptical excision," the term "fusiform excision" is generally preferred since an ellipse is oval, having rounded ends, rather than spindle-shaped with tapering ends. The fusiform excision provides the basis for more advanced surgical procedures such as skin flaps. Proper planning and technique ensure excellent cosmetic outcomes with minimal risk of complications.

The fusiform excision provides very high-quality biopsy specimens of lesions which may be too large or deep to be adequately sampled with shave or punch biopsy techniques. While shave and punch biopsies are often adequate for epidermal and superficial dermal lesions, excisional biopsy provides larger amounts of tissue for more thorough histopathologic examination and allows sampling of lesions located in the subcutaneous fat, fascia, and muscle. Additionally, pigmented lesions suspicious for melanoma are more appropriately removed when possible with an excisional biopsy to allow complete examination of the entire lesion and accurate determination of tumor depth.

Fusiform excision also facilitates complete removal of many benign and malignant lesions. Benign lesions in cosmetically important areas or those that would require removal with large punch biopsies (6–8 mm) often are best removed with fusiform excision to allow placement of subcutaneous/intradermal sutures and minimize risk of unacceptable scarring. Nonmelanoma skin cancer is also routinely treated with simple fusiform excision. While Mohs micrographic surgery is preferred for tumors that are recurrent, large, ill-defined, aggressive (infiltrating, morpheaform, metatypical), or in high-risk areas (nose, ears, eyelids, lips), tumors without these features may be removed by simple fusiform excision. Familiarity with tumor type and behavior helps determine the margin of excision of basal cell and squamous cell carcinoma.

PLANNING THE EXCISION

Patient Evaluation

Prior to performing any excisional procedure, preoperative evaluation of the patient must be undertaken (see Chap. 5). The evaluation includes review of pertinent past medical history (including abnormal wound healing and bleeding tendencies), current medications, allergies, and determination of pulse and blood pressure. Particular emphasis is placed on obtaining a history of infection (hepatitis, HIV, etc.), cardiovascular diseases (hypertension, prior myocardial infarction, arrhythmia, pacemaker), need for antibiotic prophylaxis (artificial joints, prosthetic valves and grafts, significant mitral valve prolapse), and use of anticoagulants, aspirin or aspirin-containing medications, nonsteroidal antiinflammatory drugs (NSAIDS), and alcohol. Because many patients do not spontaneously report the use of aspirin, over-the-counter NSAIDS, or alcohol, specific questions regarding their use are in order. The authors suggest discontinuation of aspirin and NSAIDS 1–2 weeks prior to surgery, when possible, and discontinuation of coumadin and alcohol 48 hr prior to surgery.

Anatomy

Before proceeding with any surgery, it is important to be familiar with the region's anatomy. Dermatologic surgeons need to familiarize themselves with superficial anatomy of the skin, subcutis, and superficial musculature including vascular and nervous structures. On the trunk and extremities, most excisions can be performed with little risk of exposing vital structures. Exceptions are the hands and feet, where nerves, vessels, and tendons can be exposed during the punch biopsy or excision (see Chap. 25). Even on the lower extremities, incision through a large vein can be a problem.

Many excisions are done on the face and neck where it is important to be aware of certain structures. The facial nerve (cranial nerve VII) is anterior to the ear but deep within the parotid gland before its branches bifurcate (Fig. 1). The facial nerve divides into five branches: temporal, zygomatic, buccal, marginal mandibular, and cervical. All of these branches exit the parotid gland but remain deep to muscle and are generally not affected by excision except when blocked by a field injection of anesthetic. An important exception is the superficial temporal branch and occasionally the zygomatic branch as it crosses the zygomatic arch. They are deep to superficial fascia but easily exposed. When transected, paralysis of the frontalis muscle and ptosis of the eyebrow with the risk of visual field deficits can occur.

Superficial vessels on the face that are of importance for excisional surgery include the superficial temporal artery and vein, which pass anterior to the ear and continue to bifurcate into the temporal and parietal regions (Fig. 2). These vessels should be palpated and identified prior to excision. It is also important to identify the anterior facial artery and vein as they cross the mandible superficially. They connect with the angular artery and vein that course along the nasolabial fold after anastomosing with the orbicularis oris artery, which circles the mouth and lies in the posterior third of the upper and lower lips. A branch of the angular artery courses across the nasal ala toward the nasal tip.

The superficial lobe of the parotid gland extends anterior to the lower third of the ear, covers the angle of the mandible, and is superficial to the posterior third of the masseter muscle (Fig. 3). The superficial lobe is connected to the deep lobe of the parotid, medial to the mandible, by a small isthmus. The parotid (Stenson's) duct extends anterior to the superficial lobe and courses superficially across the masseter muscle, where it may be palpated, before curving through the buccinator muscle entering the mouth adjacent to the second upper molar. There are, however, many small anastomosing ducts off the superficial lobe of the parotid and the parotid duct. Transection of parotid tissue results in salivary drainage that can be demonstrated by

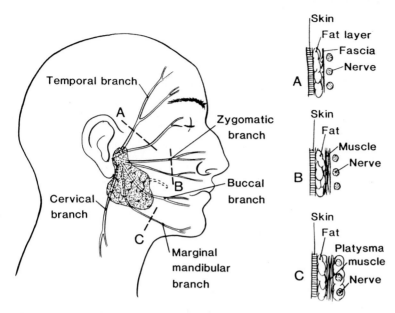

Figure 1   Distribution of the facial nerve and depths of its branches below the subcutis. (*Journal of Dermatologic Surgery and Oncology* 12(7):722–726, copyright 1986. By permission.)

measuring salivary enzymes in fluid from the surgical wound. A more simple, reliable test is to give the patient a sour food (pickle, lemon) to eat and then to observe any rapid increase in parotid secretion in the wound. Parotid secretion inhibits wound healing and can cause parotid fistulas with the skin.

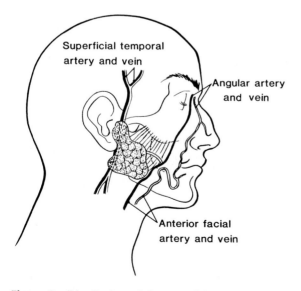

Figure 2   Distribution of the superficial vasculature of the face. (*Journal of Dermatologic Surgery and Oncology* 12(7):722–726, copyright 1986. By permission.)

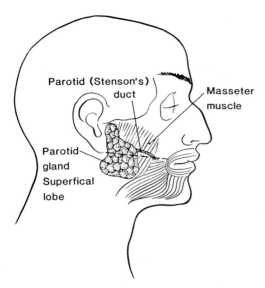

Figure 3   The superficial lobe of the parotid gland and Stenson's duct, superficial to the masseter muscle. (*Journal of Dermatologic Surgery and Oncology* 12(7):722–726, copyright 1986. By permission.)

On the neck the dermatologic surgeon should appreciate the hyoid bone, thyroid cartilage, trachea, and the sternocleidomastoid muscle (Fig. 4). All major vessels and important structures on the neck are covered by the external musculature, except the external jugular vein and the spinal accessory nerve. The external jugular vein is superficial to the sternocleidomastoid muscle until it extends deep to the fascia at the base of the posterior triangle of the neck. The posterior triangle of the neck is marked anteriorly by the posterior margin of the sternocleidomastoid, inferiorly by the clavicle, and posteriorly by the anterior margin of the trapezius muscle. When

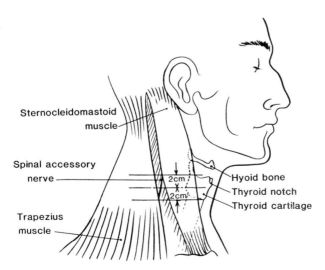

Figure 4   Superficial anatomy of the neck. (*Journal of Dermatologic Surgery and Oncology* 12(7):722–726, copyright 1986. By permission.)

the posterior triangle is exposed beneath the subcutis, the spinal accessory nerve (cranial nerve XI) can be seen coursing diagonally from behind the sternocleidomastoid muscle and entering the levator scapulae muscle beneath the trapezius muscle. Although it lies beneath fascia, it is readily visible when exposed. The spinal accessory nerve innervates the trapezius muscle. Paresthesia of this nerve results in shoulder ptosis with pain and decreased abduction.

Skin Tension Lines

One of the basic principles of excisional surgery involves proper orientation of the resulting scar. Excisions should be planned to create the least noticeable scar and not adversely affect function. This usually requires placement of scars within or parallel to the relaxed skin tension lines. Langer's lines (Fig. 5) represent relaxed skin tension lines or wrinkles that are created as a result of contraction of underlying superficial muscles, which usually occurs perpendicularly to the tension lines. Excisions made parallel to these lines create less disruption of underlying collagen fibers and are subject to less tension at the wound edges, allowing scars with higher tensile strength and less tendency to spread or hypertrophy. The resulting fine scars often blend imperceptibly into the background of tension lines, especially in patients with prominent wrinkles and when placed within major anatomic lines, such as the melolabial fold (Fig. 6a, b).

Relaxed skin tension lines become more prominent with age due to decreased elasticity of the skin, loss of subcutaneous fat, and the effects of gravity. This is particularly true of patients with chronic photodamage and of smokers. Certain regions such as the lateral margins of the chin and shoulder may have more than one set of tension lines because more than one muscle group may affect overlying skin. However, secondary wrinkle lines are caused by external factors such as sleep, accounting for vertically oriented lines on the forehead, and should not be confused with primary relaxed skin tension lines.

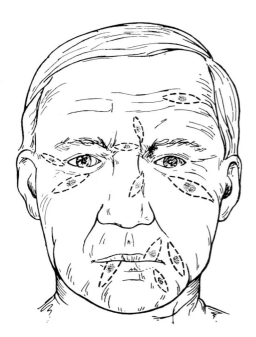

Figure 5 Lines of expression or wrinkle lines on the face. (Popkin GL, Robins P. *Workshop Manual for Basic Dermatologic Surgery.* By permission from Schering-Plough Corporation, Kenilworth, NJ.)

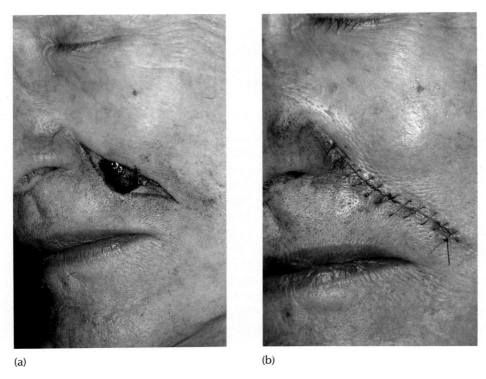

(a)   (b)

Figure 6   (a) Planned primary closure following Mohs excision. (b) Closure oriented along melolabial fold.

Since the pull of gravity on the skin may distort tension lines, determination of proper orientation of an excision should proceed with the patient in a vertical position and the extremities relaxed. Asking the patient to produce various facial expressions may accentuate tension lines, as may flexion and extension of joints (Figs. 7, 8). Pinching the skin to determine the direction

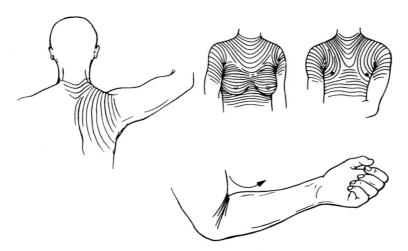

Figure 7   Tension lines on the torso and antecubital fossa. (Popkin GL, Robins P. *Workshop Manual for Basic Dermatologic Surgery.* By permission from Schering-Plough Corporation, Kenilworth, NJ.)

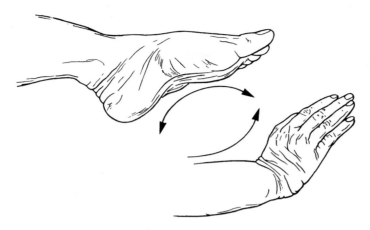

Figure 8 Tension lines on the hands and feet are more prominent when extended. (Popkin GL, Robins P. *Workshop Manual for Basic Dermatologic Surgery*. By permission from Schering-Plough Corporation, Kenilworth, NJ.)

of maximal wrinkling is also helpful. If proper orientation is not obvious after these maneuvers, the excision may be carried out in circular fashion, after which the defect will usually assume an oval configuration conforming to the proper direction of closure. The oval is then converted to a fusiform defect and closed.

Other considerations may also affect the orientation of an excision. Scars placed parallel to an underlying tendon or across a joint may cause contractures and limit range of motion. Excisions around free margins such as the eyelid or lip are usually best placed perpendicular to the free margin to avoid ectropion or eclabium. Excisions parallel to the brow on the forehead may cause permanent brow elevation.

Characteristics of the Lesion

Occasionally, the shape of the lesion determines the direction of excision. Since the final length of an excision is determined by its width, excising oval or linear lesions parallel to their long access will allow a shorter final scar length. This may or may not provide the best cosmetic outcome depending on the direction of neighboring wrinkles and location of adjacent cosmetic junction lines.

The location of the lesion also influences orientation of the excision and wound length. Lesions located near free margins are often best excised perpendicularly to the free margin to avoid distortion of the margins. Lesions located near areas of excess tissue such as the glabella, melolabial fold, preauricular cheek, and neck should be planned to utilize available excess tissue and minimize tension on wound edges. Lesions located on convex surfaces may be best excised using an S-plasty (see below) to minimize scar indentation associated with wound contraction.

Wound length is influenced by the location of a lesion in that length is in part a function of the thickness of the skin. For example, a 1-cm circular wound on the back may be closed primarily without dog ears, while the same wound on the dorsal hand may require a closure of 4–5 cm to eliminate dog ears. Skin thickness must therefore be considered when planning an excision.

Excisional biopsy of suspected malignant melanoma involves consideration of location of draining lymph nodes. If wide reexcision or lymph node dissection is anticipated, orientation of the excision should follow the direction of prevailing lymph node drainage.

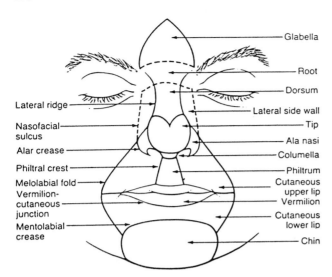

Figure 9 Cosmetic units of the central face. (Reproduced by permission from Salasche SJ, Grabski WJ. *Flaps for the Central Face*. Churchill Livingstone, New York, 1990.)

Aesthetic Considerations

The human face is composed of multiple cosmetic units and subunits (Fig. 9). These units and subunits are separated by aesthetic junction lines such as the melolabial fold, eyelid-cheek boundary, and alar groove. Excisions placed along these junction lines or within single cosmetic units may be less noticeable than excisions crossing these lines, involving more than one unit.

The standard fusiform excision has a length:width ratio of approximately 3:1, with 30° angles at the ends to avoid tissue dogears (Fig. 10). Such an excision will produce a straight scar. When a curvilinear scar would better follow relaxed skin tension lines, a "pregnant belly" type exci-

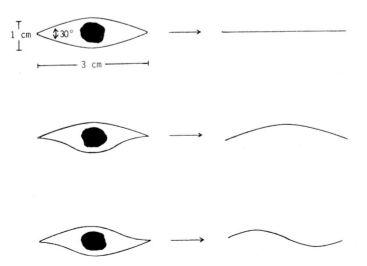

Figure 10 The standard fusiform, "pregnant belly," and S-plasty excisions, with resulting closures. (Reproduced by permission from Zalla MJ. Basic cutaneous surgery. *Cutis* 1994;53:172–186.)

sion may be used. The S-plasty is a modification of the fusiform excision that serves to increase the length of a scar and is particularly useful over convex surfaces such as the forearm. Whereas horizontal contracture of a linear scar over a convex surface leads to indentation, the increased length of the S-plasty allows for longitudinal contracture and straightening without indentation.

TECHNIQUE

Preparation

The proposed incision lines should be drawn on the skin prior to the infiltration of anesthetic to avoid distortion of skin tension lines and alteration of lesion color, which may assist in determination of appropriate margins. After cleaning the skin with 70% isopropyl alcohol, a skin-marking pen or wooden applicator dipped in gentian violet or bonnie blue may be used to mark the lines of incision. The surgical site is then anesthetized, including a wide enough margin to allow sufficient undermining, and prepared with an appropriate antibacterial scrub (chlorhexidine gluconate, povidone-iodine, etc.). All operating personnel must wear sterile gloves, and the use of masks and eye protection is recommended. The field is then draped with sterile towels and the excision carried out under sterile conditions.

Incisions

Incisions are usually made with a #15 blade, although some prefer a smaller blade such as the 6700 on a Beaver handle for small excisions. The skin is kept taut by an assistant holding two-point tension at the distal end of the incision with the operator's free hand stabilizing the proximal end. The incision is begun at the distal end with the scalpel tip perpendicular to the skin surface (Fig. 11). The blade is then lowered to a 45° angle to carry out the arc of the incision. At the proximal end, the blade is again angled perpendicularly to the surface to avoid incising beyond the tip of the excision. The remaining arc is incised similarly.

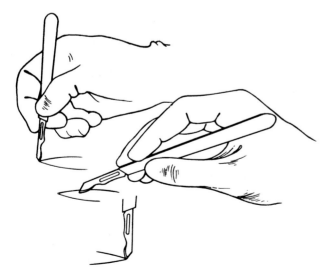

Figure 11 Proper scalpel placement when performing the initial incision. To begin, the scalpel is perpendicular to the skin; then it is angled to the beveled edge of the blade. (Popkin GL, Robins P. *Workshop Manual for Basic Dermatologic Surgery*. By permission from Schering-Plough Corporation, Kenilworth, NJ.)

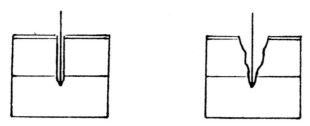

Figure 12 A fluid stroke through the dermis (left) leaves a perpendicular wound edge rather than a beveled edge created by multiple passes (right) due to retraction of incised dermis.

The incisions should be made in single, fluid strokes from tip to tip to avoid creating nicks in the skin edge, which may increase scarring. Each stroke should ideally be carried perpendicularly through the dermis into the subcutaneous fat in a single pass to avoid the inadvertent beveling of the wound edge that occurs with multiple passes (Fig. 12). A beveled incision creates a boat-shaped defect in which the deep dermal edges are closer than the epidermal edges; such an incision will leave a gap in the epidermal edge after closure unless closed under excess tension (Fig. 13).

An exception to perpendicular incisions occurs in the scalp, where both arcs are incised parallel to the hair follicles, to avoid transecting follicles and subsequent alopecia along the scar. These incisions should be carried through the subcutaneous fat and galea to reach the subgaleal plane.

Specimen Removal and Undermining

Following the incisions, the specimen is removed in a uniform plane within the subcutaneous fat using scalpel or scissors. One must be careful not to remove less tissue at the tips than in the center, or the remaining excess tissue may cause "pseudo-dog ears" (Fig. 14).

The level in the subcutis at which the lesion is removed varies by anatomic location due to skin thickness and underlying structures. Following removal, the skin is undermined around the entire defect, including the tips, at the same level as removal of the specimen. Undermining serves to minimize tension on the wound margins, facilitate wound edge eversion, and create a plate-like scar below the wound to ensure even contour without dog ears. Undermining must be carried out beyond each end of the incision to prevent tissue protrusion after closure (Fig. 15). On the face, the plane of undermining is immediately beneath the subdermal plexus in the superfi-

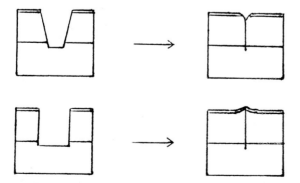

Figure 13 A beveled edge leaves an epidermal gap following closure and makes eversion difficult (above), compared to a perpendicular wound edge (below).

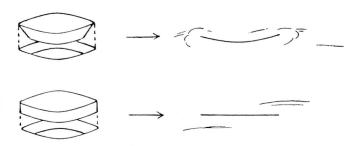

Figure 14   Removal of less tissue at the tips of the excision than in the center creates "pseudo-dog ears" (above) rather than a uniform flat closure (below).

cial subcutaneous fat. On the scalp, undermining is done in the subgaleal plane, which is easily recognized, bloodless, and avoids transection of hair follicles. On the trunk and extremities, undermining is usually done in the mid or deep subcutaneous fat superficial to muscle fascia. Undermining and suturing are best done with a skin hook rather than forceps to avoid unnecessary trauma to wound edges.

Hemostasis

Following undermining, hemostasis is obtained with electrocoagulation or suture ligature as needed. Electrocoagulation may be performed using a monopolar probe or bipolar forceps, and the patient must adequately grounded. Bipolar coagulation can also be obtained by grasping bleeding points with a forceps and touching the forceps with a monopolar probe. The operative field must be dried to allow effective electrocoagulation. To avoid unnecessary scarring, electrocoagulation should be minimized along the dermal and epidermal edge. Hemostasis of dermal capillaries is usually achieved with sutures at the time of closure. Residual capillary oozing is controlled with pressure for 5–10 min. While arterial bleeding may be treated with electrocoagulation, larger arteries should be sutured. A figure-8 ligature with absorbable suture can be secured around the proximal and distal ends of the transected artery (see Chap. 8).

Suturing

To assure optimal cosmetic results, excisional wounds are best closed in layered fashion with a buried layer of absorbable subcutaneous/intradermal sutures and a percutaneous layer, usually of nonabsorbable suture. The authors prefer polyglactin 910 (Vicryl®) subcutaneous/intradermal

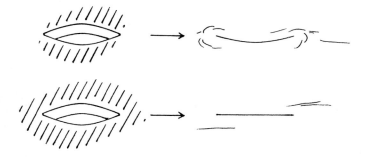

Figure 15   Inadequate undermining of the tips of the excision leaves the ends tethered and protruding after closure (above) compared to complete peripheral undermining (below).

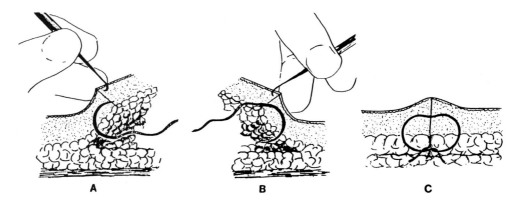

Figure 16 The buried vertical mattress suture provides eversion and prolonged support without causing suture marks. It is important to pivot the skin edge and to place the suture closes to the epidermis at a point 3-4 mm from the skin edge, and deeper in the dermis at the edge. (Reproduced with permission from Zitelli JA, Moy RC. The buried vertical mattress suture. *J Dermatol Surg Oncol* 1989;15:17–19. Copyright 1989 by Elsevier Science Publishing Co., Inc.)

sutures for facial wounds and wounds under minimal tension, while polydioxanone (PDS®) is preferred for nonfacial wounds in young patients and in areas under tension, such as the back or extensor extremities. The subcutaneous/intradermal sutures provide support and minimize spreading of the scar following removal of percutaneous sutures, when the wound has only 5% of the tensile strength of normal skin. The buried vertical mattress suture is most commonly used and provides support as well as eversion of wound edges (Fig. 16). Placement of buried sutures is usually guided by the rule of halves, such that each suture bisects the remainder of the un-closed wound. In this way, edges of unequal length can often be approximated without dog ears. When closing wounds under tension, closure may begin at either end and progress centrally, decreasing tension on the central sutures supporting the widest portion of the defect.

Ideally, closure with buried subcutaneous/intradermal sutures should provide excellent approximation of wound edge without percutaneous sutures. The epidermal edges should be free of tension and simply "fine-tuned" with percutaneous interrupted or simple running sutures (Fig. 17). Nonabsorbable sutures such as 6-0 nylon removed at 5–7 days or absorbable suture such as 6-0 fast-absorbing gut may be used for facial wounds. Nonabsorbable suture is generally preferred for trunk and extremity excisions. Wounds requiring percutaneous sutures for 10–14 days or more may be best closed with running subcuticular skin sutures to avoid risk of permanent suture marks.

Wound Dressings

Following closure, wounds are dressed with adhesive closures (e.g., Steri-Strips®), antibacterial ointment, a nonadherent dry dressing (e.g., Telfa®), gauze, and tape. Wound care with twice-daily dilute peroxide cleansing followed by antibiotic ointment is begun at 24 hr and continued for several days beyond suture removal to allow suture tracks to heal. An outer occlusive dressing such as Tegaderm® may also be applied over the remainder of the dressing and eliminates the need for wound care by the patient; this also allows for showering, swimming, etc. without fear of contaminating the wound. Additional support with Steri-strips® for several weeks following suture removal will minimize spreading of scars under tension.

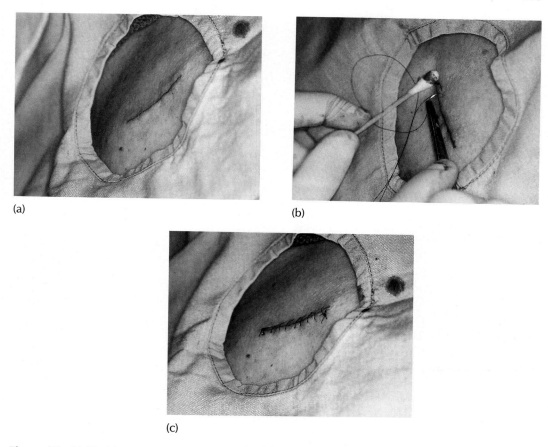

Figure 17 (a) Excision well approximated using buried sutures only. Note eversion. (b) Placement of percutaneous running suture. The needle penetrates the skin at a 90° angle (or less) from the skin edge to further enhance eversion. (c) Closed wound with everted edge.

VARIATIONS

Often a lesion cannot be excised in a traditional fusiform fashion when the natural skin tension lines or anatomic boundaries are considered. For example, when excising a lesion on the temple adjacent to the lateral canthus, the fusiform excision can be converted to an M-plasty that spares tissue and provides an excellent cosmetic result. On the dorsal surface of the hand, a 1-cm lesion may require an excision 4–5 cm long to avoid dogears. Instead of discarding that excess tissue, a modified M-plasty resembling a bilateral rotation flap can be used to spare the dogears that would be discarded and provide closure with less tension (Fig. 18a–d). The schematic in Figure 19 demonstrates that performing an M-plasty or modified M-plasty may shorten the final length of an excision from the same circular defect.

Although an excision is a basic procedure, simple modifications by the surgeon can greatly improve the cosmetic result. Lesions excised in a circular fashion can be undermined so that a variety of possible closures can be considered intraoperatively to spare the greatest amount of

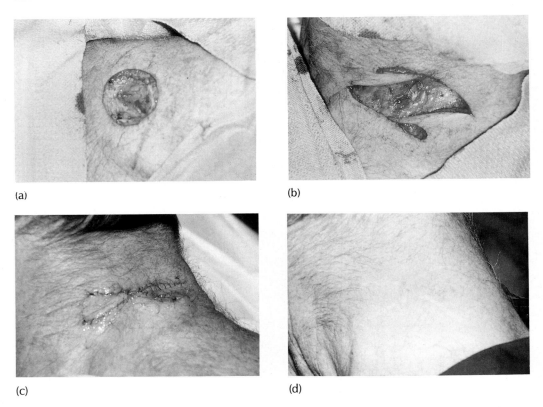

(a)

(b)

(c)

(d)

Figure 18 The lesion is removed at the level of the subcutaneous fat. The level of removal in the subcutis and subsequent undermining varies by anatomic location. (a) Circular defect. (b) Modified M-plasty incised, dog ears kept in place and rotated into the defect. (c) Sutured wound. (d) Result 1 year later.

tissue. The M-plasty and modified M-plasty, as well as some simple non–arterial-based, soft tissue flaps such as the A to T closure, are nothing more than modified excisions performed in special situations for which anatomic boundaries become obstacles, such as around the lip or nose (Figs. 20, 21a,b).

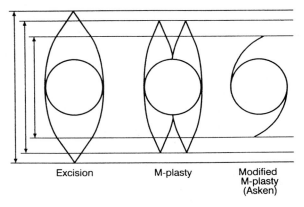

Excision   M-plasty   Modified
                                        M-plasty
                                        (Asken)

Figure 19 The final wound length of an excision can be shortened considerably with M-plasty or modified M-plasty when removing the same defect.

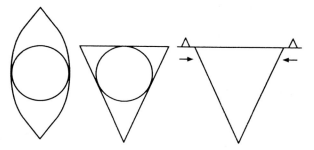

Figure 20 When excising a lesion close to an anatomic obstacle (i.e., nose, lip), converting the circular defect to an A to T advancement flap is a simple modification of the fusiform excision.

COMPLICATIONS

Fusiform excisions routinely heal with excellent results when good planning and technique have been followed. Complications are rare and include bleeding, infection, dehiscence, and necrosis (see Chap. 11). Adequate hemostasis, limiting exertion, and avoidance of aspirin, NSAIDS, and alcohol preoperatively and postoperatively (for 48 hr) will minimize risk of bleeding. Infection occurs in less than 1% of cases, and routine antibiotic prophylaxis is not necessary except in patients with conditions predisposing to endocarditis. Dehiscence is rare when subcuta-

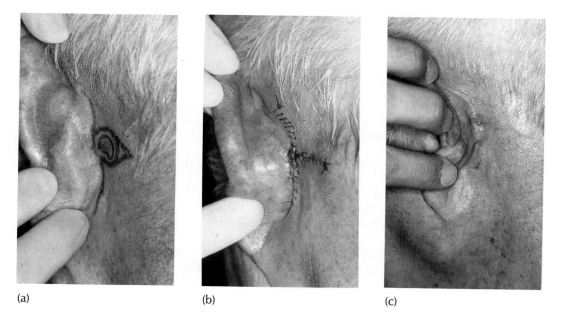

(a) (b) (c)

Figure 21 (a) Planned excision of postauricular basal cell carcinoma using A to T closure. (b) Closure with horizontal arm of T oriented along postauricular sulcus. (c) Well-healed incisions 3 weeks postoperatively.

neous/intradermal sutures are used and patients avoid stress on the wound. Necrosis is also rare when excess tension on the wound edge is avoided and undermining is done below the subdermal plexus.

BIBLIOGRAPHY

Amrein PC, Ellman L, Harris WH. Aspirin induced prolongation of bleeding time and perioperative blood loss. *JAMA* 1981;245:1825–1828.

Bennett RG. Basic excisional surgery. In *Fundamentals of Cutaneous Surgery*. RG Bennett, ed. St. Louis, CV Mosby, 1988, pp. 353–444.

Bennett RG. Cutaneous structure, function, and repair. In *Fundamentals of Cutaneous Surgery*. RG Bennett, ed. St. Louis, CV Mosby, 1988, p. 17.

Bernstein G. Surface landmarks for the identification of key anatomic structures of the face and neck. *J Dermatol Surg Oncol* 1986;12:722–726.

Bernstein L. Incisions and excisions in elective facial surgery. *Arch Otolaryngol* 1973;97:238–246.

Borges AF, Alexander JE. Relaxed skin tension lines, Z-plasties on scars, and fusiform excision of lesions. *Br J Plast Surg* 15:242–254.

Breisch EA, Greenway HT, Jr. *Cutaneous Surgical Anatomy of the Hand and Neck*. New York, Churchill Livingstone, 1992.

Courtiss EH. The placement of elective skin incisions. *Plast Reconstr Surg* 1963;31:31–44.

Cruse PJE, Foord R. The epidemiology of wound infection. A 10-year prospective study of 62,939 wounds. *Surg Clin North Am* 1980;60:27–40.

Davis TS, Graham WP III, Miller SH. The circular excision. *Am Plast Surg* 1980;4:21–24.

Hicks PD Jr, Stromberg BV. Hemostasis in plastic surgical patients. *Clin Plast Surg* 1985;12;17–23.

Jackson IT. *Local Flaps in Head and Neck Reconstruction*. St. Louis, CV Mosby, 1985.

Kneissel CJ. The selection of appropriate lines for elective surgical incisions. *Plast Reconstr Surg* 1951; 8:1–28.

Lapins NA. The cresentic ellipse revisited. *J Dermatol Surg Oncol* 1988;14:935–936.

Leshin B, McCalmont TH. Preoperative evaluation of the surgical patient. *Dermatol Clin* 1990;8:787–794.

Manstein CH, Manstein ME, Manstein G. Creating a curvilinear scar. *Plast Reconstr Surg* 1989;83:914–915.

Perry AW, McShane RH. Fine-tuning of the skin edges in the closure of surgical wounds: Controlling inversion and eversion with the path of the needle—the right stitch at the right time. *J Dermatol Surg Oncol* 1981;7:471–476.

Popkin GL, Gibb RC. Another look at the skin hook. *J Dermatol Surg Oncol* 1978;4:366–367.

Robinson JK. *Fundamentals of Skin Biopsy*. Chicago, Year Book Medical Publishers, 1982.

Salasche SJ. Acute surgical complications: Cause, prevention, and treatment. *J Am Acad Dermatol* 1986; 15:1163–1185.

Salasche SJ, Bernstein G, Senkarik M. *Surgical Anatomy of the Skin*. Norwalk, CT, Appleton & Lange, 1988.

Salzmann EW. Hemostatic problems in surgical patients. In *Hemostasis and Thrombosis: Basic Principles and Clinical Practice*. 2nd ed. Philadelphia, Lippincott, 1987, pp. 920–925.

Sharkey I, Brughera-Jones A. Evaluation of potential bleeding problems in dermatologic surgery. *J Dermatol Surg* 1975;1:41–44.

Spicer TE: Techniques of facial lesion excision and closure. J Dermatol Surg Oncol 8:551–556, 1982.

Stegman SJ. Planning closure of a surgical wound. *J Dermatol Surg Oncol* 1978;4:390–393.

Stegman SJ. Suturing techniques for dermatologic surgery. *J Dermatol Surg Oncol* 1978;4:63–68.

Swanson NA. *Atlas of Cutaneous Surgery*. Boston, Little, Brown, 1987.

Terracina JR, Wagner RF, Jr. Antibiotic use in dermatologic surgery. In *Surgical Dermatology: Advances in Current Practice*. RK Roenigk, HH Roenigk, Jr, ed. St. Louis, CV Mosby, 1993, p. 31.

Webster R, Smith RC. Cosmetic principles in surgery on the face. *J Dermatol Surg Oncol* 1978;4:397–402.

Whitaker DC, Grande DJ, Johnson SS. Wound infection rate in dermatologic surgery. *J Dermatol Surg Oncol* 1988;14:525–528.

Zitelli JA. Tips for a better ellipse. *J Am Acad Dermatol* 1990;22:101–103.

Zitelli JA. Wound healing for the clinician. *Adv Dermatol* 1987;2:243–267.

Zitelli JA, Moy RC. Buried vertical mattress suture. *J Dermatol Surg Oncol* 1989;15:17–19.

14

Scissor Surgery

Roger I. Ceilley
University of Iowa, Iowa City, Iowa

Scissors are essential instruments for performing dermatologic surgery. They are used for both cutting and blunt dissection because they allow for accurate control. Scissors stabilize tissue between the blades and allow more accurate removal of flaccid tissue than the scalpel. Scissors are designed to make use of three force vectors when cutting: closing, shearing, and torque (Fig. 1). The closing force is transferred from the operator's fingers to the shanks of the scissors, through the fulcrum to the cutting edges. Shearing force occurs when one blade slides against the other. The force that rolls the leading edge of one blade inward to the other is torque. Most scissors are designed so that a gripping motion of the right hand will combine these forces for precise cutting.

TECHNIQUE

Control of direction and accuracy depends on the stability of the tissue between the blades and the security of the operator's grip. The "tripod grip" (Fig. 2) provides the best use of the scissor's design for sharp clean cuts. The tips of the thumb and ring finger are placed through the rings of the scissors and the index finger rests on the fulcrum. This grip provides maximum control of the instrument. The thumb–index finger grip results in two-point control of the scissors and allows the cut to wander. This grip applies less torque and shearing force; therefore the blades "chew" rather than cut cleanly through the tissue.

The greatest mobility when using scissors is provided when the hand is in the pronated position. For vertical cutting, the forearm is turned midway between pronation and supination. This allows 180 degrees of pronation and 90 degrees of supination.

Scissors can be used for both sharp and blunt dissection (Fig. 3). The scissors can cut flaccid tissue better than a scalpel and provide better control of depth. Flaccid tissue is stabilized between the blades for extra control of direction. This is especially important when dissecting epidermoid cysts or undermining wound edges and flaps. The cleanest, most precise cutting

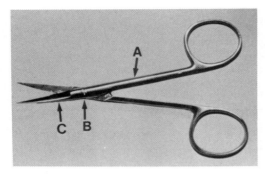
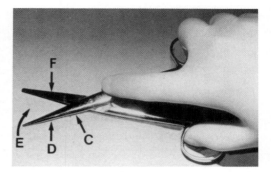

Figure 1 Scissors: (A) shank, (B) fulcrum, (C) blade. Force vectors: (D) closing, (E) shearing, (F) torque.

occurs when tissue is cut nearer to the tip of the scissors rather than close to the fulcrum. One should use just enough blade to complete the desired cut. Chewing the tissue can be avoided by taking one large bite rather than several small ones.

Blunt dissection can be performed by pushing the tips of the scissors or by spreading the scissors to separate loose subcutaneous tissue and fascia. The surgeon can alternate between sharp and blunt dissection when using a scissor with blunt tips. The rounded tips of a Metzenbaum or Stevens scissor can be used to probe the wound gently to separate subcutaneous tissue, fascia layers, and scar from normal tissue. Dissection can also be performed with or without direct vision. Blind dissection is safer with scissors than with a scalpel.

SUTURE CUTTING

Suture scissors or Metzenbaum or Gradle scissors are most useful for suture cutting. The scissor blades should be held perpendicular to the suture while the knot is kept in full view between the blades. Also, check the scissor tips to prevent damage to deeper structures. More precise cuts should be done at the outer third of the blade. Do not use fine iris scissors to cut large sutures

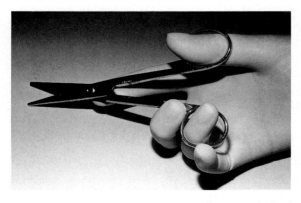

Figure 2 "Tripod grip" for most precise control of scissors.

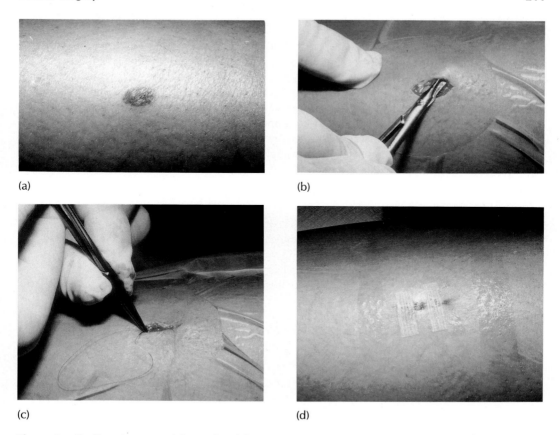

(a) (b)

(c) (d)

Figure 3 Gradle scissors used for undermining edges of wound before primary closure. (a) Congenital nevus on leg. (b) After excision, wound *edges* undermined. (c) Closing the wound with subcutaneous and subcuticular sutures. (d) Steri-Strips applied.

(especially monofilament) because this may spring the blades and damage the cutting edges. The assistant should bring the scissors into the operative field after the second hitch if three hitches are used to tie the knot. Cut the sutures deliberately and accurately. Jabbing or snapping tends to tear the suture and traumatize the tissue. When cutting sutures deep in a wound, stabilize the scissors with the other hand or on another fixed area. After cutting the suture, discard the suture material so as not to clutter the operative field and leave suture fragments in the wound.

SCISSORS

Proper instrumentation is a key factor in technically successful surgery. There are two main types of scissors: those with a straight blade and those with a curved blade.

Curved

Curved-blade scissors offer more directional mobility, visibility, and cut a smooth curve easily. They have 30–40% more mobility than straight scissors and are more useful for undermining or dissecting around epidermal cysts and lipomas.

Straight

Straight-blade scissors have greater mechanical advantage when cutting tougher tissue such as scar or nailplates. Straight scissors may be more precise for straight cutting than curved scissors.

High-quality stainless steel scissors are vital. Handle them carefully, protecting the finely honed surfaces. After use, they should be cleansed and scrubbed manually or with an ultrasonic cleaner. Before sterilizing, the instruments should be dipped in instrument milk for lubrication and to prevent rust. The choice of scissors is dictated by the function they will serve.

For most procedures performed by dermatologists, small instruments 3½–5 inches long are best. The following scissors should be considered (Figs. 4, 5).

1. Gradle: 3¾ inches, can be used for suture removal or for cutting fine, delicate tissues such as the eyelids.
2. Stevens tenotomy: straight or curved, 4½ inches, for uses similar to the Gradle.
3. Iris: straight and curved, sturdy and delicate, 4½ inches; a little bit heavier than the Stevens tenotomy or Gradle.
4. Metzenbaum: small or "baby," 5½ inches, most useful; curved blunt tips are recommended for undermining to prevent puncturing the skin surface. Larger sizes are useful for scalp reduction surgery.
5. Kilner: 5½ inches, similar to Metzenbaum but one edge is serrated.
6. Suture scissor (Spencer Litauer): used for removing sutures; do not ruin the edges of your fine tissue scissors by cutting large-caliber monofilament sutures with them.
7. General operating scissors: blunt or sharp tips, used for cutting sutures, dressing, and so on.
8. Bandage scissors: Lister.
9. Mayo: heavy-duty for cutting through thick tissue and sutures.

OFFICE PROCEDURES

Many skin lesions can be readily treated with scissors. Some lesions, like skin tags, can be removed with sharp iris scissors without anesthesia. A large number of these lesions can be snipped off in a few minutes. Elevated or pedunculated lesions such as nevi and warts are ideally suited for removal with scissors. Scissors are also important tools in removing epidermoid cysts, lipomas, punch biopsy specimens, and for excising, trimming, and undermining in more complex surgical procedures. Many nevi, seborrheic keratoses, and acrochordons can be precisely removed level with the skin. The base may then be lightly electrodesiccated or cauterized

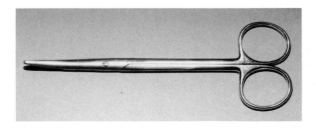

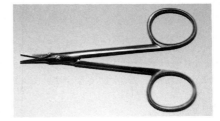

(a)   (b)

Figure 4   (a) Metzenbaum scissors. (b) Stevens scissors.

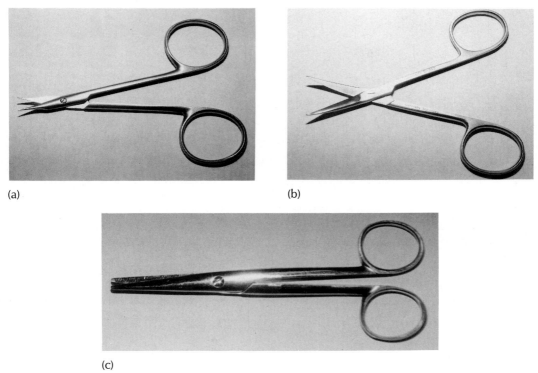

(a)

(b)

(c)

Figure 5 Types of scissors: (a) gradle; (b) iris; (c) Mayo.

to provide hemostasis. If aluminum chloride solution is used prior to cautery, less heat is needed and scar formation or hypopigmentation is less likely. In many cases, only local pressure and aluminum chloride or Monsel's solution are required. A slight elevation or irregularity of the margin is easily trimmed away. Scalpel excision with primary wound closure is preferred for active junctional nevi, dysplastic nevi, nevi with terminal hair, or for those lesions in which the diagnosis of malignant melanoma is suspected.

Cysts and Benign Tumors

Small benign lesions such as papillomas, pyogenic granulomas, fibromas, mucoceles, and small epidermoid cysts can easily be removed with scissors (Figs. 6–9). Hemostasis can be obtained by direct pressure, electrocoagulation, or by a few interrupted sutures. For larger lesions, begin the incision by stabbing one point of the scissors' blades into the edge of the lesion. Larger cysts are best treated by a small ellipse with the scalpel or by punch excision of the overlying pore attached to the skin. Then direct sharp and blunt dissection with curved scissors frees the lesion.

Warts

Filiform

These lesions may be removed with scissors usually without anesthesia. Aluminum chloride or Monsel's solution is applied to the base for hemostasis.

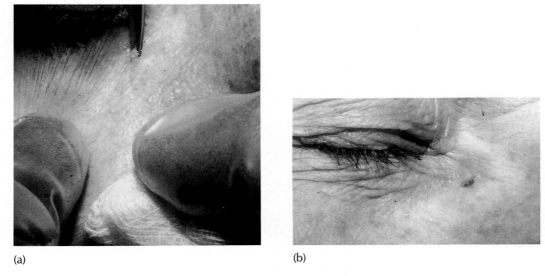

(a)   (b)

Figure 6 Removal of seborrheic keratosis with iris scissors. (a) Removal with curved iris scissors. (b) Postoperative appearance.

Periungual

Under local anesthesia, the margin between the wart and normal tissue is incised with the curved iris scissors held in the pronated position perpendicular to the skin surface. Overlying nail plate is trimmed away with a heavier scissors and the wart removed with a large-handled dermal curet. Hemostasis is obtained by pressure and application of Monsel's or aluminum chloride solution. Soft wart tissue at the margin is curetted until the gritty feel of normal tissue is obtained. The hyperkeratotic rim is then trimmed with small curved iris scissors.

Palmar and Plantar

Blunt dissection and scissor surgery are very effective for treating these often recalcitrant lesions. If carefully done, blunt dissection may atraumatically separate the wart from the dermis, mini-

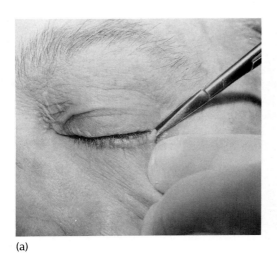
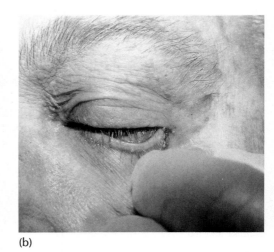

(a)   (b)

Figure 7 Removal of small epidermoid cyst. (a) Completing the cut. (b) Postoperative appearance.

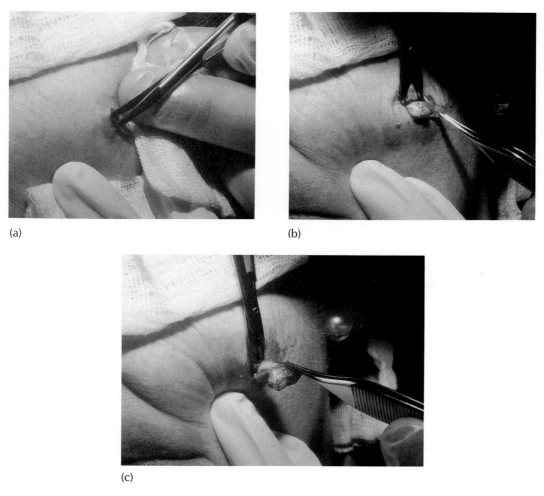

(a)

(b)

(c)

Figure 8 Removal of larger epidermoid cyst. (a) Sharp dissection around the cyst. (b) Blunt dissection by spreading the scissors. (c) Delivering the cyst.

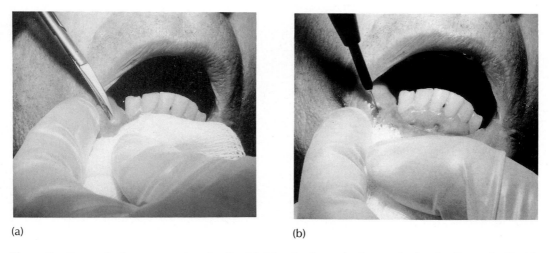

(a)

(b)

Figure 9 Removal of mucous cyst on the lip. (a) After local anesthesia, cyst is sharply dissected off with delicate iris scissors. (b) Light electrodesiccation for hemostasis.

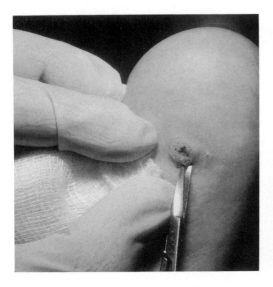

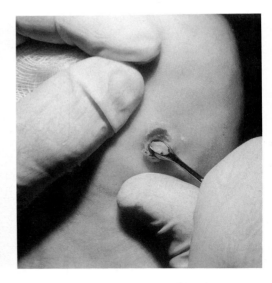

Figure 10 Scoring the surface of a hypertrophic plantar wart with iris scissors.

Figure 11 Avulsing the wart with a large curet.

mizing the risk of scarring. This technique is most effective for solitary or isolated warts of long duration (over 6 months) (Figs. 10–13).

Technique.   The area is sterilely prepped. If the wart is large or thick, it is helpful to pare the excessive stratum corneum until a sharp margin between the wart and surrounding skin is visualized. The area is then infiltrated with 1% lidocaine using a 25- to 30-gauge needle. Lidocaine with epinephrine 1:300,000 is used on the palms and soles but not on the digits. Avoid passing the needle through the wart to prevent spread along the needle tract. Injecting at an angle

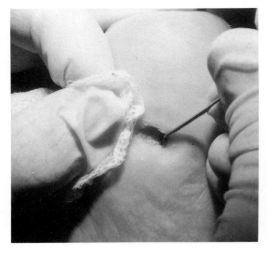

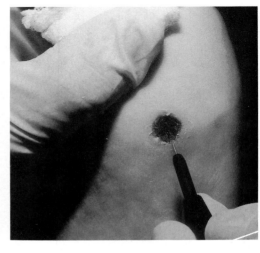

Figure 12 Curetting the margins with a small curet.

Figure 13 Light electrodesiccation of the margins.

almost parallel to the skin instead of directly perpendicular into the palm is less painful. The needle should be advanced very slowly and gently. The hyperkeratotic skin around the wart is then scored (not in the dermis) with curved scissors. The wart may then be avulsed with a large curet or separated with a nasal septum Freer elevator. Once the base is reached, the wart is carefully separated from the dermal layer. The rete ridges that make the digit dermoglyphic lines can be seen at this point. A small curet is then used to remove any remaining wart. A dull curet works well for this and ensures minimal damage to the dermis. The calloused margins of the wound are then trimmed with the scissors, and aluminum chloride or Monsel's solution is used for hemostasis and a pressure dressing is applied. Treatment of the base and margins with a low-powered, defocused beam of the CO_2 laser may also be used as the final step.

Postoperative Care. The pressure dressing is removed in 24–48 hr. The wound is cleaned with hydrogen peroxide and an antibiotic ointment applied twice daily. In 1 week, the calloused edges are trimmed, and in 21 days the wound is checked again. Early recurrences are readily removed with a small curet or frozen with liquid nitrogen. The spread of papillomavirus in patients with hyperhidrosis is well known. It is helpful to treat this to prevent recurrences.

Anogenital

Scissor excision is one of the most useful techniques in the treatment of anogenital condylomata. This technique has been utilized successfully in adults when compared to podophyllin, as reported by Khawaja, and in pediatric groups, as reported by Handley et al.

The wart is infiltrated with 1% lidocaine with epinephrine 1:300,000. This both balloons the tissue, elevating the wart, and provides hemostasis. Once blanching occurs, the warts are excised at the base with the scissors. Cutting should begin at the upper portion and finish at the most dependent area so that blood does not obscure the operative field. Hemostasis is then obtained by electrocoagulation or by suturing with an absorbant suture. Intraanal warts can be excised in the same manner using an anal retractor. If the procedure is done under general anesthesia, saline with epinephrine 1:300,000 is used to aid hemostasis. This technique is also used in conjunction with CO_2 laser surgery to "debulk" larger lesions.

SCISSOR SURGERY COMBINED WITH CRYOSURGERY

The removal of warts and nevi with the combined use of cryosurgery and scissor surgery has been reported by Biro and Brand. They recommend freezing the lesion until it is hard and easily removed with flat Converse scissors at the junction of the raised portion and the surrounding normal skin. Any raised edges are then trimmed flush and Monsel's or 35% aluminum chloride solution is used for hemostasis. They found that this helps avoid any "delling" that may be seen when local anesthesia is used or when using a scalpel or curved scissors.

BIBLIOGRAPHY

Anderson RM, Romf RF. *Technique in the Use of Surgical Tools*. New York, Appleton-Century Crofts, 1980.

Asarch RG, Ceilley RI. Cold steel surgery. *Derm Clin* 1984;2:341–351.

Biro L, Brand AJ. Cryosurgery combined with scissor excision. *J Dermatol Surg Oncol* 1983;9:185–186.

Ceilley RI. Surgical treatment of warts. In *Skin Surgery*. Epstein E and Epstein E Jr, eds. Philadelphia, W.B. Saunders, 1987, pp. 572–579.

Gollock JM, Slatford K, Hunter JM. Scissor excision of anogenital warts. *Br J Vener Dis* 1982;58:400–401.

Handley JM, Maw RD, Horner T, et al. Scissor excision plus electrocautery of anogenital warts in prepubertal children. *Pediatr Dermatol* 1991;8(3):243–245, 248–249.

Khawaja HT. Podophyllin versus scissor excision in the treatment of perianal condyloma acuminata: A pro-
 spective study. *Br J Surg* 1990;77(4):474.
Pringle WM, Helms DC. Treatment of plantar warts by blunt dissection. *Arch Dermatol* 1973;108:79–82.
Thompson JPS, Grace RH. The treatment of perianal and anal condylomata acuminata. *JR Soc Med* 1978;
 71:180–185.
Ulbrich AD. Warts: Treatment by total enucleation. *Cutis* 1974;14:582–586.

15

Electrosurgery and Electroepilation

Sheldon V. Pollack
University of Toronto, Toronto, Ontario, Canada

Roy C. Grekin
University of California, San Francisco, California

ELECTROSURGERY

Electrosurgery is one of the most important tools for performing surgery on the skin. This modality provides quick, cost-effective treatment for myriad skin lesions, both benign and malignant. In addition, electrosurgery is used as an adjunct mainly for hemostasis in surgical procedures ranging from simple excision to delicate cosmetic reconstruction.

Simply stated, electrosurgery is the destruction or removal of tissue by electrical energy. This energy, commonly in the form of high-frequency alternating current, is converted to heat as a result of tissue resistance to its passage. The heat generated is passed to the tissue while the active electrode remains "cold" throughout the procedure. This is in marked contrast to electrocautery, in which the tip is heated.

Many electrosurgical devices are available to practitioners, and over the years these have become increasingly sophisticated. A modern electrosurgical unit may generate several different electrical outputs, each with a characteristic wave form for a specific use. Use of the appropriate output allows selective incision, excision, ablation, or coagulation of tissue. If one does not fully understand the capabilities of electrosurgical devices, their efficacy may not be optimized. Moreover, the terminology is often confusing and lacks uniformity.

Historical Aspects

Electrocautery (from the Greek *kauterion*, branding iron) preceded electrosurgery. For centuries heated metal was used to cauterize (or burn) tissue to destroy microorganisms and control bleeding. Heating the metal probe was originally accomplished with fire, but later it was done with electricity, thus the term electrocautery. The metal electrode is heated by resistance to the flow of electric current. Hemostasis can be obtained even in a wet field with electrocautery, but third-degree burns may result, accounting for prolonged healing time and poor scars. It is important to realize that electrocautery with its hot electrode is not considered a form of electrosurgery.

Electrosurgery is performed with a high-frequency current through a cold electrode. Few practitioners actually utilize electrocautery today. Thus, the terms *electrocautery* and *cautery* are used inappropriately when referring to modern electrosurgical hemostasis.

In 1892 Arsene d'Arsonval noted that the application of electrical currents with frequencies greater than 10,000 cycles/sec in human subjects failed to cause neuromuscular stimulation and tetanic response. However, heat was produced. In 1899 Oudin, modifying d'Arsonval's equipment, was able to generate tissue sparks that caused superficial tissue destruction. In 1907 deForest developed the triode, a radio tube that amplified and modified electrical output. He was able to make skin incisions when the intensity of the electrical output exceeded 70 W and the frequency surpassed 2 MHz. These innovations paved the way for modern electrosurgery.

Devices

All electrosurgical instruments share certain design features required to produce electrical output suitable for electrosurgery. Power first passes through a transformer that alters the supply voltage. The current then travels through an oscillating circuit that serves to increase the frequency of the current. Finally, it enters the patient circuit.

The major difference between electrosurgical machines is the type of oscillating circuits used. The two main types of oscillating circuits most commonly used employ either a spark gap or solid-state components to increase electrical frequency. Occasionally, thermionic vacuum tubes are used. The output will vary depending on the mode by which it is produced. Some devices, for example, are useful for electrodesiccation but lack cutting current modes.

Older spark gap units such as the Birtcher Hyfrecator, the Sybron Coagulator, the Burton Electricator, and the Cameron-Miller Technicator cannot be used for electrosection. Other units including the Ellman Surgitron, Cameron-Miller 26-0345, Sybron Bantom Bovie, and Birtcher Blentome provide cutting currents by either spark gap or vacuum tube circuits. The Sybron Bovie Specialist, among others, uses solid-state circuitry (in which diodes replace spark gaps and transistors function as vacuum tubes) to produce electrodesiccation, cutting, and coagulating currents.

High-frequency power oscillators used in modern electrosurgical units produce outputs in the low radio-frequency range. They are, in effect, radio transmitters. Electrosurgical circuits differ from radio broadcasting transmitters in that the latter transmit voice- or tone-modified signals. Electrosurgical circuits are not voice-intelligence–modified (modulated). Nonetheless, any radio-frequency transmission has the potential to cause disruptive interference with other radios. Therefore, the frequency range used in electrosurgical units is assigned and regulated in the United States by the Federal Communications Commission and by similar agencies in other countries.

When looking to purchase equipment, one must first decide what function will be required from the electrosurgical unit. In general, the more expensive machines provide a variety of outputs that allow greater flexibility and can perform diverse types of electrosurgery.

How Electrosurgical Devices Work

Spark Gap Units

Electrosurgical devices consist of three major components: the power source (containing one or more transformers), the oscillating circuit (which increases the frequency), and the patient circuit (ground plate or handpiece). A transformer consists of two or more coils of wire wound onto or adjacent to each other. Electric current flowing through the first coil will induce the flow of current through the second coil (electromagnetic induction). The voltage (power) of the induced current flowing through the second coil is dependent on the number of loops in the coil. When there are fewer loops of wire on the secondary coil than on the primary coil, the voltage is lowered in direct proportion to the decreased number of turns (step-down transformer). Alternatively, if there are more loops on the secondary coil than the primary coil, the voltage will be raised (step-up transformer). A step-up transformer is used in the spark gap apparatus, while both transformers are used in the tube-type radio-frequency apparatus.

When the voltage has been raised to a suitable level for electrosurgery, it is necessary to increase greatly the frequency (oscillation) of the electric current coming from the wall outlet. This is accomplished by an electric oscillating circuit. A spark gap oscillating circuit consists of condensors (storage areas for electric energy), a small air gap (spark gap), and a transformer (inductance). The condensors (capacitors) become charged by the high-voltage current produced in the secondary coil in the high-voltage transformer. Once fully energized, the condensor releases its electrical energy across the air gap. This has an excitatory effect on the current, causing it to oscillate. Repeated charging and discharging produces a series of damped oscillating wave trains. The current then flows into a transformer (inductance coil) that sustains the oscillations and couples to the patient circuit. A blocking capacitor in the patient circuit prevents the passage of low-frequency utility supply voltage that could result in shock or burn in the event of equipment failure. Radio-frequency voltage to the patient is increased by means of an Oudin step-up transformer in the patient circuit.

Vacuum Tube Units

In vacuum tube units, a thermionic vacuum tube is used to produce oscillations instead of a spark gap. This may be a triode or tetrode tube. To illustrate how vacuum tube units work, the triode tube unit will be used as an example. The triode tube contains a plate (anode), a filament (cathode), and an interposed grid. The power source includes a step-up transformer, a step-down transformer, and a rectifier. The rectifier converts alternating current (AC) to direct current (DC).

Input current is modified, and delivered to both the plate and the filament circuits. In the case of the plate circuit, current first passes through the step-up transformer and rectifier and is delivered as high-voltage, positive direct current. The filament is heated by low-voltage current via the step-down transformer. The high voltage on the plate causes electrons to move toward it. The flow of electrons is controlled by the grid, which, when negatively charged, prevents this flow in the space between the plate and the filament. A circuit connected between the grid and the filament controls the grid polarity. All of these circuit functions and feedback phenomena combine to generate and sustain high-frequency alternating current within the oscillating circuit. This current couples into the patient circuit via appropriate capacitive and inductive control elements.

In contrast to spark gap oscillations, the oscillations produced by the vacuum tube circuit are undamped. This is due to the neutralization of internal resistance within the vacuum tube circuit and results in the generation of waves of uniform amplitude. Outputs produced in this manner have qualitative differences from those produced by the spark gap unit and may be modified for electrocoagulation, electrosection, or a combination of both.

Electrosurgical Outputs

Each electrosurgical unit produces its own unique pattern of current flow or waveform. These waveforms can be visualized on the screen of an oscilloscope or traced on an oscillograph (Fig. 1).

Oscillations produced by an electrosurgical apparatus may either be *damped* or *undamped* depending on the type of oscillating circuit used. A spark gap generator produces a *damped* wave, which consists of bursts of energy in which successive wave amplitudes gradually return to zero. This is caused by resistance from the gap. As the voltage is lowered, damping decreases and the wave trains occur closer together. Therefore, spark gap generators can be used to provide both damped and relatively undamped output that can be used for a variety of electrosurgical procedures.

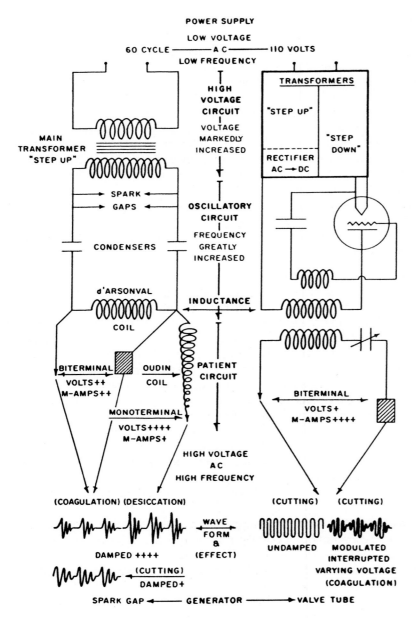

Figure 1 Diathermy circuits and wave forms produced. (Reproduced with permission from Crumay HM. Electrosurgery, ultraviolet light therapy, cryosurgery, and hyperbaric oxygen therapy. In *Dermatology*. SL Moschella, HJ Hurley, eds. Philadelphia, WB Saunders, 1985.)

Use of a thermionic tube results in a more uniform output. The valve tube circuit is able to neutralize the internal resistance responsible for the damping effect in the spark gap circuit. As a result, the amplitude of the output is unchanged. Depending on the circuitry, the output can be *partially rectified* (similar to moderately damped) or *fully rectified* (similar to slightly damped). A *filtered, fully rectified* output is essentially continuous and uniform, similar to an undamped wave. Different types of waveforms are used for different electrosurgical procedures (Table 1).

Table 1 Application of Different Wave Forms in Electrosurgery

Modality	Electrodes	Spark gap output	Tube output
Electrodesiccation	Monoterminal	Markedly damped	—
Electrofulguration	Monoterminal	Markedly damped	—
Electrocoagulation	Biterminal	Moderately damped	Partially rectified
Electrosection with coagulation	Biterminal	Slightly damped	Fully rectified
Pure electrosection	Biterminal	Undamped	Filtered, fully rectified

Electrosurgical Terminology

Several terms are often misused or poorly understood. The most commonly confused terms are monopolar, bipolar, monoterminal, and biterminal.

Monopolar and Bipolar

Monopolar and bipolar are terms used to denote the number of tissue contact points at the end of the surgical electrode. When the electrode has only one tip projecting from its end, for example, a ball electrode, it is monopolar. If two tips are used with coagulating forceps, the electrode is bipolar.

Monoterminal and Biterminal

Monoterminal and biterminal refer to the number of electrodes used during the procedure. Monoterminal means there is only one connection or electrode from the electrosurgical device delivering current to the patient. Biterminal denotes two connections or electrodes used simultaneously to deliver the current.

When biterminal electrodes are used, the second connection is often an indifferent electrode plugged into the conductive socket of the electrosurgical unit and slipped under the patient. The indifferent electrode is often referred to as a "ground plate." Rather than being a true ground, the indifferent electrode serves to complete an electrical circuit that begins and ends within the electrosurgical unit. The current from the electrosurgical device flows out of the surgical electrode, through the patient, into the indifferent electrode, and directly back to the unit's power generator.

When the indifferent electrode is not used, as in electrodesiccation, the only contact with the patient is with the surgical electrode. This is a monoterminal electrosurgery. Heat energy generated by monoterminal current is concentrated at the site of contact, producing an intense dehydrating effect on tissue. The current may have either a coagulating or volatizing effect on tissue with biterminal electrosurgery.

Clinical Applications

The simplest way to consider clinical applications of electrosurgery is by the three major capabilities of electrosurgical units. These are superficial tissue destruction (electrodesiccation), deep tissue destruction (electrocoagulation), and cutting (electrosection). Most surgical procedures done on the skin require the use of one or more of these three techniques. The objective when destroying or excising skin lesions with electrosurgery is to do so with the least amount of peripheral tissue destruction. Excessive coagulation necrosis will result in increased fibrosis. This is true of electrosurgery as well as cryosurgery or CO_2 laser surgery. Deeper penetration into the skin with a destructive modality will more likely result in an unacceptable scar. Since electrocoagulation destroys tissue more deeply then electrodesiccation, the clinician should know the histologic pathology of the lesion to be removed in order to select the correct current for treatment.

Electrodesiccation

For very superficial lesions, such as those involving the epidermis, electrosurgical destruction by electrodesiccation (from the Latin, *desiccare*, to dry up) can be done with little, if any, scarring. The damped, high-voltage current generated by spark gap units in a monoterminal (concentrative) fashion is used for electrodesiccation and electrofulguration. Low-amperage output results in superficial damage due to dehydration of the treatment site. If the electrode is held at a slight distance from the tissue, a spark is created from the electrode to the tissue. This technique, termed electrofulguration (from the Latin *fulgur*, lightning), causes very superficial destruction. This is because carbonized tissue forms an insulating barrier that protects underlying skin.

Electrodesiccation and electrofulguration are the best modalities for superficial tissue destruction. They can be used for the treatment of superficial epidermal lesions such as seborrheic keratoses, actinic keratoses, achrochordons, or plane warts. In addition, it provides hemostasis of small capillary bleeding.

To treat keratoses by this method, move the electrode slowly across the surface of smaller lesions or insert it directly into the larger lesions (Fig. 2). At a low-power setting the lesions will bubble after a few seconds as the epidermis separates from the dermis. The lesion is easily removed with a curet or simply by rubbing the site with gauze. Punctate bleeding can usually be controlled with pressure, spot electrocoagulation, or topical hemostatic agents such as aluminum chloride. Extremely small superficial lesions may be treated by fulguration, resulting in minimal adjacent tissue damage.

Local anesthesia (1 or 2% lidocaine) is used, except for small lesions that may be treated without anesthetic. The lesions should be prepared with a non–alcohol-containing skin cleanser such as Hibiclens or povidone-iodine. There is a possibility that alcohol will ignite with electrosurgery. Standard postoperative wound management is followed. Patients should be warned that delayed bleeding is possible, which can be controlled by constant direct pressure for 20–30 min. They should also be told that scarring may occur, but this is usually minimal.

Electrocoagulation

Electrocoagulation (from the Latin, *coagulare*, to curdle) uses a moderately damped (partially rectified) current applied in a biterminal manner with both concentrating and dispersing electrodes. This current has a higher amperage and lower voltage than electrodesiccation. It penetrates more deeply, potentially causing more destruction.

Electrocoagulation is useful for deep tissue destruction and surgical hemostasis. It is used for treating small, primary, uncomplicated basal cell carcinomas and squamous cell carcinomas or benign lesions such as trichoepitheliomas that extend into the dermis. The electrode is applied directly to the tissue and moved slowly across the lesion until it becomes charred. A curet is used to remove the charred tissue. When treating skin cancer, this procedure is repeated three times in an attempt to remove microscopic extensions of the tumor. A small curet is often used during the last pass to remove tiny "roots" of the tumor. Scarring is to be expected and should be considered when discussing therapeutic alternatives with the patient (Fig. 3).

Obtaining hemostasis with electrocoagulation can be achieved with either monopolar or bipolar electrodes. It is important to use a minimal exposure time and the lowest power setting possible since electrosurgical energy may be transmitted several millimeters along the vessel wall; this minimizes delayed bleeding from damaged vessels. Monopolar electrocoagulation can be used

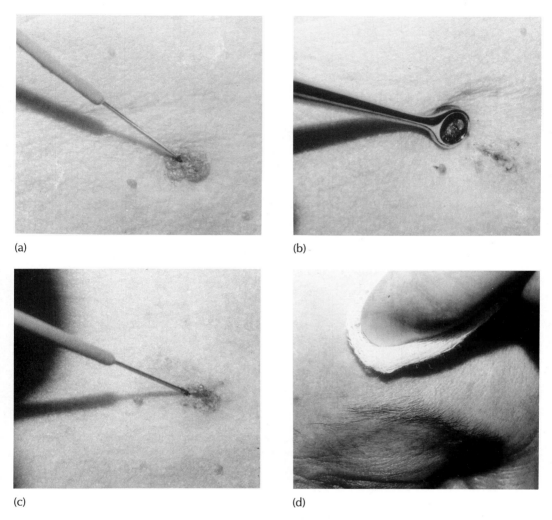

(a)

(b)

(c)

(d)

Figure 2 (a) Electrodesiccation of a seborrheic keratosis. (b) Curettage of the charred surface. (c) Spot electrodesiccation of residual bleeding. (d) Gauze is used to remove charred tissue.

by touching the electrode directly to the bleeding vessel. This may also be achieved by touching the electrode to a hemostat that has been clamped on the severed vessel. For bipolar electrocoagulation, a bipolar forceps may be used to provide more directed, pinpoint hemostasis (Fig. 4). Electrocoagulating current delivered in this latter manner will cause less adjacent tissue damage but requires a dry operative field to be effective.

Electrosection

Electrosection (cutting) is performed when slightly damped (fully rectified) current is applied in a biterminal fashion. The current has low voltage and high amperage. It vaporizes tissue, causing little lateral heat spread and peripheral tissue damage. Hemostasis and cutting occur simultaneously. The operator may perceive a slight pulsation in the handpiece, denoting a small amount of amplitude variation still present in the waveform. This slightly damped current is responsible for hemostasis.

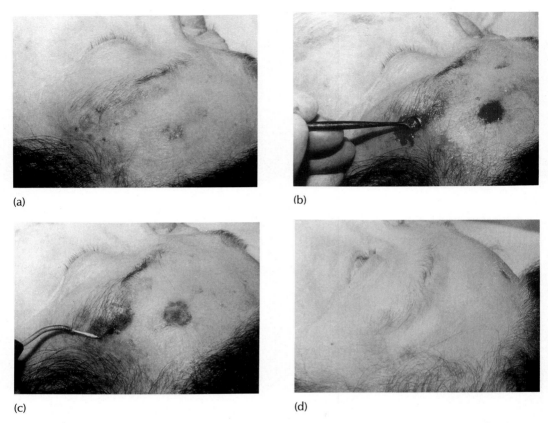

Figure 3 (a) Two superficial squamous cell carcinomas on the forehead. (b) Curettage. (c) Electroco-agulation of treatment sites. (d) Hypopigmented scar 1 year postoperatively.

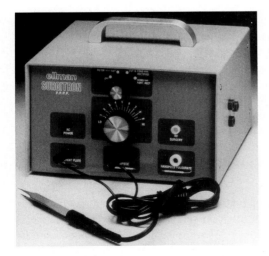

Figure 4 Bipolar forceps attached to the electrosurgical apparatus provides pinpoint hemostasis.

Pure cutting can be done using an undamped tube current (filtered, fully rectified); this minimizes the amount of lateral heat spread and causes vaporization of tissue without hemostasis. When electrosection is performed using filtered, fully rectified current, spot electrocoagulation can be achieved by changing to the partially rectified current.

Electrosection can be used for electrosurgical excision or incision in an effortless, rapid fashion. Virtually no manual pressure is required by the operator. A narrow straight electrode is used and applied to the tissue in brisk, continuous strokes. The difference between electrosection and an incision with a scalpel is readily apparent. The electrode passes through tissue smoothly, like a hot knife through butter. If sparking occurs during incision, the power setting is too high; if the electrode drags, the power setting is too low.

Slightly damped currents cause some char at the margins of excised tissue. This can be minimized by the surgeon using smooth, rapid strokes. In addition, vacuum tube units tend to provide outputs that are less destructive to adjacent tissue. However, when a specimen is required for histopathologic analysis, the filtered current should be used since this will not cause significant electrosurgical artifact. The novice in electrosection should develop technical skills by practicing on beef steak.

The major advantage of electrosection over scalpel surgery is that hemostasis is achieved as the incision is made. However, large-gauge blood vessels (over 2 mm in diameter) may require additional spot electrocoagulation. Training and familiarity with electrosectioning may expand one's use of this technique where scalpel surgery is usually preferred.

Electrosection is extremely useful for relatively bloodless excision of large, bulky lesions such as acne keloidalis nuchae and rhinophyma, in which the defect is allowed to heal by second intention (Figs. 5,6). Electrosurgery has also been used for smaller excisions in which primary closure may be done with no impairment of wound healing. In addition, this modality has been used without complication to create skin flaps, with excellent results.

Potential Hazards of Electrosurgery

Electrosurgery and Cardiac Pacemakers
Fixed rate (asynchronous) pacemakers stimulate the heart at a regular rate, independent of the intrinsic heart rate. They are resistant to external electromagnetic interference such as that caused

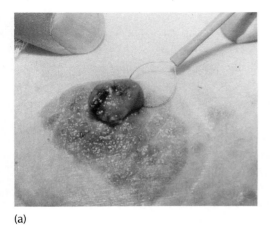
(a)

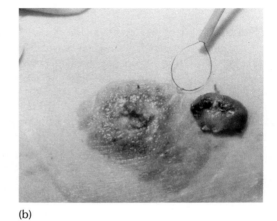
(b)

Figure 5 (a) Electrosection of an exophytic portion of a seborrheic keratosis with a loop electrode. (b) No bleeding due to the coagulating current.

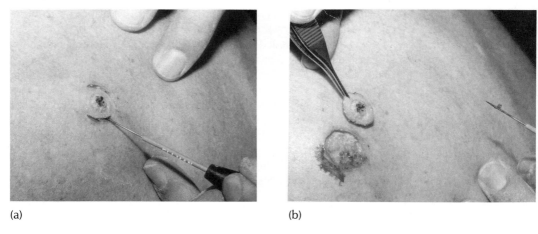

(a)   (b)

Figure 6 (a) Excision of a keratoacanthoma by electrosection. (b) The lesion is removed without significant bleeding. There will be some histologic artifact at the base of the lesion due to coagulation.

by electrosurgery. However, in recent years fixed-rate pacemakers have largely been replaced by noncompetitive demand pacemakers, which use a sensor to detect the heart's spontaneous rhythm. Triggered electrical impulses are sent to the heart when the spontaneous rhythm is slower than the preset pacemaker rate. The most commonly used ventricular-inhibited pacemaker is suppressed when impulses from normal ventricular activity are received. If no ventricular activity is detected after a preset interval, it fires at a fixed rate. Since this type of pacemaker is completely inhibited by sensed interference, asystole could occur if a patient has no spontaneous rhythm and electrical interference is prolonged. Because safety factors are built into modern units, including improved shielding and rejection circuits, magnetic and radiofrequency fields rarely cause clinical problems. Nevertheless, electrosurgery is best avoided in particularly unstable cardiac patients and for treatment of skin lesions overlying a pacemaker.

Fire

There is a risk of fire or explosion if electrosurgical procedures are conducted in the presence of alcohol, oxygen, or bowel gases (methane). Care should be taken to be certain that the operative site is free of alcohol residue. Oxygen is usually not a problem except in the operating room setting. Bowel gases are highly flammable! Use care in the perianal region.

Microorganism Transmission

The potential exists for transmission of microorganisms either via electrode or via smoke plume inhalation. Neither possibility has been investigated in sufficient depth to yield conclusive results. Practitioners should minimize the risk of possible electrode transmission by considering the use of disposable or sterilized electrodes. Adapters are available that allow disposable metal hypodermic needles to be used as electrodes.

With electrosection and extensive electrocoagulation, as with CO_2 laser surgery, a smoke plume is generated. Intact viral particles have been recovered from smoke plumes from both procedures. A smoke evacuator, with the intake held not less than 2 cm from the operative site, is indicated for extensive electrosurgical procedures in which a smoke plume is generated, particularly those involving lesions of viral origin. A variety of smoke evacuation systems is commercially available, and most include viral filters with a filtration to 0.02 μm or less.

ELECTROEPILATION

Dr. C. E. Michel is credited with the first successful use of electricity for the permanent removal of hair. In 1875 he reported the removal of eyelashes in trichiasis using direct (galvanic) current. In the 1920s, Bordier used a high-frequency alternating current to remove unwanted hair. This technique was considerably faster and generally replaced galvanic current by the 1940s. Today, depending on the technician and the caliber of hair being treated, either alternating current or a combination of alternating and direct current ("the blend") is used.

The word *electrolysis* is used by most people as a generic term to mean the electrical destruction of hair, technically, the use of direct current for hair removal. Hair destruction with an alternating current is due to heat and is designated *thermolysis*. The term *electroepilation* suggested by Richards et al. will be used as the general term for electrical hair removal.

Electroepilation is rarely performed by physicians. However, it remains the most effective modality for permanent removal of unwanted hair. Thus, it is important for the dermatologist to understand electroepilation in order to counsel patients properly.

Electrolysis

Electrolysis is done with direct current to create a destructive chemical reaction at the hair root. The negative electrode (anode) is inserted into the hair follicle. The positive electrode (cathode) is a moistened pad held in the patient's hand. When direct current is applied, a chemical reaction at the tip of the anode causes the production of sodium hydroxide (lye). The sodium hydroxide acts as a caustic to destroy the hair root. The process is slow and may take from 30 sec to 1 min.

Stainless steel needles measuring 0.002–0.005 inches in diameter are used for both electrolysis and thermolysis. The needle tips are rounded to decrease the likelihood of puncturing the hair follicle. Needle length depends on the size of the hair and the area being treated. Insertion of the needle should be parallel to the hair shaft and is performed under magnification. Excessive force should be avoided so the hair follicle is not punctured. The papilla has been reached when gentle resistance is encountered; the current is then turned on with a foot pedal. Gentle traction is applied to the hair with fine tweezers. When root destruction is complete, the hair may be lifted easily from the follicle.

Electrolysis takes longer than thermolysis. It is said by some technicians to be less painful, less likely to scar, and to result in a higher percentage of permanent hair destruction. However, this is probably technique dependent and because the technique is so tedious, it has been replaced by thermolysis or the blend.

Thermolysis

Thermolysis relies on heat to cause hair destruction. A high-frequency (13.56 MHz) alternating current is used. The generated heat is a result of tissue resistance to the flow of current. The current can be applied by the "slow" (manual) technique or the "flash" technique. A lower heat is used over 3–10 sec in the slow technique. Gentle traction of the hair allows the operator to determine when destruction is complete. The flash technique uses a higher heat delivered by a preset timer on the machine for less than 1 sec. Several pulses may be necessary to cause hair root destruction. Theoretically, the flash technique is less painful. Success rates have not been critically evaluated between the two delivery systems.

The technique of needle insertion is the same as for electrolysis. A hand-held electrode is not required since the patient is not included in an electrical circuit. The speed of thermolysis allows for treatment of much larger areas over a shorter time period. For this reason, it has replaced electrolysis as the preferred manner of electroepilation.

The Blend

The blend was developed in the 1940s in an attempt to take advantage of attributes of both electrolysis and thermolysis. It was hoped that by combining both currents an apparatus could be developed with the speed of thermolysis and the efficacy of electrolysis. The blend is slower than thermolysis but may offer some advantages in hair root destruction rate, particularly for coarser hairs.

Side Effects

Thermolysis and the blend are more painful than classical electrolysis and the risk of scarring and hair regrowth may be higher. However, highly motivated patients generally tolerate the pain and are treated with 30- to 60-min sessions once or twice weekly. Recent claims by some manufacturers state that computerization of their electroepilation equipment results in less painful hair removal. A certain amount of energy is required to successfully destroy the hair root, and it is doubtful whether computerized delivery of this energy will lessen the associated pain. Use of EMLA topical anesthetic under occlusion for 1–2 hr pretreatment has decreased the pain in some patients. Some electrologists work with physicians who can perform regional anesthesia for sensitive facial areas.

Scarring is a real risk and is operator dependent. Generally when this occurs it presents as punctate or icepicklike depressed lesions. In some cases small hypertrophic papules may be present. Most states do not regulate or certify electrologists. It is therefore very important to choose an operator carefully.

Hair regrowth has been reported at between 15 and 50%. This is also technique dependent. Regrowth may be related in part to the hair cycle. Hairs treated while in telogen phase may not experience root destruction. Some electrologists recommend shaving 2 days pretreatment so that only actively hairs will be apparent.

There may be varying degrees of erythema and edema shortly after the procedure. Post-inflammatory hypo- and hyperpigmentation have been reported. The theoretical risk of infections, both local and systemic, exists, but proper skin cleansing helps prevent this problem. It seems to be idiosyncratic in that some patients are more prone to develop folliculitis than others. Use of an antibacterial cleanser such as chlorhexidine before and after treatment may reduce this risk. Disposable needles are now the norm in the practice of permanent hair removal.

Home Use Devices

Several devices have been marketed for self-electroepilation. Those using tweezers have been found by the Food and Drug Administration to be no more effective than plucking. A hand-held electrolysis unit is available. The risk of pitted scarring and pain renders it unsatisfactory as a method of electroepilation, especially when used by unskilled operators.

BIBLIOGRAPHY

Electrosurgery

Bennett RG. *Fundamentals of Cutaneous Surgery*. Philadelphia, WB Saunders, 1987, pp. 553–590.

Blankenship ML. Physical modalities. Electrosurgery, electrocautery, and electrolysis. *Int J Dermatol* 1979; 18:443–452.

Broughton RS, et al. Electrosurgical fundamentals. *J Am Acad Dermatol* 1987;16:862–867.

Crumay HM. Alternating current: electrosurgery. In *Physical Modalities in Dermatologic Therapy*. H Goldschmidt, ed. New York, Springer-Verlag, 1978, pp. 203–227.

Jackson R. Basic principles of electrosurgery: A review. *Can J Surg* 1970;13:354–361.

Pollack SV. *Electrosurgery of the Skin*. New York, Churchill-Livingstone, 1991.

Popkin GL. Electrosurgery. In *Skin Surgery*. E Epstein, E Epstein, Jr, eds. Philadelphia, WB Saunders Co., 1987, pp. 164–183.

Sawchuk WS, Weber PJ, Lowy DR, Dzubow LM. Infectious papillomavirus in the vapor of warts treated with carbon dioxide laser or electrocoagulation: Detection and protection. *J Am Acad Dermatol* 1989; 21:41–49

Sebben JE. *Cutaneous Electrosurgery*. Chicago, Year Book Medical Publishers, Inc., 1989.

Electroepilation

Bordier H. Nouveau traitement de l'hypertrichose par la diathermie. *Vie Med* (Paris) 1924;5:561–562.

Hinkel AR, Lind RW. *Electrolysis, Thermolysis and the Blend: The Principles and Practice of Permanent Hair Removal*. Los Angeles, Arroway Publishers, 1968.

Michel CE. Trichiasis and districhiasis: Reflections upon their nature and pathology with a radical method of treatment. *St. Louis Cour Med* 1879;1:121–144.

Richards RN, McKenzie MA, Meharg GE. Electroepilation (electrolysis) in hirsutism. *J Am Acad Dermatol* 1986;15:693–697.

Wagner RF, Tomich JM, Grande DJ. Electrolysis and thermolysis for permanent hair removal. *J Am Acad Dermatol* 1985;12:441–449.

16

Suturing Techniques

Clifford Warren Lober
University of South Florida College of Medicine, Tampa, Florida

The fundamental purpose of using sutures to close wounds is to provide physical support to tissue during the early phases of wound healing. Sutures are used to eliminate dead space in subcutaneous tissues, to minimize tension that causes wound separation, and to coapt opposing edges of the wound gently. Good suturing technique cannot be substituted for basic surgical technique, such as correct wound placement with respect to relaxed skin tension lines and adequate undermining. Other factors, such as the presence of systemic diseases and the selection of suture material, also influence the ultimate surgical outcome. The surgeon must be aware of alternative methods of wound closure that may be used in conjunction with or as a substitute for sutures, such as the use of staples, tape strips, or laser skin "welding."

The specific technique used to close a given wound will depend upon the force and direction of tensions on the wound, the thickness of the tissues to be opposed, and anatomic considerations, such as the presence of vital structures (e.g., eyes) or landmarks (e.g., vermilion border of the lips). Each wound is unique, and the surgeon must use his or her judgment to determine the most advantageous suture technique for each situation.

SQUARE KNOT

The square knot is the fundamental knot used in cutaneous surgery. When properly placed, it will lie flat on the skin surface and maintain its position without slipping. It is relatively easy to construct and may be placed expediently.

To tie a square knot, the surgeon begins by taking out the slack present in the long end to be tied (that to which the needle is attached). The needle holder is then brought across the wound from the opposing shorter end toward the longer end and, with the needle holder in closed position, is looped twice around the long end of suture. The needle holder is then opened slightly, the short end of suture is grasped and pulled through the two loops, and the surgeon crosses his hands across the wound and teases the double loops onto the cutaneous surface. The loops should be placed on the skin surface gently and should not be under significant tension. The needle holder is then released and, in closed position, looped once around the long end of suture. It is then brought across the wound toward the shorter side of suture, which is subsequently grasped and pulled through the loop. The long end of suture will then be on the opposite side of the wound. The single loop is then teased into position on top of the previously placed double loops. This loop should be placed securely and may be used to adjust the tension of the underlying double loops as needed. The needle holder is then released and a second single loop of suture is constructed exactly as the first single loop was performed, except that the surgeon crosses his hands across the wound so that the second single loop will lie flat. This loop should be placed securely to assure that the knot does not slip. The final configuration of the square knot is shown in Fig. 1.

It is occasionally necessary to modify the basic surgical square knot. If, for example, significant tension exists where a square knot is placed, it may be necessary to place another single or double loop of suture to secure the knot. Alternatively, many surgeons elect to use only one single loop of suture instead of two loops to secure the initial double loops into position when closing wounds in areas such as the eyelids or genitalia.

SIMPLE INTERRUPTED SUTURE

The simple interrupted suture is the most fundamental technique of wound closure used in cutaneous surgery. It can be used to approximate large amounts of tissue when it is placed widely and deeply or for relatively fine approximation of tissue when it is placed close to wound edges and more superficially. By altering the depth or angle of the needle on one or both sides of a wound, one can use this technique to coapt wound edges of uneven thickness or make adjustments in tension.

To place a simple interrupted suture properly, the needle enters one side of the wound and penetrates well into the deep dermis or subcutaneous tissue (Fig. 2). As the needle goes deeper into the tissue, it veers slightly away from the wound edge so that it encompasses a larger volume of tissue deeper in the wound. The needle is then passed through the subcutaneous tissue to the opposing side of the wound. As it is passed through the opposing ends of the wound, the needle exits closer to the wound edge so that the final configuration of the suture is flask-shaped. A square knot may then be used to secure the suture on the skin surface.

The principal disadvantage of single interrupted sutures is that they tend to leave a series of cross-hatched linear scars on the skin surface that resemble railroad tracks. This is minimized

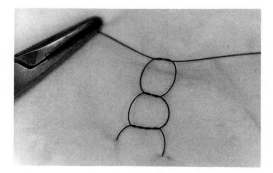

Figure 1   The final configuration of the square knot shows the initial placement of two loops of suture material followed by two single layers of one loop of suture.

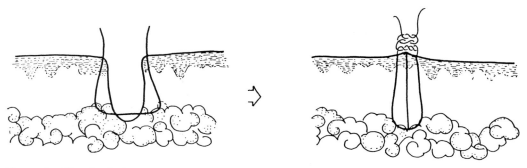

Figure 2 The simple interrupted suture, when properly placed, encompasses a greater bulk of tissue in the depth of the wound than it does more superficially. This results in eversion of the wound edges.

by using proper basic surgical technique (e.g., undermining) and subcutaneous sutures to reduce wound tension. Removing sutures as early as possible further lessens scarring. Epidermal cells begin to migrate down suture tracts approximately 5 days after sutures have been placed.

Interrupted sutures have a tendency to cause wound inversion if they are not placed correctly. Wound inversion is usually accentuated when the suture encompasses a larger bulk of tissue close to the epidermis than it does deeper in the dermis (Fig. 3). The suture effectively squeezes the epidermal edges of the wound downward. Wound inversion is minimized by placing suture in the flasklike configuration.

Placing numerous interrupted sutures may be time consuming when larger wounds are involved. Although small biopsy wounds (2–6 mm) created with circular punches are easily closed with a few interrupted sutures, larger fusiform wounds take significantly longer to close.

VERTICAL MATTRESS SUTURES

Mattress sutures are used to close dead space and provide strong support for wound closure. Vertical mattress suturing is one of the best techniques available to ensure eversion of wound edges and minimize significant wound tension simultaneously. Several vertical mattress sutures

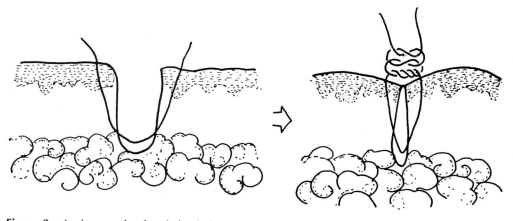

Figure 3 An incorrectly placed simple interrupted suture causes the edges of the wound to invert.

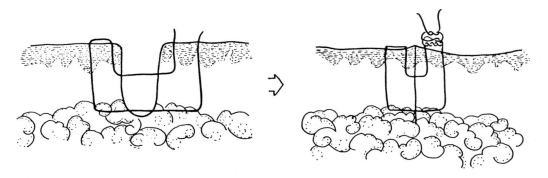

Figure 4   The vertical mattress suture is used to close dead space, thus minimizing wound tension and everting wound edges.

can be placed to close dead space, minimize wound tension, and evert the edges of a wound while interrupted sutures are placed in between to ensure finer wound edge approximation and better cosmesis.

Although vertical mattress sutures may be placed anywhere on the body, some surgeons believe that they should not be used on the face, especially when buried sutures are used to close the subcutaneous tissues. Other surgeons avoid the use of buried sutures in the face and favor vertical mattress sutures. Therefore, the use of vertical mattress sutures on the face depends upon the surgeon's preference.

The vertical mattress suture is started 0.5–1.0 cm lateral to the wound margin, with the needle inserted toward the depth of the wound to close dead space (Fig. 4). The greater the tension on the wound edge, the wider the insertion of the needle. The needle is then passed through the deep tissue to the opposing wound edge, where it exits the skin on the opposing side equidistant to the insertion. The needle is then reversed in the needle holder, and the skin is penetrated again on the side through which the suture just exited but closer to the wound edge. It is passed more superficially to the opposite side, exiting close to the wound margin. This portion of the vertical mattress suture is usually placed within 1–3 mm of the wound edge.

Placing vertical mattress sutures is time-consuming. Both the near and far skin penetrations should be equidistant from opposing wound edges. The wound is then gently teased closed to obliterate dead space and evert the epidermal edges of the wound properly. Improper placement will cause wound inversion, uneven tension, and increasing scarring. Minimal scarring depends primarily on decreased wound tension by using proper surgical technique (e.g., undermining) and removal of the sutures as early as possible, as in the case of single interrupted sutures.

If the wound is under significant tension, it is not always possible to remove vertical mattress sutures early to avoid wound dehiscence. When leaving vertical mattress sutures in the skin for prolonged periods of time, bolsters made of cardboard, rubber, or plastic may be placed between the suture and the skin. This will minimize direct contact of the suture with the epidermis. This contact can cause necrosis when postoperative edema increases pressure on the suture. Sutures can strangulate deeper tissues, especially when under significant tension. Excessive pressure at the depth of the wound may result in ischemic necrosis that is clinically evident as weak points in the healed wound. It is important to emphasize the importance of minimizing wound tension prior to the placement of mattress sutures.

NEAR–FAR VERTICAL MATTRESS SUTURES

The near–far vertical mattress suture is a modification of the standard vertical mattress suture (Fig. 5). Begin near the wound edge (1–3 mm), passing the needle into the deeper aspect of the opposing side, and exit through the epidermis wide to the incision (0.5–1.0 cm). Reverse the needle, and reenter the skin near the wound edge (1–3 mm) of the side just exited, and repeat the same procedure exiting wide to the initial penetration (0.5–1.0 cm). This technique is used primarily when one is trying to elevate the deeper tissues of the wound as well as to evert the epidermis.

HALF-BURIED VERTICAL MATTRESS SUTURES

This modification of the vertical mattress suture does not cause as much scarring as standard vertical mattress sutures, since it does not penetrate the cutaneous surface on one side of the wound. However, it is also not capable of relieving as much wound tension as a standard vertical mattress suture. Nevertheless, it usually closes more dead space and is stronger than a single interrupted suture. It is particularly useful in areas such as the face and along hairlines where suture marks can be camouflaged by hair.

The placement of a half-buried vertical mattress suture is similar to that of a vertical mattress suture, except that instead of exiting the wound on the opposing side, the needle is passed through the deeper tissue and exits the wound on the side of initial entry only (Fig. 6). Therefore, suture material does not contact the skin surface on one side of the wound.

HORIZONTAL MATTRESS SUTURES

Horizontal mattress sutures are useful for minimizing wound tension, closing dead space, and facilitating wound edge eversion. This may also provide significant hemostasis but should not be used primarily for this purpose. These sutures are quite useful for the initial placement of larger flaps, especially those that may be under a significant amount of tension. The horizontal mattress suture may be placed prior to using interrupted sutures on a wound edge.

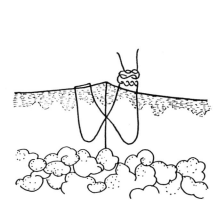

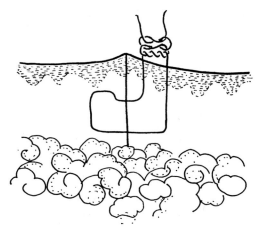

Figure 5 The near–far vertical mattress suture is useful for elevating deeper tissue and closing dead space.

Figure 6 The half-buried vertical mattress suture causes less cutaneous scarring than the standard vertical mattress suture.

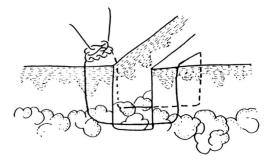

Figure 7   The horizontal mattress suture, like the vertical mattress suture, closes dead space, reduces wound tension, and everts wound edges. (Modified and reproduced with permission of Swanson NA. *Atlas of Cutaneous Surgery*. Boston, Little, Brown, 1987.)

To place a horizontal mattress suture, penetrate the skin 5–10 mm from the edge of the wound (Fig. 7). The needle is then passed dermally or subcutaneously toward the opposing wound edge where it enters at the same level in the subcutaneous or dermal tissue. Exit the opposing wound edge through the epidermis equidistant from the insertion. Reenter the skin on the same side at the same distance from the wound edge but several millimeters laterally. The needle is then passed dermally or subcutaneously to the side of initial penetration.

As in the case of vertical mattress sutures, horizontal mattress sutures may cause strangulation of underlying tissue if they are placed in wounds subject to excessive tension. Tissue hypoxia and necrosis may result in poor wound healing. Protective bolsters are useful to avoid sutures on the skin surface cutting into the skin in the presence of postoperative edema.

TIP STITCH

The tip stitch is a modification of the horizontal mattress suture in which half of the suture is buried. It is used to secure the tip of skin flaps without compressing the epidermal tissue to avoid ischemic necrosis. In the case of a single flap, the skin is initially penetrated on the side of the wound to which the flap is to be attached (Fig. 8). The needle is passed dermally or subcuta-

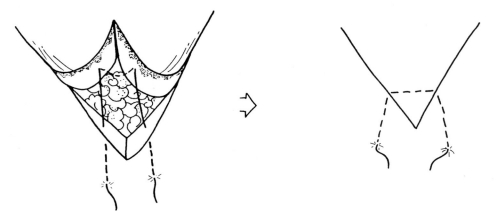

Figure 8   The tip stitch is a modification of the horizontal mattress suture.

neously toward the flap tip. It penetrates the flap tip of the dermis. The flap tip is gently positioned so that the needle can be passed along the same plane, allowing entry and exit at the same level of the dermis. The needle reenters the attachment site of the skin, still in the same dermal plane. It is passed through the skin and tied.

RUNNING SUTURE

Use of the simple running suture is a rapid way to close wounds in which the opposing edges are of approximately equal thickness and in which little or insignificant tension or dead space exists. It is useful on the eyelids, ears, and the dorsa of the hands or may also be used to secure the edges of a full or split-thickness skin graft. Running suture may be used in conjunction with subcutaneous sutures in other areas of the body. The primary advantage of the running suture is its relative ease and speed of placement.

The running suture is initiated by placing a simple interrupted suture at one end of the wound. This is tied but not cut. Simple sutures are placed down the length of the wound, repenetrating the epidermis and passing dermally or subcutaneously (Fig. 9). Tension along the suture must be adjusted continuously so that it is evenly distributed along the length of the wound. It is important to space each interval of the running suture evenly. The suture is terminated by placing a single knot between the suture material as it exits the skin at the end of the incision with the last loop of suture placed.

Simple running sutures are easily and rapidly placed. However, there is a tendency for the wound to pucker if the skin is thin or excessively loose. Furthermore, it may be difficult to adjust tension using a continuous suture as compared with interrupted sutures.

RUNNING LOCKED SUTURE

This modification of the running suture is useful for wounds closed under a moderate amount of tension or for those with regular thick edges and minimal tendency for inversion. It is particularly useful on the scalp, forehead, and back.

To place the running locked suture, begin in the same manner as for placement of simple running sutures. Instead of reentering the skin following each loop, the needle is passed through the preceding loop of suture material so that it locks into place (Fig. 10).

The running locked suture is easily and expediently placed. It provides greater strength than the simple running suture but has a greater tendency to cause strangulation of the deeper tissues. It is more difficult to adjust tension along the wound once a locked suture is placed.

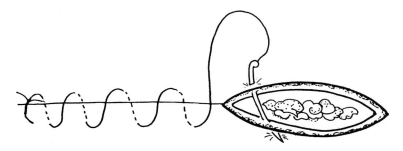

Figure 9 The running suture provides an efficient means of closing wound edges of approximately equal thickness if no significant tension is present.

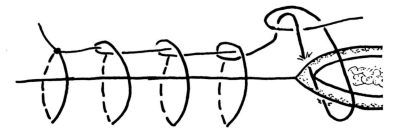

Figure 10 The running locked suture is useful for closing wounds under a moderate amount of tension.

RUNNING HORIZONTAL MATTRESS SUTURE

The running horizontal mattress suture enables one to close wounds expediently under a moderate degree of tension. It is basically a modification of the simple running suture. Instead of crossing over the wound prior to reentering the skin, the running horizontal mattress suture is done by reentering the skin on the same side through which the suture material is exited (Fig. 11).

INTERRUPTED SUBCUTANEOUS SUTURES

It is often difficult to avoid closing wounds under significant tension even when proper surgical technique is used. In certain areas of the body, such as the back and lower legs, wounds routinely enlarge due to constant tension on the skin in these areas. It is in these areas that placement of interrupted subcutaneous and dermal sutures is of considerable importance to minimize wound tension.

To place interrupted sutures in the subcutaneous and dermal tissues, the needle is inserted in the undermined wound edges close to the base of the wound (Fig. 12). It is then passed through the dermis and exits the wound edge more superficially. It reenters the opposing side of the wound superficially and is passed to the deeper aspect of the wound at the same level as the opposing side. The suture is tied so that the knot rests in the deepest aspect of the wound. If the knot is present in the upper dermis, the suture material will be absorbed more slowly and there is an increased likelihood that it will be eliminated from the wound (spit).

RUNNING SUBCUTANEOUS SUTURE

Often there is little choice but to place interrupted subcutaneous sutures for large wounds under significant tension. If the wound is relatively narrow and under less tension, a running sub-

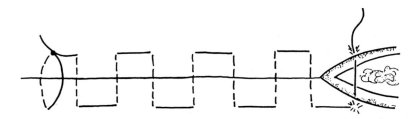

Figure 11 The running horizontal mattress suture is a modification of the horizontal mattress suture.

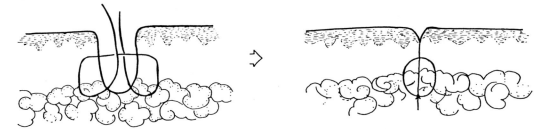

Figure 12 The interrupted subcutaneous suture. It must almost invariably be supplemented with cutaneous sutures to approximate and evert the skin surface.

cutaneous suture may be sufficient. The primary advantage of a running subcutaneous suture over interrupted sutures is the relatively rapid speed with which it can be placed. The advantage of single interrupted subcutaneous sutures over a running subcutaneous suture is that wound dehiscence following possible suture rupture is less likely.

Begin the running subcutaneous suture similarly to the single interrupted subcutaneous suture. If the wound is deep enough, a running subcutaneous suture may be initiated by placing a single subcutaneous suture with the knot tied towards the wound surface. Instead of the suture being cut, it is looped through the subcutaneous tissue by passing through opposite sides of the wound (Fig. 13). It is tied at the distal aspect of the wound, with the terminal end of the suture to the previous loop placed on the opposing side of the wound.

RUNNING SUBCUTICULAR SUTURE

The running subcuticular suture requires the most finesse. It is used primarily to enhance the cosmetic result and is useful for closing wounds with approximately equal tissue thickness on both sides and in which virtually no tension exists. Generally, the skin edges must already be closely approximated with subcutaneous sutures.

The running subcuticular suture is initiated by placing the needle through one wound edge. The opposite edge may be everted and the needle placed horizontally through the upper dermis.

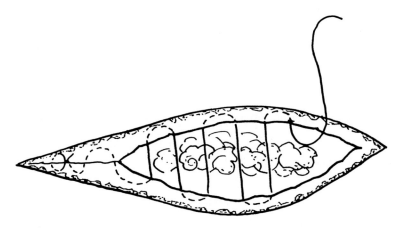

Figure 13 The running subcutaneous suture is used to minimize wound tension and close dead space before cutaneous sutures are placed.

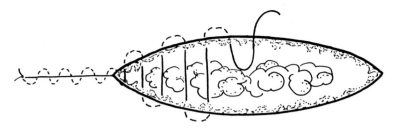

Figure 14   The running subcuticular suture is used to enhance cosmetic results in wounds under virtually no tension.

This is repeated on alternating sides of the wound (Fig. 14). The stitch is terminated similarly to the running subcutaneous suture at the distal end of the wound. Many surgeons, however, prefer to bury the entire suture. If the wound is long, one may elect to bring a loop of the suture through the skin every 1.5–2 cm to facilitate suture removal.

One may use either absorbable or nonabsorbable suture material when placing a running subcuticular suture. Absorbable subcuticular sutures may be used in children so that suture removal is avoided. If the sutures are to be left for prolonged periods of time (such as on the back), the surgeon may elect to use a nonabsorbable suture such as nylon.

COMBINATION CLOSURES

Surgeons frequently combine suture techniques to close a wound. The most common example of a combination technique is the use of interrupted or running subcutaneous sutures with interrupted or running sutures on the skin surface. An individual interrupted, vertical, or horizontal mattress suture is particularly useful to adjust tension in one area of a wound or facilitate eversion of a difficult wound edge. Only by becoming familiar with a variety of suture techniques can the cutaneous surgeon achieve optimal functional and cosmetic results.

BIBLIOGRAPHY

Albom MJ. Cutaneous surgery, including Mohs surgery. In *Dermatology*. SL Moschella, HJ Hurley, eds. Philadelphia, WB Saunders, 1992, pp. 2314–2402.

Borges AF. Techniques of wound suture. In *Elective Incisions and Scar Revision*. Boston, Little, Brown, 1973, pp. 65–76.

Cocke WM Jr, McShane RH, Silverton JS. Suture technique. In *Essentials of Plastic Surgery*. Boston, Little, Brown, 1979, pp. 17–22.

Converse JM. Plastic surgical technique. In *Reconstructive Plastic Surgery*. Philadelphia, WB Saunders, 1977, pp. 46–50.

Ethicon, Inc. Suture use. In *Wound Closure Manual*. Ethicon, Inc., ed. Sommerville, NJ, Ethicon, Inc., 1985, pp. 9–14.

McGregor IA. Technique of wound suture. In *Fundamental Techniques of Plastic Surgery and Their Surgical Applications*. New York, Churchill Livingstone, 1975, pp. 18–25.

McKinney P, Cunningham BL. Sutures. In *Handbook of Plastic Surgery*. Baltimore, Williams & Wilkins, 1981, pp. 19–25.

Nealon TF, Jr. Sutures. In *Fundamental Skills in Surgery*. Philadelphia, WB Saunders, 1979, pp. 46–54.

Odland PB, Murakami CS. Simple suturing techniques and knot tying. In *Cutaneous Surgery*. RG Wheeland, ed. Philadelphia, WB Saunders, 1994, pp. 178–188.

Popkin GL, Robins P. Closure of skin wounds. In *Workshop Manual for Basic Dermatologic Surgery*. Kenilworth, NJ, Schering, Inc., 1983, pp. 18–36.

Robinson JK. Wound closure by suturing. In *Principles of Dermatologic Plastic Surgery*. M Harahap, ed. New York, PMA Publishing Corp., 1988, pp. 35–46.

Stegman SJ. Suturing techniques for dermatologic surgery. *J Dermatol Surg Oncol* 1978;4:63–68.

Stegman SJ, Tromovitch TA, Glogau RG. Suturing techniques. In *Basics of Dermatologic Surgery*. Chicago, Year Book Medical Publishers, 1982, pp. 41–51.

Swanson NA. Basic techniques. In *Atlas of Cutaneous Surgery*. Boston, Little, Brown, 1987, pp. 26–49.

Vistnes LM. Basic principles of cutaneous surgery. In *Skin Surgery*. E Epstein, E Epstein, Jr, eds. Philadelphia, WB Saunders, 1987, pp. 51–53.

Zachary CB. Suture techniques. In *Basic Cutaneous Surgery*. CB Zachary, ed. New York, Churchill Livingstone, 1991, pp. 53–75.

17

Cryosurgical Treatment of Cutaneous Lesions

Emanuel G. Kuflik
University of Medicine and Dentistry of New Jersey–New Jersey Medical School, Newark, New Jersey

Cryosurgery is a method of therapy that uses freezing to achieve destruction of tissue. It is indicated for the treatment of various benign, premalignant, and malignant lesions. It may be used as the treatment of choice, an alternative method, or adjunctive treatment. The word cryotherapy is often used interchangeably with the word cryosurgery; however, in the United States we prefer cryotherapy for nondestructive treatment such as skin peeling.

Eradication of simple cutaneous lesions by freezing was first carried out around the turn of the century. Liquid air was applied with a cotton swab or solidified carbon dioxide was placed on the lesion, but destruction was limited. When liquid nitrogen became available it was initially applied with a cotton swab, but in the 1960s new techniques and equipment were developed that permitted deeper destruction. Thus, malignant as well as benign lesions became amenable to cryosurgical management.

MECHANISMS OF INJURY

The biologic alterations that occur in cryosurgery are caused by heat transfer with resultant freezing of tissue. Heat is removed from the skin by the application of a cryogenic agent or a cooled probe. The rate of heat transfer is a function of the temperature difference between the skin and heat sink and rapid heat flow results. The techniques of treatment have evolved from two methods of heat transfer known as boiling heat transfer and conduction. Selective destruction occurs and the stroma provides the structural framework for later repair of the cryogenic wound. This destruction varies according to the degree of freezing and the type of tissue; cellular elements and melanocytes are sensitive to freezing, while cartilage is rather resistant.

The mechanisms of injury due to freezing of tissue include direct effects, extracellular and intracellular ice formation, increased concentration of electrolytes, recrystallization, and vascular stasis. Rapid cooling of the target tissue is desirable while the rate of rewarming, or thaw, should occur slowly. Current techniques require that the tissue temperature at the base of the lesion reach at least −50°C when treating malignancies. With repeated freeze-thaw cycles, maximum destructive effects are produced.

Prior to cryosurgery a decision must be made concerning the goal of treatment, i.e., improvement, cure, or palliation. If the intent is removal of a benign lesion, the need for destruction of tissue is minimal and a lesser amount of freezing is required. However, if the intent is cure of a malignant lesion, then a greater amount of freezing, sufficient to cause complete eradication of the tumor in the first attempt, is needed.

Following freezing the tissue responds in a predictable manner, depending on the characteristics of the lesion and the duration of freezing, which leads to healing of the wound by second intention. The immediate reactions that ensue include a variable amount of erythema, vesiculation, edema, or exudation (Fig. 1). This is followed by sloughing of the necrotic tissue and eschar formation. Generally, benign and premalignant lesions heal in 2–4 weeks, malignant ones on the head and neck in 4–6 weeks. Large tumors and those located on the trunk and extremities require more time, sometimes up to 14 weeks, for complete healing.

EQUIPMENT

The equipment needed includes a cryogenic agent, cryosurgical unit, adaptable accessories, pyrometer and thermocouples, and miscellaneous protective items. Treatment can be performed in an office setting, outpatient facility, or nursing home without an elaborate surgical suite. Some available agents include carbon dioxide, nitrous oxide, chlorodifluoromethane (Verruca Freeze®), dimethyl ether and propane (Histofreezer®), and liquid nitrogen (Table 1). The latter is the coldest and is effective for either benign or malignant lesions, while the other cryogens are useful for inflammatory or benign conditions.

Liquid nitrogen cryosurgical equipment may range from a simple thermos to hand-held or tabletop units. They are filled by pouring or withdrawing liquid nitrogen from a storage tank as needed during the course of the day. A thermos should not be airtight but should allow the evaporating gas to escape. A modern safe unit is operated by a trigger mechanism that permits the liquid nitrogen, stored under pressure, to flow up a delivery tube and exit the nozzle tip as a spray. Different spray tips, cones, and probes can be attached to the unit or held against the skin. A monitoring system for measurement of the tissue temperature, consisting of thermocouple-

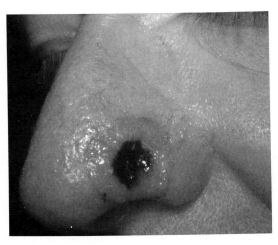

Figure 1 Exudative reaction 3 days after cryosurgery of a basal-cell carcinoma on nose of 69-year-old man.

Table 1 Boiling Points of Various Cryogens

Cryogen	Boiling point (°C)
Freon 22 (chlorodifluoromethane)	−41
Dimethyl ether, propane	−24, −42
Solidified carbon dioxide	−78.5
Nitrous oxide	−89.5
Liquid nitrogen	−196

tipped needles and a pyrometer, is sometimes employed in the treatment of certain malignant lesions. The tip of the needle is placed beneath the tumor or lateral to it. It is important to protect the eyes, ears, and nose from inadvertent sprays with a shield, goggles, or lid retractor.

Although cryosurgery poses a relatively low risk of cross-contamination, proper sterilization of any accessories should be done through dry heat or autoclaving. A small cup made of styrofoam or metal is useful for the dipstick technique. Diverse disposable plastic items are manufactured or can be improvised for treatment purposes.

NONMALIGNANT LESIONS

The types of nonmalignant lesions amenable to cryosurgical management are listed in Tables 2 and 3. The cure rates are high, and the cosmetic results are excellent. Some advantages of cryosurgery include simplicity, low cost, ability to treat multiple lesions, minimal or no scarring, no age limitations, safety during pregnancy, and ability to treat any area of the body. The use of local anesthesia is optional. Overfreezing should be avoided, since retreatment is possible.

Four treatment techniques are commonly used: dipstick, open spray, confined spray, and the cryoprobe. The choice of which one to use depends on the type of lesion and the operator's personal preference. The progress of freezing can be judged by the duration of freezing (freeze time), thawing of the lesion (thaw time), and measurement of the ice-ball beyond the target area (lateral spread of freeze).

Dipstick Technique

The dipstick technique consists of applying a cotton-tipped applicator to a lesion that is repeatedly dipped into liquid nitrogen. The depth of freezing is minimal. Separation at the dermo-epidermal junction occurs, and bulla formation that is sometimes hemorrhagic is needed for successful eradication of verruca vulgaris. Freezing lasts from 5 to 45 sec and is halted when a 1- to 2-mm white halo forms around the wart (Figs. 2–4). Undertreatment can result in recurrence of the lesion. Large verrucae can be treated segmentally. This author found a cure rate of 97.4% in the treatment of periungual warts. Although patients' pain threshold varies, they should be forewarned of pain during or shortly after treatment. It can be avoided through injection of a local anesthetic or alleviated afterwards by soaking. The blister usually dries and falls off within 3 weeks.

Spray Technique

The open-spray technique is used most frequently. Treatment can conform with the shape of the lesion, and multiple sites can be quickly frozen (Fig. 5). A spray tip is selected according to the size of the lesion, and freezing may last between 5 and 20 sec. A single freeze-thaw cycle gen-

Table 2 Benign Conditions Amenable
to Cryosurgical Management

Adenoma sebaceum
Angiokeratoma of Fordyce
Angioma
Clear cell acanthoma
Condyloma acuminata
Dermatofibroma
Epidermal nevi
Granuloma faciale
Granuloma pyogenicum
Hemangioma
Keloid
Lentigines
Lentigo simplex
Lymphangioma
Lymphocytoma cutis
Molluscum contagiosum
Mucocele
Myxoid cyst
Porokeratosis plantaris discreta
Prurigo nodularis
Rhinophyma
Sebaceous hyperplasia
Seborrheic keratosis
Trichiasis
Trichoepithelioma
Tuberous xanthoma
Varicose veins
Venous lake
Verrucae—vulgaris, periungual,
   filiform, plana

erally suffices. This technique is suitable for actinic keratosis, seborrheic keratosis, verrucae, lentigo simplex, lymphocytoma cutis, and myxoid cyst (Figs. 6–8). This author reported treatment of 57 myxoid cysts and found a cure rate of 76.7% using either the open-spray or cryoprobe technique following deroofing of the lesions.

Table 3 Premalignant Lesions
Amenable to Cryosurgical
Management

Actinic cheilitis
Actinic keratosis
Bowen's disease
Erythroplasia of Queyrat
Keratoacanthoma
Lentigo maligna

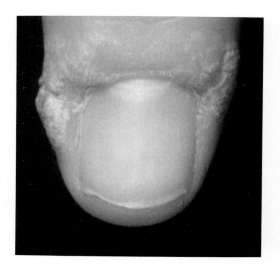

Figure 2 Periungual warts in a 12-year-old girl.

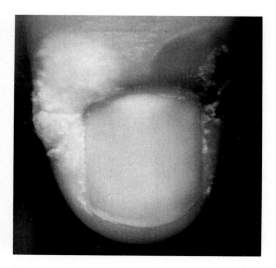

Figure 3 Freezing of second lesion with the dipstick technique in same patient. Note hemorrhagic bulla 9 days after treatment of other wart.

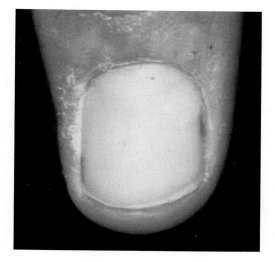

Figure 4 Excellent results 4 weeks after treatment.

Cryosurgery has been used alone, in combination with intralesional steroid injection, or combined with surgery to treat keloids and hypertrophic scars. The freeze time ranges between 10 and 30 sec, but large keloids require a longer freeze time. A single or double freeze-thaw cycle is performed, and more than one treatment session is usually needed. In a series of 65 keloids, complete flattening in 48 (73%) was achieved.

Premalignant lesions such as actinic cheilitis (Figs. 9,10), keratoacanthoma, Bowen's disease, and lentigo maligna require longer freezing than simple benign lesions. Cryosurgery is a valuable alternative method of treatment for lentigo maligna, particularly when the lesion's size or location precludes excision (Figs. 11,12). Kuflik and Gage found a recurrence rate of 6.6% in

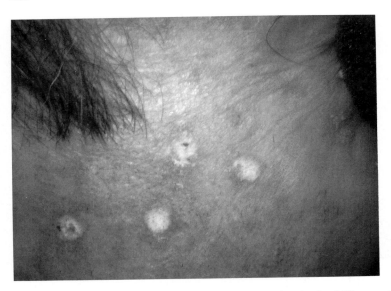

Figure 5 Freezing of multiple actinic keratoses on the cheek of 64-year-old man.

30 cases of lentigo maligna with excellent cosmetic results. The tissue temperature is monitored and should reach –40 to –50°C, a double freeze-thaw cycle is performed, and the lateral spread of freeze should extend 5–10 mm.

The confined-spray technique consists of directing a spray of nitrogen into a neoprene or otoscope cone that is held against the lesion. Freezing is thereby restricted to the size of the cone.

Cryoprobe Technique

The cryoprobe technique, also known as contact therapy, involves the use of a metal probe that is cooled internally by a circulating flow of liquid nitrogen. The probe is firmly applied to the lesion until a rim of frozen tissue is observed. The freeze time is two or three times longer than

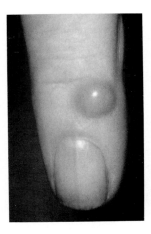

Figure 6 Myxoid cyst on index finger.

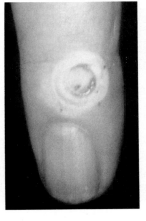

Figure 7 Cryosurgery of lesion after debulking. Note lateral spread of freeze.

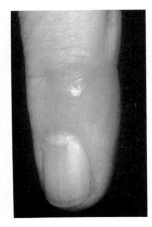

Figure 8 Complete healing 6 weeks after treatment.

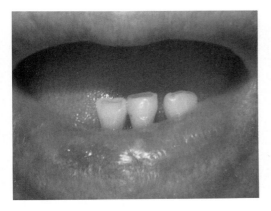

Figure 9 Actinic cheilitis at center of lower lip.

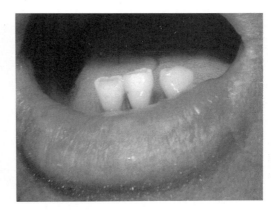

Figure 10 Excellent results 3 weeks after treatment.

the spray technique. Lesions that are suitable for treatment include condyloma acuminata, mucocele, hemangioma, sebaceous hyperplasia, dermatofibroma, myxoid cyst, keloids, and venous lake (Figs. 13,14). A single freeze-thaw cycle given one time is satisfactory for several of these conditions, but repeated treatments at 3- to 6-week intervals may be needed for condylomata, hemangioma, or keloids until the desired resolution of the lesion is achieved.

MALIGNANT LESIONS

Indications and Contraindications

Cryosurgery is effective for selected basal and squamous cell carcinomas. Tumors that are indicated for treatment should have sharply delineated or palpable margins. Cryosurgery can be used for lesions located on the scalp, face, lips, eyelids, ears, nose, neck, trunk, extremities, vulva, and penis. It is suitable for small or large tumors, multiple carcinomas, for lesions located within psoriasis or burn scars, and for selected recurrent tumors. This method is advantageous for high-risk surgical patients, for those with a pacemaker, a blood coagulopathy, the elderly, and in patients for whom other methods of treatment are impractical or undesirable. It can also serve as palliative therapy for inoperable tumors.

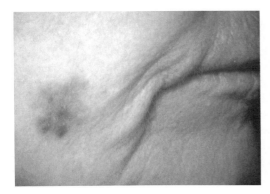

Figure 11 Lentigo maligna on cheek of 75-year-old woman.

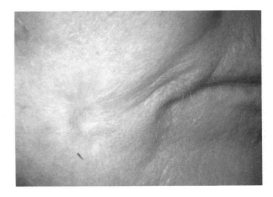

Figure 12 Good results 2 years after treatment.

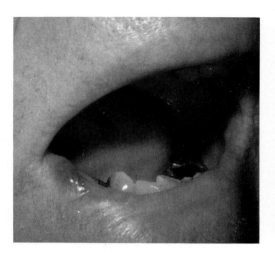

Figure 13   Venous lake on lower lip.

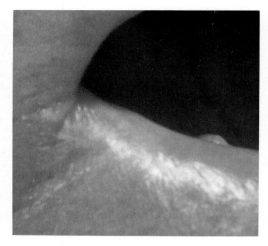

Figure 14   Excellent results 3 weeks after treatment.

There are few contraindications to the use of cryosurgery. Lesions occurring in known high-risk locations such as the inner canthi and preauricular areas should be examined carefully because of the possibility of deep penetration. Patients with cold sensitivity, cold urticaria, cryofibrinogenemia, or cryoglubulenemia may best be treated by other means. Tumors with indistinct borders are not good candidates for cryosurgery. Deep freezing is generally not recommended for lesions at the corners of the mouth, vermilion borders, and the auditory canals. Caution should be observed when treating tumors that lie over nerves, at the margins of the ala nasi, and in dark-skinned patients.

Treatment

The target area is cleansed and outlined with a skin marker prior to treatment. It is not advisable to drape the site since droplets of liquid nitrogen can accumulate below the drape and may cause inadvertent freezing. In general, treatment consists of freezing the lesion, allowing it to thaw completely for several minutes, and then subjecting it to a second freeze-thaw cycle. Curettage is often carried out prior to cryosurgery to visualize the extent and depth of the lesion, to obtain a biopsy specimen, or to convert a deep lesion to a shallower one. Since a tumor mass can modify the depth of freeze, bulky or fungating lesions can be "debulked" prior to treatment by surgical means. This facilitates placement of thermocouple needles, and freezing can be directed at the invading portion or base of the tumor. Hemostasis should be obtained prior to actual freezing. A large tumor can be successfully eradicated by dividing it into segments and treating each segment individually in either one or separate visits (Figs. 15–17).

After treatment a dry gauze dressing is applied and the patient is instructed to wash the wound three or four times daily during the exudative phase. This may last between 5 and 14 days depending on the location and volume of tissue frozen. A dry crust then develops and falls away spontaneously. Wound healing occurs within 4–6 weeks on the face and neck but takes longer for lesions on the trunk and extremities. Periorbital edema can be managed with cold compresses or a short course of systemic corticosteroids. The author reported that Celestone phosphate®, 1 ml, given IM ½ hr before treatment and followed by 20 mg prednisone daily for 3 days can minimize the edema.

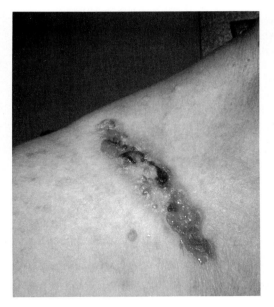

Figure 15   Linear basal cell carcinoma on shoulder of 68-year-old woman.

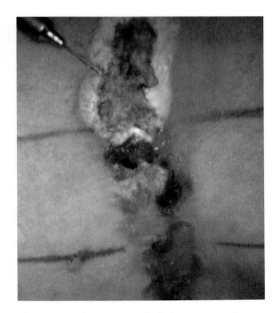

Figure 16   Cryosurgery depicting segmental treatment with freezing of upper third of lesion.

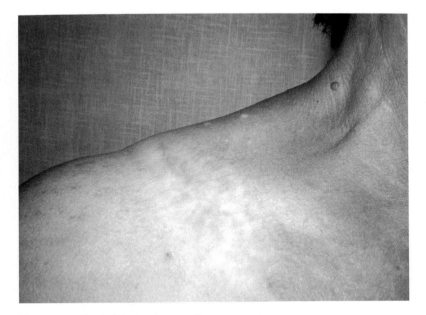

Figure 17   Healed lesion 1 year after treatment.

Techniques of Treatment

There are four techniques of treatment: open-spray, confined spray, closed spray, and the cryoprobe technique. The open-spray is most frequently used and is suitable for round or irregularly shaped lesions. The spray can be moved freely to follow the outline of the tumor and is emitted from a distance of 1–2 cm from the target site. A variation of this technique is the confined-spray method. In the closed-spray technique, the spray is directed into a cone that is attached to the cryosurgical unit and freezing is very rapid. Finally, a prechilled cryoprobe can be used for small or medium-sized lesions that are roughly round in shape. During freezing the probe is held steady since any movement will interfere with heat transfer, causing inadequate freezing of the tumor. A flat probe equal in size to the lesion or slightly larger is recommended for malignancies. Freezing is slower than the spray technique (approximately three times), since the nitrogen must first cool the probe before the tissue is frozen.

Depth Dose

It is necessary to determine the amount and depth of tissue to be frozen. The depth dose can be estimated clinically and monitored with the use of tissue temperature instrumentation. One observes and measures the lateral spread of freeze, which should reach 3–5 mm or greater. The freeze time should last between 45 and 60 sec with the open-spray technique for a carcinoma measuring up to 1.5 cm. For deeper lesions, i.e., those lying more than 3 mm from the surface, the progress of freezing can be supplemented with tissue temperature monitoring. The temperature should reach between –50 and –60°C.

Ultrasound has been used for noninvasive preoperative imaging of tumors and for diagnosis and planning. With further sophistication of equipment, ultrasonography may come into clinical use for cryosurgical management.

Results

In a series of 3540 new skin cancers, the majority of which were basal cell carcinomas, the author found an overall cure rate of 98.4%. The 5-year cure rate for 684 new tumors was 99%. As one might expect, the cure rate for recurrent tumors is lower (88.4%). The cosmetic results are good to excellent, but a variable amount of hypopigmentation occurs. There is no keloid formation, and any hypertrophic scarring that develops improves with time.

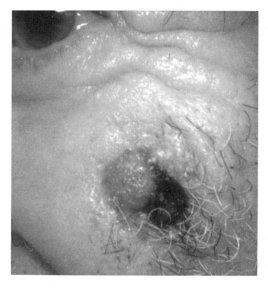

Figure 18 Nodular basal cell carcinoma on cheek of 82-year-old man.

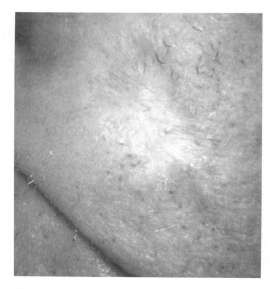

Figure 19 Complete healing 9 months after treatment.

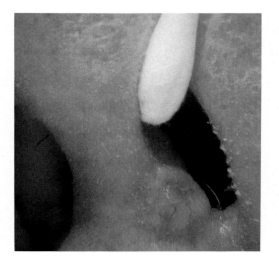

Figure 20 Nodular basal cell carcinoma at nares of 70-year-old woman.

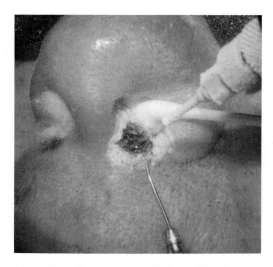

Figure 21 Cryosurgery to lesion with a thermocouple needle in place.

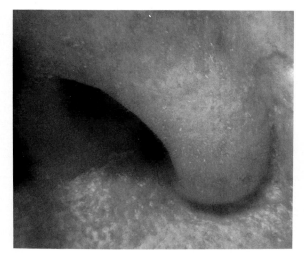

Figure 22 Complete healing 4 weeks after treatment.

Anatomic Areas

Most areas of the face can be treated with cryosurgery (Figs. 18,19). Treatment is painless, although freezing at the forehead and temples may cause mild headache. Tumors of the scalp require aggressive treatment. X-rays may be indicated to determine whether invasion of bone by cancerous tissue has occurred, and in such cases cryosurgery is not indicated. Tumors of the nose respond well to cryosurgery (Figs. 20–22). If invasion of cartilage by cancerous tissue has occurred, a depression may result. Tumors at the nasolabial folds should be treated vigorously.

Well-demarcated eyelid tumors respond well, but treatment should not be undertaken by the novice. Lesions at or away from the lid margins can be treated (Figs. 23,24). The 5-year cure rate for 95 primary basal cell carcinomas was 96.8%. Cryosurgery of lesions near the punctum

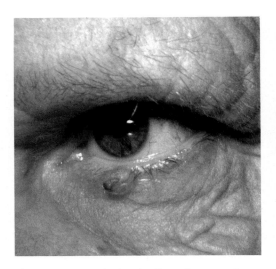

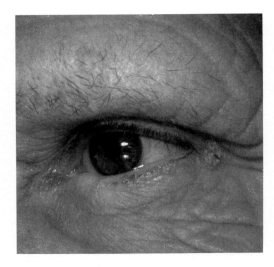

Figure 23   Nodular basal cell carcinoma on lower eyelid of 67-year-old woman.

Figure 24   Excellent results 5 years after treatment.

or lacrimal duct is advantageous since permanent damage to the lacrimal outflow system is uncommon. It is important to protect the eyes from the nitrogen spray and to avoid the formation of droplets of nitrogen at the inner canthi. Healing is excellent, and the normal function of the eyelid is retained.

All areas of the ears with the exception of the auditory canals are suitable for cryosurgical management (Figs. 25–28). In the treatment of 233 cancers of the ears, the overall cure rate was

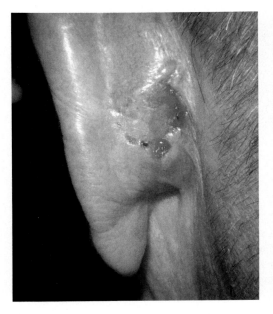

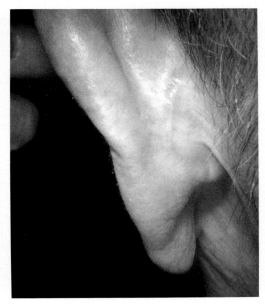

Figure 25   Ulcerative basal cell carcinoma on posterior aspect of ear.

Figure 26   Healed lesion 8 months after treatment.

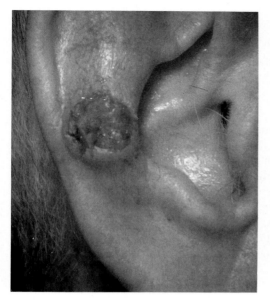

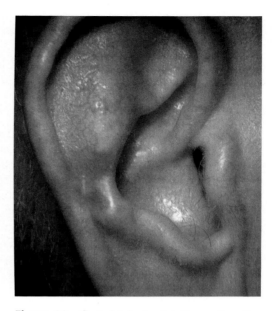

Figure 27 Nodulo-ulcerative squamous cell carcinoma on ear of 77-year-old man.

Figure 28 Completely healed 2 months after treatment.

95.7%. Management is basically the same as for facial lesions, but some modifications may be necessary due to the curvature of the ear, the presence of cartilage, and the fact that a tumor may involve both the anterior and posterior aspects of the ear. The spray technique is best since treatment can conform to the shape of the lesion, although small round ones can be treated with

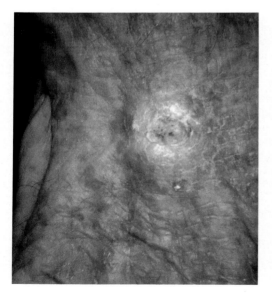

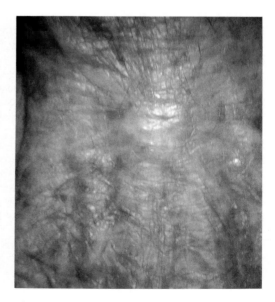

Figure 29 Squamous cell carcinoma on dorsum of hand.

Figure 30 Healed lesion 3 months after treatment.

the cryoprobe technique. The tumor can be elevated away from the cartilage (ballooning) by injection of a local anesthetic.

Tumors on the trunk and extremities heal with a flat scar. Cryosurgery is effective for superficial basal cell epitheliomas, lesions near folds and on the lower legs, and for squamous cell carcinomas on the dorsa of the hands (Figs. 29,30).

Complications

It is important to distinguish between expected sequelae and untoward results or complications. The incidence of complications after cryosurgery is low. Reactions may be unforseen or inexplicable or may arise from poor patient or lesion selection. One should not encounter similar morbidity or complications after treatment of benign lesions as compared with malignant ones. The commonly seen temporary complications are edema and throbbing pain after treatment of warts. Infrequent ones include delayed bleeding, headache, secondary infection, syncope, febrile reaction, nitrogen gas insufflation, milia, pyogenic granuloma, hypertrophic scarring, hyperpigmentation, and parasthesia. Permanent complications include retraction of tissue, neuropathy, tendon rupture, alopecia, ectropion, hypopigmentation, scarring, and tissue defect.

BIBLIOGRAPHY

Fraunfelder FT, Zacarian SA, Limmer BL, et al. Cryosurgery for malignancies of the eyelid. *Ophthalmology* 1980;87:461–465.

Gage AA. Cryosurgery for cancer of the ear. *J Dermatol Surg Oncol* 1977;2:417–421.

Gage AA. What temperature is lethal for cells? *J Dermatol Surg Oncol* 1979;5:459–464.

Graham GF. Advances in cryosurgery during the past decade. *Cutis* 1993;52:365–372.

Kuflik AS, Schwartz RA. Lymphocytoma cutis: a series of five patients successfully treated with cryosurgery. *J Am Acad Dermatol* 1992;26:449–452.

Kuflik EG. Treatment of basal and squamous-cell carcinomas on the tip of the nose by cryosurgery. *J Dermatol Surg Oncol* 1980;6:811–813.

Kuflik EG. Cryosurgery for carcinoma of the eyelids: a 12-year experience. *J Dermatol Surg Oncol* 1985; 11:243–246.

Kuflik EG. Cryosurgery in the treatment of skin cancer. In *Adjuncts to Cancer Surgery*. SG Economou, TR Witt, DJ Deziel, et al., eds. Philadelphia, Lea & Febiger, 1981, pp. 294–298.

Kuflik EG. Specific indications for cryosurgery of the nail unit: myxoid cysts and periungual verrucae. *J Dermatol Surg Oncol* 1992;18:7

Kuflik EG. Cryosurgery updated. *J Am Acad Dermatol*

Kuflik EG, Gage AA. *Cryosurgical Treatment for Skin Cancer*. New York, Igaku-Shoin, 1990.

Kuflik EG, Gage AA. The five year cure rate achieved by cryosurgery for skin cancer. *J Am Acad Dermatol* 1991;24:1002–1004.

Kuflik EG, Gage AA. Cryosurgery for lentigo maligna. *J Am Acad Dermatol* 1994;31:75–78.

Kuflik EG, Webb W. Effects of systemic corticosteroids on postcryosurgical edema and other manifestations of the inflammatory response. *J Dermatol Surg Oncol* 1985;11:464–468.

Lubritz RR, Smolewski SA. Cryosurgery cure rate of actinic keratosis. *J Am Acad Dermatol* 1982; 7: 631–632.

Rusciani L, Rossi G, Bono R. Use of cryotherapy in the treatment of keloids. *J Dermatol Surg Oncol* 1993;19:529–534.

Torre D. Cryosurgery of basal cell carcinoma. *J Am Acad Dermatol* 1986;15:917–929.

18

Complications, Indications, and Contraindications in Cryosurgery

Setrag A. Zacarian
*Tufts University Medical School, Boston, Massachusetts
and Yale University School of Medicine, New Haven, Connecticut*

Cryosurgery for malignant tumors is a rapid and safe method of treatment. Like any other physical modality, however, there are a number of complications worth considering prior to choosing this treatment. The complete list is noted in Table 1.

IMMEDIATE COMPLICATIONS

Pain

Pain is a subjective sensation that varies from patient to patient. The initial discomfort from liquid nitrogen cryosurgery ceases rapidly because of the analgesic effect of cold on the superficial sensory cutaneous nerves. A more profound and intense pain, however, returns during the thawing phase. Pain is generally more severe on the fingers, particularly in a periungual region or the fingertips. Other sites that are also painful include the helix and concha of the ear, the lips, temples, and scalp. Even patients whose tumors have been locally anesthetized for insertion of thermocouples still experience some discomfort. When the thaw cycle is complete, pain usually ceases and does not return. In rare cases, patients will complain of pain or a throbbing sensation for an hour or two after the digit has been frozen.

Headache

Freezing on the forehead, temples, and scalp invariably produces a migrainelike, throbbing discomfort. Often this is transient, but occasionally a headache will persist for several hours and may be severe. When freezing lesions on the scalp, it is advisable to keep the patient in the treatment room under observation until he or she is completely free of symptoms. Patients can rarely have such severe headaches that they can be distracted from other tasks such as driving a car home from the office. The cause for this unusual migrainelike pain is uncertain. The vascular type of pain is not always at the site of freezing. It is not unusual, for example, that a tumor

Table 1 Complications from Cryosurgery

Immediate
    Pain during the freezing and thawing period
    Headache affecting forehead, temples, and scalp
    Insufflation of subcutaneous tissue
    Intradermal hemorrhage
    Edema
    Syncope
    Vesiculobullous formation
Delayed
    Postoperative infection
    Febrile systemic reaction
    Hemorrhage from the wound site
    Pyogenic granuloma
    Pseudoepitheliomatous hyperplasia
Prolonged
    Hyperpigmentation
    Milia
    Hypertrophic scars
    Neuropathy
Permanent
    Hypopigmentation
    Ectropion and notching of eyelids
    Notching and atrophy of tumors overlying cartilage
    Tenting or notching of the vermilion border of the upper lip
    Atrophy
    Alopecia

frozen on the left temple will result in throbbing pain at the occiput or the opposing parietal area of the scalp.

Insufflation of Subcutaneous Tissue

This occurs when the refrigerant is delivered as a spray and the gaseous portion of the liquid enters an open pathway between the surface and the subcutaneous tissues and burrows through this plane. This is a rare occurrence. The portal of entry may well be a biopsy site or an eroded, ulcerated neoplastic growth. Clinically one observes an immediate swelling or bulging around the tumor site at which the refrigerant spray is directed. Insufflation of tissue is more likely to occur around the periorbital area (Fig. 1). Should this complication occur, freezing should immediately cease and treatment should be continued on another day. The nitrogenous gas is promptly absorbed, producing little or not discomfort. There have been no reports of gas emboli occurring as complications of cryosurgery.

Intradermal Hemorrhage

The areolar tissue of the eyelids is very loose, and this undoubtedly accounts for marked edema after cryosurgery. Subzero temperatures produce not only thrombosis of the microvessels of the skin but also endothelial cell separation within vessel walls, resulting in frank rupture and extravasation of blood and blood elements into the surrounding tissue interspaces (an example is the patient with a basal cell carcinoma of the right lower medial canthus shown in Fig. 2). There

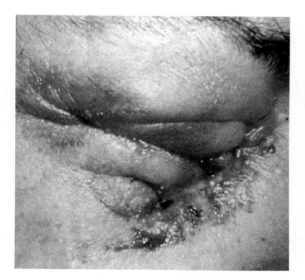

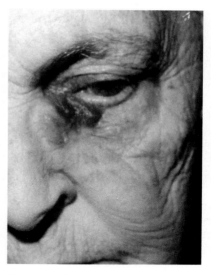

Figure 1 Insufflation of subcutaneous tissue of the periorbital area during cryosurgery. (From Elton RF. Complications from cryosurgery. *J Am Acad Dermatol* 1982;8:513.)

Figure 2 Intradermal hemorrhage of the medial canthus 30 min following cryosurgery.

is considerable swelling with the onset of subcutaneous hemorrhage 15 min after freezing. Within 30 min, a large, ecchymotic area is noted at the site of cryosurgery, which extends several centimeters at its periphery. Bleeding stops spontaneously, and there is no external hemorrhage on the cutaneous surface.

Edema

Edema following cryosurgery might not be considered a complication, rather an expected part of wound healing. The degree of edema depends not only on the degree and intensity of the freeze but also on the anatomic site and the patient's individual reaction to cold. When patients present with multiple lesions, either benign or premalignant (i.e., warts, actinic keratoses), it is reasonable to freeze only a few and ask the patient to return for further treatment. Some patients experience a marked degree of edema from the slightest amount of freezing. The greatest degree of edema is noted in the periorbital region. Figure 3 demonstrates a patient with a basal cell carcinoma of the left lower eyelid treated by cryosurgery 24 hr earlier. This type of swelling lasts from several days to a week. Occasionally one notices or palpates locular, clear fluid within the edematous site. The swelling is most prominent upon awakening in the morning and improves as the day progresses. There is no known way of circumventing this problem completely. Kuflik noticed considerable diminution of periorbital edema when a small amount of betamethasone is injected intralesionally one-half hour prior to cryosurgery. This is supplemented by oral steroids for 2 days. Kuflik also noted that this reduced the healing time by 1 week. The risk of secondary infection, however, is theoretically increased. Cyproheptadine, 5 mg orally three times a day, 1 day before and for several days after cryosurgery, is also helpful in shortening the duration of periorbital edema.

Periorbital edema can occur bilaterally after freezing of tumors on the bridge of the nose (Fig. 4) as well as after cryosurgery performed on the forehead or temple. Vigorous freezing of tu-

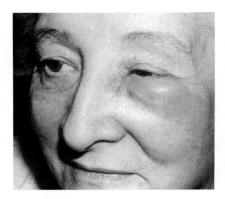

Figure 3 Lower lid 24 hr after cryosurgery of a left medial canthus carcinoma. The periorbital edema persisted for 4 days.

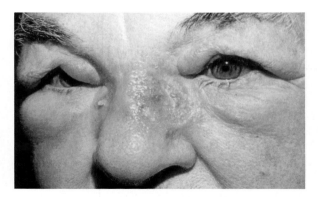

Figure 4 Bilateral periorbital edema observed following cryosurgery of a basal cell carcinoma on the bridge of the nose.

mors on the cheek may produce marked edema under the chin and particularly at the angle of the jaw, lasting for several days. It is helpful to advise patients that cryosurgery will disfigure them for a few days, so that they can plan accordingly.

Syncope

Syncope has been reported after cryosurgery. In the author's experience, this only occurs in patients who have had benign lesions frozen. Paradoxically, patients who have been subjected to vigorous freezing for malignancy of the skin tend not to have syncopal episodes. Whether syncope is induced by fear, iatrogenic factors, or histamine shock is unclear.

Vesiculobullous Formation

The occurrence of blisters after cryosurgery is common. Figure 5 demonstrates a bulla, after treatment of several adjacent warts, overlying the third and fourth knuckles of the hand. This large bulla developed within 24 hr of light freezing with a cotton swab dipped in liquid nitrogen. Drainage of the fluid within the blister provides rapid relief. Occasionally hemorrhagic vesiculobullous reactions occur and may cause the patient some concern. These too may be simply incised and drained, since they can be quite painful.

DELAYED COMPLICATIONS

Postoperative Infection

Postoperative infection following cryosurgery is extremely uncommon. This author has seen two cases on the face and several more on the lower extremities. Freezing tumors on the lower extremities is not advisable, particularly on the shins and ankles, because wound healing takes as long as several months, often leaving unsightly scars. Figure 6 shows a patient with a large nodular basal cell carcinoma of the left infraorbital region. After two thermocouple needles were inserted, the tumor was subjected to a vigorous freeze. In addition to a marked degree of edema 48 hr after cryosurgery, there was a firm indurated area below the tumor that was tender and

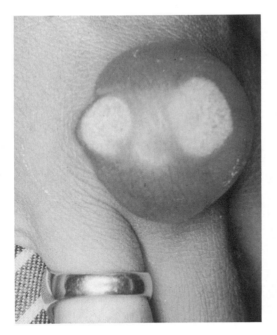

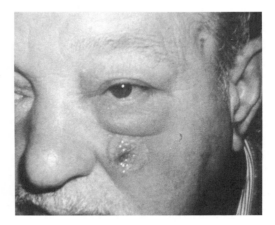

Figure 5 Large bullae 24 hr after cryosurgery of two adjacent warts overlying the knuckle. Freeze time with a cotton-tipped applicator was 10 sec.

Figure 6 Cellulitis occurring 48 hr after cryosurgery of a left lower lid carcinoma.

warm on palpation. Treatment with erythromycin, 1 g/day, resulted in resolution of the erythema and induration within 5 days. Since the rate of infection is so low, prophylactic antibiotics prior to cryosurgery are not indicated unless unusual medical circumstances dictate otherwise.

Febrile Systemic Reaction

Febrile systemic reactions after cryosurgery have been reported by Elton. They occur within the first 24 hr after freezing and promptly resolve. This is extremely rare, but the clinician should be aware of such a possibility.

Hemorrhage

Hemorrhage from the frozen tumor site is uncommon. This might be anticipated if a deep biopsy was obtained prior to freezing or if the cryosurgical procedure was preceded by extensive curettage. If hemorrhage develops, it is usually noted a few days after freezing. A simple suture or a pressure dressing often suffices. Larger vessels such as those on the temple are cryoresistant and do not reach subzero temperatures. Blood vessels lined with smooth muscle do not thrombose or occlude and appear to be resistant to cryonecrosis.

Pyogenic Granuloma

The occurrence of a pyogenic granuloma following cryosurgery is demonstrated in Figure 7. This is a rare complication and generally occurs a few weeks after cryosurgery at the wound site. Treatment with simple electrodesiccation or curettage suffices.

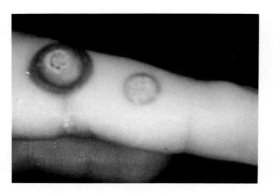

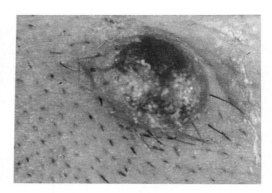

Figure 7 Pyogenic granuloma appearing at the cryosurgical wound site several weeks after freezing of a carcinoma of the skin. (Courtesy of R. F. Elton, Southfield, MI.)

Figure 8 Pseudoepitheliomatous hyperplasia appearing 6 weeks after cryosurgery. (From Elton RF. Complications from cryosurgery. *J Am Acad Dermatol* 1982;8:513.)

Pseudoepitheliomatous Hyperplasia

Pseudoepitheliomatous hyperplasia at the wound site 4–6 weeks after cryosurgery is not an uncommon finding. This can be mistaken for inadequate freezing of the neoplasm or an early recurrence. Several biopsies of this occurrence have revealed benign hyperplasia. This complication has also been noted following radiotherapy of cutaneous carcinoma, although it has not been observed after curettage and electrodesiccation. Figure 8 demonstrates classic pseudoepitheliomatous hyperplasia 6 weeks after cryosurgery.

PROLONGED COMPLICATIONS

Hyperpigmentation

Hyperpigmentation after cryosurgery is not uncommon, but, fortunately, it is transient and generally lasts just a few months, rarely as long as a year, and then resolves. Figure 9 shows a 5-year-old black child who was treated with cryosurgery for molluscum contagiosa of the face. The existing areas of hyperpigmentation disappeared within 3 months. Figure 10 demonstrates perilesional hyperpigmentation observed on the chest of a woman who was treated with cryosurgery for a superficial basal cell carcinoma 4 weeks earlier. The pigment change had resolved within 3 months. In contrast, the patient in Figure 11 still shows a distinct circular ring of hyperpigmentation 2 years after cryosurgery of a basal cell carcinoma of the right temple. This persistence of postinflammatory pigmentary change is not a common finding. The cryogen in this case was delivered with a metal cone closed-spray technique and may have affected the long-term result. Metal cones have now been replaced with plastic cones, and, as a result, this residual complication is less common.

Milia

Milia appear after cryosurgery when the freezing has been intense and particularly when a cone spray technique has been employed. Milia are uncommon when an open-spray technique or a closed probe is used. Figure 12 demonstrates the persistence of milia 3 months after open-cone cryosurgery of a basosquamous cell carcinoma of the neck. This problem can be remedied with either a comedone extractor or the application of light electrodesiccation (Fig. 13).

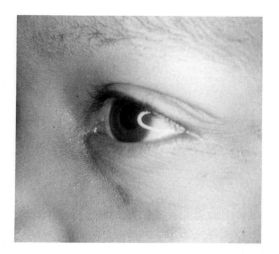

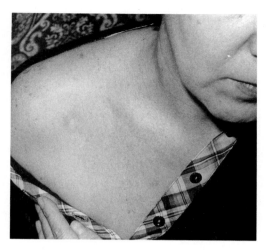

Figure 9 Hyperpigmentation 2 months following cryosurgery of molluscum contagiosa on face (left lower lid and lateral to the outer canthus).

Figure 10 Hyperpigmentation 4 weeks after cryosurgery of a basal cell carcinoma of the chest. This finally disappeared 3 months following the freezing.

Hypertrophic Scars

Hypertrophic scars occasionally appear within 4–6 weeks after freezing. These scars differ from keloids, which have not been reported after cryosurgery. The hypertrophic scars are usually thin, linear, erythematous to livid red, glossy, and threadlike lesions. The most common sites are the alae nasi, tip of the nose, upper lip, midforehead, chest, and back. Hypertrophic scars can persist for several months. They last as long as 6 months, after which they spontaneously involute. Treatment of these hypertrophic scars may include application of steroid-impregnated tape applied nightly for several weeks or intralesional injections of triamcinolone. Figure 14 shows a

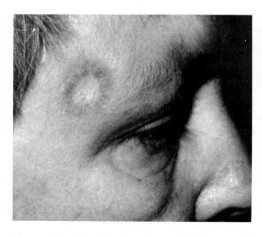

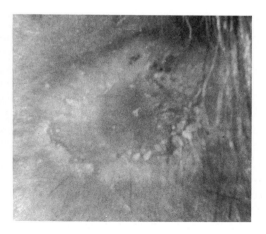

Figure 11 Persistent and marked degree of hyperpigmentation 2 years after cryosurgery using a metal ring cone.

Figure 12 Hemorrhagic vesicular bullous reaction.

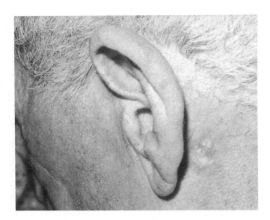

Figure 13 Milia presented infrequently following cryosurgery.

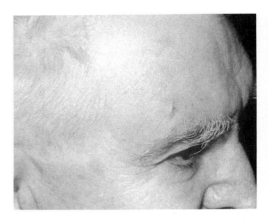

Figure 14 Hypertrophic scar 6 weeks following cryosurgery.

hypertrophic scar on the forehead above the eyebrow, which was the site of cryosurgery for a basal cell carcinoma 6 weeks earlier. Without any treatment it spontaneously resolved in 12 weeks.

Neuropathy

Neuropathy after cryosurgery is a rare complication, but when it occurs it is a serious concern for both the patient and the physician. It may persist for months and last as long as a year or more. Nerve tissue is sensitive to subzero temperatures, but, fortunately, the neural sheath is relatively cryoresistant. Nerves that lie superficially, such as the lateral aspects of fingers, anterior aspect of the tragus, postauricular area, lateral aspect of the tongue, ulnar fossa of the elbow, and the area overlying the radial aspect of the wrist, are critical sites. Freezing these areas requires particular attention to damage of subcutaneous tissues and duration of freezing and thaw time.

Studies of freezing temperatures on the sciatic and median nerves of rats demonstrated no permanent damage. The rate of regeneration to normal function varied from several days to several weeks depending on the temperature to which they were subjected (0–100°C). According to Carter and coworkers, there is no evidence to suggest that the response of sensory nerves to subzero temperatures differs significantly from that of their counterparts. The first reported cases of neuropathy were noted by Nix. In these cases, warts occurring along the lateral margins of the finger and treated with cotton-tip application of liquid nitrogen sustained sensory nerve loss. One patient recovered, but the other had some neural dysfunction after 2 years. Neither patient sustained motor nerve neuropathy. Finelli reported a patient who experienced extensive neuropathy following application of liquid nitrogen to a wart on the extensor aspect of the elbow, overlying the site of the ulnar nerve. In addition to sensory loss, the patient experienced motor weakness followed by marked atrophy of the first dorsal interosseus muscle and wasting of the hypothenar group of muscles, with weakness of all muscles of the hand innervated by the ulnar nerve. Full sensory and motor function were restored within 2 years.

Postauricular neuralgia has been reported after treatment of skin cancers close to the ear. Facial nerve paralysis was also reported following extensive cryosurgery for cancer of the ear canal. Three patients with associated nerve damage following cryosurgery have been reported. Two of the patients received treatment of lesions on the fingers and sustained nerve damage that included loss of sensation to touch, pain, temperature, and vibration distal to the treated sites. The third patient was treated for multiple warts of the fingers and feet with an open-spray technique. Within 48–72 hr she complained of a loss in sensation on the medial aspect of the right fourth finger, distal to the site of treatment. In all reported cases, the sensory loss was temporary. Sensory nerves are superficial, in contrast to motor nerves, which enter through the carpal tunnel and are protected by overlying epidermis, subcutaneous fat, and muscles. Other vulnerable sites include the fibular head (where the common peroneal nerves traverse), the medial epicondyle of the humerus, and the dorsum of the foot.

Neuropathy is a distinct complication that clinicians must be aware of and patients cautioned about. Should postcryosurgical neuropathy occur, the physician should be reassuring and supportive. Published reports to date suggest that this neuropathy will disappear within months.

PERMANENT COMPLICATIONS

Hypopigmentation

Hypopigmentation is an inevitable complication of cryosurgery. Figure 15 demonstrates a classic example of hypopigmentation evident even 5 years after cryosurgery. This complication is more prominent in patients with darker complexions but varies from patient to patient. There is a slow gradual improvement over many years, and even black patients can obtain complete repigmentation after cryosurgery, although this is uncommon. A double freeze-thaw cycle such as that used for treatment of malignancy produces a greater degree of hypopigmentation than a single freeze-thaw cycle.

Ectropion, Notching of the Eyelids, and Alopecia of Eyelashes

Ectropion and eyelash alopecia have been reported. These complications are noted when the tumor has advanced to the free margins of the lid. Cryonecrosis of the lid margin is often required because of the location of the tumor. When freezing close to the lid margin for malignant neoplasms, it is justifiable that several millimeters of uninvolved skin be frozen. Similar complications occur when other modalities are used in this same location (surgery, radiation, curettage,

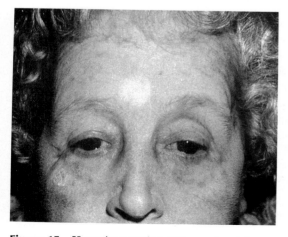

Figure 15 Hypopigmentation still prominent 5 years after cryosurgery of a basal cell carcinoma on the forehead.

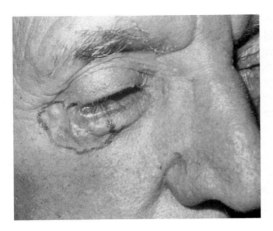

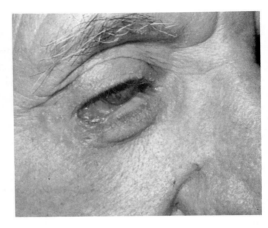

Figure 16 Patient with a second recurrence of a basal cell carcinoma of lower right eyelid following second surgical extirpation.

Figure 17 Marked degree of ectropion, notching, and eyelid eversion compounded by cryosurgery.

and electrodesiccation). Figure 16 shows a patient who has already undergone radiotherapy for a basal cell carcinoma of the right lower lid and outer canthus. Subsequent recurrence was treated with electrodessication and curettage, and then this recurrence was treated with cryosurgery. Eversion and ectropion of the right lower lid from previous treatment are already noted. Cryosurgery was performed as a palliative measure, and 2 months later, although the tumor appears to be clinically eradicated, the degree of ectropion and eversion of the lid was further compounded (Fig. 17). Mohs surgery might be an alternative approach.

Notching and Atrophy

This has been reported on the helix of the ear. Cartilaginous defects after cryosurgery occur when the tumor itself is advanced beyond the perichondrial barrier. Cancers of the skin rarely invade to this depth. Figure 18 demonstrates notching and tissue loss at the helix of the ear after vigorous freezing. This type of tissue defect is sometimes unavoidable if the underlying tumor is to be effectively frozen. Conventional surgery, radiation, and electrodesiccation may often result in similar tissue defects.

Tenting or Notching of Upper Lip

Eclabium is a distinct disfiguring complication that frequently occurs following cryosurgery of the upper lip and may be permanent. Figure 19 demonstrates an eclabium that resulted after treatment of a basal cell carcinoma measuring approximately 1.0 cm on the mid-upper lip. In this location, when freezing a tumor several millimeters beyond the visible margin of the growth, the iceball included the vermilion border of the lip. After the tumor was clinically eradicated, the eclabium persisted and has remained evident for 10 years. Extreme care must be exercised when freezing tumors of the upper lip and extending the freeze close to the vermilion border. This tends to be an uncommon problem after cryosurgery of tumors on the lower lip.

Atrophy

Atrophy following cryosurgery is inevitable if the tumor has extended down to the subcutaneous tissues. Loss of deep tissue integrity cannot be replaced simply by normal reepithelialization

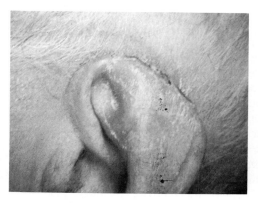

Figure 18   Moderate degree of tissue atrophy of ear after cryosurgery. (Courtesy R. F. Elton, Southfield, MI.)

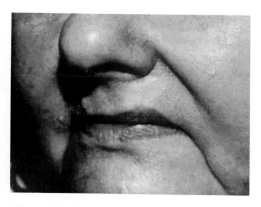

Figure 19   Permanent defect of upper lip 5 years after cryosurgery of a basal cell carcinoma. In addition, permanent hypopigmentation is noted.

of surface integument. Figure 20 shows this atrophy after cryosurgery of an invasive epidermoid carcinoma of the forehead. Atrophy is an uncommon complication; however, the forehead, tip of the nose, chest, back, and ear appear to be the anatomic sites where it is most often observed.

Alopecia

Alopecia of hair-bearing sites, such as the scalp, eyebrows, eyelashes, and sideburn areas, inevitably follows cryosurgery. Malignant tumors that advance to the epithelial sheath of hair follicles, such as a lentigo maligna and carcinoma in situ, require vigorous cryosurgery, and consequently hair follicles are sacrificed. Proper selection of patients is therefore important. If the cosmetic result is important to the patient, the cryosurgeon must respect this and recommend an alternative method of ablating the tumor.

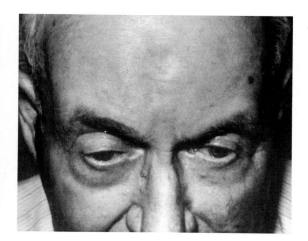

Figure 20   Marked degree of atrophy after cryosurgery of an invasive epidermoid carcinoma on the midforehead.

INDICATIONS FOR CRYOSURGERY IN MALIGNANCY

This is a subject of controversy among cryosurgeons. The author's own guidelines for indications and contraindications for cryosurgery of malignant tumors of the skin are outlined in Tables 2 and 3. General considerations prior to choosing cryosurgery for treatment include the age of the patient, the histologic type of the carcinoma, and the anatomic site of the neoplasm. An individual assessment of each patient as well as the lesion is always important.

Because of the known higher recurrence rates for skin carcinoma of the alae nasi, nasolabial fold, eyelids, and postauricular areas, think of other methods before undertaking cryosurgery in these locations. Neoplasms in these areas (with the exception of the eyelids) invade embryonal fusion planes, and their exact clinical or surgical margins are elusive. Treatment of lesions in these locations with cryosurgery would not offer the patient the greatest chance for cure with the initial treatment. When cryosurgery is chosen for tumors of higher risk, monitoring the depth of tissue freezing with thermocouple needles is recommended. When skin carcinoma appears to be adherent to underlying cartilage or periosteum, surgical intervention with Mohs micrographic surgery is the best method of treatment.

Treatment of sclerosing or morphea-type basal cell carcinoma is particularly difficult. Clinically, the borders of the tumor are often poorly defined. Because of the inferior cure rates with cryosurgery for this subtype of basal cell carcinoma, Mohs surgery is suggested as a better alternative unless there are unusual circumstances.

Carcinomas of the scalp, medial canthus of the eye, alae nasi, nasolabial fold, and postauricular areas have a recurrence rate exceeding 10%. In younger patients, cryosurgery for malignancy should not be performed in these locations. Elderly patients in whom serious medical risks or other surgical contraindications may exist would be exceptions to this rule. There is a place for

---

Table 2 Indications for Cryosurgery

Tumors with definable margins
    Nodular or ulcerated lesions
    Instrument delineation by means of a curette
    Chemical delineation by means of 5-fluorouracil
    Tumors overlying cartilage and bone
    Lentigo maligna (stage I level of invasion)
Conditions in which cryosurgery is more suitable than other modalities
    Anatomic site
        Certain neoplasms of the eyelid, nose, and ear (avoiding lachrymal obstruction and chondronecrosis)
        Tumors of the chest and back (on which hypertrophic scarring is minimal with cryosurgery, requiring no skin grafts)
        Tumors on the tip of the nose (on which surgical resection often produces marked deformity)
Nature of the neoplasm
    Infected tumors
    Recurrent tumors from previous radiotherapy
Patient characteristics
    Patients with pacemakers (electrocautery is contraindicated)
    Older patients who may be poor surgical risks
    Patients with anesthesia idiosyncrasies
Inoperable patients
    Palliation
    Removal of bulky vegetative lesions

Table 3 Contraindications for Cryosurgery

The absolute contraindications for cryosurgery are clear-cut and definitive:
  Intolerance to cold
  Cryoglobulinemia
  Cryofibrinogenemia
  Raynaud's disease
  Cold urticaria
  Pyoderma gangrenosum
  Collagen and autoimmune diseases
  Concurrent treatment with immunosuppressive drugs
  Platelet deficiency disease
  Blood dyscrasias of unknown origin
  Multiple myeloma
  Agammaglobulinemia
The following relative contraindications are based on the author's 20 years of experience in cryosurgery
  of malignant tumors of the skin:
  Morphea or sclerosing type of basal cell carcinoma
  Neoplasms of the scalp
  Neoplasms of the ala nasi and nasolabial fold
  Neoplasms of the anterior tragus of the ear
  Postauricular neoplasms
  Lesions of the free margin of the eyelid
  Tumors of the upper lip near the vermilion margin
  Tumors of the lower legs, particularly the shins
  Tumors situated on the lateral margins of the fingers and ulnar fossa of the elbow
  Lack of clinical experience and skill of the physician/surgeon
  Nodular and ulcerated lesions over 3 cm in diameter (except as a palliative measure)
  Carcinomas fixed to underlying cartilage or periosteum
  Recurrent carcinomas (in younger patients)

---

palliative cryosurgical procedures for certain patients with cutaneous malignancies. Recurrent carcinomas, particularly those following radiotherapy, are amenable to cryosurgery without any delayed or prolonged healing time.

To obtain an effective degree of cryonecrosis with an acceptable cure rate for advanced invasive tumors in critical and anatomic locations, there are several situations in which temperature monitoring with thermocouples is especially important. They are as follows:

1. The inexperienced cryosurgeon
2. Lentigo maligna
3. Carcinoma in situ (Bowen's disease)
4. Tumors situated in certain anatomic locations (medial canthus of the eyelid, alae nasi, nasolabial fold, postauricular fold, anterior to the tragus of the ear)

In the final analysis, the success or failure of cryosurgery for cutaneous cancers depends on the experience and skill of the clinician. It must not be undertaken by a physician who lacks training in cryosurgery. With the appropriate use of this technology, skin disease can be treated safely, effectively, and quickly in an office setting.

BIBLIOGRAPHY

Beard C, Sullivan JH. Cryosurgery of eyelid disorders including malignant tumors. In *Cryosurgical Advances in Dermatology and Tumors of the Head and Neck*. SA Zacarian, ed. Springfield, IL, Charles C Thomas, 1977: 265–271.

Carter DC, et al. The effect of cryosurgery on peripheral nerve function. *J R Coll Surg Edinburgh* 1972; 17:25.

Elton RF. Complications of cutaneous cryosurgery. *J Am Acad Dermatol* 1983; 8(4):513.

Elton RF. The course of events following cryosurgery. *J Dermatol Surg Oncol* 1977; 3:448.

Elton RF. Cryosurgery of advanced and difficult cancers of the skin. In *Cryosurgical Advances in Dermatology and Tumors of the Head and Neck*. SA Zacarian, ed. Springfield, IL, Charles C Thomas, 1977: 170–178.

Finelli PF. Ulnar neuropathy after liquid nitrogen cryotherapy. *Arch Dermatol* 1975; 111:1340.

Fraunfelder FT, Zacarian SA, Limmer BL, Wingfield D. Cryosurgery for malignancies of the eyelid. *Ophthalmology* 1980; 87:461–465.

Gage AA. Deep cryosurgery. In *Skin Surgery*. 4th ed. E Epstein, ed. Springfield, IL, Charles C Thomas, 1977: 471–475.

Gaster RN, et al. Comparison of nerve regeneration rates following controlled freezing or crushing. *Arch Surg* 1971; 103:378–383.

Greer KE, Bishop GF. Pyogenic granuloma as a complication of cryosurgery (letter). *Arch Dermatol* 1975; 111:1536.

Lenz H, Goertz W, Preussler H. The freezing threshold of the peripheral motor nerve: an electrophysiological and light microscopical study on the sciatic nerve of the rabbit. *Cryobiology* 1975; 12:486–496.

Levine HL, Bailin PL. Basal cell carcinoma of the head and neck: Identification of the high risk patient. *Laryngoscope* 1980; 90(6):955.

Levine H, et al. Tissue conservation in the treatment of cutaneous neoplasms of the head and neck. *Arch Otolarnygol* 1979; 105:140.

McMeekin TD, Moschella SL. Iatrogenic complications of dermatologic therapy. *Med Clin North Am* 1979; 63:441.

Millns JL, Fenske NA, Pierce D. Neurological complications of cryosurgery. *J Dermatol Surg Oncol* 1980; 6:207.

Mora RG, Robins P. Basal cell carcinoma in the center of the face: The special diagnostic, prognostic, and therapeutic considerations. *J Dermatol Surg Oncol* 1978; 4:315.

Nix TE, Jr. Liquid nitrogen neuropathy. *Arch Dermatol* 1965; 92:185.

Pollack SV, et al. The biology of basal cell carcinoma: A review. *J Am Acad Dermatol* 1982; 7(5):569.

Stewart RH, Graham GF. A complication of cryosurgery in a patient with cryofibrinogenemia. *J Dermatol Surg Oncol* 1978; 4:743.

Wood JR, Anderson RL. Complications of cryosurgery. *Arch Ophthalmol* 1981; 99:460.

Zacarian SA. *Cryosurgical Advances in Dermatology and Tumors of the Head and Neck*. Springfield, IL, Charles C Thomas, 1977.

Zacarian SA. *Cryosurgery of Tumors of the Skin and Oral Cavity*. Springfield, IL, Charles C Thomas, 1973.

Zacarian, SA. *Cryosurgery of Skin Cancer and Cutaneous Disorders*. St. Louis, MO, C.V. Mosby Co., 1985.

19

The Ear

Roger I. Ceilley
University of Iowa, Iowa City, Iowa

The external ear has obvious functional and cosmetic importance. Dermatologic surgeons frequently treat skin cancers and a variety of dermatologic diseases affecting this area. Proper selection of the method(s) of therapy depends upon many factors, including

1. Anatomy of the region
2. Pathology type of the lesion to be treated
3. Skin type and degree of solar damage
4. Age and general health of the patient
5. Surgeon's knowledge of various therapeutic modalities

ANATOMY

The auricle or pinna, formed by skin and cartilage, is dependent upon a complex cartilaginous framework for its contour and support. The auricle contains a number of prominences and depressions. The concha, anthelix and helix, and tragus and antitragus (Fig. 1) are important landmarks. The anterior one third is attached to the skull and the posterior two thirds to the scalp only. The skin is intimately attached over the surface of the cartilage except along the helix. The blood and nerve supply is abundant and complex (Fig. 2). The blood supply consists of the anterior auricular artery, a branch of superficial temporal artery supplying the lateral surface, and the posterior auricular artery supplying the medial surface and a small portion of the lateral surface. In addition, the occipital artery gives off a branch supplying the medial surface. The lymphatic drainage consists of superficial, deep cervical nodes and mastoid lymph nodes. The retroauricular area includes the mastoid process behind the ear. The medial area faces the retroauricular area, and the lateral surface is the external auricular surface.

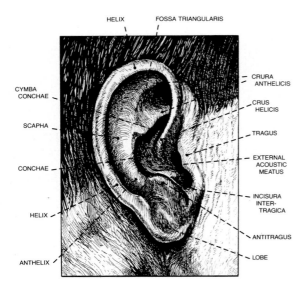

Figure 1 Topographical landmarks of the ear.

APPLIED ANATOMY FOR LOCAL ANESTHESIA

A review of the anatomy and innervation of the external ear will aid the surgeon in understanding the techniques for local anesthesia in this region. The external ear is formed by the union of tissue from the branchial arches and postbranchial regions. This is reflected in its sensory innervation, which is by branches from cranial nerves V, VII, IX, and X and C2 and C3 of the cervical plexus. There is marked overlap in the sensory distribution of adjacent cutaneous nerves and variation in the contribution from cranial nerves VII and IX.

The mandibular division of the trigeminal nerve innervates the most anterior portion of the auricle through its auriculotemporal branch. It supplies the skin of the tragus, the anterior and superior portion of the external auditory canal, and the anterior portion of the helix and its crus (Fig. 2).

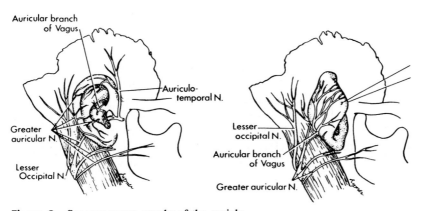

Figure 2 Sensory nerve supply of the auricle.

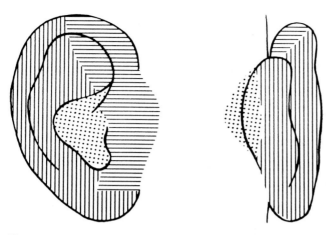

Figure 3 Sensory nerve distribution of the auricle by area. Vertical lines mark the area supplied by cervical plexus; horizontal lines mark the area supplied by auriculotemporal nerve; dots mark the arc supplied by cranial nerves VII, IX, and X.

Cranial nerves VII (facial), IX (glossopharyngeal), and X (vagal) contribute to the sensory innervation of the concha on the lateral surface of the auricle and the posterior portion of the external auditory canal (Fig. 3). A small area of skin on the postauricular sulcus and adjacent mastoid is also innervated by these cranial nerves. The auricular branch of the vagus that communicates with the glossopharyngeal and facial nerves emerges from the skull through the tympanomastoid fissure to supply the latter area.

The cervical plexus contributes to the sensory innervation of the auricle by the posterior branch of the greater auricular nerve and the lesser occipital nerve. The greater auricular nerve supplies the major portion of the medial surface of the auricle and posterior portion of the lateral surface of the auricle. There is overlap and communication with fibers from the lesser occipital nerve in the mastoid region. These nerves originate from the 2nd and 3rd cervical nerves (Fig. 2).

LOCAL ANESTHESIA OF THE AURICLE

In very apprehensive patients, intravenous sedation with diazepam and a narcotic may be beneficial. Local anesthesia is induced by field injection of 1% lidocaine with epinephrine 1:100,000 and sodium bicarbonate. The bicarbonate is added to bring up the pH of the mixture, and consequently to decrease the pain associated with the local anesthesia. The epinephrine decreases capillary bleeding by its vasoconstrictor action. The auricle has widespread and profuse vascular plexuses, and there is no danger of necrosis secondary to the use of a vasoconstricting agent in healthy individuals.

Adequate anesthesia may be obtained by a field block of the skin around the periphery of the auricle (Fig. 4). Deep infiltration anteriorly may result in temporary paralysis of the facial nerve (Fig. 5). Local infiltration of the concha and external canal at the bony cartilaginous junction is done to obtain total anesthesia of the entire auricle and canal. The field block does not anesthetize the canal, which is supplied by cranial nerves. Anesthesia of localized areas of the auricle may be obtained by regional infiltration. The advantage of a field block is less distortion of tissue and less pain from injection of the anesthetic agent. The major disadvantage is less effective vasoconstriction at the operative site.

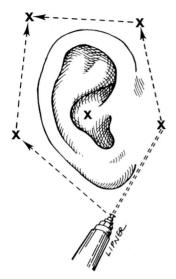

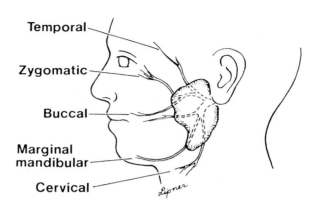

Temporal

Zygomatic

Buccal

Marginal mandibular

Cervical

Figure 4 Injection for regional anesthesia of the auricle.

Figure 5 Distribution of the five major branches of the facial nerve.

METHODS OF SURGICAL TREATMENT

The methods of therapy for carcinoma of the external ear include radiotherapy, conventional excisional surgery, electrodesiccation and curettage, cryosurgery, and Mohs micrographic surgery. All would appear to yield acceptable cure rates for primary lesions less than 1 cm in diameter that do not show an aggressive histologic pattern (Figs. 6,7). Mohs surgery should be used for more difficult tumors.

Radiation

The variability in contour of the external ear makes determining the accurate dosage of radiotherapy difficult. Because of the large amount of cartilage in the pinna, the external ear is extremely susceptible to radiation perichondritis. The frequency of recurrence appears to be higher following radiotherapy than following surgical treatment. Recurrent lesions are generally unresponsive to radiotherapy.

Cryosurgery

Cartilage is more resistant to permanent injury from freezing than is skin. This permits complete freezing of skin lesions of the external ear. Cryosurgery is more effective for lesions lateral rather than medial on the pinna. However, freezing to lethal temperatures, as is customary elsewhere, can result in necrosis of the full thickness of the external ear. This may result in chondritis and deformity of the auricle.

Elton recently reported on recurrences that follow cryotherapy of large lesions, especially deeply penetrating malignant neoplasms and sclerosing basal cell carcinomas. They appeared not only at the margins of treated malignancies but also under apparently healthy scars, much in the same way they appear under skin grafts.

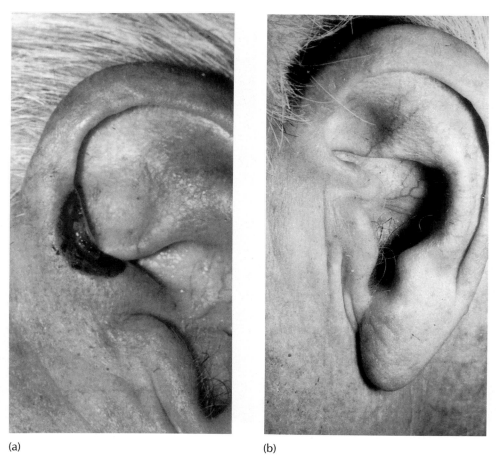

(a)   (b)

Figure 6   Result after excision and primary closure of a basal cell carcinoma.

Electrodesiccation and Curettage

Electrosurgery is effective for small primary lesions but may result in large areas of exposed cartilage. This heals very slowly because of thermal injury. The incidence of chondritis is greater, as is auricular deformity. Treatment of recurrent lesions with this method is often ineffective because the malignant tissue within the scar is not easily removed with a cruet.

Excision

Pless attempted to define adequate margins for excisional therapy, and he recommended margins of 8–10 mm, respectively, for primary basal cell and squamous cell carcinoma measuring less than 3 cm. Margins of at least 15 mm were recommended for all recurrent lesions and for primary lesions greater than 3 cm. Measurements of the preoperative size of the lesion and the postoperative surgical defect following Mohs surgery suggest that these recommendations fall short of cure in many instances, especially when one is dealing with a recurrent tumor or morphea-form basal cell carcinoma.

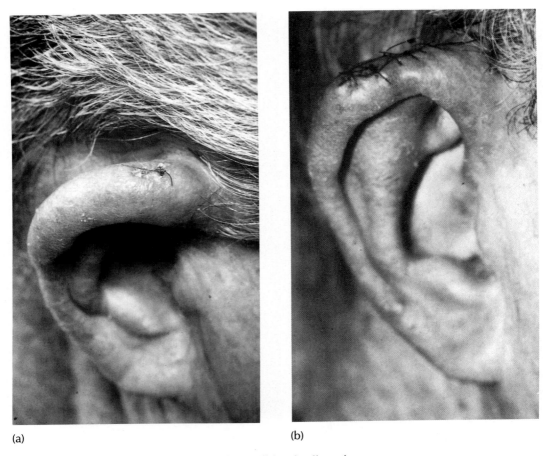

(a)   (b)

Figure 7   Excision and primary closure of a small basal cell carcinoma.

All lesions should be biopsied prior to excision with primary closure. Local anesthesia may be obtained by regional block or local infiltration of 1% lidocaine with epinephrine 1:100,000. Local infiltration provides better hemostasis than the regional block.

The proposed excision margin is outlined with skin marker before local infiltration of anesthesia is performed. A margin of 8–10 mm is suggested for basal cell carcinoma and squamous cell carcinoma. Utilizing margins of this magnitude often prevents a simple wedge excision since marked lateral protrusion of the helix will occur when the incision is closed primarily. To prevent this deformity, a stellate tension-relaxing excision is done (Fig. 8). V-shaped wedges with the long axes perpendicular to the margin of the primary excision are outlined. These are placed near the middle margins of the original wedge and may involve the antihelix. The base of the smaller relaxing wedge is approximately one third of the base of the primary wedge, while the length is also approximately one-third the length of the primary excision. It is best to make the secondary wedges smaller since they can be easily extended to obtain better closure. Tissue deficiency can be a severe problem.

Tumor and secondary wedges are excised. Skin hooks are used to approximate the margins of the helix to determine if modifications of the secondary wedges are necessary. Hemostasis may be obtained by cautery. Care is taken to minimize cauterization of the auricular cartilage to

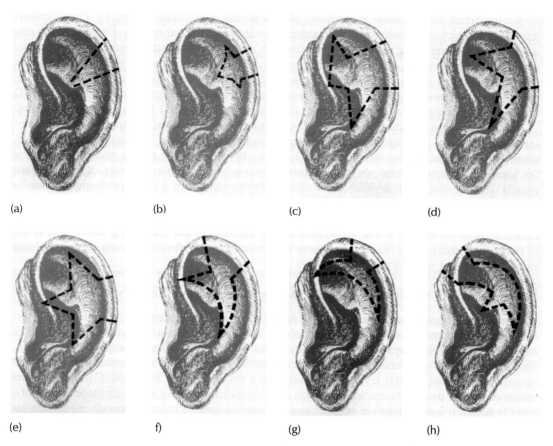

(a)   (b)   (c)   (d)

(e)   f)   (g)   (h)

Figure 8 A wedge excision can be done for small lesions on the ear. Larger lesions require tension-relaxing incisions or smaller secondary wedges to close the defect with minimal deformity.

prevent cartilage necrosis. Subcutaneous absorbable sutures, such as 5–0 Vicryl or PDS, are used to approximate the auricular cartilage. These stitches must include the perichondrium, either alone or through cartilage to induce the perichondrium on both sides. Undermining the skin along the margins may be done to facilitate eversion of the skin margin. Care must be taken to remain above the perichondrium while undermining the skin. The skin is closed with interrupted vertical mattress sutures of 6–0 synthetic material for eversion. The incision is covered with an antibiotic ointment and nonadherent gauze. A cotton ball is placed in the concha and a 4" × 4" piece of gauze placed in the postauricular region. Then a mild pressure dressing with fluffed gauze and wrapping around the head may be used. The pressure dressing is used primarily where hemostasis is a concern. This can be removed in 24–48 hr. If an open technique is used, the incision is simply covered with an antibiotic ointment.

Oral antibiotics are prescribed for 3 days. They are initiated the evening prior to surgery. For patients requiring intravenous sedation, it may be administered immediately prior to surgery. Wound care includes twice-daily cleansing with hydrogen peroxide and the application of an antibiotic ointment. This is extremely important to maximize wound healing. It prevents crust formation in the incision, which makes suture removal less traumatic in 5–7 days.

Local Flaps

Local flaps usually result in a better cosmetic result than a skin graft. There is better color and texture match while the tissue carries its own blood supply. The disadvantage of local flaps around the ear, as in all locations, is that thicker tissue may prolong detection of recurrent tumors. Recurrent tumors have the capacity to spread widely in the newly created tissue planes before appearing on the skin surface. One indication for a local flap in auricular reconstruction is the patient who wears glasses. If a skin graft is used, pressure from the bows of the glasses may cause tissue necrosis. Local flaps tolerate pressure from the bows of eyeglasses better (Figs. 10,11). The most useful flap for reconstructing the posterior or medial auricular surface would be the transposition or rhomboid flap. Given that the skin on the anterior or lateral auricle is tightly adhered to underlying cartilage and without much elasticity, a skin graft would be a better choice to repair a defect there if adequate perichondrium provides enough blood supply for grafting. For a large conchal defect, a postauricular revolving door island flap can be utilized.

Skin Grafts

Skin graft survival on cartilage or bone denuded of periosteum or perichondrium is allegedly tenuous. Dermatologic and oncologic surgeons encounter this problem frequently, and often the graft does grow directly on bone or cartilage when small areas of the perichondrium and periosteum have been removed. Split-thickness skin grafts of 0.018–0.021" were used. If a significant amount of cartilage is exposed, small holes can be made through the cartilage with a 1- to 2-mm dermal punch and the graft delayed until granulation tissue comes through these holes to cover at least half of the exposed cartilage (Fig. 12). This technique has been consistently reproduced with good cosmetic results even for large defects. Bolsters or blasting sutures are always used to hold the graft in place for a minimum of 1 week.

Meatoplasty

A meatoplasty is indicated after the removal of any tumor that involves 180 degrees or more of the external auditory canal. Skin grafts of this area have a tendency to contract. This is less common with regional flaps.

The meatoplasty is performed by excising a generous amount of conchal cartilage, which forms the posterior portion of the external canal. This opens the ear canal widely, and a skin graft is then placed on the more vascular soft tissue that remains. This technique prevents stenosis of the external auditory canal (Fig. 13).

When evaluating methods of therapy for auricular neoplasms, both the effectiveness and the functional cosmetic deformity must be considered. Auricular neoplasms, other than primary lesions smaller than 1 cm, are treated best with microscopic control of the surgical margins. Mohs surgery results in higher cure rates and decreases auricular deformity. Tumor recurrence necessitates excision of the lesion and all adjacent scar tissue. For this reason, the use of local flaps or extensive undermining of adjacent tissue should be avoided in this high-risk location. If conventional surgical excision is used, careful examination of the margins of the specimen should be done at the time of excision. If frozen sections are not readily available, the examination of permanent sections of the entire specimen should be obtained before reconstruction, except for primary lesions 1 cm or less.

TREATMENT OF BENIGN LESIONS

Surgical Treatment of Chondrodermatitis Nodularis Chronica Helicis

Chondrodermatitis nodularis chronica helicis is characterized by a painful, red nodule most commonly located on the helix of the ear. Typically the patient is male and over 40 years of

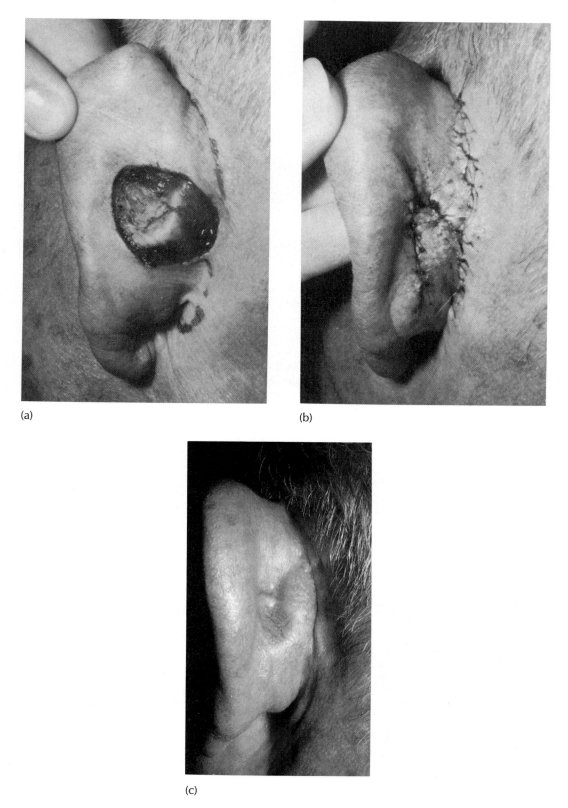

(a)

(b)

(c)

Figure 10   Inferiorly based transposition flap to repair Mohs defect after removal of a basal cell carcinoma.

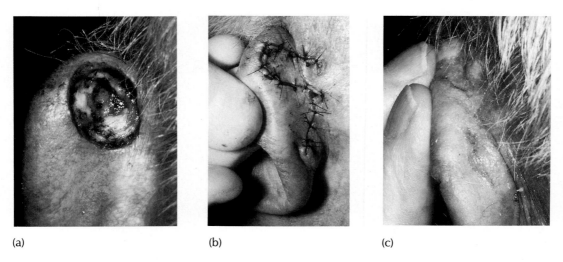

(a)   (b)   (c)

Figure 11 Laterally based transposition flap to repair Mohs defect, making it easier for patient to wear glasses.

age with a history of outdoor work. Patients may also report having had frostbite. Nodules on the tragus, antitragus, and antihelix are rare but occur most commonly in women and are often related to trauma. The lesion tends to be oval, inflamed, and fixed to underlying cartilage (Fig. 14). The cause of this condition is unclear but appears to be related to the unique anatomy of the pinna. The skin there is tightly bound to the underlying cartilage, and the circulation is poor

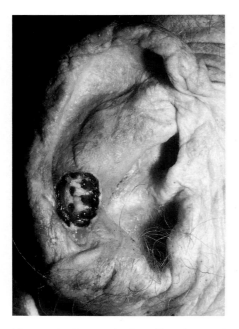

Figure 12 Removal of cartilage by punch excision will allow healing by second intention over exposed cartilage.

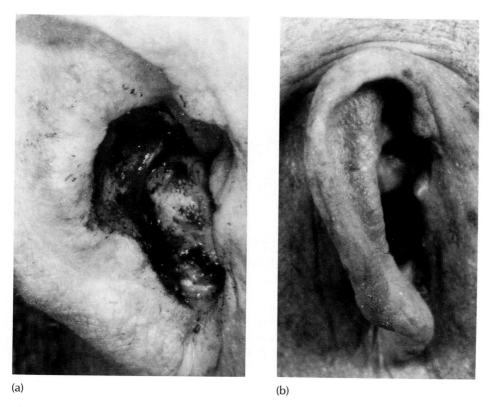

(a)   (b)

Figure 13 (a) This defect involves over 180 degrees of the external auditory canal following microscopically controlled excision of a basal cell carcinoma. (b) A patent external auditory canal 6 months after reconstructive meatoplasty and split thickness skin graft.

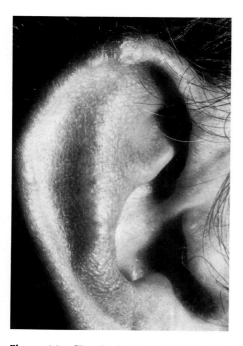

Figure 14 Chondrodermatitis nodularis helicis.

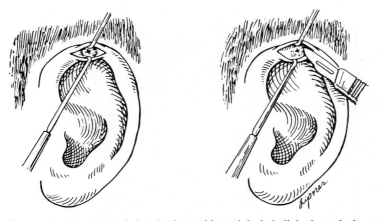

Figure 15   Excision of chondrodermatitis nodularis helicis through the cartilage.

because there is little subcutaneous tissue. Moreover, this area is frequently exposed to mechanical and environmental trauma. These factors get worse with age.

Treatment has included wedge excision and primary closure, intralesional corticosteroids, and curettage or excision allowed to heal by second intention. Recurrence after simple excision is common, probably because removal of the lesion is incomplete. Projections of damaged cartilaginous tissues may persist, or adjacent cartilage may contain foci of subclinical involvement. Nevertheless, excision is the most effective treatment because the clinical lesion is removed entirely and pain is relieved by transection of sensory nerves. With sterile technique and local anesthesia, the involved area is excised through a small incision or in an ellipse down to cartilage (Fig. 15, left). Then the clinically necrotic cartilage is removed (Fig. 15, right). Adjacent cartilage is carefully trimmed so as to contour the defect in the cartilage smoothly, free of sharp edges (Fig. 16, left). The skin is undermined just above the perichondrium, and the wound is closed with fine sutures (5-0 silk or nylon) (Fig. 16, right). The skin on the pinna heals rapidly. Sutures may be removed in 4 or 5 days and tape applied for a few more days. The preoperative and postoperative results are shown in Figures 17 and 18.

The advantages of this technique are (1) good visualization of damaged cartilage and adjacent foci of involvement, (2) contouring of adjacent healthy cartilage, eliminating sharp edges

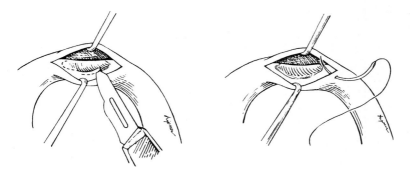

Figure 16   Closure of the defect after the cartilage is smoothed.

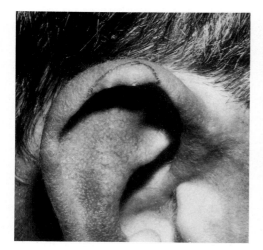

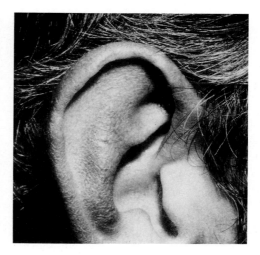

Figure 17   Chondrodermatitis nodularis helicis with projections of cartilage through the skin.

Figure 18   Postoperative results after excision and primary closure.

that may produce pain or recurrence later, (3) improved vascular supply to the overlying skin, (4) rapid and usually painless healing, and (5) excellent cosmesis. A fine linear scar is hidden within the crease of the helix.

Epidermoid Cysts

The lobule of the auricle is rich in sebaceous glands and is covered with loose skin. Epidermoid cysts commonly develop in this area. Other common locations include the concha, floor of the meatus, and the periauricular skin. Clinically they are soft, slightly fluctuant nodules that usually have a point of attachment with an overlying follicular orifice. The lesions recur if simply incised and drained, so it is essential to remove the entire cyst wall and its contents. If the cyst is acutely inflamed, incision and drainage along with systemic antibiotics should be used. Excision is then deferred until after the acute inflammation has resolved.

Keloids

Keloid formation on and around the auricle is common, especially in dark-skinned persons. Keloids often result from trauma, especially after ear piercing. Initial treatment should be pressure, cryosurgery, or intralesional corticosteroids. Larger lesions may be treated by surgical enucleation of the lesion, covering the defect with a flap created from the overlying skin (Figs. 19,20). After excising the lesion, some prefer to immediately give an intralesional Triamcinolone injection. Some prefer to excise the lesion followed by 300 R of x-ray.

Preauricular Cysts

A pitlike depression and cyst found anterior to the helix and above the tragus commonly represents embryonic remnants of the first and second branchial arches. The cyst and tracts may extend deeply and are best handled by a head and neck surgeon experienced in their treatment.

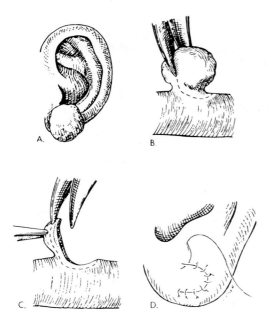

Figure 19 Keloid excision followed by flap reconstruction. (A) Preoperative appearance. (B) Excision of the bulk of the keloid. Outline a small portion of skin for a flap to cover the defect. (C) Dissection with iris scissors of residual keloidal tissue from the skin used as a flap. (D) Suture the flap in place without tension.

Preauricular Tags

Skin tags in this area may or may not contain cartilage (Fig. 21). They are the result of faulty fusion of the hillocks during embryonic development. Removal is indicated only for cosmetic reasons.

Hemangiomas and Venous Lakes

Small lesions are best treated with simple excision or electrosurgery. Larger lesions may be treated by argon laser photocoagulation. Lymphangiomas are best treated with excision, cryosurgery, or carbon dioxide laser vaporization.

Dermoid Cyst

These lesions contain squamous epithelium, hair follicles, sweat glands, and sebaceous glands. They result from faulty embryonic development and should be referred to a head and neck surgeon.

Warts and Seborrheic Keratoses

Shave excision or cryosurgery is most useful. When utilizing cryosurgery, one must be careful to avoid damaging underlying cartilage.

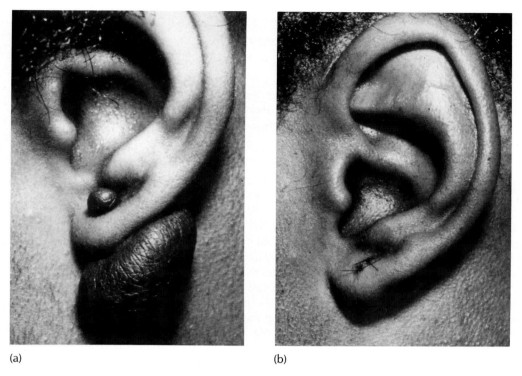

(a)   (b)

Figure 20 (a) Earlobe keloid. Preoperative injection of intralesional triamcinolone acetonide. (b) Postoperative appearance.

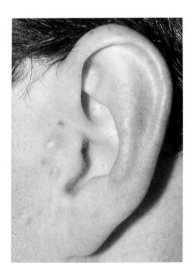

Figure 21 Accessory tragus or preauricular skin tag.

Gouty and Rheumatoid Nodules and Xanthomata

These lesions may be painful and necrotic. Treatment is directed toward the underlying disease.

Nevi

Scalpel excision is the treatment of choice. Other lesions in this area include cholesteatoma of the external auditory canal, osteoma, myomas (rhabdomyoma, leiomyoma), myxoma, and mixed tumors of salivary gland type. Rare neoplasms include adenocarcinoma, adenoid cystic carcinoma, sarcoma, and malignant melanoma.

TREATMENT OF MALIGNANT TUMORS

Malignant tumors of the external ear (which include the pinna, external auditory meatus, and periauricular structures) constitute approximately 6% of all skin cancers, with reported series ranging from 4.6 to 9.7%. The percentage of basal cell carcinomas and squamous cell carcinomas varies considerably, while other forms of malignancy of the external ear are rare.

A review of several series totaling 780 patients with malignant ear tumors demonstrated that 55% were squamous cell carcinoma, 40% basal cell carcinoma, and 5% other types of malignancy (Table 1). Malignant melanomas, sarcomas, and carcinomas derived from sudoriferous sebaceous glands and from hair follicles make up most of the remaining malignant tumors that occur as primary tumors on the external ear (Table 2).

Tumors of the external ear often begin as infiltrating growths that spread along the dermis, perichondrium, or embryonic fusion planes rather than becoming discrete and exophytic. Recurrent lesions frequently behave in this manner, often making retreatment with conventional surgical techniques or irradiation ineffective. Therefore, complete removal of malignant tumors of the external ear is often difficult. Many authors believe that the prognosis of squamous cell carcinoma of the auricle is worse than elsewhere on the body surface. Basal cell carcinoma is an unpredictable tumor with varied clinical and histologic manifestations. The sclerosing or morphea form of basal cell carcinoma is particularly resistant to nonsurgical methods of therapy.

In addition to the difficulty in achieving complete tumor removal, the auricle and ear canal play important cosmetic and functional roles. Methods of reconstruction must be varied depending on the assurance of complete tumor removal and cosmetic and functional considerations. The auricle contains a large amount of cartilage susceptible to the development of perichondritis and

Table 1 Previously Reported Series of Malignancies of the External Ear

Investigator	Basal cell carcinomas	Squamous cell carcinomas	Basosquamous	Other	Total
Mohs (1947)	55	52	0	0	107
Frederick (1956)	25	27	2	0	54
Marfatia (1966)	8	20	0	2	30
Heenan (1966)	46	32	3	2	83
Blake (1974)	51	81	3	11	146
Conway (1957)	51	42	0	7	100
Pless (1976)	79	177	0	4	260
Total	315	431	8	26	780

Table 2 Uncommon Malignancies on the External Ear

Malignant melanoma	Sarcomas
Endothelioma	Chondrosarcoma
Hemangioendothelioma	Fibrosarcoma
Lymphoendothelioma	Lymphosarcoma
Adenocarcinoma	Myxosarcoma
Adenoid cystic carcinoma	Rhabdomyosarcoma
Atypical fibroxanthoma	Ectopic salivary tissue

chondritis when the overlying skin is excised. This further complicates the therapy and reconstruction of lesions involving the auricle.

BIBLIOGRAPHY

Blake GB, Wilson JSP. Malignant tumors of the ear and their treatment. *Br J Plast Surg* 1974;27:67–76.

Bumsted RM, Ceilley RI. Local anesthesia of the auricle. *J Dermatol Surg Oncol* 1979;5(6):448–449.

Bumsted RM, Ceilley RI, Panje WR, Crumley RL. Auricular malignant neoplasms: When is chemosurgery (Mohs' technique) necessary? *Arch Otolaryngol* 1981;107:721–724.

Ceilley RI, Bumsted RM, Smith WH. Malignancies on the external ear: Ablation and reconstruction of defects. *J Dermatol Surg Oncol* 1979;5:762–767.

Ceilley RI, Lillis PJ. Surgical treatment of chondrodermatitis nodularis helicis. *J Dermatol Surg Oncol* 1979;5(5):384–387.

Conway H, Howell J. Carcinoma of the external ear. *Plast Reconstr Surg* 1957;20:45–54.

Davies J. Embryology and anatomy of the face, palate, nose, and paranasal sinuses. In *Otolaryngology*, MM Paparella, DA Schmurick, eds. Philadelphia, WB Saunders, 1973, pp. 150–178.

Elton RF. Wisdom of subsequent biopsies. *J Dermatol Surg Oncol* 1977;3(3):286.

Fredricks S. External ear malignancy. *Br J Plast Surg* 1956;9:136–160.

Gage AA. Cryosurgery for cancer of the ear. *J Dermatol Surg Oncol* 1977;3:417–421.

Hansen PB, Jensen MS. Late results following radiotherapy of skin cancer. *Acta Radiol (N.S.)* 1968;7:307.

Heenan P, Hueston JT. The distribution of skin tumors on the external ear. *Med J Aust* 1966;2:888–889.

Hollinshead WH. *Anatomy for Surgeons: The Head and Neck.* 2nd ed. Vol. 1. New York, Harper & Row, 1968, pp. 213–215, 352–358.

Marfatia PT. Malignant tumors of the ear. *Laryngoscope* 1966;76:1591–1601.

Mohs FE. Chemosurgery for skin cancer. *Arch Dermatol* 1976;112:211–215.

Mohs FE. Chemosurgical treatment of cancer of the ear. A microscopically controlled method of excision. *Surgery* 1947;21:605–622.

Noel SB, Scallon P, Meadors MC, et al. Treatment of Pseudomonas aeruginosa auricular perichondritis with oral ciprofloxacin. *J Dermatol Surg Oncol* 1989;15:633–637.

Pack GT, Conley J, Oropeza R. Melanoma of the external ear. *Arch Otolaryngol* 1970;92:106–113.

Pless J. Carcinoma of the external ear. *Scand J Plast Surg* 1976;10:147–151.

Rowe DE, Carroll RJ, Day CL. Prognotic factors for local recurrence, metastasis, and survival rates in squamous cell carcinoma of the skin, ear, and lip. *JAAD* 1992;26:976–990.

Shambaugh GE. Developmental anatomy of the ear. In *Surgery of the Ear.* Philadelphia, WB Saunders, 1967, pp. 5–39.

Shiffman MC. Squamous cell carcinomas of the skin of the pinna. *Can J Surg* 1975;18:279–283.

Thomas JM, Swanson NA. Treatment of perichondritis with a quinolone derivative—norfloxacin. *J Dermatol Surg Oncol* 1988;14:447–449.

Zimmerman MC. Chondrodermatitis nodularis helicis. *Skin Surgery.* 3rd ed. E. Epstein, ed. Springfield, IL, Charles C Thomas, 1970, pp. 641–642.

20

The Eyelid

June K. Robinson
Northwestern University Medical School, Chicago, Illinois

The orbital region presents a challenge to the dermatologic surgeon. Even though basic surgical principles still hold, this area is unique. It is necessary to preserve the functions of the eyelid, which include protecting the globe and providing a constant moist environment for the cornea. A thorough knowledge of the anatomy in this region is mandatory prior to performing any surgery. Lesions specific to the orbital region such as chalazions, hordeola, xanthelasma, and sebaceous carcinoma occur in addition to benign and malignant tumors and diseases seen in other regions. With experience in handling the skin of the eyelid and its special elasticity and properties of motion, the dermatologic surgeon can treat most lesions encountered in this region. For more advanced surgical problems, the dermatologic surgeon may wish to have the patient evaluated preoperatively by an ophthalmologist.

ANATOMY

The orbital area contains the brows and the upper and lower lids and extends medially to the root of the nose. The upper lid is limited above by the eyebrows, while the lower merges indefinitely into the cheek. Asymmetry in this region is readily noticed. The configuration of the eyes varies with race, age, and sex, and there are individual considerations such as size, roundness, slope, width, close set, or ptosis. The eyes as the "mirrors of the soul" may be the single most important facial form of expression.

The skin of the eyelids is the thinnest on the body and contains little fat. The palpebral fissures are roughly symmetrical, and the medial and lateral canthi are approximately at the same level horizontally. When the lateral canthus is higher than the medial canthus, this is termed a mongoloid slant. Transverse palpebral creases exist in both the upper and lower lids. The superior palpebral crease, 5–7 mm above the lid margin, marks the superior edge of the tarsus and is due to the attachment of the levator aponeurosis. The inferior palpebral crease varies considerably. It roughly marks the lower margin of the tarsus and is approximately 5 mm below the lash line. As with any other part of the body, the placement of surgical scars in natural creases will produce good cosmetic results (Fig. 1).

The lid structures can be divided into anterior and posterior lamellae. The anterior lamella consists of skin and orbicularis oculi muscle, while the posterior lamella consists of tarsus and conjunctiva. The lamellae are divided by a fascial plane that extends to the lid margin, where it can be identified as the gray line, a linear change in color along the lid margin that represents the mucocutaneous junction. Anterior to the gray line, the cutaneous surface is hair-bearing up to the level of the orifices of the tarsal glands. Posterior to the gray line, the conjunctiva, a thin transparent mucous membrane, lines the posterior surface of the lids and is reflected forward on the eyeball. The eyelashes are located in the anterior lamella of the lid (Fig. 2).

The orbicularis oculi, with attachments to bone medially and laterally, acts as a sphincter to close the lids and maintain muscle tone. It is divided arbitrarily into orbital and palpebral portions. The palpebral portion is further divided into pretarsal and preseptal parts (Fig. 3). In younger individuals, the skin is firmly adherent to the underlying muscle, while with age the attachment becomes loose, with more folds. The pretarsal portion is firmly attached to the underlying tarsus; the only separation is in the superior portion where the levator aponeurosis attaches the pretarsal muscle at the upper edge of the tarsus (Fig. 2). The upper and lower pretarsal muscles are attached laterally to the lateral orbital tubercle of the malar bone. The upper and lower preseptal fibers fuse over the lateral orbital tubercle laterally at the lateral palpebral raphe. Medially, both the pretarsal and preseptal muscles divide into superficial and deep heads. The superficial heads form the medial canthal tendon, which attaches to the anterior lacrimal crest in the nasal process of the maxilla. The deep heads pass depp to the lacrimal sac and attach to the lacrimal diaphragm and posterior lacrimal crest. Thus, the lacrimal sac is surrounded by muscle, and each blink will help the movement of tears down the lacrimal duct (Fig. 3).

The subcutaneous fascia is immediately posterior to the orbicularis oculi muscle, within which run branches of the facial nerve and the maxillary division of the 5th cranial nerve (Fig. 2). The tarsi are immediately beneath the fascia and are composed of dense fibrous tissue. The upper tarsus is 10 mm in vertical height in the central lid and narrows medially and laterally. The lower tarsus is the same length as the upper tarsus but is only 4–5 mm in vertical height in the cen-

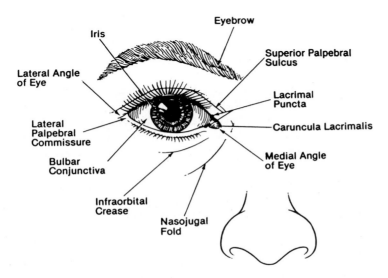

Figure 1 Surface anatomic features of the eyelid region.

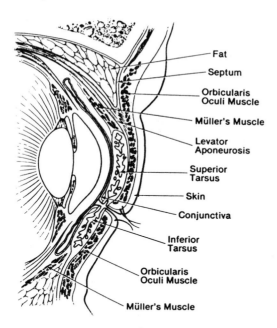

Fat
Septum
Orbicularis Oculi Muscle
Müller's Muscle
Levator Aponeurosis
Superior Tarsus
Skin
Conjunctiva
Inferior Tarsus
Orbicularis Oculi Muscle
Müller's Muscle

Figure 2 Anterior and posterior lamellae of the lid are separated by a fascial plane, which extends from the gray line at the lid margin to the tarsus, levator aponeurosis, and on up to the septum. This cross-sectional diagram of the lid structures clearly demonstrates the fascial plane of separation of the upper eyelid.

tral lid. Each tarsus contains meibomian glands arranged in parallel lines, with the meibomian duct orifices in a line along the ciliary border posterior to the gray line. The meibomian glands are specialized sebaceous glands and are responsible for a significant component of the tear film. Adherent to the posterior tarsus is the tarsal portion of the conjunctiva.

The tarsi are attached to the periosteum of the orbital rims above and below by the orbital septum, which lies in the same fascial plane with the tarsi. The tarsi represent thickened portions of the embryologically developed mesodermal layer of the lid (Fig. 2). The septum extends from the lower lid to the upper lid medially by passing under the attachment of the medial orbicularis muscle and blends in laterally with the lateral canthal tendon. The orbital septum is important in that it keeps the orbital fat in its posterior location (Fig. 4).

The retractors of the eyelids are deep to the orbital fat and their function is to open the eyelids. The upper eyelid is elevated by the levator palpebra superior, which arises as striated muscle from the apex of the orbit. It passes forward under the roof of the orbit and just under the superior orbital rim it passes vertically downward and spreads out as a thin, white, glistening tendinous sheet known as the levator aponeurosis. It fuses with the orbital septum inferiorly and attaches anteriorly to the pretarsal orbicularis muscle, where it is marked by the superior palpebral crease (Fig. 5). On the posterior surface of the levator aponeurosis lies Müller's muscle. This is a thin layer of smooth muscle that originates on the undersurface of the levator and passes down vertically 12–15 mm to insert on the upper border of the tarsus (Fig. 2).

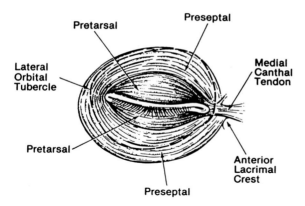

Figure 3 The pretarsal and preseptal parts of the palpebral portion of the orbicularis oculi muscle lie within the dashed line. The orbital portion of the orbicularis oculi muscle is outside of the dashed line.

The eyelids receive vascular supply from both the internal and external carotid arterial systems. The ophthalmic artery branches off the internal carotid artery, whose palpebral branches anastomose with branches from the lacrimal and transverse facial arteries, which come off the external carotid artery. These form the tarsal arcades that run between the tarsus and orbicularis

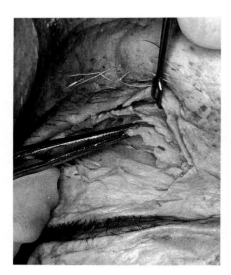

Figure 4 In a cadaver dissection, the skin and the thin orbicularis oculi muscle are elevated under the skin hook, the septum is dissected free, and the levator aponeurosis is held by the forceps. Immediately below the forceps is the superior margin of the upper tarsus. This dissection is performed at the point of fusion of the posterior-lying levator aponeurosis with the septum.

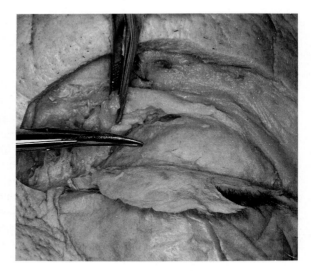

Figure 5 The septum and overlying tissues are removed. The orbital fat is dissected free and held in the clamp. The scissor tip points to the levator aponeurosis where it attaches to the pretarsal orbicularis muscle forming the superior palpebral crease. The thin pretarsal portion of the orbicularis muscle is folded down over the lashes. (Drs. June Robinson and Benjamin Raab performed these dissections.)

oculi muscle. The good vascular supply to the eyelids promotes rapid healing following surgery. The angular artery lies anterior to the medial palpebral ligament 8 mm nasal to the inner angle of the palpebral fissure. The artery is formed by the anastomosis of the dorsal nasal artery and the facial artery and is easily transected when operating in the medial canthal region.

Sensory innervation of the eyelids is via branches of the first and second division of the trigeminal nerve. The first branch gives rise to the supraorbital nerve, arising from the superior orbital fissure and supplying a major portion of the upper lid. It also gives rise to the supratrochlear and infratrochlear nerves, located medial to the eye, which innervate the medial canthal area and root of the nose, respectively. In addition, the first branch of the trigeminal nerve becomes the lacrimal nerve laterally to the eye, which supplies the lacrimal gland and lateral canthus. The lower lid is supplied by branches of the second division of the trigeminal nerve. The zygomaticofacial nerve innervates the lateral canthal area and lateral aspect of the lower lid. It exits bone approximately 1 cm inferior and lateral to the bend where the inferior rim meets the lateral orbital rim. The infraorbital nerve, which exits in the infraorbital foramen, innervates the lower lid, lacrimal sac area, side of the nose, and upper lip (Fig. 6).

The lacrimal apparatus consists of a gland that secretes the tears into the conjunctival sac and lacrimal passages. The lacrimal gland lies beneath the lateral end of the upper eyelid, covered in front by the septum orbitale, orbicularis oculi, and the skin. The gland is a mass of lobules, each about the size of a pinhead. Each lobule consists of a small mass of ramifying tubules branching into the acini of secretory cells. Accessory lacrimal glands are scattered along the conjunctival fornix.

The nasolacrimal system extends in both the upper and lower lids from the medially placed puncta. The upper and lower canaliculi traverse medially deep to the medial canthal tendon and join to form the common internal punctum that connects with the lacrimal sac. The total length of the canaliculi is about 10 mm, with an initial 1–2 mm vertical portion. Tears flow from this into the nasolacrimal duct and into the inferior turbinate of the nose. The lining membrane is continuous with that of the nose. The lacrimal sac lies in the lacrimal fossa surrounded by periosteum. The anatomy of the nasolacrimal system may be best appreciated in passing a probe though the system. The probe should enter the lower punctum and pass initially downward 2 mm,

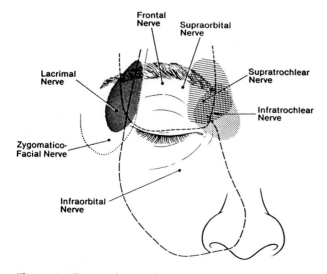

Figure 6 Sensory innervation of the eyelids.

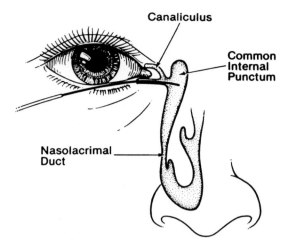

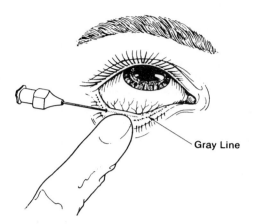

Figure 7   A probe enters the lower punctum and passes into the canaliculus before coming to rest in the lacrimal sac.

Figure 8   The lid is everted to show the gray line and anesthetic is placed between the conjunctival surface of the lid and the gray line.

then turn gently toward the nose. The lower lid may be retracted temporally to straighten the canaliculus. When the probe meets a soft bony resistance, it is in the tear sac and against the lateral wall of the nose (Fig. 7).

The eyebrows are located directly superior to the eye units and tend to extend further both medially and laterally than the eyelids. The medial brow should end at a vertical line passed perpendicularly up from the ala at the nose-cheek junction. The lateral brow should end at a point of intersection with a line passed from the ala-cheek junction to the lateral canthus of the eye. The medial and lateral ends of the brow should lie on a horizontal line. The male brow has less arch than the female. In white patients the hair of the lateral eyebrows slants upward but in Asians these hairs grow downward. While scalp hair grows for 3–10 years, the growing phase of hair in the eyebrow does not exceed 6 months.

ANESTHESIA

General anesthesia is almost never necessary for eyelid surgery unless it is expected to last many hours and involve extensive manipulation. Even extensive cases can be well managed by local anesthesia. Advantages of local over general anesthesia include: (1) greater safety of local anesthesia especially in elderly patients and those with cardiac, pulmonary, or liver disease; (2) an awake patient who will cooperate when needed; (3) a field not obstructed by endotracheal tubes, masks, inhalators, etc.; and (4) lack of dependence on the anesthesiologist for adequate and prompt anesthesia. The use of local anesthesia by the dermatologic surgeon requires thorough knowledge of the anatomy of the nervous supply to the orbital area.

Local anesthesia can be obtained by infiltration or by nerve block. Infiltration anesthesia is adequate preparation for a small portion of the eyelid. In atrophic tissue in the aged, tissue planes separate from the edema produced by local anesthesia and allow easier identification of structures. However, this can be a liability when landmarks such as palpebral creases need to be preserved. In that case, the area to be excised and anatomic landmarks can be marked with gentian violet. After injection of local anesthesia, minimal pressure to the area prevents excessive bruising.

When working with local infiltration anesthesia on small eyelid lesions, it may be advantageous to use a chalazion clamp for hemostasis and stability of the lid and to protect the cornea. The application of this clamp puts pressure on the conjunctival surface of the lid. It is necessary to infiltrate both surfaces of the lid. The hair-bearing skin of the lid is injected to the depth of the tarsal plate first. Then the lid is everted and the needle is placed between the conjunctival surface of the lid and gray line (Fig. 8).

The advantage of nerve block anesthesia is the lack of tissue distortion and the limited volume of anesthesia required. Anesthesia of the upper lid is obtained by palpating the supraorbital notch, located at the junction of the middle and medial third of the upper orbital rim, and injecting 2–3 ml anesthetic under the orbital rim in this area. This blocks the supraorbital nerve. The needle is then redirected medially and more anesthetic blocks the supratrochlear and infratrochlear nerves, which supply sensation to the medial canthus. The lower lid is anesthetized by palpating the infraorbital foramen, which lies 4–5 mm below the lower orbital margin in a vertical line with the supraorbital notch. The needle is introduced at this point and directed laterally and posteriorly, and about 2 ml of anesthetic is injected, Finally, the lateral canthal area can be anesthetized by injecting the zygomaticofacial nerve, which is located 1 cm inferior and temporal to the bend where the inferior orbital rim meets the lateral orbital rim. The lacrimal nerve also supplies the lateral canthus and can be injected by inserting the needle just above the lateral canthal tendon and directing it posteriorly for about 2 mm and then injecting 2–3 ml of anesthetic.

Lidocaine is the most commonly used agent for local anesthesia. It diffuses well through tissue and is not irritating. It is available in solutions of 0.5–2% with and without epinephrine. The maximum dose that can be safely used is 500 mg, however, this is well beyond the amount required for the eyelid. Epinephrine acts as a vasoconstrictor that slows the absorption of the lidocaine and prolongs its effect. Lidocaine 1% with epinephrine 1:100,000 is adequate for anesthesia.

Topical anesthetics are necessary when using protective corneal-scleral shields and chalazion clamps. Tetracaine can be instilled as drops directly on the cornea and conjunctiva. Its onset of action is within 26 sec and its duration ranges from 9 to 24 min. Most patients initially complain of burning that disappears once the anesthetic effect is established. Some patients require a second installation of drops a few minutes after the first. Because the drug may cause transient punctate keratopathy in high doses, the 0.5% solution is preferred.

In patients requiring premedication, meperidine (50–75 mg) with promethazine (12.5–25 mg) given intramuscularly 1 hr preoperatively is helpful. Tranquilizers are usually not needed; however, in a very anxious patient, 5–10 mg of diazepam by mouth may be used.

INSTRUMENTS

A variety of suture material is available for use in this region. The commonly used nonabsorbable sutures are silk, nylon, and Prolene. Silk has the best tying characteristics and is the most pliable but tends to cause more tissue reaction than nylon or Prolene. Braided silk (6–0) is preferred for the delicate thin skin of the eyelids. Because silk softens when moist and lies flat, it will not cause abrasions of the opposing eyelid or the unprotected cornea as may occur with monofilament nylon. However, away from the eyelids, the character of the skin changes, and for the thicker skin of the nose and brows 5–0 or 6–0 nylon should be used. Normal lid skin is so thin that subcuticular sutures are rarely indicated. Once beyond the movable lid skin, however, buried sutures are useful. The skin of the brow and zygomatic regions is well suited to subcuticular closure, and 6–0 Prolene may be considered for the skin since it tends to slide better than silk or nylon. Ideally, the wound should be closed in layers unless the excision is superficial. For deep absorbable sutures in this area, 4–0 or 5–0 gut sutures are often used.

The preferred needles for this region are the taper and reverse cutting type for skin closure and the spatula needle for suturing the tarsal plate. Skin sutures in this area can be removed between the third and fifth postoperative day. After suture removal, the wound is reinforced with sterile adhesive strips. All periorbital skin sutures should be removed by the seventh postoperative day to minimize the formation of scars or epidermal tracts.

The importance of protecting the cornea with opaque eye shields during orbital surgery cannot be overstated. They are placed on the eyeball after topical anesthesia has been obtained. They not only protect the cornea but also block the patient's view and screen the intense light used by the surgeon. They must be the appropriate size and not so large that force is necessary to close the lids over them. The spatula-shaped guard may also be used during a shave or punch biopsy of the lower lid. It is placed between the eyeball and lower lid and functions to support the lid during the procedure and ensure that the eyeball is not injured by perforation through the lid.

Two other instruments unique to this area are the chalazion clamp and the lacrimal probe. The chalazion clamp has one jaw with a round open center and another formed of a slightly curved solid plate. The open jaw surrounds the chalazion or lesion and distributes even pressure around it during excision. The back of the solid jaw is lubricated with ointment and rests lightly against the cornea. When the clamp is in place, a small nut is tightened to the desired pressure so that the surgeon can easily manipulate the end with one hand. The clamp is available in a large range of sizes (Fig. 9).

The lacrimal probe is needed when one is operating around the lacrimal duct. Identification and isolation of the lacrimal duct are performed prior to surgery in this area. A probe, such as the Johnson wire, is rotated into the horizontal plane and passed through the canaliculus to the lacrimal sac. Once surgery has been completed, a silicone stent can be placed in the lacrimal outflow system. The silicone is left in place until the scar matures and softens. The silicone tubing maintains functional patency during the healing process, which usually takes 6–8 months.

EYELID LESIONS

Practically any lesion that may occur elsewhere on the body can occur on the eyelids. In addition, certain lesions are most common in the eyelid region.

Benign Lesions

More than 75% of all eyelid lesions are benign. In addition to common lesions such as seborrheic keratoses, actinic keratoses, verrucae vulgaris, and nevi, benign tumors that occur more commonly in this region or that may produce diagnostic difficulties with malignant tumors are listed in Table 1 (Fig. 10).

A hordeolum, or sty, is an acute bacterial infection of the meibomian glands or of the accessory glands of the lash follicles. It manifests as a localized erythematous swelling but may spread to involve one or both lids. Treatment is with warm compresses and topical antibiotics. If conservative measures do not suffice, incision and drainage may be necessary (Fig. 11).

A chalazion is a chronic granuloma of a meibomian gland caused by retention of secretion. It tends to increase in size slowly, but after a while it may stabilize. It is usually painless unless secondarily infected, in which case it will clinically resemble a hordeolum, and incision and drainage are required. Noninfectious chalazions are usually removed for cosmetic reasons.

Syringoma is an adenoma of eccrine differentiation. It occurs predominantly in women at puberty or later in life. Although occasionally solitary, syringomas usually are multiple. They are small, skin-colored or slightly yellowish, soft papules usually measuring 1–2 mm. They are

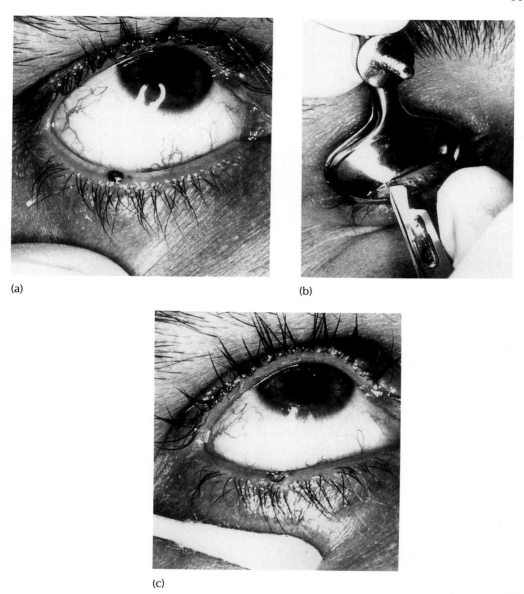

(a)

(b)

(c)

Figure 9 (a) Pigmented lesion of the lower eyelid. (b) Chalazion clamp placed on the lower lid protects the eye during the shave removal when the blade is directed towards the eye. (c) Immediately after the removal of the pigmented lesion.

usually limited to the lower eyelids but may occur on the cheeks, axillae, abdomen, and vulva. They are entirely benign.

Hidrocystoma is an adenoma that may be of eccrine or apocrine origin. It may be skin-colored or have a bluish hue. Eccrine hidrocystoma (1–3 mm) tends to be smaller than an apocrine hidrocystoma (3–15 mm) (Fig. 12).

Table 1 Common Tumors of the Eyelid Region

Benign tumors
    Seborrheic keratoses
    Actinic keratoses
    Verruca vulgaris
    Nevi
    Skin tags
Malignant tumors
    Keratoacanthoma
    Basal cell carcinoma
    Squamous cell carcinoma
    Melanoma
Inflammatory lesions
    Hordeolum (sty)
    Chalazion
Appendage tumors
    Syringoma
    Hidrocystoma
    Trichoepithelioma
    Pilomatricoma
    Sebaceous adenoma
Xanthelasma

    Trichoepithelioma is a benign epithelioma of hair follicle differentiation. It is a firm, elevated, flesh-colored nodule usually measuring less than 2 cm. Its onset is in adult life, and it is most commonly seen on the face but may occur elsewhere. Trichoepitheliomas usually occur as multiple lesions, but occasionally are solitary.

    Pilomatricoma, or calcifying epithelioma of Malherbe, is a benign epithelioma of hair follicle differentiation. It usually manifests as a firm subcutaneous nodule covered by normal skin. Its size varies from 0.5 to 3 cm, and the face and upper extremities are the most common sites.

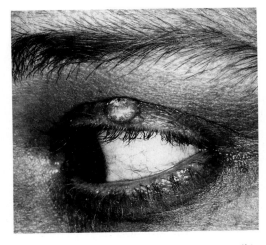

Figure 10 Keratoacanthoma of the upper eyelid.

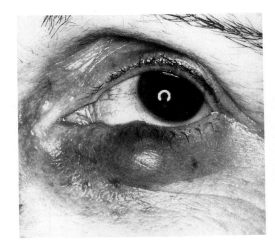

Figure 11 A hordeolum presents as an acute, tender, warm erythematous swelling.

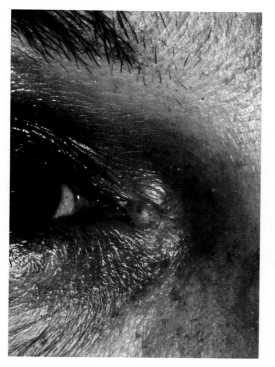

Figure 12 Apocrine hidrocystoma of the medial canthus.

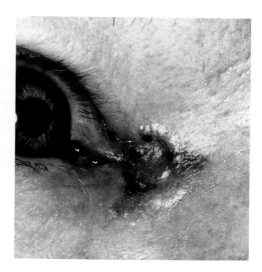

Figure 13 Basal cell carcinoma of the medial canthus with central ulceration and rolled border.

Sebaceous adenoma is a rare tumor of sebaceous gland differentiation and presents as a round, firm elevated papule that may be pedunculated. It is usually solitary and can be located on the face, especially the eyelids, or scalp of adults. The association of sebaceous adenomas of the skin with visceral carcinomas, especially of the colon, is known as Torres's syndrome.

Xanthelasma is a localized infiltrate of lipid-containing histiocytic foam cells in either the upper or lower eyelids. They are yellow, soft macules or slightly elevated papules. Although these xanthomas may suggest underlying hypercholesterolemia when occurring in patients under 40–50 years of age, less than one half of patients have elevated plasma lipid levels. In addition to excision, these can be treated with cryotherapy, electrodesiccation, and application of 25–35% trichloracetic acid.

Malignant Lesions

Basal cell carcinoma is the most common eyelid malignancy, making up more than 90% of all eyelid cancers and nearly 20% of all eyelid tumors (Fig. 13). These tumors most commonly involve the lower lid, followed by the medial canthus, upper lid, and lateral canthus. Although they often invade local tissues, they rarely metastasize. When these tumors arise near the canthi, they tend to infiltrate deeply and may involve the eye or lacrimal drainage system. Due to patient neglect and inadequate early treatment, a mortality rate of 2% was noted in one series. In the same series, enucleation or exenteration was required in 3.6% of cases.

Surgical excision with histologic control of all margins (Mohs micrographic surgery) is the most effective treatment for basal cell carcinoma in the eyelid area. Histologic examination of the margin is particularly important for morpheaform and metatypical basal cell carcinoma. In treating primary basal cell carcinoma in this area, Mohs micrographic surgery has attained cure rates of 99%. Treatment of basal cell carcinoma of the eyelids by simple excision without histologic control of the margins has a recurrence rate of 10–12%. The frequency of recurrence is probably unrelated to the size of the presenting lesion.

Curettage and electrodesiccation are not effective treatment for lesions on the eyelids, because it is difficult to immobilize the skin. Radiation therapy is effective, but results depend on the type of radiation, size of the irradiated field, duration of the tumor, its location, and the depth of penetration. The recurrence rate with radiation therapy observed by the Skin and Cancer Unit at New York University is 7.9% with a follow-up of 5 years and 12.6% after 10 years. Finally, while cryosurgical treatment of primary tumors attains cure rates equal to surgical excision as reported by Torre, many variations in the delivery of this modality in practice result in differing cure rates.

Squamous cell carcinoma, the second most common malignancy of the eyelids, is far less common than basal cell carcinoma, representing about 5% of the malignant lesions. While any part of the eyelid may be involved, the lower lid is the more common. The mortality from squamous cell carcinoma is higher than that reported with basal cell carcinoma, particularly since it has a greater predilection to metastasize to regional lymph nodes. Therefore, in addition to examination of lymph nodes, a wider resection margin is usually required around the tumor than with basal cell carcinoma. Accurate frozen-section examination of margins is mandatory.

Sebaceous gland carcinoma is a rare tumor of the eyelid and adnexa. It usually arises from meibomian glands but can also originate from the glands of Zeis, the sebaceous glands on the cutaneous surface of the eyelids, the sebaceous glands of the eyebrow, and the sebaceous glands located in the caruncle. Sebaceous carcinoma may metastasize and has a high mortality rate (30–40%), probably due to late diagnosis and multicentricity. Many sebaceous carcinomas have a yellow color and cause loss of eyelashes. They may resemble a chalazion and occasionally extend within the conjunctival epithelium by pagetoid spread and mimic blepharoconjunctivitis. Therefore, sebaceous carcinoma should be considered in the differential diagnosis of recurrent or chronic inflammation of the eyelids. Treatment of sebaceous carcinoma consists of wide surgical excision. Because of multicentricity, biopsies from various locations are important to establish the diagnosis. Treatment with Mohs micrographic surgery is the subject of controversy.

Melanoma rarely occurs on the eyelids; however, it may spread to the eyelids from the cheek. The amount of tissue removed is primarily dependent on tumor thickness. An evaluation for metastatic disease is also indicated by tumor thickness.

EXCISION OF LID LESIONS

Surgical treatment depends on the size, location, and anticipated biologic behavior of the malignancy. The main objective of oncologic ophthalmic surgery is to remove the tumor and provide the best functional and cosmetic result possible.

Tarsorrhaphy

Apposition of the margins of the two lids may be required either for protection of the cornea and globe or for immobilization of the lids, such as during healing following a graft or flap for lid reconstruction. The lid margin is deepithelialized for the distance necessary to cover the cornea. Vertical mattress sutures of 4-0 or 5-0 silk with curved needles on both ends of the suture are used. The needle enters the skin approximately 3 mm from the ciliary margin of the upper lid and passes directly into the tarsus, exiting at the lid margin posterior to the gray line. The inner lower lid is then entered at a comparable point to pass through the skin below the ciliary margin. The mattress suture is then completed by going completely through the outer lower lid and entering the inner upper lid. The suture is then tied over cotton pledgets. Usually two or three of these sutures are well tolerated for 1–2 weeks. After suture removal, the lid margins that were deepithelialized are fused.

If a lateral tarsorrhaphy is performed because of permanent loss of the blink reflex and eyelid function due to transection of the ophthalmic branch of the facial nerve, it is never released. When the lid remnants are opposed after tumor resection and prior to final reconstruction, tarsorrhaphy will only be necessary until the final reconstruction is done. Tarsorrhaphy is also done to stabilize the lid and improve survival of a full-thickness skin graft. It may prevent displacement of the lid margin due to wound contraction following full-thickness skin grafting. In this instance, the tarsorrhaphy may be released 4–6 months after the grafting procedure.

Skin Graft

When there is insufficient tissue to close a wound primarily without tension, either a skin flap or a graft can be used to provide coverage. If there is good blood supply and sufficient underlying soft tissue, a full-thickness skin graft may be applied to the base of the defect. The graft should be taken from tissue that matches closely. For the eyelids, the first choice for a donor site is eyelid skin from the opposite eye. The next choice is retroauricular or supraclavicular skin. Full-thickness grafts provide better cosmetic result and are less subject to contraction than split-thickness grafts. Split-thickness grafts are more resistant to infection, tolerate poor circulation better, and cause less disfigurement to the donor area. In eyelid repair, a common problem is avoiding ectropion; thus, full-thickness skin grafts are usually chosen. Even in this example, contracture may occur under the full-thickness skin graft and ectropion can occur.

A thin full-thickness graft for the eyelids is preferred. If retroauricular skin is used, the thinner skin of the back of the ear is placed along the aspect of the wound closest to the lash line. The thicker skin in the sulcus and non–hair-bearing scalp is oriented in the portion of the defect farthest from the lash line. When taking a full-thickness graft, a template of the shape and size of the graft needed is placed on the donor site. This is used to trace an outline of the defect. The donor area is then anesthetized with lidocaine with epinephrine, excised, undermined, and closed. Subcutaneous tissue should be removed from the graft with scissors. The dermis can be partially removed as well to produce a slightly thinner graft.

The graft is sutured into place on the recipient site with simple interrupted 6–0 silk sutures at the lid margin and 5–0 monofilament nylon sutures at other locations around the perimeter of the graft. Tacking sutures placed through the center of the graft ensure its adherence to the wound bed. The ends of several sutures are left long and lightly tied over a bulky dressing to maintain contact between the graft and the recipient site. The bolus tie-over dressing is left in place for 3–5 days and then removed. When removing the bolus dressing, pressure is applied to the graft with forceps to ensure that it remains flat against the wound bed. Most of the sutures are removed and an antibiotic ointment applied to the surface of the graft under a modest pressure dressing. This dressing and the remaining sutures are removed 10 days after surgery.

Chalazion Excision

The chalazion is the most common lid lesion requiring surgical excision. When the lesion presents on the anterior lid, the chalazion clamp is placed around the lesion and a horizontal incision is made over the mass. The cyst is evacuated and fibrous tissue is excised. The skin is closed with 6–0 silk. The horizontal scar blends well with the normal skin crease. When the lesion presents on the posterior lid surface, a chalazion clamp is applied and the lid is everted. A vertical incision is then made over the lesion. The necrotic debris is curetted and fibrosis is excised. Suturing is not necessary and bleeding can be controlled with cautery.

Simple Excision

Simple excision leaving an intact tarsus can be done for small tumors that do not cross the gray line. When possible, lid incisions should lie within the natural creases or should parallel the direction of the orbicularis oculi fibers. The defect should be small enough that no ectropion is produced when the defect is closed. Closure should be made with slight eversion of the skin edges to avoid depression when healing takes place. When closed, the edges of the wound should lie together snugly without puckering.

When the tumor lies close to the lid margin, a simple excision parallel to the orbicularis oculi fibers will produce ectropion. In this case, an intramarginal incision is made along the gray line with a #15 blade to free the mass from the tarsal plate. Two curved incisions are made with scissors, starting at the lid margin on each side of the tumor without disturbing the tarsal plate. The lesion is removed, and 6-0 silk suture is passed horizontally through the skin edges at the ciliary line to approximate the edges of the incision. The orbicularis muscle is sutured with two buried 6-0 chromic catgut sutures, and then the skin is closed with simple interrupted suture of 6-0 silk. Only about 0.5 mm of tissue should be picked up with each bite of suture. Because of the angled cuts of the incision, the skin closure will slightly overhang the tarsal edge. However, as the scar contracts, the ciliary line is reestablished and the lashes are not distorted.

Lower Eyelid Lesions

For small, raised lesions close to the lower lid border and not involving the gray line, a shave excision can be performed. This can be done for biopsy when a lesion is small and not deemed malignant, or when the lesion is not deep or large enough to require an excision. After anesthesia is induced, a backguard is inserted down into the inferior fornix. A #15 blade on a Bard-Parker handle or a #67 blade on a Beaver handle is used to shave the tumor at its base, leaving a smooth lid margin. If the lesion is flat, the scalpel is used to perforate the mass at its lateral edge. The incision is carried medially, and the medial end is cut free. The shave excision should be superficial enough to leave the hair bulbs of the eyelashes intact.

If the lesion extends beyond the gray line or if there is a question of malignancy, a full-thickness lid excision is required. After placement of the backguard or eye shield, excise in a perpendicular fashion from the lid margin on both sides of the lesion to the inferior border of the tarsus. The incisions are then extended in a V fashion to meet below the tarsus (Figs. 14,15). In older patients, direct closure is useful for central eyelid defects affecting less than 40% of the lid margin. In younger patients, because of less skin laxity, it may be possible to close a defect involving 30% or less of the lid margin.

A three-suture technique of 6-0 silk is commonly used to close a lid margin defect. One end of the suture is passed through the meibomian orifice about 1 mm from the wound margin (Fig. 16). The other end of the suture is passed through an orifice on the opposite wound margin. The lid margin should be in good opposition. A second silk suture is similarly placed posterior to the first at the junction between the skin and the conjunctiva and secured. The ends of these sutures are left approximately 2 cm long. A third lid margin suture is placed in the lash line. It is important that it not be placed anterior to the lashes: this will cause the lid margin to invert (ectropion). The long ends of the first two sutures are tied into the knot of the third suture. Three sutures are placed on the free margin of the lid to ensure that tension will be evenly distributed. If one suture ruptures, two others hold the lid in good opposition (Fig. 17).

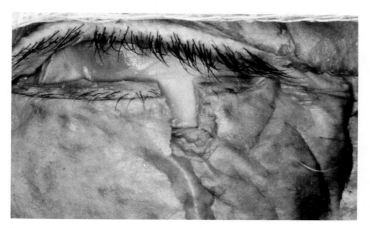

Figure 14 The incision through the lower eyelid is extended to meet in a V (cadaver procedure).

Two or three interrupted 6-0 chromic gut or vicryl sutures are placed through the tarsus in the vertical incision. Conjunctiva should not be included in these sutures. Closure of the tarsus is the most important aspect of lid repair, and great care should be taken to reapproximate the perpendicular edges precisely. If the tarsus is not closed, a notch in the lid will result. The skin is then closed with interrupted 6-0 or 7-0 silk suture. While some believe that these sutures should be placed sufficiently deep to engage the severed orbicularis muscle and reapproximate

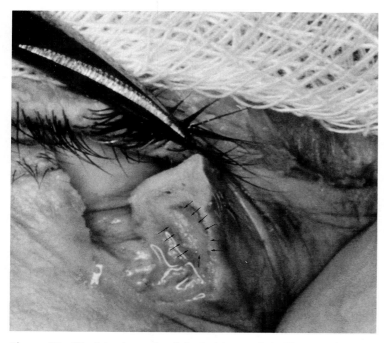

Figure 15 The lateral margin of the incision made in Figure 14 is everted to show the tarsus. Arrows delineate the tarsus (cadaver procedure).

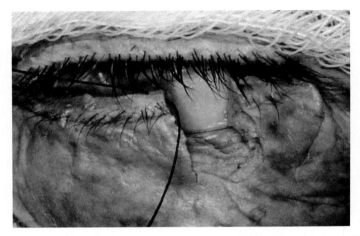

Figure 16   The first suture is placed at the gray line through the meibomian orifice, about 1 mm from the wound margin (cadaver procedure).

it, others do not place sutures into the muscle and simply allow it to reapproximate itself during wound healing (Fig. 18).

   If the initial defect is greater than 40% of the original lid margin, a lateral canthotomy will be required to reduce tension on the wound edge. This is done by making a horizontal excision at the lateral canthal angle and extending it approximately 5 mm on the skin surface. The canthotomy should be angled somewhat superiorly. A scalpel or scissors can be used for the incision. Sharp dissection is carried down to the periosteum of the lateral orbital rim, and the lower crus of the lateral canthal tendon is severed from the rim. This will allow mobilization of about

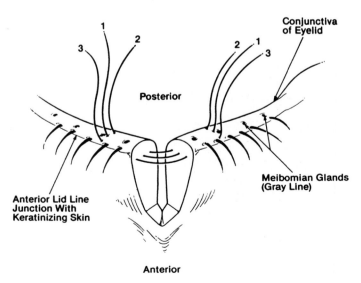

Figure 17   Diagram of the three-suture technique for closure of the lid margin (cadaver procedure).

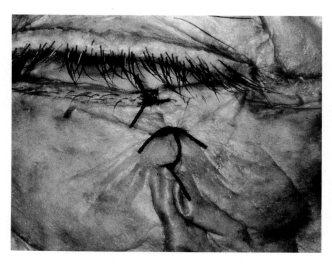

Figure 18   The tarsus is closed and finally the skin is closed.

5 mm of the lateral aspect of the lower lid, which can be moved medially. The lid margin is then closed by the three-suture technique, and the skin is closed at the lateral canthus.

Upper Eyelid Lesions

The technique for removing a lesion from the upper eyelid is similar to that described for the lower eyelid. The upper eyelid is not as conducive to shave excision as the lower eyelid, and, therefore, simple excision is often performed. As with the lower eyelid, the incision should extend in a perpendicular fashion from the lid margin to the superior border of the tarsus. At that point, the incision is extended in a V shape.

Closure is basically the same as that described for lower eyelids. If the edges cannot be easily approximated, a lateral canthotomy is also performed. However, for upper eyelid defects, the arc of the canthotomy incision curves inferiorly and the upper crus of the lateral canthal tendon is severed. Direct closure of defects up to one half of the upper lid can be performed using a canthotomy, especially in older patients. The primary defect is closed using the three-suture technique. Reapproximation of the tarsal plate is particularly important.

Medial Canthus

The simplest defect to close in this area is diamond-shaped. Defects should be fashioned in this manner whenever possible. For all types of medial canthal reconstruction, whether second intention, full-thickness skin graft, or glabella flap, the edge of the lid remnants must be attached to the posterior reflection of the medial canthal tendon to restore the normal canthal angle. This is simply done by placing a strong permanent suture, such as 4–0 silky II Polydek, through the tarsal remnant of both upper and lower lids and attaching it to the posterior reflection of the medial-canthal tendon.

In most situations, the best result is obtained by allowing defects of the medial canthus that are equal above and below the caruncle to heal by second intention. The classic teaching of covering exposed periosteum with a flap is not necessary in this location.

Lateral Canthus

In the aging face, redundancy of skin at the lateral canthus creates "crow's feet." If a lesion is benign, under 3 mm in length, and falls along one of these natural creases, a small simple ellipse may be done. This location is ideal for an M-plasty to reduce the length of the incision.

Malignant primary lesions of the lateral canthus are often deeply invasive when located at the conjunctival margin and will require a resection that disrupts the lateral-canthal tendon and invades the orbit. This should be done with Mohs micrographic surgery. This same principle is true for primary lesions of the medial canthus. Certainly all recurrent lesions of the eyelids require excision by Mohs micrographic surgery. Similarly, malignancies located along the lid margin near to the punctum will migrate along the canaliculus and require the Mohs technique to ensure adequate resection. In these extensive, invasive cases, the Mohs surgeon may work together with an ophthalmoplastic reconstructive surgeon.

One needs to consider the morbidity that will result from inadequate resection of eyelid malignancies. The residual tumor often invades deeply and affects vital structures. Recurrent cancer may require orbital exenteration and ablative craniofacial surgery for a potentially life-threatening, recurrent aggressive tumor. It is reasonable to use the technique that provides the best chance of cure as the initial resection. This technique is Mohs' micrographic surgery.

EYEBROW LESIONS

For lesions on or around the eyebrow, single and double advancement flaps are used. The length of the flap should not move more than three times the width of the base. The lesion is removed in a square or rectangular fashion. A single-advancement flap is incised and its base widely undermined for forward motion. Burow's triangles are cut at the base as the flap slides forward. The first suture is placed from the center of the advancing flap to the opposing surface. Then two corner stitches are placed at the tips of the flap, followed by the rest of the interrupted or half-buried sutures.

For eyebrow defects, double-advancement flaps or an H-plasty is performed to advance hair-bearing skin from both sides of the defect. This repair maintains continuity of the brow and prevents the cosmetically displeasing split eyebrow. After both flaps are incised, the center of each advancing limb is approximated with a single stitch and then four-point corner stitches are placed. The Burow's triangles are cut to accommodate secondary movement. The remainder of the flap is sutured with interrupted or half-buried sutures (Fig. 19).

COMPLICATIONS

An expected consequence of eyelid surgery is postoperative bruising and edema. Bleeding during surgery must be controlled before closure is performed. In addition, an adequate preoperative history must be taken to determine if the patient is taking any medications that will cause excessive bleeding. A variety of medications can affect the clotting mechanism, including aspirin, indomethacin, and anticoagulants. These should be discontinued for at least 2 weeks before

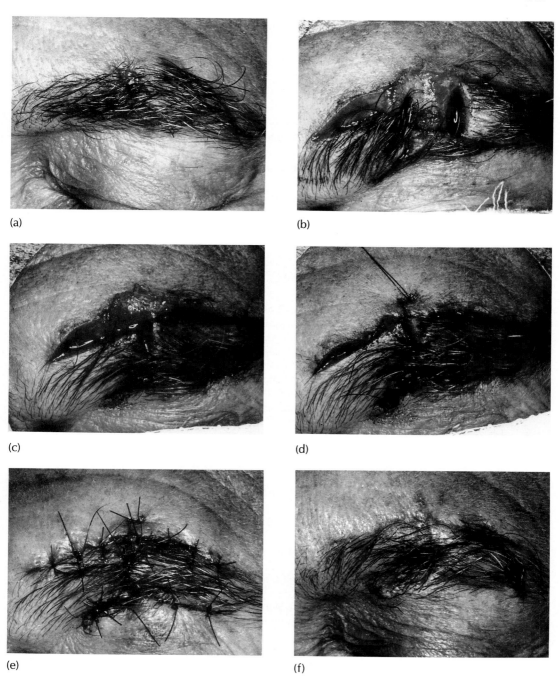

(a)

(b)

(c)

(d)

(e)

(f)

Figure 19 (a) Basal cell carcinoma of the eyebrow. (b) Tumor is excised and limbs of bilateral advancement flap are incised. (c) Advancement flaps are approximated by subcutaneous sutures. (d) The first corner suture is placed. (e) All incisions are closed with interrupted sutures and two four-point corner sutures. (f) Six weeks after surgery there is no hair loss. Incision lines are slightly erythematous.

surgery. Nevertheless, postoperative bruising is not uncommon and the patient should be made aware that this may occur.

Eyelid surgery should be done with a plastic nonconducting backguard or corneal shield to prevent abrasion of the cornea. Corneal abrasion can occur whenever an instrument is dragged across the eye when the eyelid is elevated. Inadvertent cautery of the cornea would be disastrous.

Ectropion and entropion refer to eversion and inversion of the eyelid margin, respectively. Ectropion of the lower lid results in epiphora (overflow of tears) and irritation of the skin of the lid by the tears. In addition, corneal exposure may lead to keratitis. Ectropion can occur when a large defect is produced below the lower lid and healing results in contracture. This can be prevented by excising eyelid lesions as described previously and by the use of flaps or full-thickness skin grafts.

Entropion will cause constant irritation resulting in conjunctivitis, keratitis, and corneal ulcers. The occurrence of entropion after eyelid surgery is uncommon as long as the lid margin is reapproximated properly using the three-suture technique and the edges of the tarsus are reapproximated precisely.

BIBLIOGRAPHY

Arkel S. Evaluation of platelet aggregation in disorders of hemostasis. *Med Clin North Am* 1976;60:881–911.

Bart RS, Kopf AW, Petratos MA. X-ray therapy of skin cancer: Evaluation of a "standardized" method for treating basal cell epitheliomas. Proceedings, 6th National Cancer Conference, 1970, pp.559–569.

Beard C. Observations on the treatment of basal cell carcinoma of the eyelids. *Trans Am Acad Ophthalmol Otol* 1975;79:664–670.

Brodkin RH, Kopf AW, Andrade R. Basal cell epithelioma and elastosis: A comparison of distribution. In *The Biologic Effect of Ultraviolet Radiation*. F Urbach, ed. London, Pergamon Press, 1969, pp. 581–618.

Friedman AH, Henkind P. Clinical and pathological features of eyelid and conjunctival tumors. In *Ophthalmic Plastic Surgery*. SA Fox, ed. New York, Grune & Stratton, 1976, pp. 24–63.

Grove AS, Jr. Eyelid tumors, diagnosis and management. In *Oculoplastic Surgery*. CD McCord, ed. New York, Raven Press, 1981, pp. 151–173.

Iliff CE, Iliff WJ, Iliff NI. Tumors of the ocular adnexa. In *Oculoplastic Surgery*. CE Ilif, ed. Philadelphia, WB Saunders, 1979, pp. 223–318.

Meltzer MA. *Ophthalmic Plastic Surgery for the General Ophthalmologist*. Baltimore, Williams & Wilkins, 1979.

Mohs FE. *Chemosurgery: Microscopically Controlled Surgery for Skin Cancer*. Springfield, IL, Charles C Thomas, 1978.

Mohs FE. Chemosurgical treatment of cancer of the eyelid: A microscopically controlled method of excision. *Arch Ophthalmol* 1948;39:43.

Payne JW, Duke JR, Butner R, Eifrig DE. Basal cell carcinoma of the eyelids: A long term follow-up study. *Arch Ophthalmol* 1969;81:553.

Putterman A. *Cosmetic Oculoplastic Surgery*. New York, Grune & Stratton, 1982.

Robinson JK. Prevention of intraoperative trauma to the lacrimal system. *J Dermatol Surg Oncol* 1983; 9:802–804.

Torre D. Cryosurgery treatment of eyelid tumors. In *Ocular and Adnexal Tumors*. FA Jakobiec, ed. Birmingham, AL, Aesculapius, 1978, pp. 517–524.

21

The Lips and Oral Cavity

Hubert T. Greenway
Scripps Clinic and Research Foundation, La Jolla, California

SURGERY OF THE LIPS

The lips are graceful structures that symmetrically occupy the lower third of the facial profile we present to others. The lips have been a subject of interest and decoration for societies through the ages. The original tissue expander may well have been a piece of wood inserted into the lower lip, a custom still practiced by the Suya Indian tribe in central Brazil. Once a young man is married, a small lightweight wooden disc is inserted in the lip; with time, the disc is exchanged for larger discs up to 3 inches in width and ¾ inch thick. The lip disc in this case signifies masculine self-assertion, while in the Fali tribe of northern Nigeria, women wear the lip disc as ornamentation.

The lips are perfectly symmetric structures, and many attribute certain personality traits based not only on their shape but also their use! Even the slightest movement may convey a subtle emotion, and exaggerated movements such as the protrusion of the lower lip may accentuate strong feelings. The famed smile of the "Mona Lisa" by Leonardo da Vinci has served to convey both simplistic and more complex feelings in the imagination of art lovers since 1503.

The use of lipstick allows one to dramatize the natural shape of the lips. Painting lips appears to be an ancient art practiced by highly developed civilizations for thousands of years. The original lip color, rouge, was a dye of animal or vegetable base, whereas today's formulations use lanolins, alcohols, oils, and waxes.

Anatomy

The lips represent the anterior border of the mouth. In addition to the expression of emotion, they are important for speech, intake of food, and mastication. The topical anatomy of the lips reflect the symmetric nature of all components (Fig. 1). In the midline, the philtrum and Cupid's bow contribute to the delicate symmetry of the upper lip. Laterally, the nasolabial crease denotes

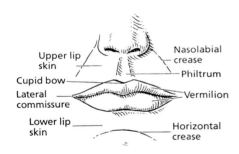

Figure 1   Topical anatomy of the lip.

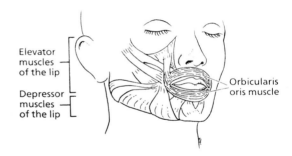

Figure 2   Basic musculature of the lip. The orbicularis oris muscle provides the bulk musculature of the lip proper.

the boundary with the cheek. The skin of the lower lip forms a horizontal crease where it contacts the chin. The skin of the lips contains hair, sebaceous glands, and eccrine glands. In the male, the entire upper lip and central portion of the lower lip are hair bearing.

The vermilion border is the mucocutaneous junction between the skin and the dry mucosa or vermilion of the lip. This border is easily visible and if violated surgically must be precisely reconstructed to preserve normal lip symmetry. The vermilion of the upper and lower lip is red in color due to a lack of keratinization and the underlying capillary plexus. Sebaceous glands are found in normal vermilion tissue 50% of the time, although normally no hairs are present. The dry vermilion becomes a wet mucous membrane proximally in the oral cavity.

The bulk of the tissue comprising the lips consists of striated muscle, primarily the orbicularis oris (Fig. 2). This is the basic muscle of the lip. The major portion, the orbicularis oris proper, consists of longitudinal fibers arranged in a sphincteric fashion about the mouth. A portion of the sphincteric fibers in the lower lip form a horizontal shelf or protrusion of the vermilion, which can be accentuated in normal expressions. The group of deep anterocaudally oriented fibers provides the compressive movement to force the lips against the teeth. In the philtral area, muscle fibers cross and intersect with vertically oriented fibers present at the philtral columns. The orbicularis oris muscle also decussates at the lateral commissures of the mouth.

Three muscles or muscle groups function in concert with the orbicularis oris muscle. The upper group of muscles, the labial elevators, consists of the zygomaticus major, the zygomaticus minor, the levator labii superioris, the levator labii superioris alaeque nasi, the levator anguli oris, and the risorius muscle. These muscles function in concert as elevators of the lips, contributing with the risorius, to the upward elevation of the corner of the mouth. Additionally, the risorius has been referred to as the "smile" or "unpleasant grin" muscle, as it assists with this function.

The lower group of muscles, the labial depressors, consists of the depressor labii inferioris, the depressor anguli oris or triangularis, and the mentalis. These muscles function in concert as depressors of the lip, acting with the orbicularis oris. The mentalis muscle also functions to force the lower lip against the gum by drawing the skin of the lip upward.

The third muscle group is the singular buccal muscle forming the majority of the muscular substance of the cheek. It arises from the maxilla, the mandible, and the pterygomandibular ligament. The buccinator acts to force the cheek against the teeth, forcing food into the oral cavity.

The commissures of the mouth (Fig. 1) form a complex area with contributions from the orbicularis oris muscle as well as insertions from the upper elevators, the lower depressors, and

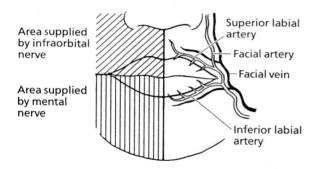

Figure 3   Vascular and nerve supply to the lip and perioral area.

the buccinator. Deficiencies in this area may be accentuated by normal actions of the contralateral commissure.

The vasculature of the lips consists mainly of the inferior and superior labial arteries, which are the main branches of the facial artery (Fig. 3). They pass deep to the elevators and depressor muscle groups to run tortuously in the orbicularis oris fibers, at times running superficially between the muscle and mucosa. With age, the tortuosity may increase and with atrophy and thinning of the orbicularis oris these vessels may be more easily palpable. Identification of the labial arteries is important in lip surgery, as ligation of these vessels is often warranted.

Nerve supply to the lips consists of a sensory and a motor portion. The sensory component to the skin and mucosa is via the trigeminal nerve, with the infraorbital nerve supplying the upper lip and the mental nerve (Fig. 3) supplying the lower lip. The facial nerve provides motor innervation to the lips mainly via buccal branches to the orbicularis oris and elevator muscles, while the marginal mandibular branch innervates the depressor muscles of the lips but also contributes to the orbicularis oris fibers. Injury to the branches of the facial nerve in the lip is rare, as innervation of the muscles is from the deep aspect.

Lymphatic drainage of the perioral area is to the submental buccal, mandibular, submandibular, superficial cervical, and upper deep cervical nodal areas. These areas should be evaluated and documented when dealing with squamous cell carcinoma as well as other tumors that can metastasize to nodal areas. In general, the lateral one third of the lip drains to the ipsilateral nodes, whereas the central one third of the lip may drain to nodes on either side.

The nasolabial folds deepen and lengthen with age. The concavity of Cupid's bow flattens, as does the entire upper lip, which is accentuated by the downward and lateral drooping of both lateral commissures. One must take the aging process into account (Fig. 4), as well as the normal anatomy, when performing surgery in this area.

Principles of Lip Surgery

Scars or imperfections after lip surgery can be a distressing problem. The following surgical principles unique to this area should be adhered to.

1.   Avoid lip distortion and unsightly scars (once a tumor-free margin is assured in the case of malignant lesions). Every attempt should be made to retain the normal contours (Fig. 1), with the philtrum and Cupid's bow contributing to the delicate symmetry of the upper lip.

2.   Be aware of the underlying anatomy. Undermining may be more difficult in the philtral area and is done superficial to the underlying muscle. Sutures may be required for vascular ligation. Damage to subdermal hair bulbs (upper lip and midline lower lip skin) should be avoided

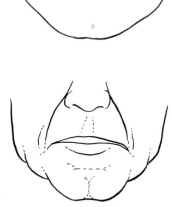

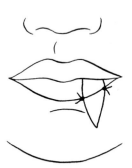

Figure 4 Changes in lip anatomy both topically and structurally with aging. There is flattening of the upper lip and drooping of the commissures.

Figure 5 Preanesthesia marking of the vermilion border with 7–0 silk suture prior to local infiltration can allow exact recreation of the border.

in male patients. Layered anatomic closure (skin, muscle, mucosa) is important to avoid dead space and restore anatomic function. Underlying architectures such as the mandible and teeth influence the closure forces as well as the final result.

3.   Incisions should be made at the junction of natural boundaries to hide their placement (i.e., vermilion border, nasolabial fold, chin horizontal crease). Intraoral incisions should also be considered. Following skin tension lines, the majority of incisions around the lip should be vertical except at the commissures. Incisions crossing the vermilion border should be planned to recreate the border exactly. Marking with 7–0 silk suture prior to administering local anesthesia (Fig. 5) can help identify the border during closure. Marking pens, "nicks" with a #11 scalpel, and careful visual approximation may also be used for this purpose. It may be necessary to close a standard fusiform excision with angles greater than 30° (i.e., 45°) in order to avoid crossing the vermilion border on either the skin or the mucosal side (Fig. 6).

4.   Nerve block anesthesia is better tolerated by patients, especially if approached intraorally following the application of topical anesthesia to the mucous membrane. Common nerve blocks performed are of the infraorbital nerve supplying the upper lip and the mental nerve supplying the lower lip. Local infiltration may then be added for hemostasis.

5.   In general, defects involving up to one third of the upper or lower lip can be closed primarily in a layered fashion (i.e., basic bilateral advancement closure) (Fig. 7). Larger defects may require local or pedicle flap closure. Nasolabial fold, cheek, and neck tissue are commonly utilized for lip reconstruction as well as scalp and forehead tissue via distant flaps. Defects of the commissure require special consideration due to the force of the underlying muscle attachments. Skin grafts may be utilized at times but may offer less acceptable cosmetic results, especially for deeper defects.

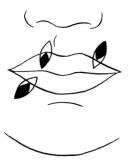

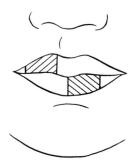

Figure 6 Compromise of the standard 30° angles of fusiform incision may be indicated (darker areas) to avoid crossing the vermilion border. Often a 45° angle will close and heal with an acceptable result, especially in older patients.

Figure 7 Defects up to one third of the upper or lower lip (shaded areas) can be closed primarily after procedures such as a wedge excision. Larger defects may require flap closure.

6. Stabilizing the lip is critical during surgical procedures and can be achieved with the help of a surgical assistant, tension suture ligatures, chalazian clamps, and dental rolls (or gauze pads), as depicted in Figure 8. These ancillary measures provide greater exposure and patient comfort. On the mucosal surface, soft, braided suture material may be preferable for the patient's comfort, such as 4–0 or 5–0 silk permanent suture or Vicryl, Dexon, or chromic absorbable suture.

Repair of Superficial Defects

Small superficial lesions around the lip removed by shave excision with a #15 blade heal well by second intention with excellent cosmetic results (Fig. 9). Stabilizing the lip is extremely important. Remember that the labial arteries may be tortuous and superficial in elderly patients.

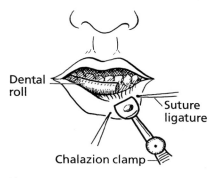

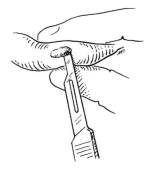

Figure 8 Stabilization of the lip may be achieved with dental rolls (or rolled gauze) between the lip and gums, suture ligatures temporarily placed, or instruments such as a chalazian clamp.

Figure 9 Shave excision of small superficial lip lesions may be allowed to heal by second intention.

Small lesions may be removed by excision or punch biopsy and will heal satisfactorily by second intention but may heal more rapidly by simple primary closure. Avoid crossing the vermilion border if possible.

Larger superficial defects may require closure with local rotation or advancement flaps (Fig. 10). Often a portion of the scar can be hidden on the inner moist mucosa, which is not normally visible.

Vermilionectomy of the lower lip may be indicated for severe solar cheilitis. This procedure is done with less frequency today due to excellent results obtained with other destructive modalities such as carbon dioxide laser vaporization. To perform the vermilionectomy, the area to be removed is precisely marked so that approximately 1 cm of dry mucosa will be removed. The incision is made with a scalpel and the vermilion excised with scissors. Underlying muscle is left intact. The vestibular wet mucosa is undermined with direct visualization prior to advancement and closure. This procedure often provides good functional and cosmetic results.

Repair of Deep and Full-Thickness Defects of the Lips

Larger defects of skin around the lips can be repaired by local flaps or skin grafts. Defects including loss of underlying muscle or full-thickness defects can often be converted to a wedge excision for primary reconstruction, providing it covers less than one third of the lip.

Defects of the upper lip skin can often be repaired by a caudally based nasolabial fold transposition flap in which cheek skin is used as the donor area (Fig. 11). At times, a superiorly or

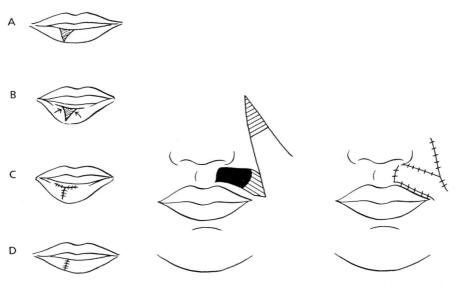

Figure 10 A-to-T closure of a mucosal defect via bilateral advancement/rotation flaps with donor incisions hidden from view. Closure is with interrupted nonirritating suture such as 5–0 or 6–0 silk.

Figure 11 Inferior or caudally based nasolabial transposition flap for upper lip defect reconstruction.

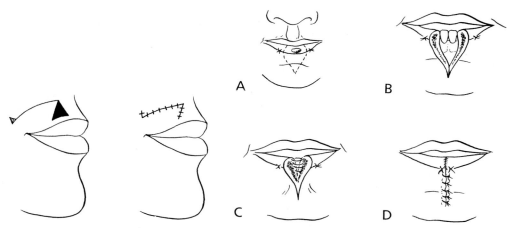

Figure 12   Rotation flap with Burow's triangle to construct upper lip defect in an older patient where a portion of the donor area laterally may be hidden in the nasolabial fold and where, because of age, the commissure is lax and maintains its normal position in spite of the primary and secondary motions of the flap.

Figure 13   Wedge excision of the lip, marking the vermilion border (A), defect with less mucosal surface removal (B), closure partially complete with mucosal surface closed and muscle being closed (C), and complete closure (D).

cranially based nasolabial fold flap may be considered. Defects of the upper lip may also be closed with a rotation flap from the nasolabial fold area with a Burow's triangle if required (Fig. 12). Avoid distorting the commissure, however. At times, perialar crescent-shaped excisions provide increased donor mobility and improve the cosmetic result. In certain cases, advancement flaps such as an A-to-T flap may be preferred, which normally do not put any upward pull on the lip. Full-thickness skin grafts can be utilized, but there can be problems with graft survival, retraction, and skin matching (i.e., color).

Wedge resection of the lip, done when the defect is less than one third of the lip, starts by marking the vermilion border as previously described. The incision or defect lines should cross the vermilion border at 90° angles if possible. On the lower lip the skin portion of the wedge should not extend below the horizontal chin crease. If necessary, an M- or W-plasty should be done to prevent this. On the mucosal side, the incision should not extend beyond the gingival-labial sulcus.

Hemostasis must be meticulous with suture ligatures normally used for the labial artery. The mucosal surface can be closed with either absorbable or nonabsorbable sutures. The orbicularis oris muscle must be closed carefully in order to prevent notching, and the anterior shelf protrusion is recreated. Interrupted sutures of 5–0 Vicryl or Dexon can be used for this. Next, the subcutaneous layer may be closed with absorbable sutures if necessary to remove tension from the surface edges. The skin and dry mucosa are closed first, carefully reapproximating the vermilion border. Monofilament sutures such as 5–0 or 6–0 nylon may be used on the lip skin; however, less irritating sutures such as 6–0 silk should be used on the dry mucosal surface. The mucosal edge may elevate slightly immediately postoperative, but this will resolve (Figs. 13–15).

An Abbe-Estlander flap can be utilized for full-thickness loss where wedge repair is inadequate. The opposing lip acts as the donor area. The pedicle based on the labial artery is divided in 3 weeks or less.

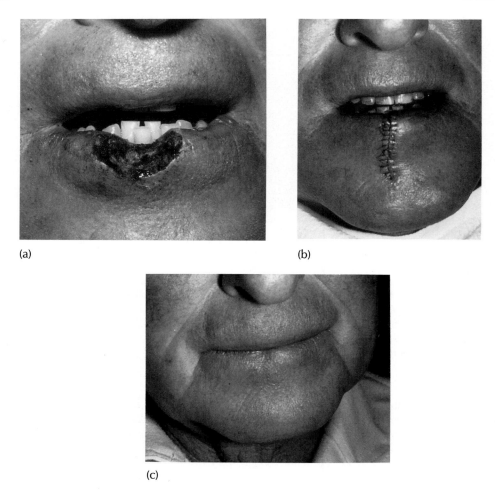

(a)   (b)

(c)

Figure 14   (a) Defect of one third of the lower lip. (b) Result after completion of layered closure. In this case the chin horizontal crease was not well defined and could be violated with a V to enhance the result. (c) Final result at 2 months.

Repair of the Lip Commissure

The commissure or angle of the mouth has several force rectors acting upon it including the underlying elevator and depressor muscles of the lip. Skin tension lines may vary. Loss of function is more noticeable because of normal function of the contralateral angle. For small defects, primary closure with an M-plasty may provide the best results (Fig. 16). Transposition flaps may be necessary for larger defects of this area in order to prevent distortion (Figs. 17, 18).

Carcinoma of the Lip

While basal cell carcinoma is the most common cancer of the skin of the lip, squamous cell carcinoma is the most common mucosal lip malignancy. Squamous cell carcinoma of the lip represents 25% of oral cancer tumors, and over 90% of these occur on the lower lip. In the past, this tumor was more common in males but today occurs in both sexes and is most common in

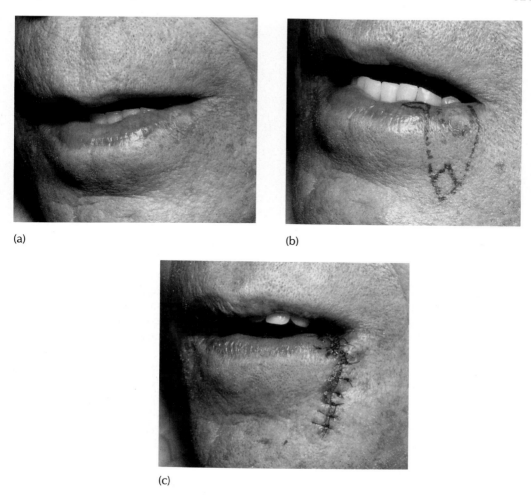

(a)   (b)

(c)

Figure 15 (a) Preoperative squamous cell carcinoma at lower lateral vermilion border after shave biopsy. (b) Wedge resection outlined providing adequate margin and utilizing a W-plasty inferiorly so as not to cross onto the chin. Note small wedge perpendicular triangle on lip proper (medially to defect), which may be of value in decreasing the thickness of the lip in certain cases. (c) W-plasty not performed. However, perpendicular medical wedge resection of adjacent lip proper allowed contouring of remaining margins at closure.

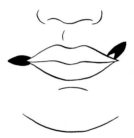

Figure 16   M-plasty closure may provide the best results for small lip commissure defects.

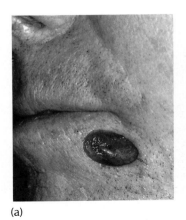
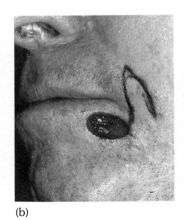
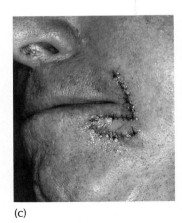

(a)   (b)   (c)

Figure 17 Defect below the lateral commissure. Reconstruction with transposition flap takes advantage of excess tissue of the nasolabial fold area in order to avoid downward pulling of the lateral commissure.

the 50- to 70-year-old group. Presenting initially as a readily visible and palpable tumor, it is usually diagnosed early. Treated at an early stage, cure rates are excellent. The two most common risk factors are solar radiation and tobacco. The upright stature of humans, as well as the normal protrusion of the lower lip, implicate the lower lip as a recipient of more solar radiation.

In addition to visual examination of suspicious scaly or nodular lesions with or without magnification, palpation allows the surgeon to determine the degree of infiltration and clinical borders. Palpation of the submental, submaxillary, and cervical lymphatics should be performed and documented. Examination of the entire perioral and oral cavity should also be performed. Biopsy confirmation requires an adequate biopsy to provide tissue for histologic examination. In certain cases, radiologic examination of the neck, jaw, sinuses, and chest may be applicable. The tumor node metastasis (TNM) classification of lip cancer categorizes tumors and assists in planning treatment (Table 1).

Treatment of squamous cell carcinoma of the lip requires surgery in most cases. Early tumor (T1 and T2) can be adequately removed and reconstructed as previously described. More extensive tumors may require specialized reconstructive techniques once the local tumor has been eliminated. Lymph nodes must be evaluated, and a decision on treatment, either surgical, irradiation, or both, must be made. Routine, close follow-up is mandatory to evaluate local and nodal extension of tumor. Cure rates for squamous cell carcinoma of the lip are good overall. As expected, this relates to the size and status of disease at the time of diagnosis. Mohs series of 1448 consecutive patients demonstrated a cure rate of 94.2%. Baker and Krause published statistics of 5-year cure rates of over 90% for small tumors, dropping to 80% for more aggressive lesions as indicated by cellular atypia, depletion of lymphocytes, and infiltration into un-

Figure 18 (a) Similar defect to Figure 17 with residual tumor. (b) Final defect with 60° transposition donor tissue inferiorly and laterally. Note flap is larger than defect to provide overcorrection and avoid downward pulling of commissure area. (c) Transposition of flap into recipient site. Closure of subcutaneous donor area first would allow flap to sit easily in defect area. (d) Repair with no downward pulling of lip or commissure. (e) Result at one month. Patient is now instructed to massage area to assist in decreasing residual swelling.

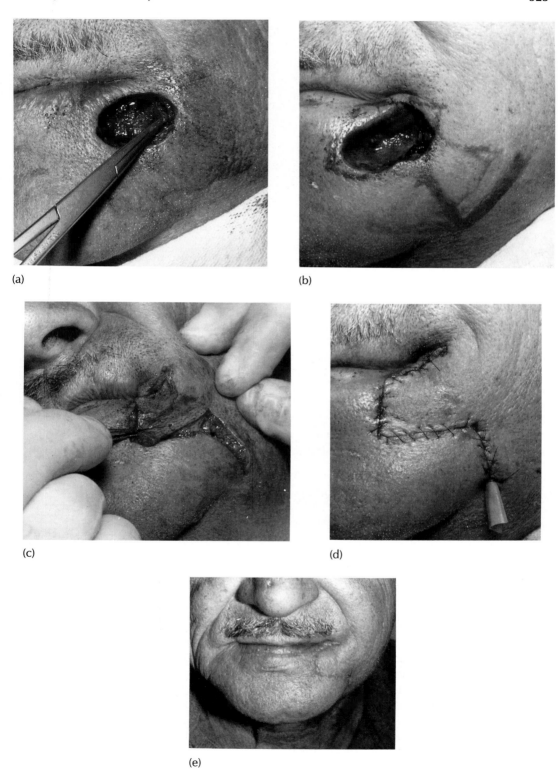

(a)

(b)

(c)

(d)

(e)

Table 1 Tumor Node Metastasis Classification for Lip Cancer

Primary tumor (T)	
TIS	Preinvasive carcinoma (carcinoma in situ)
T0	No evidence of primary tumor
T1	Tumor measuring 2 cm or less in its largest dimension, strictly superficial or exophytic
T2	Tumor measuring 2 cm or less in its largest dimension with minimal infiltration in depth
T3	Tumor measuring more than 2 cm in its largest dimension or tumor with deep infiltration, irrespective of size
T4	Tumor involving bone
Regional lymph nodes (N)	
N0	Regional lymph nodes not palpable
N1	Movable homolateral nodes
	N1a: Nodes not considered to contain growth
	N1b: Nodes considered to contain growth
N2	Movable contralateral or bilateral nodes
	N2a: Nodes not considered to contain growth
	N2b: Nodes considered to contain growth
N3	Fixed nodes
Distant metastases (M)	
M0	No evidence of distant metastases
M1	Distant metastases present

derlying muscle as well as the TNM classification at the time of diagnosis. Evaluation of the tumor for perineural invasion is important. Tumors with perineural spread may extend several centimeters beyond other negative margins. Mohs surgery combined with a course of postoperative radiation may be indicated in tumors with perineural component. Half of the cutaneous squamous cell carcinomas that metastasize have evidence of perineural invasion.

SURGERY OF THE ORAL CAVITY

Anatomy

The interior anatomy of the mouth is divided into two portions: the vestibule and the oral cavity. The vestibule is that space bounded internally by the teeth and gums and externally by the lips and cheeks. Mucous membrane lines the vestibule as well as the oral cavity proper (teeth to oropharynx) (Fig. 19). This mucous membrane must be maintained at the vestibule angle where the alveolar and buccal mucosa meet or the normal sulcus will be obliterated. The tuberculum is that area of the lip proper below the philtrum. The roof of the mouth is formed by the hard and soft palates (Fig. 20). The palatoglossal arch forms the boundary between the mouth and oropharynx. The palatine tonsil lies between this and the palatopharyngeal arch. The tongue projects from the mouth floor, and its muscle is covered only with mucous membrane. The lingual frenulum is a vertical fold of mucous membrane connecting the central undersurface of the tongue to the floor of the mouth. Stenson's duct is the opening of the parotid duct into the oral cavity located opposite the upper second molar tooth. Wharten's duct in the anterior floor of the mouth empties the submandibular gland. The orifices of these ducts should be avoided if possible during surgical procedures. Cannulization may allow precise identification during surgery.

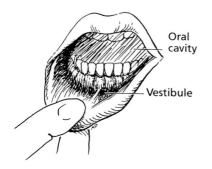

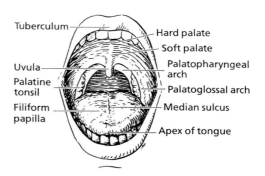

Figure 19 The mouth is divided into two portions: the vestibule and the oral cavity.

Figure 20 The oral cavity.

The inferior alveolar and lingual nerves provide sensory innervation and can be blocked readily as the two nerves are in close approximation near the mandibular foramen. The infraorbital and mental nerves may also be blocked for procedures involving the mucosa of the lips.

General Principles

1. Airway maintenance is of utmost importance both during and after surgical procedures. Postoperative edema may impair the airway.
2. Direct visualization and exposure is essential and may be different from most cutaneous procedures. Headlights, proper instrumentation, traction sutures, as well as a suction apparatus must be available.
3. Avoid critical anatomic structures (e.g., ductal orifices) whenever possible.
4. Primary closure can be accomplished in most cases and offers less morbidity than other techniques.

Repair of Surgical Defects

Biopsy or removal of cystic lesions and benign growths as well as malignant growths requires closure in most cases except for pedunculated lesions, which may be removed and allowed to heal by second intention. Primary closure can be accomplished with nonirritating sutures, which can be removed in 3–5 days in most cases.

Figure 21 demonstrates the planning and closure of an ellipse on the tongue. A 3-0 silk (braided) suture is placed in the anterior portion of the tongue to extend and stabilize it in position out of the mouth. Wrapping the tongue in gauze and grasping it with your fingers can be done, but this is less reliable. The ellipse is normally planned so the tip points toward the apex of the tongue.

Removal of oral lesions often causes brisk bleeding from the wound edges due to the excellent vascularization of the mouth. Electrocautery as well as direct pressure with gauze can be used for hemostasis prior to wound closure. Interrupted 3-0 or 4-0 silk sutures can be used for closure. Interrupted suturing provides a margin of safety over running suture as constant intraoral movement may loosen a suture. Silk is a soft braided material, which is more comfortable to

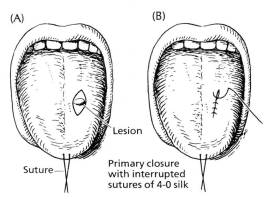

Figure 21 A silk suture through the apex of the tongue provides exposure (A). Note the correct method of elliptical excision on the tongue. Closure is accompanied with interrupted 4–0 silk sutures (B).

the patient. Alternatively, 3–0 or 4–0 Vicryl or chromic can be used, and suture removal is not necessary.

Carcinoma of the Oral Cavity

Carcinoma of the oral cavity develops due to invasion of malignant epithelial cells. Chronic irritation from tobacco, dentures, sunlight (lips), and other factors may play a role. Leukoplakia appears as a whitish, painless, shiny patch on the mucous membrane that may undergo malignant change. Biopsy of leukoplakia and, more importantly, biopsy of adjacent erythroplakia is necessary if present.

Clinical staging of carcinoma of the oral cavity is similar to the lip under the tumor nodal metasis classification (Table 2). Intraoral squamous cell carcinoma is graded 1, 2, 3, or 4 (well differentiated, moderately well differentiated, poorly or very poorly differentiated). Major initial therapeutic modalities include surgery and irradiation.

Postoperative Management and Care

Airway maintenance is of utmost importance and must not be compromised. In order to prevent bleeding and postoperative edema, stabilization of the surgical area and limitation of motion must be maintained. At times, no dressing or bandage is required (i.e., small lip or intraoral excisions); at other times a large pressure wrap (i.e., Barton's dressing) may be considered.

Infections are rare with minor lip and oral cavity procedures. They must be monitored and treated appropriately, considering the proximity of the sinuses to which the facial vein communicates.

Postoperative care in most cases includes gentle rinsing with mouthwash or saline solution several times a day. Soft diets are encouraged. Hydrogen peroxide is normally not necessary for cleansing oral cavity wounds.

The lip and oral areas normally are extremely mobile in daily activity. Movement should be decreased initially to avoid bleeding and wound edge separation. Talking may need to be minimized. The use of dentures may need to be restricted accompanied by dietary management. Dressings should be adherent as well as moisture resistant and must not interfere with underlying circulation. Dehiscence and notching of the lip can occur due to the high mobility of the area. If this occurs, conservative management may be all that is necessary; notch formation will re-

Table 2 TNM Classification for Oral Cavity Carcinoma

Primary tumor (T)

TX	Tumor that cannot be assessed by rules
T0	No evidence of primary tumor
TIS	Carcinoma in situ
T1	Tumor 2 cm or less in greatest diameter
T2	Tumor greater than 2 cm but not greater than 4 cm in greatest diameter
T3	Tumor greater than 4 cm in greatest diameter
T4	Massive tumor greater than 4 cm in diameter with deep invasion to involve antrum, pterygoid muscles, roof of tongue, or skin of neck

Nodal involvement (N)

NX	Nodes cannot be assessed
N0	No clinically positive node
N1	Single clinically positive homolateral node less than 3 cm in diameter
N2	Single clinically positive homolateral node 3 to 6 cm in diameter or multiple clinically positive homolateral nodes, none over 6 cm in diameter
	N2a: Single clinically positive homolateral node, 3 to 6 cm in diameter
	N2b: Multiple clinically positive homolateral nodes, none over 6 cm in diameter
N3	Massive homolateral node(s), bilateral nodes, or contralateral node(s)
	N3a: Clinically positive homolateral node(s), none over 6 cm in diameter
	N3b: Bilateral clinically positive nodes (in this situation, each side of the neck should be staged separately; that is, N3b: right, N2a: left, N1)
	N3c: Contralateral clinically positive node(s) only

Distant metastasis (M)

MX	Not assessed
M0	No (known) distant metastasis
M1	Distant metastasis present
	Specify site

quire surgical revision. Lip contracture with elevation of the vermilion border may be simply corrected and, if due to scar contracture, may require a Z-plasty. In females, the use of lip color may provide the finishing touch to conceal scars and provide a more pleasing appearance.

BIBLIOGRAPHY

Baker SR, Krause CJ. Cancer of the lip. In *Cancer of the Head and Neck*. Suen IY, EN Myers, eds. New York, Churchill Livingstone, 1981, p. 280.

Barrett TL, Greenway HT, Massullo V, et al. Treatment of basal cell carcinoma and squamous cell carcinoma with perineural invasion. *Advances in Dermatology*. Vol. 8. St. Louis, Mosby-Year Book, Inc., 1993

Beahrs OH, Myers MH. *Manual for Staging of Cancer*. 2nd ed. Philadelphia, JB Lippincott, 1983.

Breisch EA, Greenway HT. *Cutaneous Surgical Anatomy of the Head and Neck*. New York, Churchill Livingstone, 1991, pp. 1–133.

Calhoun, KH. *Am. J. Otolaryngol* 1992; 13:16–22.

Epstein E, Epstein E, Jr. *Skin Surgery*. 6th ed. Philadelphia, WB Saunders, 1987.

Hollinshead WH. *Anatomy for Surgeons*. Vol. 1. *The Head and Neck*. 3rd ed. New York, Harper and Row, 1982.

Mohs FE, Snow SN. Microscopically controlled surgical treatment for squamous cell carcinoma of the lower lip. *Surg Gynec-Obstet* 1985;160:37–41.

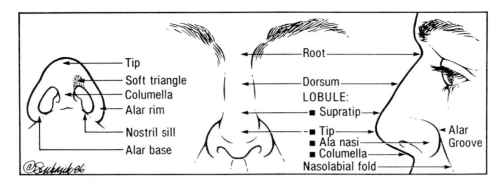

Figure 1   Topographic landmarks and regions of nose.

and upper lip at the nasolabial angle. The tip may droop several millimeters with aging, a process known as tip ptosis (Fig. 3). Laterally, the sidewalls of the nose blend with the cheek in a concave recess, the nasofacial sulcus. The ala nasi meets the face at a peculiar confluence of nose, cheek, and upper lip. The small triangle of the upper lip extends superiorly between the nose and cheek (Fig. 4). The apex of this triangle is bordered laterally by the nasolabial fold and medially by the alar crease or groove.

The concave alar groove begins at the nostril rim at the soft triangle and extends superiorly and laterally in a parabolic curve around the alar base to the sill (Fig. 5). It almost joins the nasolabial fold; before doing so, it sweeps back under the alar base.

When the nose is viewed from in front, an unbroken line seems to curve from each medial eyebrow and flow onto the dorsum of the nose in the form of parallel linear ridges. This is referred to as the radix (Fig. 6).

These bilateral ridges, known as the lateral ridges, along with the nasofacial groove, the alar crease, and the curved lines that sweep out from the supratip depression, are the contour lines of the nose (Fig. 7). These strong landmarks may be more or less pronounced, but they are

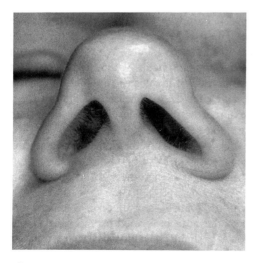

Figure 2   Base view of the infratip lobule.

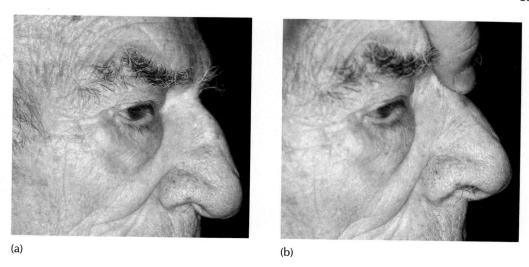

(a) (b)

Figure 3 (a) Drooping of the tip. (b) Correction of ptosis.

invariably present. They are the favored sites within which to hide scar lines. Furthermore, these contour lines wall off and define areas of the nose that share common characteristics: the regional subunits. These are the midline root, dorsum, tip, and columella, and the lateral paired sidewalls, alae nasi, and soft triangles (Fig. 8).

STRUCTURAL SUPPORT SYSTEM

The skin and muscle of the outer surface of the nose and the closely adherent interior mucosa are draped over and supported by a bony-cartilaginous infrastructure. This includes both the arched external pyramid and the supporting midline septum. This framework is responsible for

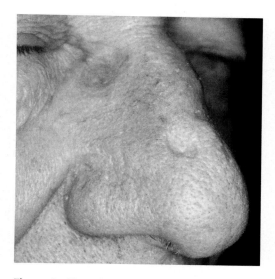

Figure 4 Extension of upper lip between ala nasi and nasolabial fold.

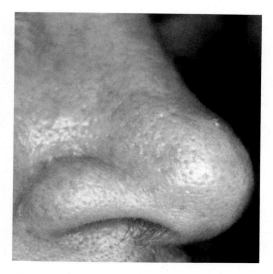

Figure 5 Alar crease.

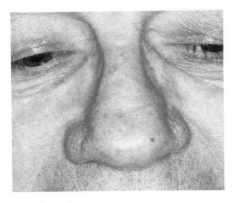

Figure 6   Radix.

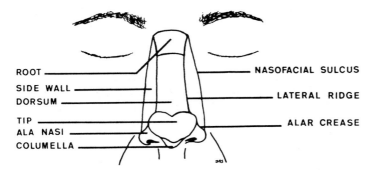

Figure 7   Contour lines and topographic subunits of the nose.

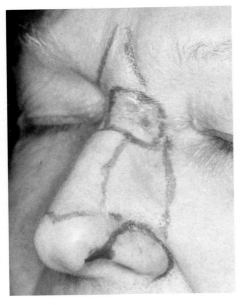

Figure 8   Demonstration of the nasal boundary lines of regional subunits.

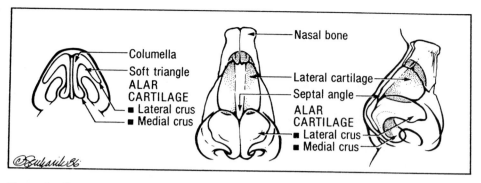

Figure 9 Support system of the nose

the shape, contour, and functional integrity of the nose. Damage to the structural system, especially the more vulnerable alar cartilages, or failure to account for their deficiencies in surgical repairs usually results in a poor outcome or an abnormality in airway patency.

The immobile, osseous components of the nose include the paired nasal bones that underlie the root and upper dorsum (Fig. 9). They also form the upper border of the pyriform aperture, the bony internal nasal opening into the skull. The remainder of the aperture is formed by the frontal process of the maxilla bone, which also underlies the sidewall.

The more pliable and movable paired lateral cartilages are, in form, a continuation of the nasal bones to which they are attached. The lateral cartilages are supported from below by the midline septal cartilage. They underlie the dorsum of the nose.

Suspended from the lateral cartilages by soft tissue ligaments are the relatively free-floating and highly movable paired alar cartilages, whose graceful, arched, wishbone design gives definition and character to the lobule. It has three well-defined components. The medial crura form the columella, while the lateral crura give shape to and support the alae. The transition or hinge area is referred to as the dome, with each side contributing to the shape of the tip (Fig. 10). It

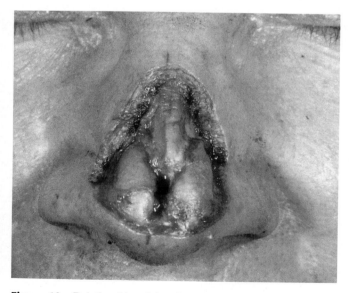

Figure 10 Relationship of the alar and lateral cartilages.

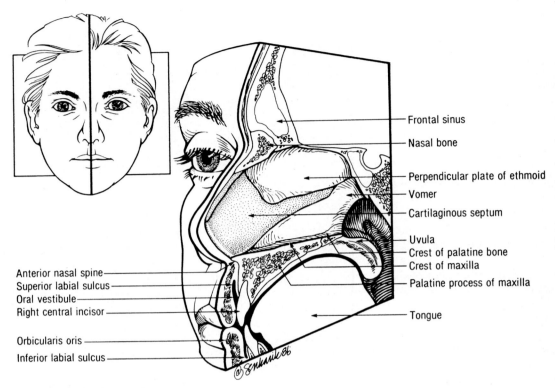

Figure 11   Nasal septum.

is important to realize that the lateral crus supports only the anterior portion of the nostril rim. The cartilage sweeps upward in a lateral and superior direction to form the support of the alae nasi. The major portion of the alae nasi subunit is fleshy, consisting of only skin, fibrofatty tissue, and muscle, but it is devoid of cartilage. This has important surgical implications.

The unpaired septal cartilage is anchored inferiorly into the bony vomer and perpendicular plate of the ethmoid bone (Fig. 11). It also attaches to the undersurface of the nasal bones and lateral cartilages but has a highly mobile free margin inferiorly in the infratip lobule. At this point in the columella, it rests between the medial crura of the alar cartilages to which it has soft tissue attachments. This highly movable arrangement allows the lobule to act as a shock absorber, preventing nasal fractures.

BLOOD SUPPLY

The nose is endowed with a particularly rich blood supply that originates from both the external and internal carotid systems. Anastomosis between these systems over the midline coupled with high-pressure vascular pedicles of large-caliber, named arteries provides blood supply for a wide variety of random and axial flaps.

The external carotid system contributes the largest proportional flow to the external nose (Fig. 12). One of the terminal branches of the external carotid system, the facial artery, branches into the inferior and superior labial arteries and continues to course along the lateral side of the nose

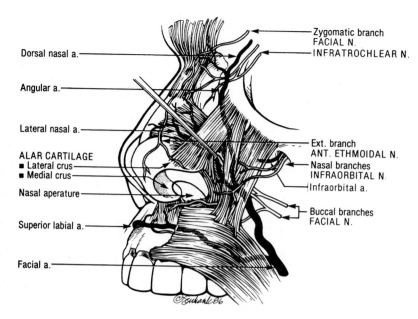

Figure 12 Vessels, nerves, and muscles of the nose.

beneath the lip elevator muscles as the angular artery. The superior labial artery sends vertical branches upward to supply the alae, the columella, and the vestibule at the base of the nose. As the angular artery courses along the side of the nose to the medial canthus, it supplies numerous lateral dorsal nasal branches to the alae, sidewalls, and dorsum. These anastomose freely with branches from the contralateral side.

The angular artery terminates at the level of the medial canthus as it connects with the dorsal nasal artery, which is a terminal branch of the ophthalmic artery of the internal carotid system. The vascular pedicle formed at this union at the level of the medial canthus extends back onto the root and dorsum of the nose. Axial flaps may be constructed based on this artery.

The supratrochlear artery, another branch of the ophthalmic artery, supplies the glabella and midline forehead and is used to construct the midline forehead flap. The external nasal artery exits onto the dorsum of the nose under the nasal bone in company with the external nasal branch of the anterior ethmoid nerve to supply the dorsum and tip. One of the terminal branches of the maxillary artery to reach the skin surface is the infraorbital artery, which anastomoses with the angular artery.

The venous drainage of the nose parallels the arterial supply. Rarely, ascending infection and thrombosis of the cavernous sinus may occur via the ophthalmic veins. Similarly, the ethmoid vein connects with the superior sagittal sinus.

SENSORY INNERVATION

The sensory innervation of the nose is complicated and includes various branches of the ophthalmic and maxillary divisions of the trigeminal nerve (5th cranial nerve) (Fig. 12). The ophthalmic division supplies tissue of the midline nose. The root, upper bridge, and upper lateral sidewalls are supplied by the infratrochlear nerve, which emerges above the medial canthal tendon to run medially onto the nose. The dorsum and tip are supplied by the paired external nasal

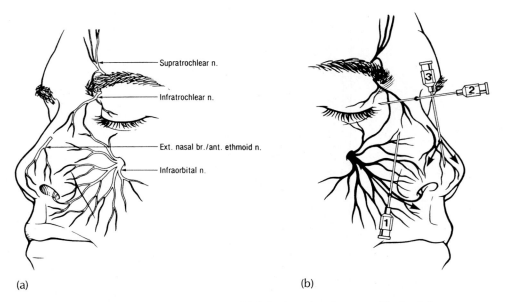

(a)   (b)

Figure 13   (a) Sensory nerves of the nose. (b) Injection sites for nerve block of the nose.

branches of the anterior ethmoid nerve, a division of the nasociliary nerve, derived from the main ophthalmic nerve trunk. The nerve emerges from between the lower nasal bone and the lateral cartilage union. Blisters on the tip of the nose in herpes zoster (Hutchinson's sign) may indicate involvement of the cornea, since the anterior ethmoid and ciliary nerves are both branches of the nasociliary nerve.

The maxillary division of the trigeminal nerve innervates the alae nasi, the lower sidewalls, and the columella via the infraorbital nerve. The nasopalatine nerve, another branch of the maxillary division, supplies the inferior nasal mucosa.

Knowledge of the sensory innervation of the nose is used to secure regional anesthetic blocks. The entire external nose may be anesthetized by a limited number of injections that block the involved nerves (Fig. 13). The infratrochlear nerve is anesthetized bilaterally by advancing the needle to either side of the root of the nose from a midline puncture site (Fig. 14). Advancing the needle superiorly and injecting along the lateral nasal wall from a puncture site opposite the lower alar base blocks the infraorbital nerve branches to the sidewall and the ala. Injecting medially to the anterior nasal spine below the columella through the same site blocks the remaining infraorbital fibers to the columella and inferior nostril rim. The dorsum and tip are blocked by anesthetizing the external nasal branch of the anterior ethmoid nerve as it exits onto the nose at the level of the junction of the nasal bones and lateral cartilages. The anesthetic is injected rapidly from a single site.

MUSCLES

The nose is relatively immobile, and the musculature there is not well developed. These muscles do not share the expressive importance of muscles located elsewhere on the face, especially those around the eyes and mouth.

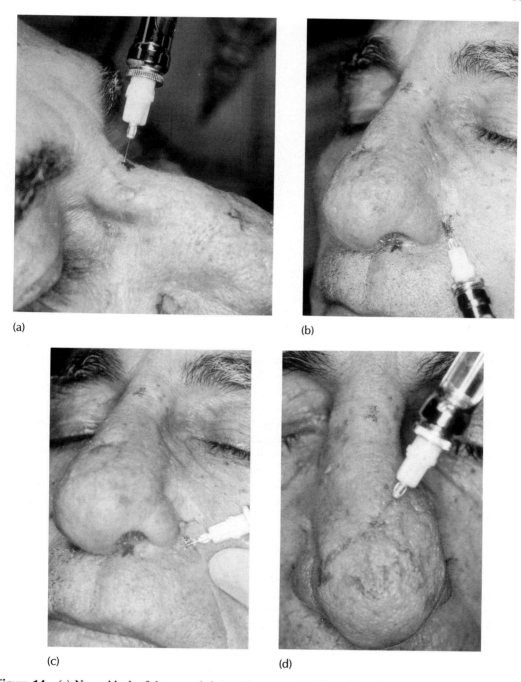

(a)

(b)

(c)

(d)

Figure 14 (a) Nerve block of the nose: infratrochlear nerve. (b) Branches of infraorbital nerve to sidewall and ala. (c) Branches of infraorbital nerve to nostril rim and columella. (d) External nasal branch of anterior ethmoid nerve.

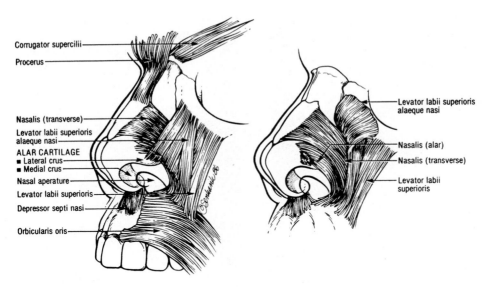

Figure 15   Muscles of the nose.

The procerus muscle extends from the paired frontalis muscles across the root of the nose in a vertical orientation to insert into the aponeurosis of the transverse portion of the nasalis muscle and the overlying skin (Fig. 15). Contraction shortens the nose and reveals the transverse skin lines across the root. The plane under this muscle is continuous with the subgaleal space of the scalp and forehead. Therefore, a bloodless dissection may be carried out from the scalp, down the forehead, and onto the midline nose between the periosteum and the overlying procerus muscle fascia. The levator labii superioris alaeque nasi arises from the maxilla and extends vertically to insert into the midline upper lip as well as the skin and lateral ala. Contraction causes flaring of the ala as well as elevation of the middle of the upper lip.

The deepest intrinsic muscles of the nose are the three paired nasalis muscles. They originate from a small crescent of the maxilla above the central incisors, below the pyriform aperture. The transverse component of the nasalis is the largest and courses over the dorsum of the nose and blends with its opposite side counterpart to form a thin aponeurosis into which the procerus blends. Contraction of this thin sheet of muscle results in tensing of the skin over the dorsum of the nose. The alar part of the nasalis muscle arches from the maxilla over the alar rim to insert onto the lateral edge of the lateral crus of the alar cartilage. It assists in dilating the nostril during inspiration. The most medial component is referred to as the depressor septi muscle. It originates from the maxilla just below the anterior nasal spine and also from some of the upper fibers of the orbicularis oris muscle to extend upward into the membranous septum to the inferior border of the septal cartilage. It acts to pull down the septum and maintain airway patency during deep inspiration. Some of the vertical fibers may contribute to the philtral column. Contraction of this muscle may also be responsible for the transverse skin lines seen beneath the columella in elderly people.

NASAL SURGERY

The nose is like a miniature face. Every few millimeters a new hump or depression is encountered, the skin texture and color changes, and the ability to undermine and mobilize the skin alters dramatically. The surgeon will be faced with a multiplicity of surgical imperatives determined by only minor differences in the site, width, and depth of the defect.

The following principles are intended as an organizational framework upon which the maze of factors to be considered may be analyzed.

Goal

The goal is to restore the area to normal. The nose occupies a preeminent location on the midface. The nose is a relatively static anatomic unit compared to other facial units and does not share their expressive ability or functional importance, but a deformity calls attention to itself disproportionately. The abnormality distracts from normal eye-to-eye focus and becomes a cosmetic burden and source of embarrassment to the patient. This is true not only of gross deformities but also of subtleties of symmetry, minor blunting of the nose-cheek or alar-cheek junctions (Fig. 16), and alterations of the normal curvatures.

Cover, Support, Lining

The nose consists of skin and muscle above and mucosa below draped over an osseous, cartilaginous infrastructure. The depth of the lesion will determine how many of these layers are affected and require replacement. Support is the most critical of these factors. If cartilage is undamaged, any number of options to cover defects including primary closure and flaps are available. Perichondrium or periosteum is required, however, if full-thickness skin grafts are expected to take successfully. Loss of cartilaginous support requires alternative and more complicated approaches to replace functional integrity. Otherwise, airway patency is endangered, and flaps will ultimately sag or droop. Ingenious techniques have been devised using the remaining nasal cartilage, cartilage containing composite grafts, pure cartilage containing composite grafts, or pure cartilage grafts from the ear combined with local skin flaps. Mucosal lining is best replaced with residual adjacent mucosa if possible. Buccal musosal grafts, turn-in flaps, and composite grafts are poor substitutes for the highly vascular and closely adherent native nasal mucosa.

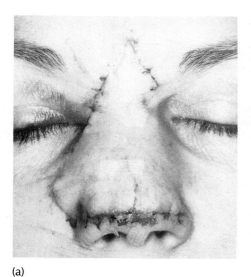
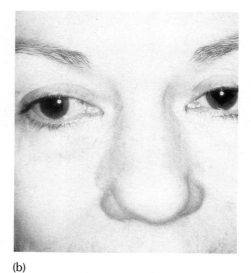

(a) (b)

Figure 16 (a) Dorsal flap covering the tip defect. (b) Obliteration of nasofacial groove due to poor flap design.

Aesthetic Subunits

The nose may be subdivided into at least 10 aesthetic units. These are the anatomic subdivisions that lie within major junction lines, have a unique contour, and share common characteristics of color, texture, and sebum production. They are also referred to as topographic, regional, or anatomic units. Nasal subunits are comprised of the root, dorsum, sidewalls, tip, alae, soft triangles, and columella (Figs. 7,8). The subunit concept is of paramount importance for repair of the nose. Scar lines placed on the borders of these units are camouflaged because, as they contract, they leave shallow depressions that cast linear shadows or ridges that reflect lines of light, both of which simulate the contour lines they are replacing. Because these scars are placed where lines are expected, they are hardly noticeable. Furthermore, defects that occupy a significant portion of the subunit may be enlarged by sacrificing normal skin in order to replace the entire subunit. The regional unit concept has overriding importance in repair and reconstruction of the nose. Much of the therapeutics portion of this chapter will be based on it.

Skin Availability for Repair

Following sound surgical technique, every effort should be made to fill defects with adjacent skin that best matches the qualities of the removed tissue. The skin of the nose is relatively mobile over the root, dorsum, and sidewalls. In adults the skin there may be lax and redundant, while in children it is more elastic. In either case, the skin may be readily undermined, either above or below the muscle plane. Once mobilized, it is available for primary closure or flap repair locally. In addition, it may be shifted inferiorly for repair of the tip or alae, where tissue is less redundant and mobile.

   If scars cannot be placed in the boundary lines between anatomic units, placing them within the relaxed skin tension lines (RSTL) is a good alternative (Fig. 17,18). On the nose the RSTL

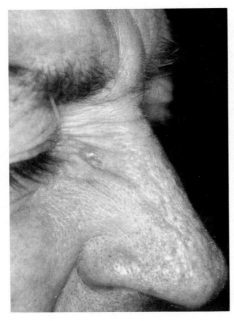

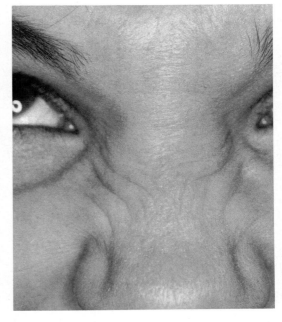

Figure 17 Skin tension lines of nose from side view.

Figure 18 Skin tension lines when viewed from in front.

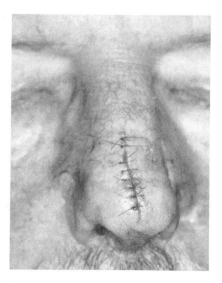

Figure 19 Midline vertical incision.

run transversely over the root and upper dorsum (due to contraction of the procerus muscle). Oblique lines emanate from the medial canthus to course across the sidewalls to the midline (levator labii superioris alaeque nasi muscle) where they become vertical over the dorsum down to the supratip (transverse portion of nasalis muscle). There are no RSTL over the tip of the nose or over the alae. Incision lines on the ala nasi should be radial to the nasal aperture. Likewise, there are no RSTL in the columella where midline incisions may be closed longitudinally. Elective transverse incisions there also do well. Midline lesions, closed vertically, in general do well over the entire nose including the tip (Fig. 19). Transverse closures, in the elderly, are aided by several millimeters of drooping of the tip (tip ptosis), which, when pulled up by closure, may improve the appearance of the nose as well as airflow.

Redundant, closely matched skin available for flap mobilization is found in the glabella, the midline forehead, and cheek skin just lateral to the nose. Skin for grafts may be harvested from the pre- and postauricular area, the nasolabial fold, the neck, and the supraclavicular area.

Preconceived Closure Plans

The long list of published local flaps that have been used on the nose may be confusing. Considerably more useful is a simplified schema that is time- and experience-tested and is consistently and repetitively applicable to common and recurring surgical defects within a range of site, size, and depth. Mastery of a single specific, reliable approach for each subunit allows the surgeon to become confident in its success. Become familiar with the flap's limitations and its ability to be adjusted for the surgical variables of a specific case.

WOUND CLOSURE

When considering a surgical plan for the nose, the simplest approach is often the best. Alternative procedures should be considered and include second intention healing, partial closure, simple primary closure, grafts, and flaps. Flaps are more complicated but are most functional and rewarding in this region. The dermatologic surgeon should master a flap for each of several commonly occurring defects. The approach must take into account size and depth of the defect as well as the regional subunit schema. Distortion or notching of the alar rim, asymmetries, or discrepancies in contour, color, and texture should be avoided. The patient must understand that repairs on the nose may take several months to heal completely, and that second procedures such as fat debulking or dermabrasion may be required.

Second Intention

Second intention healing progresses by degrees of granulation tissue formation, wound contraction, and reepithelialization. Wounds contract by the centripedal migration of myofibroblasts located at the wound edge. The amount of contraction depends largely on the laxity of the surrounding skin. Contraction proceeds until impeded by equal opposing forces.

On the nose, the skin is relatively bound to cartilage and stretched over the rigid infrastructure, so most healing is by granulation with collagen deposition and neovascularization. Any small, hollow defect will heal reasonably well, including most curettage and desiccation scars. However, second intention healing as a cosmetically acceptable alternative is limited to the concavities of the alar groove and the lateral root opposite the medial canthus (Fig. 20). In the latter location, even defects down to periosteum may heal acceptably if they are equal above and below the medial canthal tendon. Larger alar crease lesions may contract enough to draw up or notch the free margin of the nostril, resulting in a cosmetically poor scar.

Second intention healing is managed by daily dressing changes designed to keep the wound clean, moist, and covered. It is cleaned with hydrogen peroxide, followed by a thin film of antibiotic ointment, and finally a clean nonadhering dressing secured with paper tape. The main disadvantage of second intention healing is the relatively long time it takes before the wound is finally reepithelialized. The daily dressing changes are also time-consuming, and the dressings must be worn for prolonged periods of time. A superficial dermabrasion performed 6–8 weeks after reepithelialization will often improve mild differences in contour and color.

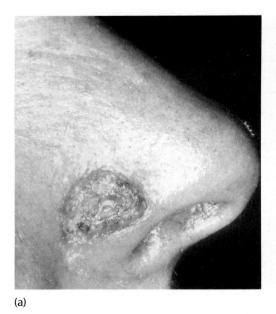
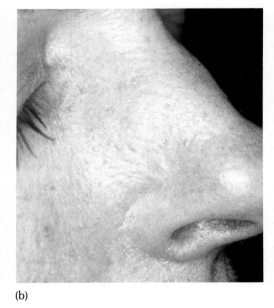

(a)   (b)

Figure 20   (a) Shallow defect of ala. (b) Second intention healing of ala nasi.

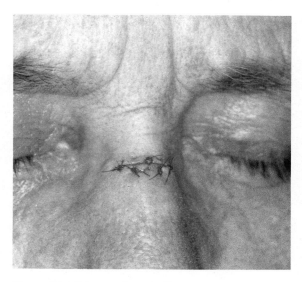

Figure 21   Primary closure of root.

Primary Closure

Simple fusiform closure is frequently the best way to treat defects on the nose. The skin over the root, dorsum, and sidewalls is relatively redundant. It is easily undermined and mobilized, especially below the muscle plane. The skin lines may be identified when the patient wrinkles the nose (Fig. 17 and 18). The long axis of the defect is oriented within the RSTL. Cosmetically acceptable results can be expected provided subcuticular sutures are placed, differences in thickness between the wound edges are adjusted, the wound is not closed under tension, and sutures are removed in about 5 days. Scars are arranged transversely on the root (Fig. 21), obliquely from the medial canthus on the sidewalls (Fig. 22), and vertically on the dorsum (Fig. 23). Scars may easily be camouflaged within the nasofacial sulcus (Fig. 24) and the alar crease (Figs. 25,26). Everting vertical mattress sutures may be used in the alar crease to prevent a deeply indented scar. Due to the thickness of the nasal skin, dog ears are often relatively large. M-plasties are helpful to reduce the length of the scar line.

The skin over the lobule (alae, tip, and columella) is thick and bound down, and primary closure often results in distortion of the nostril or septum. Vertical midline wounds of the tip, however, do well. Wounds near the nostril rim may be closed radial to the nasal aperture (Fig. 27). This may require sacrifice of normal tissue to create a full-thickness defect that is then closed. Small lesions along the rim may be closed parallel to the margin.

Grafts

A full-thickness skin graft (FTSG) can be a functional and cosmetic alternative on the nose if defect selection is appropriate. The donor and recipient site must match well for color and texture and the procedure be performed meticulously. It may be wise to enlarge some lesions so that the edge of the graft will be placed on a contour line, especially on the tip. Results are often better if the whole subunit is replaced.

The successful take of a graft depends on the ability of the recipient bed to sustain the graft. Nourishment to the graft is provided by plasma in the first 48 hr until vascular budding is noted.

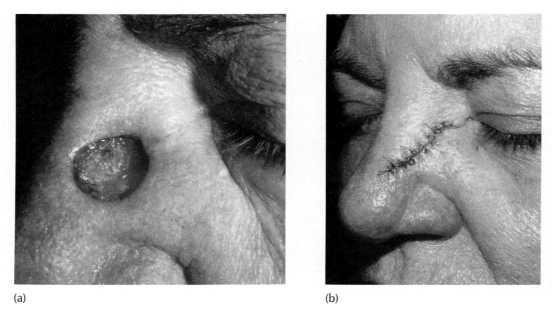

(a)   (b)

Figure 22   (a) Sidewall defect. (b) Primary closure of sidewall.

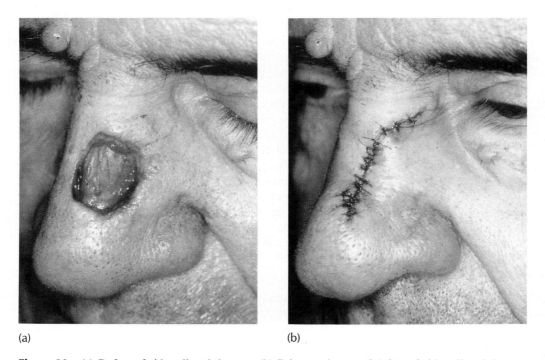

(a)   (b)

Figure 23   (a) Defect of sidewall and dorsum. (b) Primary closure of defect of sidewall and dorsum.

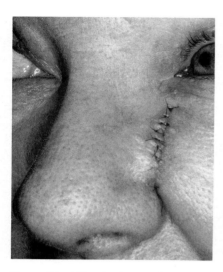

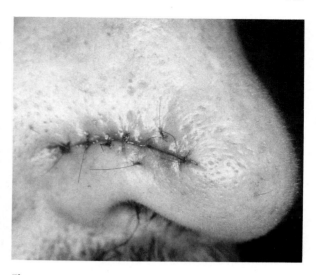

Figure 24 Primary closure of nasofacial sulcus.

Figure 25 Primary closure of alar crease.

Bare cartilage or bone will not sustain a graft. In addition, the entire graft undersurface must be trimmed of all subcutaneous fat and sutured to lie in exact opposition to the graft bed. Basting sutures and tie-over dressings are used.

The sites that benefit most from full-thickness skin grafts have been used on the lobule. The two most common sites for FTSG on the nose are for 1- to 1½-cm defects on the tip or centered in the alar crease.

If kept thin, grafts take surprisingly well on the tip (Figs. 28,29). The ideal donor site for the tip should match the pebbly quality of the region and its actinic damage while being thin

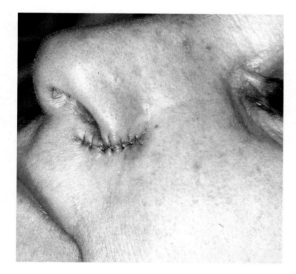

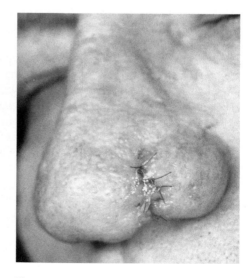

Figure 26 Primary closure of alar crease/lip junction.

Figure 27 Radial closure of nostril rim.

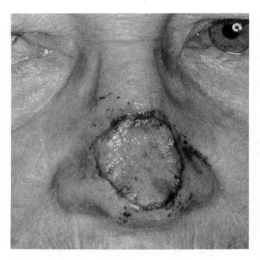

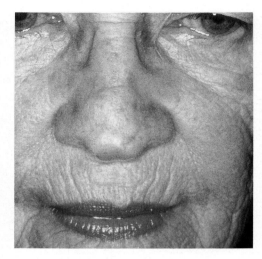

Figure 28 Full-thickness skin graft of the tip.   **Figure 29** Healing of graft at 1 year.

enough to be sustained in this location. Skin from the postauricular sulcus is best if actinic damage is minimal. The hairless preauricular skin in front of the tragus is better suited to replace skin with varying degrees of actinic damage. There is sufficient skin between the tragus and sideburn to harvest the graft and close the donor site easily. Other donor sites include the infraauricular neck, the nasolabial fold, the glabella, and the supraclavicular space. Once the graft is placed into the defect, the tip maintains its convex shape and there is close apposition of the graft to its bed. Therefore, a tie-over bolster is not required and a simple dressing with antibiotic ointment and a nonadherent pad, changed daily, is sufficient.

Defects of the alar crease usually extend onto the ala, sidewall, or tip (Fig. 30). Even when the graft is placed, the recipient site remains concave. This requires more tissue to line the defect completely. In addition, basting sutures and a tie-over bolster dressing that offers some tamponade are required to maintain intimate approximation of the graft and wound bed. Bolus dressings are fashioned from moldable petrolatum-impregnated gauze and may be changed daily. The graft may then be inspected for hematoma or seroma formation. Closely matched skin can usually be obtained from the preauricular or infraauricular area. Other choices are the postauricular skin, nasolabial fold, neck, and glabella. It is important that the graft and surrounding skin be sutured so that the edges are approximated at the same level. Uneven wound edges or differences in color or texture may be improved by superficial dermabrasion 2–3 months postoperatively.

Sites on the nose other than the lobule will accept full-thickness skin grafts, but the indications are not as great. Sufficient adjacent skin can usually be mobilized on the dorsum, root, and sidewalls for primary closure or local flaps. Flaps to the tip and alae, however, must often be mobilized and transposed from the nasolabial fold or forehead. A third, infrequent site for grafting is vertical midline closure under tension at the supratip depression. The concavity can be filled by using the dog ear that forms superiorly and placing it into the defect as an island graft (Fig. 31).

Flaps

Flaps are full-thickness portions of skin that are advanced, rotated, or transposed from an area of relative excess to fill a surgical defect. Ideally, this will not create a deformity of the donor

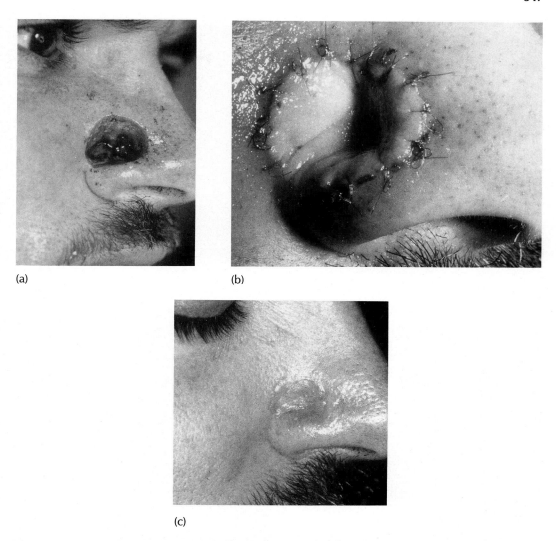

(a)

(b)

(c)

Figure 30 (a) Alar defect. (b) Full-thickness graft from preauricular site. (c) Healing at 6 months.

site. If the procedure is planned properly, the resultant scar will be camouflaged at the recipient site. Since the flap carries its own blood supply, it may be placed over poorly vascularized beds such as bone and cartilage that have been denuded of overlying periosteum and perichondrium. Unlike the linear arrangement of primary closures, flaps have more complicated scar patterns, any component of which may be less noticeable and easier to hide. Depending on the location, size, and depth of the wound, flaps may be constructed from adjacent nasal skin, or they may require more complicated transposition of skin from the adjoining forehead and cheek.

In the following discussion, each subunit will be considered independently, and defects of increasing size and depth will be considered. Several alternatives will be given for some of the more common defects to demonstrate the options available for closure. Skin cancers may not respect anatomic subunits, so many defects will occupy portions of several units. This discussion will focus on soft tissue defects. Reconstruction of support structures and mucosal lining

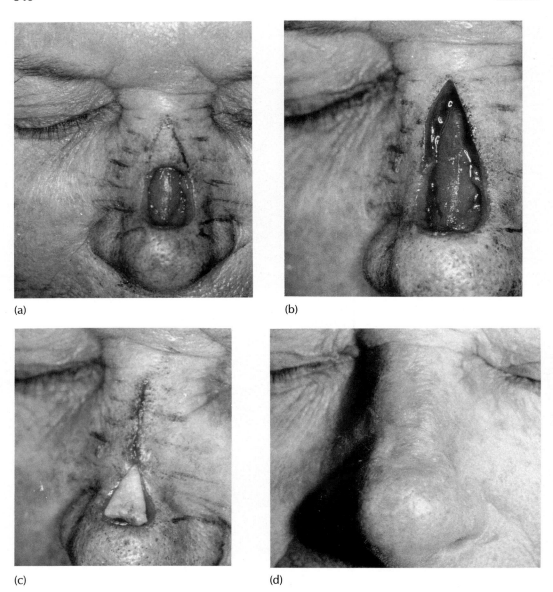

(a)

(b)

(c)

(d)

Figure 31 (a) Dorsum defect. (b) Dog ear excised. (c) Dog ear trimmed and placed as graft. (d) Healing at 1 year.

is considerably more complex and beyond the scope of this book or the skills of most dermatologic surgeons.

Root

The root is usually concave when viewed on profile, with a nasofrontal angle of approximately 120 degrees. Skin lines on the root run in a transverse direction, and most small lesions can be closed horizontally (Fig. 21). Larger lesions or those on the side wall of the root that approach

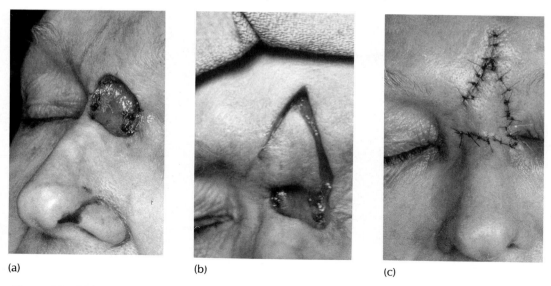

(a)   (b)   (c)

Figure 32   (a) Root defect. (b) Dorsal nasal advancement-rotation or glabellar flap. (c) Flap closed in V-Y manner.

the medial canthus can be easily filled with glabellar skin. Midline lesions, which may extend onto the dorsum, are covered easily by a sliding glabellar V-Y advancement-rotation flap. This is also referred to as the dorsal nasal flap (Fig. 32). An inverted V-like incision is begun at the level of the eyebrow to correspond with the oblique glabellar frown lines. The incision is extended down to the far side of the defect. The flap is elevated either just above or below the procerus muscle and is then advanced and rotated. The glabellar defect is closed in an inverted Y manner, which helps to push the flap down into place. This is actually a back-cut rotation flap. Creating a small transposition Z-plasty allows for less sacrifice of normal skin (Fig. 33).

If the defect is more lateral, such as on the sidewall of the root adjacent to the medial canthus, the glabellar flap may be further modified and fully mobilized as a transposition flap that is essentially a rhomboid flap (Fig. 34). The secondary defect on the glabella is closed first as the key stitch. The skin is transposed to fill the primary defect. Care should be taken with this thick flap to approximate its edges with the thinner skin of the medial canthus.

The glabellar flap, then, is really several different flaps applied in different situations. The name is applied to all of them because the glabella serves as the donor site. These three flaps— the V-Y rotation advancement flap, the Z-plasty modification, and the transposition flap—are all random pattern flaps. They are anatomically designed so that the scar lines will be easily camouflaged. It is also possible to construct an axial glabellar flap on a much narrower base utilizing the vascular pedicle at the medial canthal level. This tremendously increases the mobility of the glabellar flap and allows it to be used to correct defects much lower on the nose.

Dorsum

Lesions of the dorsum may be closed in a variety of ways depending on the size and the availability of the skin from the sidewalls. There is always skin available from the glabella or forehead (Fig. 35). If skin is available laterally, it may be mobilized with bilateral advancement flaps (Fig. 36). Scars may be placed in anatomic lines for wounds that are too large to be closed

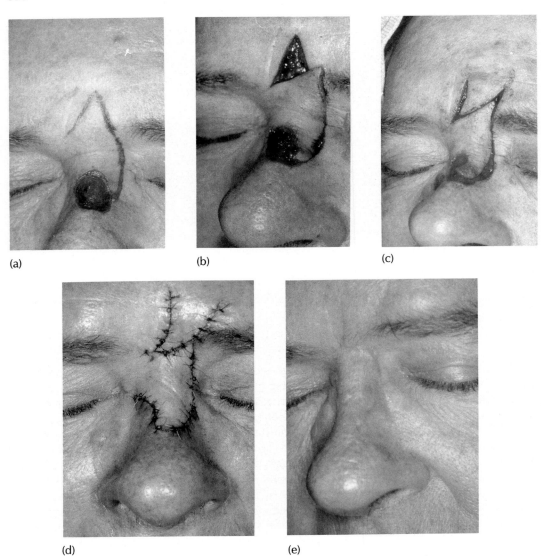

(a)

(b)

(c)

(d)

(e)

Figure 33 (a) Root-dorsum defect. (b) Glabellar flap incised. (c) Z-plasty modification. (d) Sutured in place. (e) Healing at 4 months.

primarily. As mentioned earlier, a dog ear formed superiorly may be utilized as a graft, after being defatted, to fill any midline portion of the wound that cannot be closed without tension. The Webster 30 degree transposition flap is an excellent closure method for vertically oriented dorsal lesions when half of the defect is closable with secondary movement of the surrounding tissue. An M-plasty placed inferiorly eliminates the dog ear from the tip. Bilateral 30 degree transposition flaps result in complicated scar lines but allow the skin to be borrowed from both adjacent sidewalls with a minimum of tissue movement (Fig. 37).

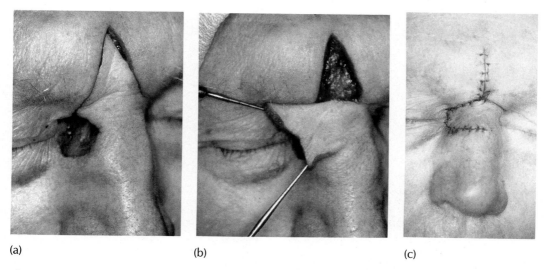

(a)   (b)   (c)

Figure 34 (a) Defect at side of root. (b) Glabellar transposition flap. (c) Final suturing.

Skin from the glabella may be brought down via the glabellar advancement-rotation flap described above, or it may be mobilized by a bilobed flap that transfers skin successively from the glabella to the nasal sidewall to the dorsal defect. Tissue may be transposed a maximum of 180 degrees, as each lobe of the flap can rotate 90 degrees. This is a remarkably versatile flap. The

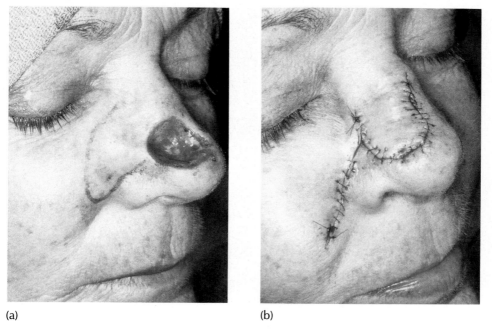

(a)   (b)

Figure 35 (a) Defect of dorsum and transposition flap design. (b) Flap transposed and sutured.

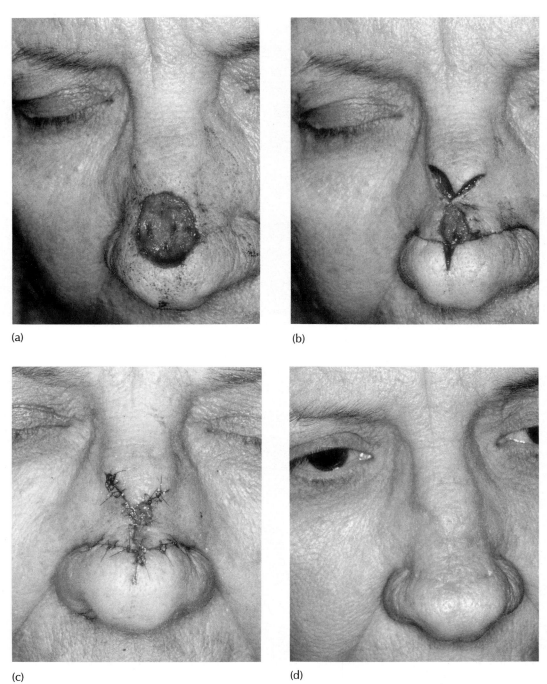

(a)

(b)

(c)

(d)

Figure 36 (a) Defect of lower dorsum. (b) A-T closure with superior M-plasty. (c) Final closure. (d) Healing at 1 year.

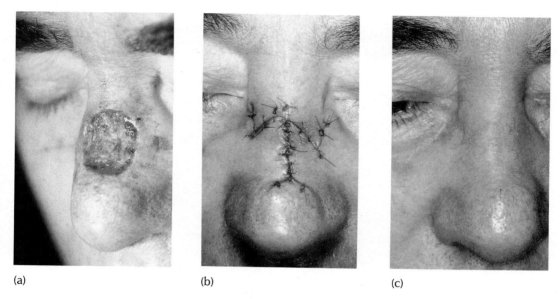

(a) (b) (c)

Figure 37 (a) Dorsum defect. (b) Bilateral 30 degree transposition flap. (c) Healing at 5 months.

disadvantages are that the scar lines are not anatomically based and remain visible. Also, since all edges are curved, the flap is prone to the trapdoor defect or bulky appearance due to fluid stasis.

Large defects of the dorsum may require tissue from several regions involving combination flaps such as the bilateral cheek advancement flap and glabellar flap illustrated in Figure 38. The midline forehead flap, a much more complicated axial flap, is designed to cover large defects of the dorsum and tip.

Tip

The skin on the tip is bound down and not very elastic; with the exception of some midline vertical closures, tissue must be brought in from elsewhere. As discussed previously, a full-thickness graft from the preauricular or postauricular region is often the best choice.

Small- to intermediate-sized defects of the upper portion of the tip may be filled by tissue from the dorsum and sidewalls. This is done with rotation flaps and various transposition flaps, including the bilobed and banner flaps (Fig. 39). The latter is a triangular-shaped flap that simulates a banner or pennant when mobilized. The more versatile and useful bilobed flap is excellent for defects of the lateral tip including those that also impinge on portions of the sidewall or ala nasi. The double transposition taps into the excess, mobile skin of the upper sidewall and successively transfers it inferiorly to fill defects up to about 1.5 cm (Fig. 40). Clues to successful flap design include preplanning the dog ear removal of the superior donor site, limiting the rotation arc of each limb to less than 90°, and ensuring that the size of each limb is equal to or slightly smaller than the recipient defect. If properly executed, the superior donor defect will close with a horizontal tension vector that does not pull up the nostril rim, and the resulting scar line will fall nicely into the RSTL emanating from the medial canthus. Closing the superior limb first

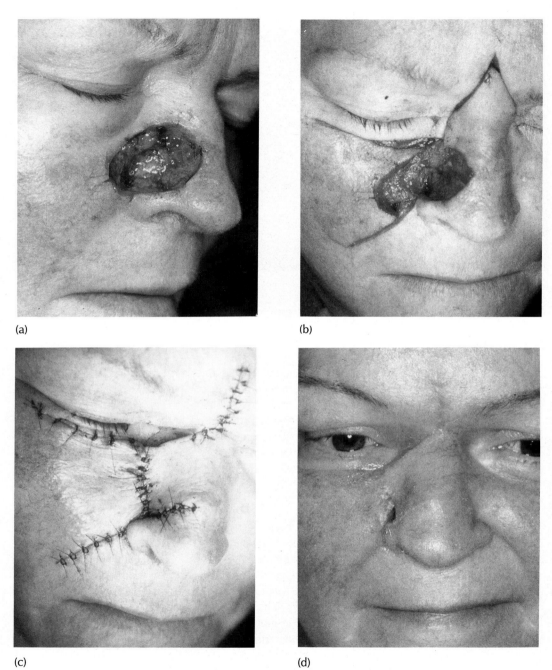

(a)

(b)

(c)

(d)

Figure 38 (a) Defect of sidewall and cheek. (b) Design for combined glabellar and cheek advancement flaps. (c) Flaps sutured. (d) After suture removal.

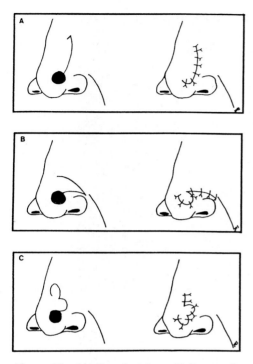

Figure 39 (A) Rotation flap. (B) Banner flap. (C) Bilobed flap.

pushes the tissue successively down into the second donor defect and then into the recipient defect.

Another excellent flap for reconstruction of small- to intermediate-sized defects of the lateral tip that do not involve the ala nasi is the "horizontal J" rotation flap (Fig. 41). This is a combination of a back-cut rotation flap and a Burow's exchange flap. A line is drawn from the inferior portion of the defect along the alar crease and continued transversely onto the cheek to a length equal to the horizontal diameter of the defect. This is incised and continued superiorly on the cheek as a relaxing incision. The flap is undermined and rotated medially to close the defect. A dog ear develops inferiorly at the superior melolabial fold, which when removed and closed completes the horizontal J.

Moderate-sized defects of the tip and ala nasi can be remodeled by a modification of the dorsal nasal or glabellar advancement-rotation flap (Rieger). This is done by converting it to an axial pattern flap from a random pattern referred to as the axial frontonasal flap (Marchac). This is accomplished by incising and mobilizing the flap at the submuscle plane between the deep muscular fascia and the periosteum of the nasal bones and perichondrium of the nasal cartilages (Fig. 42). The flap is based on the vascular pedicle at the level of the medial canthal tendon that forms at the anastomosis of the terminal branches of the ophthalmic and facial arteries: the dorsal nasal artery and the angular artery, respectively. The vascular complex allows the glabellar incision to be brought below the level of the medial eyebrow. This allows more radical rotation to slide the flap on the narrower pedicle. The incision is started at the lateral side of the defect opposite the pedicle and brought up the nasofacial groove to the sidewall of the root and into the glabellar frown lines where the depth of the incision may be more superficial above the muscle.

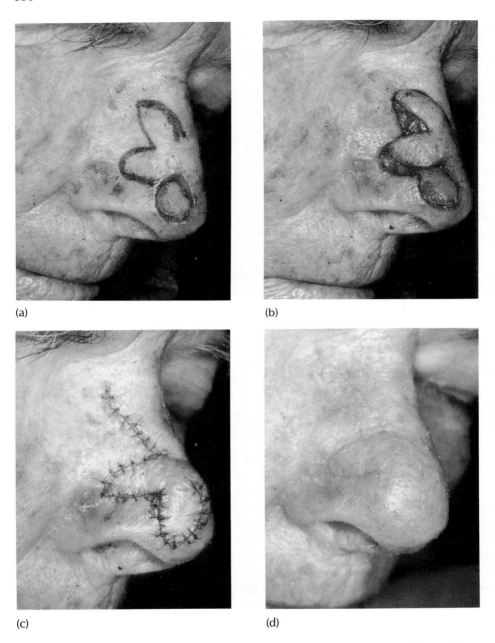

(a)   (b)

(c)   (d)

Figure 40   (a) Bilobed flap design. (b) Flap incised. (c) Sewn into place. (d) Six months postoperative.

It extends to the apex of the glabellar frown lines and then back down the opposite oblique frown line to end above the medial canthus. Undermining and elevation of the flap is done from the defect upward under the vascular pedicle. When the incision is closed, the dog ear formed on the ipsilateral side of the defect may be liberally excised since this is an axial flap. Basically all the skin on the nose and glabella is mobilized, but the flap is successful if the vasculature of the

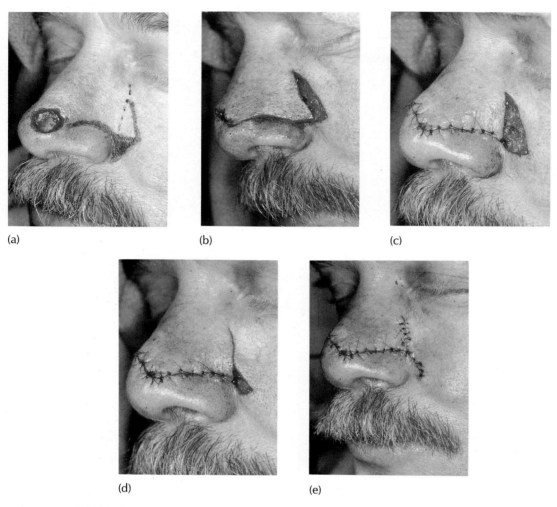

(a)   (b)   (c)

(d)   (e)

Figure 41 (a) Horizontal "J" rotation flap design. (b) Flap incised and rotated. (c) Sewn into place. (d) Back-cut sewn into place. (e) Inferior dog ear removed and sewn.

pedicle is undamaged. A good cosmetic result may be expected if the skin edges are approximated for variations in thickness between anatomic subunits and the surrounding tissue is undermined for tension-reducing secondary movement. Scar lines fall into unit boundaries and should be hidden.

The flap of choice for large defects of the tip region is the midline forehead (Fig. 43). This is a delayed, axial pattern pedicle flap based on the supratrochlear artery. Since the flap is twisted at the level of the eyebrow, the distance to the defect margin is measured from this point. A template of the defect is used to draw on the upper midforehead at a distance above the eyebrow equal to that to the defect that will allow it to be moved easily to the tip. The flap is then incised and mobilized in the subgaleal plane below the level of the frontalis muscle to ensure that the supratrochlear artery is included in the flap. The flap may be debulked distally of subdermal

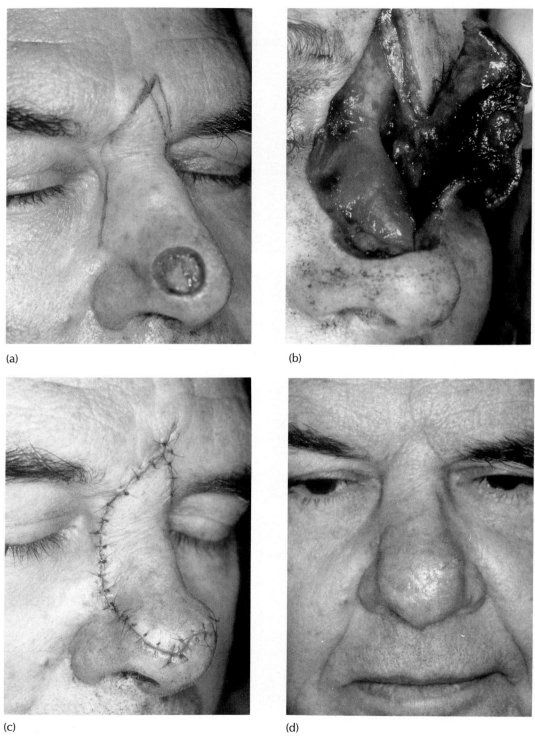

Figure 42 (a) Tip defect. (b) Large axial frontonasal flap. (c) Sutured in place. (d) Healing at 6 months.

Figure 43 (a) Tip defect. Midline forehead flap design. (b) Flap transposed. (c) Flap divided at 16 days. (d) Healing at 1 month.

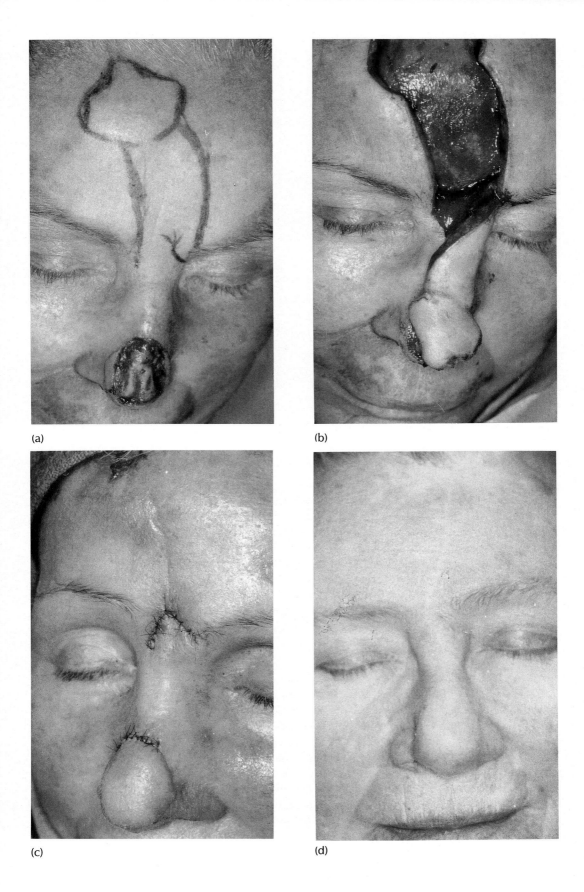

(a)

(b)

(c)

(d)

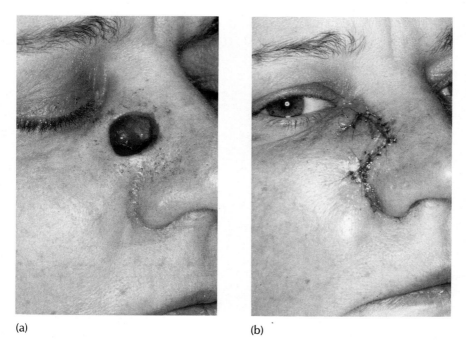

(a)   (b)

Figure 44   (a) Sidewall defect. (b) Transposition flap.

fat so that the tissue sewn into the defect is not protuberant. The flap is rotated around the pedicle at the eyebrow level and sewn into the defect. The pedicle is separated at 3 weeks and the remainder of the flap sewn in. The pedicle is also separated at the level of the eyebrow, and a triangular section placed into the inverted V of the oblique glabellar frown lines. Since there is so much tissue available in the midline forehead flap, it is often wise to enlarge the defect to include the whole subunit of the tip. Since the tip is a convex area, contraction of the flap appears normal.

A delayed pedicle flap may also be fashioned from the nasolabial fold. While this nasolabial flap is the flap of choice for alar defects, the distance to the tip makes it less applicable for this region.

Sidewall

The sidewall is the flat, sloping, concave portion of the lateral nose between the lateral ridge and nasofacial sulcus. It is frequently possible to devise small adjacent flaps for the side of the nose if primary closure is not possible. These include cleverly designed rotation, bilobed, and transposition flaps (Fig. 44). For large defects, mobilizing adjacent cheek skin via superiorly based cheek rotation flaps or full cheek advancement flaps is best. Both flaps are inordinately large for the distance that the tissue is moved, but they adhere to anatomic borders so well and the base is so broad and safe that scars are usually well camouflaged. The cheek rotation flap is incised inferiorly along the nasolabial crease until sufficient tissue is mobilized to fill the defect (Fig. 45). The incision should not be taken below the angle of the mouth since contraction of

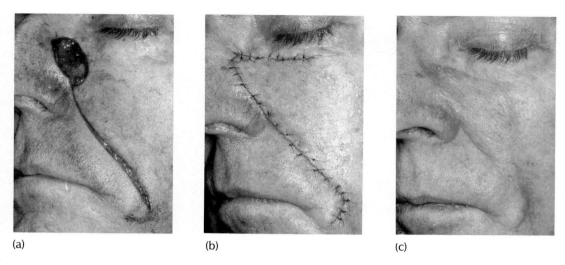

(a) (b) (c)

Figure 45 (a) Sidewall defect and rotation flap design. (b) Rotation flap sutured. (c) Short-term healing.

the final scar may cause elevation of the oral commissure. If additional movement is required, a back-cut will increase mobility. The back-cut should be done just above the angle of the mouth. A large dog ear usually forms superiorly that can be removed along the infraorbital fold. When one is closing the cheek rotation flap, a series of tension-reducing subcuticular sutures should be placed along the vector of tension starting at the low end of the nasolabial fold. This will prevent tension and necrosis of the flap tip. In the full cheek advancement flap, the lower incision is in the nasolabial fold while the upper incision is along the subciliary line just below the tarsal plate of the lower lid. The incision may be carried to the lateral canthus and then arched upward about 1 cm in one of the radial tension lines toward the temporal hairline. This elevates the heavy flap and helps prevent lid retraction and ectropion. The flap may also be suspended from the periosteum of the lateral orbital rim.

Both flaps cross the concavity of the nasofacial groove, tenting or obliterating this junction. This may be prevented by tacking the undersurface of the flap to the periosteum of the maxilla.

Either flap may be combined with a dorsal nasal (glabellar) flap to cover defects of the dorsum and sidewalls (Fig. 38). Anatomic subunits of the nose are retained if these flaps meet at the lateral ridges or nasofacial groove.

Ala Nasi

The fleshy ala nasi is a frequent site of basal cell carcinoma and one of the regions at high risk for recurrence. It is a convex subunit devoid of cartilaginous support. The thick, sebaceous skin is intimately interwoven with the underlying levator labii superioris alaeque nasi and nasalis muscles. Consequently, it is firmly bound and inelastic, which generally precludes primary closure except along the alar crease. Primary closure along the alar crease must be done without elevating the nostril rim. Small, deep defects near the nostril rim may be converted into wedge defects and closed primarily, as is done on the tip or helix. The line of closure is radial to the nostril. Maintaining a patent nasal airway is the primary concern. Second intention healing is frequently

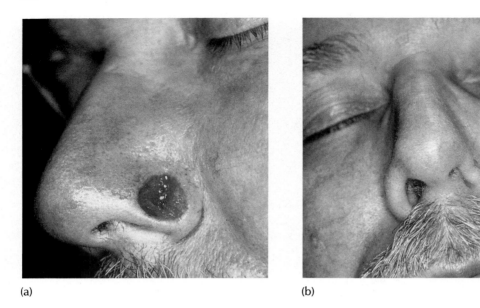

Figure 46   (a) Alar defect. (b) Nostril collapse on inspiration.

acceptable in the broad, shallow lesions, especially when they extend into the concave alar crease. When the defect is deeper, it may heal with loss of the natural convexity. This may draw up the nostril rim, or, if thin enough, collapse on inspiration (Fig. 46).

Full-thickness skin grafts, when the texture and color match, are often the closure of choice for larger, broad lesions that abut the alar crease. Superficial dermabrasion is required at 2–3 months to improve color, texture, and contour inequities between the graft and surrounding tissue.

Cheek skin next to the nasolabial fold is frequently mobilized to fill alar defects. This may be done with a subcutaneous island pedicle advancement flap if the alar base-cheek junction is involved (Fig. 47). Deeply placed subcuticular tacking sutures are required to obliterate dead space and recreate the concave alar rim.

The most useful closure for defects of the ala nasi is the superiorly based nasolabial fold flap, which may be transposed as a rhomboid flap (Fig. 48) or as the classic transposition flap (Fig. 49). The transposition flap is usually made longer than anticipated to account for the dog ear in the donor site. This extra tissue may be trimmed once the donor defect is closed and the flap is transposed. The trapdoor defect is a common complication of this flap. To minimize this, the flap should be defatted just below the subdermal plexus and the tissue surrounding the recipient bed undermined several millimeters. Everting sutures may be helpful too. On occasion, either of the axial pattern flaps—the midline forehead flap or the frontonasal flap—may be the best solution for an alar lesion.

Some small, full-thickness wounds involving the alar rim may be treated with cartilage-containing composite auricular grafts (Fig. 50). Alternatively, a large nasolabial flap whose distal tip has been deepithelialized and sewn back on itself to create a lining surface and a new alar rim can be used (Fig. 51).

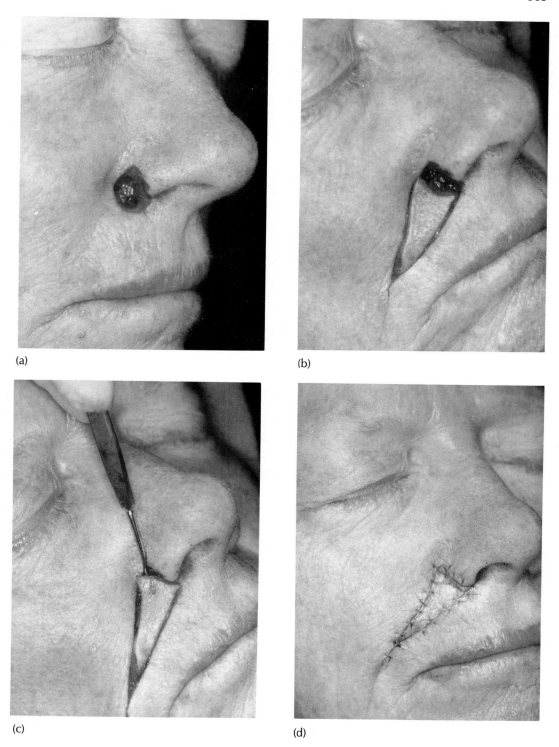

(a)

(b)

(c)

(d)

Figure 47 (a) Alar base defect. (b) Island pedicle flap incised. (c) Flap advanced. (d) Flap closed in V-Y manner.

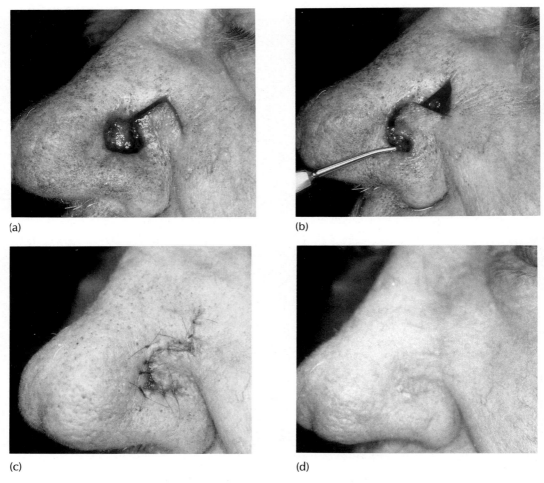

(a)

(b)

(c)

(d)

Figure 48 (a) Alar defect and rhomboid flap design. (b) Flap transposed. (c) Sutured in place. (d) Healing at 7 months.

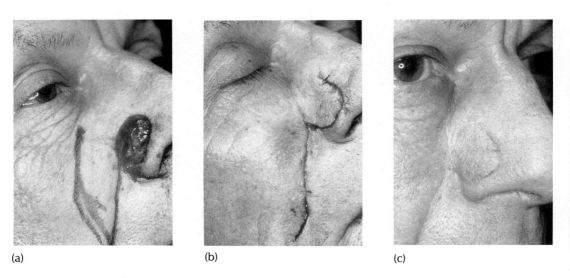

(a)

(b)

(c)

Figure 49 (a) Nasolabial flap design. (b) Trimmed and transposed. (c) Healing at 1 year.

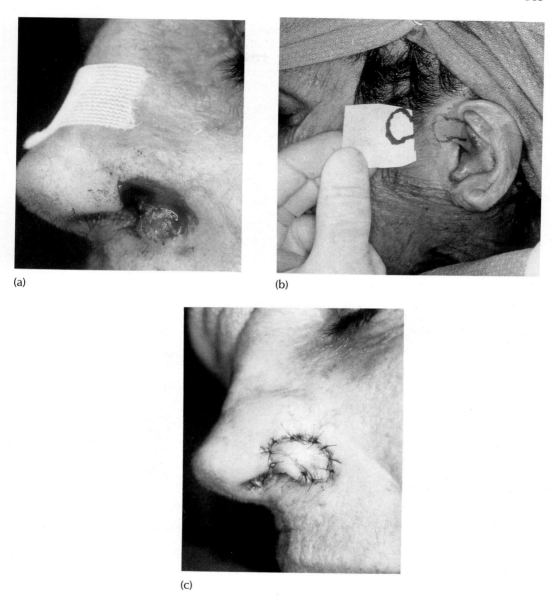

(a)

(b)

(c)

Figure 50 (a) Alar defect: full-thickness. (b) Auricular donor site. (c) Composite graft sutured in place.

DRESSINGS

Dressings serve the same function on the nose as elsewhere, but because the nose is a midface projection, dressings are difficult to fashion and secure. Cutting a nonadherent gauze pad like a shield will roughly conform to the pyramidal shape of the nose (Fig. 52). Loose gauze is then added as an absorbent layer. Securing the dressing is done by placing a few transverse tape strips

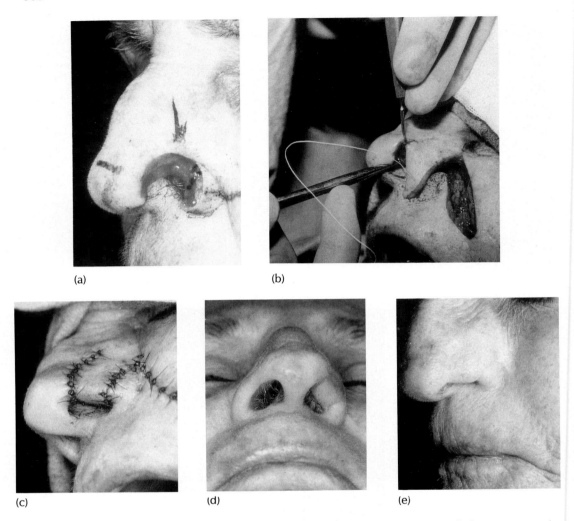

(a)   (b)

(c)   (d)   (e)

Figure 51 (a) Full-thickness alar defect. (b) Nasolabial flap sutured in place. (c) Nostril rim reconstructed with distal flap sutured back on itself. (d,e) Healing at 1 year.

across the dorsum of the nose to hold the dressing down. It is then secured by crisscrossing tape from the forehead to the nasolabial fold bilaterally. Tamponade may be added to the dressing by strategically placed, rolled 2 × 2 gauze pads or dental rolls either within the nostril or on the side of the nose (Fig. 53). Tension on wounds of the tip or dorsum may be reduced or a tip elevation dressing (Fig. 54). Tape strips are placed along the sidewalls and draped over the

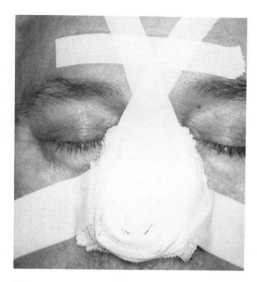

Figure 52 Nasal dressing.

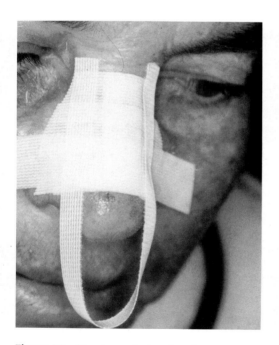
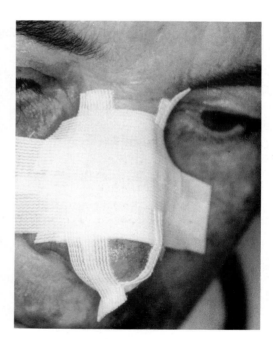

Figure 53 Tension-reducing dressing.

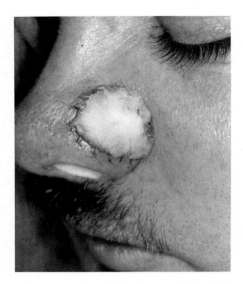

Figure 54 Nasal plug in nostril aids in hemostasis.

nostril rim. The tip is then pushed up by pinching the sticky loose ends of the tape together under the tip.

ACKNOWLEDGMENT

The author is grateful to Appleton and Lange, Publishers for permission to reprint Figures 2, 3, 11, 13, 14, 19, 22, 29, 42, and 43 from Salasche SJ, Bernstein G, Senkarik, M; *Surgical Anatomy of the Skin.*

BIBLIOGRAPHY

Antia NHY, Daver BM. Reconstructive surgery for nasal defects. *Clin Plast Surg* 1981;8:535–563.

Baker SR, Swanson NA. Regional and distant skin flaps in nasal reconstruction. *Facial Plast Surg* 1984; 2:33–44.

Baker SR, Swanson NA. Oblique forehead flap for total reconstruction of the nasal tip and columella. *Arch Otolaryngol* 1985;111:425–429.

Barton FE. Aesthetic aspects of partial nasal reconstruction. *Clin Plast Surg* 1981;8:177–191.

Bennett JE. An adjunct to nasolabial flap transfers. *Plast Reconstr Surg* 1981;67:236.

Bennett JE. Reconstruction of lateral nasal defects. *Clin Plast Surg* 1981;8:587–598.

Bernstein L. Surgical anatomy in rhinoplasty. *Otolaryngol Clin North Am* 1975;8:549–558.

Bray DA, Eichel BS. Closure of the large nose-cheek groove defects. *Arch Otolaryngol* 1977;103:29–31.

Breach NM. Repair of a full-thickness nasal defect with an ear lobe "sandwich" graft. *Br J Plast Surg* 1979; 32:94–95.

Brent B. The versatile cartilage autograft: Current trends in clinical transplantation. *Clin Plast Surg* 1979; 6:163–180.

Burget GC. Aesthetic restoration of the nose. *Clin Plast Surg* 1985;12:463–480.

Burget GC, Menick FJ. The subunit principle in nasal reconstruction. *Plast Reconstr Surg* 1985;76:239–247.

Burget GC, Menick FJ. Nasal reconstruction: Seeking a fourth dimension. *Plast Reconstr Surg* 1986;78:145–157.

Chester EC. Closure of a surgical defect in a nose using island grafts from the nose. *J Dermatol Surg Oncol* 1981;8:790–791.

Cronin TD. The V-Y rotational flap for nasal tip defects. *Ann Plast Surg* 1983;11:282–288.

Dingman RO, Natvig P. Surgical anatomy in aesthetic and corrective rhinoplasty. *Clin Plast Surg* 1977;4:111–120.

Elliot RA, Jr. Rotation flaps of the nose. *Plast Reconstr Surg* 1969;44:147–149.

Field LM. Skin grafts to the distal parts of noses using dual vertical W-plasties. *J Dermatol Surg Oncol* 1982;8:735.

Field LM. Nasal alar rim reconstruction utilizing the crus of the helix, with several alternatives for donor site closure. *J Dermatol Surg Oncol* 1986;12:253–258.

Harahap M. Some useful flaps for covering some defects in the nose. *J Dermatol Surg Oncol* 1982;8: 126–131.

Herbert DC. A subcutaneous pedicled cheek flap for reconstruction of alar defects. *Br J Plast Surg* 1978;31:79.

Jackson IT, Reid CD. Nasal reconstruction and lengthening with local flap. *Br J Plast Surg* 1978;31:343.

Jost G, Walter C, Bull TR, et al. Nasal defect repair. *Facial Plast Surg* 1983;1:75–80.

Kotler R. The midline forehead flap for resurfacing the nose. *J Dermatol Surg Oncol* 1981;7:57–66.

Lipman SH, Roth R. Composite grafts from earlobes for reconstruction of defects in noses. *J Dermatol Surg Oncol* 1982;8:135–137.

McGregor JC, Soutar DS. A critical assessment of the bilobed flap. *Br J Plast Surg* 1981;34:197–205.

Marchac D, Toth B. The axial frontonasal flap revisited. *Plast Reconstr Surg* 1985;76:686–694.

Masson JK, Mendelson BC. The banner flap. *Am J Surg* 1977;134:419–423.

Monheit GD. Nasal reconstruction with full thickness skin graft; a cosmetic procedure. *Adv Dermatol* 1987;2:229–239.

Natvig P, Sether LA, Gingrass RP, et al. Anatomical details of the osseous-cartilaginous framework of the nose. *Plast Reconstr Surg* 1971;48:528–532.

O'Quinn B, Thomas JR, Patton TJ. Classification of nasal defects. A practical guide for reconstruction. *Otolaryngol Head Neck Surg* 1986;95:5–9.

Patton TJ, Thomas JR. Classification and etiology of nasal defects. *Facial Plast Surg* 1984;2:9–15.

Peck GC. The onlay graft for nasal tip projection. *Plast Reconstr Surg* 1983;71:27.

Renner G, Davis WE. Adjacent flaps for nasal reconstruction. *Facial Plast Surg* 1984;2:17–32.

Rieger RA. A local flap for repair of the nasal tip. *Plast Reconstr Surg* 1967;40:147–149.

Rigg BM. The dorsal nasal flap. *Plast Reconstr Surg* 1973;52:361–364.

Rintala AE, Asko-Seljavaara S. Reconstruction of midline skin defects of the nose. *Scand J Plast Surg* 1969;3:105–108.

Rybka FJ. Reconstruction of nasal tip using nasalis myocutaneous sliding flap. *Plast Reconstr Surg* 1983;71:40–44.

Sawhney CP. Reconstruction of partial loss of nose. *Clin Plast Surg* 1981;8:521–534.

Snow SN, Mohs FE, Olansky DC. Nasal tip reconstruction: The horizontal "J" rotation flap using skin from the lower lateral bridge and cheek. *J Dermatol Surg Oncol* 1990;16:727–732.

Symonds FC, Crikelair CF. Auricular composite grafts in nasal reconstruction. *Plast Reconstr Surg* 1966;37:433–437.

Tardy ME, Sykes J, Kron T. The precise midline forehead flap in reconstruction of the nose. *Clin Plast Surg* 1985;12:481–494.

Thomas JR. Problem-specific analysis in nasal reconstruction. *Facial Plast Surg* 1984;2:1–8.

Vieira RC. Reconstruction of the nose with malignant disease. *Clin Plast Surg* 1981;8:603–613.

Webster RC, Smith RC, Smith KF, et al. Local flaps for the middle third of the face. *Facial Plast Surg* 1983;1:1–30.

Weerda H. Bilobed and trilobed flaps in head and neck defect repair. *Facial Plast Surg* 1983;1:51–60.

Winton GB, Salasche SJ. Use of rotation flaps to repair small surgical defects on the ala nasi. *J Dermatol Surg Oncol* 1986;12:154–158.

Yanai A, Nagata S, Tanaka H. Reconstruction of the columella with bilateral nasolabial flaps. *Plast Reconstr Surg* 1986;77:129–132.

Zide BM, Nasal anatomy: The muscles and tip sensation. *Aesth Plast Surg* 1985;9:193–196.

Zitelli JA. The bilobed flap for nasal reconstruction. *Arch Dermatol* 1989;125:957–959.

23

Male and Female Genitalia

Lawrence E. Gibson
Mayo Clinic and Mayo Medical School, Rochester, Minnesota

Harold O. Perry
Mayo Clinic/Foundation, Rochester, Minnesota

ANATOMY

Diseases of the genitalia encompass those problems unique to this area, as well as problems that are part of a generalized process. To surgically manage diseases of the genitalia, it is necessary to review the pertinent anatomy to facilitate proper biopsy, as well as anesthetic delivery and surgical technique. A basic knowledge of the lymphatic drainage of the genitalia is a prerequisite before treatment of malignancies of this area.

Starting with the male genitalia, the lymphatic drainage of the penis is largely into vessels that lie in the subcutaneous region and along dorsal vessels that run approximately to the base, where they diverge and pass into the superficial inguinal lymph nodes (Fig. 1). Some lymphatics from the glans penis as well as the distal urethra drain to the deep inguinal nodes. The superficial blood supply and venous drainage to the scrotum and penis is derived from the external pudendal artery and vein. The penis is drained by two primary sets of veins: the deep dorsal vein and the superficial dorsal vein. The latter, easily visible on the surface, which drains the skin and subcutaneous tissue of the penis, proceeds to the superficial external pudendal vein and then to the long saphenous vein. The deep dorsal vein drains the three corporeal bodies and is located beneath the fascia (Fig. 2). The deep dorsal vein goes beneath the pubic symphysis to the prostatic and perivesical plexus. The plexus of small veins proximal to the glans drains into the superficial dorsal vein of the penis. This plexus may be the site of phlebitis of the superficial dorsal vein (Mondor's disease). Possible causes for Mondor's disease include trauma, use of constrictive devices, infection, and intravenous drug injection. This process is painful and responds to local infiltration with bupivacaine.

The female genitalia have a very similar arteriovenous supply and lymphatic drainage (Fig. 3). The perineal artery continues as posterior labial arteries. The internal pudendal artery divides into two terminal branches: the deep and the dorsal arteries of the clitoris. The deep dorsal veins drain primarily into the vesicle plexus. The lymphatics from the lowest part of the vagina join

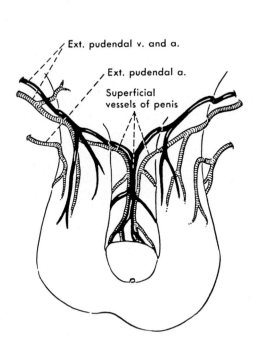

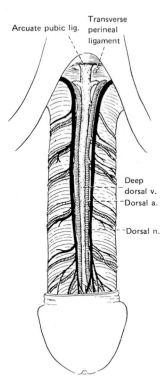

Figure 1 Superficial blood supply of the male genitalia. (From Hollinshead, 1974, p. 732. By permission of Mayo Foundation.)

Figure 2 Dorsal view of the penis after removal of the penile fascia. (From Hollinshead, 1974, p. 738. By permission of Mayo Foundation.)

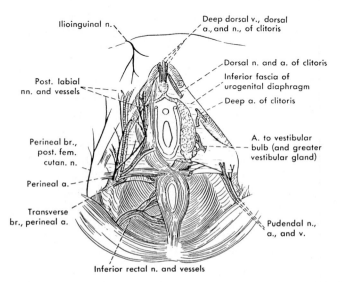

Figure 3 Blood supply and nerves of the female perineum. (From Hollinshead, 1974, p. 747. By permission of Mayo Foundation.)

the lymphatics from the vestibule in the labia and drain into the superficial inguinal lymph nodes. In the area around the anal canal internally to the dentate or pectinate line, which is the muco-cutaneous junction, lymphatic drainage is to the superficial femoral nodes. Proximal to the pectinate line, lymphatic drainage is to the pelvic lymph nodes.

ANESTHESIA

Lidocaine, 1 or 2% injected subcutaneously, provides adequate anesthesia for most biopsies. As a rule, it is best to avoid the use of epinephrine when injecting the penis, and in particular to avoid direct infiltration of the foreskin, as this on occasion has resulted in tissue necrosis. If a procedure is planned for which a large surface area in the genital region needs treatment, use of a local block may be considered. A basic knowledge of the innervation of the genital area is necessary before attempting a regional block. The penis is innervated by the left and right dorsal nerves, which are deep divisions of the pudendal nerves, which are in turn divisions of S2 through S4 (Fig. 2). The glans and the dorsal penis are supplied by the dorsal nerves, and the ventral or underside of the penis is supplied by smaller branches. The skin around the base of the penis, as well as the scrotum, is innervated by the genital branch of the genitofemoral nerve, and at the more proximal aspect of the scrotum and penis the skin is supplied by the anterior scrotal nerve, which is a branch of the ilioinguinal nerve (L1) (Fig. 4). Regional anesthesia can be obtained by the use of lidocaine, which will result in anesthesia for 1¼–3 hr. The use of tetracaine (Pontocaine) or bupivacaine (Marcaine) will provide anesthesia for 3½–6 hr. The anesthetic solution is injected in the dermis and subcutaneous tissue at the base of the penis in a fanlike fashion to the penile fascia. Although not common, cases of impotence following injection of anesthetic solution beneath the deep penile fascia have been noted. The penile block requires meticulous attention to injection around the entire circumference of the penis or small areas may be left without anesthesia; therefore, a caudal block is the most often used regional anesthetic for this area.

For anesthesia of a large area of the female perineum or labia, a pudendal block may be required. The pudendal nerve derives its fibers from the ventral branches of the 2nd, 3rd, and 4th sacral nerves. The pudendal nerves reenters the pelvis through the lesser sciatic foramen and

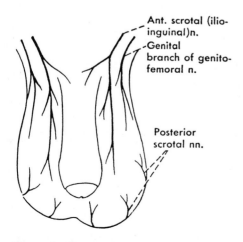

Ant. scrotal (ilio-
inguinal)n.
Genital
branch of genito-
femoral n.

Posterior
scrotal nn.

Figure 4   Cutaneous nerves of the scrotum. (From Hollinshead, 1974, p. 732. By permission of Mayo Foundation.)

accompanies the internal pudendal blood vessels along the lateral wall of the ischiorectal fossa. Branches of the pudendal nerve are the dorsal nerve of the clitoris, the perineal nerve, and the inferior rectal or hemorrhoidal nerve. The ilioinguinal (L1) and genitofemoral nerves (L1, L2) supply the skin and subcutaneous tissue over the mons area, as well as anterior portions of the labia majora. The pudendal block can be carried out with either lidocaine or bupivacaine, depending on the duration of the procedure planned. These regional blocks have associated risks, such as intravascular injection, ecchymosis formation, and puncture of the rectum, and should only be performed after adequate training in the technique.

BIOPSY

For most purposes, the use of a dermal punch biopsy 4 mm in diameter is best for tissue sampling of the genitalia. Once adequate anesthesia has been obtained, a punch biopsy can be obtained with little or no discomfort to the patient. It is essential to use a sharp punch, so disposable punches are best used in this area. A moderate amount of traction placed on the skin and subcutaneous tissue will allow penetration of the punch without distortion of the overlying epidermis. The use of a dull punch or inadequate traction will result in damage to the epidermis as the punch is passed through this layer to the subcutaneous tissue. It is important to obtain a biopsy specimen of adequate depth for proper fixation and orientation, especially when one is dealing with a malignancy. The biopsy site is cleansed several times per day with either saline or betadine solution diluted 1:5. The biopsy site is closed with sutures placed perpendicular to the long axis of the penis to prevent traction during erection. When removing nonmalignant cystic structures or papillomatous lesions, the scissors technique is good for removal of tissue for histologic examination. A slight amount of traction is applied to the lesion with forceps. This allows dissection beneath the lesion with the curved scissors pointed down. These wounds can be lightly electrocoagulated, or hemostasis can be obtained with aluminum chloride or pressure and allowed to heal by second intention. Excisional biopsies can also be done in the genital area.

CONDYLOMATA, VULVAR INTRAEPITHELIAL NEOPLASIA, BOWENOID PAPULOSIS

The approach to treatment of genital verrucae is evolving, with a rapid accumulation of evidence implicating various types of human papilloma virus (HPV) as the cause of condylomata, linking this same virus to other conditions of the genital area, including vulvar intraepithelial neoplasia (VIN), bowenoid papulosis, Bowen's disease, verrucal carcinoma, and squamous cell carcinoma. The development of DNA hybridization techniques along with radioactive probes has expanded our knowledge of the role of human papilloma virus in verrucae, as well as carcinomas. The most common types of human papilloma virus in genital warts are HPV6 and HPV11, accounting for approximately 90% of all condylomata acuminata and for approximately one third of oral papillomas. HPV16 and, less often, HPV18 have been associated with bowenoid papulosis and Bowen's disease. Infection with human papilloma virus resulting in verrucae followed by the development of neoplasia is a concept receiving a great deal of support. It is thought that the incidence of human papilloma virus infection has increased sixfold in the last decade, and it is estimated that approximately 3% of women under 30 years of age are infected by this virus. Also, 60-85% of sexual partners of persons infected with HPV will develop lesions within 2-3 months. In a recent study, warts were present in the sexual partner of 60-80% of women with vulvar intraepithelial neoplasia.

Human papilloma virus is also multifocal. Several studies have shown that if vulvar lesions are present, vaginal or cervical lesions may be present in approximately 70% of cases. An appreciation for the multifocal nature of this infection, as well as accumulating evidence that HPV infections may be the forerunners of neoplasia, has altered the approach to therapy for this problem. For initial evaluation, it is essential that a complete gynecologic and cutaneous examination be done. This includes a careful external inspection, as well as inspection of the distal portion of the anus and a speculum examination of the vagina and cervix. A Pap smear for cytologic examination should be done on all patients presenting with genital verrucae. It is also essential to examine the sexual partners of these patients, and treatment must be carried out in a simultaneous fashion to prevent rapid recurrence. It is a good idea to submit at least one of the condylomata for microscopic examination to rule out intraepithelial neoplasia or verrucous carcinoma. Visualization of the verrucae may be difficult, so pretreatment of the area with liberal quantities of a low concentration of acetic acid (3–5%) is helpful. A colposcope also aids in visualization of small lesions. For examination of the penis it is best to dip the penis into a cup of acetic acid solution for several minutes, and then examine very carefully with the aid of a magnifying glass or colposcope. Since genital verrucae are sexually transmitted, evaluation for concomitant sexually transmitted diseases is advised.

Several techniques for the treatment of condylomata are available, including cryotherapy or applications of podophyllin resin. There have been reports of cure rates of 70% when condylomata are injected with bleomycin (1 mg/ml solution). However, should these forms of therapy fail to clear the lesions, either electrodesiccation or vaporization with the CO_2 laser should be attempted. Side effects from this therapy include soreness in the area, itching, and some spot bleeding. Treatment of minute lesions can be accomplished with electrodesiccation without the use of analgesia. However, local or regional anesthesia should be accomplished prior to the treatment of more extensive lesions or laser therapy. The cure rate for condyloma acuminatum in the genital area treated by CO_2 laser approaches 90% in experienced hands. The specifics of laser therapy for this condition are discussed elsewhere in this volume.

Intraepithelial neoplasia should be considered when one is evaluating verrucal lesions. The singular designation includes several entities: hyperplastic vulvar dystrophy with atypia, mixed vulvar dystrophies, bowenoid papulosis, Bowen's disease, erythroplasia of Queyrat, and carcinoma in situ of the vulva. This same concept of intraepithelial neoplasia applies to the male genitalia. It is clear that human papilloma virus is involved in the development of genital intraepithelial neoplasia (GIN). DNA sequences hybridizing to HPV16 have been detected in 84% of intraepithelial neoplastic lesions and in 73% of DNA samples from clinically and histologically normal tissues from these patients with cancer. Nine of 11 vulvar tumors were positive for HPV16. There is a strong association between HPV16 genomes and genital tumors, and between HPV16 and histologically normal tissue within 2–5 cm of these tumors. In fact, it appears justified to summarize that the majority of cervical, vulvar, and penile cancers contain HPV DNA. Because of this clinical and histologic spectrum of lesions progressing from condylomata to intraepithelial neoplasia and squamous cell carcinoma, it is essential to biopsy lesions when treating these conditions. Close follow-up and repeat biopsies are warranted for lesions that do not resolve. Because of a tendency to have histologically banal areas with small samples, several punch biopsies or an excisional biopsy are recommended when evaluating vulvar intraepithelial neoplasia (VIN).

Bowenoid papulosis should be discussed in the context of human papilloma virus infection and GIN. Bowenoid papulosis was first described by Lloyd in 1970. It is characterized by multiple lesions located in the genital area of both sexes, usually occurring in younger people. There may be several clinical variants, including macular, papular, leukoplakic, and verrucal lesions (Fig. 5). Bowenoid papulosis is distinguished from Bowen's disease or squamous cell carcinoma in situ by involvement of young adults, multiplicity of lesions, lack of associated symptoms, smaller size of lesions, and occurrence in circumcised men. History of antecedent condylomata acuminata

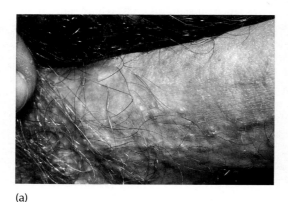

(a)

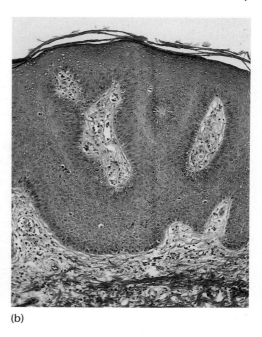

(b)

Figure 5   Bowenoid papulosis. (a) Small papules on the shaft of the penis. (b) Crowded and hyperchromatic nuclei plus several mitoses in a biopsy specimen (hematoxylin & eosin, × 160).

of the genital area was present in 12 of 34 patients. HPV16 has been identified in 6 of 10 cases of Bowen's disease (4 of 5 from genital sites) and 8 of 10 biopsies of bowenoid papulosis. While this condition has been reported to regress spontaneously, a case has been reported to progress to Bowen's disease. Treatments for bowenoid papulosis include cryotherapy, electrodesiccation, and 5-fluorouracil. Some very favorable results have been obtained with CO_2 or neodymium-YAG laser for leukoplakic or papillomatous lesions. Argon laser treatment for pigmented lesions has been tried. Laser treatment results in high cure rate and good cosmetic and functional results. Interferon therapy may have a role in treatment in the near future. Since progression to squamous cell carcinoma in situ has been reported, optimal management of this lesion consists of treatment, close follow-up for recurrence, and repeated biopsies. One must remember when submitting specimens for histopathologic examination that previous use of podophyllin resin causes changes in nuclear morphology, including mitotic figures with dispersion or clumping of the chromatin, pyknotic nuclei, and cytoplasmic swelling and vacuolization. These changes can persist as long as 2 weeks and may be mistaken for squamous cell carcinoma.

SQUAMOUS CELL CARCINOMA

The incidence of squamous cell carcinoma in the United States in 1 per 100,000. The site of origin in most cases is the preputial cavity. Circumcision in the neonatal period may lower the risk of invasive SCC. In addition to infection with HPV, other risk factors include exposure of the genitalia to ultraviolet light and cigarette smoking. Squamous cell carcinoma of the genital area can have varied clinical morphology. Giant condyloma acuminatum is now considered to be synonymous with verrucous carcinoma of the genital area. This concept of verrucous carcinoma includes other similar lesions, including oral verrucous carcinoma or carcinoma canniculatum on the extremities. Verrucal carcinoma can involve the inner lip and mouth (where it is most common—33%), the larynx, perianal area, cervix, vulva, scrotum, penis, and extremities. In the Mayo Clinic experience there were 19 cases of verrucous carcinoma out of a total of 169 cases of penile carcinoma. Fifty-seven percent of these cases were deeply invasive, although not metastatic. It is well known that the histologic morphology of verrucous carcinoma varies, depending on the location of the biopsy. Therefore, it is essential to either excise the lesion entirely or take several deep biopsies to ensure adequate histologic examination. Despite the somewhat banal cytologic appearance of the keratinocytes, these carcinomas are notorious for their tendency to invade deeply the underlying tissues and for formation of fistulous tracts. Other diseases should be considered when dealing with verrucal carcinoma of the genitalia. Because the histologic pattern may closely resemble pseudocarcinomatous hyperplasia, one should consider unusual infectious or inflammatory diseases, such as deep fungal infections or pemphigus vegetans. In this type of pemphigus, acantholysis may not be apparent, but other histologic clues such as eosinophilic spongiosis may be present.

While cryosurgery of verrucous carcinoma of the penis has been reported, most authors recommend complete excision of the tumor with systematic histologic examination (Mohs micrographic surgery). Radiation therapy is not recommended, because transformation to a much more aggressive tumor has occurred. There have been cases of giant condylomata treated successfully by excision combined with intralesional injection with bleomycin sulfate.

Other types of squamous cell carcinoma of the genitalia include erythroplasia of Queyrat, which is much more common in uncircumcised men and presents clinically as shiny, red, velvety plaques, usually involving the glans and foreskin, as well as the coronal sulcus and urethral meatus. Occasionally these lesions may be papillary and most often are asymptomatic unless ulcerated. It is important to note that urethral involvement can be present and cystoscopy is mandatory for all patients with carcinoma in situ of the distal urethra. Lymph node metastasis has been reported in patients with erythroplasia of Queyrat; careful clinical examination of the inguinal lymph nodes is needed. Treatment for this condition has included the use of 5-fluorouracil and electrodesiccation and curettage. The use of 5-fluorouracil is difficult when one is trying to limit application to the lesion. Significant inflammation of the surrounding tissues may result. Electrodesiccation and curettage has a high failure rate. Good results have been obtained using cryotherapy for the treatment of this condition. Circumcision is recommended in the management of this problem, as well as either conservative excision, the use of CO_2 laser vaporization, or Mohs micrographic surgery.

Bowen's disease is also a form of squamous cell carcinoma in situ, and while histologically the cytologic atypia is confined to the epidermis, there have been cases of nodal metastasis (Fig. 6). As with the approach to verrucous carcinoma of the genitalia, Bowen's disease requires careful examination and the use of multiple biopsies to ensure adequate sampling for histologic examination. Due to the high failure rate with the use of electrodesiccation and curettage, Mohs micrographic surgery or CO_2 laser surgery is recommended for treatment of squamous cell carcinoma in situ. Surveillance for systemic malignancies is warranted: up to one third of patients with Bowen's disease are reported to develop systemic malignancies.

Invasive squamous cell carcinoma of the genitalia is less common, but 95% of invasive carcinomas in this area are the squamous cell type. Squamous cell carcinoma usually develops in the background of chronic disease, which clinically resembles lichen sclerosus et atrophicus or leukoplakia (Fig. 7). Leukoplakia connotes a white lesion and is a clinical term that does not imply histologic atypia. Since histologic changes associated with leukoplakia can range from inflammation to squamous cell carcinoma, this term should not be used without modifiers describing the associated histologic findings. The most common locations of squamous cell carcinoma are the labia majora and the preputial area of the penis, but other areas may be involved. As a rule these lesions have been present for a considerable length of time and are most common in the seventh decade of life. It is not uncommon for an ulcer or nodule with associated

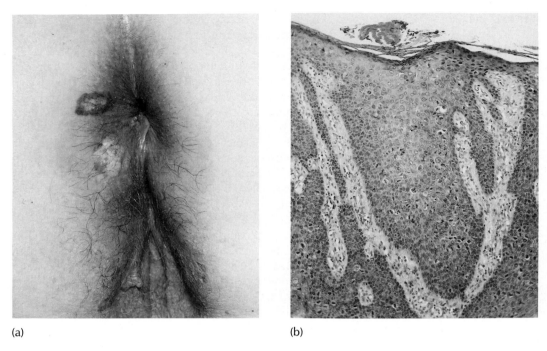

(a)   (b)

Figure 6   (a) Verrucal lesions of the perianal area. Biopsy showed squamous cell carcinoma in situ or Bowen's disease. (b) Bowen's disease. Extremely irregular, crowded arrangement of keratinocytes with many atypical mitoses (hematoxylin & eosin, ×160).

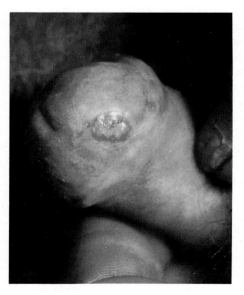

Figure 7   Asymptomatic erosive lesion of glans evolving in background of atrophic changes. Biopsy specimen showed squamous cell carcinoma with superficial invasion of dermis.

bleeding and pain to be present. The treatment of these conditions should be reserved for those familiar with surgical expertise in this area, including the ability to carry out nodal dissection, should this be required.

LICHEN SCLEROSUS ET ATROPHICUS

Lichen sclerosus et atrophicus is an inflammatory disease that results in atrophy of the genitalia. In older postmenopausal women, the term *kraurosis vulvae* has been applied to these same changes. Histologically, vascular changes consisting of intimal and vascular wall thickening are found, but these changes may be age related and not part of the disease process. In the male, this disease is known as *balanitis xerotica obliterans* or *kraurosis penis*, the latter term used in males without regard to age.

The early lesions consist of pearly white papules clustered in plaques over the genitalia or in diffuse, shiny, and atrophic plaques. The histologic changes of an atrophic epidermis and a band of middermal inflammation are characteristic and diagnostic. In the male, the glans is most commonly involved, although involvement of the shaft may also occur. Infrequently, the atrophying and scarring process compromises the urethral meatus so that dilation of the urethral orifice or a meatotomy must be done. Infrequently, circumcision is required because of phimosis.

In the female, the atrophy may result in effacement of the vulvar and clitoral tissues. Commonly the process also involves the perineal tissue, producing the "inverted keyhole" appearance of these areas. In the female, pruritus may be a major problem. Topical therapies, including corticosteroid creams and antipruritic lotions, gives some degree of symptomatic relief. Three-month treatment cycles with clobetasol propionate have shown promise in recent studies. Topical testosterone seems to break the cycle of itching in some female patients, but be aware of the masculinizing effects of the drug. The antimalarials given systemically have been most efficacious when used in the inflammatory stage of disease (Fig. 8).

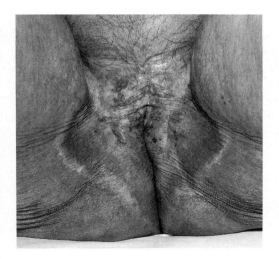
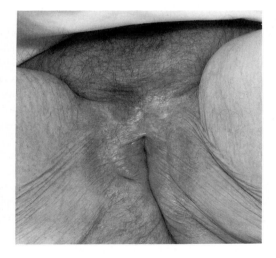

(a)   (b)

Figure 8   (a) Lichen sclerosus et atrophicus in a middle-aged woman whose major complaint was pruritus. Hydroxychloroquine therapy was given for 6 months. (b) Except for effacement of the vulvae, the tissues appear normal 15 years later.

Wallace has emphasized the development of carcinoma as a sequela in these patients with severe atrophic disease. If crateriform ulcers, nodules, or thickened areas with crusts and fissures occur in these patients, biopsies should be done to rule out carcinoma. Vulvectomy under these circumstances is indicated for the management of the carcinoma, but vulvectomy is not indicated in the usual patient as routine therapy. HPV infection has been suspected as a risk factor for squamous cell carcinoma in some cases of lichen sclerosus et atrophicus.

BASAL CELL CARCINOMA

While basal cell carcinoma is usually present in sun-exposed areas, it also occurs in areas shaded from sun exposure including the genital and perianal areas. Reports of basal cell carcinoma in the vulvar area are unusual; these lesions are thought to represent approximately 2% of vulvar malignancies. As with basal cell carcinoma elsewhere, the clinical lesion may present as a nodule, a superficial erosive plaque, or an ulceration. Basal cell carcinomas are not associated with leukoplakia. These tumors are most often present on the labia majora, but they may also involve the labia minor or the clitoris and the perianal region. They occur more commonly in patients in the sixth, seventh, or eighth decade of life; however, they have been reported in persons as early as the fourth decade. Approximately three fourths of the patients will complain of a "mole," nodule, or ulceration; however, approximately one fourth present with complaints of pruritus, rash, or irritation. The time between onset of symptoms and diagnosis averages over 10 months. These tumors are rare in blacks (3.3% of patients). Most often the lesions are solitary, but multiple vulvar basal cell carcinomas have been reported.

The treatment of choice appears to be excision, with microscopic examination to ensure adequate margins. Radiotherapy may be helpful, but because of the problems with radiodermatitis, it is best reserved for patients in whom surgery is not feasible. This condition should not be confused with baseloid carcinoma of the anal canal, which has a similar histologic appearance consisting of solid and circumscribed clumps of tumor cells containing baseloid, round, or oval nuclei. There are several differences between baseloid carcinoma and basal cell carcinoma of the skin. For the most part, baseloid carcinoma arises above the dentate line, but may occur adjacent to this line separating the endodermal and ectodermal mucosa. There is a greater tendency for baseloid carcinoma of the anal canal to contain keratin pearls and eosinophilic necrosis. There is also a tendency for greater variation in the shape and size of the nuclei than occurs with basal cell carcinoma. While baseloid carcinoma is a rare type of rectal carcinoma, there is a tendency for metastasis if not treated properly. Most of those patients in a large series who developed metastasis or died had either moderately differentiated or poorly differentiated and anaplastic tumors. This tumor represented 18% of 206 cases of squamous cell types of carcinoma of the anus and anal canal in one series.

PIGMENTED LESIONS

The spectrum of pigmented lesions of the genital area is similar to that occurring elsewhere. Simple hyperpigmentation of the genital skin may be due to various injuries or as a result of a drug reaction, including a fixed reaction, use of antimalarials, or bismuth intake. Lentigines in the genital area most often present as solitary or multiple asymptomatic, hyperpigmented macules of uniform color and varying size on the glans or shaft of the penis. Biopsy reveals hyperpigmentation of the basal layer of the epidermis, with varying numbers of dermal melanophages and hyperplasia of melanocytes. True nevi can also be present in the genital area, most often seen in the vulvar area, but also in the introitus.

Malignant Melanoma

Over 300 cases of vulvar melanoma have been reported. This represents 3–7% of all melanomas in women, and approximately 9% of malignant vulvar processes. The mean age of patients with vulvar melanoma is 54 years, the range being 17–84 years. Approximately one third of the patients are less than 50 years of age. In a series of 44 patients, only three noted changes in preexisting moles as the presenting complaint. Approximately one third of the patients noted a lump in the vulva, but one fourth of the patients had a nodule in the groin as their sole initial complaint (Fig. 9). The presenting symptom is bleeding in approximately one fourth of the patients, and pruritus in approximately 20%. The labia majora are the most often cited location for melanoma. However, approximately one third of the tumors occurred on the labia minora alone, while others occurred on both the labia minora and the clitoris or the clitoris alone. Slightly more than half of the melanomas initially involve mucosal sites. Amelanotic melanomas make up approximately 5% of melanomas in this area. The 5-year survival rate is 40% or less in most series for this type of melanoma. As in other melanomas, the prognosis appears to be dependent upon the level of invasion at the time of treatment, with those patients who have melanomas limited to the epidermis or the superficial papillary dermis showing a much better prognosis than those patients with lesions invading to the reticular dermis or the subcutaneous fat. The best method of treatment is surgical excision. It is not clear whether lymph node dissection is of value in the long-term survival for those patients with melanoma extending to the deep dermis or panniculus.

Melanomas of the penis are less common than vulvar melanomas, with the most common site being the glans and foreskin, respectively. The usual age of incidence is between 50 and 80 years, and these lesions most commonly present as enlarging, ulcerated, pigmented tumors. The rec-

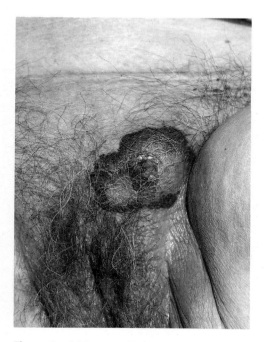

Figure 9   Melanoma. This lesion developed in 2 months. Biopsy specimen showed superficial spreading malignant melanoma.

ommended treatment for melanoma of the penis is surgical removal, including amputation. Since there is often a delay between onset of pigmented lesions in the genital area and treatment, it is recommended that pigmented lesions, including nevi, be excised when found in these areas. Because the histologic interpretation of recurrent nevi is difficult and can be confused with melanoma, it is recommended that nevi be totally excised or the entire lesion be removed by punch biopsy.

EXTRAMAMMARY PAGET'S DISEASE

Extramammary Paget's disease is most often located in the anogenital region, but can develop in any apocrine gland–bearing area, including the axillae, eyelids, and external auditory canal. Clinically, this process most often presents as a slowly enlarging, pruritic, erythematous, eczematous patch with serous crust (Fig. 10). Most commonly, these plaques are considered to represent areas of neurodermatitis. Diagnosis first requires an index of suspicion sufficient to warrant biopsy. Histologically, these lesions are characterized by the presence of Paget's cells within the epidermis. Paget's cells are large, round cells with pale-staining cytoplasm lacking intercellular bridges, which often show a positive reaction with stains for neutral and acid mucopolysaccharides, such as the Alcian blue, periodic acid–Schiff stain, or Hale's colloidal iron. Generally, mucin is more abundant than in mammary Paget's disease, which involves the areolar area of the breast. Once the diagnosis has been confirmed, management requires a thorough examination to rule out contiguous or simultaneous adenocarcinoma. Carcinoma of the rectum is the most common malignancy associated with extramammary Paget's disease of the perineum. However,

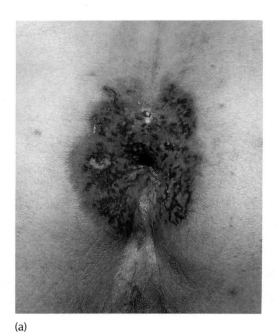

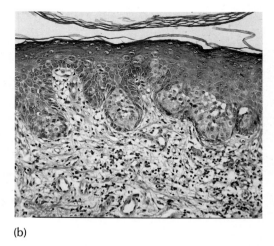

(a)   (b)

Figure 10 (a) Extramammary Paget's disease, perianal area. Lesion developed over several years, associated with pruritus. One recurrence was reexcised 3 years after initial surgery. (b) Many Paget's cells are present in the epidermis, both singly and in groups. These cells have ample pale-staining cytoplasm (hematoxylin & eosin, ×250).

Table 1 Malignancies Reported in Patients with Extramammary Paget's Disease

Apocrine gland carcinoma
Eccrine gland carcinoma
Carcinoma of Moll's glands
Ceruminal gland carcinoma
Bartholin's gland carcinoma
Perianal gland carcinoma
Adenocarcinoma of rectum
Carcinoid of ileum
Adenocarcinoma of breast
Carcinoma of ureter, bladder, urethra
Adenocarcinoma of prostate
Carcinoma of cervix
Adenocarcinoma of ovary
Carcinoma of pancreas

Source: Powell et al., 1985.

several other malignancies have also been reported in patients with extramammary Paget's disease, including apocrine gland carcinoma, eccrine gland carcinoma, and carcinoma of Bartholin's glands and perianal glands (Table 1). The exact cause of extramammary Paget's disease is still not settled, despite the use of newer peroxidase stains including CEA and keratin stains, that confirm the Paget's cells to be adenocarcinoma. It is important to note that in addition to an associated or underlying adenocarcinoma, pagetoid spread of malignancies in the perineal area is also possible. A recent report of eight cases of extramammary Paget's with associated transitional cell carcinoma of the bladder demonstrates this point (Fig. 11). In two of these cases there was contiguous spread of bladder carcinoma to the genital skin. One must do a thorough and

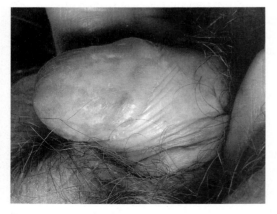

Figure 11 Transitional cell carcinoma (TCC). Pagetoid involvement of the glans 13 years following cystectomy for TCC of the bladder and 3 years posturethrectomy for TCC in situ.

careful examination of the rectum, as well as the vagina, cervix, uterus, and urethra and bladder, to rule out pagetoid spread of a contiguous carcinoma. Another management point is the clinically silent or inapparent peripheral extensions of extramammary Paget's disease that extend in an unpredictable fashion away from the lesion. Local recurrences following surgical excision of extramammary Paget's disease are well known and occur at rates of 31–61%. The mean time for recurrence has been approximately 45 months. The use of Mohs micrographic surgery has been reported with five cases of extramammary Paget's disease. Because of the high rate of recurrence with excision, microscopically controlled surgical techniques are the treatment of choice for this problem.

VASCULAR LESIONS

Vascular lesions may be present in the genital region, either as isolated phenomena or as part of a systematized process. Examples of the latter include cavernous hemangiomas as part of blue rubber bleb nevus syndrome or of angiokeratomas of Fabry's disease. One of the most common lesions seen in the scrotum is the angiokeratoma of Fordyce: usually a small papulonodular lesion, 2–4 mm in diameter, arising in midlife and not associated with any systemic disease. Angiokeratomas can also be present in the vulva, usually occur in women less than 50 years of age, and may be related to increased venous pressure secondary to pregnancy or hemorrhoids. Glomus tumors may involve the genital region and have been a reported cause of dyspareunia.

Often, hemangiomas or angiokeratomas of the genital area require no treatment; however, should there be a question about diagnosis or if lesions are of functional or cosmetic concern, removal can be accomplished. If one desires tissues for diagnosis, use of the punch biopsy or small excisional biopsy is adequate. If the diagnosis is not in doubt, angiomatous lesions can be treated with either electrocoagulation or, if larger, with the argon laser. The argon laser decreases the size or eliminates the vascular lesions and usually does not result in scarring or functional impairment. Lymphangiomas can also be present in the genital area. When present in this area, they most often involve the groin or the scrotum and present as a subcutaneous swelling. A lymphangioma may involve deeper structures and can be misdiagnosed as a hernia. Most of these lesions are present in patients less than 10 years of age. Possible complications include chronic lymphedema, elephantiasis, fistula formation, infection, and chronic leakage of lymph fluid. With chronic lymphedema, one must be aware of the development of angiosarcoma (Stewart-Treves syndrome) in the edematous extremity. These tumors may develop in lymphedematous extremities of congenital origin, as well as those secondary to surgical procedures. The treatment of choice for larger lymphangiomas is surgical excision. However, small lesions can be treated adequately by electrosurgery. CO_2 laser vaporization has also been advocated. Malignant vascular tumors such as Kaposi's sarcoma can present in the genital area, especially in patients with acquired immunodeficiency virus.

MISCELLANEOUS CONDITIONS

Cysts

The median raphe cyst is one of the most common cystic lesions of the male genitalia. Clinically these cystic structures arise in the midline at any point along the genital fold extending from the anus to the urethra. Histologically, they are cystic spaces with no connection to the urethra or to the overlying epidermis. The epithelium is usually of a pseudostratifed columnar type, but occasionally can be cuboidal or fusiform. Mucin stains of the contents are usually negative, but mucin-containing clear cells can be seen in the wall of the cyst. The median raphe cyst is postulated to be due to epithelial rests incidental to incomplete closure to the urethral or genital folds, or development from outgrowths of embryologic epithelium after primary closure of these folds. The treatment of choice is excision with primary closure of the wound.

Other cysts include the well-known Bartholin's gland cyst, the surgical treatment of which is described in several texts of gynecologic surgery. Perhaps less well known is the mucous cyst of the vulvar vestibule. Such cysts are usually asymptomatic and located in the vestibular portion of the vagina and vulva. They are usually solitary and range in size from 0.2 to 3 cm. As with median raphe cysts the lining is columnar epithelium and there are mucin-positive cells in the cyst wall. Once again, treatment is simple excision with primary closure. Epidermoid cysts may occur in the genital region, labia majora, or scrotum. Treatment is identical to that for cysts located elsewhere and is indicated if the cyst if painful, draining, infected, or of cosmetic or functional concern. Scrotal calcifications may resemble cysts, but do not show a cyst wall histologically. These calcifications are not associated with systemic disease and can be removed if they are draining or if they become large.

Papillary Hidradenoma

This is a tumor unique to the vulvar area and rarely found in other apocrine areas. In a series of 69 cases these lesions were solitary in all but three patients. The peak age of onset is the fifth and sixth decade. Approximately 40% are located in the area of the labia majora and another 25% are located in the area of the labia minora. Two thirds of these lesions are asymptomatic; however, bleeding is reported in approximately 10% of cases. The differential diagnosis includes epidermoid cyst or leiomyoma. The histologic characteristics of this tumor include an apocrine papillomatous growth encapsulated in the dermis surrounded by a fibrous capsule, in most instances showing no connection to the overlying epidermis. These tumors have rarely been reported to occur on the nipple or the eyelid. One case of associated squamous cell carcinoma has been reported. Treatment consists of simple excision using local anesthesia and primary closure.

Leiomyoma

Leiomyomas are known to occur in the genital area, most often in the scrotum or labia majora. These lesions tend to be asymptomatic and histologically are identical to leiomyomas seen elsewhere in the skin. There has been a case report of leiomyoma involving the clitoris. Treatment if needed consists of simple excision and primary closure.

Syringoma

Syringomas may involve the genitalia. This most commonly occurs outside the genital area in women (neck, face, chest, and supraclavicular regions). Cases involving the male genitalia are rare, but tend to be multiple and involve the dorsum and lateral aspects of the shaft of the penis. Multiple syringomas involving the vulva have also been reported.

Trichoepithelioma

This lesion is usually located on the face, but there have been case reports involving the genital area. In a recent report of three giant solitary trichoepitheliomas of the perianal area, two were in the natal cleft. These tumors differed from the usual trichoepithelioma in that they were very large and deep, extending to the subcutaneous fat. All of these lesions were excised, with no recurrence.

Zoon's Balanitis

An inflammatory condition of the glans, seen almost entirely in uncircumcised men, Zoon's balanitis is clinically characterized by velvetlike erythema and, rarely, erosions of the glans with a tendency to bleed. It can be confused with several other conditions, including Bowen's disease or erythroplasia of Queyrat. This same condition can occur in the vulvar area. Synonyms include *balanitis circumscripta plasmacellularis* and *vulvitis circumscripta plasmacellularis*. There are also reports of plasma cell inflammation involving other mucous membranes, such as the mouth and tongue, and *circumorificial plasmacytosis* has been used to describe this process. Histologically there is thinning of the overlying epidermis, with ulceration on occasion. The epidermis is characterized by thin or "lozenge-shaped" keratinocytes and may be separated from the underlying dermis. The infiltrate in the upper dermis is characterized by numerous plasma cells. There have been several reports of treatment by circumcision with excellent results in all cases (follow-up of up to 3 years). Other forms of medical therapy have been less successful. It is essential to biopsy this condition to rule out squamous cell carcinoma in situ or other malignancy.

BIBLIOGRAPHY

Asarch RG, Golitz LE, Sausker WF, Kreye JM. Median raphe cyst of the penis. *Arch Dermatol* 1979; 115:1084–1086.

Baggish MS. Condylomata acuminata genital infections treated by the CO_2 laser. In *Basic Advanced Laser Surgery in Gynecology*. MS Baggish, ed. Norwalk, CT, Appleton Century Crofts, 1985.

Banner EA, Winkelmann RK. Glomus tumor of the vagina. Report of a case. *Obstet Gynecol* 1957;9:326–328.

Barth JH, Dawber RPR. Letter to the editor: Cryosurgery as alternative treatment [for erythroplasia of Queyrat]. *J Dermatol Surg Oncol* 1986;12:1144.

Bean SF, Becker FT. Basal cell carcinoma of the vulva: A case report and review of the literature. *Arch Dermatol* 1968;98:284–286.

Berger BW, Hori Y. Multicentric Bowen's disease of the genitalia. Spontaneous regression of lesions. *Arch Dermatol* 1978;114:1698–1699.

Bernstein G, Forgaard DM, Miller JE. Carcinoma in situ of the glans penis and distal urethra. *J Dermatol Surg Oncol* 1986;12:450–455.

Bhawan J, Cahn T. Atypical penile lentigo. *J Dermatol Surg Oncol* 1984;10:99–100.

Blair C. Angiokeratoma of the vulva. *Br J Dermatol* 1970;83:409–411.

Bracco GL, Carli P, Maestrini G, DeMarco A, Taddei GL, Cattaneo A. Clinical and histological effects of topical treatments of vulvar lichen sclerosis. A critical evaluation. *J Reprod Med* 1993;38(1):38–40.

Buecker JW, Heaton C. Residents corner: Bleomycin sulfate—postoperative intralesional usage for giant condylomata. *J Dermatol Surg Oncol* 1985;11:972–973.

Carneiro SJC, Gardner HL, Knox JM. Syringoma of the vulva. *Arch Dermatol* 1971;103:494–496.

Chung AF, Woodruff JM, Lewis JL. Malignant melanoma of the vulva: Report of 44 cases. *Obstet Gynecol* 1975;45:638–646.

Collins PS, Farber GA, Hegre AM. Basal-cell carcinoma of the vulva. *J Dermatol Surg Oncol* 1981;7:711–714.

Connors RC, Ackerman AB. Histologic pseudomalignancies of the skin. *Arch Dermatol* 1976;112:1767–1780.

DeVillez RL, Stevens CS. Bowenoid papules of the genitalia: A case progressing to Bowen's disease. *J Am Acad Dermatol* 1980;3:149–152.

Elliott GB, MacDougall JA, Elliott JDA. Problems of verrucose squamous carcinoma. *Ann Surg* 1973; 177:21–29.

Ferenczy A, Masaru M, Nagai N, Silverstein SJ, Crum CP. Latent papillomavirus in recurring genital warts. *N Engl J Med* 1985;313:784–788.

Ferrandiz C, Ribera M. Zoon's balanitis treated by circumcision. *J Dermatol Surg Oncol* 1984;10:622–625.

Figueroa S, Gennaro AR. Intralesional bleomycin injection in treatment of condylomata acuminatum. *Dis Colon Rectum* 1980;23:550–551.

Friedrich EG, Wilkinson EJ. Mucous cyst of the vulvar vestibule. *Obstet Gynecol* 1973;42:407–414.

Goldberg D. Multiple basal cell carcinomas of the vulva. *J Dermatol Surg Oncol* 1984;10:615–617.

Graham JH, Helwig EB. Bowen's disease and its relationship to systemic cancer. *Arch Dermatol* 1959; 80:133–159.

Gross G, Roussaki A, Papendick U. Efficacy of interferons on Bowenoid papulosis and other precancerous lesions. *JID* 1990;95(6 suppl):152S–157S.

Gueukdjian SA. Lymphangioma of the groin and scrotum. *J Int Coll Surg* 1955;24:159–170.

Hanash KA, Furlow WL, Utz DC, Harrison EG. Carcinoma of the penis. Clinicopathologic study. *J Urol* 1970;104:291.

Hollinshead WH. *Textbook of Anatomy*. 3rd ed. Hagerstown, MD, Harper & Row, 1974.

Hughes PSH. Cryosurgery of verrucous carcinoma of the penis (Buschke-Lowenstein tumor). *Cutis* 1979; 24:43–45.

Ikenberg H, Gissmann L, Gross G, Grussendorf-Conen E-I, Zur Hausen H. Human papillomavirus type 16 related DNA in genital Bowen's disease and in bowenoid papulosis. *Int J Cancer* 1983;32:563–565.

Jackson R. Melanosis of the vulva. *J Dermatol Surg Oncol* 1984;10:119–121.

Keine P, Milde-Langosch K, Loning T. Papillomavirus infection in vulvar lesions of lichen sclerosis et atrophicus. *Arch Dermatol Res* 1991;283(7):445–448.

Khan SA, Smith NL, Hu K-N. New perspectives in diagnosis and management of thrombophlebitis of the superficial dorsal vein of the penis. *J Dermatol Surg Oncol* 1982;8:1063–1067.

Kopf AW, Bart RS. Tumor Conference Number 38. Lymphangioma of the scrotum and penis. *J Dermatol Surg Oncol* 1981;7:870–872.

Kopf AW, Bart RS. Tumor Conference Number 43. Penile lentigo. *J Dermatol Surg Oncol* 1982;8:637–639.

Kopf AW, Bart RS. Tumor Conference Number 54. Laser treatment of penile hemangiomas. *J Dermatol Surg Oncol* 1985;11:20–22.

Kraus EW. Perianal basal cell carcinoma. *Arch Dermatol* 1978;114:460–461.

Landthaler M, Haina D, Brunner R, Waidelich W, Braun-Falco O. Laser therapy of bowenoid papulosis in Bowen's disease. *J Dermatol Surg Oncol* 1986;12:1253–1257.

Levine RU, Crum CP, Herman E, et al. Cervical papillomavirus infection and intraepithelial neoplasia: A study of male sexual partners. *Obstet Gynecol* 1984;64:16–20.

Lopansri S, Mihm MC Jr. Clinical and pathologic correlation of malignant melanoma. *J Cutan Pathol* 1979;6:180–194.

MacNab JCM, Walkinshaw SA, Cordiner JW, Clements JB. Human papillomavirus in clinically and histologically normal tissue of patients with genital cancer. *N Engl J Med* 1986;315:1052–1058.

Malek RS, Goellner JR, Smith TF, Espy MJ, Cupp MR. Human papillomavirus infection and intraepithelial in situ and invasive carcinoma of penis. *Urology* 1993;42:159–170.

Meisels A, Morin C, Casas-Cordero M. Human papillomavirus infection of the uterine cervix. *Int J Gynecol Pathol* 1982;1:75.

Mohs FE, Blanchard L. Microscopically controlled surgery for extramammary Paget's disease. *Arch Dermatol* 1979;115:706–708.

Moore DC. Regional block. 4th ed. Springfield, IL, Charles C Thomas, 1981.

Ordonez NG, Awalt H, MacKay B. Mammary and extramammary Paget's disease: An immunocytochemical and ultrastructural study. *Cancer* 1987;59:1173–1183.

Pang LSC, Morson BC. Baseloid carcinoma of the anal canal. *J Clin Pathol* 1967;20:128–135.

Powell FC, Bjornsson J, Doyle JA, Cooper AJ. Genital Paget's disease and urinary tract malignancy. *J Am Acad Dermatol* 1985;13:84–90.

Ridley CM. Lichen sclerosus et atrophicus. *Arch Dermatol* 1987;123:457–460.

Roy M, Meisels A, Fortier M, et al. Vaginal condylomata: A human papillomavirus infection. *Clin Obstet Gynecol* 1981;24:461–483.

Sanchez-Conejo-Mir J, Moreno-Gimenez JC, Camacho-Martinez F. Genitoperineal cyst of the median raphe. *J Dermatol Surg Oncol* 1984;10:451–454.

Shapiro L, Platt N, Torres-Rodriguez VM. Idiopathic calcinosis of the scrotum. *Arch Dermatol* 1970;102: 199–204.

Sonnex TS, Dawber RP, Ryan TJ, Ralfs IG. Zoon's (plasma cell) balanitis: Treatment by circumcision. *Br J Dermatol* 1982;106:585–588.

Stenchever MA, McDivitt RW, Fisher JA. Leiomyoma of the clitoris. *J Reprod Med* 1973;10:75–76.

Stern RS and Members of the Photochemotherapy Study Group. Genital tumors among men with psoriasis exposed to psoralens and ultraviolet A radiation (PUVA) and ultraviolet B radiation. *N Engl J Med* 1990;322:1093–1097.

Strauss RJ, Fazio VW. Bowen's disease of the anal and perianal area: A report and analysis of 12 cases. *Am J Surg* 1979;138:231–234.

Sullivan M, King LS. Effects of resin of podophyllum on normal skin, condylomata acuminata and verruca vulgaris. *Arch Dermatol Syphilol* 1947;56:30–47.

Tatnall FM, Wilson-Jones E. Giant solitary trichoepitheliomas located in the perianal area: A report of 3 cases. *Br J Dermatol* 1986;115:91–99.

Taylor PT, Stenwig JT, Klausen H. Paget's disease of the vulva: A report of 18 cases. *Gynecol Oncol* 1975;3:46–60.

Wade TR, Kopf AW, Ackerman AB. Bowenoid papulosis of the genitalia. *Arch Dermatol* 1979;115:306–308.

Wallace HJ. Lichen sclerosus et atrophicus. *Trans St. John's Hosp Dermatol Soc* 1971;57:9–30.

Williams SL, Rogers LW, Quan SHQ. Perianal Paget's disease: A report of seven cases. *Dis Colon Rectum* 1976;19:30–40.

Woodworth H, Dockerty MB, Wilson RB, Pratt JH. Papillary hidradenoma of the vulva: A clinicopathologic study of 69 cases. *Am J Obstet Gynecol* 1971;110:501–508.

Zalla JA, Perry HO. An unusual case of syringoma. *Arch Dermatol* 1971;103:215–217.

24

The Nail

Richard K. Scher
Columbia University College of Physicians and Surgeons,
New York, New York

The important functions of the nails must be taken into account when one is considering performing nail surgical procedures: (1) they protect the distal digit; (2) they enhance fine touch so that small objects can be picked up more efficiently; (3) they have important cosmetic attributes. It is estimated that over $5 billion a year are spent on nail cosmetics.

Nail problems may make up 5% of the conditions seen by physicians in general and perhaps twice that number are seen by dermatologists. As many as 1 patient in 10 seeks dermatologic care for a nail disorder. Therefore, it is essential that a knowledge of nail anatomy be clearly understood. About half of all nail problems are due to fungal disease and the rest to psoriasis, lichen planus, tumors, ingrown nails, and a large miscellaneous group. Once a diagnosis is established, the most effective form of treatment, whether medical or surgical, can be initiated. However, the spectrum of clinical expression for nail conditions is extremely limited. Unlike the skin, where diagnoses are facilitated by changes in color, size, shape, and so on, these changes are limited in the nail unit. Consequently, a number of diagnostic procedures must be performed more frequently on the nail than on the skin. Thus evolves the area of nail surgery and the nail biopsy. Tumors of the nail unit as well as the sequelae of trauma are best treated by reliable surgical methods. The hand, orthopedic, or plastic surgeon, though well trained in advanced techniques of this site, may be unwilling or unable to handle the simple diagnostic and therapeutic methods that are best left to the dermatologist with a particular interest in this area.

ANATOMY

Prior to performing satisfactory nail surgery, a thorough knowledge of the anatomic structure of the nail unit with its blood and nerve supply is essential. The nail appendage consists of the following components: matrix, proximal and lateral folds, plate, bed, hyponychium, and four grooves—proximal, distal, and two lateral (Fig. 1).

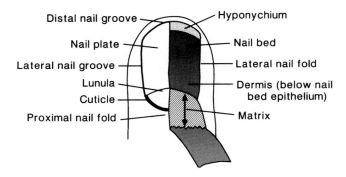

Figure 1   Anatomy of the nail unit.

The nail matrix lies deep in the fingertip, below the proximal nail fold, and is the manufacturing center that produces the nail plate, its horny end product. Any defect at this site will be reflected in onychodystrophy of the evolving nail plate. The distal portion of the matrix is called the lunula, and this may be seen in some digits lying beneath the proximal portion of the nail plate distal to the cuticle. The proximal portion of the matrix abuts the bony terminal phalanx. There is no granular layer in the matrix, so keratohyaline granules are absent. The proximal portion of the matrix produces the upper portion of the nail plate. The distal portion of the matrix (lunula) produces the underportion of the nail plate. Extreme care must be exercised when performing surgery in the vicinity of the proximal nail matrix. A defect after surgery will produce a deformed nail plate surface. The split nail is an example of such a defect.

The proximal nail fold is a modified extension of the finger that forms a fold over the matrix. It is continuous with the lateral nail fold that forms the side borders of the nail plate. The cuticle is the horny end product of the proximal nail fold. It is deposited on the surface of the newly formed nail plate and desquamates shortly thereafter. Unlike the matrix, the nail fold does have a granular layer with keratohyaline granules.

The nail plate extends about 5 mm proximal to the cuticle where it fits into the proximal nail groove, the roof of which is the undersurface of the proximal nail fold; the floor is the matrix. That portion of the nail plate in the proximal groove is often referred to as the nail root. The nail plate fits laterally into the lateral nail grooves formed by the junction of the lateral nail folds to the nail bed.

The nail bed begins at the distal portion of the lunula (matrix) and extends distally to terminate at the hyponychium. The epidermis of the nail bed is arranged in longitudinal grooves and ridges overlying the dermis and contains no granular layer. Splinter hemorrhages occur when a small amount of blood enters a longitudinal groove and is trapped by the overlying adherent nail plate, assuming the longitudinal configuration of this natural trough. The dermis contains both capillaries and glomus bodies.

The hyponychium commences with the termination of the nail bed at a point where the nail plate separates to its free end. A granular layer is present at this site. A transverse groove demarcates the end of the hyponychium. The hyponychium then becomes continuous with the volar epidermis of the digit. This site is often the point at which fungal organisms enter to produce the most common fungus infection of the nails: distal subungual onychomycosis.

The dermis of the nail appendage is limited by the underlying phalanx upon which it rests. There is no subcutaneous tissue below the nail unit dermis. Consequently, when one is cutting through this structure, the underlying periosteum of the distal phalanx may be exposed. The distance from the surface of the nail plate to the periosteum is no more than several millimeters.

The blood and nerve supply of the nail unit run approximately the same course. Two lateral digital arteries and nerves on either side of the finger give rise to dorsal branches at the junction of the middle and terminal phalanges (Fig. 2). The branches subdivide to form distal and proximal arches with a ramus to both the matrix and the proximal nail fold. It is important to remember this circulatory and neural pattern when anesthetizing and operating on the nail unit.

PREOPERATIVE CONSIDERATIONS

Objectives of nail surgery include diagnostic biopsy, excision of both benign and malignant tumors, relief of pain, treatment of infection, and improvement of both hereditary and acquired anatomic deformities. Prior to the surgical procedure itself, a careful medical history must be obtained from the patient. Nail surgery should be avoided, if possible, in those who have peripheral vascular disease, diabetes mellitus, or connective tissue disorders that compromise circulation. This includes Raynaud's phenomenon, particularly when surgery in the toenails is considered. Taking an allergy history is important. If the patient is taking anticoagulant drugs or aspirin, surgery should be postponed.

If there is evidence of active infection, elective procedures should be deferred until these are treated with antibiotics and soaks for 2 or more weeks. When the nail plate punctures the skin, as in ingrown toenail, it may not be possible to postpone surgery. Removing a nail spicule could be done initially. In this situation, the nail plate pierces the epithelium of the lateral nail groove, resulting in a foreign body reaction. Nail surgery should be performed only under aseptic conditions. The surgical site should be thoroughly scrubbed with an antiseptic surgical cleanser. Many nail surgeons prefer to administer systemic antimicrobial agents prior to surgery.

Standard surgical instruments are used in procedures on the nail. Several bear special mention. These include the dual-action nail nipper, which permits close and accurate nail cutting in an atraumatic manner (Fig. 3). It is also helpful for excision of the onycholytic nail plate without anesthesia. The ordinary nail clipper should only be used for routine nail trimming because it is rigid and requires the patient's nail to conform to the instrument; this often produces pain. The nail nipper has a flexible neck that conforms to the patient's nail and allows simple proce-

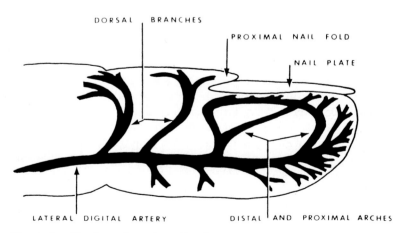

Figure 2 Blood supply to the nail unit.

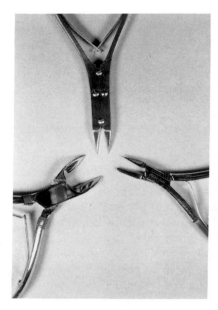

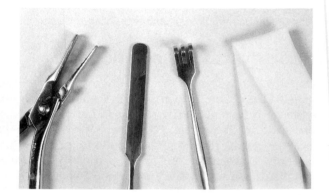

Figure 3 Top: Dual-action nail nipper. Left: Nail clipper. Right: Nail splitter.

Figure 4 Left to right: nail-pulling forceps, dental spatula, rake retractor, wide Penrose drain.

dures to be done painlessly without anesthesia. The nail splitter is particularly effective for removal of a longitudinal strip of nail plate in the patient with ingrown toenails. It has two teeth: the lower one, flat and anvil-like, is pushed beneath the nail plate for separation; an upper cutting tooth is used to incise the plate prior to removal. A nail-pulling forceps (Fig. 4) is practical for gripping the plate prior to avulsion once it has been separated from its attachments. The latter may be accomplished with a dental spatula or Freer elevator. The ingrown nail scissors allows removal of skin-piercing nail spicules from ingrowing toenails with minimal discomfort. A variety of rake retractors are used to retract the proximal nail fold when one is performing matrix surgery.

ANESTHESIA

A plain solution of 1 or 2% lidocaine hydrochloride is most commonly used as a local anesthetic. Mepivacaine hydrochloride, 1 or 2%, has also been used as an anesthetic. It may be used in patients sensitive to lidocaine and has the added advantage of longer action and better hemostasis. For more extended anesthesia bupivacaine is recommended. Tourniquets, digital blocks, and general and regional anesthesia are usually unnecessary for the simple nail procedures and should be avoided. Some surgeons use epinephrine with the local anesthetic; in my opinion, it is rarely required and adds an undesirable element of risk. Digital blocks are preferred by some operators. However, in most situations, a local block suffices. The tourniquet may be essential for matrix visualization when surgery is done in this area. A wide Penrose drain should be used to avoid the constricting effect of a rubber band. Keeping in mind the vascular anatomy of the nail unit, simply pinch both digital arteries between the thumb and forefinger to limit bleeding to continue with the procedure. A 30-gauge needle is used to inject at the junction of the proximal and lateral nail fold (Fig. 5). If a cryogen such as ethyl chloride or fluoroethyl is sprayed

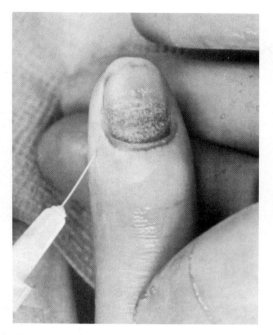

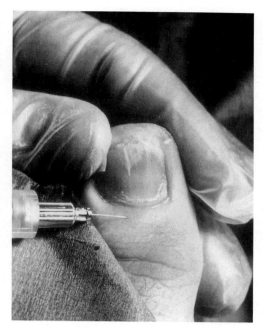

Figure 5   Injection of anesthetic at junction of lateral and proximal nail folds.

Figure 6   Injection of anesthetic at site of branch of lateral digital nerve in the proximal nail fold.

prior to injection, the pain is diminished. The injection proceeds distally and inferiorly to include the lateral digital nerve and its branches. The injection then goes across the proximal nail fold to block the transverse nerve branch at this site and then to the other side of the digit (Fig. 6). Place each subsequent injection into a previously anesthetized site. Finally, after anesthesia is complete, additional anesthetic may be injected into the tip of the digit, particularly for procedures on the distal portion of the nail unit. A sufficient quantity of anesthetic may cause moderate blanching, which aids in hemostasis.

If the patient has a history of peripheral vascular disease, is elderly, or has diabetes mellitus, vasospasm due to excess anesthetic must be avoided. To ensure painless nail surgery, a 3- to 5-min waiting period should precede the procedure.

NAIL AVULSION

As a therapeutic adjunct to various pathologic processes of the nail unit, it is often necessary to perform either chemical avulsion with 40% urea ointment or salicylic acid or surgical avulsion. Indications for surgical avulsion include the relief of pain from subungual hematoma after failure to evacuate a fresh hematoma by puncture aspiration. Acute bacterial infection as well as chronic mycotic disease are sometimes indications for nail avulsion. For long-standing onychomycosis of the toenails, removal of the nail may be combined with topical or systemic therapy. Toenail onychomycosis of short duration (less than 1 year) as well as fingernail onychomycosis usually do not require avulsion. Other indications for nail avulsion include anatomic abnormalities or excision of nail unit tumors.

The nail plate is attached to the digit at two locations: the nail bed on its inferior surface and the proximal nail fold on its superior surface. Therefore, the undersurface of the nail plate may

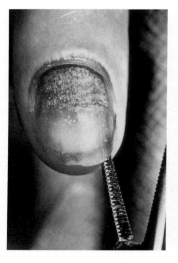

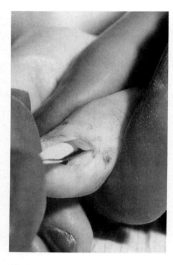

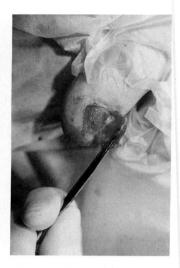

Figure 7 Separation of under-surface of nail palate from nail bed. (From Scher RK, *J Dermatol Surg Oncol* 1980;6:805, with permission.)

Figure 8 Separation of superior surface of nail plate from proximal nail fold.

Figure 9 Removal of nail plate with curving motion.

be separated with a nail spatula or mosquito clamp (Fig. 7). Then separate the superior surface of the nail plate from the proximal nail fold with the same instrument (Fig. 8). When using the mosquito clamp (Kelly), the serrated portion of the instrument should abut the nail plate surface rather than the soft tissue. A clamp is then applied to one side of the plate and, with a simple curving motion, it is easily peeled off (Fig. 9). Bleeding is minimal and the patient has little discomfort after the anesthetic has worn off (Fig. 10).

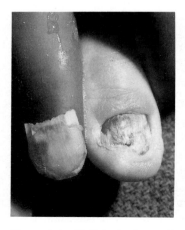

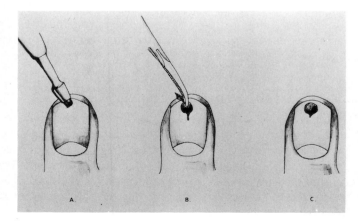

Figure 10 Nail bed after nail avulsion.

Figure 11 Diagram of nail punch bed biopsy.

PUNCH BIOPSY OF THE NAIL BED

Punch biopsy of the nail bed is the most commonly performed procedure on the nail unit. It should be done more frequently to provide accurate diagnoses and better treatment. Dermatologists should not be hesitant to perform a punch biopsy of the nail bed (Fig. 11). A 3- or 4-mm disposable punch is used to bore directly through the nail plate into the nail bed or hyponychium. Disposable punches are preferred because they are sharp, and nail plate penetration is less difficult. The nail plate may damage stainless steel punches that are used for other purposes. Biopsy of the matrix should be avoided to prevent the formation of a permanently dystrophic nail. If matrix tissue is required, an elliptical excision or longitudinal biopsy, which is then sutured, is preferable. The nail plate should not be removed because to do so may distort the histopathologic appearance. Often, the procedure will dislodge the nail plate, in which case both specimens should be examined by the dermatopathologist. When the punch reaches the underlying periosteum, it is withdrawn. A fine scissors, such as an iris or gradle, is then used to remove the specimen (Fig. 12). There generally is little bleeding since the anesthetic bolus tends to compress the arteries in the operative field.

After the specimen is removed (Fig. 13), Monsel's solution or 35% aluminum chloride in 50% isopropyl alcohol is applied to the site for hemostasis. Occasionally, absorbable gelatin sterile sponges, oxidized cellulose, or absorbable collagen may be required. Suturing is not necessary since the biopsy site granulates quickly without nail distortion. A small, temporary focus of onycholysis occasionally may result.

A periodic acid–Schiff (PAS) or Gomori methenamine silver stain is required on all nail biopsy specimens. In the presence of onychomycosis, there may be few fungal elements that can easily be missed if stained only with hematoxylin and eosin.

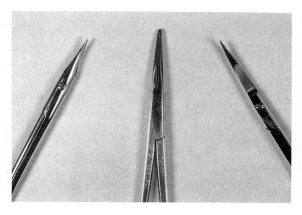

Figure 12 Left to right: iris scissors, Kelly clamp, gradle scissors.

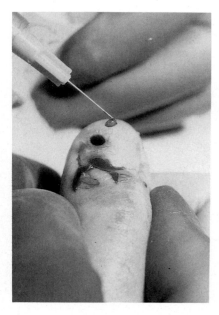

Figure 13 Punch biopsy specimen of the nail bed on needle tip.

For narrow (3 mm or less) longitudinal pigmented bands in the nail plate (melanonychia striata in longitudinum), a small punch biopsy from the matrix is acceptable. Be careful to avoid bisecting the matrix; a permanently split nail may result.

INGROWN TOENAIL

Ingrown toenail is a common affliction. Predisposing factors include (1) hyperhidrosis, a situation most commonly encountered in adolescents, (2) excess external pressure, due to poor stance and gait, ill-fitting shoes, trauma, (3), excess internal pressures from subungual growths, malformed phalanges, inflammatory processes, arthropathies, (4) associated systemic disease, e.g., geriatric nail changes (subungual hyperkeratosis, onychauxis), obesity, diabetes mellitus, and (5) incorrectly trimmed nails. Any one or combination of these factors produces one or more of the three features that characterize ingrown toenails: increased transverse overcurvature of the nail plate (Fig. 14), hypertrophy of the lateral nail wall (Fig. 15), perforation of the lateral nail groove epithelium with a spicule of nail plate (onychocryptosis) that results in a foreign body type reaction.

Prior to corrective surgery for ingrown toenails, simple techniques should be attempted. Removal of skin-piercing nail spicules may be curative. Placing cotton beneath the nail plate allows it to grow out straight. It is advisable to trim the nail plate straight across. Partial or complete avulsion alone may be used, but this may worsen pain when the digit abuts the regrowing nail plate. When conservative measures fail, one method that is successful is longitudinal resection of the lateral nail fold including the adjacent portion of the hyponychium, bed, and matrix. Many surgeons prefer to do this in two stages. The first includes removal of nail spicules with curettage followed by ablation of the hypertrophic granulation tissue from the nail folds (Fig. 16). About 1 month later, the more definitive resection of the lateral nail fold is done.

The nail unit is anesthetized and the nail plate partially avulsed. Two longitudinal incisions are made approximately 4 mm apart beginning distally at the hyponychium and proceeding proximally through the bed, proximal fold, and matrix. The wedge is removed with a fine scissors after the proximal nail fold is reflected to allow one to visualize the matrix. When the wedge is

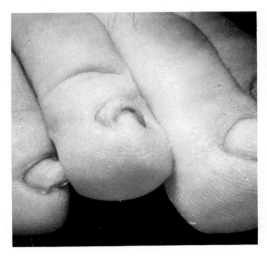

Figure 14 Ingrown toenail: transverse overcurvature of the nail plate.

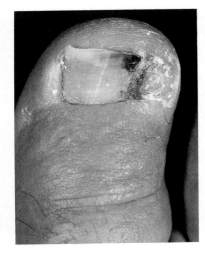

Figure 15 Ingrown toenail: hypertrophy of the lateral nail wall.

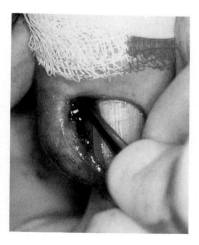

Figure 16 Curettage of lateral nail groove granulation tissue secondary to ingrown toenail.

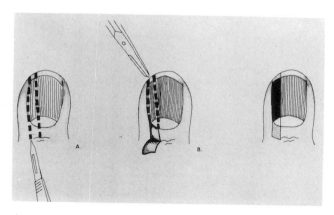

Figure 17 Diagram of longitudinal resection of the nail unit for recalcitrant ingrown toenail.

extricated, being certain to include the lateral horn of the matrix, the nail fold is returned to its original position. The defect is then permitted to heal by second intention. The end result is a cosmetically acceptable digit without ingrowth of the nail plate. It is narrower due to partial matrix removal.

Longitudinal resection in an elliptical fashion may be used to include any individual components of the nail unit for biopsy (Fig. 17). This technique is applicable for excision of small neoplasms in the nail bed itself (Fig. 18). After the specimen is removed, the defect is sutured (Fig. 19). Special care is taken to approximate the matrix to avoid a split nail (Fig. 20). 3–0 to 5–0 absorbable suture material is usually used in nail surgery.

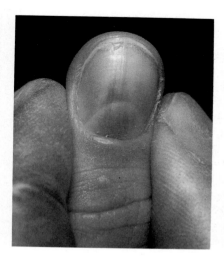

Figure 18 Glomus tumor of the nail bed prior to longitudinal resection.

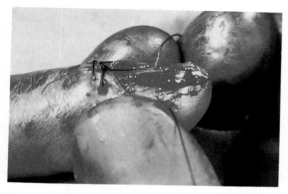

Figure 19 Suturing of nail bed after longitudinal resection.

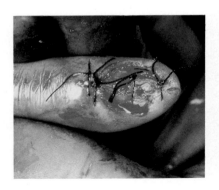

Figure 20 Approximated nail unit after longitudinal resection. (From Scher RK. *J Dermatol Surg Oncol* 1980;6: 805, with permission.)

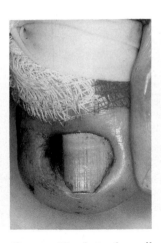

Figure 21 Lateral nail groove thoroughly cleansed and dried prior to phenolization.

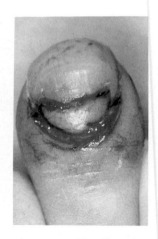

Figure 22 Crescent-shaped excision of cuticle-proximal nail fold for evaluation of connective tissue disease.

Phenol may also be used for permanent nail matrix destruction either to narrow the nail plate by partial phenolization or totally destroy the nail plate with total matrix cauterization. Application of phenol to the nail matrix is simple and may be used in preference to the longitudinal resection. After anesthesia and curettage of the lateral nail groove from hyponychium to proximal matrix, a wide tourniquet is applied to dry the wound base and matrix thoroughly (Fig. 21). A supersaturated solution of phenol is applied to the matrix including the lateral horn. Three 30-sec applications with a wisp of cotton on an applicator stick are all that is required. After the third application, the area is neutralized with alcohol and thoroughly cleansed before the dressing is applied.

PROXIMAL NAIL FOLD SURGERY

Crescent excision of the proximal nail fold and cuticle has been described for the study of patients with connective tissue disorders. This or a modified technique has been used as treatment for intractable chronic paronychia and focal mucinosis (myxoid cyst) of the proximal nail fold. The nail unit is anesthetized as previously described using 1% lidocaine without epinephrine in a local perionychial block fashion. No digital block or tourniquet is necessary. A crescent-shaped area of the cuticle–proximal nail fold is marked with skin marker. The crescent usually measures 10 × 4 mm. A mosquito hemostat is used to separate the undersurface of the proximal nail fold from the superior surface of the proximal nail plate (nail root). The serrated portion of the instrument must be against the nail plate and not the nail fold to avoid distortion of the specimen. A dental spatula or Freer elevator may also be used. When the nail fold crescent is separated, it is cut with a scalpel along the outline. Care must be taken not to penetrate the nail plate: this would risk matrix injury and possible permanent nail dystrophy. A dental spatula may be placed beneath the nail fold to prevent this. The excision is completed by removing the tissue with fine scissors and sending it for histologic study (Fig. 22). Monsel's or aluminum chloride solution suffices for hemostasis: if needed, hemostatic gauze may be applied. No sutures are required, and the excised area heals by second intention, giving an excellent cosmetic result.

When such connective tissue disease is present, histopathologic sections reveal the presence of amorphous eosinophilic globules in the cuticle–proximal nail fold area, visible with the PAS stain. Diffuse staining of the ground substance is also noted. Primary Raynaud's disease unassociated with systemic disorders may be differentiated from Raynaud's phenomenon secondary to a connective tissue syndrome, since the former has no deposits. Immunofluorescent studies may also be performed on a portion of the tissue.

DRESSINGS

It is difficult to keep dressings in place on the digits, but they are important. Various dressings are available that are specifically designed for digits, such as Surgitube. The dressing must not constrict the digit. Adhesive tape should not be applied completely around the digit. This may result in vasoconstriction and compromise of the blood supply with edema. The adhesive is placed in a longitudinal direction rather than transversely. If unusual pain, edema, throbbing, or bluish discoloration is noted, the dressing should be removed at once and the surgeon contacted immediately. A thick and bulbous dressing will absorb external trauma and reduce excessive movement. The use of prophylactic oral antibiotics following nail surgery is the subject of controversy and should be decided on a case-by-case basis.

ACKNOWLEDGMENTS

Portions of this chapter have been reproduced with permission from the author's contributions to Epstein E, Epstein E, Jr, eds. *Techniques in Skin Surgery*. Philadelphia, Lea & Febiger, 1979; Demis DJ, ed. *Clinical Dermatology*. New York, Harper & Row, 1985; Callen JP, Dahl MV, Golitz LE, Rasmussen JE, Stegman SJ, eds. *Advances in Dermatology*, Vol. 1. Chicago, Year Book Medical Publishers, 1986.

BIBLIOGRAPHY

Achten G. Histopathology of the nail. In *The Nail*. M Pierre, ed. Edinburgh, Churchill Livingstone, 1981, p. 1.

Baran R, Bureau H. Surgical treatment of recalcitrant chronic paronychias of the fingers. *J Dermatol Surg Oncol* 1981;7:106–107.

Boll OF. Surgical correction of ingrowing nails. *J Am Podiatr Assoc* 1945;35:8–9.

Cornelius C, Shelley WB. Pincer nail syndrome. *Arch Surg* 1968;96:321.

Crandon JH. Lesser infections of the hand. In *Hand Surgery*. 3rd ed. JE Flynn,ed. Baltimore, Williams & Wilkins, 1982, p. 676.

Farber EM, South DA. Urea ointment in nonsurgical avulsion of nail dystrophies. *Cutis* 1978;22:689.

Fosnaugh RP. Surgery of the nail. In *Skin Surgery*. Vol. 2. 5th ed. E Epstein, E Epstein, Jr., eds. Springfield, IL Charles C Thomas, 1982, pp. 981–1007.

Lloyd-Davies RW, Brill GC. The management etiology and outpatient of ingrowing toenails. *Br J Surg* 1963;50:592–597.

Maricq HR. Nailfold biopsy in scleroderma and related disorders. *Dermatologica* 1984;168:73–77.

Norton LA. Disorders of the nails. In *Dermatology*. 2nd ed. SL Moschella, HJ Hurley, eds. Philadelphia, WB Saunders, 1985, pp. 1415–1417.

Runne U. Nail surgery: Indications and contraindications (translation). *Z. Hautkr* 1982;58:324–332.

Salasche SJ. Myxoid cysts of the proximal nail fold: A surgical approach. *J Dermatol Surg Oncol* 1984; 10:35–39.

Samman, PD, Fenton DA. *The Nails in Disease*. 4th ed. London, Heinemann Medical Books, 1986.

Scher RK. Biopsy of the matrix of a nail. *J Dermatol Surg Oncol* 1980;6:19–21.

Scher RK. Longitudinal resection of nails for purposes of biopsy and treatment. *J Dermatol Surg Oncol* 1980;6:805–807.

Scher RK. Nail surgery. In *Advances in Dermatology*. Vol 1. JP Callen, MV Dahl, LE Golitze, JE Rasmussen, SG Stegman, eds. Chicago, Year Book Medical Publishers, 1986, pp. 191–209.

Scher RK. Nail surgery. *J Dermatol Surg Oncol* 1992;18:665–758.

Scher RK. Nail surgery. In *Techniques in Skin Surgery*. E Epstein, E Epstein, Jr, eds. Philadelphia, Lea & Febiger, 1979, p. 164.

Scher RK. Punch biopsies of nails: A simple, valuable procedure. *J Dermatol Surg Oncol* 1978;4:528.

Scher RK, Ackerman AB. The value of nail biopsy for demonstrating fungi not demonstrable by microbiologic techniques. *Am J Dermatopathol* 1980;2:55–57.

Scher RK, Daniel CR III. Surgery of the nails. In *Clinical Dermatology*. Vol. 1. Section 3–15. DG Demis, J McGuire, eds. New York: Harper & Row, 1985;1, pp.1–10.

Scher RK, Daniel CR, III. *Nails: Therapy, Diagnosis, Surgery*. Philadelphia, W. B. Saunders, 1990.

Scher RK, Tom DWK, Lally EV, et al. The clinical significance of periodic acid-Schiff positive deposits in cuticle-proximal nail fold biopsy specimens. *Arch Dermatol* 1985;121:1406–1409.

Schnitzler L, Baran R, Civatte J, et al. Biopsy of the proximal nail fold in collagen diseases. *J Dermatol Surg Oncol* 1976;2:313–315.

Siegle RL, Harkness J, Swanson NA. Phenol alcohol technique for permanent matricectomy. *Arch Dermatol* 1984;120:348–350.

Thompson RP, Harper PE, Matze JC, et al. Nail fold biopsy in scleroderma and related disorders: Correlation of histologic capillaroscopic and clinical data. *Arthritis Rheum* 1984;27:97–103.

Zaias N. The longitudinal nail biopsy. *J Invest Dermatol* 1967;49:406–408.

Zaias N. *The Nail in Health and Disease*. 2nd ed. Connecticut, Appleton and Lange, 1990.

25

The Hand

John Louis Ratz
*Tulane University, Louisiana State University,
and The Ochsner Clinic, New Orleans, Louisiana*

Jefferson J. Kaye
The Ochsner Clinic, New Orleans, Louisiana

Randall J. Yetman
Cleveland Clinic, Cleveland, Ohio

The hand is a unique structure on which dermatologic surgeons often work. Intricate in design and function, its use is vital in our daily lives. Its importance cannot be overstated, and, because of this, any anticipated surgical procedure in this area should be carefully considered with regard to underlying anatomy, innervation, circulation, function, and cosmesis.

A reasonable approach to skin surgery of the hand is discussed here, but it is beyond the scope of the dermatologic surgeon to perform extensive excisional and reconstructive procedures; these are more appropriately left to the hand surgeon. Discussion will be limited here to procedures done with the scalpel. Cryosurgery, electrosurgery, and laser surgery, as they apply to the hand, are discussed in other chapters.

ANATOMY

The anatomy of the hand is complex. Full details of its anatomy are described in appropriate texts on the subject. However, it is not possible to discuss surgery of the hand without understanding some of its important anatomic landmarks.

Surface Anatomy

The surface anatomy of the hand is relatively simple (Fig. 1). There is a dorsal and ventral surface and a radial and ulnar aspect. The five digits are named or numbered, and the fingers are subdivided into distal, middle, and proximal phalanges. Common creases are all named. The volar muscular eminences, which are present proximally, are the thenar radially and hypothenar on the ulnar aspect.

From a surgical standpoint, the anatomy of the dorsal surface of the hand is unique because many of the large veins are superficial due to the relative paucity of subcutaneous fat (Fig. 2). Care should be taken to avoid transecting these vessels during surgery. Punch biopsies can be

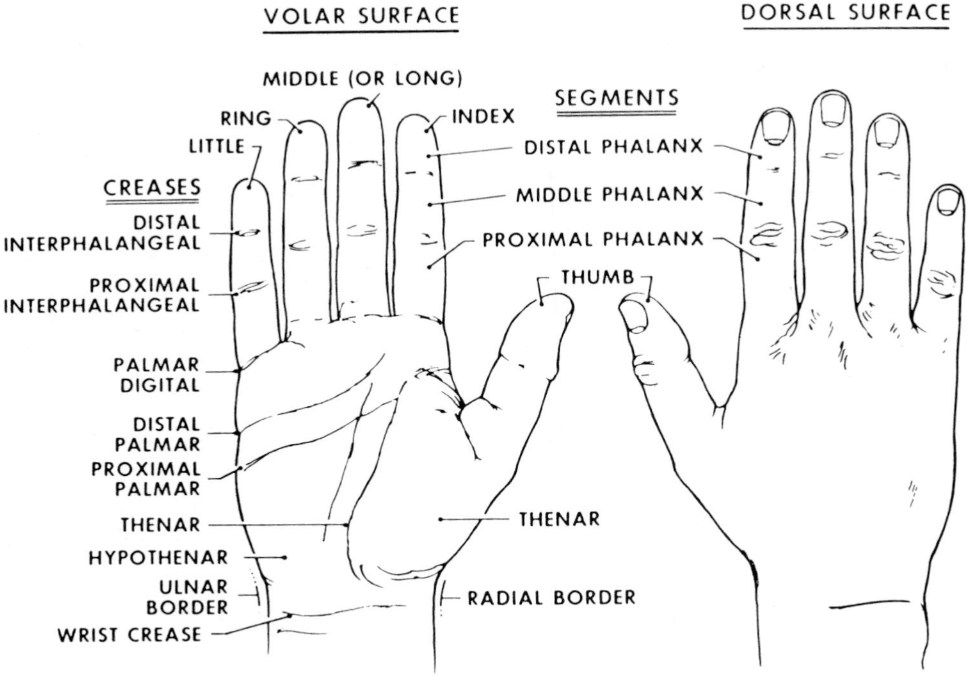

VOLAR SURFACE   DORSAL SURFACE

MIDDLE (OR LONG)

RING   INDEX   SEGMENTS

LITTLE   DISTAL PHALANX

CREASES   MIDDLE PHALANX

DISTAL
INTERPHALANGEAL   PROXIMAL PHALANX

PROXIMAL
INTERPHALANGEAL   THUMB

PALMAR
DIGITAL

DISTAL
PALMAR
PROXIMAL
PALMAR

THENAR   THENAR

HYPOTHENAR

ULNAR
BORDER   RADIAL BORDER

WRIST CREASE

Figure 1   Surface anatomy of the hand.

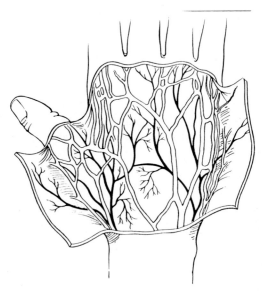

Figure 2   There is very little subcutaneous fat underlying the skin of the dorsal surface of the hand. Large veins in this area are superficial and subject to possible trauma during surgery.

safely performed in this area by applying pressure only until the instrument has penetrated the skin. Without further downward pressure, a continuous clockwise rotation of the punch will draw up the subcutaneous tissue and minimize the risk of injury to underlying vessels.

Deeper Anatomy

The skeleton of the hand consists of three phalanges for each finger, with the exception of the thumb, which has two. The phalanges are attached to the metacarpals, which, in turn, are attached to the system of carpal bones, each of which is named (Fig. 3). The intrinsic muscles of the hand are the lumbricals and interossei, all of which have their origins and insertions on the skeletal structures of the hand itself (Fig. 4). However, the majority of hand movement is due to muscles in the forearm, and their attachments to the hand are complex. This elaborate system of flexor and extensor tendons and tendon sheaths is demonstrated in Figures 5–7. Further details are available from texts on the subject.

The blood supply of the hand is derived from a superficial and deep palmar arch system that arises jointly from the radial and ulnar arteries (Fig. 8). The digital and interosseous arteries arise from the arch system and form a collateral network about each digit. Patency of both ulnar and radial arteries should be established prior to any surgery to avoid vascular compromise. At no time during surgery on the hand should any vessel be ligated. It is also important that arteries not be entered during administration of local or digital anesthesia. Knowledge of the anatomy for this purpose is important. The syringe plunger should be withdrawn prior to injection of digital anesthesia to ensure that a vessel has not been entered.

It is reasonable to assess motor and sensory status prior to surgery and note any deficits so they cannot be attributed to the procedure. Motor function of most intrinsic muscles of the hand,

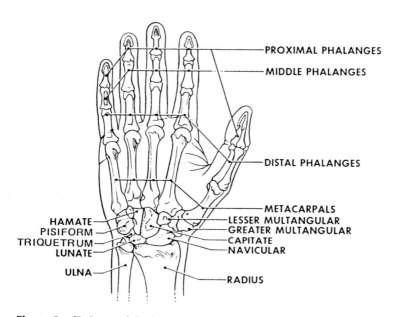

Figure 3 Skeleton of the hand.

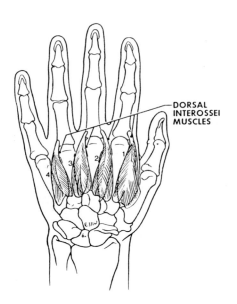

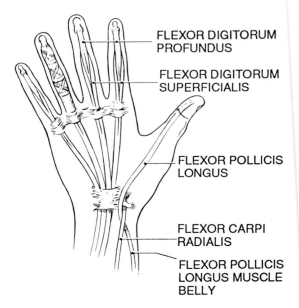

Figure 4 Dorsal interossei: all intrinsic muscles of the hand have their origins and insertions on the skeletal structures of the hand itself.

Figure 5 Deep flexor tendon and tendon sheath structures.

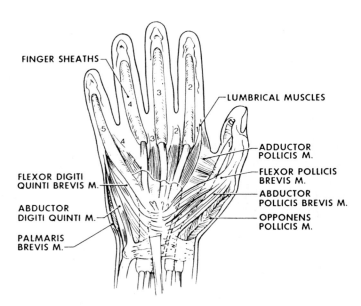

Figure 6 Superficial flexor tendon and tendon sheath structures.

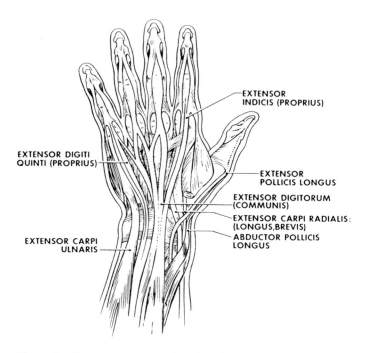

Figure 7 Extensor tendon and tendon sheath structures.

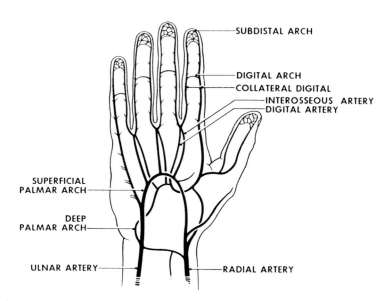

Figure 8 The blood supply of the hand arises jointly from the radial and ulnar arteries through a complex double arch system. The deep arch generally is supplied mostly by the dorsal branch of the radial artery crossing over the radial side of the base of the thumb. The digital and collateral systems, in turn, arise from the superficial and deep palmar arches.

as well as several of the flexors, is supplied by the ulnar nerve (Fig. 9). The remainder of the intrinsic musculature and flexors receive their innervation from the median nerve (Fig. 10), while all of the extensors are supplied by the radial nerve (Fig. 11). Note that the radial nerve supplies none of the intrinsic musculature of the hand.

Sensory innervation is supplied by a combination of the ulnar, median, and radial nerves (Fig. 12). The radial nerve generally supplies the radial aspect of the dorsal two-thirds of the hand but notably not the distal aspects of the index, middle, or ring fingers. The ulnar third of the dorsal surface is supplied by the ulnar nerve, with the exception of the distal ring and little fingers. The ulnar nerve also supplies the palmar third to the hand on the ulnar aspect. The median nerve is responsible for the remainder of the sensation, most of which is on the palmar aspect of the hand. Knowledge of sensory innervation is important, particularly when regional or digital anesthesia is being considered.

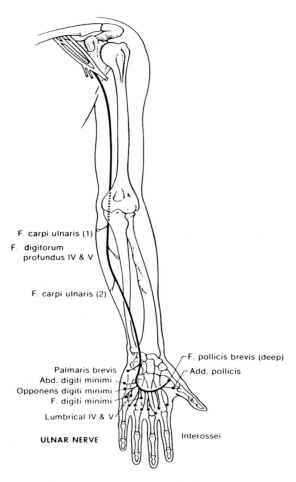

Figure 9   Muscles supplied by the ulnar nerve.

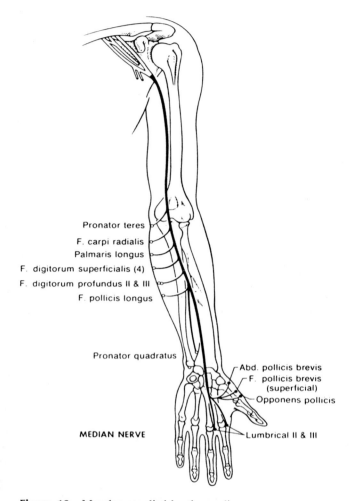

Pronator teres

F. carpi radialis

Palmaris longus

F. digitorum superficialis (4)

F. digitorum profundus II & III

F. pollicis longus

Pronator quadratus

Abd. pollicis brevis

F. pollicis brevis (superficial)

Opponens pollicis

MEDIAN NERVE

Lumbrical II & III

Figure 10   Muscles supplied by the median nerve.

Lines of Tension

An understanding of the skin tension lines is important when one is planning incisions. Naturally occurring tension in the skin of the hand, as well as other parts of the body, is due to elastic fibers in the dermis. These elastic fiber bundles are arranged along "lines of tension." These lines of tension were first noted by Dupuytren in describing wounds of the skin made by penetrating instruments. He noted that when round instruments were used to puncture the skin, the wounds became linear. Langer found that when round incisions of the skin were made, there was a tendency for these wounds to extend along lines of tension. He considered the skin to be less extensible in the direction of the lines of tension than across them.

Experience has shown that incisions heal better when they are made parallel to these naturally occurring skin tension lines. These lines of minimal tension are often at right angles to the

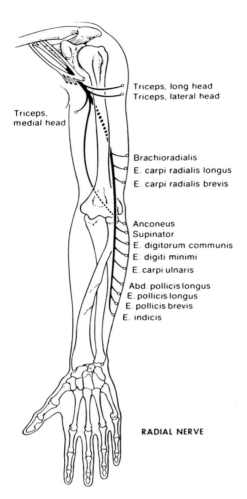

Triceps, long head
Triceps, lateral head

Triceps,
medial head

Brachioradialis
E. carpi radialis longus
E. carpi radialis brevis

Anconeus
Supinator
E. digitorum communis
E. digiti minimi
E. carpi ulnaris

Abd. pollicis longus
E. pollicis longus
E. pollicis brevis
E. indicis

RADIAL NERVE

Figure 11 Muscles supplied by the radial nerve. Note that no intrinsic muscles are innervated by the radial nerve.

long axis of the underlying muscles. An incision parallel to these lines is not subject to the same tension from underlying musculature.

On the hand these lines of skin tension (Fig. 13) result from the movement of the flexor and extensor muscles. Since flexion and extension take place perpendicular to these tension lines, there is a redundancy of skin parallel to these lines that allows motion to occur. Therefore, skin can be excised parallel to these lines without unduly increasing the amount of tension when the wound is closed.

PLANNING THE PROCEDURE

It is essential to plan the incision carefully. The direction of an elective incision should always be chosen in relation to the lines of minimal tension. A marking pencil is a helpful guide. There are significant differences in the character of the skin between the dorsal and palmar surfaces

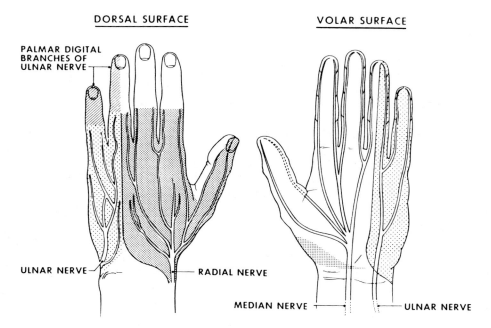

DORSAL SURFACE   VOLAR SURFACE

PALMAR DIGITAL BRANCHES OF ULNAR NERVE

ULNAR NERVE — RADIAL NERVE

MEDIAN NERVE — ULNAR NERVE

Figure 12 Common pattern of sensory innervation of the hand.

of the hand. Incisions perpendicular to the skin tension lines on the palmar surface of the hand are tolerated much less well than those on the dorsal surface. Scar contracture and functional impairment are common when incisions are made perpendicular to the crease lines on the palmar surface. Incisions must not cross the flexion creases in a perpendicular fashion. Incisions parallel to crease lines are perpendicular to underlying nervous and vascular structures; therefore, care must be taken to avoid injuring these structures.

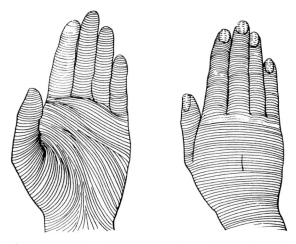

Figure 13 Lines of minimal tension on the hand, as elsewhere, are related to the underlying musculature of its movements.

ANESTHESIA

Detailed knowledge of the anatomy of the hand is essential if one is to administer direct nerve blocks appropriately for anesthesia. Wrist blocks are commonly used to produce anesthesia. These blocks are simple to perform and provide 20–30 min of anesthesia.

The median nerve can be blocked at the wrist (Fig. 14), where it lies between the palmaris longus and flexor carpi radialis tendons. Occasionally, the palmaris longus is congenitally absent. A 25-gauge needle is inserted between the two tendons until very light paresthesias are encountered. At that point approximately 5 ml local anesthetic without epinephrine is injected.

In a similar fashion, the ulnar nerve can be blocked at the wrist where it lies just radial to the flexor carpi ulnaris tendon. A 25-gauge needle is inserted just radial to the flexor carpi ulnaris tendon at the level of the proximal wrist crease (Fig. 15). When very light paresthesias are elicited, 5 ml local anesthesia without epinephrine is injected.

For anesthesia of one finger only, it is best to use a digital block. The dorsal approach is the preferred method since it is less painful than the palmar approach. This allows block of the dorsal nerves. A 25-gauge needle is inserted just proximal to the web space. A skin wheal is made, and approximately 1 ml anesthetic solution is injected. The needle is advanced in a palmar direction, and another 1 ml local anesthetic is injected. This is repeated in the other web space. Avoid using more than 3 ml on each side to prevent a circumferential pressure increase at the base of the finger, which may result in vascular compromise.

HEMOSTASIS

The hand has a richly endowed vascular supply, and appropriate hemostasis is often important. However, the use of the epinephrine as a hemostatic agent should be avoided. Accidental or inadvertent injection of epinephrine into the arterial circulation could have disastrous results and lead to ischemic necrosis of the digit. A bloodless field is the best means of minimizing potential injury to underlying structures. This can be achieved with the use of a tourniquet. When operating on an individual finger, several methods can be used to obtain hemostasis. The use of a Penrose drain to exsanguinate the finger, in addition to use of the drain as a tourniquet at the base of the finger, allows one to make incisions safely and efficiently (Fig. 16). Use the minimum pressure needed to achieve hemostasis.

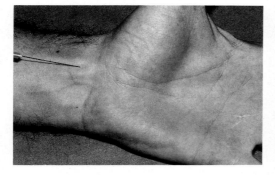

Figure 14 The median nerve block. The nerve can best be approached at the wrist, where it lies between the palmaris longus and flexor carpi radialis tendons.

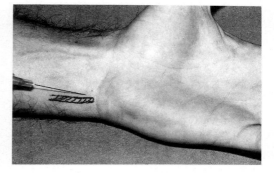

Figure 15 The ulnar nerve can be blocked at the wrist where it lies radial to the flexor carpi ulnaris tendon.

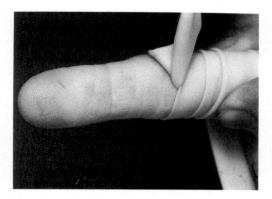

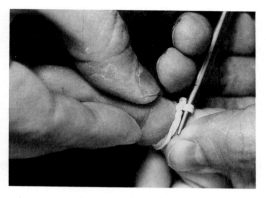

Figure 16 Penrose drain tourniquet: a small Penrose drain is wound tightly around the finger distally to proximally. The drain is unwound beginning at the distal end.

Figure 17 Rubber band tourniquet: a rubber band is looped over the base of the finger and doubled or tripled. A hemostat is placed between the loops and wound to provide the desired minimal tension required.

Alternatively, hemostasis of the digit can be achieved by using a rubber band tourniquet at the base of the finger. The rubber band can be looped several times and then tightened further by placing the tip of a hemostat under one of the loops and winding the hemostat. Applying pressure distally to proximally (milking the finger) to create a blanche removes blood that will not return until the tourniquet is released (Fig. 17).

A third method of hemostasis is to fit the patient with a sterile surgical glove in which a small incision is made at the tip of the finger that will be operated on. That portion of the glove can then be rolled down to the base of the finger. This both milks out the blood and provides tourniquet action in one simple maneuver (Fig. 18).

When operating on the palm or dorsum of the hand, a proximal forearm tourniquet is usually necessary. Hemostasis with this tourniquet can be maintained for 25–30 min. Beyond this

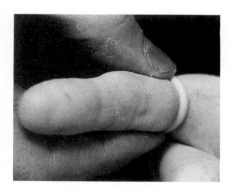

Figure 18 Glove tourniquet: a sterile glove is placed on the hand and a hole cut in the tip of the finger. The glove finger can be rolled proximally to the base of the digit. Sterility of the entire field can be easily maintained.

the tourniquet causes significant pain. A general guideline is 100 mm Torr above systolic pressure.

Should bleeding occur during the surgical procedure, electrocautery or chemical cautery can be used. This is most effectively accomplished with a bipolar electrocautery device. Under no circumstance should hemostasis be achieved with ligature. This could result in ischemic necrosis.

WOUND CLOSURE

Once an excision is completed, there are various methods of wound closure. Most skin incisions or small excisions can be closed by direct approximation using fine suture material. The use of subcutaneous sutures is generally not necessary on the hand. Wounds should be repaired with fine nonabsorbable suture material, such as 5-0 nylon, using a simple everting technique. In general the sutures are removed on the seventh postoperative day.

If the wound is not amenable to direct suture approximation, a free skin graft is the method of choice in most situations. When replacing skin on the palmar surface of the hand, it is important to use tissue of similar histologic architecture. It is also important to use a full-thickness graft to maximize the return of sensation to this area.

A convenient source of tissue on the palmar surface is the hypothenar eminence (Figs. 19,20). Small defects can be easily replaced with a full-thickness graft from this area. Once the skin graft has been obtained, it is important to remove all subcutaneous tissue to maximize revascularization. Five days of splinting will help revascularization.

In general, use glabrous skin to replace glabrous palmar hand or foot skin, especially in dark-skinned individuals. If the skin is used on the palmar aspect of the hand, significant hyperpigmentation of the graft may result (Fig. 21).

When repairing defects on the dorsum of the hand, either split-thickness or full-thickness grafts can be used. For small defects, full-thickness grafts taken from the antecubital fossa work well but can leave cosmetic defects in that area. For larger defects, a split-thickness skin graft harvested from the groin will cover these wounds. Once the graft is in place with interrupted sutures, the dressing is applied. This is particularly important. Compression must be applied by the dressing in order to prevent fluid accumulation between the graft and its underlying bed. A bolus or tie-over dressing is recommended. As long as there is no drainage or sign of infection, the dressing is left undisturbed for approximately 1 week.

If, after the excisional part of the procedure is completed, bone, blood vessel, or tendon is exposed, a skin graft is not adequate coverage. A variety of local or regional flaps can be used to achieve coverage for these situations. The V-Y advancement or island pedicle (kite) flap can be used for a number of small defects on both the palmar and dorsal aspects of the hand. These flaps are simple to develop and quite reliable (Figs. 22,23). In addition, skin retains its normal sensation.

After wound closure has been achieved, immobilization of the hand is important. The dressing should apply uniform pressure to the entire hand. It should be snug enough to control capillary oozing, but not restrict venous return. Web spaced should be separated to prevent maceration of these areas. A palmar plaster splint may be used to immobilize the hand.

In general the hand is immobilized in the positions of function. The wrist should be moderate dorsiflexion (30–45 degrees). The metacarpophalangeal joints should be flexed 70–80 degrees. The interphalangeal joints are only slightly flexed (10 degrees or less). In this position the collateral ligaments are at almost maximal extension. This will prevent contracture of these important ligaments and subsequent joint stiffness.

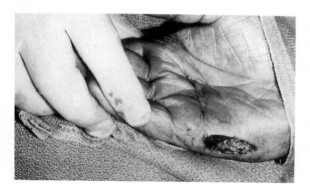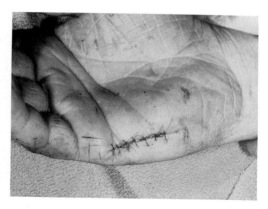

Figure 19,20 The hypothenar eminence is a convenient source of full-thickness skin graft replacement for other locations on the palmar surface of the hand. Generally the donor site can be closed primarily with little or no difficulty.

COMPLICATIONS

Skin surgery of the hand has attendant risks. Several postoperative complications are possible. The risk of postoperative infection and wound dehiscence is no greater than for any other cutaneous site. However, because of its anatomy and because of the proximity of vascular and nervous elements, several complications more unique to the hand may be encountered.

Ischemia and ischemic necrosis have already been mentioned. These can result from the use of epinephrine as a hemostatic agent, ligation of a functional component of the arterial system, or inadvertent compression of an artery through deep closure, which may have encompassed the vessel. This can be avoided by not using epinephrine and ligature during surgery. Evaluation of the entire hand postoperatively to ensure vascular competence is mandatory.

Decreased or altered mobility is a possible complication of cutaneous hand surgery and can have many causes. The alteration or decrease in mobility may be due to damage to muscle, tendon, or tendon sheath structures. Such damage may be repaired but should only be attempted

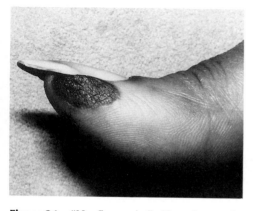

Figure 21 "Nonfingerprint" skin, when used as donor tissue for palmar surface defects, should be avoided, particularly in black individuals. Significant hyperpigmentation of the graft can occur, leaving an unacceptable cosmetic result.

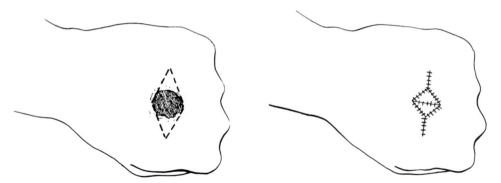

Figure 22,23 The V-Y advancement or island pedicle (kite) flap is useful in repairing small defects on both the palmar and dorsal aspects of the hand. This is a simple procedure to perform, has a high degree of success, and allows for normal sensation in the area postoperatively.

by a qualified hand surgeon. Damage to a motor nerve can also cause decreased mobility but may be a more difficult situation to remedy, and evaluation by a hand surgeon is suggested. Mobility can be decreased by edema or hemorrhage. These should be relatively easy to detect and appropriate measures undertaken to remedy them. If hemorrhage is the problem, care should be taken when achieving hemostasis to avoid compromising the blood supply to any area of the hand.

Decreased sensation immediately following surgery may be transient and should be evaluated several days after the procedure. Proper evaluation of decreased sensation can only be done if sensation was evaluated preoperatively. Any sensory deficit present prior to surgery is not likely to have been altered by the surgical procedure. Sensory deficits present several days after the procedure are most likely due to nerve damage and may be irreversible. Digital nerves are approximately 1 mm beneath the skin surfaces at flexion creases of the fingers and are very easily injured during skin closures and surgical procedures unless extreme care is used during the entire surgical procedure.

Because of the flexibility and mobility of the hand, delayed healing is likely, particularly if the procedure is performed over the extensor aspect of a flexing joint. The usual cause of delayed healing is increased mobility and can be remedied by appropriate immobilization measures. Careful preoperative planning is important to avoid tension on lines of closure.

SURGICALLY AMENABLE CONDITIONS SPECIFIC TO THE HAND

Although numerous cutaneous entities can occur on the hand, few are truly peculiar to this location. Common lesions such as nevi and epidermal cysts are not particularly common on the hand, but when they do occur, they are more likely to be present dorsally rather than on the palmar aspect. Removal of such lesions is generally uncomplicated, and the principles established in this chapter should be followed.

Verruca vulgaris is common on the hand. Its treatment, however, is usually topical, cryosurgical, electrosurgical, or with the use of a laser, and rarely by excisional surgery. Excision of a small wart should follow the parameters already mentioned.

Actinic keratoses, like warts, are common on the hands, and their treatment is usually by other modalities. Squamous cell carcinoma, however, is best removed as an intact specimen so that surgical margins can be evaluated histologically. Mohs micrographic surgery should be considered. Whether excision is done conventionally or by the Mohs technique, the size, location, and orientation of the tumor will dictate the lines of closure. Because complete histologic tumor-free margins are important, it may be difficult to adhere to rules regarding tension lines. Difficult wounds may result, leading to complicated closure or repair techniques.

Vascular lesions such as glomus tumor and pyogenic granuloma can occur on the hand. All vascular extensions must be removed to avoid recurrence. Occurrence of such lesions subungually or in the nail fold entail special considerations, which are discussed in another chapter.

Of all cutaneous lesions, the most specific to the hand are the ganglion and cutaneous myxoma or mucinous cyst. Although these lesions can occur in other locations, they are most common on the hand and often are attached to deeper structures, which complicates their effective removal. Failure to remove these lesions completely will often result in a recurrence.

A mucous cyst is a small lesion located on or about the distal interphalangeal joint of the finger. It often causes a groove in the adjacent fingernail due to pressure on the nail matrix (Fig. 24). Osteoarthritis in the joint is associated with these cysts. These osteophytes should be excised with the cyst (Fig. 25). If they are not removed with the cyst, recurrence of the cyst is likely.

A slightly curved incision is used (Fig. 26). The cyst is dissected down to its origin on the joint capsule and excised with the joint capsule. The accompanying osteophytes can be removed with fine rongeur. Care must be taken to not injure the extensor mechanism. Skin closure often requires a rotation flap or a full-thickness skin graft (Fig. 27).

Although wrist ganglia appear to be quite superfacial, they usually have extensions down to the deeper ligament of the wrist. Simple incision of ganglia is discouraged because there is a high recurrence rate with this procedure. The cyst must be dissected down to its origin on the wrist scapholunate ligament (Fig. 28). Since an arthrotomy is required to excise these ganglia of the wrist properly, this type of surgery should be done by someone with experience in hand sur-

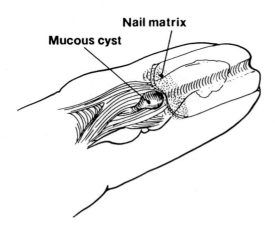

Figure 24 A mucous cyst can cause grooving of the fingernail because of direct pressure on the nail matrix.

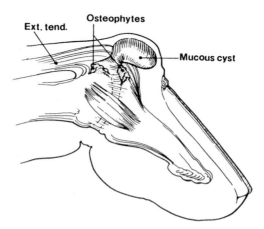

Figure 25 Osteophytes, which commonly accompany mucous cysts, must be excised during the procedure to minimize chances for recurrence.

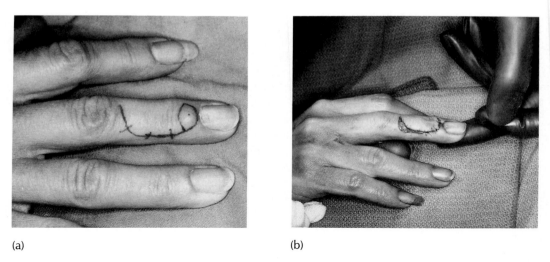

(a)   (b)

Figure 26 (a) A slightly curved incision is a reasonable approach to the mucous cyst. (b) Such an incision can usually be closed by means of a rotation flap. Alternatively, a full-thickness skin graft can be used.

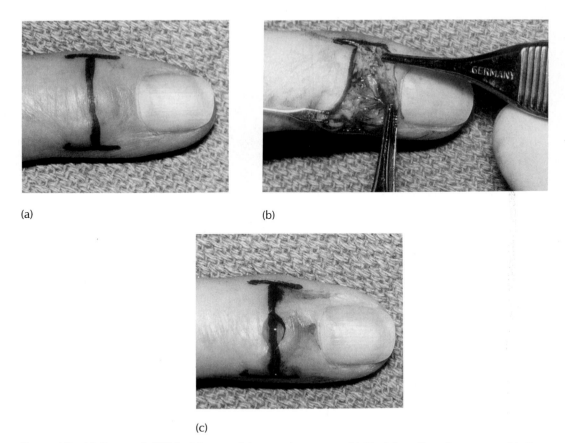

(a)   (b)

(c)

Figure 27 (a) Proposed "H"-incision overlying mucinous cyst. (b) Excision of mucinous cyst. (c) Cyst removal (H-incision) just before closure.

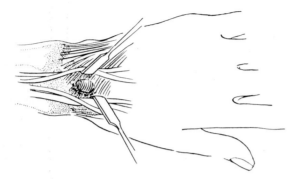

Figure 28 A dorsal wrist ganglion generally has its deepest attachments at its origin on the scapholunate interosseous ligament. An anthrotomy may be required for complete removal.

gery. Alternatively, wrist arthroscopy may be used to excise the ganglion yet minimize the size of the scar.

BIBLIOGRAPHY

Angelides AC, Wallace PF. The dorsal ganglion of the wrist. Its pathogenesis, gross and microscopic anatomy and surgical treatment. *J Hand Surg* 1976;1:228.

Bauer BS, Vicari FA, Richard ME, Schwed R. Expanded full-thickness skin grafts in children: case selection, planning, and management. *Plast Reconstr Surg* 1993;92(1):59–69.

Bean DJ, Rees RS, O'Leary JP, Lynch JB. Carcinoma of the hand: A 20-year experience. *South Med J* 1984;77(8):998–1000.

Beasley RW. Local flaps for surgery of the hand. *Orthop Clin North Am* 1970;1:219.

Boyes JH. Incisions in the hand. *Am J Orthop* 1962;4:308.

Eaton RG, Dobranski AI, Littler JW. Marginal osteophyte excision in treatment of mucous cysts. *J Bone Joint Surg* 1973;55A:570.

Heim U et al. Subungual glomus tumors. Value of the direct dorsal approach. *Ann Chir Main* 1985;4(1):51–54.

Hutton K, Podolsky A, Roenigk RK, Wood MB. Regional anesthesia of the hand for dermatologic surgery. J Derm Surg Oncol 1991;17:881–888.

Langer K. Zur anatomic and physiologic der hant. Z Die Spanning der Cutis SB Akad. Wiss, Wien 1862;45:133.

LeWinn LR (guest ed.). Perspectives in hand surgery. *Clin Plast Surg* 1986;13(2).

Micks JE, Wilson JN. Full-thickness sole skin grafts for resurfacing the hand. *J Bone Joint Surg* 1967;49A:1128.

Miller PK, Roenigk, RK, Amadio PC. Focal muscinosis (myxoid cyst) surgical therapy. J Derm Surg Oncol 1991;18:716–719.

Reigstad A, Hetland KR, Bye K, Rokkum M. Free flaps in the reconstruction of hand and distal forearm injuries. *J Hand Surg (Br)* 1992;17(2):185–188.

Robotti EB, Edstrom LE. Split-thickness plantar skin grafts for coverage in the hand and digits. *J Hand Surg (Am)* 1992;17(1):182.

Salasche SJ. Myxoid cysts of the proximal nail fold: A surgical approach. *J Dermatol Surg Oncol* 1984;10(1):35–39.

Salem MZA. Simple finger tourniquet. *Br Med J* 1973;1:779.

26

Epidermal Tumors

Glenn Kolansky and Duane C. Whitaker
University of Iowa Hospitals and Clinics, Iowa City, Iowa

Barry Leshin
*Bowman Gray School of Medicine, Wake Forest University,
Winston-Salem, North Carolina*

There is a wide clinicopathologic spectrum of epidermal tumors. Some, such as seborrheic keratoses, have a characteristic appearance that can be easily recognized. Others, such as the dermatitic appearance of extramammary Paget disease, can be more difficult. There is also great histologic variability expressed by these epidermal growths. The keratin-filled sac of an epidermoid cyst is diagnosed at low power with a rapid glance. However, the proliferation of atypical keratinizing squamous epithelium can make differentiation of a keratoacanthoma from a squamous cell carcinoma more subtle.

The biologic spectrum of epidermal tumors is also vast. The explosive onset of inflammatory seborrheic keratoses, or the sign of Leser-Trélat, may signal the presence of an occult malignancy. Bowen's disease of the penis is a potentially invasive, life-threatening squamous cell carcinoma. Extramammary Paget disease may be a cutaneous marker of underlying carcinoma.

Just as the clinical, histologic, and biologic nature of epidermal tumors varies, treatment options for these tumors are similarly varied. Simple electrodesiccation and curettage or cryosurgery may be sufficient in many cases, while wide excision and work-up for internal disease may be indicated for others.

SEBORRHEIC KERATOSIS

Seborrheic keratosis are benign epidermal tumors that occur on the skin of middle-aged and older individuals. Clinically the lesions appear as one or more exophytic light brown to brown-black plaques with slightly raised and sharply demarcated borders. They are verrucous papules with a characteristic "stuck-on" appearance with dirty, friable scale. Close inspection may show keratotic follicular plugging of the surface (Fig. 1). A variant termed dermatosis papulosa nigra is frequently seen in blacks and Asians. These lesions consist of multiple small, heavily pigmented papules that usually develop on the face, especially on the upper cheeks and orbital areas, usually arising in adolescence. They are primarily of cosmetic importance and are asymp-

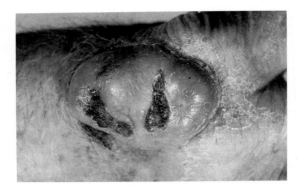

Figure 1 Seborrheic keratosis on back.

tomatic unless the lesions are irritated. Malignant melanoma, basal cell carcinoma, and squamous cell carcinomas have been reported to arise within a seborrheic keratosis. In a prospective study of 4310 tumors clinically diagnosed as seborrheic keratosis, 60 (1.4%) proved to be squamous carcinoma in situ. The majority of these were on sun-exposed areas of the head and neck.

Occasionally, a deeply pigmented seborrheic keratosis is clinically indistinguishable from malignant melanoma. This warrants removal by excisional biopsy. The sudden eruptive appearance of multiple seborrheic keratosis, known as the sign of Leser-Trélat, may suggest an internal malignancy. Traditionally, the sign of Leser-Trélat is associated with adenocarcinomas of the stomach. However, hematopoietic malignancies as well as several cases of patients with mycosis fungoides and Sézary syndrome have been described.

Histologically, seborrheic keratoses are benign epithelial growths with no malignant potential. There are five histologic types: acanthotic, hyperkeratotic, adenoidal (reticulated), clonal, and inflamed (irritated or inverted follicular). A few cases of seborrhic keratosis with focal acantholysis have been reported. Separation of intraepidermal epithelioma (IE) and the clonal type of seborrheic keratosis is based on histological grounds, with IE showing atypical nests of keratinocytes, nuclear pleomorphism, atypia, malignant dyskeratosis, and mitosis within the epidermis. These lesions are regarded as premalignant—about 9% may invade the underlying dermis and subcutaneous tissue—whereas the clonal variant of seborrheic keratosis is benign.

These common tumors are primarily of cosmetic importance. When histologic confirmation is not required, these lesions are easily removed in several ways.

Liquid Nitrogen Cryotherapy

Depending on the size of the lesion, either a spray apparatus or a cotton-tipped applicator may be used. The entire lesion with a 1- to 2-mm halo of surrounding skin is treated with a 30- to 45-sec freeze-thaw cycle. Several lesions can be treated at a time without anesthesia. Lesions will persist if inadequately frozen, and thick lesions may require additional treatment. However, deeper freezes my result in hypopigmentation or scar. The patient feels a burning sensation initially, which increases in intensity as the area thaws. Instructions for local wound care are given, and the area heals with minimal to no scarring. Curettage is an effective supplement to cryotherapy. After freezing lightly with liquid nitrogen or skin refrigerants (Frigiderm), the seborrheic keratosis can be easily curetted off the underlying normal skin.

The fast curette method consists of holding the skin taut and with a firm grasp of the instrument, sweeping the lesion off the skin with a single motion. Pedunculated lesions can be removed with a small scissor. These small lesions may shrink down and char quickly when touched by the hyfrecator tip. This is followed by curettage. As many of these patients have dark skin, avoidance of cryotherapy decreases the risk of hypopigmentation.

Electrodesiccation and Electrofulguration Plus Curettage

The acanthotic epidermis of a seborrheic keratosis can be ablated by electrosurgery. Electrodesiccation and electrofulguration cause the most superficial type of tissue destruction. This type of treatment usually requires local anesthesia. For electrodesiccation, touch the lesion gently and move the electrode across the lesion with low power current. Thicker lesions may require direct insertion of the electrode into multiple points for 1–2 sec. The destroyed tissue is easily removed with a piece of gauze or a curette for adherent lesions. Punctate bleeding is controlled with spot electrocoagulation, pressure, or aluminum chloride solution. Use of Monsel's solution on the face is avoided because of the risk of permanent brown staining. Extremely small lesions can be treated with electrofulguration, during which the electrode does not touch the lesion. A few sparks are dispersed across the lesion, minimizing the extent of adjacent tissue damage.

Shave Excision

Seborrheic keratoses can be easily removed with a superficial shave excision. This technique is particularly effective and offers the advantage of a specimen for histologic examination, should the clinical diagnosis be in doubt. Shave excision should not be used when melanoma is in the differential diagnosis. In this instance, a full-thickness excision is the treatment of choice to provide a specimen for complete histological examination and measurement of depth if melanoma is discovered. Shave excision requires the use of local anesthesia and has the potential for scarring.

Dermabrasion and Chemical Peel

Superficial dermabrasion can be used for the treatment of giant seborrheic keratosis and for patients with multiple lesions. Mild hypertrophic scarring without evidence of recurrence has been described. Trichloroacetic acid (25–50%) can be used as a treatment by carefully painting the surface of the lesion with acid and repeating the application at a later date if necessary.

SEBACEOUS HYPERPLASIA

Sebaceous hyperplasia is a common disorder, occurring in adults with increasing frequency with age. These lesions usually occur in middle age, however, lesions arising at puberty have been well documented. The lesions are cream- to yellow-colored papules with a central area of umbilication and are 2–6 mm in size located on the forehead, cheeks, lower eyelids, and nose.

Histologically, numerous sebaceous glands are arranged around a central follicle. There are clearly too many normal glands for the central, single follicle.

Treatment is often performed for cosmetic reasons. When basal cell carcinoma cannot be ruled out, excision is the treatment of choice. Excision, deep curettage, or hot cautery are effective but may leave a visible scar. Trichloroacetic acid 50% or 1% bichloroacetic acid is applied directly to the lesion with a cotton tip or pointed wooded applicator for a few seconds, until the lesion turns white. This is followed with antibiotic ointment for 1 week.

Cryosurgery with a cotton-tipped applicator for a freezing time of 10–15 sec with a 1-mm frost halo around the lesion results in resolution without discernible scarring. Systemic administration of isotretinoin has been reported as successful, however, lesions returned 3 weeks after discontinuation of therapy.

EPIDERMOID CYSTS

Epidermoid cysts arise from implantation and proliferation of the epidermis within the dermis or subcutaneous tissue. They commonly occur on the face, scalp, neck, or trunk and range from 1 to 5 cm. Uncommon cases of a giant epidermoid cyst on the chest as well as an epidermoid cyst arising on the sole of the foot have been reported. They may arise from occlusion of pilosebaceous follicles or from implantation of epidermal cells into the dermis following penetrating injury. Clinically they appear as spherically shaped, slowly enlarging firm to fluctuant nodules. A small central punctum connecting to the cyst cavity representing the plugged orifice of the pilosebacous unit can often be observed. Malodorous, cheesy-white keratinous material may be expressed from this punctum. Lesions are asymptomatic unless they become inflamed after rupture of the cyst wall or become infected. Clinically, infected epidermoid cysts exhibit bacterial growth predominantly with *Staphylococcus aureus*. The presence of human papillomavirus antigen has been reported, but the association between the virus and the epidermoid cyst remains obscure. Rare instances of cyst-derived Bowen's disease, basal cell carcinoma, and squamous cell carcinoma have been reported. The cyst is lined by a stratified squamous epithelium with a well-formed granular layer. Within the cyst, a thick, compact, keratinous material is organized into laminated layers. Foreign-body reaction with giant cells may occur due to trauma or infection in response to spillage of cyst contents to the surrounding dermis (Fig. 2).

The removal of epidermoid cysts is a common problem. Procedures for the treatment of epidermoid cysts include different modes of surgical excision, incision, and drainage, and some have suggested electrocautery, cryosurgery, and the injection of chemical irritants. We favor incision and thorough drainage or surgical excision.

Excision

Noninflamed, uninfected cysts are easily removed. To prevent recurrence, the complete removal or destruction of the cyst wall is necessary. Before cyst removal, simple palpation is used to define the dimensions of the cyst and to determine how freely mobile the cyst is. The area is

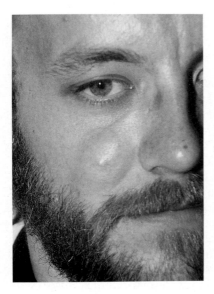

Figure 2 Epidermoid cyst on cheek. Note puncta.

prepared in a surgical manner, and the surgical site is marked with gentian violet. The skin overlying the cyst and the surrounding skin needs to be anesthetized. Anesthesia is injected between the skin and around the cyst wall in a ringlike manner, taking care to avoid injection into the cyst itself, as this will increase the likelihood of rupture. Supplemental injections may be required into the surrounding tissue and deep to the cyst. It is recommended that the dermatologic surgeon wear a protective cap and protective eyewear to shield the eyes from the occasional "eruption" of cyst contents.

Minimal Surgery Technique

A small to medium-sized cyst may be excised by making a single 2- to 3-mm linear excision over the cyst. Pressure is applied to the base of the cyst for delivery of the contents. The cyst wall may evert as the cyst contents are expressed or extracted with a hemostat. It is then identified and completely removed. The wound is carefully inspected to ensure complete removal of the capsule and irrigated with sterile saline to remove any retained fragments of the wall to prevent cyst recurrence. The surgical wound is closed with suture, and hemostasis is with electrocautery.

After palpation, a freely movable cyst with little attachment to its surroundings can be excised with a #15 scalpel blade. The top of the cyst is incised along the maximal skin tension lines to the level of the glistening white capsule wall. This incision should be through the punctum or directly to the side of it. A small amount of tissue enclosing the punctum is removed with it. Continue as above, removing cyst contents and then the capsule.

Elliptical excision should include the punctum overlying the cyst. A small ellipse overlying the cyst is excised up to the capsule overlying the cyst with a #15 scalpel blade. The epidermis attached to the cyst can be elevated with an Allis clamp and using blunt-tipped dissection scissors (tenotomy scissors or baby Metzenbaum scissors) or hemostat, carefully dissect around the cyst, and the cyst can usually be delivered intact. The standard elliptical excision is closed in the usual manner; if the defect left by the cyst is small, skin sutures of only 4.0–6.0 monofilament nylon may be necessary. Vertical mattress sutures assist in opposing wound edges and decreasing dead space. For a large defect, buried absorbable 4.0 or 5.0 suture is used.

Substituting a biopsy punch for a scalpel provides a simple, rapid method for removal of epithelial cysts. The cyst is anesthetized with a needle inserted superficially into the opening of the cyst and then deeply into the cyst itself. Squeezing the base of the cyst firmly, a 2- to 4-mm biopsy punch is inserted perpendicular to the cyst over the visible pore until it penetrates the cyst wall. The contents of the cyst are squeezed out with firm pressure through the hole until no more of the contents appear. Then a curet or a small scissor is inserted to dislodge the wall from the surrounding stroma, and it is grasped with a small hemostat and removed. To reduce wound care requirements and afford a superior cosmetic result, the wound is closed with suture only if the surgeon is confident that the cyst wall is completely removed. If there are any retained contents, the wound is not closed and the wound heals by secondary intention aided by moist warm compresses. It should be emphasized that this method works well for small cysts of the face and is not to be used for severely inflamed or fibrosed cysts.

An epidermoid cyst can be easily removed unless the cyst wall has become fibrosed to the adjacent tissue from trauma or infection. Acutely inflamed cysts should be allowed to "cool down." Treatment is with an oral antibiotic that provides good staphylococcus coverage, such as dicloxacillin, azithromycin, or a cephalosporin, followed by a small amount of intralesional triamcinolone (5–10 mg/ml) into the cyst cavity can be employed. The cyst may contract in 3–4 weeks and then it can be excised.

Fluctuant cysts are treated with a central stab incision to drain the cyst contents, followed by gauze packing. Local anesthesia may be necessary, and the walls of the cyst can then be curetted to assist in removing contents and breaking up lobulations. Before packing the defect, generously place antibiotic ointment inside the cavity for local antibacterial effect and to allow easy removal of the gauze packing without adhesion. The packing is removed slowly at 24–72 hours and an appropriate antibiotic is prescribed. If the area is acutely inflamed, a modest amount of intralesional triamcinolone can be injected into the surrounding area. Excision can be performed in 4–6 weeks.

TRICHILEMMAL CYSTS (PILAR CYSTS)

Trichilemmal cysts occur most commonly on the scalp and are often referred to as a "wen" or sebaceous cyst. Clinically they are similar to epidermoid cysts, however, trichilemmal cysts occur on the scalp 90% of the time, comprising 15% of surgically excised cysts. There is an autosomal dominant genetic disposition. They are produced from budding off of the external root sheath in the region of the follicular isthmus. Individual cysts enlarge, and some of the central keratin may disintegrate to produce a pseudo-calcareous mass. True calcification is found in 25% of cysts. There is a tendency for trichilemmal cysts to recur after excision, when only the parent cyst is removed and one or more daughter cysts are left behind. Budding of new cysts occurs de novo from the cyst wall or directly around areas of calcification.

Histologically trichilemmal cysts are rarely connected to the epidermis. The cyst wall is composed of stratified squamous epithelium with a palisaded outer layer resembling the outer root sheath of the hair follicle. The inner layer of pale-staining cells keratinizes without a granular layer, consequently without keratohyalin granules in contradistinction to an epidermoid cyst. The keratin lining the cyst is dense, pink, and homogeneous, in contrast to the delicate loose keratin of an epidermoid cyst. Calcium is displayed in 24% and cholesterol clefts in 92% of cysts.

Excision of trichilemmal cysts is similar to epidermoid cysts. The wall of the cyst is firmer and more likely to remain intact. A shallow incision is made over the cyst, scissors are used to dissect surrounding tissue bluntly, and the cyst is expressed easily intact.

Moderate-sized cysts may be removed using the punch excision method. After obtaining superficial anesthesia, a 4- to 5-mm punch of skin is removed to the depth of the capsule. Anesthetic is injected deeper around the cyst. Pressure is applied around the punch site until the cyst is visible. The cyst is then grasped by a small hemostat and dissected out intact. The defect is closed by simple wound closure.

This can often be accomplished on the scalp without hair removal, since the hair can be taped with paper tape or clipped with hair clips out of the operative field. Wound care consists of moist sterile compresses twice daily followed by antibiotic ointment dressing.

PROLIFERATING TRICHILEMMAL TUMOR

Proliferating trichilemmal tumor is an uncommon variant of trichilemmal cysts. It is usually a solitary lesion occurring on the scalp of elderly women. However, this tumor has occurred in individuals in their twenties and thirties. They may arise from trauma or inflammation of common trichilemmal cysts. The possibility of malignant transformation should be considered in longstanding cystic and nodular scalp lesions that show rapid growth or exophytic enlargement.

Histologically the tumor represents a proliferation of the outer root sheath epithelium composed of irregularly shaped, well-circumscribed lobules of squamous epithelium in a palisading pattern. Trichilemmal keratinization without a granular layer, foci of calcification may be present in areas of amorphous keratin, and squamous epithelium may contain squamous pearls and eddies. In some tumors' foci of cytological atypia, nuclear pleomorphism and numerous mitoses can produce a picture difficult to distinguish from squamous cell carcinomas.

The tumor should be excised with a margin of normal tissue to prevent recurrence. Routine follow-up of patients is recommended, especially in tumors with a malignant appearance.

MILIA

Milia are small, 1- to 3-mm, white papular lesions. Primary lesions occur on the face and are seen in adults or children. Secondary lesions occur in diseases associated with subepidermal bullae such as porphyria cutanea tarda, epidermolysis bullosa, bullous pemphigoid, bullous lichen planus, and lichen sclerosis et atrophicus. Histologically both forms resemble tiny epidermoid cysts. Milia may connect to the epidermis or to an eccrine sweat duct or to a hair follicle.

Milia commonly appear during the healing phase of dermabrasion, chemical peel, or incisional surgery, and may result from fragments of detached epidermis that continue to keratinize. The incidence of milia may be reduced by scrubbing the face after dermabrasion with a "gauze pad with copious amounts of saline."

Milia are treated by incising the overlying dermis with the tip of a #15 blade, a 25 needle, or surgical lancet. The contents are expressed by simple finger pressure or a comedone extractor. Electrocautery or electrosurgery with an epilating needle set at low current touched lightly to the top of the milia for a fraction of a second will break the cyst sac. The contents may boil out or be removed as above.

KERATOACANTHOMAS

Keratoacanthoma (KA) is a proliferation of squamous epidermis characterized clinically by dome-shaped nodules 1–2.5 cm in diameter with a keratotic plug in the center. Keratoacanthomas usually arise on sun-exposed, hair-bearing skin. This is usually followed by a slow involution over 3–6 months without metastases. The appearance of keratoacanthomas can be divided into three stages: proliferative, fully developed, and involuting.

In the early proliferative stage, a horn-filled invagination of the epidermis arises from contiguous hair follicles, from which epidermal strands may extend into the dermis. The lesion shows mild hyperkeratosis, acanthosis, and premature keratinization with atypical mitotic cells (Figs. 3 and 4).

A fully developed lesion shows a crateriform nodule with a central depression filled with keratin. The epidermis buttresses over the sides of the crater. Irregular epidermal proliferations extend upward into the crater and downward below its base. These epidermal proliferations may appear atypical but less so than during the initial stage. Keratinization of the squamous cells is marked, producing an eosinophilic glassy appearance. Horn pearls are present, and the base in mature lesions appears regular and well demarcated and usually does not extend below the level of the sweat glands.

In the involuting stage, proliferation has concluded and most of the cells at the base of the lesion have undergone keratinization. A mixed dermal infiltrate with granulation tissue may be present with fibrosis. The lesion flattens and finally disappears, leaving an atropic scar in its place.

Keratoacanthomas have characteristic histologic features that are best observed in a section cut through the center of a mature lesion. Although the histologic diagnosis is usually possible when an adequate and properly oriented biopsy specimen includes the lateral and lower margins of the lesion, the final diagnosis must be based on clinicopathologic correlation. A rapidly growing lesion exhibiting features of a well-differentiated squamous cell carcinoma is likely to be a keratoacanthoma, whereas a slowly enlarging tumor with similar histologic features but without regression is likely to be a squamous cell carcinoma.

Although a solitary lesion that occurs spontaneously and regresses is the classic prototype of keratoacanthoma, there are other clinical variants of the tumor that follow an unconventional clinical behavior. The Ferguson-Smith or self-healing lesion begins in adolescence or early adult life with hundreds of lesions on exposed and nonexposed areas. These familial lesions persist throughout the patient's life, suddenly appearing, fading and recurring, tending to be deeper and

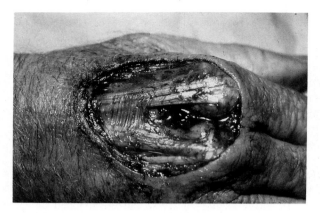

Figure 3 Surgical defect following Mohs micrographic surgery. Deep extent of tumor necessitated removal of peritenon overlying extensor tendons.

more destructive. Eruptive or Grzybowski lesions occur after the fourth decade of life and are characterized by hundreds to thousands of small pruritic papules on exposed and nonexposed areas.

Keratoacanthomas may be extremely aggressive, causing local tissue destruction, or may disappear spontaneously, leaving scarring that may have adverse effects. A tumor such as on the upper eyelid or an invasive giant keratoacanthoma variant greater than 3 cm occurring on the middle face requires active intervention. It is critical to recognize keratoacanthomas that behave in an atypical manner. These must be differentiated from squamous cell carcinoma. Cases have been reported that were initially diagnosed as keratoacanthoma, but recurred after conservative therapy with rapidly spreading metastatic cutaneous lesions resulting in death.

In practice, it is often difficult to pathologically differentiate a well-differentiated squamous cell carcinoma from a keratoacanthoma. Keratocanthomas usually have intraepithelial elastic fibers, eosinophilic, ground glass cytoplasm with glycogen in a cup-shaped lesion with a well-defined border along with microabscesses—features that assist in differentiation.

Excision is the treatment of choice because it removes the specimen in its entirety. Complete excision including the deep margin allows the pathologist to evaluate the architectural pattern of

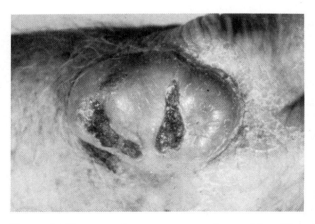

Figure 4 Keratoacanthoma, recurrent after excision. Unresponsive to intralesional fluorouracil.

the tumor to distinguish it from a squamous cell carcinoma. When differentiation between them cannot be made with certainty, an assessment of surgical margins is made to assess the adequacy of resection. The scar resulting from an excisional biopsy is more acceptable than that resulting from ablative techniques or the atrophic scar that can follow spontaneous resolution. A razor blade excision, starting a few millimeters outside the lesion and down to mid-dermis centrally, creates a convex defect. This simple technique provides material for histopathologic examination with minimal scarring.

Incisional biopsy is a limited procedure that is useful for a large keratoacanthoma or one that is in a location that would make excision technically difficult. Incisional biopsy frequently triggers spontaneous involution. To ensure adequate sampling, the incisional biopsy specimen should be large enough that the architecture of the tumor can be assessed. A proper biopsy specimen may be obtained by performing a wedge or an elliptical incisional biopsy through the center of the lesion, making certain to include the deep margin of the lesion. A punch biopsy does not allow evaluation of the overall configuration of the tumor.

Mohs Micrographic Surgery

Keratoacanthomas arising at sites of functional or cosmetic importance, particularly the nasal bridge, canthi, and periauricular regions, are appropriately treated by Mohs surgery. Giant keratoacanthoma threatening critical underlying structures is best treated by this technique as well. In a series of 43 treated lesions by Mohs surgery, there was only one recurrence after a follow-up period of 6 months to 2 years.

Destructive Procedures

Destructive procedures such as curettage and electrodesiccation or cryotherapy do not provide a specimen for histologic analysis and margin determination. Such therapy applied to a squamous cell carcinoma with a keratoacanthomalike appearance might result in the local recurrence of a problematic tumor and allow an interval time for tumor invasion. Finally, the scars resulting from these procedures are often depressed and hypopigmented, which are no more desirable than the scar resulting from spontaneous involution.

Radiotherapy

A keratoacanthoma may be treated with radiotherapy in a dosage and fractionation similar to that used to treat squamous cell carcinoma. Radiotherapy may afford effective therapy in the elderly patient or in a patient with general poor health. Skin changes with radiation include telangiectasia and atrophy. These must be weighed against the disfiguring appearance and/or sequelae of an aggressive lesion. Lesions should be treated before they damage underlying cartilage, creating a less favorable cosmetic defect. Radiotherapy is useful for treating keratoacanthomas not amenable to conventional treatment. However, there is a risk of developing a malignant lesion within the treatment field in later years.

Intralesional Chemotherapy

Surgical excision can result in functional and cosmetic defects when large or strategically located lesions are treated. A nonsurgical approach may be desirable in these cases.

Intralesional fluorouracil has displayed effectiveness in the treatment of keratoacanthomas. Intralesional injection of 0.1–0.2 ml of 50 mg/ml 5-fluorouracil using a 27–30 gauge needle in a series of weekly injections for 5–9 weeks was effective for small keratoacanthomas. Large keratoacanthomas treated with 1–2 ml at 1- to 4-week intervals for 2–6 treatments responded favorably without recurrence of lesions. However, intralesional 5-fluorouracil may be effective only in rapidly proliferating lesions. Topical 5% 5-fluorouracil has also been effective.

Intralesional interferon-α injected into the borders and into the base of large keratoacanthomas (>2 cm) was successful in five out of six patients treated. The starting treatment was 3 × 3 million units per week increased to 3 × 6 M units per week for 4–7 weeks. The main side effects were pain during injection and transitory fever, which responded to acetaminophen. Regression was obtained with good cosmetic results.

Treatment with intralesional methotrexate, infiltrated into the shoulder of the keratoacanthoma, into four quadrants at a depth of 2–8 mm with a 30 gauge needle in a way to blanch the entire rim of the lesion has been reported to be successful in the treatment of keratoacanthomas. The dose was 0.4–1.5 ml of 12.5 or 25 mg/ml of methotrexate and was repeated in 2 weeks at follow-up if any portion of the lesion remained. The lesions responded with complete resolution after one or two injections with minimal scarring. No side effects were noted, and discomfort with injection was minimal with or without lidocaine. Intralesional therapy may be considered in patients with multiple lesions, relatively inaccessible locations, large lesions on the head and neck, and in cosmetically sensitive areas for lesions with histories and morphologies characteristic of keratoacanthoma.

Retinoids

Retinoids have been used in the treatment of keratoacanthomas. Although the exact mechanism of action is unknown, these agents may act by regulating gene expression. Retinoids have been shown to be modulators of epithelial cell differentiation and can suppress carcinogenesis in a variety of epithelial tissues.

A few case reports have documented successful treatment of keratoacanthoma with oral retinoids. Etretinate has been used to treat patients with multiple keratoacanthomas of the Ferguson-Smith type. Dosages of 1 mg/kg/day resulted in resolution of lesions, but new papular lesions reappeared when the dose was titrated down to 0.25 mg/kg/day. A maintenance dose of 0.75 mg/kg/every other day resulted in complete resolution of lesions. In a patient with eruptive keratoacanthomas, etretinate 40 mg/day titrated down to 10 mg/day resulted in a gradual decrease in lesions over one month. Maintenance therapy of 10 mg/day was stopped, and a few lesions reappeared. Isotretinoin (13-*cis* retinoic acid) for solitary and multiple keratoacanthomas has been documented in doses ranging from 0.5 to 1.0 mg/kg/day for 4–12 weeks with resolution of lesions. Also, a dosage of 1.5 mg/kg/day followed by a lower maintenance therapy resulted in clearing of lesions and prevention of new lesions.

Retinoid therapy is associated with multiple dose-related side effects. Mucocutaneous side effects, arthralgias, and elevation of serum cholesterol, triglycerides, and elevation of liver enzymes may occur. Retinoid therapy may be indicated for patients with multiple lesions, aggressive lesions, and in those cases where surgery would result in severe disfigurement. It may also be used as adjunctive therapy to maintain remission.

The single disadvantage of retinoid therapy and intralesional therapy is the lack of histological confirmation of the lesion before treatment. Therefore, it would be best to reserve this treatment for lesions verified by biopsy or for those that remain or recur postoperatively. A complete excision of the lesion should not be delayed if a response is not obtained promptly.

EPIDERMAL NEVUS

The epidermal nevus is an uncommon epidermal hamartoma present at birth or arising during childhood. It consists of wartlike and scaling overgrowths of the epidermis without nevus cells. It is often characterized by light brown, closely set hyperkeratotic papules in a linear distribution. Lesions tend to occur on the trunk and extremities. There is substantial clinical variation in the form of ichthyosis hystrix, nevus unius lateris, nevus verrucous, inflammatory linear verrucous nevus, and epidermal nevus syndrome. Extensive lesions may be associated with skeletal deformities, seizures, mental retardation, and neural deafness. In the epidermal nevus syndrome, there are associated abnormalities of the central nervous, vascular, and musculoskeletal systems. Malignant degeneration of epidermal nevi is unusual and usually consists of a basal cell carcinoma. Keratoacanthoma has been reported to develop in some lesions, while in others malignant transformation beginning as Bowen's disease and becoming an invasive, well-differentiated squamous cell carcinoma has been described. Usually, cutaneous lesions occur without associated abnormalities, but they become a substantial cosmetic problem when located in exposed areas. Histologic patterns vary, displaying epidermal hyperplasia and papillomatous thickening, hypertrophy of the granular and cornified layers, with spotty areas of parakeratosis. Normal or abnormal appendages may appear or be distinctively inflammatory and psoriasiform or may show epidermolytic hyperkeratosis.

The variety of reported treatments for epidermal nevi are evidence of the adversity encountered treating these lesions. The treatment of epidermal nevi is often unsatisfactory, and treated lesions tend to recur within weeks to months. There are a collection of treatment case reports describing effective therapy in a very limited group of patients.

Nonsurgical treatments have consisted of keratolytics, topical or intralesional steroids, and topically applied tars. Steroid ointments as well as Dermojet injections have produced remission or pruritus and cutaneous lesions, but after a few months the lesions recur. Weekly application of 0.125–.75% podophyllin ointment under occlusion for 9 months resulted in a complete cure during a 3-month follow-up period in one case report. However, the application of podophyllin ointment over a large area of skin or in areas of maceration may lead to systemic absorption and is associated with central nervous system toxicity, renal damage, thrombocytopenia, and death. For these reasons, treatment with topical podophyllin is not recommended (Figs. 5–7).

Excision

Surgical excision has been cited as the treatment of choice. However, to avoid recurrence, a full-thickness excision is necessary and may be impractical for large lesions.

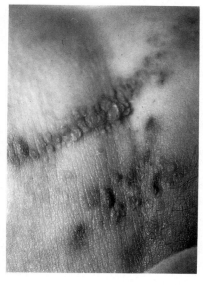

Figure 5 Epidermal nevus involving the medial thigh of a 30-year-old woman.

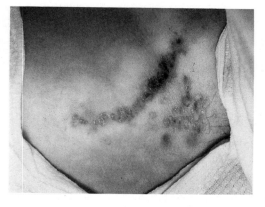

Figure 6 Epidermal nevus immediately following vaporization by carbon dioxide laser.

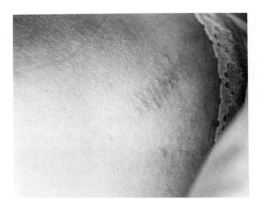

Figure 7 Scar 6 months following carbon dioxide laser ablation of epidermal nevus.

Dermabrasion

The treatment of epidermal nevi by dermabrasion is effective in removal of epidermal nevus lesions but usually produces scarring. Recurrence of lesions after dermabrasion has been reported. Success depends on complete removal of the epidermis and dermal component. Scarring depends on the depth of the lesion's involvement in the dermis.

Cryosurgery

Cryosurgery employing a freeze-thaw cycle of 1–2 min thawing time and repeating this cycle one time has been described as effective. Local anesthetic is necessary because a deep freeze with liquid nitrogen produces a significant amount of discomfort. Scarring results, and it is often more prominent than scarring resulting from carbon dioxide laser vaporization. There is also some limitation on the amount of nevus treated by cryotherapy in a single session.

Carbon Dioxide Laser

The carbon dioxide laser is used at low wattage in the defocused mode to vaporize the abnormal epidermis. Two to three passes over the treatment area are necessary before normal-appearing dermis is achieved. A curet is useful between passes to help define a normal dermal plane. Residual epidermal nevus has a characteristically darker appearance than adjacent, uninvolved tissue. It is often beneficial to treat large lesions in segments at 6-week intervals. This may minimize the risk of hypertrophic scar formation. Even with laser surgery, some degree of scarring may result. Treatment of verrucous nevi with argon laser requires multiple treatments and may result in hypopigmentation.

Surgical excision, dermabrasion, cryotherapy, carbon dioxide laser, and argon laser may produce acceptable cosmetic results in some patients, but there is the risk of recurrence. When a surgical procedure is selected, it should be the one that will afford the highest chance of success with the least amount of morbidity for the patient.

Recently a linear verrucous epidermal nevus was treated using a combination of topical tretinoin 0.1% and 5% 5-fluorouracil for 3–6 months twice a day under occlusion. The lesions resolved with minimal postinflammatory hyperpigmentation. Recurrence of the lesions after 3–4 weeks prompted reinitiation of therapy on a twice-weekly basis, with apparent good results.

WARTS (VERRUCA)

Warts are benign epidermal tumors of the skin occurring in adults and children. They are induced by the human papilloma virus (HPV). The human papillomavirus is a double-stranded DNA virus enclosed in an icosahedral capsid. Clinical lesions of warts include common warts (verruca vulgaris), filiform warts, flat warts (verruca plana), plantar warts (including myrmecia and mosaic types), anogenital warts, and bowenoid papulosis. Extracutaneous lesions occur on mucous membranes and include oral common warts, oral condylomata acuminata, focal epithelial hyperplasia, oral florid papillomatosis, nasal papillomas, conjunctival papillomas, laryngeal papillomatosis, and cervical warts.

Common warts are rough keratotic papules that occur on the dorsal hands, fingers, or knees of children. Butcher's warts are commonly caused by HPV-7 and are found on the hands and fingers of meat cutters. Flat warts are slightly elevated flesh-colored to gray or brown smooth papules. The Koebner phenomenon is common in flat warts. Plantar warts are covered with a thick hyperkeratotic surface with punctate black dots or thrombosed capillaries. A mosaic wart is the result of multiple warts coalescing into a large plaque. Condyloma acuminatum or anogenital warts consist of hyperplastic, verrucous papules, which may coalesce into cauliflowerlike lesions.

Small, macular, and slightly elevated lesions have been defected on normal-appearing penile skin after the application of 5% acetic acid. Bowenoid papulosis consists of multiple, small, velvety pigmented papules in the anogenital region. HPV-16 and HPV-18 virus have been demonstrated in lesions of bowenoid papulosis.

Histologic features of common warts are acanthosis, papillomatosis, hyperkeratosis, and parakeratosis with acanthotic rete ridges. There are foci of vacuolated cells, referred to as koilocytes, and foci of clumped keratohyalin granules. Plantar warts (myrmecia) contain large eosinophilic inclusions within the cytoplasm of keratinocytes. Flat warts have a diffuse zone of vacuolated cells in the upper stratum corneum but, unlike verrucae vulgaris, have no papillomatosis or areas of parakeratosis. Anogenital warts show considerable acanthosis, with thickening and elongation of the rete ridges. Bowenoid papulosis shows changes of carcinoma in situ of Bowen's disease with an irregular, "wind-blown" arrangement of nuclei.

Although warts are often of cosmetic importance, they can also be painful or even disabling. They are common in immunosuppressed patients. There are many effective treatments for warts. The treatment choice should be based on the size and location of lesions, patient compliance, effectiveness of previous treatments, and cost factors. Common treatment of warts involves physically destroying the cells infected with virus. Keratolytic agents such as salicylic, lactic, and trichloroacetic acids cause simple destruction of the epithelial cells infected with papilloma virus. Destruction of the wart can be accomplished by cryosurgery, curettage, or electrocautery. However, to be effective, any form of therapy must remove the entire wart and eradicate all of the virus, otherwise recurrences are common. Chemotherapeutic agents such as podophyllin, bleomycin, and 5-fluorouracil are reported to be effective. When traditional forms of therapy prove to be ineffective, surgical removal with the carbon dioxide laser is often performed.

Salicylic Acid

Salicyclic acid is topically applied in concentrations of 15–40%. It is usually a simple first-line treatment with few complications. Patients are instructed to soak the wart in warm water for approximately 5 min and to remove any loose tissue with a pumice stone or an emery board. The salicylic acid is then applied to the wart surface, which may be covered with an adhesive bandage. The procedure is repeated once or twice daily as tolerated. Vaseline may be placed around the wart to minimize irritation to unaffected tissue. Hand warts treated with salicylic acid or liquid nitrogen alone had similar cure rates, whereas combination therapy showed higher cure rates. However, keratolytic agents applied every second day under occlusive dressing proved to be more beneficial than daily application alone.

Cryotherapy

One of the most common office procedures for the treatment of warts is cryosurgery. Liquid nitrogen is applied to the wart surface with a cotton-tipped applicator or with a liquid nitrogen spray. Before treatment, excessive keratin is removed with a #15 scalpel blade, as this acts as an insulator. This is necessary for plantar warts, but plane warts and anogenital warts with scant keratin freeze more readily. The liquid nitrogen is applied to the wart until a 1- to 2-mm halo surrounds the wart base, indicating that the full depth has been frozen. Usually two freeze-thaw cycles are performed. The interval between treatments should be no longer than 3 weeks, and less if response is not obtained. A salicylic acid preparation may be applied between treatments. Patients experience a burning sensation while warts are being frozen and may have throbbing pain afterwards. Patients with a low pain threshold can be helped by taking an analgesic one-half hour before treatment or at bedtime if the throbbing persists. There are generally few complications with cryosurgery. However, side effects include edema, necrosis, blister formation, hypopigmentation, and a slight risk of superficial nerve damage. Periungual verrucae using a cotton-tipped applicator should encompass the lesion plus a small rim of normal tissue. The intent of freezing is necrosis with the development of a bulla, usually hemorrhagic because of the dermal-epidermal separation. Large or multiple warts that encircle the nail should be treated in sections. Healing occurs without scarring, but retraction of the nail can rarely occur. Recalcitrant warts or those that extend beneath the nail plate are not good candidates for cryosurgery.

Caustic Acids

The application of acids, such as trichloroacetic acid 50%, destroys cellular protein, which causes inflammation and cell death. It is applied to the wart surface after excessive keratin is removed. Therapy is repeated at weekly intervals until the wart resolves.

Glutaraldehyde

Glutaraldehyde is used topically as a freshly prepared buffered solution. It fixes keratin and has a success rate analogous to topical salicylic acid. Side effects are drying and fissuring of the skin, possible sensitization to glutaraldehyde, and brown staining of skin.

Surgery

Simple surgical excision of warts may be effective when few warts are present. The area is infiltrated with local anesthetic. The wart is dissected away from the surrounding tissue, and any remaining wart is removed by curettage. The base and the sides of the wound are treated with electrodesiccation to stop the bleeding, and a dry dressing is applied. However, there is still a significant risk of recurrence with surgery and the potential risk of scarring.

Bleomycin

Intralesional bleomycin has been used in the treatment of recalcitrant warts. Bleomycin inhibits DNA synthesis and repair causing tissue necrosis and a hemorrhagic scar. The agent is diluted with 0.9% sodium chloride to 1 U/ml. Small amounts of 0.05–0.1 ml are injected into individual warts. The solution is stable for 4 months under refrigeration. However, James et al. found that bleomycin 1 mg/ml stored at –20°C in glass containers led to no significant loss of immunore-activity in 27 months. The use of intralesional bleomycin in the treatment of warts may result in systemic drug exposure and this treatment should be avoided in pregnant women or women of childbearing age. However, intralesional bleomycin has not been associated with any systemic toxicity.

A dose of 0.1–0.2 ml is injected into the wart with a 30-gauge syringe to achieve blanching. In one study the cure rate was 77% for warts on the extremities, 71.4% for periungual warts, and 47.6% for plantar warts after one or two treatments.

The multiple puncture technique using a bifurcated vaccination needle resulted in elimination of 92% of warts after a single treatment. The wart is soaked for 10 min in warm water to hy-drate the keratin, and plain lidocaine is injected. Bleomycin solution (1U/ml) is dropped onto the wart surface with a tuberculin syringe. The wart surface is punctured 40 times per 5 mm of wart surface and the needle must penetrate to the wart base. A dry dressing is applied, and patients may experience local pain.

The bifurcated needle technique uses less than one tenth of the amount of bleomycin than the intralesional technique. Therefore, it may introduce bleomycin more uniformly into the wart and lead to lower peak blood levels. Intralesional bleomycin is associated with moderate to severe pain and may require prior local anesthesia. Tenderness or pain at the treatment site can occur from 1 to 7 days after injection. Patients may need to take aspirin or acetaminophen, and some patients may require a codeine-containing analgesic for a day or two. Extreme caution is nec-essary when treating periungual warts, since loss of nails or permanent nail dystrophy may occur. Scarring or local urticaria has been reported. It is judicious to refrain from treating patients with symptoms of unusual sensitivity to cold suggestive of Raynaud's disease, as isolated reports of Raynaud's phenomenon developing after intralesional injection of finger warts have been de-scribed.

Interferon Therapy

Interferons are a family of proteins and glycoproteins, which occur naturally in the body and are now able to be produced by recombinant biotechnology. These naturally occurring hormones have antiviral, antiproliferative, antitumor, and immunomodulatory activities.

Interferon (1 million units) injected into genital warts (condylomata acuminata) three times a week for 3 weeks cleared 36% of patients and produced a reduction in mean wart area of 39.9%. The most common adverse effects of recombinant interferon-alpha therapy for warts are fever, chills, headache, myalgia, and pain at the injection site. These effects are usually mild, with decreasing intensity during treatment, and rarely interfere with daily routines. Interferon-α in-jected with a Dermo-Jet twice a week produced clearance of hand and plantar warts. This method enhances patient acceptance by significantly reducing local pain at the injection site. While some studies have shown promising results for condyloma acuminata, plantar warts have displayed no response in some reports. The role of interferon in the treatment of verruca remains to be elu-cidated.

Podophyllotoxin

Genital warts have been successfully treated using a 0.5% solution of podophyllotoxin. The solution is applied twice a day by the patient for 3 days for a cycle of 3 weeks. This prepara-tion can be applied by the patient and has a greater safety profile than the resin. Side effects are generally well tolerated and consist of mild erythema, burning, and tenderness.

Carbon Dioxide Laser

Carbon dioxide laser is a therapeutic technique reserved for the treatment of recalcitrant warts. In the defocused mode, the carbon dioxide laser can vaporize tissue in a relatively bloodless field. Local anesthesia is injected into the area being treated. A power setting of 3–10 W, depending on the thickness of the tissue, is used. After each pass, the resultant charred tissue is removed with a curette or gauze pad. The laser beam is moved slowly over the wart surface in a series of passes. The first pass should include a 5-mm border beyond the visible edge of the wart, as papillomavirus has been demonstrated in apparently normal tissue. Three to four passes are continued until all visible signs of warts tissue are removed. The cessation of treatment is based on clinical judgment. The patient is advised to perform local wound care until reepithelialization takes place. Healing may take 4–8 weeks to occur. During the procedure, the patient and the staff should wear protective goggles, and safety masks, and the immediate perioperative area should be protected by moist surgical drapes. The smoke and vapor plume should be extracted with a vacuum system. This is necessary to minimize hazard to both patient and staff, as papillomavirus has been detected in the vapor of warts treated with carbon dioxide laser and electrocoagulation.

Carbon dioxide laser treatment may eradicate recalcitrant warts after other therapeutic methods have failed. Cure rates of 56% for hand and foot warts that have failed prior treatments and cure rates of 71% for periungual warts with one or two treatments have been reported. In another study 81% of recalcitrant hand and foot warts were cured during a 6-month follow-up with one treatment, 15% required a second treatment, and 4% three treatments.

Side effects include postoperative pain after laser treatment, scarring, and loss of function. Pain can vary from mild to moderate in severity. In the treatment of periungual warts, there was significant pain in some patients as well as changes such as distal onycholysis, nail thickening, nail curvature, and grooves.

The reappearance of warts can occur after any treatment. This may be due to incomplete treatment, latent infection in normal-appearing tissue, or reexposure to the papillomavirus.

BIBLIOGRAPHY

Altman J, Mehregan AH. Inflammatory linear verrucose epidermal nevus. *Arch Dermatol* 1971;104:385–389.

Amer M, Diab N, Ramadan A, Galal A, et al. Therapeutic evaluation for intralesional injection of bleomycin sulfate in 143 resistant warts. *J Am Acad Dermatol* 1991;17:234–236.

Barrasso R, DeBrux J, Croissant O, et al. High prevalence of papillomavirus-associated penile intraepithelial neoplasia in sexual partners of women with cervical intraepithelial neoplasia. *N Engl J Med* 1987;317: 916–923.

Benoldi D, Alinovi A. Multiple persistant keratoacanthomas: Treatment with oral etretinate. *J Am Acad Dermatol* 1984;10:1035–1038.

Brook I. Microbiology of infected epidermoid cysts. *Arch Dermatol* 1989;125:1658.

Bunney MH. *Viral Warts: Their Biology and Treatment.* Oxford, Oxford University Press, 1982.

Bunney MH, Nolan MW, Williams DA. An assessment of methods of treating viral warts by comparative treatment trials based on a standard design. *Br J Dermatol* 1976;94:667–676.

Burgdorf WHC. Tumors of sebaceous gland differentiation in *Pathology of the Skin.* Farmer ER, Hood AF, eds. Norwalk, CT, Appleton and Lange, 1990, p. 617.

Burton CS, Sawchuk WS. Premature sebaceous gland hyperplasia: successful treatment with isotretinoin. *J Am Acad Dermatol* 1985;12:182–184.

Cassidy DE, et al. Podophyllin toxicity: Report of a fatal case and review of literature. *J Toxicol Clin Toxicol* 1982;19:35–44.

Cohen BH. Prevention of postdermabrasion milia (letter). *J Dermatol Surg Oncol* 1988;14(11):1301.

Cohen JH., Lessin SR. Vowels BR, et al. The sign of Leser-Trelat in associated with Sezary syndrome:

simultaneous disappearance of seborrheic keratosis and malignant T-cell clone during combined therapy with photopheresis and interferon alpha. *Arch Dermatol* 1993;129:1213-1215.

De Villez RL, Roberts LC. Premature sebaceous gland hyperplasia. *J Am Acad Dermatol* 1982;6:933-935.

Donohe B, Cooper JS, Rush S. Treatment of aggressive keratoacanthomas by radiotherapy. *J Am Acad Dermatol* 1990;23:489-493.

Epstein E. Intralesional bleomycin and Raynaud's phenomenon (letter). *J Am Acad Dermatol* 1991;24: 785-786.

Epstein W, Kligman AM. The pathogenesis of milia and benign tumors of the skin. *J Invest Dermatol* 1956;26:1-11.

Eron LJ, Judson F, Tucker S, Prawer S, et al. Interferon therapy for conylomata acuminata. *N Engl J Med* 1986;315:1059-1064.

Eubanks SW, Gentry RH, Patterson JW, May DL. Treatment of multiple keratoacanthomas with intralesional fluorouracil. *J Am Acad Dermatol* 1982;7:126-129.

Fisher BK, Macpherson M. Epidermoid cyst of the sole. *J Am Acad Dermatol* 1986;15:1127-1129.

Fox BJ, Lapins NA. Comparison of treatment modalities for epidermal nevus: a case report and review. *Dermatol Surg Oncol* 1983;9(11):879-885.

Garb J. Nevus verrucosus unilateris cured with podophyllin ointment. *Arch Dermatol* 1960;81:606-609.

Goldberg LH, Rosen T, Becker J, Knauss A. Treatment of solitary keratoacanthomas with isotretinoin. *J Am Acad Dermatol* 1990;23:934-936.

Golitz LE, Poomeechaiwong S. Cysts. In *Pathology of the Skin*. Farmer ER, Hood AF, eds. Norwalk, CT, Appleton & Lange, 1990, pp. 516-517.

Golitz LE, Western WL. Inflammatory linear verrucous epidermal nevus associated with epidermal nevus syndrome. *Arch Dermatol* 1979;115:1208-1209.

Grob JJ, Suzini F, Weiller RM, Zarour H, Noe C, Munoz MH, Bonerandi JJ. Large keratoacanthomas treated with intralesional interferon alfa-2a. J Am Acad Dermatol 1993;29:237-241.

Hayes ME, O'Keefe EJ. Reduced dose of Bleomycin in the treatment of recalcitrant warts. *J Am Acad Dermatol* 1986;15:1002-1006.

Hodak E, Jones RE, Ackerman AB, et al. Controversies in dermatology. Solitary keratoacanthoma is a squamous cell carcinoma: three examples with metastasis. *Am J Dermatopathol* 1993;15:332-352.

Hodge SJ, Barr JM, Owen LG. Inflammatory linear verrucose epidermal nevus. *Arch Dermatol* 1978;114: 436-438.

Holdiness MR. On the classification of the sign of Leser-Trelat. *J Am Acad Dermatol* 1988;19:754-757.

Hong WK, Lippman SM, Itri LM, Karp DD, et al. Prevention of second primary tumors with isotretinoin in squamous-cell carcinoma of the head and neck. *N Engl J Med* 1990;323:795-801.

Hurwitz S. Epidermal nevi and tumors of epidermal origin. *Ped Clin North Am* 1983;30:483-494.

James MP, Collier PM, Aherne, Hardcastle A. Histologic, pharmacologic and immunocytochemical effect of injection of bleomycin into viral warts. *J Am Acad Dermatol* 1993;28:933-937.

Johannesson A. Razor blade surgery of keratoacanthoma. *J Dermatol Surg Oncol* 1986;12:1056-1057.

Kao GF. benign tumors of the epidermis. In *Pathology of the Skin*, Farmer ER, Hood AF, eds. Norwalk, CT, Appleton & Lange, 1990, pp. 537-546.

Kettler AH, Goldberg LH. Seborrheic keratosis. *Am Fam Phys* 1986;34(2):147-152.

Klin Baruch, Ashkenazi. Sebaceous cyst excision with minimal surgery. *Am Fam Phys* 1990;41(6): 1746-1748.

Kopf AW. Keratoacanthoma. In *Cancer of the Skin*. Andrade R, Gumport SL, Popkin GL, Rees TD, eds. Philadelphia, W.B. Saunders Co, 1976, pp. 755-781.

Kuflik EG. Specific indications for cryosurgery of the nail unit. *J Dermatol Surg Oncol* 1992;18:702-706.

Landthaler M, Haina D, Waidelich W, et al. Argon laser therapy of verrucous nevi. *Plast Reconstr Surg* 1984;74:108-111.

Laing V, Knipe RC, Flowers FP, Stoer CB, Ramos-Caro FA. Proliferating trichilemmal tumor: report of a case and review of the literature. *J Dermatol Surg Oncol* 1991;17:295-298.

Larson PO. Keratoacanthomas treated with Mohs micrographic surgery (chemosurgery): a review of forty cases. *J Am Acad Dermatol* 1987;16:1040-1044.

Leppard BJ, Sanderson KV. The natural history of trichilemmal cyst. *BJD* 1976;94:379-389.

Lever WF, Schaumburg-Lever G, eds. *Histopathology of the Skin*. Philadelphia, JB Lippincott, 1990, pp. 411–418, 535–536.

Lieblich LM, Geronemus RG, Gibbs RC. Use of a punch for removal of epithelial cyst. *J Dermatol Surg Oncol* 1982;8(12):1059–1062.

Logan RA, Zachary CB. Outcome of carbon dioxide laser therapy for persistent cutaneous viral warts. *Br J Dermatol* 1989;121:99–95.

Maeda M. Mori Shunji M. Seborrheic keratosis with focal acatholysis. *J Dermatol* 1989;16:79–81.

Mahler D, Ben-yaker, Rosenberg L. Linear verrucous nevus. *J Dermatol Surg Oncol* 1981;7:262–265.

Manz LA, Pelachyk JM. Bleomycin-lidocaine mixture reduces pain of intralesional injection in the treatment of recalcitrant verrucae. *J Am Acad Dermatol* 1991;25:524–526.

Martin H, Strong E, Spiro RH. Radiation-induced skin cancer of the head and neck. *Cancer* 1970;2:61–71.

McBurney, EI, Rosen DA. Carbon dioxide laser treatment of verrucae vulgares. *J Dermatol Surg Oncol* 1984;10:145–148.

McGavran MN, Binnington B. Keratinous cysts of the skin. Identification and differentiation of pilar cyst from epidermal cysts. *Arch Dermatol* 1966;94:499–508.

Mehregan AH, Lee KC. Malignant proliferating trichilemmal tumors—report of three cases. *J Dermatol Surg Oncol* 1987;13(12):1339–1342.

Melton JL, Nelson BR, Stough DB, Brown MD, Swanson NA, Johnson TM. Treatment of keratoacanthomas with intralesional methotrexate. *J Am Acad Dermatol* 1991;25:1017–1023.

Morag C, Metzker A. Inflammatory linear verrucous epidermal nevus: report of seven new cases and review of the literature. *Pediatr Dermatol* 1985;3:15–18.

Morison WL. Viral warts, herpes simplex and herpes zoster in patients with secondary immune deficiencies and neoplasms. *Br J Dermatol* 1975;92:625.

Naples SP, Brodell RT. Verruca vulgaris. *Arch Dermatol* 1993;129:698–700.

Nelson BR, Kolansky G, Gillard M, et al. Management of linear epidermal nevus treated with topical 5-fluorouracil 5% and tretinoin. *J Am Acad Dermatol* 1994;30:287–288.

Oliveira AS, Picoto AS, Verde SF, Martins O. A simple method of excising tricholemmal cysts from the scalp. *J Dermatal Surg Oncol* 1979;5(8):625–627.

Orth G, Jablonska S. Favre M, et al. Identification of papillomavirus in butcher's warts. *J Invest Dermatol* 1981;76:97–102.

Parker CM, Hanke CW. Large keratoacanthomas in difficult locations treated with intralesional 5-fluorouracil. *J Am Acad Dermatol* 1986;14:770–777.

Pepper E. Dermabrasion for the treatment of a giant seborrheic keratosis. *J Dermatol Surg Oncol* 1985;11(6):646–647.

Pollack SV. *Electrosurgery of the Skin; Electrodesiccation and Electrofulguration*. New York, Churchill Livingstone, 1991, pp. 31–35.

Popkin GL, Brodie SJ, Hyman AB, Andrade R, Kopf AW. A technique of biopsy recommended for keratoacanthomas. *Arch Dermatol* 1966;94:191–193.

Rapaport J. Giant keratoacanthoma of the nose. *Arch Dermatol* 1975;111:73–75.

Ratz JL, Bailin PL, Wheeland RG. Carbon dioxide laser treatment of epidermal nevi. *J Dermatol Surg Oncol* 1986;12:567–570.

Requena L, Romero E, Sanchez M, Ambrojo P, Yus ES. Aggressive keratoacanthoma of the eyelid: "malignant" keratoacanthoma or squamous cell carcinoma. *J Dermatol Surg Oncol* 1990;16:564–568.

Rios, AS, Ocampo CJ. Giant epidermoid cyst: clinical aspect and surgical management. *J Dermatol Surg Oncol* 1986;12(7):734–736.

Rosen T. Keratoacanthomas arising within a linear epidermal nevus. *J Dermatol Surg Oncol* 1982;8:878–880.

Rosian R, Goslen JB, Brodell RT. The treatment of benign sebaceous hyperplasia with the topical application of bichloracetic acid. *J Dermatol Surg Oncol* 1991;17:876–879.

Sawchuk WS, Weber PJ, Lowry DR, Dzubow LM. Infectious papillomavirus in the vapor of warts treated with carbon dioxide laser of electrocoagulation: detection and protection. *J Am Acad Dermatol* 1989;21:41–49.

Schwartz RA. The keratoacanthoma: a review. *J Surg Oncol* 1979;12:305–317.

Shaw JC, White CR. Treatment of multiple keratoacanthomas with oral isotretinoin. *J Am Acad Dermatol* 1986;15:1079–1082.

Shelley WB, Shelly D. Intralesional bleomycin sulfate therapy for warts. *Arch Dermatol* 1991;25:524–526.

Sloan JB, Jawoesky, C. Clinical misdiagnosis of squamous cell carcinoma in situ as seborrheic keratosis, a prospective study. *J Dermatol Surg Oncol* 1993;17:413–416.

Solomon LM, Fretzin DF, Dewald RL. The epidermal nevus syndrome. *Arch Dermatol* 1968;97:273–285.

Stadler R, Mayer da Silva, Bratzke B, et al. Interferons in dermatology. *J Am Acad Dermatol* 1989;20: 650–656.

Stegman SJ, Tromovitch TA, Glogau RG, *Cosmetic Dermatologic Surgery*; 2nd ed. Chicago, Year Book Medical Publishers, 1990, pp. 20–21.

Stegman SJ, Tromovitch TA, Glogau RG. Benign facial lesions. In *Cosmetic Dermatologic Surgery*. 2nd ed., Chicago, Year Book Medical Publishers, 1990, p. 26.

Street ML, Roenigk RK. Recalcitrant periungual verrucae: the role of carbon dioxide vaporization. *J Am Acad Dermatol* 1990;23:115–120.

Strong EW. Treatment of head and neck cancers. *J Dermatol Surg Oncol* 1983;19:644–646.

Swint RB, Klaus SN. Malignant degeneration of an epithelial nevus. *Arch Dermatol* 1970;101:56–58.

Vance JC, Bart BJ, Hansen RC, Reichman RC. Intralesional recombinant alpha-2 interferon for the treatment of patients with condyloma acuminatum or verruca plantaris. *Arch Dermatol* 1986;122:272–277.

Veien NK, Madsen SM, Avrach W, et al. The treatment of plantar warts with a keratolytic agent and occlusion. *J Dermatol Treat* 1991;2:59–61.

Wheeland RG, Wiley MD. Q-tip cryosurgery for the treatment of senile sebaceous hyperplasia. *J Dermatol Surg Oncol* 1987;13:729–730.

Winer LH, Levin GH. Pigmented basal cell epitheliomas arising in a linear nevus. *Arch Dermatol* 1961;83: 114–118.

Winkelmann RK, Brown J. Generalized eruptive keratoacanthoma. *Arch Dermatol* 1968;97:615–623.

Yoshikawa K, Hirano S, Kato T, Mizuno N. A case of eruptive keratoacanthoma treated by oral etretinate. *Br J Dermatol* 1985;112:579–583.

27

Premalignant Lesions

Jeffry A. Goldes
Associated Dermatology, Helena, Montana

Grace F. Kao
University of Maryland School of Medicine, Baltimore, Maryland

Several skin disorders commonly affecting the sun-exposed skin and mucocutaneous junction exhibit a natural history for the development of invasive carcinoma and malignant melanoma. Invasive neoplasms arising in association with an underlying premalignant lesion will be discussed. Solar keratosis, actinic cheilitis, radiation keratosis, Bowen's disease, and arsenical keratosis all show microscopic features of squamous carcinoma in situ. These lesions affect the epidermis, the pilosebaceous adnexal structures, or both. Arsenical keratosis is discussed with Bowen's disease, since they share similar clinical and histopathologic features. Lentigo maligna and acquired melanosis are discussed together because both demonstrate atypical melanocytic proliferation at the dermoepidermal junction.

Each premalignant tumor has characteristic clinicopathologic features and progresses into a malignant tumor in a significant percentage of patients. The diagnosis of malignant disease is made based on cytologic and biologic characteristics of each tumor. Recognition of premalignant disease of the skin is important since these lesions can be treated less aggressively at the in situ stage. Early clinical detection and microscopic examination of premalignant disease are important for prevention of aggressive malignant neoplasms.

SOLAR KERATOSIS AND ACTINIC CHEILITIS

Synonyms for these conditions include actinic keratosis, solar precancerosis, senile keratosis, senile keratoma, and solar cheilitis.

Clinical Features and Gross Pathologic Appearance

Solar keratoses develop in sun-exposed, aging skin that is often dry, wrinkled, and atrophic with irregular mottled hyperpigmentation (actinic melanosis). Lesions are flat, round, or irregularly shaped papules and plaques with adherent scale and are usually less than 1 cm in diameter. Their color varies from red to gray-brown (Fig. 1). They slowly enlarge with time and may become horny or nodular and show a warty configuration resembling a cutaneous horn. The term *cutaneous horn* should be used descriptively, not as a diagnostic term, since in addition to solar keratosis and squamous cell carcinoma, other epidermal neoplasms such as seborrheic keratosis, inverted follicular keratosis, trichilemmoma, basal cell carcinoma, and verruca may present as a cutaneous horn. Solar keratoses are more often multiple than single and are usually located on the face, particularly the forehead, cheeks, nose, and sideburns as well as on other sun-exposed areas such as the ear, neck, dorsum of the hands, forearms, anterior chest, back, and balded scalp.

The average patient is in his early 60s when first diagnosed. In recent years with more leisure-time sun exposure, young people are developing solar keratosis. Solar keratosis develop more energetically in patients who have had a range of sun exposures dating from early childhood. They occur in both sexes, but affect primarily fair-complexioned (types I,II) individuals who have had significant sun exposure over many years. Patients with solar keratoses may also have other cutaneous premalignant lesions such as actinic cheilitis (Fig. 1) or malignant lesions such as squamous cell carcinoma, basal cell carcinoma, lentigo maligna, and malignant melanoma. So-

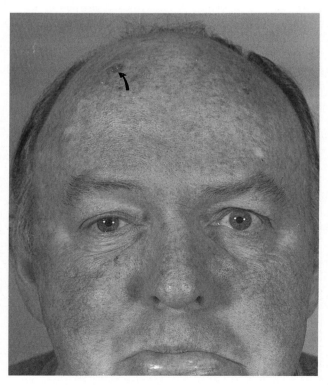

Figure 1   A flat, erythematous to brown, scaly papule of solar keratosis (arrow) on the face of a middle-aged man. Note also the actinic cheilitis involving the lower lip.

lar keratosis is also associated with other cutaneous sun damage, such as solar elastosis and solar lentigines. Within 5–10 years of onset, solar keratoses and actinic cherilitis tend to spread peripherally with loss of skin markings. Spontaneous bleeding and induration signal degeneration to squamous cell carcinoma.

Immunosuppressed patients tend to show accelerated evolution of solar keratoses to squamous cell carcinoma. In addition, malignancy in these patients tends to behave more aggressively with frequent metastases. Patients with xeroderma pigmentosum develop solar keratoses in the first year of life. The incidence of solar keratoses and squamous cell carcinoma increases in patients after prolonged psoralen/ultraviolet A (PUVA) treatment.

Porokeratoses are known to give rise to squamous cell carcinoma and basal cell carcinoma. It has been shown that failure of keratinocytes in prokeratoses to mature and differentiate normally may be related to the increased incidence of carcinoma associated with these lesions.

Actinic cheilitis is similar to solar keratoses but involves the sun-exposed mucous membrane and mucocutaneous junction of the lips (Fig. 1), particularly the lower lip margin. Squamous cell carcinoma of the lip has a higher incidence of metastases.

Microscopic Features

Five histologic types of solar keratosis and actinic cheilitis are recognized: hypertrophic, atrophic, bowenoid, acanthoyltic (Fig. 2), and pigmented. The epidermis and mucous membrane epithelium show hyperkeratosis, parakeratosis, hypergranulosis, frequent irregular acanthosis, and sometimes atrophy. The palisaded basal layer of the epidermis and the pilar epithelium above the sebaceous gland level are replaced by small buds and broad or elongated rete ridges containing atypical keratinocytes, sometimes associated with liquefaction degeneration or acantholysis (Fig. 2). The atypical keratinocytes are characterized by hyperchromatic nuclei, prominent nucleoli, vacuolated cytoplasm, malignant dyskeratosis, multinucleate giant cells, and abundant mitoses. In the hypertrophic type of solar keratosis, papillomatosis is prominent and sometimes forms a cutaneous horn (Fig. 3). Atrophic solar keratoses exhibit thinned, atrophic epidermis with liquefaction degeneration of the dermoepidermal junction. The bowenoid type shows a windblown pattern of atypical keratinocytes and frequently clumped nuclei. Unlike Bowen's disease, atypical keratinocytic proliferation in bowenoid solar keratosis spares the outer root sheath of the hair follicle and the upper layers of the epidermis. The basal epidermis in acantholytic solar keratosis shows prominent acantholysis with suprabasal lacunae containing malignant dyskeratotic cells. Pigmented solar keratosis (actinic melanosis) contains prominent pigmented melanocytes in the epidermis and melanophages in the dermis. In all types of solar keratosis there is evidence of solar damage: moderate to severe elastosis of dermal collagen and a dense, chronic inflammatory infiltrate composed of lymphocytes, histiocytes, and plasma cells. In some instances, the infiltrate lies close to the base of the lesion and shows a lichenoid pattern.

Solar Keratosis and Actinic Cheilitis with Squamous Cell Carcinoma (Solar Carcinoma)

Without treatment, approximately 13% of patients with solar keratoses develop one or more lesions that invade the dermis as squamous cell carcinoma. The invasive lesions appear as flesh-colored, pink, red, or brown keratotic papules, and nodules with scale and elevated pearly margins (Fig. 4). Patients complain about nonhealing, enlarging lesions that bleed with trauma and are pruritic and rarely painful. Microscopically, these lesions are seen to invade the dermo-epidermal junction with atypical keratinocytes that extend into the dermis at various depths. Adenoid squamous cell carcinoma arising in the acantholytic type of solar keratosis demonstrates a pseudoglandular pattern (Fig. 5). Solar keratosis degenerating into squamous cell carcinoma

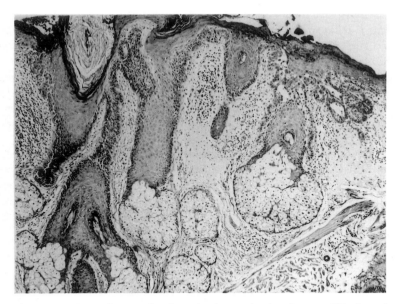

Figure 2 Photomicrograph of a solar keratosis showing small buds and diffuse basal epidermal and pilary outer root sheath involvement by the atypical keratinocytes. Note acantholysis and elastosis of dermal collagen (hematoxylin & eosin, × 160).

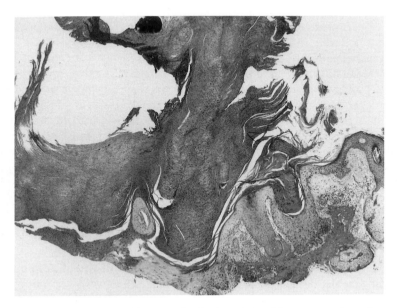

Figure 3 A hypertrophic type of solar keratosis with cutaneous horn formation (hematoxylin & eosin, ×25).

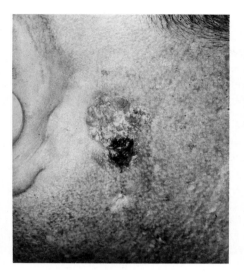

Figure 4 A crusting, hyperkeratotic papule of squamous carcinoma arising in a solar keratosis on the retroauricular skin of an elderly man. Note the elevated pearly margin and focal hemorrhage.

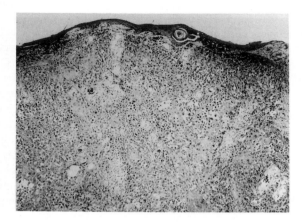

Figure 5 An adenoid squamous cell carcinoma arising in an acantholytic type of solar keratosis showing prominent acantholysis (hematoxylin & eosin, ×60).

is considered a low-grade malignancy, and studies indicate that this tumor almost never develops metastasis unless neglected. Adenoid squamous cell carcinoma may metastasize when the tumor is larger than 2.5 cm. These tumors are rare in blacks.

Recent advances in molecular pathology have shown that mutation of certain tumor suppressor genes is linked to carcinogenesis. Mutations of the p53 gene are the most common genetic abnormality described in human cancer. A 53 kd nuclear phosphoprotein, p53, is believed to play an important role in controlling proliferation of neoplastic and normal cells. A significant number of lesions of solar keratosis (SK) (50%) and squamous cell carcinoma arising in solar keratosis (SK-SCC) (57%) have demonstrated mutated p53. Using the immunoperoxidase method, anti-p53 decorates the nuclei of the atypical keratinocytes located at the basal layer of the epidermis and in the infiltrating carcinoma cells in the dermis. Expression of p53 protein is an early event in UV light–induced cutaneous squamous cell carcinogenesis, and it precedes tumor invasion in squamous cell neoplasia of the skin.

Squamous cell carcinoma arising in actinic cheilitis has been associated with a higher rate of metastasis (10–30%). Therefore, excision with microscopically controlled margins (Mohs micrographic surgery) and an evaluation for lymph node metastasis are indicated.

Differential Diagnosis

The distinction of solar keratosis from seborrheic keratosis can be made on a clinical basis. The latter is more discrete and elevated from the surrounding epidermis. It has a typical stuck-on appearance with comedonal openings of the skin surface.

The hypertrophic type of solar keratosis should be distinguished from squamous cell carcinoma arising in solar keratosis, the de novo type of squamous cell carcinoma, and keratoacanthoma. Because of the clinical similarity of these lesions, a biopsy should include the lateral margins and the base of the lesion for definitive histopathologic diagnosis. Squamous cell carcinoma lacking marginal changes of solar keratosis should be classified as the de novo type. A superficial multicentric type of basal cell carcinoma may resemble solar keratosis clinically, but a rolled, translucent, telangiectatic edge characterizes the former.

An atrophic solar keratosis may be mistaken for discoid lupus erythematosus, but lupus usually contains follicular plugging and has easily detachable scale. The microscopic lack of atypical keratinocytes, prominent liquefaction degeneration of the dermoepidermal junction, and a patchy periappendageal lymphocytic infiltrate are features that favor discoid lupus erythematosus. Localized forms of poikiloderma, atrophic lichen planus, and lichenoid drug eruption should also be considered in the microscopic differential diagnosis of atrophic solar keratoses. These lesions, however, do not show atypia or pleomorphism of the keratinocytes.

Unlike bowenoid solar keratoses, Bowen's disease on sun-exposed areas usually has more irregular contour and a red base. Microscopic examination shows full-thickness involvement of epidermis and pilar epithelium with atypical keratinocytes.

The acantholytic type of solar keratosis must be distinguished from the following diseases microscopically: isolated dyskeratosis follicularis (warty dyskeratoma), keratosis follicularis (Darier's disease), familial benign chronic pemphigus (Hailey-Hailey disease), transient acantholytic dermatosis, and pemphigus vulgaris. Cellular pleomorphism, disorderly arrangement of keratinocytes, malignant dyskeratosis, and absence of corps ronds and grains characterize solar keratosis with acantholysis.

A pigmented solar keratosis may resemble lentigo maligna (melanotic freckle of Hutchinson), an acquired precancerous pigmented melanosis that frequently degenerates into lentigo maligna melanoma or sometimes desmoplastic and neurotropic malignant melanoma. In lentigo maligna there is more flattening of the epidermis than in pigmented solar keratoses, and, more importantly, atypical melanocytic cells, not keratinocytes, are present at the dermoepidermal function.

Benign lichenoid keratosis may be mistaken for solar keratosis or actinic cheilitis on low-power examination. However, it does not demonstrate keratinocyte atypia.

Treatment

The treatment of patients with solar keratoses and related squamous cell carcinoma should be conservative. Complete ablation is the treatment of choice. Several modalities are available depending on the size, number, and anatomic location of the lesions.

Cryosurgery is the most common method used for scattered solitary lesions. A cotton-tipped applicator or cryostat spray is used to freeze the lesion and a thin rim of surrounding skin for 5–15 sec. Repeated two to three times, this will be sufficient to ablate these lesions. Bullae followed by an exudative crust may supervene; healing occurs in 1–3 weeks. Complications include secondary infection, especially if the wound is occluded without proper dressing changes.

Full face liquid nitrogen cryospraying or cryopeeling has been described to remove a generally unsightly or large areas of involved skin surface with multiple actinic keratoses and large lentigines.

Larger, multiple solar keratoses may be treated by applications of 1–5% 5-fluorouracil (5-FU) cream or solution twice daily. Five percent 5-FU is the standard concentration used; however, lower concentrations have been advocated by some for patients with more sensitive facial skin. This treatment causes clinical and subclinical lesions to be more pronounced (Fig. 6) and culminates in acute erythema and tender erosions after 1–4 weeks. Symptoms are improved by the application of 1% hydrocortisone cream (Fig. 7). The time span of this mode of therapy averages 6 weeks. A weekly pulse-dosing regimen for topical 5-FU therapy has been proposed to diminish the severe irritation that can occur. Scarring is a rare complication when secondary infection has supervened. Injection of 5-FU (50 mg/ml) at 0.1–0.5 ml/plaque has been advocated

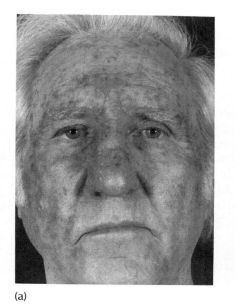

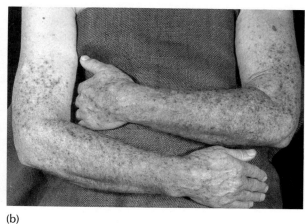

(a)   (b)

Figure 6   Solar keratoses of the (a) face and (b) arms of a 60-year-old man showing reddening and prominence of the plaques, 2 weeks after 5% 5-FU cream application.

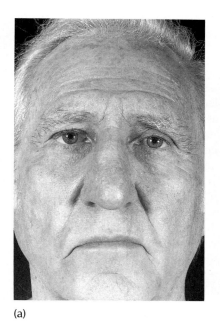

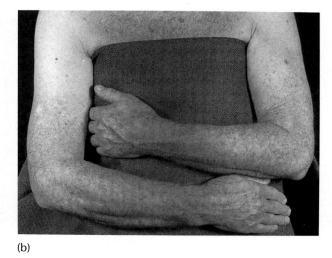

(a)   (b)

Figure 7   Clinical improvement of solar keratoses on the (a) face and (b) arms of patient illustrated in Figure 6, noted 4 weeks after initiation of treatment. The therapy consisted of 2 weeks of 1% hydrocortisone cream twice daily following 2 weeks of 5% 5-FU.

for larger lesions, solar keratoses, and associated squamous cell carcinoma. However, recurrences are common. Combining 5-FU with pyruvic acid (an alpha-hydroxy acid) has been shown to diminish the required exposure time to 5-FU and thus improve patient acceptance.

Masoprocol cream has been evaluated in the treatment of actinic keratoses in the last several years. Twice-daily treatment from 2 to 4 weeks decreases actinic keratoses with diminished irritation.

Topical tretinoin has been shown to help reverse solar damage to the skin including actinic keratoses. The use of various strengths of tretinoin may also enhance the use of 5-FU, particularly in the treatment of solar keratoses on the extremities.

Topical interferon gel, 30,000,000 IU/g, failed to show statistically significant improvement with actinic keratosis after 4 weeks of application.

Dermabrasion is a popular alternative to 5-FU to treat groups of multiple solar keratoses. Wound healing is rapid, generally 2 weeks. Furthermore, recurrences are less frequent and make this alternative more cost-effective. Chemical peel with trichloroacetic acid has also been described.

Excision, as well as curretage and electrodesiccation, is used to treat lesions of solar keratosis suspicious for squamous cell carcinoma. It is useful to obtain a biopsy to assess dermal invasion before ablating the lesion with curettage and electrodesiccation. The defocused CO_2 laser is used to vaporize cutaneous neoplasms and verrucae and is especially successful for the treatment of actinic cheilitis. Carbon dioxide laser oblation of the vermilion has been shown to be associated with fewer postoperative complications than either a lip shave or a trichloracetic acid peel. Retinoids (Accutane and Tegison) may be used to prevent the development of new solar keratoses and squamous cell carcinomas. They are not effective for treating well-established lesions. Radiation therapy is reserved for established neoplasms and should not be used for solar keratosis. Further radiation damage to solar-damaged skin may be counterproductive. An alternative treatment for solar keratoses is the use of endogenous porphyrins followed by radiation with visible light after the application of exogenous 5-amino levulinic acid.

Prognosis and Prevention

The prognosis of solar keratosis–derived squamous cell carcinoma is excellent. The biologic potential for metastasis is rare, with the exception of the adenoid subtype, in which about 2–3% of patients with tumors larger than 2 cm develop metastasis.

Consistent sun screen use has been shown to reduce the development of lesions of solar keratoses. The best protection is offered by agents that contain para-aminobenzoic acid and benzophenones. Water-resistant formulations are available that require less frequent application when swimming. Sun protection factor (SPF) is defined as the protection required to prevent erythema after a minimal erythema dose (MED) of sunlight on a sunscreen-treated site. Each factor unit protects for one MED, so that SPF 15 protects for 15 MEDs and is generally adequate for a full day of erythemogenic sun exposure. A high SPF combined with protective clothing constitutes effective sunscreening in conjunction with avoidance of midday sun, which contains the highest proportion of ultraviolet B (UVB). SPFs of greater than 30 tend to be less accurate and are probably not as useful in predicting sun protection. Opaque sunscreens with zinc oxide ointment and red petrolatum are an effective block, but they are difficult to apply over large areas and are cosmetically unappealing.

The use of topical tretinoin has been shown to reduce solar keratoses and by implication to reduce onset of new lesions; thus it may be helpful in prevention. It is not clear at what age the use of topical tretinoin would be considered useful to help prevent solar keratoses. Further studies are pending at the present time. A custom lip shield has been described that protects the lower lip in vulnerable individuals. Finally, diet has been suggested to help prevent solar keratoses.

Diets rich in beta-carotene may reduce the numbers of lesions. Beta-carotene may be obtained in foods or via supplements.

RADIATION KERATOSIS

Synonyms for this condition include x-ray keratosis, postirradiation keratosis, irradiation dermatitis, x-ray burns, x-ray dermatitis, and roentgen dermatitis.

Clinical Data and Gross Pathologic Appearance

Radiation keratosis may occur in a scar following radiation therapy or excessive fluoroscopy. People at high risk, such as radiologists, radiotherapists, dentists, surgeons, and patients exposed to radiation for a variety of disorders, including acne, basal cell carcinoma, and squamous cell carcinoma, may be exposed to small doses of x-rays and develop postirradiation keratoses. Such cases are now becoming rare. Chronic radiation dermatitis and radiation keratosis may occur several months to many years after the exposure. The skin is atrophic with telangiectasia and irregular hyperpigmentation and hypopigmentation. Ulceration and foci of hyperkeratotic scale may be seen in areas of atrophy. Cutaneous malignancy frequency develops in these areas.

Microscopic Features

The epidermis is irregular, showing both atrophy and variable hyperplasia. There is hyperkeratosis, and the squamous cells show disorderly maturation, pleomorphism with individual cell keratinization, and atypia. Degeneration of the cells in the stratum malpighii and scanty lymphocytic exocytosis may be present.

In the dermis, the collagen bundles are enlarged and often show hyalinization. The deep dermal blood vessels often show fibrous thickening of their walls. Some of the vessels show thrombosis and recanalization. In contrast, the upper dermal vessels may be dilated. Lymphedema in the subepidermal region may be seen. Pilosebaceous units and sweat glands are usually preserved.

Carcinoma Arising in Radiation Keratosis (Radiation Carcinoma)

Squamous cell and basal cell carcinoma are the most common malignancies attributed to irradiation. In most cases, the tumor develops either within hyperkeratotic areas of chronic radiodermatitis or in a persistent ulcer. There is a long latent period between irradiation and carcinoma, varying from 4 to 39 years, with a median of 7–12 years. Before 1940 most reported cases of radiation carcinoma were squamous cell carcinoma occurring on the hands, feet, and occasionally, the face. An increasing number of basal cell carcinomas have been reported since 1951. In cases of radiation dermatitis, basal cell carcinoma develops almost exclusively on the head and neck, while in all other areas squamous cell carcinoma is more common. Many cases of radiation carcinoma seen in recent years have been due to treatment of acne or other benign disorders. Due to a general awareness of the potential dangers of repeated low-dose x-ray irradiation, it can be expected that the incidence of radiation carcinoma will decrease.

Squamous cell carcinoma arising in radiation keratosis is frequently of the spindle cell type. Large columns of atypical keratinocytes are connected to the overlying epidermis, and interlacing spindle-shaped cells with hyperchromatic nuclei, frequent mitoses, and abundant eosinophilic, sometimes vacuolated, cytoplasm are present. The dermal changes are similar to those seen in chronic radiodermatitis or radiation keratosis. Histologic differential diagnoses of spindle cell squamous cell carcinoma should include spindle cell amelanotic malignant melanoma, desmoplastic malignant melanoma, lentigo maligna melanoma, and atypical fibroxanthoma. Immunoperoxidase staining for cytokeratin is usually positive, and electron microscopic demonstration of intercellular desmosomes and cytoplasmic tonofilaments confirms the diagnosis.

Treatment

Radiation keratoses should be treated in the same way as solar keratoses. Radical surgical extirpation with skin grafting was standard treatment for radiation carcinoma in the past. Topical treatment with 5-FU has been effective for superficial tumors. Cryosurgery and Mohs micrographic surgery should be considered. Prevention or minimization of chronic x-ray exposure remains of paramount importance.

BOWEN'S DISEASE

Synonyms for this condition include Bowen's dermatosis, epithelioma of Bowen, precancerous dermatosis of Bowen, dyskeratose lenticulaire et en disque (Darier), squamous carcinoma in situ, and vulvar intraepithelial neoplasia.

Clinical Data and Gross Pathologic Appearance

Bowen's disease occurs in both sexes, but predominantly in fair-complexioned men; only one-fifth of patients are women. Sun-sensitive, predominantly older persons are affected most often. Bowen's disease is relatively rare. It is estimated to occur in less than 1% of the population. The average age at onset is 48 years. About one-third of cases involve the head and neck, particularly the face.

Bowen's disease is a slowly enlarging, reddish-brown, annular or polycyclic, scaly, fissured, crusty, eroded plaque (Fig. 8). The lesions are devoid of hair and are sharply demarcated from normal skin. Areas of normal-appearing skin may occur within the boundaries of larger plaques. The average duration to diagnosis is 6.4 years. Lesions of short duration appear as small, scaly, nonelevated keratoses. In the anogenital area, they are often verrucous and pigmented.

The criteria for referring to Bowen's disease as a precancerous lesion are based on microscopic carcinoma in situ involving the epidermis and the pilosebaceous epithelium. The association with extracutaneous malignancy has been controversial since Bowen first reported that a patient died of gastric carcinoma after having had Bowen's disease for 34 years. Similar observations have been made by several others. A recent study, however, showed no direct cause and effect relationship between Bowen's disease and internal malignancy.

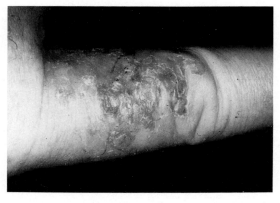

Figure 8 A focally pigmented, scaly plaque of Bowen's disease is sharply demarcated from the surrounding normal skin.

Microscopic Features

Typical microscopic features of Bowen's disease are hyperkeratosis, parakeratosis, hypergranulosis, acanthosis, and a chronic inflammatory infiltrate in the upper corium. The epidermis exhibits total or focal loss of normal polarity and progression of keratinocyte maturation. The loss of normal epidermal architecture is characterized by a windblown appearance of atypical keratinocytes, hyperchromatism, vacuolated cells, multinucleate cells, malignant dyskeratosis, and abnormal mitoses (Fig. 9). These changes occur at all epidermal levels but may be focal and are confined by an intact dermoepidermal basement membrane. Examination of lesions from hair-bearing areas shows involvement of the pilary acrotrichium, infundibulum, and sebaceous gland. The atypical cellular proliferation involves all levels of the outer root sheath and eventually replaces the sebaceous gland cells. In some lesions, the majority of the atypical epithelial cells appear vacuolated. Hyperchromatic undifferentiated keratinocytes replace the epidermal basal layer and the pilary outer root sheath. This gives the appearance of cellular nesting. The acrosyringium generally is not involved. The inflammatory infiltrate of lymphocytes, histiocytes, and sometimes plasma cells is seen in the upper corium. In the upper dermis there is capillary endothelial proliferation and some ectatic small vessels. Lesions located on the sun-exposed areas of the body show prominent solar elastosis.

The atypical vacuolated keratinocytes are routinely negative for cytoplasmic mucin; however, some contain glycogen. Melanin is present in the atypical cells in most lesions. The abnormal keratinizing cells are intensely reactive with glucose-6-phosphatase dehydrogenase.

Precancerous lesions of the genital skin, such as Bowen's disease (carcinoma in situ) and bowenoid papulosis, are associated with human papillomavirus (HPV) of the high-risk types (HPV types 16,18,31,33, and 35). The mechanism of malignant transformation of keratinocytes in these lesions has been shown to involve E6 and E7 segments of oncoprotein of these high-risk HPVs. HPVs possess multiple capabilities to promote tumorigenesis by defeating intracellular defense

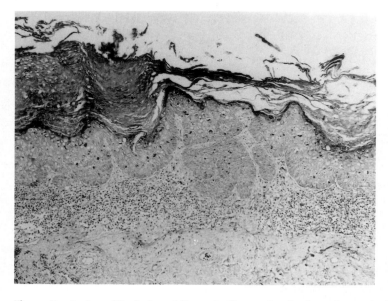

Figure 9 A plaquelike lesion of Bowen's disease showing hyperkeratosis, hypergranulosis, absent normal keratinocyte maturation, and atypical keratinocytes replacing the entire thickness of the epidermis (hematoxylin & eosin, ×75).

mechanisms against neoplastic proliferation. The most critical is the double inactivation of the two antioncogene products p53 and pRB. This causes failure to eliminate, through programmed cell death (apoptosis), cells that have incurred DNA damage. These events lead to the persistence of cells that may have initiated neoplastic alterations. With contribution from additional internal and external cofactors, malignant transformation of the keratinocytes is then set into motion.

Nongenital Bowen's disease has been less well investigated for the presence of HPV. Clinical factors associated with the presence of HPV's in nongenital lesions of Bowen's disease included black skin, location of the palmar surface and the feet, young age, and verrucous or hyperkeratotic clinical appearance.

Ultrastructural changes include abnormal cell division of dyskeratotic cells, abnormal mitotic figures, decrease in tonofilament-desmosomal attachments, absence of keratohyalin, and aggregate tonofilaments and nuclear substances.

Bowen's Disease and Invasive Adnexal Carcinoma

Without treatment, about 3–5% of patients with Bowen's disease develop invasive carcinoma. This commonly presents as a rapidly growing, ulcerating or nodular tumor in a preexisting patch of many years' duration (Fig. 10). In a study of 100 such cases from the Armed Forces Institute of Pathology, the patients ranged from 29 to 91 years with a male/female ratio of 3:1 and a white/black ratio of 20:1. The extremities, face, and anogenital areas were common sites of involvement. The size of the tumor varied from 1 to 12 cm. Histopathologic evidence of Bowen's disease was identified in all cases. The cytologic changes of invasive adnexal carcinoma showed basaloid, squamoid, pilar, pilosebaceous (Fig. 11), and occasionally glandular differentiation favoring interpretation of the invasive lesion as a form of adnexal carcinoma. Mitoses and malignant dyskeratosis are commonly seen.

Differential Diagnosis

Bowenoid solar keratosis differs from Bowen's disease. The former is usually smaller, occurring almost exclusively on sun-exposed areas. On microscopic examination the atypical squamous keratinocytes do not involve the entire thickness of the epidermis or pilary epithelium as seen

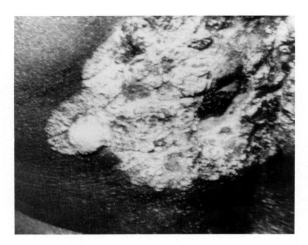

Figure 10   An invasive carcinoma module (arrow) arising in a large plaque of Bowen's disease of prolonged duration on the back of an African man.

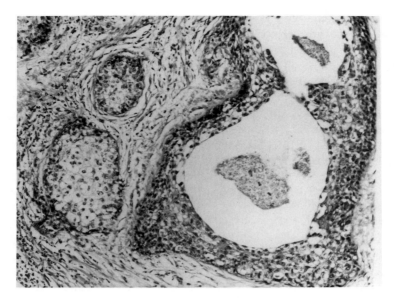

Figure 11 Invasive adnexal carcinoma arising in Bowen's disease shows prominent pilar and epilosebaceous differentiation (hematoxylin & eosin, ×250).

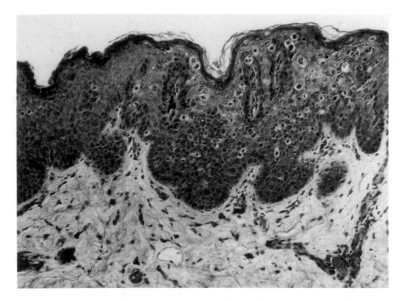

Figure 12 A section of vulvar bowenoid papulosis showing mild hyperkeratosis, vacuolated cells, acanthosis, and scattered dysplastic and dyskeratotic keratinocytes (hematoxylin & eosin, ×160).

in Bowen's disease. Mammary and extramammary Paget's disease may share with Bowen's disease the presence of vacuolated cells, but in contrast there is no dyskeratosis. In addition, the cytoplasm of Paget's cells often contains sialomucin. The material in vacuolated cells of Bowen's disease is glycogen. The cellular nesting of vacuolated pageotoid cells in some lesions of Bowen's disease can cause confusion with malignant melanoma and intraepidermal epithelioma.

Bowenoid papulosis shares some histologic similarity with Bowen's disease, particularly the presence of keratinocyte atypia and mitoses. Therefore, Bowen's disease involving the genitalia must be differentiated from bowenoid papulosis, which shows an orderly background with scattered dysplastic, dyskeratotic cells and mitotic figures in a salt-and-pepper fashion (Fig. 12). Atypical keratinocytes are seen in full thickness in epidermis, pilosebaceous epithelium, and mucosal epithelium in Bowen's disease and carcinoma in situ and not in bowenoid papulosis. Plasma cells are rare in the dermal and submucosal infiltrate in bowenoid papulosis, in contrast to Bowen's disease.

The clinical presentation of bowenoid papulosis is quite different from that of Bowen's disease. Bowenoid papuloses predominantly affect patients under the age of 46 and are typically small, dome-shaped papules or plaques located on the external genitalia (Fig. 13). Bowenoid papulosis is considered benign, and spontaneous regression is common (Fig. 14). Condyloma acuminatum with epithelial atypia may sometimes be mistaken for Bowen's disease. Superficial keratinocyte maturation and prominent koilocytotic atypia with vacuolated cells in the parakeratotic layer typify condylomata. The role of human papillomavirus in all these lesions as a precursor of malignancy has yet to be clarified.

Treatment

The origin of Bowen's disease from pilary outer root sheath cells at the sebaceous gland level helps explain the high recurrence rate after treatment with superficial x-ray, curettage and desiccation, and topical 5-FU. Mohs micrographic surgery should be considered. Liquid nitrogen cryotherapy and topical chemotherapy with 5-FU are less effective. Ionizing radiation using soft x-rays is suitable for elderly patients who are poor candidates for surgery. CO_2 laser vaporization has been used but is limited because of the lack of histologic margin control.

Thus, excision of Bowen's disease is the best modality. This allows complete microscopic evaluation of the surgical margins. Acetowidening has been described as assisting in the enhancement of clinical margins of Bowen's disease. Photodynamic therapy may be used as an adjuvant therapy for Bowen's disease occurring in various difficult anatomic sites or lesions of unusually large size. Photofrin 1.0 mg/kg is administered intravenously and laser treatment given 48 hr later with the argon dye laser. Light is administered at a wavelength of 630 nm and the dosage ranges from 185 to 250 J/cm^2. Treatment is given by surface radiation only.

ARSENICAL KERATOSIS AND ARSENICAL CARCINOMA

Arsenical keratoses frequently present as cornlike, punctate papules on the extremities, characteristically affecting the palms and soles (Fig. 15). The microscopic features and subsequent carcinoma are indistinguishable from Bowen's disease and subsequent adnexal carcinoma. Intake of arsenic in small amounts for long periods produces a general neoplastic tendency. It is possible that arsenic is a cause of Bowen's disease. There is an affinity of arsenic for keratinizing epithelium.

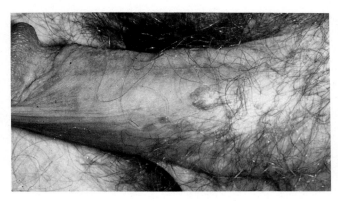

Figure 13 Flesh-colored, grouped papules of bowenoid papulosis on the penile shaft of a 28-year-old man.

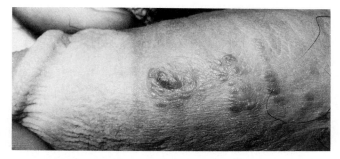

Figure 14 Spontaneous regression of bowenoid papulosis in a 26-year-old man, noted 2 weeks after biopsy.

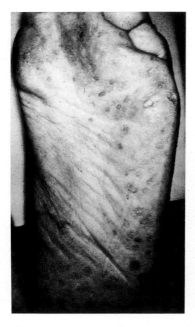

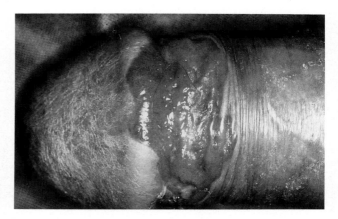

Figure 15 Cornlike, punctate, arsenical keratosis on the soles of a patient with a history of chronic arsenism.

Figure 16 A well-demarcated, focally eroded plaque of erythroplasia of Queyrat involving the penile skin, mucosa of the glans penis, and corona sulcus.

Differential Diagnosis

Arsenical keratoses must be differentiated from punctate keratoderma. Darier's disease, and lichen planus. Plantar warts are more papillomatous and are easily differentiated microscopically.

Treatment

The multiplicity of the lesions makes radical treatment and complete removal impractical. Frequent monitoring for clinical evidence of carcinoma is important. Keratolytics such as salicyclic acid, urea, and lactic acid as well as physical debridement are helpful.

ERYTHROPLASIA OF QUEYRAT

Synonyms include carcinoma in situ and Bowen's disease of the glans penis.

Clinical Data and Gross Pathologic Appearance

Erythroplasia of Queyrat is a distinct clinicopathologic entity: carcinoma in situ involving the penile skin, mucosa, and mucocutaneous junction of the glans penis. The clinical and histologic features of erythroplasia of Queyrat are similar to Bowen's disease, particularly involving the vulva. The disease occurs almost exclusively in uncircumcised men. It typically manifests as an asymptomatic, well-demarcated, red, velvety plaque with yellow crusted flecks on the glans penis, in the coronal sulcus (Fig. 16), or on the inner surface of the prepuce. Ulceration, crusting, and erosion are sometimes observed. The disease more commonly affects middle-aged and older men. The average duration to diagnosis is about 3 years, and the median lesion size is 1.0 cm.

Microscopic Features

Erythroplasia of Queyrat shows thickening of the epidermis and mucosa with increased cellularity, hypokeratosis, and focal erosion. The normal keratinocytes are entirely replaced by nonkeratinizing basaloid cells with mild nuclear hyperchromatism and pleomorphism. The microscopic features are those of carcinoma in situ.

Adnexal Carcinoma Arising in Erythroplasia of Queyrat

Without adequate treatment, up to 30% of patients may develop invasive carcinoma. Squamous, basaloid, and ductal differentiation are frequently observed. About 20% of those with invasive carcinoma develop metastasis.

Surgical excision is the treatment of choice. Electrodesiccation and curettage and topical 5-FU are effective. A 1–2% 5-FU cream is applied. If no reaction occurs with twice-daily application after 1 week, 5% 5-FU should be used. Application under occlusion may be more effective. Phallectomy with inguinal lymph node dissection is reserved for cases of invasive carcinoma. When ionizing irradiation is used as the only treatment, a high recurrence rate (up to 80%) has been noted. Mohs micrographic surgery may be the best approach.

INTRAEPIDERMAL EPITHELIOMA

Synonyms for this condition include intraepidermal epithelioma of Borst-Jadassohn, intraepidermal basal cell epithelioma, combined intraepidermal basosquamous carcinoma, intraepidermal acanthoma, intraepidermal nevus, hidroacanthoma simplex, eccrine poroepithelioma, and intraepidermal eccrine poroma.

Clinical Data and Gross Pathologic Appearance

Intraepidermal epithelioma occurs as a single gray to tan-brown, keratotic, scaly, flat, sometimes verrucous, round to irregularly shaped papule, plaque, or nodule varying from 0.5 to 10 cm in diameter. The plaque usually is sharply demarcated from the adjacent skin. Differentiation from seborrheic keratosis requires microscopic examination. Papillary lesions are uncommon, and erosion and ulceration sometimes occur. Lesions occur on all parts of the body except the palms and soles. About 25% occur on the head and neck, particularly the face (17%), 46% on the lower extremities, and the rest on other parts of the body; in decreasing order of frequency: the buttocks, chest, back, upper extremity, abdomen, and feet. They predominantly occur in white patients aged 40–79 years and more commonly in women than men. The duration to diagnosis varies from less than 1 month to more than 30 years, but more than half are present for less than 3 years.

There is controversy about the cell of origin. Some conclude that the lesion represents a benign epidermal proliferation. The cells of origin are acrosyringial keratinocytes or multipluripotential adnexal cells. When the dermoepidermal basement membrane is disrupted and atypical keratinocytes invade the corium, intraepidermal epithelioma is considered to represent an adnexal eccrine carcinoma. Support for eccrine histogenesis is based on histopathologic features and immunohistochemical studies, particularly evidence of carcinoembryonic antigen and enzyme reactivity of discrete cell nests. Intraepidermal epithelioma may represent the premalignant counterpart of eccrine porocarcinoma. Long-term follow-up shows that 15% of patients develop local recurrences, in most cases due to incomplete removal.

Microscopic Features

Intraepidermal epithelioma is characterized by hyperkeratosis, spotted parakeratosis, hypergranu-losis, occasional horn cysts, and plaquelike acanthosis, with discrete nests of uniform and dys-plastic keratinocytes composed of basaloid or squamoid cell types within the stratum malpighii (Fig. 17). Some lesions show prominent papillomatosis and verrucous acanthosis. Spindle-shaped, pigmented cells are sometimes present. Some keratinocytes form squamous eddies reminiscent of inflamed seborrheic keratosis, inverted follicular keratosis, and epidermal nevus. The pig-mented lesions have melanin pigment associated with discrete nests of keratinocytes. Capillary-endothelial proliferation, ascular ectasia, and fibrosis are present in the upper dermis of most lesions. The dermoepidermal basement membrane remains intact for long periods of time in most cases.

Intraepidermal Epithelioma and Invasive Carcinoma

Eight percent of patients show clinical and microscopic evidence of invasive carcinoma in the primary lesion. In general, these lesions are larger and appear papillary with areas of erosion and ulceration (Fig. 18). There are intraepidermal cell nests with marked cellular atypia, pleo-morphism, malignant dyskeratosis, vacuolated cells, mitotic figures, and occasionally multinucle-ate cells and disruption of the dermoepidermal basement membrane with atypical keratinocytes invading the dermis. The tumor cells infiltrating the dermis and those at metastatic sites show some tendency to nesting, as seen in the epidermis. This tumor should be regarded as a form of adnexal carcinoma. Metastasis occurs in 6% of patients. The potential for distant metastasis requires consideration of intraepidermal epithelioma along with other cutaneous premalignant neoplasms.

Differential Diagnosis

Cutaneous epithelial neoplasms with cellular nesting can be confused with intraepidermal epi-thelioma; these include seborrheic keratosis, epidermal nevus, inverted follicular keratosis, lichenoid benign keratosis, Bowen's disease, mammary and extramammary Paget's disease, spindle cell nevus, and precancerous-acquired melanosis (melanoma in situ). Epidermal nevi demonstrate squamous eddy formation when inflamed and are often confused with intraepidermal epithelioma.

Treatment

Excision, curettage, and desiccation are acceptable methods of treatment.

LENTIGO MALIGNA (MELANOTIC FRECKLE OF HUTCHINSON)

Synonyms for this condition include senile freckle, lentigo malin des vieillards, melanese cir-conscrite precancereuse, premalignant lentigo, malignant freckle, precancerous melanosis, and acquired melanosis.

Clinical Data and Gross Pathologic Appearance

Lentigo maligna or melanotic freckle of Hutchinson is a multicentric melanocytic disorder of the epidermal melanocytes, the clinical features of which were described by Hutchinson in the early 1890s. It begins as a small brown pigmented macule that slowly extends in an irregular fashion. The lesion is composed of small spots and lines of pigment. The color varies, producing a var-iegated pigmented macule. Individual lesions are light to dark brown or gray and black (Fig. 19).

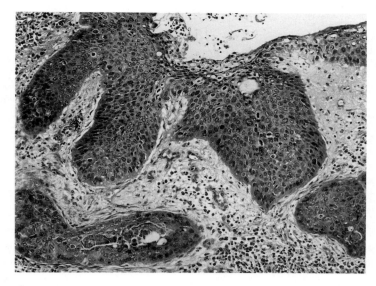

Figure 17 Photomicrograph of adnexal carcinoma shows full thickness of mucosal epithelial dysplasia and an invasive adnexal carcinoma showing prominent ductal differentiation (hematoxylin & eosin, ×250).

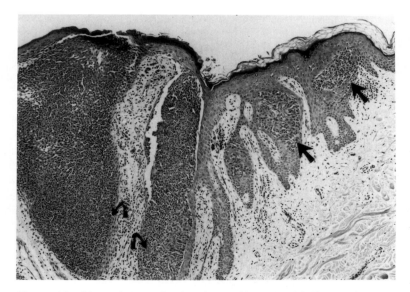

Figure 18 Photomicrograph of an intraepidermal epithelioma with focal invasive adnexal carcinoma exhibits intraepidermal nests of keratinocytes with mild pleomorphism (straight arrows). These cell nests are distinct from the subjacent epidermal keratinocytes. Focal upper dermal invasion is present (curved arrows) (hematoxylin & eosin, ×160).

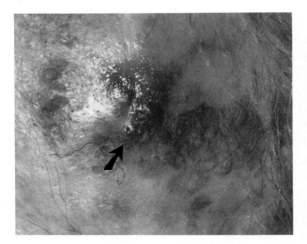

Figure 19 A pigmented macule of lentigo maligna with irregular border on the temple of an elderly man. Nodules of lentigo maligna melanoma that developed from lentigo maligna (arrow) are noted.

The clinical appearance of the surrounding skin is unremarkable; however, elderly patients with lentigo maligna on sun-exposed skin occasionally have other sun-induced lesions in the vicinity. Lentigo maligna occurs exclusively in whites, while men and women are equally affected. It is predominantly a disease of the middle-aged and elderly; patients' ages average 57 years. Only 10% of cases are found in patients younger than 40 years. The average duration is 14 years. The most common location is the head, particularly the face (over 50%) and neck, but other areas including the back, upper extremity, chest, and abdomen are also affected. The size varies from 1 to 3 cm. Larger lesions, particularly those greater than 4 cm, are more likely to develop lentigo maligna melanoma.

Microscopic Features

A single layer of pleomorphic, hyperchromatic, frequently spindle-shaped, atypical melanocytes replaces the dermoepidermal junction (Fig. 20, left). The junctional change is extensive and frequently extends along the outer root sheath of the hair follicle. Nests and theques of similar cells are sometimes present. The atypical melanocytes are often vacuolated with clear cytoplasm and irregular, hyperchromatic nuclei resembling Paget's cells. Spindle-cell forms of typical melanocytes are common; however, multinucleate cells and mitoses are rare. A bandlike inflammatory infiltrate in the upper dermis is usually present.

PRECANCEROUS ACQUIRED PIGMENTED MELANOSIS

Synonyms for this condition include premalignant melanocytic dysplasia, atypical melanocytic hyperplasia, malignant melanoma in situ, precancerous melanosis of the compound nevus type, and malignant melanoma, Clark's level I.

Clinical Data and Gross Pathologic Appearance

Precancerous melanosis is a melanocytic disorder of the epidermal melanocytes. The clinical features of this neoplasm are similar to lentigo maligna. The clinical location, however, includes

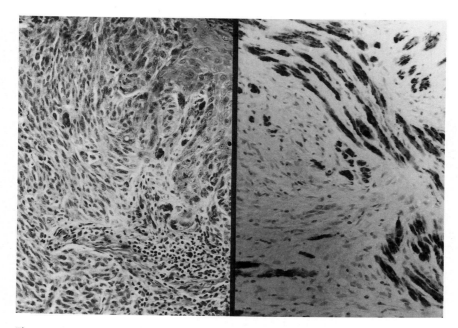

Figure 20 Photomicrograph of a lentigo maligna showing diffuse spindle-shaped melanoma cells at dermo-epidermal junction (left) (hematoxylin & eosin, ×160). Adjacent desmoplastic melanoma consists of prominent fibrous stroma separating fascicles of spindle-shaped melanoma cells with strongly positive S-100 protein stain (right) (immunoperoxidase stain, ×250).

both sun-exposed and non-exposed skin. The brown pigmented macule slowly extends laterally with an irregular border and variegated pigmentation (Fig. 21). The color varies from dark brown to gray or black. The adjacent skin is usually unremarkable. The patients are middle-aged or older. Without treatment, lesions progress to become nodules and increase in size, which are signs of malignant melanoma. Lesions vary in size from a few millimeters to 2–3 cm. An adequate excisional specimen is essential for accurate distinction from melanoma.

Microscopic Features

The histologic findings include nests, theques, or individual atypical melanocytes present at the dermoepidermal junction or scattered in all layers of the epidermis (Fig. 22). The junctional change is extensive and frequently extends into the pilary epithelium. Nuclear pleomorphism with large epithelioid cells, spindle-shaped atypical melanocytes, and mitoses is characteristic. Dyskeratotic cells and eosinophilic bodies (apoptotoic cells, Kamino bodies) are sometimes seen. Pre-existing benign nevocellular nevus cells can be identified in about one-third of lesions.

Prognosis and Treatment

Precancerous melanosis is treated by complete surgical excision. The lesions will recur following incomplete excision. Lack of treatment will eventually result in invasion of the dermis.

Lentigo maligna is often treated with superficial therapies that are associated with high recurrence rates. The high recurrence rates are a result of incomplete destruction or removal of tumor from clinically inapparent but histopathologically positive areas. The problem with super-

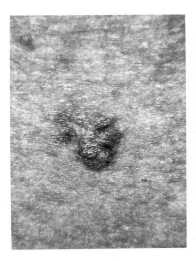

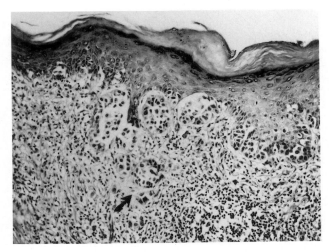

Figure 21 An enlarging precancerous melanosis with irregular border and pigmentation present on the arm of a 30-year-old man for 6 months.

Figure 22 Photomicrograph of a precancerous melanosis of the compound nevus type illustrates extensive dermoepidermal junction involvement by nests of pleomorphic, atypical melanocytes with focal superficial malignant melanoma (arrow) (0.45 mm in depth; Clark's level II) (hematoxylin & eosin, ×250).

ficial therapies is that the atypical melanocytes often infiltrate along the pilosebaceous epithelium and extend deep into the dermis. These cells are protected from superficial therapy and are the foci of recurrences.

Mohs micrographic surgery with rapid permanent sections is effective for the complete removal of this melanocytic neoplasm. Topical azelaic acid has been used in patients unable to undergo surgery with close clinical monitoring and treatment of recurrences. Cryotherapy has also been used to treat lesions of lentigo maligna and lentigo maligna melanoma. However, because of the problems related to superficial removal of the lesions as discussed above, this modality should be used with caution.

BIBLIOGRAPHY

Ackerman AB. Histopathologists can diagnose malignant melanoma in situ correctly and consistently. *Am J Dermatopathol* 1984;6:103–107.

Ackerman AB, Godomski J. Neurotropic malignant melanoma and other neurotropic neoplasms in the skin. *Am J Dermatopathol* 1984;6:63–80.

Anderson, NP, Anderson HE. Development of basal cell epithelioma as a consequence of radiodermatitis. *Arch Dermatol Syphilol* 1951;63:586.

Arbesmain H, Ransohoff DF. Is Bowen's disease a predictor for the development of internal malignancy? A methodological critique of the literature. *JAMA* 1987;257:516–518.

Baker EJ, Hobbs ER. Enhancement of the clinical margins of Bowen's disease by acetowidening. *J Dermatol Surg Oncol* 1990;16:846–850.

Berger P, Baughman R. Intraepidermal epithelioma. *Br J Dermatol* 1979;9:343.

Berger TG, Graham JH, Goette DK. Lichenoid benign keratosis. *J Am Acad Dermatol* 1984;11:635–638.

Bettley FR, O'Shea JA. The absorption of arsenic and its relation to carcinoma. *Br J Dermatol* 1975;92:563.

Bowen JT. Precancerous dermatoses: The further course of 2 cases previously reported. *Arch Dermatol Syphilol* 1920;1:23.

Braverman IM. *Skin Signs of Systemic Disease*. 2nd ed. Philadelphia, WB Saunders, 1981, pp. 67–77.

Brownstein MH, Rabinowitz AD. The precursors of cutaneous squamous cell carcinoma. *Int J Dermatol* 1979;18:1.

Callen JP. *Cutaneous Aspects of Internal Disease*. Chicago, Year Book Medical Publishers, 1981, pp. 209–212.

Callen JP, Headington J. Bowen's and non-Bowen's squamous intraepidermal neoplasia of the skin. *Arch Dermatol* 1980;116:422.

Campbell C, Quinn AG, et al. p53 mutations are common and early events that precede tumor invasion in squamous cell neoplasia of the skin. *J Invest Dermatol* 1993;100:746–748.

Chiarello SE. Full-face cryo- (liquid nitrogen) peel. *J Dermatol Surg Oncol* 1992;18:329–332.

Clark WH, From L, et al. Histogenesis and biologic behavior of primary human malignant melanomas of the skin. *Cancer Res* 1969;29:705–727.

Clark WH, Mihm MC. Lentigo maligna and lentigo maligna melanoma. *Am J Pathol* 1969;55:39.

Collins P, Rogers S, et al. Cryotherapy for lentigo maligna. *Clin Exp Dermatol* 1991;16:433–435.

Conley J, Lattes R, Orr W. Desmoplastic malignant melanoma (a rare variant of spindle cell melanoma). *Cancer* 1971;28:914.

Cook MG, Ridgway HA. The intraepidermal epithelioma of Jadassohn: a distinct entity. *Br J Dermatol* 1979;101:659.

Costello MJ, Fisher SB, DeFeo CP. Melanotic freckle—lentigo maligna. *Arch Dermatol* 1959;80:753.

Cox FH, Becker FF. Metastatic potential of biologic variants of skin squamous cell carcinoma. *J Fla Med Assoc* 1982;69:516.

Dhawan SS, Wolf DJ, et al. Lentigo maligna. The use of rush permanent sections in therapy. *Arch Dermatol* 1990;126:928–930.

Dubrenich MW. Lentigo malin des vieillards. *Bull Soc Fr Dermatol Syphiligr* 1984;460.

Edwards L, Levine N, et al. The effective topical interferon Alpha 2 b. on actinic keratoses. *J Dermatol Surg Oncol* 1990;16:445–449.

Goette DK. Erythroplasia of Queyrat. *Arch Dermatol* 1974;110:271–273.

Goette DK. Topical chemotherapy with 5-fluorouracil. *J Am Acad Dermatol* 1981;4:633–649.

Goltz RW, Fusaro RM, Sweitzer SE. Borst-Jadassohn epithelioma. *Arch Dermatol* 1957;75:117.

Graham JH. Is Bowen's disease a marker of internal cancer? In *Controversies in Dermatology*. E. Epstein, ed. Philadelphia, WB Saunders, 1984, pp. 86–95.

Graham JH. Selected precancerous skin and mucocutaneous lesions. In *Neoplasms of the Skin and Malignant Melanoma*. Chicago, Year Book Medical Publishers, 1976, pp. 86–99, 118–121.

Graham JH, Helwig EB. Premalignant cutaneous and mucocutaneous diseases. In *Dermal Pathology*. JH Graham, WC Johnson, EB Helwig, eds. Hagerstown, MD, Harper & Row, 1972, pp. 561–581.

Graham JH, Helwig EB. Erythroplasia of Queyrat. A clinicopathologic and histochemical study. *Cancer* 1973;32:1396–1414.

Gray MH, Sandler BS, et al. Carcinogenesis in porokeratosis. Evidence for a role relating to chronic growth activation of keratinocytes. *Am J Dermatopathol* 1991;13:438–444.

Griffin TD, Van Scott EJ. Use of pyruvic acid in the treatment of actinic keratoses: a clinical and histopathologic study. *Cutis* 1991;47:325–329.

Haber H. Intraepidermal epithelioma (Borst–Jadassohn). *Trans St. Johns Hosp Dermatol Soc* 1954;33:46.

Haber H. Intraepidermal acanthoma. *Dermatologica* 1958;117:304.

Haber H, Seville RH. Borst–Jadassohn intraepidermal epithelioma. *Proc R Soc Med* 1953;46:171.

Holman CD, Armstrong BK, et al. Relationship of solar keratosis and history of skin cancer to objective measures of actinic skin damage. *Br J Dermatol* 1984;110:129–138.

Holubar K, Wolff K. Intraepidermal eccrine poroma. *Cancer* 1969;23:626.

Ikenberg H, Gissmann L, et al. Human papillomavirus type 16 related DNA in genital Bowen's disease and in bowenoid papulosis. *Int J Cancer* 1983;32:563–565.

Ishikawa K. Malignant hidroacanthoma simplex. *Arch Dermatol* 1971;104:529.

Jackson R, Williamson GS, Beattie WG. Lentigo maligna and malignant melanoma. *Can Med Assoc J* 1966;95:846.

Johnson WC, Helwig EB. Adenoid squamous cell carcinoma (adenocanthoma). *Cancer* 1966;19:1639.

Jones CM, Mang T, et al. Photodynamic therapy in the treatment of Bowen's disease. *J Am Acad Dermatol* 1992;27:979–982.

Kamino Hm, Ackerman AB. Malignant melanoma in situ. The evolution of malignant melanoma within the epidermis. In *Pathology of Malignant Melanoma*. AB Ackerman, ed. New York, Masson, 1981, pp. 59–91.

Kao GF. Carcinoma arising in Bowen's disease (editorial). *Arch Dermatol* 1986;122:1124–1126.

Kao GF, Graham JH. Premalignant cutaneous disorders of the head and neck. In *Otolaryngology*. Vol. 5. GM English, ed. Philadelphia, Harper & Row, 1987, 58, pp. 1–20.

Kao GF, Kao WH. Malignant transformation of keratinocytes by human papillovavirus. *J Cutan Pathol* 1994.

Kettler AH, Rutledge M, et al. Detection of human papillomavirus in nongenital Bowen's disease by in situ DNA hybridization. *Arch Dermatol* 1990;126:777–781.

King CM, Yates VM, Dave VK. Multicentric pigmented Bowen's disease of the genitalia associated with carcinoma in situ of the cervix. *Br J Vener Dis* 1984;60:406–408.

Lane CW. Senile freckle. *Arch Dermatol* 1930;21:494.

Lever WF, Schaumburg-Lever G. Tumors and cysts of the epidermis. In *Histopathology of the Skin*. WF Lever, G Schaumburg-Lever, eds. Philadelphia, JB Lippincott, 1983, pp. 489–493, 498.

Maiorana A, Nigrisoli E, Papotti M. Immunohistochemical markers of sweat gland tumors. *J Cutan Pathol* 1986;13:187–196.

Marks R, Jolley D, et al. The role of childhood exposure to sunlight in the development of solar keratoses in nonmelanocytic skin cancer. Med J Aust 1990;152:52–66.

Mehregan AH, Levson DN. Hidroacanthoma simplex. *Arch Dermatol* 1969;100:303.

Mehregan AH, Pinkus H. Intraepidermal epithelioma: a critical study. *Cancer* 1964;17:609.

Mikhail GR. Cancers, precancers and pseudocancers on the male genitalia. *J Dermatol Surg Oncol* 1980;6:1027–1035.

Miki Y, Kawatsu T, Matsuda K, et al. Cutaneous and pulmonary cancers associated with Bowen's disease. *J Am Acad Dermatol* 1982;6:26.

Misiewicz J, Sendagorta E, et al. Topical treatment of multiple actinic keratoses of the face with arotinoid methyl sulfone (Ro 14-9706) cream versus trentinoin cream: a double-blind, comparative study. *J Am Acad Dermatol* 1991;24:448–451.

Mishima Y. Epitheliomatous differentiation of the interepidermal eccrine sweat duct. *J Invest Dermatol* 1969;52:233.

Mitchell RE. Squamous cell carcinoma developing in the Jadassohn phenomenon: a case report. *Australas J Dermatol* 1975;16:79.

Nagano T, Ueda M, et al. Expression of p53 protein is an early event in UV-light induced cutaneous squamous cell carcinoma. *Arch Dermatol* 1993;129:1157–1161.

Nazzaro-Porro M, Passi S, et al. Ten years' experience of treating lentigo maligna with topical azelaic acid. *Acta Dermato-Venereol* (suppl) 1989;143:49–57.

Nelson MA, Janine E, et al. Mutations in the p53 and H-ras gene in human actinic keratosis lesions and squamous cell cancers. *Proc Am Assoc Cancer Res* 1994;35:622.

Ollstein RN, Kaplan HS, Crikelair GF, et al. Is there a malignant freckle? *Cancer* 1966;19:767.

Olsen EA, Abernethy ML, et al. A double-blind vehicle controlled study evaluating Masoprocol cream in the treatment of actinic keratoses on the head and neck. *J Am Acad Dermatol* 1991;24:738–743.

Patterson JW, Kao GF, et al. Bowenoid papulosis. A clinicopathologic study with ultastructural observations. *Cancer* 1986;57:823–836.

Pearlman DL. Weekly pulse dosing: effective and comfortable topical 5 Fluorouracil treatment of multiple facial actinic keratoses. *J Am Acad Dermatol* 1991,25:665–667.

Penneys NS, Nadji M, Morales A. Carcinoembryonic antigen in benign sweat gland tumors. *Arch Dermatol* 1982;118:225.

Pinkus H. Keratosis senilis. *Am J Clin Pathol* 1958;29:193.

Reed RJ, Clark WH Jr, Mihm MC. Premalignant melanocytic dysplasias. In *Pathology of Malignant Melanoma*. AB Ackerman, ed. New York, Masson, 1981, p. 178.

Reed RJ, Leonard DD. Neurotropic melanoma: A variant of desmoplastic melanoma. *Am J Surg Pathol* 1979;3:301–311.

Reese AB. Precancerous and cancerous melanosis. *Am J Ophthalmol* 1966;61:1272.

Reese AB. Precancerous melanosis and the resulting malignant melanoma (cancerous melanosis) of the conjunctiva and lids. *Arch Ophthalmol* 1943;29:737.

Robinson JK. Actinic cheilitis. A prospective study comparing four different treatment methods. *Arch Otolaryng* 1989;115:848–852.

Rywlin AM. Malignant melanoma in situ, precancerous melanosis, or atypical intraepidermal melanocytic proliferation. *Am J Dermatopathol* 1984;6:97–100.

Sachs W. Intraepidermal nevus. *Arch Dermatol* 1952;65:110.

Sagebiel RW. Histopathology of borderline and early malignant melanomas. *Am J Surg Pathol* 1979;3: 543–552.

Saunders TS, Montgomery H. Chronic roentgen and radium dermatitis. *JAMA* 1938;110:23.

Scheffner M, Werness, BA, Hulbregtse JM, et al. The E6 oncoprotein encoded by human papillomavirus types 16 and 18 promotes the degeneration of p53. *Cell* 1990;63:1129–1136.

Siegel JM. Intraepidermal epithelioma of Jadassohn. *Arch Dermatol* 1974;110:478.

Sims, CF, Parker RL. Intraepidermal basal cell epithelioma. *Arch Dermatol* 1949;59:45.

Sims CS, Slater S, McKee PH. Mutant p53 expression in solar keratosis: an immunohistochemical study. *J Cutan Pathol* 1992;19:302–308.

Smith JLS, Coburn JG. Hidroacanthoma simplex. *Br J Dermatol* 1956;68:400.

Stanley RJ, Roenigk RK. Actinic cheilitis: Treatment with the carbon dioxide laser. *Mayo Clin Proc* 1988;63: 230–235.

Steffen C, Ackerman AB. Intraepidermal epithelioma of Borst-Jadassohn. *Am J Dermatopathol* 1985;7:5–24.

Sturm HM. Bowen's disease and 5-fluorouracil. *J Am Acad Dermatol* 1979;1:513–522.

Subrt P, Jorizzo JL, Apisarnthanarax P, et al. Spreading pigmented actinic keratosis. *J Am Acad Dermatol* 1983;8:63–67.

Thompson SC. Reduction of solar keratoses by regular sun screen use. *N Engl J Med* 1993;329:1147–1151.

Urback F. Reactions to physical agents. In *Dermatology*, Vol. 2, SL Moschella, DM Pillsbury, HJ Hurley Jr., eds. Philadelphia, WB Saunders, 1975, pp. 1452–1455.

Vitasa BC, Taylor HR, et al. Association of nonmelanoma skin cancer in actinic keratosis with cumulative solar ultraviolet exposure in Maryland Waterman. Cancer 1990;65:2811–2817.

Wade TR, Ackerman AB. The many faces of solar keratoses. *J Dermatol Surg Oncol* 1978;4:730–734.

Wayte DM, Helwig EB. Melanotic freckle of Hutchinson. *Cancer* 1968;21:893.

Winton GB, Salasche SJ. Dermabrasion of the scalp as a treatment for actinic damage. *J Am Acad Dermatol* 1986;14:661–667.

Wolf P, Rieger E, Kerl H. Topical photodynamic therapy with endogenous porphyrins after application of 50aminolevulinic acid. An alternative treatment modality for solar keratoses, superficial squamous cell carcinomas, and basal cell carcinomas? *J Am Acad Dermatol* 1993;28:17–21.

Wu YL, Casey DM. Custom lip shield for chronic actinic cheilitis. *J Prosthet Dent* 1991;65:284–286.

Yeh S. Cancer in chronic arsenicism. *Hum Pathol* 1973;4:469–485.

28

Dermal and Subcutaneous Tumors

Richard M. Rubenstein
Northwestern University Medical School, Chicago, Illinois

DERMATOFIBROMAS

Dermatofibromas are benign dermal tumors that usually present as a papule or nodule on the lower extremities (Fig. 1). They are generally solitary, although multiple lesions do occur. Women are affected more frequently than men, and often there is a history of trauma or insect bite.

The typical lesion is a 0.5–1-cm dome-shaped, firm brown nodule attached to the overlying skin, but freely movable and unattached to the subcutaneous tissues. Lateral compression on the tumor produces a depression or characteristic dimple sign. These tumors may grow rapidly in a short period, then reach a maximal size and persist. Regression occurs uncommonly.

Histologically, dermatofibromas are composed of fibroblasts, mature collagen, capillaries, and histiocytes. They may appear fibrous if they are composed mainly of fibroblasts and collagen or cellular if histiocytes predominate. The epidermis is spared, but the tumor can involve much of the dermis and extend into the subcutis.

Treatment of dermatofibromas is not necessary. Reassuring the patient of the benign nature of the lesion is frequently all that is required. If treatment is requested, surgical excision is the method of choice. Since the tumor can extend into the deep layers of the subcutis, a deep elliptical excision is recommended with removal of all tissue to the fascial layer. The lateral margins need only encompass the nodule itself. The defect created is usually not large and can be closed after careful undermining with subcutaneous and skin sutures. Because these lesions are usually on the lower extremity, risks inherent to that location, such as wound separation, infection, or slower healing, must be considered during the postoperative care. Recurrence is less than 5% and is probably related to the incomplete removal of the deepest layers.

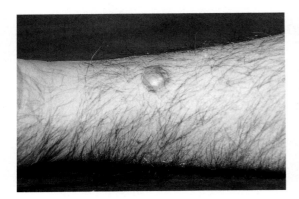

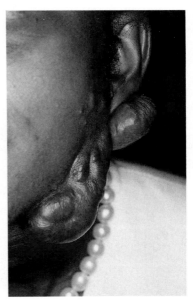

Figure 1 Dermatofibroma.   **Figure 2** Keloid.

KELOIDS

Hypertrophic scars, or keloids, are proliferations of fibrous tissue, usually occurring in sites of tissue injury. By definition, a hypertrophic scar remains in the boundary of the site of initial trauma, while keloids grow beyond this area. Keloids are firm, slightly tender or pruritic, hyperpigmented nodules or tumors (Fig. 2). They tend to occur in areas where skin tension from underlying musculature pulls across the wound, such as the deltoid region or on the anterior chest. There is a rapid growth phase lasting several weeks or months after the inciting event, followed by a more stable period of growth. There is a genetic predilection, especially in black patients. Histologically, there is a fibroblastic proliferation, with formation of new collagen bundles.

Both hypertrophic scars and keloids have increased cellularity compared to normal dermis. There is an abundance of extracellular material, primarily chondroitin 4-sulfate. Collagen synthesis is both increased and abnormal while collagen degradation may also be altered.

The treatment of keloids includes the combination of surgery and intralesional corticosteroids. There is a high risk of recurrence with most forms of therapy, which is sometimes greater than the risk from the original lesion. Smaller keloids may be excised entirely, but it is important that the wound be closed without tension. This is done with wide undermining and closure in skin tension lines. Larger keloids may be shaved with the scalpel and allowed to heal by second intention. Hemostasis is obtained with pressure, using as little cautery as possible to avoid damage to the dermis and subsequent fibroblast proliferation. The base of the wound is injected with intralesional corticosteroids at the time of surgery and at 2-week intervals. The dose of triamcinolone acetonide is diluted with physiologic saline to concentrations of 5–40 mg/ml. A 30-gauge needle is used for injections. Intradermal or intralesional injections through the base of the lesion should result in significant blanching. Larger-gauge needles are required for thick, fibrous lesions. The concentration of glucocortoid is titrated with the clinical response. Recurrence of keloid may occur up to 2 years after treatment.

Cryotherapy has been used in the treatment of keloids. Repeated vigorous freezes at 2- to 3-week intervals may be helpful, but will probably not result in complete resolution. Cryotherapy preceding intralesional steroids may yield better results. Edema following a freeze–thaw cycle of cryotherapy may make intralesional injections easier.

Pressure is useful to prevent recurrences of keloids after surgical excision. Pressure must be maintained for 4–6 months, and can be in the form of elastic garments, corsets, or adhesive wraps. A spring pressure device has been reported to be effective to prevent recurrences of earlobe keloids.

Carbon dioxide lasers with a wavelength of 10,600 nm have been used to treat hypertrophic scars and keloids. The carbon dioxide laser produces precise destruction with little peripheral thermal injury to the surrounding tissue. Small capillaries are sealed, providing "bloodless" surgery. Tissue is sterilized by the laser and peripheral nerve endings are sealed, thus reducing postoperative discomfort. For keloids, the beam is usually focused and used as a cutting tool. The tumor is removed by shave excision until normal tissue is reached or is simply excised down to subcutaneous tissue. The wound can be left to heal by second intention without tension. Minimizing tissue injury helps prevent recurrence, although the mechanism is not fully understood. Results have been favorable, with 50–70% cure rates.

Radiation therapy has been used in combination with excision for single keloids but should only be used by those with experience.

LIPOMAS

Lipomas are benign tumors of adipose tissue, usually solitary and encapsulated. They occur commonly on the trunk, nape of the neck, and forearms. They most frequently arise in subcutaneous tissue, but can occur in deeper soft tissue. Histologically, lipomas are surrounded by a connective tissue capsule, but the fat cells contained within are indistinguishable from normal adipose tissue.

Angiolipomas are a variant of lipoma consisting of adipose tissue and clusters of thin-walled vessels. These tumors are often painful, and there may be several. Liposarcomas are pleomorphic neoplasms that infiltrate surrounding tissues. Atypical lipoblasts are found histologically.

The standard treatment for lipomas is excision. The length of the incision need only by one-fourth to one-half of the tumor itself and should be made the full thickness of the skin and upper subcutis. Gentle but firm pressure around the lipoma will express the tumor through the incision, often intact. Blunt dissection with scissors is usually needed to separate the lipoma from both the underlying fat and fascia.

There can be a significant dead space after excision of larger lipomas. Hemostasis must be obtained to avoid a hematoma or seroma. The dead space should be closed with subcutaneous sutures. If the overlying epidermis is atrophic and redundant, it can be trimmed.

Large lipomas can be treated with liposuction (Figs. 3,4). The lipoma is infiltrated with dilute lidocaine and epinephrine and the skin injected only at the insertion of the cannula. A 1-cm incision is made in the base of the tumor. A standard liposuction cannula and suction machine are passed into the body of the tumor, with the openings in the cannula directed away from the skin to avoid injury to epidermal structures. Manual pressure with the operator's free hand is necessary at the periphery of the tumor to facilitate suctioning. Scissors and forceps may also be necessary to free fatty tissue from the surrounding stroma. This method is useful for giant lipomas (> 8 cm), for which a large surgical excision has greater risk of hematoma and requires an extensive multilayered closure. While some fat cells may remain, the tumor can be considerably reduced, giving an excellent cosmetic result with little chance of recurrence.

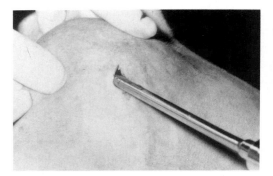

Figure 3 Lipoma, treated by liposuction.

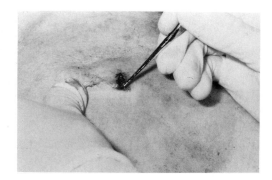

Figure 4 Lipoma. Forceps and manual pressure are used to assist in removal of fat.

VASCULAR TUMORS

Vascular tumors comprise a range of lesions including pyogenic granulomas, hemangiomas, cherry angiomas, and angiokeratomas.

Pyogenic Granulomas

Pyogenic granulomas are solitary, slightly pedunculated soft nodules with a dull red color (Fig. 5). They usually grow rapidly for a short period of time and then stabilize. The surface may be smooth, but often there is crusting or ulceration due to the tendency to bleed easily. Pyogenic granulomas occur at sites of trauma or mechanical irritation and are usually found on the fingers or face. There is a slightly increased incidence during pregnancy. Histologically, these

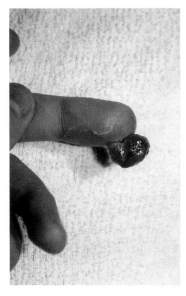

Figure 5 Pyogenic granuloma.

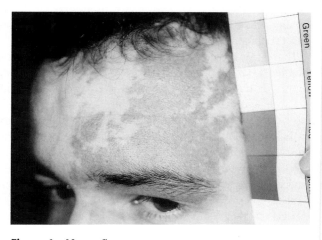

Figure 6 Nevus flammeus.

lesions show a proliferation of capillaries embedded in an edematous stroma. The lesion is neither pyogenic nor a granuloma, but this misnomer has persisted.

A simple method of removal is shave excision to the deep dermis. Only the visible borders of the lesion need to be removed. Alternatively, the lesion can be shelled out with a curet. Since these tumors are vascular, brisk bleeding should be anticipated. On the finger, a tourniquet may be applied to minimize bleeding and provide a dry field for electrocautery. Vigorous manual pressure for 5–10 min may still be required to control bleeding adequately. The wound can then heal by second intention.

The entire lesion can be excised and closed primarily. Cryosurgery may be attempted in difficult areas such as beneath the nail plate, or in young children. Freezing is less reliable, however, especially in larger lesions, and does not provide tissue to confirm the diagnosis histopathologically. Both the argon and carbon dioxide laser have been used successfully. Recurrent pyogenic granuloma may occur with satellite lesions in rare cases. These usually resolve with or without treatment in months.

Hemangiomas

Hemangiomas are vascular anomalies that occur sporadically but can be associated with widespread cutaneous or systemic disease. They can be either flat or raised. The elevated variety includes capillary (65%), cavernous (15%), and mixed lesions (20%) (Table 1). Flat lesions such as the nevus flammeus or port-wine stain (Fig. 6) are sharply demarcated pink, red, or purple patches present at birth. Blanching on diascopy suggests the lesion is thin with minimal deep dermal involvement. Lesions generally persist into adult life. The most common hemangioma is the asymptomatic, rarely noticed, "stork bite." These usually occur on the nape of the neck and are covered by the patient's hair.

A common hemangioma of infancy is the capillary hemangioma (Fig. 7). These may become quite large, occasionally obstructing such vital functions as vision or smell when in these vital areas. These hemangiomas undergo a rapid growth phase followed by spontaneous involution over several years.

Surgery is best avoided unless the lesion persists into puberty or obstructs vital function; however, controversy over when to treat persists. Cavernous hemangiomas are a variant of the capillary type, with a predominance of dilated vessels and less tendency for resolution. The combined lesions have features of both.

Oral prednisone may be of value during active growth phases. Dosages may begin at 1 mg/kg, with gradual tapering as the growth phase slows or stops. X-ray therapy is not a viable option, because of the long-term damage to underlying structures. Cryotherapy and sclerosing agents have been tried with varying rates of success.

Surgical treatment of large hemangiomas is advised if the lesion interferes with vital structures such as the eyes, mouth, or ears. Large cavernous hemangiomas may cause extensive

Table 1 Hemangiomas

Elevated
  Capillary
  Cavernous
  Mixed
  Nevus flammeus
Flat
  Nevus flammeus (port-wine stain)

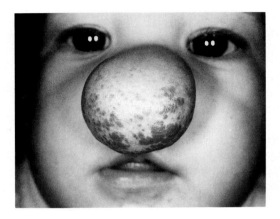

Figure 7 Capillary hemangioma.

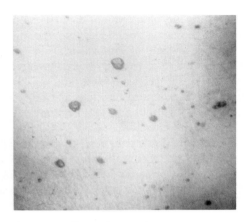

Figure 8 Cherry hemangioma.

regional tissue destruction. Preoperative arteriography helps one to evaluate the extent of these lesions. Selective embolization of feeder vessels significantly aids in surgery. These procedures are best performed by physicians with extensive experience in these areas. The pulsed dye laser is effective in the treatment of superficial hemangiomas, but is of limited value in larger lesions. The depth of injury to blood vessels is only 1.2 mm, requiring other modalities for treatment of larger capillary or cavernous hemangiomas.

Port-wine stains are hemangiomas that may be relatively flat early on but often become more cavernous and thick with age. Growth does not extend beyond the original boundaries of the tumor, however. They may be small tumors often limited to dermatomal distribution, especially on the face when they usually follow the sensory distribution of the trigeminal nerve unilaterally. Some port-wine stains may be quite large and occasionally are associated with underlying abnormalities such as seizures and intracranial calcification as seen in Sturge–Weber syndrome, or abnormalities of the upper extremities as seen in Klippel–Trenauney–Weber syndrome. Small port-wine stains can be treated by excision and primary closure. In the past, larger areas required serial excision and closure with flaps or grafting. Dermabrasion may be of value when the port-wine stain is limited to the superficial dermis, determined clinically by blanching with diascopy. A biopsy may also help determine the depth of the lesion.

The pulsed dye laser has become the most favored modality for port-wine stains. This laser causes selective photothermolysis of the dilated blood vessels while sparing normal tissue. It achieves excellent results with minimal anesthesia, though it usually requires multiple treatment sessions. Unlike previous continuous-wave lasers, which were associated with pigment and textural change, the pulsed dye laser has a very low incidence of scarring.

Cherry Angiomas

These common lesions, also called senile hemangiomas or cherry red spots, are small persistent red papules that present on the trunk, neck, and face of middle-aged patients (Fig. 8). Often dozens of these occur. Histologically, they are a variant of capillary hemangiomas with fewer vascular spaces and more abundant stroma.

Treatment is unnecessary except for cosmetic purposes. Superficial electrodesiccation or cryotherapy is generally adequate. Another method is fluoroethyl refrigerant spray followed by curettage with a firm brush stroke. Several lesions can be removed with minimum discomfort.

Table 2   Angiokeratoma

Solitary
Angiokeratoma circumscriptum
Angiokeratoma of Mibelli
Angiokeratoma of Fordyce
Fucosidosis
Angiokeratoma corporis diffusum (Fabry's disease)

Alternatively, shave excision with local anesthesia and light electrodesiccation will remove lesions with minimal scarring. The pulsed dye laser is also very effective in the treatment of these lesions.

Angiokeratomas

These are round, elevated, purplish papules, which may become hypekeratonic (Fig. 9). There are six clinically recognizable types (Table 2). The solitary angiokeratoma presents in childhood, often on the arms or legs. Angiokeratoma circumscriptum is present at birth as a warty growth in bands or streaks. Angiokeratoma of Mibelli occurs as hemorrhagic keratotic papules in adolescence. Angiokeratoma of Fordyce presents as multiple red-purple papules seen primarily on the scrotum. The last two types of angiokeratomas are associated with enzyme deficiencies. In fucosidosis, multiple angiokeratomas appear on the trunk and legs in association with mental retardation. In Fabry's disease (angiokeratoma corporis diffusum), the lesions are also on the trunk, in association with defective function of the enzyme galactosidase A. Histologic examination reveals dilated capillaries surrounded by a thickened epidermis. Lipid stains can detect deposits associated with Fabry's disease. No treatment is necessary for angiokeratomas, but punch excision, shave biopsy, electrodesiccation, cryotherapy, or pulsed dye laser will give acceptable results.

XANTHELASMA

Xanthelasma are soft, yellow-orange plaques on the eyelids, and are the most common form of xanthomas (Fig. 10). They start as small growths but may become large nodules. They generally present in the fourth to fifth decade of life, and approximately 50% will result from an

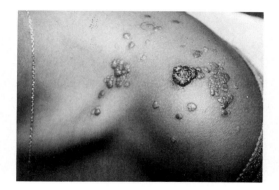

Figure 9   Angiokeratoma.

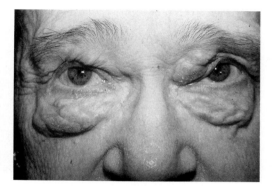

Figure 10   Xanthelasma.

underlying serum lipoprotein disorder. Histologic examination reveals collections of lipid-laden histiocytes in the upper levels of the dermis.

The treatment of xanthelasma is essentially cosmetic. Small lesions can be excised and the wound closed with fine, nonabsorbable sutures, which are removed after 3–4 days. Alternatively, these may be treated with light electrodesiccation and curettage to remove the viscous fatty material. Cryosurgery can also be used.

Other methods include trichloroacetic acid applied directly to the lesions. Start with a 20–25% solution and increase to 50% as needed. The acid is applied for approximately 30 sec and a white frost is noted. The solution is then removed with moist cotton gauze or alcohol.

SEBACEOUS HYPERPLASIA

Sebaceous hyperplasia is a benign condition occurring on the forehead and cheeks of middle-aged patients. It presents as elevated, soft, yellowish papules 2–3 mm in diameter (Fig. 11). This must be differentiated from basal cell carcinoma, which can look similar. The histologic examination of sebaceous hyperplasia reveals a greatly enlarged sebaceous gland with numerous lobules grouped around a wide duct.

The surgical treatment is essentially cosmetic, and any superficial destructive method can be used. One or two lesions may be removed by shave or circular punch excision. Larger areas can be treated with cryotherapy, or light electrodesiccation and curretage. A linear incision allows easier curettage. These areas heal in several weeks with minimal scarring.

ACROCHORDONS

Acrochordons, or skin tags, are benign flesh-colored pedunculated tumors that occur in several forms. The most common is the 1- to 2-mm soft furrowed papule that occurs on the trunk, axilla, and face coalesced in body folds (Fig. 12). Acrochordons also present as single or multiple filiform growths, usually measuring 2–5 mm. The large solitary pedunculated tags may be 1 cm or larger.

Histologically, these lesions are composed of loose collagen fibers and dilated capillaries, with varying degrees of fatty tissue. The epidermis ranges from flattened to acanthotic.

Small skin tags are easily removed with a sharp curved scissors cut flush to skin level, often without local anesthesia. The minor bleeding is controlled with pressure, chemical cautery, or light electrodesiccation. Larger skin tags require local anesthesia and can be shaved with a #15 blade.

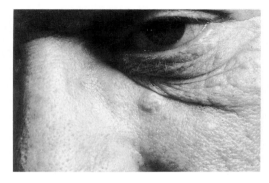

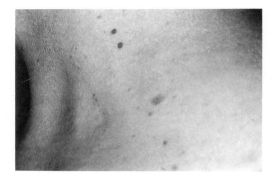

Figure 11 Sebaceous hyperplasia.   **Figure 12** Acrochordon.

Alternative methods include light electrocautery or liquid nitrogen. The lesions will usually fall off within several days.

ACKNOWLEDGMENT

A special thanks to Dr. Jerome Garden for supplying the clinical photographs.

BIBLIOGRAPHY

Aversa AJ, Miller OF III. Cryo-curettage of cherry angiomas. *J Dermatol Surg Oncol* 1983;9:930–931.

Bailin PL. Lasers in dermatology—1985. *J Dermatol Surg Oncol* 1985;11:328–334.

Brent B. The role of pressure therapy in management of earlobe keloids. *Ann Plast Surg* 1978;1:579–581.

Ceilley RI, Babin RW. The combined use of cryosurgery and intralesional injections of suspensions of fluorinated adrenocorticosteroids for reducing keloids and hypertrophic scars. *J Dermatol Surg Oncol* 1979; 5:54–56.

Griffith BH, Monroe CW, McKinney P. A follow up study on the treatment of keloids with triamcinolone acetonide. *Plast Reconstr Surg* 1970;46:145–150.

Henderson DL, Cromwell TA, Mes LG. Argon and carbon dioxide laser treatment of hypertrophic and keloid scars. *Lasers Surg Med* 1984;3:271–277.

Hruza GJ, Geronemus RG, Dover JS, Arndt KA. Lasers in dermatology—1993. *Arch Derm* 1994;129:1026–1035.

Kantor GR, Wheeland RG, Bailin PL, et al. Treatment of earlobe keloids with carbon dioxide laser excision: a report of 16 cases. *J Dermatol Surg Oncol* 1985;11:1063–1067.

Levy DS, Salter MM, Roth RE. Postoperative irradiation in the prevention of keloids. *Am J Roentgenol* 1976;127:509–510.

Rubenstein R, Roenigk HH Jr, Garden JM, et al. Liposuction for lipomas. *J Dermatol Surg Oncol* 1985; 11:1070–1074.

29

Benign Pigmented Lesions

Darrell S. Rigel and Robert J. Friedman
New York University School of Medicine, New York, New York

Patients with problems related to pigmented lesion disorders are among the most commonly evaluated for dermatologic surgery. The vast majority of these lesions are benign and are often treated surgically. However, recent data suggest that some of these lesions may be both markers for and precursors to malignant melanoma. It is, therefore, important that patients with pigmented lesions be carefully evaluated and treated appropriately.

ATYPICAL MOLE (DYSPLASTIC NEVUS) SYNDROME

Perhaps the most controversial topic in dermatology currently is the management of patients with dysplastic nevus syndrome. In the past, a syndrome of familial malignant melanoma has been described, but it was not until 1978 that Clark et al. noted that certain individuals in these high-risk families had atypical moles. At that time, the designation "B-K mole syndrome" was used to describe two affected families whose last names began with the letters "B" and "K." Subsequently, Lynch et al. coined the term "familial atypical multiple mole melanoma syndrome" (FAMMMS). In 1980 Greene et al. introduced the term "dysplastic nevus syndrome" because of the disorderly growth pattern of melanocytes, the histologic hallmark of these lesions. Recognition of the dysplastic nevus syndrome in the nonfamilial setting was later noted. In 1983 Kraemer et al. developed a classification of dysplastic nevus syndrome. The five risk groups are based upon whether the nevi are familial or whether there is a personal or family history of malignant melanoma (Table 1). The National Institutes of Health Consensus Conference on Early Melanoma in 1992 suggested the term "atypical mole" as being more appropriately descriptive of this entity.

Familial atypical mole syndrome (AMS) [dysplastic nevus syndrome (DNS)] is a worldwide problem. Estimates of prevalence range from 2 to 8%. Crutcher et al. estimated a prevalence in California of approximately 4.9%. Projecting these data, it is estimated that approximately 10–12 million people in the United States have at least one lesion. More recently, Kopf et al. showed

Table 1 Classification of Types of Atypical Mole (AM) Syndromes by Risk of Melanoma

Type	Description	Personal or family history of MM	Family history of AM	MM risk	Number of afflicted individuals
A	Sporadic AM	–	–	Lowest	Highest
B	Familial AM	–	+	Low	High
C	Sporadic AM	+	–	High	Low
D–1	Familial with MM	+	+	Higher	Lower
D–2	Familial AM with MM in 2 or more family members	+ +	+	Highest	Lowest

that there is an increased incidence of atypical mole in the fairer skin types (I–II) compared with the darker types (III–IV). The association of atypical mole with fair skin types might partially explain the increased risk these individuals have of subsequently developing malignant melanoma.

Clinical Features

One of the most striking features of atypical moles is their heterogeneity. Most lesions differ significantly from one another by marked variations in size, shape, and color. However, several critical clues can regularly be used to differentiate atypical moles from common acquired nevi (Fig. 1). In general, dysplastic nevi tend to be more oval than acquired nevi. They are usually slightly larger (>5 mm) and have borders that seem to blend gradually into the surrounding normal skin (shoulder phenomenon). Patients may have as few as one or as many as several hundred nevi (Fig. 2). The lesions may be mamillated, papular, nodular, or sessile.

Friedman et al. classified atypical moles into eight clinical types (Table 2). The most common clinical variant of atypical mole is the dark target/centrally elevated type (Fig. 3). This is characterized by a darkly pigmented papular component centrally, surrounded by a lighter, tan-brown, macular periphery. The macular pigmented halo gradually diffuses into the surrounding normal skin. The second most prevalent type of atypical mole is the dark target/macular variety. This is similar to the dark target/centrally elevated variety but lacks the central papular component.

Next in prevalence is the mamillated variety (Fig. 4). This lesion is slightly elevated, with a barely perceptible macular "shoulder." The surface of the lesion is best described as "cobblestoned," and, with careful observation, occasional tiny "milialike" structures may be seen. The halo is minimal.

A less common variant is the erythematous type (Fig. 5), which is characterized by a prominent red-orange component. There is also the light target variety. This lesion is characterized by a more deeply pigmented light to dark brown macular periphery and a less pigmented, centrally located, tan to light brown papular component. This type of nevus may also have a central macular area (Fig. 6).

The least common varieties include the lentiginous type and melanoma simulant. The lentiginous type has clinical features similar to simple lentigo. However, it is generally larger and often has a more striking reticulated pigment pattern. The melanoma simulant has many of the early features of a malignant melanoma. However, these features are not as striking as would be seen in a clinically apparent early malignant melanoma.

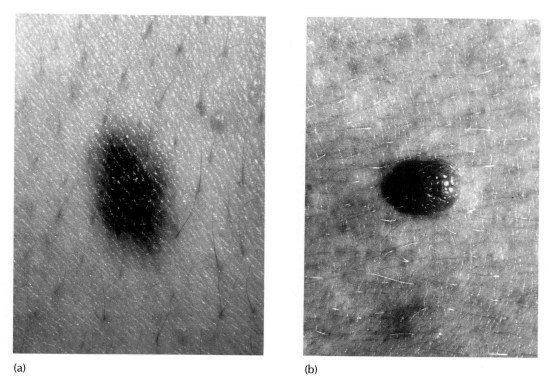

(a)   (b)

Figure 1 (a) Atypical mole showing oval shape, gradual peripheral "diffusing" of pigment with poorly circumscribed margins. (b) Common acquired atypical mole showing uniform color, round shape, and crisp border demarcation.

Although it has been suggested that atypical nevi be clinically identified as a specific entity, it is not always a simple task to differentiate them from early malignant melanoma. It is, therefore, important that lesions suspected of being malignant melanoma be biopsied and evaluated. Recently, the use of epiluminescence microscopy has been proposed as a better way to differentiate atypical nevi from melanoma and other pigmented lesions.

Atypical moles are predominantly anatomically distributed on the trunk and upper extremities. In addition, it has been suggested that atypical moles are larger and more numerous on relatively sun-exposed compared to sun-protected sites. Since these sites correlate somewhat with the anatomic distribution of cutaneous melanoma, the increased risk for melanoma might partially be explained by these findings.

Histologic Features

The specific histologic features of atypical moles are currently being debated. Both architectural and cytologic features are used by dermatopathologists to differentiate these lesions from malignant melanoma in situ. Typical histologic features of an atypical mole are generally superimposed on those of a junctional or compound nevus. They include the following:

1. Basalar melanocytic hyperplasia along elongated rete ridges
2. Random cytologic atypia with hyperchromatic nuclei often present

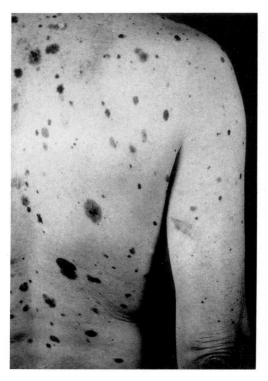

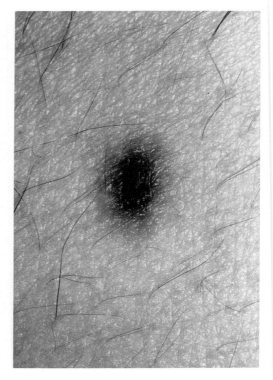

Figure 2   Patient with florid AMS, who previously had two melanomas.

Figure 3   Atypical mole: dark target, centrally elevated type. Note the raised dark center with trailing lighter peripheral pigment.

3. Melanocytes that may be spindle shaped and arranged horizontally or occasionally in nests of variable size; may lie between adjacent rete ridges to produce bridging
4. Lamellar and concentric dermatofibroplasia
5. Lymphocytes in patchy or diffuse superficial dermal infiltrate

Because these histologic changes may be focal, several histopathologic sections may be required to identify the diagnostic features of a dysplastic nevus.

Table 2   Clinical Types of Atypical Moles

Most common
   Dark target/Centrally elevated
   Dark target/Macular
   Papillated/Mamillated
   Erythematous
Less common
   Light target/Centrally elevated
   Light target/Macular
   Lentiginous
   Melanoma simulant

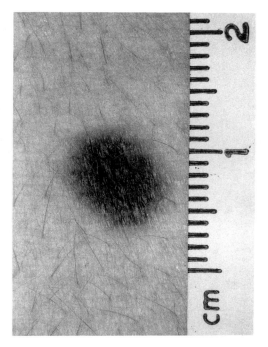

Figure 4 Atypical mole: mamillated variety. Note prominent center with fine mamillation and minimal shoulder.

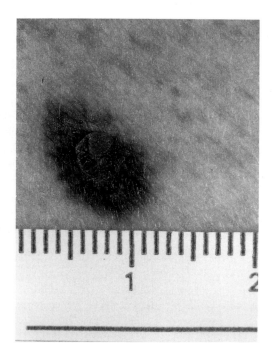

Figure 5 Atypical mole: erythematous variety. The superior one-third of the lesion had an erythematous/orange component.

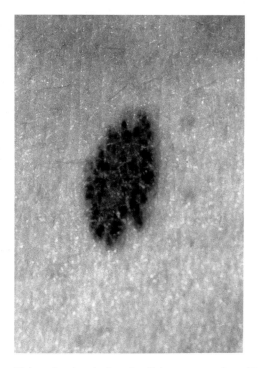

Figure 6 Atypical mole: light target variety. Note the central light brown area with an irregularly marginated darker periphery.

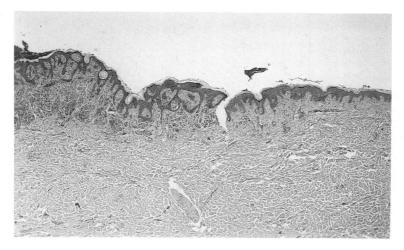

Figure 7   Photomicrograph of atypical mole shows nests of nevus cells in the center with a trailing off of the nests to the periphery at the dermal-epidermal junction (×100).

Perhaps the most important histologic feature for clinical management of these patients is the distribution of the nevus cells. Typically, there is a cluster of cells in the center of the lesion with nests trailing off along the periphery (Fig. 7). This distribution of nevus cells correlates clinically with the dark center and the halo of pigment diffusing out to the ill-defined margin.

In an attempt to evaluate the histologic spread of atypical mole cells and determine clinical margins required to remove atypical moles, 53 of these lesions were etched with a #11 scalpel blade at their clinical borders. The lesion was then excised with a wide zone of perilesional skin. It was found histologically that dysplastic cells were seen microscopically as far as 2 mm beyond the clinical margin of the lesion (Fig. 8).

Monoclonal antibodies have been developed that bind with atypical mole cells. However, the stain is not completely specific. A refined immunochemical stain may be the key to identifying these lesions histologically in the future.

Management

Atypical moles can be both precursors for malignant melanoma and markers for increased risk of melanoma. This difference has important implications for medical or surgical management. If these lesions are true precursors, the appropriate management would be to remove them all. However, if they are merely markers, removing the lesion would provide no direct benefit to the patient.

To demonstrate that atypical moles are precursors of malignant melanoma, they must be contiguous with the tumor histologically. There is marked variation in the percentage of malignant melanomas reported to be associated histologically with dysplastic nevi. This association has ranged from 40% to less than 1%. The variance in observations is probably due to differences in histologic criteria used to make the diagnosis of atypical moles.

Calculations of the precursor risk of atypical moles are based on three assumptions:

1. Histologic criteria for the identification of precursor lesions must be agreed upon and reliably evaluated by different observers of the same lesion.

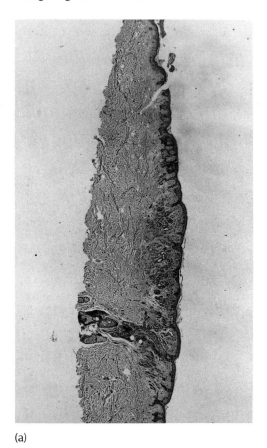

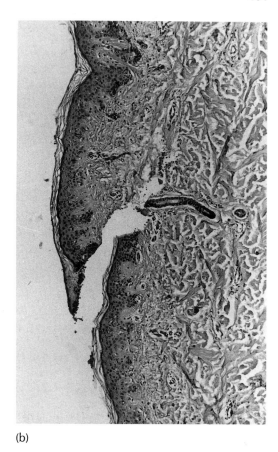

(a)   (b)

Figure 8 (a) Atypical mole shows central aggregation of nevus cells with surgical etching at clinically apparent margin (×100). (b) Higher-power view (×400) shows nests of nevus cells extending lateral to clinically etched margin.

2. Calculations must be based on data with little variation between observers.
3. Malignant melanoma and the precursor lesions must be equally and randomly distributed over the entire cutaneous surface.

None of these premises has been substantiated by previously reported calculations. Therefore, the magnitude of the risk that atypical moles are precursors of malignant melanoma has yet to be determined.

The data establishing these lesions as markers for malignant melanoma are much more straightforward. Among white persons in the United States today, the risk for developing malignant melanoma in a lifetime is approximately 1%. For patients with atypical moles, (who constitute a heterogeneous group), the risk for developing melanoma in a lifetime has been estimated at 6–10%.

The risk is greater for patients with a family history of melanoma. The risk of developing melanoma in a lifetime may approach 100% for patients with atypical moles who are from melanoma-prone families (that is, families with two or more first-degree relatives with cutaneous melanoma). In this case, melanoma may arise within the atypical moles or de novo.

Table 3 Increased Risk of Persons Developing Melanoma by Types of AM Syndrome

Type	Description	Number of patients evaluated	Increased risk for MM detected
A	Sporadic AM	224	35×
B	Familial AM	56	250×
C	Sporadic AM with MM	104	166×
D	Familial AM with MM	45	460×
D–2	Familial AM with MM in 2 or more family members	23	1575×
All	—	452	205×

Rigel et al. attempted to quantify the increased risk of melanoma in patients with atypical moles based on Kraemer's classification by following 452 patients for an average of 14 months. Malignant melanoma was found 205 times more frequently in this group than would be expected in the general population. The relative risk for developing melanoma increased according to the Kraemer scale. The risk was 35-fold greater for type A patients and up to 1575-fold greater for the type D-2 patients (Table 3). The management of these patients is, therefore, based on the magnitude of increased risk for developing malignant melanoma.

The entire skin surface should be examined closely with a good light. Careful examination of the scalp and eye should be included. At least one of the more atypical appearing levi should be subjected to excisional biopsy. The lesion should be removed with a 2- to 3-mm margin to ensure complete excision. The family history should be obtained with special attention given to such items as "moles," "skin cancer," and melanoma.

If the family history suggests melanoma, an effort should be made to examine first-degree relatives. If any family members have melanoma, all blood relatives should be examined to determine the incidence of melanoma in the kindred.

For patients with atypical moles and a family history of melanoma, additional lesions should be removed if they are suspected as early melanoma. Follow-up examinations should be conducted every 3–6 months. Photography may be helpful for the evaluation of changes in lesions during follow-up examinations of patients with atypical moles.

In patients with atypical moles and no family history of melanoma, the risk of developing melanoma is uncertain. Existing lesions should be evaluated for evidence of progression and biopsied if a change is noted.

All patients with atypical moles should be taught about the need for regular follow-up. Self-examination of the skin is encouraged to detect changes in existing nevi or the appearance of new ones. Educational materials demonstrating the changes to watch for in nevi are helpful. Avoidance of excessive exposure to the sun and the use of sunscreens should be encouraged (Table 4).

CONGENITAL NEVI

A congenital nevus is a melanocytic nevus present at birth. Not all pigmented lesions present at birth represent melanocytic nevi. Congenital nevi have been classified into three groups according to size: (1) small (less than 1.5 cm in diameter); (2) medium (1.5–20 cm in diameter); (3) large (greater than 20 cm in diameter).

Nevi classified by size occupy different proportions of the body surface at different ages. The size of the lesion has different implications for diagnosis, treatment, and prognosis.

Table 4 Management Guidelines for Patients with Atypical Mole Syndrome

Diagnosis
  Careful skin examination
  Biopsy
  Family history
Familial screening
  Examination of first-degree relatives
Treatment and follow-up
  With family history: full body photographs (if possible), 3- to 6-month follow-up
  Without family history: evaluate lesions for progression, remove changing lesions
Patient education
  Self-examination
  Educational material
  Sun avoidance

Congenital nevi have a much lower prevalence than dysplastic nevi. It has been estimated that approximately 1–2.5% of the white United States population have congenital nevi at birth.

Clinical Appearance

The clinical appearance of congenital nevi is variable and somewhat dependent on their size. Large (greater than 20 cm) congenital nevi can vary greatly in size. Some occupy a major portion of the body surface and are called giant congenital, bathing trunk, or garment nevi. Clinical features include a grossly irregular surface, increased pigmentation with varying shades of brown, and hypertrichosis.

Medium-sized (1.5–20 cm) congenital nevi share the above clinical features and are almost always easily identified as congenital nevi. Small (less than 1.5 cm) congenital nevi may not be recognized as such if not apparent at birth. The clinical appearance often may not differ from the acquired nevocytic nevi because these smaller lesions may have a smooth surface, more uniform pigmentation, and lack hair.

Histologic Features

The classic histologic description of congenital nevi includes nevus cells in the lower two-thirds of the dermis, occasionally extending into the subcutis; between collagen bundles distributed as single cells, or cells in single file, or both; and on the lower two-thirds of the reticular dermis or subcutis associated with appendages, nerves, and vessels. However, many congenital nevi do not have these microscopic features.

Large congenital nevi usually have characteristic features in some areas, but elsewhere they may be indistinguishable from acquired nevi. Medium-sized congenital nevi may or may not show all these microscopic features. Small congenital nevi, in many cases, do not show the classic microscopic features. Often, they may be indistinguishable from acquired nevi. In many cases, the typical microscopic picture of a congenital nevus may be seen in acquired nevi.

Management

Melanoma can develop in congenital nevi. The giant congenital nevus is most likely to undergo malignant change (Fig. 9). The incidence of melanoma arising in large congenital nevi has been estimated as between 5 and 20% over the lifetime of the patient. The risk of medium- and small-

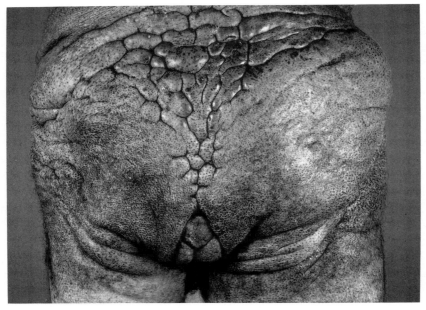

(a)

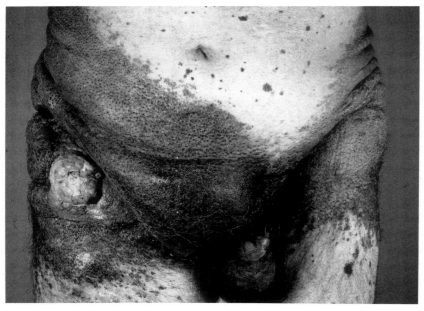

(b)

Figure 9 (a) Giant "bathing trunk" congenital nevus. (b) Note melanoma arising on right lateral thigh. (Courtesy of NYU Skin and Cancer Clinic.)

sized congenital nevi evolving into malignant melanoma remains in doubt. The aforementioned problems related to determining the risk of dysplastic nevi acting as markers or precursors of malignant melanoma are also true for congenital nevi. Therefore, the exact magnitude of their precursor risk remains in doubt.

Table 5 Management Guidelines for Patients with Congenital Nevi

Large
Surgical removal/debulking (if feasible)
Balance risk of malignant melanoma against surgical procedure
Medium or small
Conservative management
Self-examination
Biopsy if alteration is noted

Congenital nevi appear to be markers for increased risk of malignant melanoma. However, the magnitude of risk is much less than that for dysplastic nevi. Kopf et al. have estimated that persons with small congenital nevi have approximately 2.5 times the risk of the general population for developing melanoma in their lifetime (not necessarily histologically associated with the congenital nevus itself).

The management of congenital nevi depends primarily on their size and the perceived risk of developing malignant melanoma (Table 5). Large congenital nevi, which have the highest risk for developing melanoma, are the rarest. Their management is complex. Nevus cells can extend deeply into the subcutis and, in some cases, have been reported to penetrate the muscle. With this in mind, in most cases, surgical excision or dermabrasion will at best only debulk the lesion. The defect is often repaired with a large graft or flap. Recently, tissue expanders have been used to augment the reconstruction.

Because of the uncertain incidence of melanoma arising in congenital nevi, conservative management usually is recommended. The lesion should periodically be documented, measured, and observed for alterations in size, shape, color, and topography. Should the patient desire removal, a simple excision is usually adequate. In children, it is recommended that this procedure be deferred until an age at which general anesthesia is no longer required because of an estimated morbidity of 7:100,000.

There are insufficient data at present to recommend prophylactic excision of all congenital nevi. Patients should be examined periodically and, when appropriate, taught supplementary self-examination. A biopsy is indicated if, after examination by a physician, a significant alteration in the nevus has occurred.

COMMON ACQUIRED NEVI

One of the most common requests made of the dermatologist is to remove a common acquired nevus. On average there are about 25 nevi per person, so there are approximately 6 billion common acquired nevi in the United States.

The risk of an acquired nevus evolving into melanoma is somewhat greater than in de novo skin. However, it is significantly less than that of a dysplastic or congenital nevus. Thus, no group of acquired nevi can be objectively singled out on the basis of histologic type (compound, intradermal, junctional) or anatomic site as being at increased risk for malignant change. For that reason, the management of common acquired nevi is usually predicated on maximizing the cosmetic result.

In most cases, the lesion can be removed by shave excision with closure by second intention. Often these lesions will partially recur after treatment as a hyperpigmented macule or papule. Repeat biopsy may yield pseudomelanoma histologically. Therefore, it is important to warn the patient of this possibility if a clinical recurrence occurs in case of rebiopsy at a later date. A deeper excision closed primarily with sutures usually results in a more definitive removal. The cosmetic result is as good but the procedure takes longer and is slightly more expensive.

Although these lesions appear to have little precursor potential, two recent studies have suggested an association of common acquired nevi as markers for an increased risk of malignant melanoma. It may be that patients with large numbers of acquired nevi should be evaluated more closely than average to allow detection of melanomas as early as possible.

BIBLIOGRAPHY

Ackerman AB, Mihara I. Dysplasia, dysplastic melanocytes, dysplastic nevi, the dysplastic nevus syndrome, and the relation between dysplastic nevi and malignant melanomas. *Hum Pathol* 1985;16:87–91.

Cage GW. Small congenital nevi (letter). *J Am Acad Dermatol* 1982;7:685–687.

Chun K, Vazquez M, Sanchez JL. Malignant melanoma in children. *Cancer* 1989;63:386–389.

Clark WH, Reimer RR, Greene M. Origin of familial malignant melanomas from heritable melanocytic lesions. *Arch Dermatol* 1978;114:732–738.

Cook MG, Robertson I. Melanocytic dysplasia and melanoma. *Histopathology* 1985;9:647–658.

Crutcher WA, Sagebiel RW. Prevalence of dysplastic naevi in a community practice (letter). *Lancet* 1984;1:729.

Elder DE, Goldman LI, Goldman SC et al. Dysplastic nevus syndrome: A phenotypic association of sporadic cutaneous melanoma. *Cancer* 1980;46:1787–1794.

Elder DE, Green MH, Guerry D et al. The dysplastic nevus syndrome: Our definition. *Am J Dermatopathol* 1982;4:455–460.

Friedman RJ, Heilman ER, Rigel DS, Kopf AW. The dysplastic nevus: Clinical and pathologic features. *Dermatol Clin* 1985;3(2):239.

Friedman RJ, Rigel DS, Kopf AW. Early detection of malignant melanoma. The continued role of physician examination and self-examination of the skin. *CA* 1991;40:130–151.

Greene MH, Clark WH, Tucker MA et al. Precursor naevi in cutaneous malignant melanoma: A proposed nomenclature (letter). *Lancet* 1980;2:1024.

Holly EA, Kelly JW, Shpall SN et al. Number of melanocytic nevi as a major risk factor for malignant melanoma. *J Am Acad Dermatol* 1987;17:459–468.

Kang S, Barnhill RL, Mihm MC Jr, Fitzpatrich TB, Sober AJ. Melanoma risk in individual with clinically atypical nevi. *Arch Dermatol* 1994;130:999–1001.

Kopf AW, Gold RS, Rogers GS et al. Relationship of lumbosacral nevocytic nevi to sun exposure in dysplastic nevus syndrome. *Arch Dermatol* 1986;122:1003.

Kopf AW, Levine LJ, Rigel DS. Prevalence of congenital-nevus-like nevi, nevi spili and café-au-lait spots in patients malignant melanoma. *J Dermatol Surg Oncol* 1985;11:275–279.

Kopf AW, Lindsay AC, Rogers GS et al. Relationship of nevocytic nevi to sun exposure in dysplastic nevus syndrome. *J Am Acad Dermatol* 1985;12:656–662.

Kraemer KH, Tucker M, Tarone R et al. Risk of cutaneous melanoma in dysplastic nevus syndrome type A and B (letter). *N Engl J Med* 1986;315:1615.

Kraemer KH, Greene MH, Tarone R et al. Dysplastic nevi and cutaneous melanoma risk (letter). *Lancet* 1983;2:1076–1077.

Kuflik JH, Janniyen CK. Congenital melanocytic nevi. *Cutis* 1994;53:112–114.

Lynch HT, Frichot BC, Lynch JF. Familial atypical melanocytic mole-melanoma syndrome. *J Med Genet* 1978;15:352–356.

Maeda K, Jimbow K. Development of MoAb HMSA-2 for melanosomes of human melanoma and its application to immunohistopathologic diagnosis of neoplastic melanocytes. *Cancer* 1987;59:415–423.

Manghoob AA, Kopf AW, Riger DS, Bart RS, Friedman RJ, Yadav S, Abadia M. Risk of cutaneous malignant syndrome. *Arch Dermatol* 1994;130:993–998.

Manghoob AA, Onlow SJ, Kopf AW. Syndromes associated with melanocyte nevi. *J Acad Dermatol* 1993;29:373–388.

Mark GJ, Mihm MC, Liteplo M. Congenital melanocytic nevi of the small and garment type. Clinical, histologic, and ultrastructural studies. *Hum Pathol* 1973;4:395–418.

NIH Consensus Conference Report in the detection of treatment of early melanoma. *JAMA* 1992;268: 1314–1319.

Metcalf JS, Maize JC. Melanocytic nevi and malignant melanoma. *Dermatol Clin* 1985;3:217.

Nakanishi T, Hashimoto K. The differential reactivity of benign and malignant nevolmelanocytic lesions with mouse monoclonal antibody TNKH1. *Cancer* 1987;59:1340–1344.

Prepkorn MW, Barnhill RC, Cannon-Albright LA, Elden DE, Goldgar DE, Lewis CW, Maize JC, Meyer LJ, Sagebiel RW. A multiobserver, population based analysis of histologic dysplasia in melanocytes nevi. *J Am Acad Dermatol* 1994;30:707–714.

Rhodes AR. Acquired dysplastic melanocytic nevi and cutaneous melanoma: Precursors and prevention. *Ann Intern Med* 1985;102:546–548.

Rhodes AR, Sober AJ, Day CL et al. The malignant potential of small congenital nevocellular nevi. An estimate of association based on a histologic study of 234 primary cutaneous melanomas. *J Am Acad Dermatol* 1982;6:230.

Rigel DS, Friedman RJ. The management of patients with dysplastic and congenital nevi. *Dermatol Clin* 1985;3:251–255.

Rigel DS, Friedman RJ, Kopf AW. Surgical margins for removal of dysplastic nevi (abstract). *J Dermatol Surg Oncol* 1985;11:745.

Rigel DS, Friedman RJ, Kopf AW. Precursors of malignant melanoma. Problem in computing the risk of malignant melanoma arising in dysplastic and congenital nevocytic nevi. *Dermatol Clin* 1985;3:361–365.

Rigel DS, Rivers JK, Kopf AW. Dysplastic nevi. Markers for minimal risk for melanoma. *Cancer* 1989; 63:386–389.

Roush GC, Burnhill RC, Duray PH et al. Diagnosis of the dysplastic nevus in different populations. *J Am Acad Dermatol* 1986;14:419–425.

Steiner A, Pehamberger H, Wolff K. In vivo epiluminescence microscopy of pigmented skin lesions. *J Am Acad Dermatol* 1987;17:584–591.

Swerdlow AJ, English J, Mackie RM et al. Benign naevi associated with high risk of melanoma (letter). *Lancet* 1984;2:168.

Swerdlow AJ, Green A. Melanocytic naevi and melanoma: An epidermiological perspective. *Br J Dermatol* 1987;117:137–146.

Williams ML, Sargebiel RW. Melanoma risk factors and atypical moles. *West J Med* 1994;160:343–350.

basal cell carcinoma to be more common in male than in female patients, but more recent studies have shown this gap to be narrowing.

Basal cell carcinoma is most typically found on sun-exposed areas of fair-skinned individuals. The prevalence of basal cell carcinoma is highest in sun-exposed areas of the body. In spite of this, correlation with sun exposure is not complete, since up to one-third of all basal cell carcinomas occur on relatively sun-protected areas of the face such as the medial canthus or postauricular areas. Studies evaluating basal cell carcinoma and adjacent solar elastosis show that 7% of tumors arise on skin without evidence of solar damage. Another 26% of tumors arise in areas with only mild solar elastosis. The most common predisposing factor is a history of having had a basal cell carcinoma. Having had one tumor, there is a 40% chance of developing a second primary lesion in the ensuing 10 years.

Basal cell carcinoma may also result from exposure to other external carcinogens, such as ionizing radiation. Patients who have been treated with irradiation for facial acne are at increased risk of developing basal cell carcinoma in those areas. Trivalent inorganic arsenic, once commonly used as an insecticide and medicinal (Fowler's solution), is also recognized as a predisposing factor. Most basal cell carcinomas associated with chronic arsenic exposure are the superficial erythematous type. Recently, it has been suggested that a papular form of basal cell carcinoma may result from industrial exposure to tar compounds.

Basal cell carcinoma develops more frequently in a number of inherited syndromes (Table 1). However, aside from these syndromes, basal cell carcinoma is not associated with an increased risk for other malignancies. Basal cell carcinoma may arise within or in close proximity to other cutaneous tumors, such as epidermal nevi, nevus sebaceous of Jadassohn (organoid nevus), other common adnexal tumors, seborrheic keratosis, dermatofibroma, and junctional nevi. Basal cell carcinoma may also occur in scars secondary to burns, blunt trauma, sharp trauma, and vaccination.

Table 1 Syndromes Associated with Basal Cell Carcinoma

Syndrome	Other prominent findings	Inheritance
Basal cell nevus (Gorlin's)	Pitting of palms and soles Mandibular cysts Bifid ribs Hypertelorism Other neoplasms	Autosomal dominant or sporadic
Albinism	Reduced or absent melanin formation Squamous cell carcinoma	Multiple patterns
Xeroderma pigmentosum	Sun sensitivity Photophobia Freckling Abnormal DNA repair Other neoplasms	Autosomal recessive
Rombo	Vermiculate atrophoderma Milia, hypotrichosis Trichoepithelioma Peripheral vasodilation with cyanosis	Autosomal dominant
Bazex	Follicular atrophoderma Localized anhidrosis Hypotrichosis	Autosomal dominant
Cancer family (Muir-Torre)	Sebaceous neoplasms Internal malignancy	Autosomal dominant

BIOLOGY

Although much is known about the progression of basal cell carcinoma, explaining this behavior on a basic biologic level has been difficult. Only fragments of the mechanism underlying the behavior of basal cell carcinoma are known.

The average cell cycle time of basal cell carcinoma is 217 hr, which translates into a doubling time of 9 days. However, basal cell carcinoma is clinically a slow-growing tumor. This discrepancy is accounted for in several ways. First, there is a large resting component in each basal cell carcinoma. Many cells are arrested in the G_2 or G_0 stages. Furthermore, the rapidly dividing cells are located primarily at the periphery of tumor nodules. The cells in the center do not divide as rapidly. Thus, only a small percentage of cells are actively dividing. Growth is also showed by individual cell death and regression in portions of the tumor. Apoptic cells with colloid bodies and amyloid deposition represent cell death.

Basal cell carcinoma has a complex relationship with its surrounding stroma. Parallel bundles of connective tissue are arranged around basal cell tumor masses, suggesting a dependent interaction, and it is indeed dependent upon its stroma for survival in many circumstances. When basal cell carcinoma is transplanted without its surrounding stroma into experimental animals, it does not survive well. Autotransplantation of basal cell carcinoma in humans without accompanying stroma also results in poor survival. In addition, the tumor appears less malignant histologically when grown without its stroma. Therefore, it appears that basal cell carcinoma interacts in some way with the dermis rather than occurring independently.

Local invasion of basal cell carcinoma has been postulated to occur via three stages: adhesion, enzymatic modification, and migration. Adhesion of tumor cells to the extracellular matrix and to the underlying basement membrane occurs first and is thought to be mediated by a family of proteins called integrins, which bind to matrix ligands. Next, activation of proteolytic enzymes occurs in the connective tissue stroma adjacent to tumor islands. These enzymes are known as matrix metalloproteinases and include interstitial collagenase, type IV collagenase, stromelysin-1, -2, and -3, and other enzymes capable of breaking down collagen, elastin, fibronectin, and other connective tissue components. These enzymes digest the extracellular matrix surrounding the tumor, thereby facilitating tumor growth and invasion.

The basement membrane zone of basal cell carcinoma has been studied extensively, as basement membrane characteristics appear to be linked to tumor invasiveness. While nodular, superficial, and circumscribed tumors are surrounded by an intact, sometimes thickened, basement membrane, aggressive growth pattern basal cell carcinomas have a discontinuous basement membrane. Defects in the basal lamina, loss of basement membrane type IV collagen, and the presence of type IV collagenase are noted in aggressively growing tumors but not in nodular, superficial, or circumscribed tumors. It is possible that the basement membrane defects noted in desmoplastic basal cell carcinomas may underlie their more aggressive growth characteristics, but this hypothesis has not yet been proven.

Growth factors and cytokines seem to play a role in tumor development, but the role that they play is not yet clear. Basal cell carcinoma has been found to produce both tumor angiogenic factor and fibronectin. Both of these factors may be important in local tumor growth.

Finally, local and systemic immune responses may play a role in the clinical and histologic appearance of basal cell carcinomas. The majority of cells that infiltrate these tumors are activated T lymphocytes, which may be consistent with a delayed type hypersensitivity reaction. It is interesting to note, however, that T lymphocytes and natural killer cells have been found to exhibit decreased activity in extracts of tumor cells. It may be that these cells play a role in tumor surveillance and that their effectiveness within this role decreases over time. It is also possible that an age-related decline in global immune function plays a permissive role in tumor development.

CLINICAL PRESENTATION

The classic rodent ulcer of basal cell carcinoma is easily recognized. Unfortunately, most lesions are not as clear and present with a combination of features. Features common to many basal cell carcinomas include scaling with erosion or ulceration, surrounding erythema with telangiectases, and a slow but relentless growth pattern.

Maintaining a high index of suspicion is essential to making the diagnosis. Any chronic, nonhealing lesion must be carefully evaluated. Patients with a history of basal cell carcinoma or evidence of chronic sun damage need thorough periodic skin examinations. Basal cell carcinoma may be classified into several characteristic types, but almost any combination of features may appear in any individual tumor.

Noduloulcerative Basal Cell Carcinoma

The noduloulcerative basal cell carcinoma is the classic rodent ulcer. In its early stages, the tumor is a small, smooth-surfaced nodule (Fig. 1). Fine telangiectases may be present at the periphery. As the lesion slowly expands, the central portion may ulcerate and bleed. This area may become crusted and depressed centrally. The borders of the papule may become pearly or rolled, typical of the rodent ulcer (Fig. 2). As the tumor enlarges and ulceration continues, pink or violaceous, fleshy nodules of tumor may appear in the central portions (Fig. 3). The tumor may become very friable and bleed easily.

Morpheaform or Sclerosing Basal Cell Carcinoma

The morpheaform or sclerosing basal cell carcinoma may be the most difficult to detect. Often it presents as a solitary flat or slightly depressed plaque that is slightly indurated. The surface is often smooth or shiny and white or slightly yellow in color (Fig. 4). Ulceration or erosion may occur in long-standing, large lesions (Fig. 5). Telangiectases may be present at the periphery. Atrophy or healing that appears atrophic may occur in the central portions of the lesion. As the name implies, these lesions often resemble a plaque or morphea or scar.

Because these lesions often appear innocuous, they are often quite extensive by the time the patients seeks treatment. This tumor is easily misdiagnosed because of its appearance, unless a

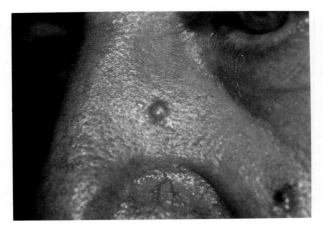

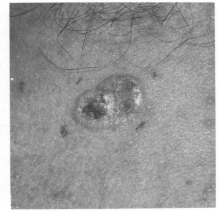

Figure 1 Noduloulcerative basal cell carcinoma; early lesion with smooth domed surface.

Figure 2 Noduloulcerative basal cell carcinoma with central ulceration and rolled border with telangiectasia.

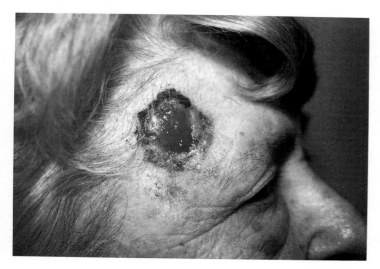

Figure 3 Noduloulcerative basal cell carcinoma: long-standing lesion with central fleshy nodule.

high index of suspicion is maintained. Furthermore, these lesions must be treated aggressively, since recurrence after conservative treatment is common. Unfortunately these lesions often occur on the nose, eyebrow, or forehead, causing cosmetic problems when removed.

Superficial Basal Cell Carcinoma

Superficial basal cell carcinoma is an erythematous, scaly, slightly indurated plaque. It may spread with a fine, threadlike border with small telangiectases (Fig. 6). Superficial ulceration and crust commonly develop in the central portion. This may heal, resulting in an atrophic appearance. Nodules of basal cell carcinoma may develop within these plaques.

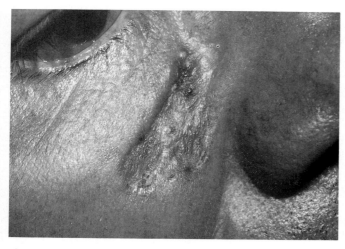

Figure 4 Morpheaform basal cell carcinoma; early lesion may resemble a scar.

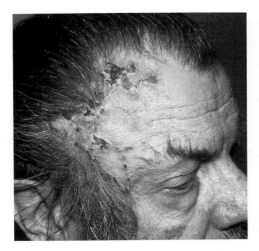

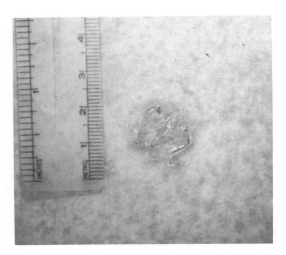

Figure 5 Morpheaform basal cell carcinoma. This long-standing lesion is extensive and has ulcerated.

Figure 6 Superficial erythematous basal cell carcinoma; erythematous plaque with advancing threadlike border.

Superficial basal cell carcinoma often occurs as several lesions on sun-damaged shoulders, back, or upper chest (Fig. 7). The clinical appearance may mimic psoriasis or eczema.

Pigmented Basal Cell Carcinoma

Melanin pigment may be present in any basal cell carcinoma in varying amounts. Deeply pigmented lesions are referred to as pigmented basal cell carcinoma. Noduloulcerative basal cell carcinomas may at times be so pigmented that they are confused with malignant melanoma (Fig. 8). Pigmented superficial basal cell carcinomas have a black or brown serpiginous advancing border.

Metastatic Basal Cell Carcinoma

Metastatic basal cell carcinoma is very rare. The incidence has been estimated as 0.0028% of dermatologic patients. The spread is most often to local lymph nodes, lungs, and bone. The median survival of patients with metastatic basal cell carcinoma is only 8 months. However, the time between diagnosis of the primary tumor and the diagnosis of metastatic disease averages 9 years.

The extremely low incidence of metastatic basal cell carcinoma may be due to the stromal dependence of the tumor. Basal cell carcinoma experimentally transplanted with the stroma survived, while basal cell carcinoma without the stroma did not. Therefore, basal cell carcinoma has diminished autonomy and little metastatic potential.

The occurrence of squamous metaplasia in basal cell carcinoma does not seem to play a role in the development of metastatic disease. Factors that seem to be important are the neurophilic response and intravascular invasion. Recurrence of basal cell carcinoma after treatment with radiation has also been associated with metastatic disease.

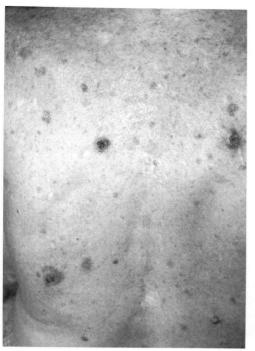

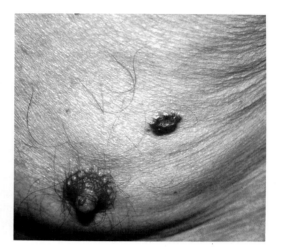

Figure 7 Superficial erythematous basal cell carcinoma often occurs as multiple lesions.

Figure 8 Pigmented basal cell carcinoma; deeply pigmented nodular basal cell carcinoma may mimic melanoma.

Nevoid Basal Cell Carcinoma Syndrome

The nevoid basal cell carcinoma syndrome is inherited in an autosomal dominant fashion with variable penetrance. Approximately 75% of patients develop dozens of multiple basal cell carcinomas at an early age. They may first occur in childhood but continue to develop into adulthood, commonly totaling hundreds of basal cell carcinomas.

Patients with the nevoid basal cell carcinoma syndrome may be genetically predisposed to develop basal cell carcinomas, due at least in part to increased sensitivity to the carcinogenic effects of ultraviolet radiation. The genetic mutation permits additional mutations by ultraviolet light that would otherwise be repaired in the normal host. The biologic behavior of the basal cell carcinomas in the nevoid basal cell carcinoma syndrome is highly variable: some act in a benign fashion, while others may be aggressively destructive.

Nevoid basal cell carcinoma syndrome is associated with a multiplicity of other growths, including fibromas, ovarian sarcomas, and fibrosarcomas of the sinuses and jaw. Odontogenic jaw cysts, calcification of the falx cerebri, and pitting of the palms and soles also occur. Abnormal facies with frontal bossing, a broad nasal root, and hypertelorism as well as other skeletal abnormalities such as bifid ribs and bone cysts are frequently seen as well.

Treatment of the tumors in nevoid basal cell carcinoma syndrome is by modalities used to treat solitary basal cell carcinoma, including cryosurgery, curettage, excision, and Mohs micrographic surgery. Radiation should only be used as palliative treatment for advanced carcinoma because of the genetic predisposition to develop more tumors. Photodynamic therapy with hematoporphyrin derivative and laser radiation as well as interferon have shown promise in early trials.

The prevention of the development of new tumors is of crucial importance in these patients. Sunscreens and sun protective clothing are essential. A twice-daily regimen of topical 5-fluorouracial and 0.1% tretinoin cream has been reported to be effective in controlling the development of new superficial tumors in one young patient. A large multicenter clinical trial of low-dose isotretinoin in the prevention of basal cell carcinomas in patients with the nevoid basal cell carcinoma syndrome found this form of therapy to be ineffective.

HISTOPATHOLOGIC FINDINGS

Even though there are several well-recognized subtypes of basal cell carcinoma, most tumors have several features in common. These are best illustrated by the most common variant, the solid basal cell carcinoma (Fig. 9). It consists of irregular masses of basaloid cells, often connected with the epidermis and invading the superficial or deep dermis. The cells resemble epidermal basal cells. They are small, tightly packed polymorphic cells composed of a basophilic nucleus without a discernible nucleolus and scanty cytoplasm. Frequently, there is a palisading arrangement at the periphery of the tumor nodule. Intercellular bridges are not observed. Mitotic activity and cellular atypia are characteristically rare or absent. Necrosis and ulceration may be noted in the superficial aspects of larger tumors. The surrounding stroma changes with increased numbers of fibroblasts, as well as increased amounts of collagen and connective tissue mucin. Typically, stromal retraction separates the tumor and dermis, which is an artifact of histologic processing. Acute and chronic inflammation of varying intensity may be present in the dermis adjacent to the tumor nodules.

While the solid or nodular basal cell carcinoma may be the most common histologic subtype, there is no obvious correlation between the clinical and histopathologic patterns. Frequently, several subtypes can be present histologically in one lesion. Adenoid, keratotic, and, more rarely, the cystic histologic patterns may be present in the noduloulcerative tumor. The adenoid type (Fig. 10) exhibits glandlike structures. The central aspect in the keratotoic type (Fig. 11) undergoes keratinization, forming horn cysts. The cystic type is hollow in the central portion of large tumor lobes, probably as a consequence of cell necrosis.

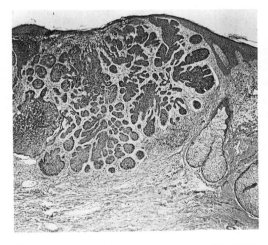

Figure 9 Solid basal cell carcinoma. Irregular masses of basaloid cells invade the dermis. Palisading arrangement of peripheral tumor cells can be seen.

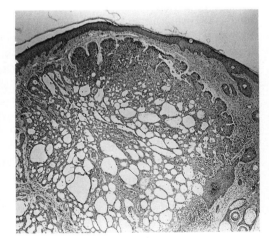

Figure 10 Adenoid basal cell carcinoma. Note glandlike structures of various sizes.

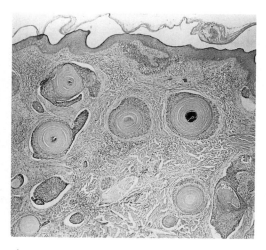

Figure 11 Keratotic basal cell carcinoma. Tumor is composed of foci of basaloid cells at the periphery with concentric whorls of keratin (horn cysts) in the center. Retraction of tissue causes an artifactual separation between tumor and stroma.

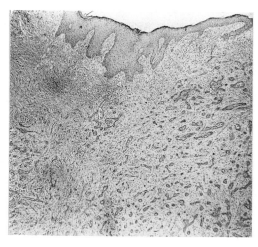

Figure 12 Morpheaform basal cell carcinoma. Small, thin, elongated, branching tumor cell aggregates fill the dermis amid a fibrous stroma.

The morpheaform or sclerosing (fibrosing) basal cell carcinoma (Fig. 12) is composed of very small tumor cell aggregates arranged in thin strands, often single cell layers (Fig. 13) embedded in a fibrotic stroma. Sometimes it is extremely difficult to determine the extent of invasion by these tumors. It frequently extends along perineural, perivascular, perichondrial, and other tissue fascial planes.

Superficial basal cell carcinoma is composed of several independent (multifocal) buds of tumor cells attached to the epidermis (Fig. 14). Biologically this tumor spreads horizontally, so

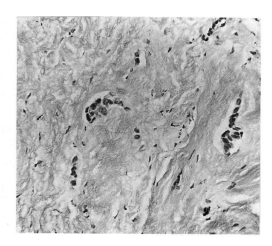

Figure 13 Single-cell invasion by basal cell carcinoma. Small tumor aggregates and even single tumor cells appear surrounded by fibrous stroma in this example of morpheaform basal cell carcinoma.

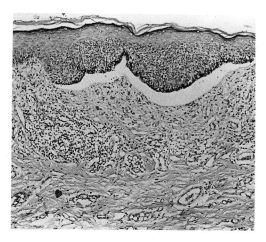

Figure 14 Superficial basal cell carcinoma. Two confluent buds of basaloid cells with peripheral palisading invade the superficial dermis. Retraction is prominent between the tumor and fibrotic dermis with sparse chronic inflammation.

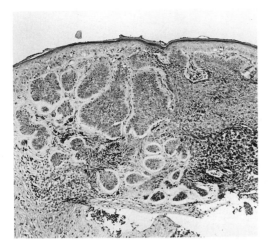

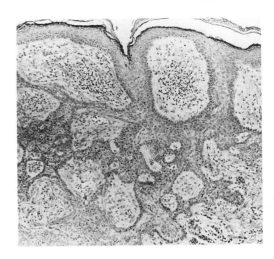

Figure 15 Pigmented basal cell carcinoma. The pattern is that of a solid basal cell carcinoma mixed with melanocytes and melanin pigment in the tumor cells. Pigment is abundant in the surrounding stroma, where it may be loose or contained in macrophages.

Figure 16 Fibroepithelioma of Pinkus. Anastomosing strands and aggregates of tumor cells with peripheral palisading are surrounded by fibrous stroma.

the superficial margins may be difficult to assess. This is because some of the tumor buds may be small and composed of as little as a single row of cells, which can be clinically indistinct.

Pigmented basal cell carcinoma (Fig.15) results from the presence of melanocytes and melanin admixed with the tumor cells. In most instances, the melanin accumulates in the stroma immediately adjacent to the tumor. Treatment is unaffected by the presence of melanin, aside from the need to rule out melanoma.

Many more histologic subtypes of basal cell carcinoma have been described and are reviewed in dermatopathology textbooks. Of note, the fibroepithelioma of Pinkus is not unanimously considered a subtype of basal cell carcinoma. This tumor consists of anastomosing strands and aggregates of tumor cells surrounded by fibrous stroma (Fig. 16).

In most instances, the diagnosis of basal cell carcinoma and its subtypes can be made readily by the trained observer. However, basal cell carcinoma may resemble elements of skin appendages, and it may be difficult to distinguish between these variants and appendageal neoplasms. For example, keratotic and solid basal cell carcinomas resemble rudimentary hair follicles and should be distinguished from trichoepitheliomas. Morepheaform basal cell carcinoma may resemble desmoplastic trichoepithelioma, and adenoid basal cell carcinoma may mimic sweat gland tumors. Basal cell carcinoma may exhibit sebaceous gland differentiation and must be distinguishable from squamous cell carcinoma and has been called the basosquamous carcinoma (metatypical basal cell carcinoma). Furthermore, basal cell carcinoma may also be difficult to distinguish from some cases of breast cancer, adenoic cystic tumors, and metastatic tumors.

Basal cell carcinomas do not show a distinct pattern when associated with the syndromes listed in Table 1. Likewise, it is not possible to predict the biological behavior of a basal cell carcinoma based on its histologic appearance. However, certain features, frequently encountered in recurrent tumors, are indicative of a more ominous prognosis. These features include stroma invasion by the tumor in small strands or even single cells (Fig. 13) and the invasion of the tumor along nerve sheaths (Fig. 17). In both instances, the extent of invasion may be unpredictable.

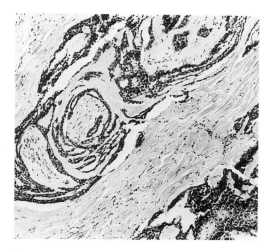

Figure 17 Perineural invasion of basal cell carcinoma. Layers of tumor cells invade perineural spaces, often in single-cell rows.

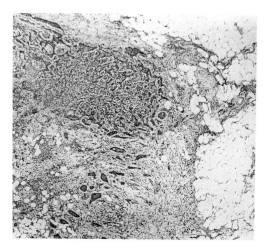

Figure 18 Metastatic basal cell carcinoma. Small aggregates of basal cell carcinoma have replaced a small lymph node and extend into the surrounding fat.

The most obvious sign of the malignant potential of basal cell carcinoma is the presence of metastasis (Fig. 18).

TREATMENT

The goal of treatment is to eradicate the tumor such that the likelihood of recurrence is as low as possible. While the majority of basal cell carcinomas are small, low-risk tumors that are easily treated, there is a high-risk population of tumors that must be treated more carefully, as their frequency of recurrence is greater. High-risk basal cell carcinomas include tumors that are recurrent, located in a site with a high rate of recurrence (such as the eyelid, lip, or nose), have an aggressive or morpheaform pattern of growth on biopsy, are clinically characterized by ill-defined borders, multicentricity, or radiation changes, or are large (i.e., >2 cm).

Small low-risk basal cell carcinomas may be treated by excision, electrodesiccation and curettage, cryosurgery, or electrosurgery. Recurrence rates for basal cell carcinomas treated with these modalities range from 4 to 10%. Patients who are poor surgical candidates or who have tumors in areas that are difficult to treat surgically, such as the eyelid, may be treated with radiation. Intralesional interferon-alpha has been used in the treatment of small nodular or superficial basal cell carcinomas with some success.

The treatment of choice for the high risk basal cell carcinoma is Mohs micrographic surgery. This is the only technique that permits a complete examination of the deep and peripheral margins via horizontal sectioning at the time of surgery. Advantages of this technique include its cure rate of 98–99% for primary tumors, its ability to conserve the maximal amount of normal tissue, and the fact that it provides an optimal tumor-free defect for repair.

BIBLIOGRAPHY

Adamson HG. On the nature of rodent ulcer: Its relationship to epithelioma adenoides cysticum of Brooke and to other trichoepitheliomata of benign nevoid character, its distinction from malignant carcinoma. *Lancet* 1914;1:810–814.

Barsky SH, Grossman DA, Bhuta S. Desmoplastic basal cell carcinomas possess unique basement membrane-degrading properties. *J Invest Dermatol* 1987;88:324–329.

Boring CB, Squires TS, Tong T. Cancer Statistics. *CA* 1993;43:7–26.

Cancer Statistics. *CA* 1993;43:18–19.

Cooper M, Pinkus H. Intrauterine transplantation of rat basal cell carcinoma as a model for reconversion of malignant to benign growth. *Cancer Res* 1977;37:2544–2552.

Cornell RC, Greenway HT, Tucker SB, Edwards L, et al. Intralesional interferon therapy for basal cell carcinoma. *J Am Acad Dermatol* 1990;23:694–700.

Cox NH. Basal cell carcinoma in young adults. *Br J Dermatol* 1992;127(1):26–29.

Diffey BL, Tate TJ, Davis A. Solar dosimetry of the face: The relationship of natural ultraviolet radiation exposure to basal cell carcinoma localization. *Phys Med Biol* 1979;24:931–939.

Domarus H, Stevens PJ. Metastatic basal cell carcinoma. *J Am Acad Dermatol* 1984;10:1043–1060.

Drake LA, Ceilley RI, Cornelison RL, Dobes WA, et al. Guidelines of care for basal cell carcinoma. The American Academy of Dermatology Committee on Guidelines of Care. *J Am Acad Dermatol* 1992;26(1): 117–120.

Foot NC. Adenexal carcinoma of the skin. *Am J Pathol* 1947;23:1–27.

Gallagher RP, MA B, McLean DI, Yang CP et al. Trends in basal cell carcinoma, squamous cell carcinoma, and melanoma of the skin from 1973 through 1987. *J Am Acad Dermatol* 1990;23(3 Pt 1):413–421.

Gerstein W. Transplantation of basal cell epithelioma to the rabbit. *Arch Dermatol* 1963;88:834–836.

Geschickter CF, Koehler HP. Ectodermal tumors of the skin. *Am J Cancer* 1935;23:804–836.

Goldstein AM, Bale SJ, Peck GL, DiGiovanna JJ. Sun exposure and basal cell carcinomas in the nevoid basal cell carcinoma syndrome. *J Am Acad Dermatol* 1993;29(1):34–41.

Gosten JB, Eisen AZ, Bauer EA. Stimulation of skin fibroblast collagenase production by a cytokine derived from basal cell carcinomas. *J Invest Dermatol* 1986;86:161–164.

Grimwood RE, Ferris CF, Mercill DB, Huff JC. Proliferating cells of human basal cell carcinomas are located on the periphery of tumor nodules. *J Invest Dermatol* 1986;86:191–194.

Grimwood RE, Ferris CF, Nielsen LD, Huff JC, Clark RAF. Basal cell carcinoma grown in nude mice produce, and deposit fibronectin in the extracellular matrix. *J Invest Dermatol* 1986;87:42–46.

Guillen FJ, Day CL Jr, Murphy GF. Expression of activation antigen by T-cells infiltrating basal cell carcinomas. *J Invest Dermatol* 1985;85:203–206.

Hernandez AD, Hibbs MS, Postlethwaite AE. Establishment of basal cell carcinoma in culture: Evidence of a basal cell carcinoma-derived factor(s) which stimulates fibroblasts to proliferate and release collagenase. *J Invest Dermatol* 1985;85:470–475.

Howell JB. Nevoid basal cell carcinoma syndrome. *J Am Acad Dermatol* 1984;11:98–104.

Jacob A. Observations respecting an ulcer of peculiar character which attacks the eyelids and other parts of the face. *Dublin Hosp Rep* 1827;4:231–239.

Kraemer KH. Xeroderma pigmentosum. In *Clinical Dermatology*, Vol. 4. DJ Demis, ed. Philadelphia, Harper & Row, 1986;19(7):1–33.

Kripke ML. Impact of ozone depletion of skin cancers. *J Dermatol Surg Oncol* 1988;14:853–857.

Krompecher E. *Der Basalzellenkrebs*. Jena, Gustav Fischer, 1903.

Lever WF, Schaumburg-Lever G. *Histopathology of the Skin*, 7th ed. Philadelphia, JB Lippincott, 1983, pp. 622–634.

Lever WF. Pathogenesis of benign tumors of cutaneous appendages and of basal cell epithelioma. *Arch Dermatol Syphilol* 1948;57:679–724.

Lowe L, Rapini RP. Newer variants of simulants of basal cell carcinoma. *J Dermatol Surg Oncol* 1991;17(8): 641–648.

Lynch HT, Fusaro RM, Roberts L, Voorhees GJ, Lynch JF. Muir-Torre syndrome in several members of a family with variant of the cancer family syndrome. *Br J Dermatol* 1985;113:295–301.

Mallory FB. Recent progress in the microscopic anatomy and differentiation of cancer. *JAMA* 1910;55:1513–1516.

Maloney ME, Jones DB, Sexton FM. Pigmented basal cell carcinoma developing after treatment of a basal cell carcinoma. *J Am Acad Dermatol* 1993;27(1):74–78.

Marghoob A, Kopf AW, Bart RS, Sanfilippo L et al. Risk of another basal cell carcinoma developing after treatment of a basal cell carcinoma. *J Am Acad Dermatol* 1993;28(1):22–28.

Michaelsson G, Olsson E, Westermark P. The Rombo syndrome: A familial disorder with vermiculate atrophoderma, milia, hypotrichosis, trichoepitheliomas, basal cell carcinomas and peripheral vasodilation with cyanosis. *Acta Derm Venereol (Stockh)* 1981;61:497–503.

Millard LG. Multiple pigmented papular basal cell carcinomas: A new pattern of industrial tar-induced skin tumors. *Br J Int Med* 1986;43:134–136.

Miller SJ. Biology of basal cell carcinoma (Part I). *J Am Acad Dermatol* 1991;24(1):1–13.

Miller SJ. Biology of basal cell carcinoma (Part II). *J Am Acad Dermatol* 1991;24(II):161–175.

Mulay DM. Skin cancer in India. *Natl Cancer Inst Mongr* 1963;10:215–223.

Noodleman FR, Pollack SV. Trauma as a possible etiologic factor in basal cell carcinoma. *J Dermatol Surg Oncol* 1986;12:841–846.

Oettle AG. Skin cancer in Africa. *Natl Cancer Inst Mongr* 1963;10:197–214.

Paver K, Poyzer K, Burry N, Deakin M. The incidence of basal cell carcinoma and their metastases in Australia and New Zealand. *Australas J Dermatol* 1973;14:53.

Pawlowski A, Haberman HF. Heterotransplantation of human basal cell carcinomas in "nude" mice. *J Invest Dermatol* 1979;72:310–313.

Pinkus H. Epithelial and fibroepithelial tumors. *Bull NY Acad Med* 1965;41:176–189.

Pinkus H. Premalignant fibroepithelial tumors of the skin. *Arch Dermatol Syphilol* 1953;67:598–615.

Robinson JK, Salasche SJ. Isotretinoin does not prevent basal cell carcinoma. *Arch Dermatol* 1992;128:975–976.

Sandstrom A, Larsson L-G, Damber L. Occurrence of other malignancies in patients treated for basal cell carcinoma of the skin: A cohort study. *Acta Radiol Oncol* 1984;23:227–230.

Silverman MK, Kopf AW, Grin CM, Bart RS, Levenstein MJ. Recurrence rates of treated basal cell carcinomas. Part 1: Overview. *J Dermatol Surg Oncol* 1992;17(9):713–718.

Smith SP, Grande DJ. Basal cell carcinoma recurring after radiotherapy: A unique, difficult treatment subclass of recurrent basal cell carcinoma. *J Derm Surg Oncol* 1991;17(1):26–30.

Stanley JR, Beckwith JB, Fuller RP, Katz SI. A specific antigenic defect of the basement membrane is found in basal cell carcinoma but not in other epidermal tumors. *Cancer* 1982;50:1486–1490.

Strange PR, Lang PG. Long-term management of basal cell nevus syndrome with topical tretinoin and 5-fluorouracil. *J Am Acad Dermatol* 1992;27(5 Pt 2):842–845.

Synkowsky DR, Schuster P, Orlando JC. The immunobiology of basal cell carcinoma: An in situ monoclonal antibody study. *Br J Dermatol* 1985;113:441–446.

Terz J, Lawrence W Jr, Cox B. Analysis of the cycling and noncycling cell populations of human solid tumors. *Cancer* 1977;40:1462–1470.

Traenkle HL. X-ray-induced skin cancer in man. *Natl Cancer Inst Monogr* 1963;10:423–432.

Urbach F, Davies RE, Forbes PD. Ultraviolet radiation and skin cancer in man. In *Advances in Biology of Skin*, Vol. III. W Montagna, RL Dobson, eds. Oxford, Pergamon Press, 1955, pp. 195–214.

Urbach F, Rose DB, Bonnem M. Genetic and environmental interactions in skin carcinogenesis. In *Environment and Cancer*. Baltimore, William & Wilkins, 1972, pp. 355–371.

Van Scott EJ, Reinertson RP. The modulating influence of stromal environment on epithelial cells studied in human autotransplants. *J Invest Dermatol* 1961;36:109–117.

Viksnins P, Berlin A. Follicular atrophoderma and basal cell carcinomas: The Bazex syndrome. *Arch Dermatol* 1977;113:948–951.

Weinstein GD, Frost P. Cell proliferation in human basal cell carcinoma. *Cancer Res* 1970;30:724–728.

Wilson BD, Mang TS, Stoll H, Jones C, et al. Photodynamic therapy for the treatment of basal cell carcinoma. *Arch Dermatol* 1992;128(12):1597–1601.

Yeh S. Skin cancer in chronic arsenicism. *Hum Pathol* 1973;4:469–485.

Zaynoun S, Ali LA, Shaib J, Kurban A. The relationship of sun exposure and solar elastosis to basal cell carcinoma. *J Am Acad Dermatol* 1985;12:522–525.

31

Squamous Cell Carcinoma

Jeffrey L. Melton
Loyola University of Chicago, Maywood, Illinois

C. William Hanke
Indiana University School of Medicine, Indianapolis, Indiana

Squamous cell carcinoma (SCC) of the skin and mucous membranes often arises on actinically damaged skin. Solar keratoses are the precursor, premalignant lesions, but occasionally SCC develops in clinically normal skin. Urbach demonstrated that nearly all SCC occurs in sun-exposed areas, while only two-thirds of all basal cell carcinomas are similarly distributed. SCC is, therefore, more directly related to ultraviolet radiation than is basal cell carcinoma. Approximately one-quarter of all nonmelanoma skin cancers are squamous cell carcinoma. In 1994, the incidence of nonmelanoma skin cancer was projected to be approximately 1,000,000. Therefore, the current incidence of SCC is approximately 250,000 cases per year, the majority of which are due to SCC. Interestingly, the incidence of SCC may be increasing even faster than that of other cutaneous malignancies. An Australian survey indicated an 11% increase in the incidence of basal cell carcinoma, and a striking 51% increase in the incidence of SCC over the 5-year period from 1985 to 1990. Statistics for morbidity due to SCC are sketchy or nonexistent; however, it is clear that substantial morbidity due to SCC exists.

METASTATIC SPREAD

SCC has a metastatic potential intermediate between that of basal cell carcinoma and melanoma. The actual metastatic rate of SCC is controversial, and a wide range of metastatic rates (0.5–31%) appear in the literature. Metastatic rate can be characterized with somewhat more accuracy when certain host factors are taken into account. SCC occurring in actinically damaged skin may have a lower incidence of metastasis than SCC arising in nonactinically damaged skin. However, many now feel that the estimated 0.5% incidence of metastasis for SCC arising in actinically damaged skin may be much too low. SCC arising in certain specific sites are more likely to metastasize. The most notable example is SCC of the lip, which has an 11% rate of metastasis (Fig. 1). The eyelid, ear, oral mucous membranes, glans penis, and vulva are the other high-risk sites for metastasis.

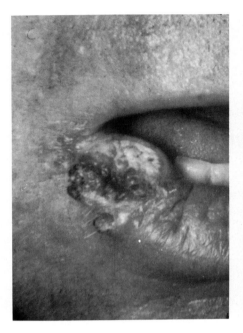

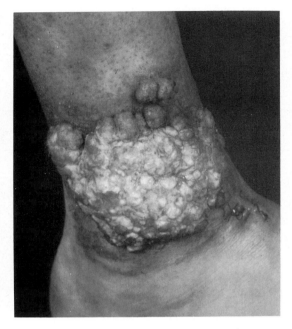

Figure 1 Ulcerated nodule on the lower lip. This is a common presentation of squamous cell carcinoma.

Figure 2 A draining sinus in a patient with chronic osteomyelitis. An exophytic squamous cell carcinoma developed after several years.

The larger the clinical size of the tumor, the more likely metastasis is to occur. In the review by Rowe et al., 9% of lesions smaller than 2 cm metastasized, while 30% of lesions larger than 2 cm metastasized. Histologic depth is also predictive of metastasis, with lesions penetrating to Clark's level IV or V being much more likely to metastasize. Histologically poorly differentiated SCC are more likely to metastasize. In studies reporting degree of differentiation, the metastatic rate was 9% for well-differentiated tumors vs. 33% for poorly differentiated tumors.

SCC arising in sites of chronic injury or scars have a notably high rate of metastasis. For example, 31% of SCC arising in foci of chronic osteomyelits metastasize (Fig. 2). Similarly, 20% of SCC that result from radiation injury and 18% of those arising in old scars will metastasize (Figs. 3–5). SCC occurs more frequently and is more aggressive in immunocompromised patients. In such cases SCC is often more prevalent than is basal cell carcinoma (BCC). Clinical settings include HIV infection and AIDS, status postrenal transplantation, and status post-PUVA treatment. Previously treated SCC has a higher rate of metastasis, ranging from 25 to 45%, depending upon the site of the lesion.

CAUSE AND PATHOGENESIS

Ultraviolet Light Carcinogenesis

Ultraviolet (UV) radiation is the most important cause of SCC of the skin. UV light, especially UVB (290–320 nm), causes photochemical alterations in DNA resulting in abnormal nucleotide pairing and carcinogenesis. UV exposure also induces immunologic defects in the skin and lymphocytes that may predispose to malignancy.

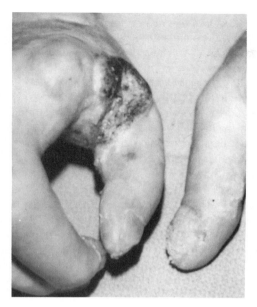

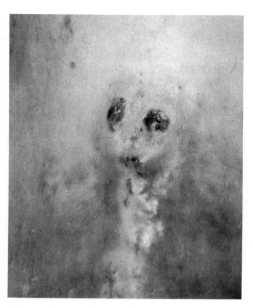

Figure 3 After superficial x-ray treatment for hand eczema 30 years previously, the patient now has an infiltrating recurrent squamous cell carcinoma involving the right metacarpal head and proximal thumb.

Figure 4 An ulcerated squamous cell carcinoma in an old burn scar on the leg.

Sun exposure was first implicated as a carcinogenic factor during the late 1800s. In 1906, Hyde observed that some people had a greater sensitivity to sunlight than others. He recognized that skin pigmentation provided some protection from the sun's effects.

Later studies showed that the incidence of skin cancer was associated with certain physical characteristics. Skin type and skin color are the most important factors affecting the frequency

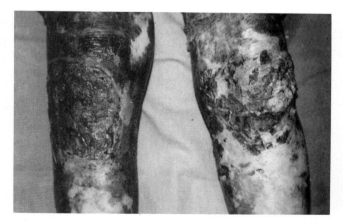

Figure 5 Extensive scarring due to epidermolysis bullosa dystrophica. Large squamous cell carcinomas developed below the knees.

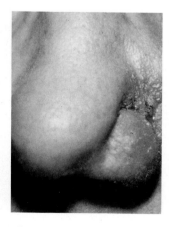

Figure 6 A painful, indurated subcutaneous nodule in the nasofacial sulcus due to poorly differentiated squamous cell carcinoma.

of skin cancer. SCC occurs most commonly in people with fair skin who sunburn easily and do not tan well (skin types I and II). These individuals usually have blue eyes and red or blond hair. Irish, Scottish, and English ancestry is associated with an especially high risk of SCC as well as other forms of skin cancer.

The amount of UV exposure is another factor that influences the incidence of skin cancer. The intensity of UV light that reaches the skin is determined in part by latitude. Ratzer and Strong found that each 3°45' latitude closer to the equator doubled the frequency of skin cancer. In the United States, the incidence of SCC of the skin is much higher in the south than the north.

Altitude, air pollution, meteorologic conditions, and the stratospheric ozone layer also affect the intensity of UV radiation. The ozone layer absorbs many of the carcinogenic wavelengths of UV light. However, the ozone layer has been damaged by pollutants and is not as effective a barrier as it once was.

Occupation and leisure activity influence the amount of UV exposure that the skin receives. Unna observed changes in sailors' skin due to excessive sun exposure. People who work outdoors, such as farmers, sailors, construction workers, and some professional athletes, have a higher incidence of skin cancer than people who work indoors.

In light-skinned people, most SCC occurs on areas of the body chronically exposed to UV radiation. These include the head, neck, dorsal hands, and forearms (Fig. 6,7). The ears and scalp (in balding men) are also particularly susceptible (Fig. 8). PUVA treatment also appears to put patients at increased risk for SCC.

Chemical Carcinogenesis

SCC of the skin may also result from contact with chemical carcinogens. Arsenic and organic hydrocarbons are the most common offenders. Exposure is frequently occupational; however, chemical carcinogens are found in many settings. The cancers are produced by the direct action of the chemical on the skin. The incidence of chemically induced skin cancer is proportional to the duration of exposure to the carcinogen.

The Englishman Percivall Pott was the first to describe chemical carcinogenesis. In 1755 he reported that the high frequency of scrotal cancer in chimney sweeps was due to chronic expo-

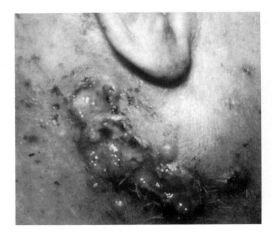

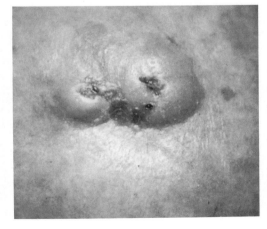

Figure 7   Squamous cell carcinoma of the neck.

Figure 8   A nodular squamous cell carcinoma on the bald scalp of a 70-year-old man.

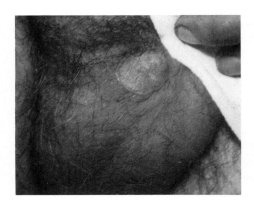

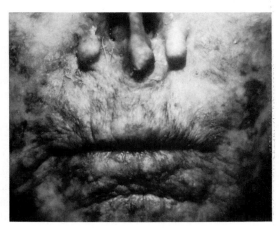

Figure 9 Chronic exposure to oils. Squamous cell carcinoma of the scrotum in a textile worker.

Figure 10 Chronic radiodermatitis secondary to superficial x-ray treatment for facial acne. The patient now has pigment changes as well as multiple basal cell and squamous cell carcinomas in this area.

sure to soot. Since then other environmental carcinogens have been identified including coal tar, paraffin oil, shale oil, creosote oil, petroleum oil, and asphalt (Fig. 9).

Arsenic is another chemical carcinogen. Industrial exposure occurs in the smelting of metal ores and the manufacture and agricultural use of insecticides. In the environment, carcinogenic amounts of arsenic can be found in drinking water in several parts of the world. During the nineteenth and early twentieth centuries, arsenic was used medicinally. Fowler's solution (AS_2O_3), Donovan's solution (ASI_3 plus HgI_2), and Asiatic pills (AS_2O_3) are arsenic-containing medications commonly used to treat many different common diseases.

Ionizing Radiation Carcinogenesis

Ionizing radiation may produce SCC of the skin as a result of fractionated, small doses of radiation. The cancers appear following a lag period of 10–30 years. Several occupational groups are frequently exposed to radiation including physicians, dentists, nurses, technicians, and engineers. Exposure may also be therapeutic. Radiation used to treat malignancies as well as benign conditions such as acne, hirsutism, and hemangiomas is associated with cutaneous malignancy (Fig. 10).

In 1902, soon after the discovery of x-rays, Frieben first reported roentgen-radiation–induced SCC. He reported SCC in people working with roentgen machines. Shortly thereafter, cutaneous carcinoma was observed in patients who had received roentgen radiation thereapeutically.

Today ionizing radiation is responsible for very little cutaneous carcinoma. The treatment of benign skin lesions with radiation has largely been abandoned, and occupational and industrial exposure are better controlled. Radiation therapy for malignancy has advanced and the technology improved to minimize this problem.

HUMAN PAPILLOMAVIRUS

Human papillomavirus (HPV) has been increasingly implicated as having an important role in the development of cervical, and more recently, cutaneous, SCC. Most cervical and penile SCC contain HPV DNA. DNA of HPV type 16 is the HPV type DNA most strongly associated with malignancy in these lesions. Moy et al. first reported the presence of HPV-16 DNA in nongenital SCC, in periungual lesions. HPV-16 DNA was present in five of seven SCC of the finger. HPV DNA has also been demonstrated in keratoacanthomas. HPV is much less likely to be present or involved in SCC of nongenital, nonperiungual sites. The exact role of HPV in oncogenesis is not yet known, but the role of the HPV E6 and E7 genes appears to be important.

PREMALIGNANT FORMS OF SQUAMOUS CELL CARCINOMA

SCC has premalignant forms (actinic keratosis, radiation keratosis, actinic cheilitis, arsenical keratosis, thermal keratosis, hydrocarbon keratosis, and cutaneous horn) and in situ forms (Bowen's disease, erythroplasia of Queyrat) that are confined to the epidermis. Bowen's disease may involve hair follicles and extend to the level of subcutaneous tissue (Fig. 11). Actinic keratoses are macules and papules with variable degrees of scaling on sun-exposed areas. Hyperkeratotic actinic keratoses require biopsy to rule out invasive SCC. When a large number of actinic keratoses are present in an area, the potential for the development of invasive SCC is increased (Fig. 12).

Bowen's Disease

Bowen's disease presents as a sharply circumscribed scaling erythematous patch that is generally larger than the usual actinic keratosis (Fig. 13). The plaque may be slightly elevated and

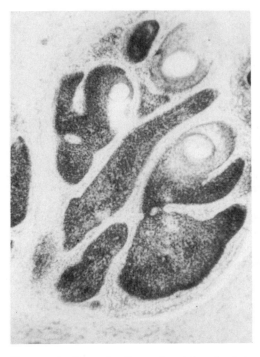

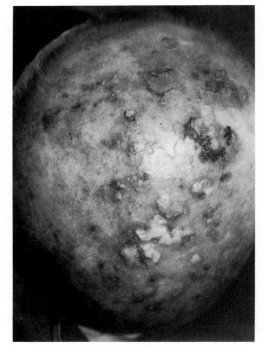

Figure 11 Bowen's disease involving the hair follicle epithelium deep in the scalp (hematoxylin & eosin, ×200).

Figure 12 Multiple hypertrophic actinic keratoses on the bald scalp of a 75-year-old man.

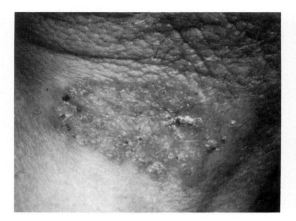

Figure 13 Bowen's disease.

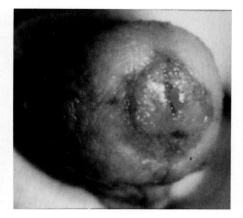

Figure 14 Erythroplasia of Queyrat in an uncircumcised man. Surgical resection revealed involvement of the distal third of the urethra.

mimic eczema or psoriasis. Most cases of Bowen's disease are on sun-exposed sites and may be related to solar exposure. Bowen's disease on non–sun-exposed areas may be caused by inorganic arsenic exposure or may be a marker for internal malignancy. Bowen's disease may develop into invasive SCC in 11% of cases. Bowen's disease in blacks occurs three times more frequently on non–sun-exposed areas. Mora et al. reported on black patients with Bowen's disease who developed invasive SCC and internal malignancy.

Erythroplasia of Queyrat

Erythroplasia of Queyrat is squamous cell carcinoma in situ localized to the glans penis, more commonly occurring in uncircumcised men. Clinically it is characterized as a well-marginated, shiny, red plaque (Fig. 14). The histopathologic appearance is identical to that of Bowen's disease. Thirty percent of patients with erythroplasia of Queyrat develop invasive SCC within the lesion and 20% of these metastasize.

CLINICAL FEATURES

The clinical features of SCC vary. Commonly SCC appears as an ulcerated nodule or a superficial ulceration on the skin or lower lip (Fig. 15). Another common presentation is as a verrucous papule or plaque with a thick cornified layer. Less commonly, a large verrucous nodule may develop. The typically rolled pearly border with overlying telangiectases seen in basal cell carcinoma easily differentiates this from SCC. When a rolled border is present, it usually does not have overlying telangiectasia. Peripheral margins of the tumor are not well defined, as in basal cell carcinoma. The tumor may fix to the deeper structures as it invades. Perineural invasion is an uncommon finding that is usually indicative of a poor prognosis (Figs. 16,17).

HISTOPATHOLOGIC FINDINGS

SCC consists of proliferating masses of epidermal cells that extend into the dermis. The most malignant varieties of SCC contain a larger proportion of atypical cells.

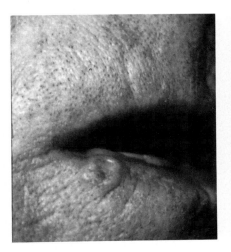

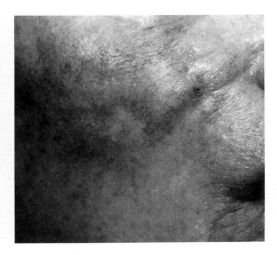

Figure 15 A biopsy specimen from this nodule on the vermilion border of the lip demonstrated a well-differentiated squamous cell carcinoma.

Figure 16 Preoperative photograph of a squamous cell carcinoma (with extensive perineural invasion) on the central right cheek that had recurred many times.

Well-differentiated SCC is composed of large polygonal cells with intercellular bridges, round nuclei, and eosinophilic cytoplasm (Fig. 18). Horn pearls are common, composed of concentric layers of keratin and characterized by incomplete keratinization in the center. Poorly differentiated SCC is characterized by nuclear atypia and mitotic figures (Fig. 19). Tumor cells vary in shape from polygonal to stellate or fusiform (i.e., spindle cells).

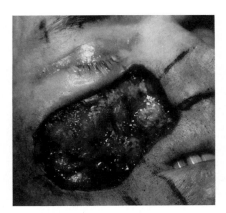

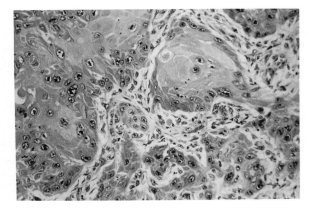

Figure 17 Extensive perineural invasion was evident after three stages of Mohs micrographic surgery. This is the immediate postoperative wound. The tumor ultimately invaded the brain stem and caused the patient's death (same patient shown in Fig. 16).

Figure 18 Well-differentiated squamous cell carcinoma with horn pearls (hematoxylin & eosin, ×200).

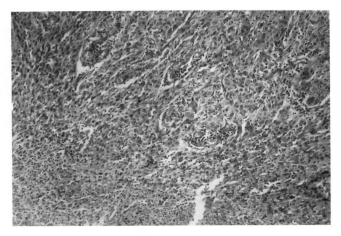

Figure 19 Poorly differentiated squamous cell carcinoma with sheets of anaplastic cells without horn pearl formation (hematoxylin & eosin, ×200).

Broders' classification of the degree of malignancy of SCC is based on the proportion of differentiated squamous cells to undifferentiated squamous cells. SCC grade I contains greater than 75% well-differentiated cells; grade II, 50–74%; grade III, 25–49%; grade IV, less than 25%. Thus, histologically SCC represents a continuum based on cytologic characteristics. Well-differentiated SCC has a good prognosis while, at the other end of the spectrum, poorly differentiated SCC has a poorer prognosis. The majority of SCC are low-grade tumors with a high degree of cellular differentiation and superficial depth of invasion.

Another feature that affects prognosis is depth of invasion. Invasion to the level of the eccrine sweat glands or below is predictive of poor prognosis. Perineural invasion is uncommon but is an ominous sign when it occurs (Fig. 20). Weidner and Foucar reported SCC associated with epithelial mucin production and considered that it was a sign of more aggressive behavior.

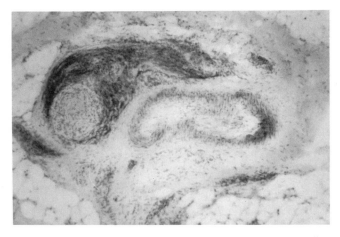

Figure 20 Chronic inflammation and tumor cells surrounding cutaneous nerves (hematoxylin & eosin, ×300).

It is sometimes difficult to know if an actinic keratosis has progressed to SCC. Atypical cells, dyskeratosis, and downward epidermal proliferation occur in both conditions. In SCC, however, the dermis is invaded by a tumor mass. Often step sectioning a hypertrophic actinic keratosis reveals invasive SCC in other parts of the lesion.

The adenoid or pseudoglandular variant of SCC occurs predominantly on sun-exposed areas in elderly patients. It may arise from actinic keratoses or de novo. Clinically, it is impossible to distinguish from other types of SCC. Metastases occur rarely. Acantholytic actinic keratoses may overlie adenoid SCC. Tubular lumina and alveolar formations are lined by several layers of tumor cells (Fig. 21). The luminal spaces are filled with acantholytic cells, some of which are keratinized. The process of acantholysis in adenoid SCC is similar to that seen in acantholytic actinic keratoses. An additional feature of acantholytic SCC is a proliferation of sweat duct epithelium induced by the inflammatory infiltrates surrounding the tumor.

Spindle cell SCC occurs largely on sun-damaged or radiation-damaged skin. The cells are spindle-shaped and sometimes difficult to differentiate from malignant melanoma, atypical fibroxanthoma, and fibrosarcoma. Differentiation is more difficult when there is no evidence of keratinization, intercellular bridges, or epidermal connection. Immunoperoxidase staining with anti-keratin antibodies and electron microscopy may be necessary.

KERATOACANTHOMA

Although keratoacanthoma has been considered a benign lesion by some, it is considered by most to be a variant of SCC. It is often difficult to differentiate the two clinically or histopathologically. Both entities occur on sun-exposed skin of older patients. HPV-16 DNA has been found in keratoacanthomas as well as in classical SCC. Immunocompromised patients have a higher incidence of keratoacanthomas and classical SCC. Multiple lesions are common in this clinical setting. Keratoacanthoma is a dome-shaped verrucous nodule with a central keratin-filled crater. Keratoacanthomas characteristically are faster growing than most SCC. The key feature that differentiates keratoacanthoma from SCC is its tendency to involute and resolve spontaneously. Regression usually occurs over a 6-month period. However, keratoacanthomas do not always follow the prototypical course. They may continue to grow rapidly and become quite large.

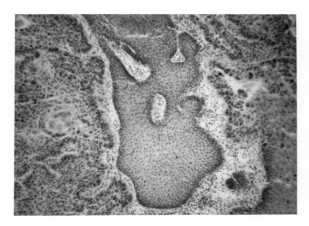

Figure 21 An adenoid squamous cell carcinoma with atypical cells and clefts containing acantholytic cells (hematoxylin & eosin, × 200).

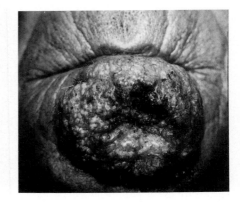

Figure 22 A giant keratoacanthoma rapidly enlarged over 6 weeks.

Considerable deformity and destruction of tissue may occur, particularly when keratoacanthomas occur in the nasal area (Fig. 22). A keratoacanthoma may also remain static for several years, followed by renewed rapid growth. Metastases have been reported.

An excisional biopsy of the entire lesion provides the best material for histopathologic diagnosis. Alternatively, a pie-shaped wedge biopsy may be helpful if taken to adequate depth. Intracytoplasmic glycogen and intraepithelial elastic fibers are more abundant in keratoacanthoma than in SCC. Immunohistochemical stains have not been helpful in differentiating keratoacanthoma from SCC. Resolution of the lesion, either spontaneously or in response to intralesional chemotherapy, is perhaps the most reliable diagnostic criterion, albeit a retrospective one. Both 5-FU and methotrexate have been successfully used as intralesional agents. Two to four injections are usually required. Careful follow-up is important if intralesional treatment is used, and a post-treatment biopsy to confirm tumor eradication should be considered. If there is any question regarding the diagnosis, the lesion should be treated as if it were SCC.

VERRUCOUS CARCINOMA

Verrucous carcinoma is a low-grade SCC that occurs in the oral cavity, anogenital region, and on the plantar aspect of the foot. It was first described by Ackerman in 1948 in the oral cavity. Verrucous carcinoma presents as an exophytic verrucous mass that grows slowly (Fig. 23). The diagnosis is made both on clinical and microscopic grounds.

In the oral cavity, verrucous carcinoma is also called oral florid papillomatosis. Large areas of the oral mucosa are involved with white cauliflowerlike vegetations. In the anogenital region, it is called giant condyloma of Buschke and Loewenstein. Papillomatous vegetations most commonly occur on the glans penis of uncircumcised men, and the urethra may also be involved. Verrucous carcinoma has also been described in the anovulvar areas. On the plantar surface, verrucous carcinoma is also called epithelioma cuniculatum and may be confused with a large plantar wart. Deep crypts develop on the tumor surface as it enlarges. In late stages, the plantar fascia and metatarsal bones may be involved.

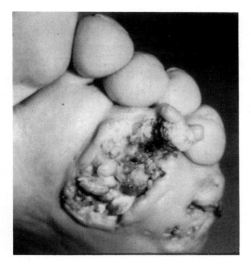

Figure 23 Verrucous carcinoma of the plantar surface.

A large excisional biopsy is important to the diagnosis. Features of verrucous carcinoma in common with warts include hyperkeratosis, parakeratosis, and acanthosis. Some portions of verrucous carcinoma demonstrate broad proliferations of well-differentiated keratinocytes and keratin-containing cysts that compress normal collagen. Nuclear atypia is absent even at the depth of the tumor. HPV viral particles have been identified by DNA hybridization techniques in some patients with plantar verrucous carcinoma.

Verrucous carcinoma has low metastatic potential but can penetrate deeply into local tissues. Metastasis occurs in rare cases. It has been suggested that radiation therapy for verrucous carcinoma may increase metastatic potential. The first case of verrucous carcinoma from the foot with extranodal metastases was reported by McKee et al. One patient with plantar verrucous carcinoma seen by the author had not received radiation yet developed regional lymph node metastases.

TREATMENT

Treatment of SCC is based on several factors including the size, location, and degree of histologic differentiation of the tumor, as well as the age and physical condition of the patient. Preoperative biopsy is essential to reveal the degree of cellular differentiation and the depth of penetration. These facts aid in the selection of the most appropriate treatment and the proper degree of aggressiveness of the treatment.

Surgical excision, radiation, curettage and electrodesiccation, and cryosurgery are standard methods of primary treatment. Mohs micrographic surgery is best-suited for recurrent lesions or tumors in critical anatomic sites. Any of the standard methods will suffice for primary, superficial, well-differentiated tumors. However, when SCC demonstrates an infiltrating pattern with narrow microscopic strands of tumor cells, Mohs micrographic surgery is a better alternative.

When metastases develop, wide excision is usually indicated (Fig. 24). Radiation may be given as the primary treatment, or following surgery to increase the cure rate. Radiation and chemotherapy are useful as palliative measures.

Surgical Excision

The efficiency and simplicity of surgical excision are distinct advantages for the patient and physician. The procedure can be performed on an outpatient basis with local anesthesia. A fusiform excision closed primarily without distortion of adjacent anatomic structures is used for small and moderate-sized lesions. For larger tumors, a skin flap or graft may be performed.

Based upon a prospective study of subclinical tumor extension, Brodland and Zitelli have proposed guidelines for surgical margins for excision of SCC. Four-millimeter margins were proposed for all but high-risk SCC, for which a minimum margin of 6 mm was recommended. High-risk features associated with greater risk of subclinical extension included size of 2 cm or larger, histologic grade 2 or higher, invasion of subcutaneous tissue, and location in high-risk areas.

For recurrent or large aggressive SCC, reconstruction of the defect should not be done until there is confirmation of clear margins. A split-thickness skin graft or healing by second intention may be a better alternative. Delayed closure should be considered when the risk of recurrence is high. Recurrent tumor after complete reconstruction may be camouflaged.

Curettage and Electrodesiccation

Curettage and electrodesiccation (C & E) is useful for tumors less than 1 cm in diameter that do not extend to the subcutaneous fat. This method is used to treat small, well-defined SCC in

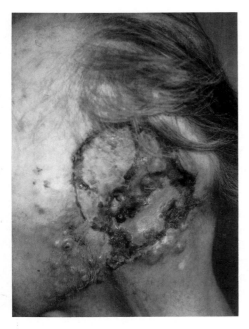

Figure 24 Metastatic nodules around a skin graft 6 weeks after excision of squamous cell carcinoma from the auricle.

patients with chronic radiation dermatitis. The procedure is quick and simple, it avoids suturing, and the scars are acceptable. When treating SCC, it is important to electrodesiccate the wound bed thoroughly at the end of the procedure to destroy viable tumor cells on the surface of the wound that may implant.

A disadvantage of C & E compared to surgical excision is that no specimen is sent for margin examination. However, the cure rates for C & E indicate that this is not significant when the appropriate tumors are treated in this fashion. The cure rate for uncomplicated superficial SCC with C & E is greater than 90%. Physicians with skill and experience in this method obtain significantly higher cure rates than physicians in training. Curettage is not recommended for recurrent, fibrosing, or deeply invasive tumors.

Cryosurgery

Cryosurgery with liquid nitrogen (–196°C) is used to destroy the tumor cells. A biopsy for diagnosis is done first because the procedure does not provide a specimen for pathologic examination. Most leading cryosurgeons have developed their own liquid nitrogen delivery apparatus. The most popular devices deliver a liquid nitrogen spray to the skin surface. Solid probes are also used.

The clinical limits of the tumor are determined visually, and 2- to 5-mm margin of normal skin is treated. The liquid nitrogen spray is directed at close range to the central portion of the tumor. Spray until the ice ball spreads to the desired margin and then for an additional 30 sec. More precise monitoring of the depth of freeze can be done with thermocouple needles inserted at the margin of the tumor. A temperature of –40°C should be obtained at the depth of the tumor. The treatment site should take 90–120 sec to thaw if freezing has been adequate. A slow thaw is more damaging to tumor cells than a rapid thaw. A second freeze–thaw cycle is recommended for treating cutaneous malignancy.

Cure rates greater than 90% are reported with cryosurgery. The cure rate for cancer of the scalp is less, due to the rich vascular supply that thaws the ice ball. Cryosurgical treatment of cancers on the legs or thighs is avoided because of the prolonged wound healing time (6 months).

Radiation

Radiation may be a good alternative to surgery, especially in elderly patients with several medical problems. Also, local anesthetic injections are avoided. Large exophytic SCC on the ears and nose in elderly patients may be treated without a significant resultant deformity. The cure rate for primary SCC is approximately 90%. This is similar to cure rates for primary BCC with radiation.

Smaller SCC may be clinically well defined. Lesions of this type can be treated with 3- to 5-mm margins. Larger or infiltrative tumors must be treated accordingly, and margins may reach 2–3 cm. Once the area to be treated has been determined, a lead cutout is prepared to protect surrounding skin and is taped in place during each treatment session.

Large SCC is often treated with surgical removal of as much tumor as possible followed by postoperative radiation. The effectiveness of postoperative radiation is improved by the surgical debulking of gross tumor.

Radiation is given in fractional doses over several days or weeks. Radiation given in a single dose will not allow the tissue to recover adequately. This results in poor healing and a lower cure rate. SCC less than 10 mm in diameter may be treated with a single dose of 2200 rads. Larger lesions may require up to 6000 rads in fractionated doses. Proper fractionation reduces the potential for osteonecrosis, chondronecrosis, and unnecessary damage to the dermis and other structures. Best results are achieved with 10 fractions for lesions up to 20 mm and 15 fractions when lesions are larger.

If a SCC involves an area immediately adjacent to a regional lymph node group, the group can be included in the radiation field. This is easily accomplished in the parotid, preauricular, and postauricular areas. The radiation field is also enlarged when perineural invasion has occurred. These patients must be evaluated carefully for paresthesias as a sign of recurrence.

Various types of radiation have been used to treat SCC including electron beam, radionucleotide implants, superficial x-ray therapy (photon beam), and contact x-ray therapy. Contact x-ray therapy is ideal for lesions less than 35 mm in diameter and less than 5 mm in thickness. This method allows a minimal number of fractions and leaves minimal radiation change in the skin. Deeper SCC is treated with more penetrating orthovoltage or megavoltage radiation.

Electron beam therapy is used for the control of extensive SCC when surgery may be unsuitable. Electron beam (3–18 MV) therapy has the advantages of a high-surface dose with a rapid reduction in dose several millimeters into the dermis.

Implants of radium, cesium, tantalum, or iridium are used when other forms of radiation cannot be given. Implant treatment is complex and usually requires hospitalization. Approximately 1000 rads are given daily, to a total dose of 6000–7000 rads.

The scar that develops in areas of radiation treatment worsens with time. If patients are 65 years or older when treated, this may not be a practical concern.

Radiation is not the treatment of choice for cancers of the lips and eyelids. Considerable morbidity can occur on the eyelids due to conjunctival keratinization that occurs from the radiation. Excisional surgery is a better alternative.

SCC in hair-bearing areas is best treated with methods other than radiation because permanent hair loss can result. SCC that arises in chronic sinuses or scars are usually treated surgically because of poor tolerance to radiation in these areas. Similarly, radiation is not the preferred treatment for SCC of the penis and anogenital area.

Tumors invading bone are not well suited to radiation because of the potential for necrosis of the bone. Devitalized bone must be removed surgically to allow the area to heal. When SCC occurs in an area of previous radiation damage, a modality other than radiation is usually chosen. Skin can only tolerate a finite amount of radiation before ulcers and necrosis develop.

Mohs Micrographic Surgery

Mohs micrographic surgery is more precise than any of the previously described standard methods. Mohs involves surgical excision of tumors in thin layers that are color-coded, mapped, and prepared for microscopic horizontal frozen section examination of deep and peripheral margins. The Mohs surgeon excises and reexcises cancerous tissue until no residual tumor is left microscopically. The advantage of this method includes the highest cure rates, maximum conservation of normal tissue, and preservation of important anatomic structures.

Mohs micrographic surgery is indicated for recurrent tumors, tumors with a high likelihood of recurrence, tumors with indistinct margins, and tumors that may require disfiguring surgery (Figs. 25,26). Mohs is also cost-effective since it markedly reduces the likelihood of future treatment for the same tumor.

The cure rate for difficult SCC with Mohs is more than 94%. Dzubow et al. reported a 93.3% 5-year cure rate in a series of 414 primary SCC treated with Mohs. Risk factors for local recurrence include male patients less than 50 years old, requiring more than five layers of Mohs, and patients with SCC on the lower extremity. In spite of use of the Mohs technique, SCC larger than 5 cm is more likely to recur than smaller tumors. In their extensive review of the literature, Rowe et al. found a local recurrence rate of 10% for recurrent SCC treated by Mohs technique vs. 23% for those treated by other modalities.

Chemotherapy

Partial and complete remissions have been obtained in three patients with extensive SCC receiving chemotherapy with cisplatin and doxorubicin. An 83-year-old woman with multiple kerato-

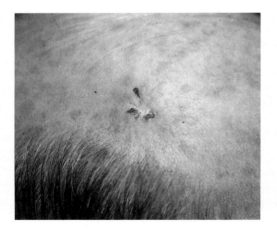

Figure 25 Recurrent squamous cell carcinoma presenting as a superficial ulceration on the scalp.

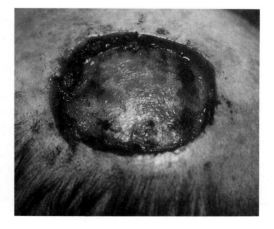

Figure 26 The tumor-free defect following Mohs surgery for the patient in Figure 25. The galea was involved but not the periosteum.

acanthomas and SCC on the legs was treated successfully with oral isotretinoin, with complete regression over 6 months. Partial response has been reported after the treatment of SCC and actinic keratoses with oral retinoids. Four of fourteen patients with advanced SCC have been reported to undergo complete remission following treatment with systemic retinoids. Twenty-eight patients with advanced inoperable cutaneous SCC were treated with 13 *cis*-retinoic acid and interferon-alpha-2a. Sixty-eight percent responded and seven (25%) had a complete response. Response rates were better with an advanced local disease (93%) than with regional disease (67%) or distant metastasis (25% response rate). Chemotherapy in the setting of distant metastasis has generally met with poor results.

BIBLIOGRAPHY

Ackerman LV. Verrucous carcinoma of the oral cavity. *Surgery* 1948;23:670.

Anderson SLC, Nielsen A, Reymann F. Relationship between Bowen disease and internal malignant tumors. *Arch Dermatol* 1973;108:367.

Arhelger SW, Kremen AJ. Arsenical epitheliomas of medicinal origin. *Surgery* 1951;30:977.

Arons MS, Lynch JB, Lewis SR, et al. Scar tissue carcinoma. I. A clinical study with special reference to burn scar carcinoma. *Ann Surg* 1965;161:170.

Barr RJ, Wuerker RB, Graham JH. Ultrastructure of atypical fiboxanthoma. *Cancer* 1977;40:736.

Blau S, Hyman AB. Erythroplasia of Queyrat. *Acta Derm Venereol (Stockh)* 1955;35:341.

Borelli D. Aspetti pseudoglandolari nell'epithelioma discheratosico: "Adenoacanthoma of sweat glands" di Lever. *Dermatologica* 1948;97:193.

Broders AC. Squamous cell epithelioma of the skin. *Ann Surg* 1921;73:141.

Brodland DG, Zitelli JA. Surgical margins for excision of primary cutaneous squamous cell carcinoma. *J Am Acad Dermatol* 1992;27(2 part 1):241.

Callen JP, Headington J. Bowen's and non-Bowen's squamous intraepidermal neoplasia of the skin. *Arch Dermatol* 1980;116:422.

Chuang TY, Heinrick LA, Schultz MD, et al. PUVA and skin cancer. The historical cohort study on 492 patients. *J Am Acad Dermatol* 1992;26(2 part 1):173.

Cottel WI. Moh's surgery for carcinomas of the skin. *Dallas Med J* 1977;63:176.

Cottel WI. Perineural invasion by squamous cell carcinoma. *J Dermatol Surg Oncol* 1982;8:589.

Cottel WI, Proper S. Mohs surgery, fresh-tissue technique: Our technique with a review. *J Dermatol Surg Oncol* 1982;8:576.

Crum CP, Mitao M, Levine RU, et al. Cervical papillomaviruses segregate within morphologically distinct pre-cancerous lesions. *J Virol* 1985;54:675.

Dawson DF, Duckworth JK, Bernhard H, et al. Giant condyloma and verrucous carcinoma of the genital area. *Arch Pathol* 1965;79:225.

Delacrétaz J, Madjedi AS, Loretan R. Epithelioma spino-cellulare segregans. Über die sogennannten "Adeno-acanthome der Schweissdrüen" (Lever). *Hautarzt* 1957;8:512.

DiLuca DR, Pilotti S, Stanfanon B, et al. Human papillomavirus type 16 in genital tumors; a pathological and molecular analysis. *J Gen Virol* 1986;67:583.

Dzubow LM, Rigel DS, Robins P. Risk factors for local recurrence of primary cutaneous squamous cell carcinomas. *Arch Dermatol* 1982;118:900.

Elierzri YD, Silverstein SJ, Nuovo GJ. Occurrence of human papillomavirus type 16 DNA in cutaneous squamous and basal cell neoplasms. *J Am Acad Dermatol* 1990;23:836.

Elliott JA, Welton DG. Epithelioma: Report on 1742 treated patients. *Arch Dermatol Syphilol* 1946;53:307.

Epstein EE, Epstein NN, Bragg K, et al. Metastases from squamous cell carcinoma of the skin. *Arch Dermatol* 1968;97:245.

Evans HL, Smith JL. Spindle cell squamous carcinomas and sarcoma-like tumors of the skin. *Cancer* 1980;45:2687.

Forman AB, Roenigk HH, Caro WA. Long-term follow-up of skin cancer in the PUVA-48 cooperative study. *Arch Dermatol* 1989;125:515.

Frieben A. Cancroid des rechten Handrückens nach langdauernder Einwirkung von Röntgenstrahlen. *Fortschr Roentgenstr* 1902;6:106.

Ghadially FN. The role of the hair follicle in the origin and evolution of some cutaneous neoplasms of man and experimental animals. *Cancer* 1961;14:801.

Graham JH, Helwig EB. Bowen's disease and its relationship to systemic cancer. *Arch Dermatol* 1959; 80:133.

Graham JH, Helwig EB. Erythroplasia of Queyrat. In *Dermal Pathology*. JH Graham, WC Johnson, EB Helwig, eds. Hagerstown, MD, Harper & Row, 1972, pp. 597–606.

Grier WRN. Squamous cell carcinoma of the body and extremities. In *Cancer of the Skin*, Vol. 2. R Andrade et al., eds. Philadelphia, W. B. Saunders, 1976, pp. 916–932.

Grinspan D, Abulafia J. Oral florid papillomatosis (verrucous carcinoma). *Int J Dermatol* 1979;18:608.

Grupper CH, Beretti B. Cutaneous neoplasia and etretinate. In: Sptizy KH, Karrer K, eds. *Proceedings of the 13th International Congress of Chemotherapy*. Vienna, Egermann VH, 1983, pp. 204–207.

Guthrie TH Jr, McElveen LJ, Porubsky ES, et al. Cisplatin and doxorubicin. *Cancer* 1985;55:1629.

Hanke CW, Zollinger TA, O'Brien JJ, Bianco L. Skin cancer in professional and amateur women golfers. *Phys Sportsmed* 1985;13(8):51.

Haynes HA, Mead KW, Goldwyn RM. Cancers of the skin. In *Cancer: Principles and Practice of Oncology*, 2nd ed. VT DeVita Jr, Hellman S, Rosenberg SA, eds. Philadelphia, J. B. Lippincott, 1985.

Hodak E, Jones RE, Ackerman AB. Solitary keratoacanthoma is a squamous cell carcinoma: Three examples with metastases. *Am J Dermatopathol* 1993;15(4):332.

Honigsmann H, Wolff K, Gschnait F, et al. Keratoses and nonmelanoma skin tumors in long-term photo-chemotherapy (PUVA). *J Am Acad Dermatol* 1980;3:406.

Hoxtell EO, Mandel JS, Murray SS, et al. Incidence of skin carcinoma after renal transplantation. *Arch Dermatol* 1977;113:436.

Hueper WC. *Occupational Tumors and Allied Diseases*. Springfield, IL, Charles C Thomas, 1942.

Hyde JN. On the influence of light in the production of cancer of the skin. *Am J Med Sci* 1906;131:1.

Immerman SC, Scanlon EF, Christ M, et al. Recurrent squamous cell carcinoma of the skin. *Cancer* 1983; 51:1537.

Johnson WC, Helwig EB. Adenoid squamous cell carcinoma (adenocanthoma). *Cancer* 1966;19:1639.

King DF, Barr RJ. Intraepithelial elastic fibers and intracytoplasmic glycogen: Aids in differentiating kerato-acanthomas from squamous cell carcinoma. *J Cutan Pathol* 1980;7:140.

Kingston T, Gaskell S, Marks R. The effects of a novel potent oral retinoid (R013–6298) in the treatment of multiple solar keratoses and squamous cell epithelioma. *Eur J Cancer Clin Oncol* 1983;19:1201.

Kochevar IE, Pathak MA, Parrish JA. Photophysics, photochemistry, and photobiology. In *Dermatology in General Medicine*, 3rd ed. TB Fitzpatrick et al., eds. New York, McGraw-Hill, 1987.

Kripke ML, Fisher MS. Immunologic parameters of ultraviolet carcinogenesis. *J Natl Cancer Inst* 1976; 57:211.

Kripke ML. Ultraviolet radiation and tumor immunity. *J Reticuloendothel Soc* 1977;22:217.

Lever WF. Adenocanthomas of sweat glands. *Arch Dermatol Syphilol* 1947;56:157.

Levine H, Bailin P, Wood B, et al. Tissue conservation in the treatment of cutaneous neoplasms of the head and neck. *Arch Otolaryngol* 1979;105:140.

Levine N, Miller RC, Meyskens FL. Oral isotretinoin therapy. *Arch Dermatol* 1984;120:1215.

Lippman SM, Meyskens FL. Treatment of advanced squamous cell carcinoma of the skin with isotretinoin. *Ann Intern Med* 1987;107:499.

Lippman SM, Parkinson DR, Itrilm, et al. 13-*cis*-Retinoic acid and interferon-2A: effective combination therapy for advanced squamous cell carcinoma of the skin. *J Natl Cancer Inst* 1992;84(4):235.

Lund HZ. How often does squamous cell carcinoma of the skin metastasize? *Arch Dermatol* 1965;92:635.

MacDonald EJ. The epidemiology of skin cancer. *J Invest Dermatol* 1959;32:379.

Magee KL, Rapini RP, Duvic M. Human papillomavirus associated with keratoacanthoma. *Arch Dermatol* 1989;125:1587.

Martin HT, Strong E, Spiro RH. Radiation-induced skin cancer of the head and neck. *Cancer* 1970;25:61.

McKee PH, Wilkinson JD, Black MM, et al. Carcinoma (epithelioma) cuniculatum. *Histopathology* 1981; 5:425.

McKee PH, Wilkinson JD, Corbett MF, Davey A, Sauven P, Black MM. Carcinoma cuniculatum: A case metastasizing to skin and lymph nodes. *Clin Exp Dermatol* 1981;6:613.

Melton JL, Nelson BR, Stough DB, et al. Treatment of keratoacanthomas with intralesional methotrexate. *J Am Acad Dermatol* 1991;25:1017.

Meyskens FL, Gilmartin E, Alberts DS, et al. Activity of isotretinoin against squamous cell cancers and preneoplastic lesions. *Cancer Treat Rep* 1982;66:1315.

Mikhail GR. Chemosurgery in the treatment of skin cancer. *Int J Dermatol* 1975:14:33.

Mikhail GR. Cancers, precancers, and pseudocancers on the male genitalia. *J Dermatol Surg Oncol* 1980; 6:1027.

Miller RA, Spittle MF. Electron beam therapy for difficult cutaneous basal and squamous cell carcinoma. *Br J Dermatol* 1982;106:429.

Miller DL, Weinstock MD. Nonmelanoma skin cancer in the United States: Incidence. *J Am Acad Dermatol* 1994;30:7/4.

Mohs FE. Chemosurgery: Microscopically controlled surgery for skin cancer: Past, present, and future. *J Dermatol Surg Oncol* 1978;4:41.

Mohs FE. *Chemosurgery: Microscopically Controlled Surgery for Skin Cancer.* Springfield, IL, Charles C Thomas, 1978.

Mohs FE. Chemosurgery for the microscopically controlled excision of cutaneous cancer. *Head Neck Surg* 1978;1:150.

Møller R, Reymann F, Hou-Jensen K. Metastases in dermatological patients with squamous cell carcinoma. *Arch Dermatol* 1979;115:703.

Mora RG, Perniciaro C. Cancer of the skin in blacks. I. A review of 163 black patients with cutaneous squamous cell carcinoma. *J Am Acad Dermatol* 1981;5:535.

Mora RG, Perniciaro C, Lee B. Cancer of the skin in blacks. III. A review of nineteen black patients with Bowen's disease. *J Am Acad Dermatol* 1984;11:557.

Muller SA, Wilhelmj CM Jr, Harrison EG Jr, et al. Adenoid squamous cell carcinoma (adeonoacanthomas of Lever). *Arch Dermatol* 1964;89:589.

Nikolowski W. Zur Problematik des Keratoakanthoms. *Dermatol Monatsschr* 1970;156:148.

Parker CM, Hanke CW. Large keratoacanthomas in difficult locations treated with intralesional 5-fluorouracil. *J Am Acad Dermatol* 1986;14(5):770.

Perez CA, Kraus FT, Evans JC, et al. Anaplastic transformation in verrucous carcinoma of the oral cavity after radiation therapy. *Radiology* 1966;86:108.

Potter M. Percivall Pott's contribution to cancer research. *Natl Cancer Inst Monogr* 1963;10:1. *Protection Against Depletion of Stratospheric Ozone by Chlorofluorocarbons*, Washington, DC, National Academy of Sciences, 1979.

Ratzer ER, Strong EW. Squamous cell carcinoma of the scalp. *Am J Surg* 1967;114:570.

Robins P. Chemosurgery: My 15 years of experience. *J Dermatol Surg Oncol* 1981;7:779.

Robins P, Dzubow LM, Rigel DS. Squamous cell carcinoma treated by Mohs surgery. *J Dermatol Surg Oncol* 1981;7:800.

Roenigk HH Jr, Caro WA. Skin cancer in the PUVA-48 cooperative study. *J Am Acad Dermatol* 1981; 4:319.

Rowe DE, Carroll RJ, Day CL. Prognostic factors for local recurrence, metastasis, and survival rate in squamous cell carcinoma of the skin, ear, and lip. *J Am Acad Dermatol* 1992;26:976.

Rundel RD, Nachtwey DS. Projections of increased non-melanoma skin cancer incidence due to ozone depletion. *Photochem Photobiol* 1983;38:577.

Rundel RD. Promotional effects of ultraviolet radiation on human basal and squamous cell carcinoma. *Photochem Photobiol* 1983;38:569.

Sage HH, Casson PR. Squamous cell carcinoma of the scalp, face, and neck. In *Cancer of the Skin*, Vol. 2. R Andrade et al., eds. Philadelphia, W. B. Saunders, 1976.

Sedlin ED, Fleming JL. Epidermal carcinoma arising in chronic osteomyelitic foci. *J Bone Joint Surg (Am)* 1963;45:827.

Sheild AM. A remarkable case of multiple growths of the skin caused by exposure to the sun. *Lancet* 1899; 1:22.

Sommers SC, McManus RG. Multiple arsenical cancers of skin and internal organs. *Cancer* 1953;6:347.

Stern RS, Laird N, Melski J, et al. Cutaneous squamous cell carcinoma in patients treated with PUVA. *N Engl J Med* 1984;310:1156.

Stern RS, Thibodeau LA, Kleinerman RA, et al. Risk of cutaneous carcinoma in patients treated with oral methoxsalen photochemotherapy for psoriasis. *N Engl J Med* 1970;300:809.

Stoll HL Jr, Schwartz RA. Squamous cell carcinoma. In *Dermatology in General Medicine*. 3rd ed. TB Fitzpatrick, ed. New York, McGraw-Hill, 1987.

Sullivan JJ, Donoghue MF, Kynaston B, et al. Multiple keratoacanthomas. *Australas J Dermatol* 1980;21:16.

Ten Seldam REJ. Skin cancer in Australia. *Natl Cancer Inst Monogr* 1963;10:153.

Traenkle HL. X-ray induced skin cancer in man. *Natl Cancer Inst Monogr* 1963;10:423.

Turner JE, Callen JP. Aggressive behavior with squamous cell carcinoma in a patient with preceding lymphocytic lymphoma. *J Am Acad Dermatol* 1981;4:446.

Unna PG. *Die Histopathologie der Hautkrenkheiten*. Berlin, Hirschwald, 1984.

Urbach F, Epstein JH, Forbes RD. Ultraviolet carcinogenesis: Experimental, global, and genetic aspects. In *Sunlight and Man*. TB Fitzpatrick, ed. Tokyo, University of Tokyo Press, 1974, p. 249.

Urbach F. Ultraviolet radiation carcinogenesis. *J Dermatol Surg Oncol* 1983;9:597.

Urbach F, Forbes PD. Photocarcinogenesis. In *Dermatology in General Medicine*, 3rd ed. TB Fitzpatrick et al., eds. New York, McGraw-Hill, 1987, p. 1477.

Van der Leun JC, Daniels F Jr. Biologic effects of stratospheric ozone decrease: A critical review of assessments. In *Impacts of Climatic Change on the Biosphere*. AJ Grobecker, ed. CIAP Monograph 5, Chapter 7, DOT-TST-75-55. Washington, DC, Department of Transportation, 1975.

Von Essen CF. Roentgen therapy of skin and lip carcinoma: Factors influencing success and failure. *Am J Roentgenol* 1960;83:556.

Weidner N, Foucar E. Adenosquamous carcinoma of the skin. *Arch Dermatol* 1985;121:775.

32

Keratoacanthoma

Robert A. Schwartz
University of Medicine and Dentistry of New Jersey–New Jersey Medical School, Newark, New Jersey

The keratoacanthoma (KA) is a common and distinctive epidermal neoplasm that demonstrates a growth pattern of rapid enlargement combined with histology often indistinguishable from that of an ordinary cutaneous squamous cell carcinoma (SCC). For this reason, it may be viewed as the prototype of cutaneous pseudomalignancies. The diagnosis of a KA requires that the clinician rule out the highly malignant de novo type of SCC. The solitary KA usually appears on sun-exposed regions of light-complected persons of middle age or older. I regard it as an aborted cancer that only rarely progresses into an aggressive SCC. Nevertheless, the KA is quite unique in many ways, mandating a management approach that is often different from that of a SCC.

HISTORICAL ASPECTS

In 1889, the renowned British surgeon Sir Jonathan Huchinson made the first description of the KA, calling it "the 'crateriform ulcer of the face,' a form of acute epithelial cancer." He illustrated the tumor in an atlas a year earlier and described its histologic features a few years later. Hutchinson wrote, "It is a disease of very rapid growth. . . . I have for many years been in the habit of calling it the 'crateriform ulcer,' a name more or less appropriate on account of its taking on the form of a large elevated boil (or beehive), and then breaking down into a deep hollow in the center. Microscopic examination, which has been made in at least four cases, has always revealed conditions considered characteristic of epithelial cancer." He noted that ". . . it occurs on the same parts and under very similar conditions" as does the rodent ulcer. All eight of his patients had a KA excised without recurrence; he did not mention spontaneous resolution. Similar descriptions followed, notably by Dupont and by Gourgerot. Shaw Dunn and Ferguson Smith in 1934 called the solitary KA a "self-healing primary squamous cell carcinoma of the skin." A report on the morphologic and biologic behavior of KA by MacCormac and Scarff in 1936 described how KA "develops rapidly to its maximum in four to six weeks and remains stationary." They described 10 patients, each with a solitary KA, usually on the middle of the face.

They named it molluscum sebaceum, as they thought the KA's "microscopic architecture bears a resemblance to molluscum contagiosum." Freudenthal is credited with suggesting the name "keratoacanthoma," observing that sebaceous glands were not usually involved, and one of the tumor's most impressive histological changes is acanthosis. Rook and Whimster used this designation in their 1950 report of 29 cases. Synonyms for KA include kyste sébacé atypique, molluscum pseudocarcinomatosum, verrucome avec adénite, self-healing primary squamous carcinoma, tumorlike keratosis, multiple self-healing epithelioma, familial primary self-healing squamous epithelioma of the skin, and keratocarcinoma.

Although most early descriptions emphasized the solitary KA, others recognized multiple KAs. Poth in 1939 described multiple "tumor-like keratoses" on the dorsal hand of a man after a severe sunburn. The multiple familial type of keratoacanthomas was described by the British dermatologist and long-time head of dermatology at the Glasgow Royal Infirmary, John Ferguson Smith in 1934. The generalized eruptive type of KAs was described by the Polish patriot Marian Grzybowski in 1950. By the time of this publication, Grzybowki, professor and head of dermatology at Warsaw University, who had risked his life to teach dermatology during the German occupation, had already been murdered as a part of a notorious Stalinist action, the General Tartar Purge of 1949. An expanding massive tumor form, keratoacanthoma centrifugum, was described in 1962 by the Polish dermatology professors Franciszek Miedziński (professor and head of dermatology at the Medical Academy in Gdańsk and Grzybowski's former student) and Jerzy Kozakiewicz. In 1959 Dąbska and Madejczykowa studied the histopathology of 60 KAs, emphasizing the need for representative skin biopsies for diagnosis, with specimen taken by incisional biopsy to include peripheral and central tumor.

Historically, KA has sometimes been diagnosed as a clinically aggressive SCC, resulting at times in inappropriate therapy. The KA does share clinical and histological features with an aggressive type of SCC, especially an initial period of rapid growth. The best test of distinction is often spontaneous resolution. However, this would mandate anxiety-filled months of waiting and often a cosmetically unacceptable final result due to an atrophic and even disfiguring scar.

CLINICAL FEATURES

Keratoacanthoma (KA) occurs mainly on sun-exposed areas of the skin of elderly persons. Actinic skin damage is often evident, including solar elastosis, actinic keratoses, solar lentigines, and at times sun-induced cutaneous cancers such as basal cell carcinomas or ordinary squamous cell carcinomas. The KA is best considered an abortive malignancy that only rarely progresses into an invasive SCC. Its peak incidence is between 50 and 69 years of age. Most KAs occur on the face, forearms, and hands. Baer and Kopf noted a predilection for sites where resting hair is found, such as the upper cheeks, nose, ears, forehead, eyelids, temples, forearms, and dorsa of hands and wrists. KAs of the hand occur more commonly in men, and KAs of the calf and anterior tibial area are more frequent in women (and are very uncommon in men). However, a KA may develop on any cutaneous surface, including the male nipple. It is more frequent in light-complected persons and much less so in more darkly pigmented individuals. Several studies indicate that the incidence of KA is about one-third that of SCC. Jackson and Williamson found KA to be much less common, with 355 cutaneous SCCs versus 9 KAs in their series from Ottawa, Canada. Yet a South African study found KA to be 1.8 times more frequent. Because the KA is either often presumptively or mistakenly treated as a SCC, its true incidence is often unavailable or difficult to determine. A recent study from Kauai, Hawaii, showed an incidence among whites of 104 per 100,000 residents, virtually the same as that of SCC in that population. The incidence of KA has been said to plateau after the age of 55 years, although a recent report suggests it increases with advancing age. The familial type of multiple KAs often has its onset in adolescence. Most studies of solitary KAs have shown that men are affected more often, up to three times more frequently as women. Baer and Kopf observed both sexes to be affected equally. Beare found a higher incidence in women. A Belgian study by Piérard-Franchimont and Piérard showed an overall men-to-women ratio of 1.11, with the rate of estimated prevalence increasing steadily in women but not men over the age of 70 years, so that the KA was more common in women than men over the age of 80 years. Multiple eruptive keratoacanthomas of Ferguson Smith show a three-to-one male predominance, with generalized eruptive KAs of Grzybowski of roughly equal incidence in men and women.

There are three clinical stages (Table 1) in the natural history of the keratoacanthoma: proliferative, mature, and resolving (Figs. 1–4). The proliferative stage produces a firm hemispheric, smooth, enlarging papule that grows rapidly for 2–4 weeks, often achieving a size of 2 cm or greater. The border is skin-colored or slightly erythematous. Fine telangiectasias may be evident. The mature form is a bud-, dome-, or berry-shaped, skin-colored or erythematous nodule with a central, often umbilicated, keratinous core (Figs. 1,2,4). It is firm, but without induration at its base or fixation to underlying structures. If the keratotic core is partially removed, the KA may appear crateriform. Involution tends to take place after a few months with tumor resorption and expulsion of the central keratotic plug, leaving a typical slightly depressed puckered often hypopigmented unattractive looking scar. Some lesions persist for a year or more. In its resolving phase, it appears as a keratotic necrotic nodule (Fig. 3). The keratotic debris gradually becomes detached, healing with scar formation. The entire process from origin to spontaneous resolution usually takes about 4–6 months.

The morphologic features of the mature keratoacanthoma are distinctive. Ghadially's studies classified the KA into three clinicopathologic types: type 1, or bud-shaped; type 2, or dome-shaped; and type 3, or berry-shaped. He considered the latter two patterns to represent lower follicular origin and the former upper follicular derivation. Histologically typical KAs are encountered in practice that are bud-shaped or berry-shaped, resemble a hypertrophic actinic keratosis, a digitate verruca vulgaris, or at times even a seborrheic keratosis.

TYPES OF KERATOACANTHOMA

The KA is usually solitary. In one report from the private referral practice of a distinguished dermatology professor, Kingman and Callen found that 84 of 90 patients had a solitary lesion.

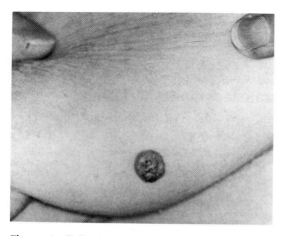

Figure 1 Fully developed crateriform keratoacanthoma in a patient with florid cutaneous papillomatosis and gastric adenocarcinoma. (From Schwartz, 1979.)

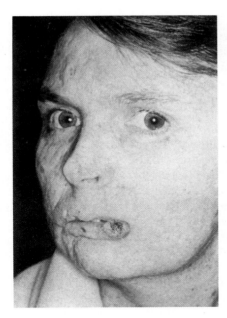

Figure 2 Mature bud-shaped keratoacanthoma, lower lip, in an adolescent with xeroderma pigmentosum.(From Schwartz, 1979.)

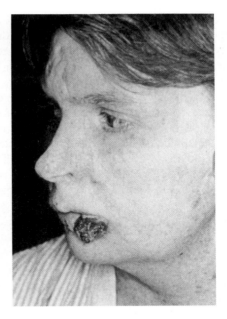

Figure 3 Resolving keratoacanthoma of the lower lip, showing abundant green-black keratotic debris, in this adolescent with xeroderma pigmentosum. (From Schwartz, 1979.)

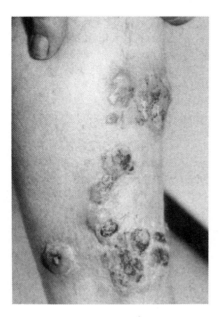

Figure 4 Keratoacanthomas, in various stages of development on the leg of a patient with multiple persistent keratoacanthomas. Solitary dome-shaped nodule on the left is an early proliferative lesion. To its right are mature and resolving keratoacanthomas, adjacent to a large skin graft site. (From Schwartz, 1979.)

However, multiple lesions may be present (Table 2). In fact, two solitary KAs in that study were seen in each of four patients; two patients had more than two KAs and could be classified as having the Ferguson Smith type of multiple KAs. The KA may have many morphologic forms. In some, no central core is evident clinically. Rarely, the hyperkeratosis is massive so that the KA resembles a cutaneous horn. There are, in addition, several special morphologic or syndromic types:

1. *Agglomerated keratoacanthomas.* This type is composed of several nodules that coalesce to form a large keratotic tumorous plaque. These plaques persist for almost 6 months and then spontaneously involute. Some show ulceration before healing. Stevanovic coined the name "keratoacanthoma dyskeratoticum et segregans" based upon the histologic findings in his one patient.

2. *Keratoacanthoma centrifugum.* This form of KA exhibits peripheral growth up to 20 cm in diameter with concurrent central healing. A small KA of 1 cm or less may expand to more than 5 cm in diameter. New KAs may form peripherally. There may be no spontaneous resolution, or it may heal in 6–12 months rather than the 2–6 months for the common KA. It affects men and women of middle age or older (range 41–92 years) and involves the face, trunk, or extremities. Only about 25 cases have been reported. This variant has been reported as aggregated keratoacanthoma, coral-reef keratoacanthoma, nodulo-vegetating keratoacanthoma, multinodular keratoacanthoma, keratoacanthoma centrifugum marginatum, and keratoacanthoma centrifugum of Miedziński and Kozakiewicz. It was first described by Miedziński and Kozakiewicz, who coined the term "keratoacanthoma centrifugum." A similar case had been described earlier by Puente Duany.

3. *Giant keratoacanthoma.* This tumor may grow to 9 cm or larger. Although the KA usually does not invade below the level of the eccrine sweat glands, in some giant KAs there may be destruction of underlying tissue and cartilage. Some of these patients might be better viewed as having a verrucous carcinoma. Keratoacanthoma centrifugum is in a sense a giant KA, but its growth characteristics and morphologic features distinguish it.

4. *Subungual KA.* This form can be persistent, painful, and locally destructive to underlying bone. It originates in the nail bed, growing at times to destroy the distal phalanx. Twenty-three subungual KAs in 19 patients have been reported, 80% of whom were men, usually between the third and seventh decade of life (average age, 49 years). The thumb or little finger was involved in 70% of cases. There is one report of an interdigital KA with osteolysis of the proximal and middle phalanges. Shatkin and coworkers reported two siblings with both subungual KA and incontinentia pigmenti. According to McKee et al., the infiltrating nature and other findings suggest that many of these cases may be better classified as verrucous carcinoma (epithelioma cuniculatum).

5. *Intraoral and other mucous membrane KAs.* KA can occur on the hard palate, lips, and other oral sites, and also on the bulbar conjunctiva, nasal mucosa, and genitalia. Because there are no hair follicles in oral mucosa, the Ka may develop from ectopic sebaceous glands. A rare type of KA, generalized eruptive KAs of Grzybowski, has a tendency to involve the mucosal surfaces. Solitary ones with localization on the lips and nose are most often derived from skin rather than mucosa.

6. *Multiple eruptive KAs of Ferguson Smith type.* This disorder, also called familial primary self-healing squamous epithelioma of the skin, is characterized by several to many KAs that suddenly erupt, slowly involute, and periodically reappear for many years. Each lesion starts as an erythematous macule, becomes papular, and then grows rapidly into an ordinary solitary KA. The number of KAs vary from only a few to hundreds; they may heal with deep unslightly scars, especially on the face, unless each lesion is treated at an early stage. They usually begin in childhood, adolescence, or early adulthood. They may even begin in infancy. The mean age

of onset in women is 25.5 years (standard deviation 11.1 years); in men the mean age of onset is 26.9 years (standard deviation 12.4 years). They persist throughout life, mainly on sun-exposed areas, but the scalp and external genitalia may be involved. This type of KA affects both sexes with equal severity, but its distribution differs in men and women because of differences in sun-exposure patterns. It also tends to develop at sites of trauma, such as the edge of a donor site of a graft or in a fingertip puncture site. Muliple KAs remained unilateral in three patients, who had involvement of the face and upper extremities. One patient had a moderate elevation of the T-helper/T-suppressor ratio. This disorder appears to be inherited in an autosomal dominant manner. One patient with Ferguson Smith–type eruptive KAs was reported by Weber et al. to have an adenocarcinoma of the fallopian tube plus a stem cell leukemia. In another patient an eruption of over a dozen typical KAs was associated with a poorly differentiated laryngeal SCC.

7.   *Multiple persistent KAs.*   These are slow healing and nonfamilial. The conjunctivae, palms, soles, and penis can be involved (Fig. 4). In one case, the KAs continued to develop for 35 years, becoming a painful mass that extended around the underlying tendon.

8.   *Generalized eruptive KAs of Grzybowski.*   Literally, thousands of tiny disseminated 2- to 3-mm KAs are present. Grzybowski observed the lesions to be "varying in size from a nearly invisible point to the size of a bean." Jaber et al. calculated that the 22 patients reported tended to be middle-aged or older, with an age of onset ranging from 32 to 84 years (mean age, 57 years). Of these, 13 were women and 9 were men. No familial pattern has been shown, with the cases being sporadic. Most patients are white, but it has been described in one black American and two Japanese. Individual lesions resolve spontaneously with scarring in about 6 months. Pruritus is common, as is ectropion caused by KAs of the eyelids. Corrective blepharoplasty may be required to prevent a serious keratopathy. The face may become so involved as to produce a masked facies. Individual nodules may coalesce to become tumors cherry-sized or larger. Köbnerization may be evident. An unexplained hepatomegaly may be noted. KAs may appear as multiple papulonodules on the palms and soles, oral mucosa and palate, larynx, and glans penis. Adenocarcinoma of the ovary has been reported by Snider and Benjamin in one patient with generalized eruptive KAs. Another patient was reported to have a lymphoma.

9.   *KA in Torre syndrome (Muir-Torre syndrome).*   An eruption of KAs may appear in association with sebaceous neoplasms and one or more low-grade visceral cancers usually of gastrointestinal or urogenital origin. The association of KAs and sebaceous neoplasms may be explained by their common derivation from pilosebaceous glands. Almost half of the patients with this syndrome have at least one KA. The KAs tend to be 0.5–1.0 cm in diameter, 3 to 10 in number, and scattered on the head and trunk. Patients may have one or multiple KAs, no sebaceous tumors, and an internal cancer, possibly—in at least some of them—a manifestation of this syndrome. However, Kingman and Callen found that patients with a solitary KA (and no sebaceous tumors) do not have an increased risk of concurrent or subsequent internal cancer. I believe that every patient with multiple KAs should be evaluated for the presence of sebaceous neoplasms, the absence of which still requires consideration of this syndrome. It is inherited as an autosomal dominant trait.

10.   *KA in xeroderma pigmentosum.*   This defect of DNA repair is associated with development at an early age of basal cell carcinomas, SCCs, melanomas, and KAs on sun-exposed sites (Figs. 2,3). A keratocanthoma in a child should suggest consideration of this syndrome. A 3-year-old Bantu child with probable xeroderma pigmentosum had a KA.

11.   *KA in florid cutaneous papillomatosis and an underlying cancer.*   Multiple papillomas and a keratoacanthoma were noted in the original report. This disorder is believed to be caused by a malignancy-secreted growth factor.

12. *KA in nevus sebaceus of Jadassohn.* This type of epidermal nevus tends to occur on the scalp in infants, proliferate at puberty, and contain a wide variety of neoplasms within it. Most are a basal cell epithelioma or a benign appendageal tumor such as a syringocytostadenoma papilliferum, but occasionally a keratoacanthoma or a SCC develops. One series of 150 cases had 52 tumors, four of which in adults were a KA. The KA can also occur in childhood within a nevus sebaceus. The KA may also occur with an ordinary linear epidermal nevus.

13. *Pseudorecidive KA.* Pseudorecidives are defined as pseudoepitheliomatous reactions that occasionally develop after radiotherapy for skin and other cancers. These are rapidly developing early sequelae of radiation therapy that may be confused with a recurrence of the original skin cancer, hence the name "pseudorecidive." They occur when the initial radiation reaction is subsiding and evolve rapidly, sometimes in a few days, at other times in a few weeks. They tend to appear granulomatous or wartlike. These histologic pattern varies from acanthomatous (wartlike) to closely resemble or be indistinguisable from a KA. Pseudorecidives may lack the typical central keratotic plug of the KA, and their exact categorization is still unclear. Lesions with both clinical and histological features considered "classical" for KAs have been described that developed in cutaneous radiotherapy sites several years after treatment of a basal cell carcinoma.

14. *Reactive keratoacanthomas.* KAs have been noted to appear at the site of scar formation (Fig. 5), recently healing herpes zoster sites, in hypertrophic lichen planus, in discoid lupus erythematosus, and in other benign inflammatory disorders, including psoriasis, pemphigus foliaceus, and epidermolysis bullosa dystrophica. Some of these KAs may have been associated with the underlying therapy used, such as tar. Just as crops of KAs may occur after an outbreak of dermatitis, multiple KAs were reported to suddenly appear three weeks after a thermal burn from a gasoline explosion. With multiple eruptive KAs of the Ferguson Smith type, KAs tend to develop at sites of trauma.

15. *Chemical-induced (mainly tar) keratoacanthomas.* In humans as well as in animals, contact with tar or pitch enhances the chance of KA formation. There is a significantly increased incidence of KAs in tar and pitch workers. Often the occupational exposure occurs in machin-

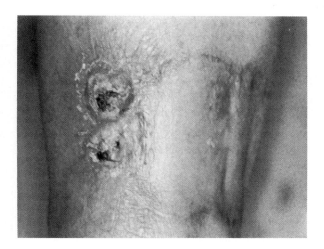

Figure 5 Multiple keratoacanthomas developing at the site of a previous excision and graft. (From Schwartz, 1979.)

ists as chronic contact with machine oil. Typical KA has been described after topical podophyllin therapy.

16. *The KA in an immunosuppressed patient.* The immunocompromised patient may be at increased risk for KAs as well as for skin cancers. There seems to be no significantly increased incidence of KAs with the use of cyclosporine. At least some skin neoplasms and possibly KA may show increased aggressive potential in immunosuppressed patients. Eruptive KAs in an immunosuppressed transplantation recipient have been described.

HISTOGENESIS

The probable derivation of KAs from hair follicles has been well-documented in humans and in animals by Ghadially and by others. In fact, the pioneer study in chemical carcinogenesis by Yamagiwa and Ichikawa in 1918 produced a number of growths that these investigators labeled folliculoepitheliomas. Many were undoubtedly KAs. They observed the histologic evolution of these tumors as follows: "The epithelium, and especially that at the periphery of the hair follicles, gradually undergoes hyperplasia: 1) each layer increases considerably in thickness; 2) many symmetrical mitoses are found in its basal layer; 3) the hair follicles become cystic; 4) the basal layer grows irregular in outline, owing to the projection of processes which ramify in the surrounding subcutaneous tissues."

The role of hair follicles and epidermis in the origin and evolution of cutaneous tumors in humans and animals has been elucidated and summarized by Ghadially. Ridgon found a chemical-induced KA-like lesion arising from a feather follicle in a white Pekin duck. Ghadially noted that the usual description of most benign cutaneous growths produced during experimental carcinogenesis has been as a "papilloma," an inadequate term for a variety of tumors. He illustrated diagrammatically and histologically how some of these benign neoplasms are of sebaceous gland origin, and others of epidermal or hair follicle origin. The latter began as striking cellular growth and keratinization in the upper part of the hair follicle and evolved into a keratoacanthoma. He also described a type of KA derived from the hair follicle below the attachment of the erector pili muscle. Although this lower hair follicle histogenesis is not universally accepted, it serves as a model for the histogenesis of the three distinct morphologic types of keratoacanthomas. These deeper types of KAs displayed a consistent and rapid resolution and were derived from the cyclically evanescent hair germ rather than the permanent upper portion of the hair follicle.

ETIOLOGY

The etiology of the KA is uncertain. Its usual occurrence on sun-exposed areas in elderly persons suggests that ultraviolet light (UVL) may be of etiologic significance in the common solitary type of KA. In England and Australia, the incidence of both KA and SCC show parallel increases with increased sun exposure (1). The occurrence of KAs in patients with xeroderma pigmentosum is also consistent with solar induction (Figs. 2,3). The defective deoxyribonucleic acid repair in xeroderma pigmentosum after UVL injury has been well characterized. The role of higher electromagnetic frequencies in tumorigenesis is suggested by the possible induction of KAs by cutaneous x-ray therapy.

Chemical tumorigenesis has been documented in KAs in several animal models (rabbit, rat, hamster, mouse, hedgehog, duck, chicken) by painting the skin with tar derivatives. KAs induced in rabbit skin in this way and human KAs both show a relatively high frequency of an activated H-*ras* oncogene. Human KAs were shown to display p53 oncoprotein expression in 16 of 20 (80%) KAs examined by Kerschmann and associates. In animal studies, two main types of tumors have been noted: papillomas derived from surface epithelium and keratoacanthomas of hair follicle origin. The latter were both clinically and histologically indistinguishable from the Ka of humans. A somewhat greater tendency for continued local growth was observed in mice and hamsters than in rabbits. In humans a study of 250 KAs in 238 patients showed a significantly increased incidence of these tumors among pitch and tar workers compared to matched controls. A larger proportion of the 238 patients were smokers than would be anticipated in the control group. There have also been a number of patients who worked as machinists in constant contact with oil. Crude coal tar, which enhances UVL carcinogenesis in animals, has been used in conjunction with UVL to treat psoriatic patients for many years. The development of multiple KAs in six psoriatic patients has been reported, although this is rather unusual. There is also a description of two psoriatic patients with multiple keratoacanthomas possibly induced by oral psoralens and ultraviolet light (PUVA). However, the risk of developing a KA after PUVA therapy is less than the risk of developing a SCC or basal cell carcinoma.

A viral etiology for KA has been postulated by Koziorowska and Dux and by many others. This idea is suggested by the fact that Shope virus–induced tumors of rabbits are similar to KA. In 1961 viral-like particles were observed within the nucleus of 40–60% of KA tumor cells; however, others believe these intranuclear particles are nonviral in origin, and inoculation experiments, including those by Koziorowska and Duz, have been negative. Nevertheless, DNA related to human papillomavirus (HPV) 25 has been found in solitary KAs. In one study, HPV 25–related DNA was detected in 14 of 32 KAs. However, the role of HPV in the development of KA remains unclear; as Höpfl and associates pointed out, even its association with HPV 25 requires more refined techniques than nonisotopic in situ hybridization for confirmation. A study among renal transplant recipients by Euvrard and associates found benign and oncogenic human papillomaviruses detected within keratoacanthomas.

It is possible that there is a relationship between genetic predisposition and other cofactors such as ultraviolet light, infrared radiation, x-rays, chemical agents, and viral infections together with trauma or immunosuppression in the pathogenesis of KA. Clearly, trauma plays a role because KAs tend to occur at or near skin graft sites. Ghadially's experiments demonstrated that trauma to the chemically pretreated experimental animal produced KAs. The appearance of KAs after bone marrow transplantation or during cyclosporine therapy suggests the possibility of immunosuppression as a contributory factor.

Genetics is also important in a number of ways. A light-complected person has a relatively high risk of UVL-induced tumors, including KA. One study of 43 cases of solitary KAs claimed an increased incidence of HLA-B16 and HLA-B18 antigens. The Ferguson Smith type of multiple KAs was studied in 62 persons from 11 Scottish families. It seemed probable that these were the result of a single mutation occurring before 1790. The same mutation was probably responsible for some cases in Canada and the United States as members of affected families immigrated to North America.

HISTOPATHOLOGIC FINDINGS

The histologic appearance of KA has been reviewed by many, including Kwittken, Lever and Schaumburg-Lever, Dąbska and Madejczykowa, Milewski and Chorzelski, Ghadially and Ghadially, and Ackerman and associates. It can be divided into three stages: proliferative, fully developed, and involuting.

Proliferative Stage

In the early, rapidly growing phase there is a horn-filled invagination of the epidermis arising from contiguous hair follicles, from which epidermal strands may extend into the dermis (Figs. 6,7). This incipient lesion shows mild hyperkeratosis, acanthosis, and premature keratinization

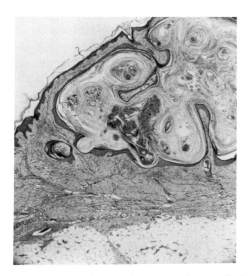

Figure 6 Early development of a keratoacanthoma, displaying keratin-filled invagination of the epidermis and a few epidermal stands extruding into the dermis (hematoxylin-eosin, original magnification ×30). (From Schwartz, 1979.)

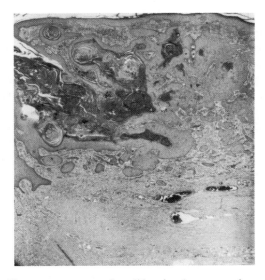

Figure 7 Glassy appearance of proliferating keratoacanthoma (hematoxylin-eosin, original magnification ×30). (From Schwartz, 1979.)

characterized by enlarged cells of the lower portion of the malphigian layer reportedly often with a thick granular layer with prominent keratohyalin granules. There may or may not be a central depression. The hyperkeratosis forms a crenulated border with the acanthotic epidermis. The epidermal strands may be carcinomalike, containing atypical-appearing squamous cells with multiple mitotic figures as the KA enlarges and extends downward toward the level of the eccrine sweat glands (Fig. 7). Some of these mitotic figures may appear atypical. Tripolar mitosis was described by Giltman; Ghadially and Ghadially believe that abnormal mitoses in general and tripolar ones in particular strongly indicate a carcinoma. Some tumor regions may show pronounced keratinization, with the abundant and pale-staining cytoplasm producing an eosinophilic "glassy" appearance. Eosinophils and neutrophils may be present, probably causing some of the keratinocytes to be come necrotic and others to disassociate as evidenced by acantholysis. One variant, keratoacanthoma dyskeratoticum et segregans, was named for its marked dyskeratosis and acantholysis. Collagen and elastin fiber fragments may be trapped within the expanding tumor. A sparse dermal inflammatory infiltrate may be present at the tumor interface with the dermis. Perineural invasion may occasionally be seen at this stage and should not be interpreted as a sign of malignancy. Likewise, intravascular extension and deep invasion below the eccrine glands can be present, but these are considered benign phenomena. Nests of squamous cells can be seen in medium-size veins. However, deep invasion below the level of the eccrine glands is considered by this author to be an ominous sign.

Fully Developed Stage

The fully developed dome-shaped crateriform nodule contains a central depression composed of a keratotic central core (Fig. 8). The epidermis extends around the crater sides, forming a lip. Irregular epidermal proliferations protrude both into the crater and below its base. In the ma-

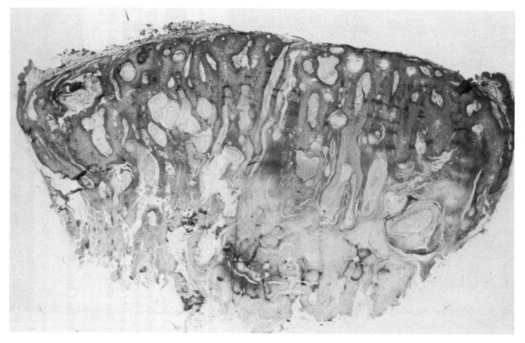

Figure 8 Mature keratoacanthoma, with large keratin-filled core, epidermal lip, and tumor cells extending into dermis (hematoxylin-eosin, original magnification ×25) (From Schwartz, 1979.)

ture KA the individual squamous cells may appear somewhat atypical; but atypia is more pronounced in the rapidly growing stage. However, carcinomalike foci appear either focally or diffusely in almost three fourths of established KAs and are more common in them than in early or regressing lesions. Keratinization of these squamous cells is marked, producing an eosinophilic and glassy appearance. Many keratinocytes have undergone necrosis. Microabcesses may be evident, composed of neutrophils and often eosinophils. Horn pearls, also characteristic of cutaneous SCC, are present (Fig. 9). These are concentric layers of squamous cells with central keratinization that increases centripetally. Lateral tumor strands projecting between collagen bundles can also be seen. There is a focally dense, mixed dermal infiltrate composed of lymphocytes, histiocytes, eosinophils, neutrophils, and plasma cells. In carcinomalike foci, the infiltrate is prominent at its advancing margins but does not infiltrate the tumor. Atypical eccrine sweat duct hyperplasia may be present.

Involutional Stage

During involution, the lesion becomes flattened and less crateriform, as most cells at the crater base have become keratinized. There may be shrunken cells staining intensely with eosin adjacent to tumor cells nearby and within the stroma. A mixed dermal infiltrate is usually evident, sometimes containing multinucleated histiocytes, probably best considered a foreign body granuloma to keratin. Beneath the KA, granulation tissue may be evident, with fibrosis at its base. Fibroblasts at the KA base proliferate, with resultant fibrosis pushing the neoplastic remnants through the crater to the surface. A lichenoid reaction may be seen at the epidermal-dermal interface lining the regressing crater. The crater slowly becomes flat and heals with the formation of an irregularly shaped atrophic scar.

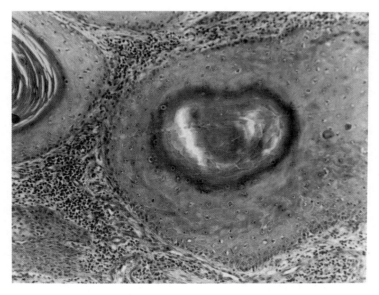

Figure 9 Keratoacanthoma, showing somewhat glassy appearance of keratinocytes, which are arranged in concentric layers with increasing keratinization centrally. Note collection of neutrophils (hematoxylin-eosin stain; ×160). (From Schwartz, 1979.)

Ultrastructural Pathology

Electron microscopy analysis of the keratoacanthoma has been performed on both human KAs and experimental animal ones. There appears to be a greater number of desmosomes in a KA than in normal skin. They may be seen within abnormally keratinized cells. Intranuclear inclusions may sometimes be evident; these viruslike particles may actually be perichronmatin granules and nuclear bodies. The main morphologic features distinguishing the KA from the SCC are the desmosomes and the intracellular space. Both the number and surface density of desmosomes are smaller than in normal skin; in well-differentiated SCC these are significantly smaller than in a KA. The intercellular space, a reflection of keratinocyte cohesiveness, is significantly larger in a SCC than in a KA.

Cellular and Basement Membrane Features

Two important pathologic features commonly used to separate benignity from malignancy require consideration for KAs: individual cell cytology and invasiveness below the basement membrane. Premalignant tumors can usually be distinguished from malignant ones by whether or not the tumor has invaded below the basement membrane. However, a number of exceptions, as in the case of the verrucous carcinoma, have reduced the value of this generalization. Immunologic, histochemical, and electron microscopic studies of KA have shown conflicting results. Also, the degree of cellular atypia may be useful in separating benign from malignant neoplasms. Studies demonstrated aneuploidy in some KAs, although to a lesser extent than in well-differentiated SCC. The majority of both were diploid. One DNA image cytometry study showed a significant difference in peak DNA index and highest DNA content between KA and SCC.

DIFFERENTIAL DIAGNOSIS

The most frequent consideration in the clinical and histological differential diagnosis of KA is SCC. Clinically, rapid tumor growth may suggest a de novo cutaneous SCC, a relatively rare, aggressive tumor that produces regional or distant metastases in at least 8% of patients. A series of four such patients illustrated this point. Each de novo SCC was initially diagnosed as KA, but each had an early recurrence after conservative therapy. In three of the four patients, rapidly spreading metastatic cutaneous SCC occurred, resulting in the death of two. Other examples exist. Occasionally, an unusual type of cutaneous squamous cell carcinoma, verrucous carcinoma, requires distinction. This slow-growing tumor may produce a bulky locally destructive mass that may necessitate distinction from a giant keratoacanthoma or from a subungual keratoacanthoma. However, our main discussion focuses on the differences between the ordinary type of SCC and its de novo form.

Fortunately, the morphologic features and growth pattern of a KA are sufficiently distinctive to be diagnostic in most cases. In short, the diagnosis of a KA is based upon its architecture rather than its cytologic features. Although the cellular characteristics of KA and SCC are often similar, the tumor architecture usually provides the distinction. Thus, as Dąbska and Madejczykowa pointed out, it is important to obtain a representative tissue specimen. It is done with a biopsy specimen down to subcutaneous fat, achieved either by total excision or by a fusiform partial excision through the entire KA to include its center and both sides. In this way both the tumor architecture and the presence or absence of tumor invasiveness into underlying tissue can be analyzed. Incision through a KA is not associated with an increased risk of aggressive behavior. The presence of deep invasion mandates therapy for a SCC.

as part of a generalized eruption such as florid cutaneous papillomatosis or the Torre syndrome, both of which are markers for internal malignancy. The KA may also occur with xeroderma pigmentosum.

TREATMENT

Although KA usually involutes spontaneously, biopsy and treatment are undertaken for several important reasons. Biopsy establishes the diagnosis and serves to rule out SCC. Treatment provides hastened resolution or cure, prevention of rapid enlargement or impingement on important structures, and improvement in overall cosmetic result. Solitary KAs should usually receive complete conservative excision, which also provides an optimal biopsy specimen and in most patients a greater likelihood of a favorable cosmetic outcome than one would anticipate with spontaneous resolution. A fusiform partial excision cut symmetrically through the center so as to include normal lateral tissue and underlying normal fat also provides an adequate specimen to distinguish SCC from KA. If this is done, it is important that the pathologist is informed so that appropriate sections showing the lateral aspects as well as deep margins of the lesions be visualized microscopically. Although the fusiform partial excisional biopsy was initially thought to possibly hasten resolution of a KA, time has not shown this observation to be valid in my experience or in that of the senior author of the original report. Shave and incisional punch biopsy specimens are not acceptable forms of biopsy when one is considering the diagnosis of a KA. Excision of a subungual KA may require amputation of a digit when underlying bone is involved and other options fail. Micrographic surgery may be used to preserve to a maximum of normal tissue in selected patients. With the Smith Ferguson type of multiple eruptive KA, limited surgical excision, cryosurgery, curettage, or other options should be considered for use on early lesions to avoid the disfigurement that may ensure with spontaneous resolution.

Simple curettage may be employed, as may blunt dissection. Curettage is usually used together with electrodesiccation. An 8% recurrence rate was found for solitary KA treated mostly in this manner. Radiotherapy with superficial x-ray, orthovoltage radiation, or electron beam may be used primarily or after the recurrence of a KA following excision or curettage and electrodesiccation. The same tumoricidal doses as employed for a SCC should be used. Large facial KAs may be treated by radiotherapy with acceptable cosmesis. Laser surgery has also been employed with good success for small solitary KAs in tough to treat locations. Kuflik and Kuflik have noted that cryosurgery with liquid nitrogen is of value, especially for small early KAs. For larger ones, it is usually used as adjunctive therapy to the base after the KA has been removed by excisional biopsy or curettage. The base is frozen completely with at least a 3-mm halo of healthy tissue after hemostasis is achieved. Topical podophyllin has been used alone, in combination with curettage and electrodesiccation, or in combination with radiotherapy. Curiously, topical podophyllin may also produce KA formation.

Intralesional and topical 5-fluorouracil (5-FU) for KAs was introduced by Klein and associates in 1962. It may be administered by either daily or every-other-day focal injections of 0.1 ml of a 5% solution directly into the base of the KA or by topical application of 5-FU cream or ointment up to five times daily, with or without occlusion. Therapy is continued for about 2½ weeks. Others used 50 mg/ml of 5-FU injected with a 27- or 30-gauge needle inserted tangentially into the slopes of the KA in three or four sites and 0.1 to 0.3 ml injected circumferentially and 0.1–0.2 ml sublesionally. This approach was performed weekly until the KA size was decreased by 60–80%. It took up to 8 weeks, with an average of 3 weeks, for each KA to resolve. Only one of 26 KAs in 14 patients did not respond. This modality provides an excellent therapeutic result and has proven valuable for large KAs in difficult-to-treat locations. It may be ineffective in a KA that is not rapidly proliferating. Intralesional bleomycin may also be used instead of 5-FU. Intralesional injection of oil bleomycin, with a depot effect, has been suggested. Intralesional methotrexate may also be employed. Systemic chemotherapy including methotrexate has been used for multiple KAs.

Other therapies may have value in treating keratoacanthomas. Transfer factor was found effective in two patients with the Ferguson Smith type of familial multiple eruptive keratoacanthomas. Etretinate, 1 mg/kg/day for 2 months, may be valuable for multiple KAs, including the Ferguson Smith eruptive-type, and for the generalized eruptive type of Grzybowski. Intralesional injections of triamcinolone have also been employed, with impressive benefit in 10 patients with a total of 17 KAs. One report claims that normalization of a moderately elevated T-helper/T-suppressor ratio with thymic hormone was associated with regression of multiple KAs in one patient. Another study by Grob and associates suggested that intralesional interferon alpha-2a may also be of value, especially with large keratoacanthomas, promoting regression while facilitating good cosmetic healing.

THE KERATOACANTHOMA—AN OVERVIEW

The keratoacanthoma is a common skin tumor that tends to occur on sun-exposed sites in light-skinned persons of middle age or older. It is best viewed as an aborted SCC that only rarely evolves into a progressively invasive SCC. Sometimes labeled a typical pseudomalignancy, the KA may paradoxically merit the alternative designation as a pseudobenignity. It is most likely derived from hair follicle cells. Its etiology is unknown, although ultraviolet light, viruses, and chemical carcinogens have been considered. Its diagnosis should be made by complete conservative excision or by a properly performed fusiform partial excision designed to provide an adequate biopsy specimen to distinguish a KA from an SCC. The Ferguson Smith type of multiple eruptive KAs is particularly important to recognize and treat to avoid natural healing, which can lead to disfigurement.

BIBLIOGRAPHY

Ackerman AB, Ragaz A. *The Lives of Lesions. Chronology in Dermatopathology.* New York, Masson, 1984, pp. 102–109.

Ahmed AR, Sofen H, Saxon A. Detection of an antisquamous antibody in multiple keratoacanthoma. *Clin Immunol Immunopathol* 1982;22:20–31.

Akiyama M, Hata Y, Nishikawa T. Keratoacathoma with glandular proliferation. *J Dermatol (Tokyo)* 1993; 20:109–113.

Allen JV, Callen JP. Keratoacanthomas arising in hypertrophic lichen planus. A case report. *Arch Dermatol* 1981;117:519–521.

Baer RL, Kopf AW. Complications of therapy of basal cell epitheliomas (based on 1,000 histologically verified cases). *Year Book of Dermatology.* (1964–1965 series). Chicago, Year Book Medical Publishers, 1965, pp. 7–26.

Baer RL, Kopf AW. Keratoacanthoma. *Year Book of Dermatology.* (1962—1963 series). Chicago, Year Book Medical Publishers, 1963, pp. 7–41.

Banse-Kupin L, Morales A, Barlow M. Torre's syndrome: report of two cases and review of the literature. *J Am Acad Dermatol* 1984;10:803–817.

Beare JM. Molluscum sebaceum. *Br J Surg* 1953;41:167–172.

Belisario JC. Brief review of keratoacanthomas and description of keratoacanthoma centrifugum marginatum, another variety of keratoacanthoma. *Aust J Dermatol* 1965;8:65–72.

Benest L, Kaplan RP, Salit R, et al. Keratoacanthoma centrifugum marginatum of the lower extremity treated with Mohs micrographic surgery. *J Am Acad Dermatol* 1994;31:501–502.

Benoldi D, Alinovi A. Multiple persistent keratoacanthomas: treatment with oral etretinate. *J Am Acad Dermatol* 1984;10:1035–1038.

Berenblum I, Haran-Ghera N, Trainin N. An experimental analysis of the "hair cycle effect" in mouse skin carcinogenesis. *Br J Cancer* 1958;12:402–413.

Berndt R, Grouls V. Keratoakanthom mit Infiltration von Nervenscheiden. *Pathologe* 1993;14:47–50.

Binkley GW, Johnson HH, Jr. Keratoacanthoma (molluscum sebaceum). *AMA Arch Dermatol Syphilol* 1954;71:66–72.

Blitstein-Willinger E, Haas N, Nürnberger F, et al. Immunological findings during treatment of multiple keratoacanthoma with etretinate. *Br J Dermatol* 1986;114:109–116.

Blohmé I, Larkö O. No difference in skin cancer incidence with or without cyclosporine—a 5-year perspective. *Transplant Proc* 1992;24:313.

Bogdanowski T, Rubisz-Brzezińska J, Macura-Gina M, et al. Ocena chirurgicznego leczenia rogowiaka kolczystokomórkowego. *Przegl Dermatol* 1990;77:29–33.

Bonnetblanc JM, Gualde N, Bonnetblanc F. Hypocomplementemia in keratoacanthoma. *Arch Dermatol Res* 1981;270:189–191.

Bönniger F, Burg G. Multiple keratokanthome. *Hautarzt* 1979;30:92–94.

Borum K. The role of the mouse hair cycle in epidermal carcinogenesis. *Acta Pathol Microbiol Scand* 1954;34:542–553.

Brothers WS, New WN, Nickel WR. Keratoacanthoma. A review of histopathological specimens previously diagnosed as keratoacanthomas or as squamous cell carcinoma of the skin. *AMA Arch Dermatol* 1960; 81:369–372.

Bryant J. Basal cell carcinoma associated with keratoacanthoma. *J Dermatol Surg Oncol* 1985;11:1230–1231.

Buescher L, DeSpain JD, Diaz-Arias AA, et al. Keratoacanthoma arising in an organoid nevus during childhood: case report and literature review. *Pediatr Dermatol* 1991;8:117–119.

Burgdorf WHC, Pitha J, Fahmy A. Muir-Torre syndrome: histologic spectrum of sebaceous proliferations. *Am J Dermatopathol* 1986;8:202–208.

Cabotin PP, Vignon-Pennamen MD, Miclea JM, et al. Kérato-acanthomes multiples éruptifs révélateurs d'un lymphome. *Ann Dermatol Venereol (Paris)* 1989;116:860–862.

Calonje E, Wilson Jones E. Intravascular spread of keratoacanthoma. An alarming but benign phemonenon. *Am J Dermatopathol* 1992;14:414–417.

Chapman RS, Finn OA. Carcinoma of the larynx in two patients with keratoacanthoma. *Br J Dermatol* 1974;90:685–688.

Chuang T-Y, Reizner GT, Elpern DI, et al. Keratoacanthoma in Kauai, Hawaii. The first documented incidence in a defined population. *Arch Dermatol* 1993;129:317–319.

Cipollaro VA. The use of podophyllin in the treatment of keratoacanthoma. *Int J Dermatol* 1983;22:436–440.

Claudy A, Thivolet J. Multiple keratoacanthomas: association with deficient cell mediated immunity. *Br J Dermatol* 1975;93:593–595.

Cockerell CJ. Cutaneous manifestations of HIV infection other than Kaposi's sarcoma: clinical and histologic aspects. *J Am Acad Dermatol* 1990;22:1260–1269.

Cooper PH, Wolfe JT III. Perioral keratoacanthoma with extensive perineural invasion and intravenous growth. *Arch Dermatol* 1988;124:1397–1401.

Corominas M, Sloan SR, Leon J, et al. *ras* activation in human tumors and in animal model systems. *Environ Health Perspect* 1991;93:19–25.

Corominas M, Leon J, Kamino H, et al. Oncogene involvement in tumor regression: *H-ras* activation in the rabbit model. *Oncogene* 1991;6:645–651.

Currie AR, Ferguson Smith J. Multiple primary spontaneous-healing squamous-cell carcinomata of the skin. *J Pathol Bacteriol* 1952;64:827–839.

Dąbska M, Madejczykowa A. Rogowiak kolczastokomórkowy—keratoacanthoma (molluscum sebaceum, molluscum pseudocarcinomatosum). Studium patologiczno-kliniczne. *Nowotwory* 1959;9:1–23.

De Moragas JM. Multiple keratoacanthomas. Relation to Jamarsan therapy for pemphigus foliaceus. *Arch Dermatol* 1966;93:679–683.

De Moragas JM, Montgomery H, McDonald JR. Keratoacanthoma versus squamous-cell carcinoma. *AMA Arch Dermatol* 1958;77:390–395.

Dogliotti M, Caro I. Keratoacanthoma in a Bantu child. *Int J Dermatol* 1976;15:524.

Donahue B, Cooper JS, Rush S. Treatment of aggressive keratoacanthomas by radiotherapy. *J Am Acad Dermatol* 1990;23:489–493.

Drut R. Solitary keratoacanthoma of the nipple in a male. Case report. *J Cutan Pathol* 1976;3:195–198.

Dupont A. Kyste sébacé atypique. *Bull Soç Belge Dermatol Syphiligr* 1930;177–179.

Eliezri YD, Libow L. Multinodular keratoacanthoma. *J Am Acad Dermatol* 1988;19:826–830.

Epstein EH Jr, Epstein EH. Keratoacanthoma recurrent after surgical excision. *J Dermatol Surg Oncol* 1978;4:524–525.

Ereaux LP, Schopf-Locher P, Fournier CJ. Keratoacanthomata. *AMA Arch Dermtaol* 1955;71:73–83.

Ereaux, LP, Schopflocher P. Familial primary self-healing squamous epithelioma of skin. Ferguson-Smith type. *Arch Dermatol* 1965;91:589–594.

Euvrard S, Chardonnet Y, Pouteil-Noble C, et al. Association of skin malignancies with various and multiple carcinogenic and noncarcinogenic human papillomarviruses in renal transplant patients. *Cancer* 1993;72:2198–2206.

Fanti PA, Tosti A, Peluso AM, Bonelli U. Multiple keratoacanthoma in discoid lupus erythematosus. *J Am Acad Dermatol* 1989;21:809–810.

Fathizadeh A, Medenica MM, Soltani K, et al. Aggressive keratoacanthoma and internal malignant neoplasm. *Arch Dermatol* 1982;118:112–114.

Ferguson Smith J. A case of multiple primary squamous-celled carincomata of the skin in a young man, with spontaneous healing. *Br J Dermatol Syph* 1934;46:267–272.

Ferguson Smith J. Multiple primary, self-healing squamous cell carcinomas of the skin. *Br J Dermatol Syph* 1948;60:315–318.

Ferguson-Smith MA, Wallace DC, James ZH, Renwick JH. Multiple self-healing squamous epithelioma. In *Birth Defects: original article series. The Third Conference on the Clinical Delineation of Birth Defects. Part XII: Skin and nails.* D. Bergsma, ed. Baltimore, Williams and Wilkins, 1971, pp. 157–163.

Fisher AA. Subungual keratoacanthoma: possible relationship to exposure to steel wool. *Cutis* 1990;46: 26–28.

Fisher ER, McCoy MM II, Wechsler HL. Analysis of histopathological and electron microscopic determinants of keratoacanthoma and squamous cell carcinoma. *Cancer* 1972;29:1387–1397.

Flannery GR, Muller KH. Immune response to human keratoacanthoma. *Br J Dermatol* 1979;101:625–632.

Fléchet ML, Barba L, Beltzer-Garelly E, et al. Kérato-acanthomes multiples sous-unguéaux. *Ann Dermatol Venereol (Paris)* 1989;116:862–864.

Foschini MP, Magnani P, Marconi F, et al. Multiple keratoacanthomas: a case report with evidence of regression with thymic hormone. *Br J Dermatol* 1991;124:479–482.

Friedman RP, Morales A, Burnham TK. Multiple cutaneous and conjunctival keratoacanthomata. *Arch Dermatol* 1965;92:162–165.

Furukawa M, Hamada T, Shibata H, et al. Keratoacanthoma ensuing from bone marrow transplantation for chronic myeloid leukemia. *Osaka City Med J* 1992;38:83–88.

Gassenmaier A, Pfister H, Hornstein OP. Human papillomavirus 25-related DNA in solitary keratoacanthoma. *Arch Dermatol Res* 1986;279:73–76.

Ghadially FN, Barton BW, Kerridge DF. The etiology of keratoacanthoma. *Cancer* 1963;16:603–611.

Ghadially FN. A comparative morphological study of kerato-acanthoma of man and similar experimentally produced lesions in rabbit. *J Pathol Bacteriol* 1958;75:441–453.

Ghadially FN. The experimental production of kerato-acanthomas in the hamster and the mouse. *J Pathol Bacteriol* 1959;77:277–282.

Ghadially FN. The role of the hair follicle in the origin and evolution of some cutaneous neoplasms of man and experimental animals. *Cancer* 1961;14:801–816.

Ghadially FN. *Ultrastructural Pathology of the Cell and Matrix. A Text and Atlas of Physiological and Pathological Alterations in the Fine Structure of Cellular and Extracellular Components.* 3rd ed. London, Butterworths, 1988, pp. 66–68, 1110.

Ghadially R, Ghadially FN. Keratoacanthoma. In *Dermatology in General Medicine.* TB Fitzpatrick, AZ Eisen, K Wolff, et al., eds. New York, McGraw-Hill, 1993, pp. 848–855.

Gheeraert P, Goens J, Schwartz RA, et al. Florid cutaneous papillomatosis, malignant acanthosis nigricans, and pulmonary squamous cell carcinoma. *Int J Dermatol* 1991;30:193–197.

Giltman LI. Tripolar mitosis in a keratoacanthoma. *Acta Derm Venereol (Stockh)* 1981;61:362–363.

Goette DK. Keratoacanthoma and its treatment. *J Assoc Milit Dermatol* 1984;10(1):3–10.

Goldschmidt H, Sherwin WK. Radiation therapy of giant aggressive keratoacanthomas. *Arch Dermatol* 1993;129:1162–1165.

Gougerot H. Verrucome avec adénite, à structure épithéliomatifome, curable par le 914. *Arch Dermato-Syphiligr Clin Saint-Louis* 1929;1:374–385.

Graham JH. Selected precancerous skin and mucocutaneous lesions. In *Neoplasms of the Skin and Malignant Melanoma*. Chicago, Year Book Medical Publishers, 1976, pp. 69–121.

Graham RM, MacFarlane AW, Curley RK, et al. β₂-Microglobulin expression in keratoacanthomas and squamous cell carcinoma. *Br J Dermatol* 1987;117:441–449.

Green WS, Underwood LJ, Green R. Multiple keratoacanthomas on upper extremities. *Arch Dermatol* 1977;113:512–513.

Grinspan D, Abulafia J. Idiopathic cutaneous pseudoepitheliomatous hyperplasia. Verrugoma (Gougerot), molluscum sebaceum (MacCormac and Scarff), self-healing, primary, squamous-cell carcinoma (Ferguson Smith), and keratoacathoma (Rook and Whimster). *Cancer* 1955;8:1047–1056.

Grinspan Bozza NO, Totaro II, Pocovi M, et al. Queratoacanthoma centrífugo de Miedzinski y Kozakiewicz. *Med Cutan Ibero-Latin-America* 1989;17:234–238.

Grob JJ, Suzini F, Weiller RM, et al. Large keratoacanthomas treated with intralesional interferon alpha-2a. *J Am Acad Dermatol* 1993;29:237–241.

Grzybowski M. A case of peculiar generalized epithelial tumours of the skin. *Br J Dermatol Syph* 1950;62:310–313.

Guillot B, Fesneau H, Mourad G, et al. Kératoacanthomes multiples sous ciclosporine. *Presse Med* 1990;19:1286.

Habel G, O'Regan B, Eissing A, et al. Intra-oral keratoacanthoma: an eruptive variant and review of the literature. *Br Dental J* 1991;170:336–339.

Habif TP. Extirpation of keratoacanthomas by blunt dissection. *J Dermatol Surg Oncol* 1980;6:652–654.

Hackel H, Burg G, Lechner W, et al. Keratoacanthoma centrifugum marginatum. *Hautarzt* 1989;40:763–766.

Haider S. Keratoacanthoma in a smallpox vaccination site. *Br J Dermatol* 1974;90:689–690.

Hashimoto Y, Matsuo S, Iizuka H. A flow cytometric study of the DNA content from paraffin-embedded samples of keratoacanthoma and squamous cell carcinoma. *Jpn J Dermatol* 1991;101:701–705.

Hellier FF, Rowell NR. Giant keratoacanthoma complicating dermatitis. *Arch Dermatol* 1962;85:485–487.

Hendricks WM. Sudden appearance of multiple keratoacanthomas three weeks after thermal burns. *Cutis* 1991;47:410–412.

Henseler T, Christophers E, Hönigsmann H, et al. Skin tumors in the European PUVA study. Eight-year follow-up of 1,643 patients treated with PUVA for psoriasis. *J Am Acad Dermatol* 1987;16:108–116.

Herold WC, Nelson LM. Pseudoepitheliomatous reaction (pseudorecidive) following radiation therapy of epitheliomata. In *The Eleventh International Congress of Dermatology Stockholm 1957 Proceedings*, Vol. 2. Hellerström S, Wikström K, Hellerström A-M, eds. Lund, Håkan Ohlssons Boktryckeri, 1959, pp. 426–432.

Herzberg AJ, Kerns BJ, Pollack SV, et al. DNA image cytometry of keratoacanthoma and squamous cell carcinoma. *J Invest Dermatol* 1991;97:495–500.

Heslop JH. The histogenesis of experimental molluscum sebaceum. *Br J Cancer* 1958;12:553–560.

Higuchi M, Tanikawa E, Nomura H, et al. Multiple keratoacanthomas with peculiar manifestations and course. *J Am Acad Dermatol* 1990;23:389–392.

Ho T, Horn T, Finzi E. Transforming growth factor α expression helps to distinguish keratoacanthomas from squamous cell carcinomas. *Arch Dermatol* 1991;127:1167–1171.

Hodak E, Jones RE, Ackerman AB, et al. Controversies in dermatopathology. Solitary keratoacanthoma is a squamous-cell carcinoma: three examples with metastases. with responses by Grant-Kels JM, From L, Reed RJ, et al. *Am J Dermatopathol* 1993;15:332–352.

Höpfl RM, Schir MM, Fritsch PO. Keratoacanthomas: human papillomavirus associated? *Arch Dermatol* 1992;128:563–564.

Hoxtell EO, Mandel JS, Murray SS, et al. Incidence of skin carcinoma after renal transplantation. *Arch Dermatol* 1977;113:436–438.

Hundeiker M, Otto H, Gerozissis C. Plattenepithelkarzinom oder Keratoakanthom? *Internist Prax* 1990;30:329–334.

Hutchinson J. A peculiar form of cancer of the skin. In *Illustrations of Clinical Surgery Consisting of Plates, Photographs, Woodcuts, Diagrams, etc. Illustrating Surgical Diseases, Symptoms and Accidents Also Operative and Other Methods of Treatment with Descriptive Letterpress.* Philadelphia, P. Blakiston & Son, 1888, Vol. 2, plate 92.

Hutchinson J. Demonstrations at the clinical museum. The crateriform ulcer—microscopic examination. *Arch Surg* 1896;7:88–89.

Hutchinson J. Morbid growths and tumours. 1. The "crateriform ulcer of the face," a form of acute epithelial cancer. *Trans Pathol Soc London* 1889;40:275–281.

Inoshita T, Youngberg GA. Keratoacanthoma associated with cervical squamous cell carcinoma. *Arch Dermatol* 1984;120:123–124.

Jaber PW, Cooper PH, Greer KE. Generalized eruptive keratoacanthoma of Grzybowski. *J Am Acad Dermatol* 1993;29:299–304.

Jablonska S, Schwartz RA. Giant condyloma acuminatum of Buschke and Lowenstein. In *Clinical Dermatology.* 18th ed. DJ Demis, ed. Philadelphia: JB Lippincott, 1991, Unit 14–14, pp. 1–5.

Jackson IT. Diagnostic problem of keratocanthoma. *Lancet* 1969;1:490–492.

Jackson IT, Alexander JO'D, Verheyden N. Self-healing squamous cell epithelioma: a family affair. *Br J Plast Surg* 1983;36:22–28.

Jackson R, Williamson GS. Keratoacanthoma: incidence and problems in diagnosis and treatment. *Can Med J* 1961;84:312–315.

Janecka IP, Wolff M, Crikelair GF, et al. Aggressive histologic features of keratoacanthoma. *J Cutan Pathol* 1978;4:342–348.

Janniger CK, Kapila R, Schwartz RA, et al. Histoid lepromas of lepromatous leprosy. *Int J Dermatol* 1990;29:494–496.

Job CK. Keratoacanthoma associated with leprosy. *Indian J Pathol Bacteriol* 1963;6:160–162.

Jolly HW, Jr, Carpenter CL, Jr. Multiple keratoacanthomata. A report of two cases. *Arch Dermatol* 1966;93:348–353.

Jordan RCK, Kahn HJ, From L, et al. Immunohistochemical demonstration of actinically damaged elastic fibers in keratoacanthomas: an aid in diagnosis. *J Cutan Pathol* 1991;18:81–86.

Jung-Grimm H. Pseudo-Rezidive nach Röntgenbestrahlung der Haut. *Dermatol Wochenschr* 1957;135:210–215.

Kanitakis J, Hoyo E, Hermier C, et al. Nucleolar organizer region enumeration in keratoacanthomas and squamous cell carcinomas of the skin. *Cancer* 1992;69:2937–2941.

Kannon G, Park HK. Utility of peanut agglutinin (PNA) in the diagnosis of squamous cell carcinoma and keratoacanthoma. *Am J Dermatopathol* 1990;12:31–36.

Kerschmann RL, McCalmont TH, LeBoit PE. p53 oncoprotein expression and proliferation index in keratoacanthoma and squamous cell carcinoma. *Arch Dermatol* 1994;130:181–186.

Kestel JL, Jr, Blair DS. Keratoacanthoma treated with methotrexate. *Arch Dermatol* 1973;108:723–724.

King DF, Barr RJ. Intraepithelial elastic fibers and intracytoplasmic glycogen: diagnostic aids in differentiating keratoacanthoma from squamous cell carcinoma. *J Cutan Pathol* 1980;7:140–148.

Kingman J, Callen JP. Keratoacanthoma: a clinical study. *Arch Dermatol* 1984;120:736–740.

Klein E, Helm F, Milgrom H, et al. Tumors of the skin-II: keratoacanthoma: local effect of 5-fluorouracil. *Skin* 1962;1:153–156.

Klein-Szanto AJP, Barr RJ, Reiners JJ, et al. Filaggrin distribution in keratoacanthomas and squamous cell carcinoma. *Arch Pathol Lab Med* 1984;108:888–890.

Kopf AW, Bart RS. Development of more keratoacanthomas following skin testing with nitrogen mustard in a patient with the multiple keratoacanthoma syndrome. *J Dermatol Surg Oncol* 1979;5:450–451.

Kopf AW, Bart RS. Giant keratoacanthoma. *J Dermatol Surg Oncol* 1978;4:444–445.

Kopf AW. Multiple keratoacanthomas. *Arch Dermatol* 1971;103:543–544.

Korenberg R, Penneys NS, Kowalczyk A, et al. Quantitation of S100 protein-positive cells in inflamed and non-inflamed keratoacanthoma and squamous cell carcinoma. *J Cutan Pathol* 1988;15:104–108.

Koziorowska J, Dux K. Poszukiwanie etiologicznego czynnika w keratoacanthoma. *Nowotwory* 1959;9:269–273.

Kuflik EG, Kuflik AS. Cryosurgery. In *Clinical Dermatology.* 20th ed. DJ Demis, ed. Philadelphia, JB Lippincott, 1993, Unit 37–5, pp. 1–5.

Kuflik EG. Cryosurgery updated. *J Am Acad Dermatol* 1994;31:925-944.

Kvedar JC, Fewkes J, Baden HP. Immunologic detection of markers of keratinocyte differentiation. Its use in neoplastic and preneoplastic lesions of skin. *Arch Pathol Lab Med* 1986;110:183-188.

Kwittken J. A histologic chronology of the clinical course of the keratocarcinoma (so-called keratoacanthoma). *Mt Sinai J Med* 1975;42:127-135.

Kwittken J. Dermatologic pseudobenignities. *Mt Sinai J Med* 1980;47:34-37.

Laaff H, Mittelviefhaus H, Wokalek H, et al. Eruptive Keratoakanthome Typ Grzybowski und Ektropium. Ein therapeutisches Problem. *Hautarzt* 1992;43:143-147.

Larson PO. Keratoacanthoma treated with Mohs' micrographic surgery (chemosurgery). A review of forty-three cases. *J Am Acad Dermatol* 1987;16:1040-1044.

Lawrence N, Reed RJ. Actinic keratoacanthoma. Speculations on the nature of the lesion and the role of cellular immunity in its evolution. *Am J Dermatopathol* 1990;12:517-533.

Lejman K, Starzycki Z. Giant keratoacanthoma of the inner surface of the prepuce. *Br J Venereol Dis* 1977;53:65-67.

Lever WF, Schaumburg-Lever G. *Histopathology of the Skin.* 7th ed. Philadelphia, JB Lippincott, 1990, pp. 560-563.

Levy EJ, Cahn MM, Shaffer B, et al. Keratoacanthoma. *J Am Med Assoc* 1954;155:562-564.

Lloyd KM, Madsen DK, Lin PY. Grzybowski's eruptive keratoacanthoma. *J Am Acad Dermatol* 1989; 21:1023-1024.

Lyell A. John Ferguson Smith (1888-1978). *Am J Dermatopathol* 1986;8:525-528.

MacCormac H, Scarff RW. Molluscum sebaceum. *Br J Dermatol Syph* 1936;48:624-627.

Maddin WS, Wood WS. Multiple keratoacanthomas and squamous cell carcinomas occurring at psoriatic treatment sites. *J Cutan Pathol* 1979;6:96-100.

Markey AC, Churchill LJ, MacDonald DM. Altered expression of major histocompatibility complex (MHC) antigens by epidermal tumours. *J Cutan Pathol* 1990;17:65-71.

Markey AC, MacDonald DM. Identification of CD16/NKH-1[+] natural killer cells and their relevance to cutaneous tumour immunity. *Br J Dermatol* 1989;121:563-570.

Marshall J, Pepler WJ. Mollusca pseudocarcinomatosa. Discussion of a case of the Ferguson Smith type of unilateral distribution. *Br J Cancer* 1954;8:251-254.

Marshall V. Premalignant and malignant skin tumours in immunosuppressed patients. *Transplantation* 1974; 17:272-275.

Maxwell TB, Lamb JH. Unusual reaction to application of podophyllum resin. *AMA Arch Dermatol Syphilol* 1954;70:510-511.

McGlashan JA, Rees, G, Bowdler DA. Solitary keratoacanthoma of the nasal vestibule. *J Laryngol Otol* 1991;105:306-308.

McGregor JM, Yu CC, Dublin EA, et al. Aberrant expression of p53 tumour-suppressor protein in non-melanoma skin cancer. *Br J Dermatol* 1992;127:463-469.

McKee PH, Wilkinson JD, Black MM, et al. Carcinoma (epithelioma) cuniculatum: a clinico-pathological study of nineteen cases and review of the literature. *Histopathology* 1981;5:423-436.

McNairy DJ. Intradermal triamcinolone therapy of keratoacanthomas. *Arch Dermatol* 1964;89:136-140.

Mehregan AH, Fabian L. Keratoacanthoma of nailbed: a report of two cases. *Int J Dermatol* 1973;12: 149-151.

Mehregan AH, Pinkus H. Life history of organoid nevi. Special reference to nevus sebaceus of Jadassohn. *Arch Dermatol* 1965;91:574-588.

Mehta VR. Keratoacanthoma with osteolysis (a case report with an isolated interdigital lesion). *Indian J Dermatol Venereol Leprol* 1980;46:360-363.

Melato M, Cecovini G, Perazza L, et al. Perineural invasion in solitary keratoacanthoma: a malignant feature? *Acta Dermatovenerol APA* (Ljubljana) 1995;4:60-62.

Melton JL, Nelson BR, Stough DB, et al. Treatment of keratoacanthomas with intralesional methotrexate. *J Am Acad Dermatol* 1991;25:1017-1023.

Michałowski R. Program tajnego nauczania dermatologii w klinice dermatologicznej w Warszawie podczas niemieckiej okupacji. *Arch Histor Filozof Med* 1988;51:439-447.

Miedziński F, Dratwiński Z, Brzozowski J, et al. Ein Beitrag zur nosologischen Stellung des Keratoakanthoma centrifugum. *Hautarzt* 1973;24:120-123.

Miedziński F, Kozakiewicz. J. Das Keratoakanthoma centrifugum—eine besondere Varietät des Keratoakanthoms. *Hautarzt* 1962;13:348–352.

Miedziński F. Keratoacanthoma as a pathogenic and clinico-histological problem, its 40th anniversary. In *Postępy Dermatologii. Annals in Polish and English. Rocznik pod redakcja VII.* J Bowszyc, ed. Poznań, Akademia Medyczna Im. Karola Marcinkowskiego w Poznaniu, 1990, pp. 61–70.

Milewski B, Chorzelski T. Vergleichende histologische und histochemische Untersuchungen von Keratoakanthomen und höber differenzierten spinocellulären Epitheliomen. *Hautarzt* 1962;13:7–12.

Miracco C, De Santi MM, Lio R, et al. Quantitatively evaluated ultrastructural findings can add to the differential diagnosis between keratoacanthoma and well differentiated squamous cell carcinoma. *J Submicrosc Cytol Pathol* 1992;24:315–321.

Mittal RR, Popli R, Parsad D. Multiple keratoacanthoma in a female infant. *Ind J Dermatol Venereol Leprol* 1992;58:227–228.

Molochkov VA, Ilyin II, Dolgushin II, et al. Histocompatibility antigens and solitary keratoacanthoma. *Voprosy Onkology* 1989;35:286–288.

Morita H, Sagami S. Analysis of lymphocyte subpopulations using monoclonal antibodies in a case of keratoacanthomas. *Acta Dermatol (Kyoto)* 1985;80:209–211.

Muir EG, Bell AJY, Barlow KA. Multiple primary carcinomata of the colon, duodenum, and larynx associated with kerato-acathomata of the face. *Br J Surg* 1967;54:191–195.

Muller HK, Flannery GR. Epidermal antigens in experimental keratoacanthoma and squamous cell carcinoma. *Cancer Res* 1973;33:2181–2186.

Musso L, Gordon H. Spontaneous resolution of a molluscum sebaceum. *Proc R Soc Med* 1950; 43: 838–839.

Nedwich JA. Evaluation of curettage and electrodesiccation in treatment of keratoacanthoma. *Australas J Dermatol* 1991;32:137–141.

Nelson LM. Self-healing pseudocancers of the skin. *Calif Med* 1959;90:49–54.

Neumann RA, Nobler RM. Argon laser treatment of small keratoacanthomas in difficult locations. *Int J Dermatol* 1990;29:733–736.

Odom RB, Goette DK. Treatment of keratoacanthomas with intralesional fluorouracil. *Arch Dermatol* 1978; 114:1779–1783.

Odom RB. Keratoacanthoma. *J Assoc Milit Dermatol* 1980;6(1):2–5.

Oettlè AG. Skin cancer in Africa. *Natl Cancer Inst Monogr* 1963;10:197–214.

Pagani WA, Lorenzi G, Lorusso D. Surgical treatment for aggressive giant keratoacanthoma of the face. *J Dermatol Surg Oncol* 1986;12:282–284.

Parker CM, Hanke CW. Large keratoacanthomas in difficult locations treated with intralesional 5-fluorouracil. *J Am Acad Dermatol* 1986;14:770–777.

Patel MR, Desai SS. Subungual keratoacanthoma in the hand. *J Hand Surg* 1989;14A:139–142.

Pavithran K. Multiple keratoacanthomas on the mons pubis and labia majora. *Indian J Dermatol Venereol Leprol* 1988;54:262–263.

Pellicano R, Fabrizi G, Cerimele D. Multiple keratoacanthomas and junctional epidermolysis bullosa. A therapeutic conundrum. *Arch Dermatol* 1990;126:305–306.

Peteiro MC, Caeiro JL, Toribio J. Keratoacanthoma centrifugum marginatum versus low-grade squamous cell carcinoma. *Dermatologica (Basel)* 1985;170:221–224.

Piérard-Franchimont C, Piérard GE. Rates of epidermal carcinomas in the Mosan region of Belgium. *Dermatologica (Basel)* 1988;177:76–81.

Pfister H, Gassenmaier A, Fuchs PG. Demonstration of human papillomavirus DNA in two keratoacanthomas. *Arch Dermatol Res* 1986;278:243–246.

Phillips P, Helm KF. Proliferating cell nuclear antigen distribution in keratoacanthoma and squamous cell carcinoma. *J Cutan Pathol* 1993;20:424–428.

Pillsbury DM, Beerman H. Multiple keratoacanthoma. *Am J Med Sci* 1958;236:614–623.

Poleksic S, Yeung K-Y. Rapid development of keratoacanthoma and accelerated transformation into squamous cell carcinoma of the skin. A mutagenic effect of polychemotherapy in a patient with Hodgkin's disease. *Cancer* 1970;41:12–16.

Poleksic S. Keratoacanthoma and multiple carcinomas. *Br J Dermatol* 1974;91:461–463.

Popkin GL, Brodie SJ, Hyman AB, et al. A technique of biopsy recommended for keratoacanthomas. *Arch Dermatol* 1966;94:191–193.

Poth DO. Tumor-like keratoses: report of a case. *AMA Arch Dermatol Syphilol* 1939;39:228–238.

Prutkin L. An ultrastructure of the experimental keratoacanthoma. *J Invest Dermatol* 1967;48:326–336.

Puente Duany N. Squamous cell pseudoepithelioma (keratoacanthoma). A new clinical variety, gigantic, multiple, and localized. *Arch Dermatol* 1958;78:703–709.

Ramselaar CG, van der Meer JB. Non-immunological regression of dimethylbenz(A) anthracene-induced experimental keratoacanthomas in the rabbit. *Dermatologica (Basel)* 1979;158:142–151.

Ramselaar CG, van der Meer JB. The spontaneous regression of keratoacanthoma in man. *Acta Derm Venereol (Stockh)* 1976;56:245–251.

Ramselaar CG. Spontaneous regression of keratoacanthoma. Doctoral thesis, Amsterdam, Rodopi, 1980.

Randall MB, Geisinger KR, Kute TE, et al. DNA content and proliferative index in cutaneous squamous cell carcinoma and keratoacanthoma. *Am J Clin Pathol* 1990;93:259–262.

Rapaport J. Giant keratoacanthoma of the nose. *Arch Dermatol* 1975;111:73–75.

Reder PA, Neel HB, 3rd: Blastomycosis in otolaryngology: review of a large series. *Laryngoscope* 1993:103:53–58.

Reid BJ, Cheesbrough MJ. Multiple keratoacanthomata. A unique case and review of the current classification. *Acta Derm Venereol (Stockh)* 1978;58:169–173.

Reid E, Grosshans E, Lazrak B, et al. Keratoacanthoma centrifugum marginatum. *Ann Dermatol Venereol (Paris)* 1979;106:367–370.

Reiffers J, Laugier P, Hunziker N. Hyperplasies sébacées, kérato-acanthomes, épithéliomas du visage et cancer du côlon. Une nouvelle entité? *Dermatologica (Basel)* 1976;153:23–33.

Requena L, Romero E, Sánchez M, et al. Aggressive keratoacanthoma of the eyelid: "malignant" keratoacanthoma or squamous cell carcinoma. *J Dermatol Surg Oncol* 1990;16:564–568.

Reymann F. Treatment of keratoacanthomas with curettage. *Dermatologica (Basel)* 1977;155:90–96.

Ridgon RH. Histopathologenesis of "keratoacanthoma" induced with methylcholanthrene. Lesions in the skin of chicken. *AMA Arch Dermatol* 1960;81:381–387.

Ro YS, Cooper PN, Lee JA, et al. p53 protein expression in benign and malignant skin tumours. *Br J Dermatol* 1993;128:237–241.

Rook A, Champion RH. Keratoacanthoma. *Natl Cancer Inst Monogr* 1963;10:257–273.

Rook A, Moffatt JL. Multiple self-healing epithelioma of Ferguson Smith type. Report of a case of unilateral distribution. *Arch Dermatol* 1956;74:525–532.

Rook A, Whimster I. Keratoacanthoma—a thirty year retrospect. *Br J Dermatol* 1979;100:41–47.

Rook A, Whimster I. Le kérato-acanthome. *Arch Belg Dermatol Syphiligr* 1950;6:137–146.

Rosen T. Keratoacanthoma arising within a linear epidermal nevus. *J Dermatol Surg Oncol* 1982;8:878–880.

Rossman RE, Freeman RG, Knox JM. Multiple keratoacanthomas. *Arch Dermatol* 1964;89:374–381.

Roth AM. Solitary keratoacanthoma of the conjunctiva. *Am J Ophthalmol* 1978;85:647–650.

Rothenberg J, Lambert WC, Vail JT, Jr, et al. The Muir-Torre (Torre's) syndrome: the significance of a solitary sebaceous tumor. *J Am Acad Dermatol* 1990;23:638–640.

Samochocki Z. Rogowiak kolczystokomórkowy (keratoacanthoma). *Przegl Dermatol* 1984;71:177–180.

Sanchez Yus E, Requena L. Keratoacanthoma within a superficial spreading malignant melanoma in situ. *J Cutan Pathol* 1991;18:228–292.

Santa Cruz DJ, Clausen K. Atypical sweat duct hyperplasia accompanying keratoacanthoma. *Dermatologica (Basel)* 1977;154:156–160.

Santa Lucia P, Wilson BD, Allen HJ. Localization of endogeneous β-galactoside-binding lectin as a means to distinguish malignant from benign skin tissue. *J Dermatol Surg Oncol* 1991;17:653–655.

Sayama S, Tagami H. Treatment of keratoacanthoma with intralesional bleomycin. *Br J Dermatol* 1983;109:449–452.

Schaumburg-Lever G, Alroy J, Gavris V, et al. Cell-surface carbohydrates in proliferative epidermal lesions: distribution of A, B, and H blood group antigens in benign and malignant lesions. *Am J Dermatopathol* 1984;6:583–589.

Schwartz RA, Burgess GH. Florid cutaneous papillomatosis. *Arch Dermatol* 1978;114:1803–1806.

Schwartz RA, Flieger FN, Saied NK. The Torre syndrome with gastrointestinal polyposis. *Arch Dermatol* 1980;116:312–314.

Schwartz RA, Torre DP. The Muir-Torre syndrome: a 25-year retrospective. *J Am Acad Dermatol* 1995;33:90–104.

Schwartz RA, Goldberg DJ, Mahmood F, et al. The Muir-Torre syndrome: a disease of sebaceous and colonic neoplasms. *Dermatologica (Basel)* 1989;178:23–28.

Schwartz RA, Klein E. Ultraviolet light-induced carcinogenesis. In *Cancer Medicine*, 2nd ed. JF Holland, E. Frei III, eds. Philadelphia, Lea & Febiger, 1982, pp. 109–119.

Schwartz RA, Stoll HL, Jr. Squamous cell carcinoma. In *Dermatology in General Medicine*, 4th ed. TB Fitzpatrick, AZ Eisen, K Wolff, et al., eds. New York, McGraw-Hill, 1993, pp. 821–839.

Schwartz RA. Multiple persistent keratoacanthomas. *Oncology (Basel)* 1979;36:281–285.

Schwartz RA. *Skin Cancer Recognition and Management.* New York, Springer-Verlag, 1988, pp. 48–56.

Schwartz RA. The keratoacanthoma: a review. *J Surg Oncol* 1979;12:305–317.

Schwartz RA. Keratoacanthoma. *J Am Acad Dermatol* 1994;30:1–19.

Schwartz RA. Verrucous carcinoma.In *Clinical Dermatology.* 18th ed. DJ Demis, ed. Philadelphia, JB Lippincott, 1991, Unit 21–22, pp. 1–8.

Seidman JD, Berman JJ, Moore GW, et al. Multiparameter DNA flow cytometry of keratoacanthoma. *Anal Quant Cytol Histol* 1992;14:113–119.

Shatkin BT, Hunter JG, Song IC. Familial subungual keratoacanthoma in association with ectodremal dysplasia. *Plast Reconstr Surg* 1993;92:528–531.

Shaw Dunn J, Ferguson Smith J. Self-healing primary squamous cell carcinoma of the skin. *Br J Dermatol Syphil* 1934;46:519–523.

Shaw JC, Storrs FJ, Everts E. Multiple keratoacanthomas after megavoltage radiation therapy. *J Am Acad Dermatol* 1990;23:1009–1011.

Shellito JE, Samet JM. Keratoacanthoma as a complication of arterial puncture for blood gases. *Int J Dermatol* 1982;21:349.

Shewmake SW. Keratoacanthoma arising in a nevus sebaceus of Jadassohn. *J Assoc Milit Dermatolog* 1978; 4(2):50–52.

Shimm DS, Duttenhaver JR, Doucette J, Wang CC. Radiation therapy of keratoacanthoma. *Int J Rad Oncol Biol Phys* 1983;9:759–761.

Silberberg I, Kopf AW, Baer RL. Recurrent keratoacanthoma of the lip. *Arch Dermatol* 1962;86:92–101.

Sina B, Adrian RM. Multiple keratoacanthomas possibly induced by psoralens and ultraviolet A photochemotherapy. *J Am Acad Dermatol* 1983;9:686–688.

Smoller BR, Kwan TH, Said JW, et al. Keratoacanthoma and squamous cell carcinoma of the skin: immunohistochemical localization of involucrin and keratin proteins. *J Am Acad Dermatol* 1986;14:226–234.

Snider BL, Benjamin DR. Eruptive keratoacanthoma with an internal malignant neoplasm. *Arch Dermatol* 1981;117:788–790.

Sommerville J, Milne JA. Familial primary self-healing squamous epitheliomna of the skin (Ferguson Smith type). *Br J Dermatol Syphil* 1950;62:485–490.

Spitler LE, Levin AS, Fudenberg HH. Transfer factor II: results of therapy. In *Birth Defects: Original Article Series. Part I. Immunodeficiency in Man and Animals.* Bergsma D, Good RA, Finstad J, eds. Sunderland, MA, Sinauder Assoc, 1975, pp. 449–456.

Sródka A. Akademickie nauczanie dermatologii i wenerologii w Warszawie w latach 1869–1939. *Przeg Dermatol* 1989;76:188–193.

Starzycki Z. Zastosowanie maści Efudix w leczeniu rogowiaka kolczystokomórkowego (keratoacanthoma). I. Kliniczna ocena wyników leczenia. *Przegl Dermatol* 1980;67:469–474.

Starzycki Z. Zastosowanie maści Efudix w leczeniu rogowiaka kolczystokomórkowego (keratoacanthoma). II. Obserwacje histologiczne w przebiegu leczenia. *Przegl Dermatol* 1980;67:475–479.

Stephenson TJ, Royds JA, Bleehen SS, et al. 'Anti-metastatic' nm23 gene product expression in keratoacanthoma and squamous cell carcinoma. *Dermatology (Basel)* 1993;187:95–99.

Stephenson TJ, Royds J, Silcocks PB, et al. Mutant p53 oncogene expression in keratoacanthoma and squamous cell carcinoma. *Br J Dermatol* 1992;127:566–570.

Sterry W, Steigleder G-K, Pullmann H, et al. Eruptive keratoakanthome. *Hautarzt* 1981;32:119–125.

Stevanovic DV. Keratoacanthoma dyskeratoticum and segregans. *Arch Dermatol* 1965;92:666–669.

Stevanovic DV. Keratoacanthoma in xeroderma pigmentosum. *Arch Dermatol* 1961;84:53–54.

Stevanović DV. Keratoacanthoma. Mucous membranes as the site of its localization. *Dermatologica (Basel)* 1960;121:278-284.

Stevanović DV. Pseudocarcinomatous hyperplasia. In *Proceedings of the XII International Congress of Dermatology September 1962/Washington D.C.* Vol. 2. DM Pillsbury, CS Livingood, eds. Amsterdam, Excerpta Medica Foundation, 1963, pp. 1577-1578.

Stewart W-M, Lauret P, Hemet J, et al. Kérato-acanthomes multiples et carcinomes viscéraux: syndrome de Torre. *Ann Derm Venereol (Paris)* 1977;104:622-626.

Stone OJ. Non-immunologic enhancement and regression of self-healing squamous cell carcinoma (keratoacanthoma)—ground substance and inflammation. *Med Hypothesis* 1988;26:113-117.

Street ML, White JW Jr, Gibson LE. Multiple keratoacanthomas treated with oral retinoids. *J Am Acad Dermatol* 1990;23:862-866.

Strumia R, Venturini D, Califano AL. Seasonality of presentation of keratoacanthoma. *Int J Dermatol* 1993;32:691.

Svirsky JA, Freedman PD, Lumerman H. Solitary intraoral keratoacanthoma. *Oral Surg Oral Med Oral Pathol* 1977;43:116-122.

Takaki Y, Masutani M, Kawada A. Electron microscopic study of keratoacanthoma. *Acta Derm Venereol (Stockh)* 1971;51:21-26.

Tanigaki T, Endo H. A case of squamous cell carcinoma treated with intralesional injection of oil bleomycin. *Dermatologica (Basel)* 1985;170:302-305.

Tarnowski WM. Multiple keratoacanthomata: response of a case to systemic chemotherapy. *Arch Dermatol* 1966;94:74-80.

Tham SN, Lee CT. Condyloma latum mimicking kerato-acanthoma in patient with secondary syphilis. *Genito-Urinary Med* 1987;63:339-340.

Toh BH, Muller HK. Smooth muscle-associated antigen in experimental cutaneous squamous cell carcinoma, keratoacanthoma, and papilloma. *Cancer Res* 1975;35:3741-3745.

Torre D, Lubritz RR, Kuflik EG. *Practical Cutaneous Cryosurgery*. Norwalk, CT, Appleton & Lange, 1988, p. 76.

Torre D. Multiple sebaceous tumors. *Arch Dermatol* 1968;98:549-551.

Trowell HE, Dyall-Smith ML, Dyall-Smith DJ. Human papillomavirus associated with keratoacanthomas in Australian patients. *Arch Dermatol* 1990;126:1654.

Van De Staak WJBM, Bergers AMG. Intranuclear particles in keratoacanthoma: possible association with malignant degeneration. *Dermatologica (Basel)* 1979;158:413-416.

Venkei T, Sugár J. Precancerous and cancerous varieties of keratoacanthoma. *Acta Unio Int Cancum (Louvain)* 1960;16:1454-1457.

Vickers CFH, Ghadially FN. Keratoacanthomata associated with psoriasis. *Br J Dermatol* 1961;73:120-124.

Washington CV, Jr, Mikhail GR. Eruptive keratoacanthoma en plaque in an immunosuppressed patient. *J Dermatol Surg Oncol* 1987;13:1357-1360.

Webb AJ, Ghadially FN. Massive or giant keratoacanthoma. *J Pathol Bacteriol* 1966;91:505-509.

Weber G, Stetter H, Pliess G, et al. Assoziiertes Vorkommen von eruptiven Keratoacanthomen, Tubencarcinom und Paramyeloblastenleukämie. *Arch Klin Exp Dermatol* 1970;238:107-119.

Whiting DA. Skin tumours in white South Africans. *S Afr Med J* 1978;53:98-102, 131-136, 162-170.

Wick MR, Manivel JC, Millns JL. Histopathologic considerations in the management of skin cancer. In *Skin Cancer Recognition and Management*. Schwartz RA, ed. New York, Springer-Verlag, 1988, pp. 246-275.

Wilkinson SM, Tan CY, Smith AG. Keratoacanthoma arising within organoid naevi. *Clin Exp. Dermatol* 1991;16:58-60.

Wiss K, McNeely C, Solomon AR, Jr. Chromoblastomycosis can mimic keratoacanthoma. *Int J Dermatol* 1986;25:385-386.

Witten VH, Zak FG. Multiple, primary, self-healing prickle-cell epithelioma of the skin. *Cancer* 1952; 5:539-550.

Yamagiwa K, Ichikawa K. Experimental study of the pathogenesis of carcinoma. *J Cancer Res* 1918;3:1-29.

Yell JA. Grzybowski's generalized eruptive keratoacanthoma. *J R Soc Med* 1991;84:170-171.

Zalewska-Kubicka L. DNA cytophotometry as a method for differentiation between keratoacanthoma and spinocellular carcinoma. In *Congressus Dermatologiae 24th Polish Dermatologic Congress 1992 Gdańsk Summaries*. Gdańsk, Akademii Medycznej, 1992, pp. 256–257.

Zelickson AS, Lynch FW. Electron microscopy of virus-like particles in a keratoacanthoma. *J Invest Dermatol* 1961;37:79–83.

33

Malignant Melanoma

Robert J. Friedman, Darrell S. Rigel, Sarah Silverman, and Robert Nossa
New York University School of Medicine, New York, New York

The most serious cancer of the skin, malignant melanoma, will account for more than 6900 deaths this year in the United States. Approximately 32,000 new cases of malignant melanoma will occur. About 1 in 100 Americans will develop malignant melanoma in 1994, and it is estimated that the number will increase to 1 in 75 by the year 2000. A recent report by Salopek et al. calculates the incidence of malignant melanoma in the United States to be approximately 80,000 new cases per year as of 1992 (in situ and invasive malignant melanoma). The incidence of malignant melanoma has been increasing at a rate of 4% per year. Despite these dismal statistics, malignant melanoma is almost always curable when it is discovered and removed in its early stages.

Malignant melanoma is best defined as a malignant neoplasm comprised of atypical melanocytes that almost always begin within the epidermis. A wholly intraepidermal ("in situ") malignant melanoma is a biologically benign neoplasm that does not metastasize and this is 100% curable if completely removed. The identification of such neoplasms is important since the incidence of metastases increases in direct proportion to the thickness of the neoplasm once the atypical melanocytes of the malignant melanoma penetrate into the dermis. Early malignant melanoma can be readily identified by using the mnemonic "ABCDs of melanoma" (Fig. 1).

HISTOPATHOLOGY

Almost all malignant melanomas have their origin within the epidermis of the skin. Under the light microscope and with routine staining, they initially appear as a small proliferation of foci of melanocytes, increased in number and apparently cytologically normal (Fig. 2). In time, some of the melanocytes begin to appear cytologically atypical with somewhat hyperchromatic pleomorphic nuclei, some with prominent eosinophilic staining nucleoli (Fig. 3). To this point, most, if not all, of the singly arranged melanocytes are found along the dermoepidermal junction. The evolving in situ malignant melanoma is next characterized by a few single melanocytes proliferating upward within the epidermis as well as single melanocytes coalescing within the lower

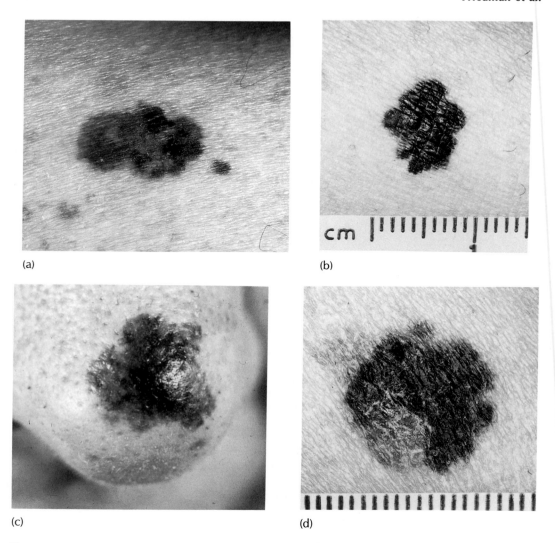

(a)   (b)

(c)   (d)

Figure 1   ABCDs of early malignant melanoma. (a) Asymmetry. (b) Border irregularity. (c) Color variegation. (d) Diameter greater than 6 mm.

epidermis into collections, or nests, which become somewhat irregular in size and shape (Fig. 4). Some of these nests are seen not only along the dermoepidermal junction but at higher levels of the epidermis. Maize and Ackerman state that an important criterion for the diagnosis of very small (less than 3 mm in diameter) evolving malignant melanomas is the predominance of a proliferation of *single* atypical melanocytes (compared to nests) within the epidermis. Over time, the epidermis may be filled with atypical melanocytes, at all levels, including the cornified layer. These melanocytes are usually arranged both singly and in irregularly shaped nests, many of which may be confluent (Fig. 5).

In many instances, the epithelial adnexal structures demonstrate similar proliferation of atypical melanocytes. By the time the malignant melanoma measures approximately 4 or 5 mm in diameter, it may infiltrate into the dermis. However, some malignant melanomas never progress into

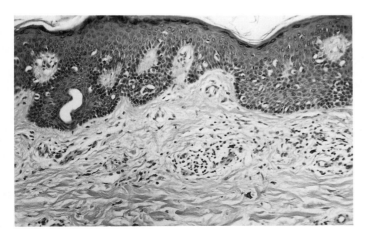

Figure 2 Malignant melanoma in situ evolving early, showing an increased number of cytologically normal-appearing melanocytes focally arranged, predominantly as single cells along the dermoepidermal junction and slightly above it.

the "invasive" phase and may remain "in situ" for decades (e.g., lentigo maligna melanoma). Others may infiltrate into the dermis early in their development (Figs. 6, 7). Once the atypical melanocytes of malignant melanoma infiltrate into the dermis, they begin to extend deeper into the reticular dermis and subcutis unless they are surgically removed.

It is thought that once the neoplasm exceeds a certain size or volume, new blood vessels must form (neovascularization) to sustain a nutrient supply for continued growth. Metastases occur when the atypical melanocytes penetrate into local lymphatic and vascular channels. This event is directly proportional to both the thickness and volume of the neoplasm.

Some authors have defined the following as common histologic features of malignant melanoma, regardless of size or anatomic site:

1. Diameter usually greater than 6 mm when readily identifiable.
2. Asymmetrical proliferation of melanocytes.

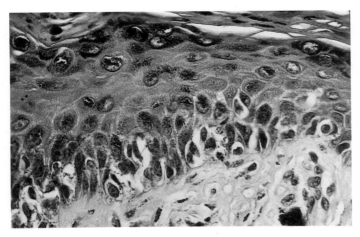

Figure 3 Malignant melanoma in situ: early changes show an increased number of cytologically atypical melanocytes arranged as single cells along the dermoepidermal junction and slightly above it.

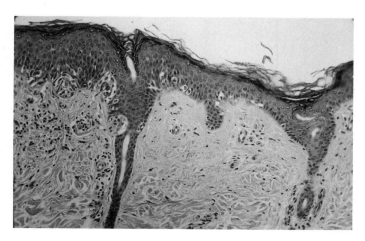

Figure 4   Malignant melanoma in situ showing an increased number of cytologically atypical melanocytes arranged both singly and in confluent nests within the epidermis and at somewhat higher levels of the epidermis.

3. Poorly circumscribed melanocytic proliferation.
4. When involving the epidermis alone, a proliferation of single atypical melanocytes within the epidermis and adnexal structures; often single melanocytes within the epidermis predominate over nests of melanocytes.
5. Melanocytes usually present at all levels of the epidermis ("buck-shot" scatter of melanocytes throughout the epidermis).
6. Irregular nests of melanocytes not equidistant from each other.
7. Nests of melanocytes vary in size and shape and tend to be confluent.
8. Nuclei of atypical melanocytes tend to be the same or larger in size with progressive descent into the dermis (in contrast to melanocytic nevi, in which nuclear size tends to decrease with progressive descent into the dermis).

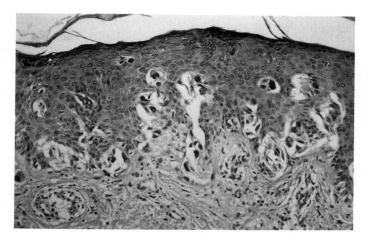

Figure 5   Malignant melanoma in situ showing an increased number of atypical melanocytes arranged both singly and in confluent nests throughout the epidermis.

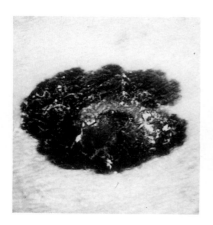

Figure 6 Malignant melanoma involving the epidermis and dermis.

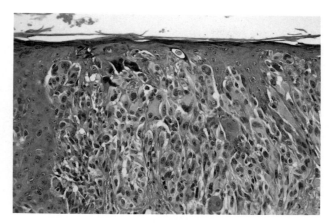

Figure 7 Malignant melanoma involving the epidermis and dermis.

9. Deposition of melanin pigment tends to be nonuniform and patchy.
10. Atypical melanocytes are usually present far down into epithelial structures of adnexae.
11. The inflammatory cell infiltrate tends to be asymmetrically distributed in varying densities at the base of the neoplasm.
12. Nuclear atypia, including pleomorphic and hyperchromatic nuclei.
13. Melanocytic necrosis (variable).
14. Melanocytes in mitosis (some atypical) (variable).

The histopathologic diagnosis of malignant melanoma requires the identification of a number of features common to malignant melanoma. Identifying the classic architectural pattern is essential to the diagnosis of this neoplasm. Cytological features, though important, appear to be secondary, particularly in early evolving lesions. Most of the histopathologic features mentioned above have clinically apparent counterparts. Clinical features are essential in the early diagnosis of curable lesions of malignant melanoma.

CLINICOPATHOLOGIC CORRELATIONS

If one recalls the mnemonic for the early diagnosis of malignant melanoma ("ABCDs"), each of the clinical features has its histologic counterpart. The clinical asymmetry ("A") of an early malignant melanoma is due to the asymmetrical proliferation of atypical melanocytes, both singly and in nests within the epidermis. The irregular growth pattern of these melanocytes causes the jagged or notched border irregularity ("B"). Color variability ("C") seen in early malignant melanoma is secondary to the presence of irregular amounts of melanin pigment within at all levels of the epidermis. Melanin pigment within the cytoplasms of atypical melanocytes in the lower half of the epidermis gives the clinical colors of various shades of tan and brown. Once the melanin pigment is present at higher levels of the epidermis, and particularly within the cornified layer, the color becomes black. Thus early malignant melanomas present as small, asymmetrical, irregularly shaped pigmented macules with nuances of tan and brown first, and later with areas of dark brown and black. The peripheral growth or diameter ("D") of malignant melanoma provides the fourth letter of the mnemonic. Usually a diameter ("D") greater than

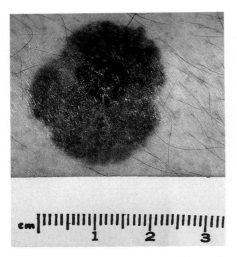

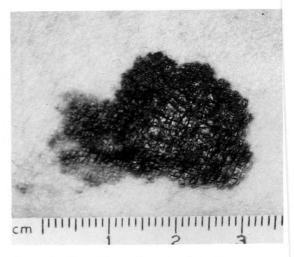

Figure 8 Malignant melanoma with small invasive component.

Figure 9 Plaquelike malignant melanoma.

6 mm (about the size of a pencil eraser) is a common feature of early malignant melanoma (Fig. 1).

As the neoplasm continues to grow and the atypical melanocytes infiltrate into the dermis, the previously flat malignant melanoma in situ becomes elevated. If the typical melanocytes infiltrate into the dermis focally, a small papule or nodule may appear superimposed on the macule (Fig. 8). If the atypical melanocytes broadly infiltrate into the dermis, a plaquelike lesion may be seen (Fig. 9). If the neoplasm infiltrates into the dermis early, the macular (in situ) component may be obscured; a nodular variant of malignant melanoma may become manifest. Later clinical variations of malignant melanoma include the presence of ulceration (Fig. 10).

At times, the immune system may partially or, rarely, completely destroy the malignant melanoma manifesting itself clinically and histologically as focal or complete regression. Histologically, these changes are characterized by the finding of a thickened fibrotic papillary dermis with a few scattered lymphocytes and melanophages (Fig. 11). Clinically, such areas are seen as focal zones of white or pink within (or at the site of) a malignant melanoma (Fig. 12). The earliest histologic feature of regression is a dense bandlike infiltrate of lymphocytes, often followed by broad zones of histiocytes laden with melanin (melanophages) resulting in so-called melanosis (Fig. 13).

PROGNOSIS

Malignant melanoma, when advanced, often will result in death from widespread metastases. During the last century, malignant melanoma was uniformly fatal. Forty years ago, only 43% of patients with malignant melanoma survived for 5 years. By the beginning of this deade, the percentage of individuals with malignant melanoma surviving 5 years or more after diagnosis and treatment of their disease has increased to over 80%. Despite these encouraging statistics, the death rate from malignant melanoma has doubled over the past 30 years. While the cause of malignant melanoma has yet to be elucidated, the fact remains that certain persons with this disease survive, while others die. Thus, important prognostic factors must play a role in the

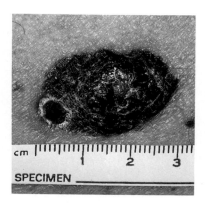

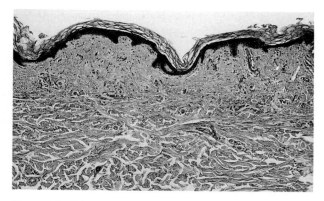

Figure 10 Malignant melanoma, ulcerated.

Figure 11 Histopathologic appearance of partially regressed melanoma shows a thickened fibrotic papillary dermis with a few scattered lymphocytes and melanophages.

biologic behavior of this neoplasm. These factors not only are helpful in the clinical management of patients with malignant melanoma, but they may also be key to unlocking the mysteries of the pathobiology of this neoplasm.

By far the most important of the factors related to prognosis in patients with malignant melanoma is the thickness of the neoplasm. Clark et al. noted that the depth of penetration of the neoplasm into the dermis was directly proportional to biologic behavior. Five levels of microinvasion have been repeatedly found to redict prognosis accurately. The NYU Melanoma Cooperative Group data have found 5-year survival to be 99% for level II lesions (melanoma penetrating into the papillary dermis) compared with 75% and 30%, respectively, for level IV (melanoma penetrating into the reticular dermis) and level V (melanoma penetrating in to the subcutis) lesions. Breslow further refined the concept of microinvasion using ocular micrometry to measure the precise thickness of the neoplasm in millimeters. The thickness of a malignant melanoma, as measured vertically from the stratum granulosum to the deepest penetration of the

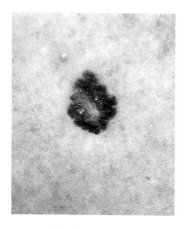

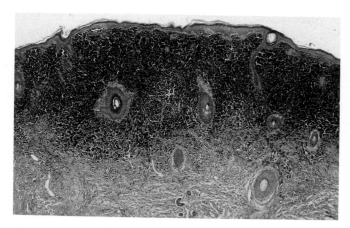

Figure 12 Malignant melanoma shows changes of partial regression.

Figure 13 Histopathologic appearance of the early features of histologic regression shows a dense bandlike infiltrate of lymphocytes and melanophages.

Table 1 5-Year Survival of Melanoma Patients
Based on Breslow's Thickness

Thickness (mm)	5-Year Survival (%)
≤0.85	97
0.86–1.69	92
1.7–3.59	76
≥3.60	48

neoplasm in the dermis or subcutis, is a more accurate predictor of biologic behavior than Clark's level of invasion.

The relationship between the thickness of the neoplasm and prognosis does not appear to be linear. Certain ranges of thickness seem to correlate well with survival. These ranges and the respective 5-year survivals are as follows: <0.85 mm, 97% 5-year survival; 0.86–1.69 mm, 92% 5-year survival; 1.7–3.59 mm, 76% 5-year survival; and 3.60 mm, 48% 5-year survival (Table 1).

The staging of patients with malignant melanoma is an important prognostic factor. Patients with only local cutaneous disease (stage 1) have an 87% 5-year survival overall. Those patients with involvement of regional lymph nodes (stage II) have a 53% 5-year survival. Stage III patients (disseminated disease) had a 0% 5-year survival in the NYU study group. It is of interest that in stage I disease (clinically negative regional lymph nodes) patients who underwent an elective lymph node dissection and were subsequently found to have histologically positive lymph nodes, the 5-year survival dropped to 42%. This group could be further classified into two subgroups. The first included those with a primary lesion thicker than 4 mm or with the product of lesion thickness times percent of positive lymph nodes greater than 20. This group had an 18% 5-year survival. In the second group, the remaining patients had a 91% 5-year survival. Further, in stage II patients, the number of positive lymph nodes related in a direct fashion to poorer prognosis in a manner similar to that seen in breast cancer. Patients with one positive lymph node had a 53% 5-year survival; those with two or three positive lymph nodes had a 39% 5-year survival; while those with four or more positive lymph nodes had a 31% 5-year survival.

Anatomic site appears to play a role in prognosis. In general, patients with malignant melanoma on the head and neck, trunk, hands and feet had a poorer 5-year survival than those with malignant melanomas on the remaining areas of the arms and the legs (78% vs. 92%).

Age also is an important prognostic variable. Patients older than 50 years of age have worse 5-year survivals (80%) than those younger (88%). Female patients have a better prognosis than males (88% 5-year survival vs. 80% 5-year survival). Ulcerated malignant melanoma has a poorer 5-year survival than a nonulcerated lesion (62% vs. 89%).

In the presence of histologic evidence of a preexisting melanocytic nevus, thickness for thickness, patients with those malignant melanomas arising in association with a preexisting nevus had better 5-year survival than those not having an associated melanocytic nevus. The number of mitoses noted on histologic examination correlates directly with 5-year survival. Those having 0–1 mitoses/high power field have a 91% 5-year survival compared to those having 2 or more mitoses/high power field, which yield a 69% 5-year survival rate. These findings have been confirmed and refined by Schmoeckel et al. using the concept of the "mitotic index."

The presence of so-called "intraspecimen metastasis" or "local satellitosis" has been found to be an important prognostic factor. Patients with malignant melanoma demonstrating "local satellitosis" have a 54% 5-year survival vs. 85% in patients lacking this histologic finding.

The "volume" of the neoplasm calculated mathematically may be an important prognostic variable. Lesions with a "tumor volume of greater than 200 cu mm have an 11% 5-year survival vs 89% in those having a tumor volume of 200 cu mm or less."

MANAGEMENT

The first step in the management of the patient with malignant melanoma is biopsy of the suspicious lesion. Clinical suspicion for malignant melanoma is guided by the clinical presentation ("ABCD" changes), along with history. In its early evolving stages, even the astute dermatologist often has difficulty making an unequivocal diagnosis. A properly obtained biopsy specimen and expert histologic interpretation are vital for the definitive diagnosis.

Biopsy Technique

The best way to biopsy a malignant melanoma is by total excision. Exceptions to this include lesions that are so large that their complete removal would result in a significant surgical procedure or those in difficult anatomic locations for which the deformity, if the lesion were benign, would be unacceptable. In such cases, an incisional biopsy is permissible. Many practitioners find that procedures such as punch biopsy, curet biopsy, and needle biopsy are not acceptable when the possibility of malignant melanoma is seriously entertained. It is important to emphasize that the histologic diagnosis of malignant melanoma requires the pathologist to assess breadth, circumscription, and depth of the lesion. Any biopsy technique that does not permit the assessment of the above features may lead to a misdiagnosis.

Excisional biopsy of most malignant melanomas is an office or outpatient procedure. The patient should be made aware of the fact that often the excisional biopsy of a malignant melanoma is only one part of the treatment. Generally, a margin of at least 2 mm around the clinically suspicious pigmented lesion is sufficient for an excisional biopsy (Fig. 14). Local anesthesia is generally administered in a field block outside of the 2-mm margin. The incision should be directed such that the long axis of the ellipse is placed in the direction of the probable pathway

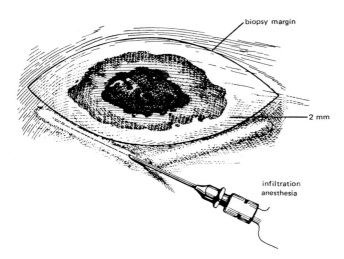

Figure 14 Biopsy in toto of a malignant melanoma. (Reproduced with permission from Roses DF, Harris MN, Ackerman AB. *Diagnosis and Management of Cutaneous Malignant Melanoma*. Philadelphia, WB Saunders, 1983.)

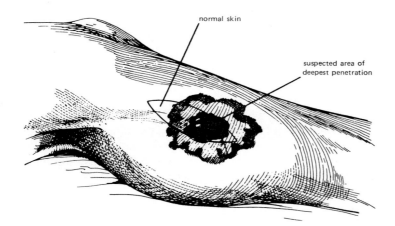

normal skin

suspected area of
deepest penetration

Figure 15 Biopsy in part for large malignant melanoma. (Reproduced with permission from Roses DF, Harris MN, Ackerman AB. *Diagnosis and Management of Cutaneous Malignant Melanoma*. Philadelphia, WB Saunders, 1983.)

of lymphatic drainage for that anatomic site. The incision should extend through the skin and into the subcutaneous adipose tissue but not to the level of the underlying fascia. The wound can be closed easily with simple, interrupted sutures. The specimen should be placed in 10% formalin solution for transport to the pathology laboratory. It is essential that an adequate clinical description of the lesion accompany the specimen, including the size of the lesion.

An incisional biopsy of a malignant melanoma (Fig. 15) should be done to include tissue that clinically contains the thickest portion of the lesion. The surgical technique is otherwise the same. The incisional specimen should include the thickest portion of the lesion and extend to include some of the surrounding normal skin. There appears to be evidence that a biopsy specimen obtained by incision into a malignant melanoma has a detrimental influence on the survival of patients.

Handling and Processing Specimens Suspected of Being Malignant Melanoma

Specimens submitted to be evaluated for malignant melanoma should be placed in neutral buffered 10% formalin solution in a bottle containing 20 times as much volume of fixative as specimen. "Grossing" of the specimen by the laboratory can be as important as the biopsy technique. The size of the excision, as well as the dimensions of the pigmented lesion, should be properly recorded as part of the gross description of the specimen. The specimen should be step-sectioned at 2-mm intervals (Fig. 16). An alternative method is to section the specimen on the long axis of the specimen. This method may permit a better assessment of the breadth of the neoplasm.

In most instances, an accurate diagnosis can be obtained using routine hematoxylin and eosin staining. At times, specialized silver stains, S-100, and HMB45 immunoperoxidase stains may be helpful.

Clinical Evaluation

A properly performed history and physical examination should include careful questioning concerning the pigmented lesion in question, sun exposure history, personal and family history of malignant melanoma or dysplastic nevi, as well as a history of other medical illnesses. The

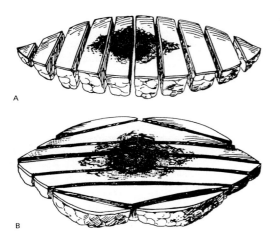

Figure 16 Laboratory preparation of a specimen of malignant melanoma. (Reproduced with permission from Roses DF, Harris MN, Ackerman AB. *Diagnosis and Management of Cutaneous Malignant Melanoma*. Philadelphia, WB Saunders, 1983.)

physical examination should be comprehensive. All patients, including those with malignant melanoma, should be completely undressed and the entire cutaneous and mucocutaneous surfaces examined. Examination of the site of the melanoma, including careful palpation for any subcutaneous satellite lesions, should be performed. A complete examination of the regional lymph nodes should be done as well as examination for organomegaly.

The definitive treatment for malignant melanoma is wide and deep excision along with, in some instances, an elective lymph node dissection. The routine evaluation of a patient with malignant melanoma at our institution includes, in addition to a thorough history and physical examination, a complete blood count, urinalysis, chest x-ray, electrocardiogram, serum chemistry screen, and, when indicated, a computed tomographic (CT) scan of the chest and abdomen. Additional tests are confined to the work-up of specific symptoms. Serum lactate dehydrogenase (LDH) has been shown to be of primary importance in the detection of liver metastases. Serum gamma glutamyl transpeptidase (GGTP) may be used to monitor progression of malignant melanoma.

The definitive surgical procedure for cutaneous malignant melanoma varies somewhat from surgeon to surgeon. In general, however, Table 2 best summarizes the definitve treatment for malignant melanoma at New York University Medical Center.

The question regarding lymph node dissection as part of the surgical management of primary cutaneous malignant melanoma remains controversial. In the absence of disseminated disease with clinically palpable nodes, most investigators consider that a therapeutic node dissection is indicated. While an in-depth discussion of the efficacy of elective lymph node dissection in the management of patients with malignant melanoma is beyond the scope of this chapter, the following summarizes the general approach at New York University: Elective lymph node dissections should not be performed in the following instances: (1) patients with primary malignant melanoma less than 1.0 mm in thickness; (2) patients with primary malignant melanoma in the midline of the head and neck and the trunk; (3) elderly patients or those with serious underlying diseases, unless the primary cutaneous malignant melanoma directly overlies its nodal group; (4) patients with evidence of disseminated disease. For the remainder of patients, the question as to the efficacy of an elective lymph node dissection is best answered by considering the anatomic location of the primary lesion and its nodal drainage. For head and neck lesions, histo-

Table 2 Surgical Treatment of Melanoma

Malignant melanoma in situ	Malignant melanoma less than 1 mm in thickness	Malignant melanoma greater than 1 mm in thickness
A wide and deep excision with subcutaneous fat and 5-mm borders around lesion, with primary closure	A wide and deep excision with subcutaneous fat and primary closure; width of excision 1 cm around lesion	A wide and deep excision with margins no less than 2 cm and a depth that includes all subcutaneous fat and underlying fascia; some lesions on anatomic sites such as the face, etc. are exceptions—in these situations, smaller margins may be taken; primary closure is desirable when possible

logically positive lymph nodes are associated with an extremely grave prognosis. Furthermore, it has been shown that nodal metastases in head and neck melanomas follow specific and predictive patterns. Thus a selective rather than a radical approach to an elective lymph node dissection in the head and neck region will allow for accurate histologic staging and the possibility for cure in patients with microscopic disease, with the least morbidity and deformity. The benefit from elective lymph node dissection from malignant melanomas of the trunk is quite modest. The presence of positive regional lymph nodes is, however, one of the most important prognostic signs for the potential development of disseminated disease. For malignant melanomas of the extremities, several studies have supported a discernible benefit of elective lymph node dissection when no nodes are palpable clinically but turn out to be positive microscopically. The value of the elective lymph node dissection is most pronounced in intermediate-thickness lesions.

Prevention of death from malignant melanoma is not only a possibility but should also be a reality and the goal of each and every physician managing diseases of the skin throughout the world. Through early detection of malignant melanoma, no human being should die from this disease. Learn to recognize malignant melanoma when it is small, flat, and curable. Teach those around you to do the same.

"But what is the black spot, Captain?" I asked.
"That's a summons, mate . . ."

Treasure Island
Robert Louis Stevenson

BIBLIOGRAPHY

Ackerman AB, Su WPD. The histology of cutaneous malignant melanoma. In *Malignant Melanoma*. AW Kopf, RS Bart, RS Rodriguez-Sains, AB Ackerman, eds. New York, Masson Publishing Company, 1979, p. 25.

Breslow A. Prognosis in stage I cutaneous melanoma: Tumor thickness as a guide to treatment. In *Pathology of Malignant Melanoma*. AB Ackerman, ed. New York, Masson Publishing Company, 1981.

Breslow A. Thickness, cross-sectional area, and depth of invasion in the prognosis of cutaneous melanoma. *Ann Surg* 1970;172:902.

Clark WH Jr. From L, Bernardino EA, Mihm MC, Jr. The histogenesis and biologic behavior of primary human malignant melanoma of the skin. *Cancer Res* 1969;29:705.

Einhorn LH, Burgess MA, Vallejos C et al. Prognostic correlations and response to treatment in advanced metastatic malignant melanoma. *Cancer Res* 1974;34:1995–2004.

Friedman RJ, Rigel DS, Kopf AW. Early detection of malignant melanoma: the role of physician examination and self-examination of the skin. *CA* 1985;35:130.

Friedman RJ, Rigel DS, Kopf AW. Tumor volume in malignant melanoma: A superior prognostic indicator to lesion thickness. Cited in DS Rigel, RJ Friedman, Prognosis of malignant melanoma. *Dermatol Clin* 1985;3:309.

Friedman RJ, Rigel DS, Kopf AW, et al. Favorable prognosis for malignant melanoma associated with acquired melanocytic nevi. *Arch Dermatol* 1983;119:455.

Kamino H, Ackerman AB. Malignant melanoma in situ: The evolution of malignant melanoma within the epidermis. In *Pathology of Malignant Melanoma*. AB Ackerman, ed. New York, Masson Publishing Company, 1981, p. 59.

Maize JC, Ackerman AB. Malignant melanoma. In *Pigmented Lesions of the Skin*. JC Maize, AB Ackerman, eds. Philadelphia, Lea & Febiger, 1987, pp. 165–223.

National Institute of Health Consensus Conference on Early Melanoma. *JAMA* 1992;268:1314–1319.

Rigel DS, Friedman RJ. Symposium on melanoma and pigmented lesions. *Dermatol Clin* 1985;3(2).

Rigel DS, Rogers GS, Friedman RJ. Prognosis of malignant melanoma. *Dermatol Clin* 1985;3:309.

Roses DF, Harris MN, Ackerman AB. *Diagnosis and Management of Cutaneous Malignant Melanoma*. Philadelphia, WB Saunders, 1983.

Salopek TG, Rigel DS, Kopf AW. The incidence of malignant melanoma in the United States-Is it under-reported? *J Am Acad Dermatol* (in press).

Schmoeckel C, Braun-Falco O. Prognostic index in malignant melanoma. *Arch Dermatol* 1978;114:871.

Silverberg E, Lubera J. Cancer statistics, 1986. *CA* 1986;36:9.

34

Cutaneous Soft Tissue Sarcomas

Marc D. Brown
University of Rochester, Rochester, New York

INTRODUCTION

Compared to other skin malignancies, cutaneous soft tissue sarcomas (STS) are relatively rare. The average annual age-adjusted incidence rate of STS is estimated at 2 per 10,000 population, and less than 1% of adults admitted to a hospital with a diagnosis of cancer have a STS. The fact that STS are uncommon leads to delays in correct diagnosis and makes difficult the determination of optimal treatment plans and overall prognosis. In 1994, it was estimated that approximately 6000 new cases of STS would be diagnosed in the United States and upwards of 50% of these patients will die from their disease. Soft tissue sarcomas account for 1% of all cancers and 2% of all cancer deaths. Although STS can develop at any anatomic site, they are most common in the extremities (especially large skeletal muscles of the leg), trunk, retroperitoneum, and mediastinum (Table 1). Only 10% of STS involve the head and neck. Most STS present as an enlarging mass in the subcutaneous tissue or muscle. The tumors tend to be large, often greater than 5 cm in size at initial presentation. Intracavitary STS, due to their inaccessibility, can be massive in size before symptoms develop. On the other hand, STS that arise in the subcutis are more easily palpable and recognized at an early stage of growth. The majority of STS encountered by dermatologic surgeons will be those arising in the dermis and subcutis. Soft tissue sarcomas are more common in males and in older patients. There is no proven racial variation.

The pathogenesis of most STS is unknown. Implicated environmental factors include previous trauma or injury, exposure to carcinogens (polycyclic hydrocarbons, dioxin, asbestos), and previous radiation exposure. In most instances, a specific environmental cause cannot be clearly established. Immunodeficiency and immunosuppression can influence the development of STS, as they do other types of cutaneous malignancies. Genetic factors may play a role in the development of STS but have been established for only a small number of these tumors.

Table 1 Anatomic Location: Soft Tissue Sarcomas

Location	Occurrence (%)
Leg	40
Arm	20
Chest and abdominal wall	20
Retroperitoneum	10
Head and neck	10

PROGNOSIS, GRADING, AND STAGING

The most important prognostic indicator for STS is the histologic grade of the tumor. The grade is determined by several factors, including the degree of cellularity, cellular pleomorphism, mitotic activity, necrosis, and tumor growth pattern (infiltrative or invasive). The significance and prognostic value of these histologic parameters differ from the various types of STS. For example, mitotic activity is important for grading leiomyosarcomas but is of little significance for malignant fibrous histiocytomas. Soft tissue sarcomas are typically graded as well, moderately, and poorly differentiated, corresponding to low-, moderate- and high-grade malignancies. There is a direct correlation between grade, risk of recurrence, metastatic rate, and overall survival.

In addition to histologic grade, other prognostic factors include tumor size, anatomic location, and evidence of lymph node involvement or distant metastases. Tumors less than 5 cm in size have a better prognosis than larger tumors. Anatomic location is important, with retroperitoneal and intracavitary tumors having a poor prognosis. Extremity sarcomas show a better survival, and distal extremity tumors generally do better than more proximal tumors. Superficial tumors above the muscle fascia have a better prognosis than more deeply situated STS.

The current American Joint Committee on Cancer Staging of STS is based on grade, size, and evidence of metastatic disease. Stages I, II, and III are localized STS that are either well differentiated (I), moderately differentiated (II), or poorly differentiated (III). Each of these stages is further classified based on tumor size: A $\leq$ 5 cm and B $\geq$ 5 cm in greatest dimension. Stage IV is defined by the presence of metastatic disease, Stage IVA denoting regional lymph node metastases (any grade or size), and Stage IVB distant metastases (any grade or size) (Table 2).

Table 2 Staging of Soft Tissue Sarcomas

Stage	Description
Stage I	Well differentiated, localized
A	$\leq$ 5 cm
B	$\geq$ 5 cm
Stage II	Moderately differentiated, localized
A	$\leq$ 5 cm
B	$\geq$ 5 cm
Stage III	Poorly differentiated, localized
A	$\geq$ 5 cm
B	$\leq$ 5 cm
Stage IVA	Regional lymph node metastases
Stage IVB	Distant metastases

TREATMENT

Surgical excision, with or without adjuvant radiation therapy, is the primary treatment for STS. Low-grade sarcomas (grade I, well differentiated) rarely metastasize, but can be locally aggressive with a significant rate of local recurrence. High-grade sarcomas (II and III) are locally aggressive and frequently metastasize. A major challenge with the surgical treatment of STS is to obtain local control and thus prevent recurrence. STS often enlarge in a centrifugal fashion, compressing normal tissue and give the appearance of "encapsulation." However, islands of tumor project outside of the pseudocapsule and give rise to satellite lesions. STS will also locally invade and infiltrate along nerves, vessels, fascia, and muscle bundles. Thus, even with a wide local excision utilizing a 2- to 3-cm margin, the local recurrence rate can still be in the range of 30–50%. With limb amputation or complete skeletal muscle compartment excision, the local recurrence drops to about 20%. A more recent trend in management has been the use of adjuvant radiation to reduce the rate of local recurrence and metastases while avoiding limb amputation. The use of adjuvant radiation has allowed a high rate of limb salvage for STS, with amputations decreasing from 50 to 5%. Most STS are removed with a maximum margin that attempts to preserve maximum function. In general, the larger the margin, the lower the recurrence. Adjuvant chemotherapy has been of little value. Only 5% of patients with STS develop regional node metastases at any point during the course of their disease; therefore, elective lymph node resection is not routinely recommended. Most STS that recur will do so within 2 years of initial treatment.

Unfortunately, about 50% of patients with high-grade sarcomas die of their disease. These tumors generally spread hematogenously, usually to the lungs. The initial evaluation of patients with high-grade STS should therefore include a CT of the chest. Determination of metastatic disease may alter the treatment plan of the primary tumor. The vast majority of patients with STS do not present with clinical evidence of metastasis; these patients harbor occult micrometastases that only later become clinically evident.

CLASSIFICATION

Classification of STS has been one of ongoing evaluation. Most recent classifications have been based on the type of tissue formed by the tumor (rather than the type of tissue from which the tumor arose). Malignant fibrous histiocytomas (MFH) and liposarcomas are the most common histologic subtypes in adults. Together, they account for 35–45% of all sarcomas. Interestingly, MFH was a rare diagnosis in the past; however, with clarification of histologic criteria, it is now the most common adult STS. Table 3 presents a partial listing of STS (based on tissue type) that

Table 3 Cutaneous Soft Tissue Sarcomas

Fibrohistiocytic:
    Atypical fibrous xanthoma/Malignant fibrous histiocytoma
    Dermatofibrosarcoma protuberans
Adipose
    Liposarcoma
Muscle
    Leiomyosarcoma (striated)
    Rhabdomyosarcoma (striated)
Blood vessel
    Angiosarcoma
    Kaposi's sarcoma

may be encountered by dermatologic surgeons. Most STS encountered by dermatologists will be those in a subcutaneous location. Fortunately, these have a better prognosis, with an overall metastatic rate closer to 10%. Nonetheless, these tumors can be highly aggressive with local tissue destruction and frequent recurrence. The focus of this chapter will be to discuss those STS encountered by dermatologists, with a special emphasis on the fibrohistiocytic tumors. Liposarcomas and rhabdomyosarcomas are typically deeply situated tumors rarely seen in the skin or superficial soft tissue, and therefore will be excluded from discussion.

FIBROHISTIOCYTIC TUMORS

Fibrohistiocytic tumors are a heterogeneous group of soft tissue neoplasms composed of cells that resemble fibroblasts and/or histiocytes. Historically fibrohistiocytic tumors were designated as such to imply their tissue origin from a pleuropotential tissue histiocyte that could assume fibroblastic properties. To date the histogenesis of fibrohistiocytic tumors remains uncertain, although more recent immunohistochemical studies provide evidence that the fibroblast is the probable cell of origin.

Fibrohistiocytic tumors can be classified according to their malignant potential. For example, the most common fibrohistiocytic neoplasm is the benign dermatofibroma, which has no invasive or malignant potential and rarely requires surgical intervention. The dermatofibroma is considered to be a cutaneous form of the benign fibrohistiocytoma. There is a deeper fibrohistiocytoma, which is seen less commonly but at times does exhibit a more locally aggressive growth pattern. The dermatofibrosarcoma protuberans (DFSP) is considered to be a fibrohistiocytic sarcoma of intermediate malignancy. It has histologic similarity to the benign fibrohistiocytoma but grows in a more infiltrative fashion and has a marked tendency for local recurrence. In rare instances, a DFSP can metastasize. The malignant fibrohistiocytoma (MFH) is the most aggressive of the fibrohistiocytic tumors, with a high local recurrence rate and a significant metastatic rate associated with a poor prognosis. The prognosis and survival of MFH tumors appears to be in part related to tumor depth and anatomic location. Deeply situated skeletal muscle and retroperitoneal MFH tumors have a grave prognosis, whereas MFH tumors confined to the subcutis have a much better prognosis. Fortunately, most dermatologic surgeons deal primarily with the more superficial of the MFH tumors. The atypical fibroxanthoma (AFX) represents the most superficial or limited form of an MFH tumor. Due to its more superficial intradermal location, the AFX pursues a relatively benign course with a low recurrence rate and an excellent prognosis. Table 4 outlines the fibrohistiocytic tumors based on malignant potential.

Dermatofibrosarcoma Protuberans

The DFSP is a relatively uncommon spindle cell neoplasm with a marked propensity for local recurrence but a low incidence of metastatic spread. It accounts for about 0.1% of all malignan-

---

Table 4   Fibrohistiocytic Tumors

Benign
  Dermatofibroma
Intermediate malignancy
  Dermatofibrosarcoma protuberans
  Atypical fibrous xanthoma
Low- to high-grade malignancy
  Malignant fibrous histiocytoma

---

cies. The DFSP was initially described in 1924 as a "progressive and recurring dermatofibroma." The term dermatofibrosarcoma protuberans was coined in 1925. The DFSP typically presents as a nodular cutaneous tumor more common during early or midadult life. The DFSP is slightly more common in males than in females and is most frequently seen on the trunk and proximal extremity. Typical anatomic areas of involvement include the thigh, groin, abdomen, back, and chest. About 15% of all DFSP tumors occur in a head and neck location. The initial DFSP lesions may be plaquelike and/or sclerotic with a surrounding red to blue discoloration. Differential diagnosis includes a keloid, dermatofibroma, or even localized scleroderma. There is a slow but relentless growth over a period of several years, eventually giving rise to a more accelerated growth phase with the development of one or more nodules. Satellite lesions can appear around the original tumor. This gives the clinical "protuberant" appearance (Fig. 1). Patients will tend to stay relatively asymptomatic. The tumor is firm to palpation, sometimes freely movable but at times fixed to the underlying muscle fascia. The Bednar tumor is a pigmented variant to the DFSP occurring primarily in blacks. Melanin-containing cells cause a black discoloration of the tumor. Electron microscopic studies suggest that the fibroblast is the cell from which a DFSP arises.

Histologically, the DFSP is characterized by a uniform storiform pattern of plump spindle fibroblasts. It may assume a classic cartwheel appearance. Mitotic activity is low, and nuclear pleomorphism is minimal. Occasional tumors may show myoxid areas characterized by the interstitial accumulation of hyaluronic acid ground substance. Myxoid foci are more commonly seen in recurrent tumors. Infrequently, a DFSP tumor may show areas that closely resemble a fibrosarcoma or MFH. However, the fibrosarcoma or MFH usually has significantly more necrosis, pleomorphism, and marked mitotic activity.

The DFSP tumor diffusely infiltrates the dermis and subcutis. It interdigitates with subcutaneous fat lobules and spreads along connective tissue septa and between adnexal structures (Fig. 2). The tumor infiltrates outward and downward, sending off tentacle or fingerlike projections from the central mass. It does spread well beyond obvious clinical margins. The tumor tends to follow the path of least resistance, including muscle fascia, nerves, vessels, and adenxial. Recurrent tumors are more likely to invade deeper structures such as skeletal muscle.

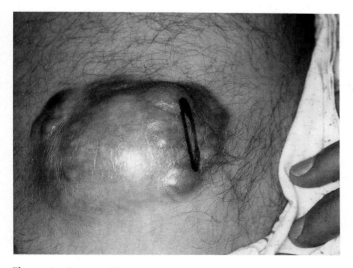

Figure 1 Dermatofibrosarcoma protuberans on upper leg of 28-year-old male. Note incisional biopsy site.

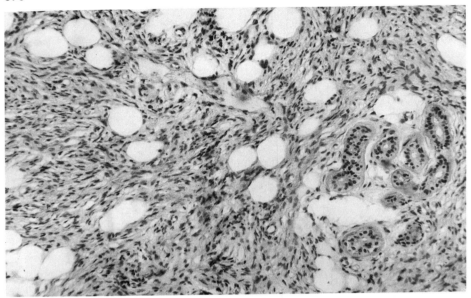

Figure 2 Dermatofibrosarcoma protuberans invading in subcutis.

Metastases are rare, occurring in 1–4% of patients. In a review of 913 cases of DFSP, 11 cases (1%) had regional node metastases and 37 cases (4%) developed distant metastic disease. The lung is the most common site of distant metastases, but they can also be seen in the brain, bone, and heart. Most cases of metastatic DFSP represent recurrent tumors (often multiple recurrences) with an interval of several years between initial diagnosis and the development of metastases. Fibrosarcomatous foci are seen in recurrent DFSP and may be partly responsible for the eventual development of metastatic spread. Unfortunately, the development of distant metastases is a poor prognostic sign, with most patients dying within 2 years.

Although the DFSP closely resembles the benign fibrous histiocytoma, it shows a marked tendency for locally aggressive growth, with local recurrence occurring in up to 50% of patients. The high recurrence is due to its extensive subcutaneous infiltration and initial inadequate surgical excisional margins. Most recurrences will be seen in the first 2–3 years, with 50% occurring within the first year. However, recurrences have been described as long as 20 years after surgical removal. Therefore, long-term follow-up is necessary. The recurrence rate correlates well with the surgical margin. The wider the excision, the lower the recurrence: a 2-cm margin will give a recurrence of 40–50%, whereas a 3-cm margin will give a local recurrence of 10–20%. Recurrences remain highest for DFSP tumors of the head and neck (50–75%), reflecting the difficulty in achieving an adequate wide local excision.

The primary treatment of DFSP is complete surgical excision. Current recommendations are for a wide excision with a 3-cm margin down to and including the muscle fascia. Due to the very low incidence of regional node involvement, elective lymph node dissection is not recommended. Radiation appears to be of minimal benefit, and chemotherapy has no proven value.

Due to functional and cosmetic concerns, a 3-cm excisional margin is not always feasible. Even then, a recurrence rate of 20% is not acceptable. Recent evidence strongly suggests that Mohs micrographic surgery achieves a high cure rate due to the ability of the procedure to carefully and meticulously track out the subclinical extensions of the DFSP tumor. The precise margin control of Mohs surgery (with simultaneous examination of the entire deep and peripheral margins) allows for complete tumor extirpation while preserving maximum normal tissue. Arbitrary margin guidelines thus become unnecessary. Initial reports utilizing Mohs surgery for DFSP occurred in the mid to late 1980s, with studies reporting only a few patients. The largest series of patients (10) was reported from the Cleveland Clinic. Seventeen cases were examined at the University of Michigan (Neil Swanson, personal communication). In all of these reports, local recurrences and/or metastases were not seen, despite the fact that these tumors were often large and recurrent, having failed non-Mohs surgical treatment. In recurrent lesions, the collagen of the DFSP can blend into the previous scar tissue, making histologic diagnosis difficult. Myxomatous areas can also be encountered. Therefore, complete removal of the scar is recommended to help ensure clear margins. Certainly, recurrences of DFSP treated with Mohs surgery will occur, as they do with other cutaneous carcinomas. However, the reports to date as well as the ongoing experience gained by Mohs surgeons in treating these tumors indicates that the Mohs procedure may become the treatment of choice for DFSP.

Atypical Fibroxanthoma

The AFX is probably best thought of as a superficial MFH or "MFH in situ." This tumor is histologically indistinguishable from pleomorphic forms of MFH, but it does not invade deeper subcutaneous tissue, fascia, or muscle. Initially, the AFX was interpreted as a benign reactive lesion but most dermatopathologists now view the AFX as a superficial or early form of the MFH. Previously, the AFX had been referred to as pseudosarcoma of the skin, pseudosarcomatous dermatofibroma, and paradoxical fibrosarcoma. The term AFX has been retained not only for historic reasons, but also to distinguish it from the deeper, more invasive MFH, which necessitates a more radical surgical approach. Due to the superficial location and typically small size of the AFX, it pursues a relatively benign course. However, in rare instances this tumor can metastasize to regional lymph nodes and an apparent AFX can progress to a MFH. Thus, the AFX is best thought of as a fibrohistiocytic neoplasm of low-grade malignancy.

Clinically the AFX is typically seen on the actinically damaged skin of the elderly patient. It appears as an asymptomatic solitary nodule or nodular ulcer, most commonly on the nose, cheek, or ear (Fig. 3). Typically an AFX tumor is less than 2 cm in size; its clinical appearance is not distinctive and must be differentiated from a squamous cell carcinoma, basal cell carcinoma, or a necrotic pyogenic granuloma. As the tumor enlarges, it may erode, ulcerate, and bleed. Less commonly, the AFX tumor will present on the extremities and trunk of younger persons. These lesions are often larger, less well demarcated, and more nodular in appearance with extension into the subcutaneous tissue.

The etiology of the AFX is uncertain, but ultraviolet exposure has to be a prime consideration given the common occurrence of this tumor on the actinically damaged face of elderly persons. Other actinic-related neoplasms are often associated with an AFX. In some cases previous x-ray therapy has been proposed as an etiologic factor, although this is not consistently documented. The AFX is thought to be a mesenchymal-derived neoplasm (like the MFH) rather than a spindled carcinoma. Electron microscopic studies have demonstrated fibroblastic and histiocyticlike cells and no features specifically suggesting epithelial differentiation.

Microscopic findings under low-power magnification show an expansile dermal nodule that often abuts the epidermis. Dilated vessels are commonly seen adjacent to the tumor. Occasionally, dilatation of the subepidermal vessels may lead to the separation of the epidermis from the underlying tumor. The AFX tumor can extend into the superficial subcutis, but by definition does not invade more deeply. Histologically the AFX resembles a pleomorphic MFH. There is a dense cellular infiltrate with pleomorphic hyperchromatic nuclei in an elongated irregular arrangement. A characteristic feature is that of large bizarre multinucleated cells arranged in a vague fascicular pattern. There can be marked nuclear atypicality with many mitoses. Cells will vary from

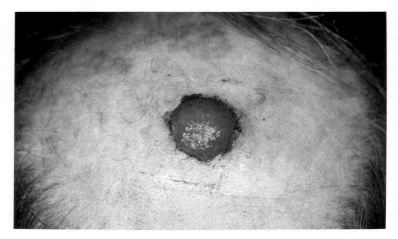

Figure 3 Atypical fibroxanthoma on sun-exposed forehead in 70-year-old male.

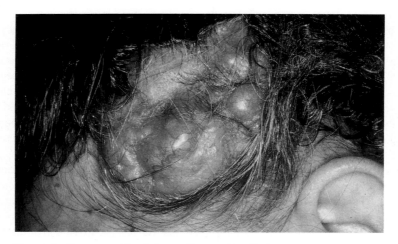

Figure 4 Large, multinodular malignant fibrohistiocytoma.

plump spindled cells to large rounded cells. A scattered inflammatory infiltrate can sometimes be seen. The histologic differential diagnosis of an AFX includes that of a spindle cell squamous cell carcinoma, melanoma, or metastatic cancer. Mucin and melanin stains are helpful, as are immunostains for cytokeratin and S-100 protein. The MFH differs from the AFX only by its deeper location in the subcutis or muscle and its often larger size. Necrosis is also a prominent feature in MFH but is rarely seen in AFX. Because AFX is considered to be an early form of MFH the distinction of the two is somewhat arbitrary; nonetheless, it is important to distinguish them because of their differing natural histories and recommended surgical treatment. Deeper involvement, necrosis, and vascular or perineural invasion strongly suggests a diagnosis of MFH instead of AFX. An adequate biopsy is very important to distinguish AFX from MFH; if only a portion of the entire tumor is submitted for pathologic interpretation, it may be difficult to assess the true depth and nature of invasion.

The AFX has a very good prognosis. Due to its "in situ" dermal location, the risk of recurrence and/or metastatic disease is quite low. In one review, only 9 out of 140 patients developed a recurrence, and no metastatic lesions were found. In rare instances the AFX tumor can metastasize to regional lymph nodes and an apparent AFX can progress to a MFH.

Recommended surgical treatment of an AFX should include complete excision and margin control. Due to the possible extension into superficial subcutaneous tissue, curettage and electrodesiccation or other superficial distinctive modalities are not recommended. It would seem unnecessary to utilize excisional margins of greater than 1 cm in order to achieve tumor-free peripheral margin control. Dissection should be carried well into the subcutaneous tissue in order to ensure a free deep margin. Mohs micrographic surgery can be utilized to treat AFX allowing for horizontal frozen section control. Swanson treated five patients with AFX. All tumors were less than 2 cm in size, none were recurrent, and all excised easily with only one stage of Mohs surgery. Although a conservative excision may be sufficient treatment for AFX, Mohs surgery does offer the advantage of tissue conservation in important facial areas as well as assurance of tumor-free margins at the time of surgery. If an AFX does recur in a deeper subcutaneous location, then it should be considered a MFH and treated accordingly.

Malignant Fibrohistiocytoma

The malignant fibrohistiocytoma (MFH) is the most common soft tissue sarcoma of late adult life. Tumors previously described as pleomorphic variants of liposarcoma, fibrosarcoma, or rhabdosarcoma were probably mislabeled examples of MFH. Malignant fibrohistiocytoma tumors can be classified as either superficial or deep. Superficial MFH tumors tend to be confined to the subcutaneous tissue but may be attached to the fascia. Most MFH tumors presenting to the dermatologic surgeon will be of this superficial type and overall will have a more favorable prognosis. However, the majority of MFH tumors are deeper lesions with approximately twice as many deeply situated tumors as superficial tumors. The deep MFH tumors can extend from subcutaneous tissue through fascia and into muscle. At times the tumor can be situated entirely within the muscle; this is especially true when MFH involves limb skeletal muscles.

Although there are several histologic subtypes of MFH, the clinical features are relatively similar. This neoplasm typically appears between the ages of 50 and 70. The MFH tumor is extremely rare in patients under the age of 20. The tumor is slightly more common in males, and Caucasians are affected more frequently than blacks or Orientals. Clinically, the MFH presents as a painless enlarging mass of several months' duration. At times, growth of the tumor may be rapid. Accelerated growth has been observed during pregnancy. The tumor is usually solitary, can be multinodular, and may often be as large as 5–10 cm in size at the time of diagnosis (Fig. 4). The more superficial of the MFH tumors are usually smaller at the time of diagnosis. The extremities are the most common site of involvement, especially the thigh, buttocks, and limb skeletal muscles. The lower extremity is affected more commonly than the upper extremity. Any area of the body may be involved, and approximately 10% of MFH tumors are on the head and neck region. Those MFH tumors located in the retroperitoneum are the largest because early diagnosis is difficult. If a malignant fibrohistiocytoma presents with evidence of metastatic disease, a primary source is usually readily diagnosable. This is in contrast to some other spindle squamous cell tumors, such as melanoma and spindle cell carcinomas where there may be an unknown primary.

Most patients with MFH are asymptomatic. On occasion there may be an associated fever and leukocytosis, which seems to resolve after the tumor is removed. Patients with retroperitoneal tumors may develop fatigue, weight loss, anorexia, and abdominal pain. The etiology of the MFH is unclear. There are sporadic reports suggesting that previous radiation exposure may be a predisposing factor, but this would explain only a minority of cases. Unlike AFX, sun exposure does not appear to be an important factor.

The MFH manifests a broad range of histologic appearances and is divided into five subtypes, which are not mutually exclusive (Table 5). The most common subtype is the *storiform-pleomorphic* type (Fig. 5). This highly cellular tumor is composed of plump pleomorphic spindle cells, histiocytes, and frequent multinucleated giant cells. The morphologic pattern is highly variable with frequent transitions from storiform to pleomorphic areas. Mitotic figures are common and often atypical. Although the storiform-pleomorphic MFH may resemble a DFSP, there are distinctive histologic differences. The numerous atypical mitotic figures, less prominent storiform pattern, marked pleomorphism, and typical foamy giant cells seen with MFH are all key differential elements (Table 6). The storiform-pleomorphic pattern would be the most common subtype presenting to the dermatologic surgeon. This shows the closest resemblance to its superficial counterpart, the atypical fibroxanthoma.

The *myxoid variant* of MFH is the next most frequent subtype, comprising approximately 25%. Histologically there is a prominent myxoid change of the stroma. Large areas appear hypocellular with widely spaced bizarre spindle-shaped cells in a myxoid matrix rich in acid mucopolysaccharides. For unclear reasons, the myxoid variant can be a slower-growing tumor and has a slightly better prognosis. The last three histologic subtypes are much less common. In the *inflammatory type*, there is a diffuse neutrophilic infiltrate with numerous foam and xanthoma cells. The retroperitoneal MFH tumor is usually of the inflammatory type. The *giant cell* subtype shows osteoclasticlike giant cells. The *angiomatoid* variant is the least common subtype. This tumor occurs in a younger population and combines features of both a fibrohistiocytic and a vascular neoplasm. Patients are 20 years of age or younger, and the tumor usually has a more superficial location in the subcutis. Gross examination of the angiomatoid MFH shows characteristic cystic areas of hemorrhage. Of all of the histologic subtypes, the angiomatoid has the best prognosis. The histologic differential diagnosis of MFH includes pleomorphic variants of liposarcoma and rhabdomyosarcoma, pleomorphic carcinoma, histiocytic lymphoma, leiomyosarcoma, and epithelioid sarcoma.

Although the MFH has a clinical appearance of being a circumscribed tumor, it often spreads for considerable distances along fascial planes or between muscle fibers. Previously the MFH

Table 5   MFH: Histologic Subtypes

Storiform-pleomorphic
Myxoid
Giant cell
Inflammatory
Angiomatoid

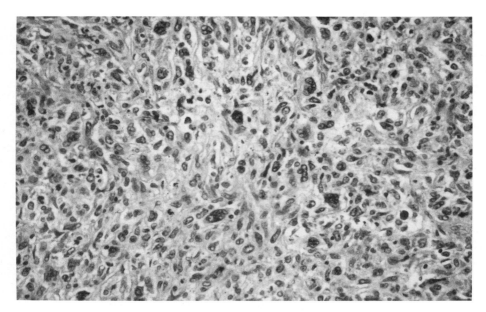

Figure 5 Malignant fibrohistiocytoma, storiform pleomorphic pattern.

was considered a low-grade form of sarcoma. Invasive behavior of the MFH accounts for its high rate of local recurrence, estimated to be 40–50% even after wide local excision. Unfortunately, the metastatic rate is also in the range of 40–45% with a high associated mortality. The 2-year survival is only about 60%. Metastic disease occurs early (usually within 2 years of diagnosis) and most frequently affects the lung, liver, lymph nodes, and bone.

Prognosis appears to correlate best with the depth of the MFH tumor (not unlike other aggressive cutaneous tumors such as melanoma, squamous cell carcinoma, and Merkel cell cancers). For example, less than 10% of MFH tumors confined entirely to the subcutis without deeper fascial or muscle involvement will metastasize. When tumor does involve the fascia, the rate of metastatic disease increases to almost 30%. Tumors involving the skeletal muscle will metastasize 40–45% of the time. The size of the tumor also correlates with the risk of metastatic disease, but this may be a covariable with tumor depth. Anatomic location of the tumor also correlates with prognosis. Distally located MFH tumors have a better prognosis than proximally located tumors. Histologic features, including degree of anaplasia and the number of mitoses, appear to have little prognostic value. However, the histologic subtypes of the myxoid and angiomatoid variant appear to do slightly better. There is some evidence that tumors with a significant inflammatory response may have an improved prognosis, but the metastatic rate for the

Table 6 MFH: Key Histologic Features

Focal storiform pattern
Marked pleomorphism
Prominent atypical mitotic figures
Necrosis
Myxoid foci
Prominent foam cells and giant cells

Table 7 Prognostic Variables for MFH

Good	Poor
Superficial	Deep
intradermal	skeletal muscle
subcutis	retroperitoneal
Small tumor size	Large tumor size
Distal extremity	Proximal extremity
Myxoid or angiomatoid variant	

inflammatory subtype is still in the range of 30–35%. Table 7 outlines the prognostic variables for MFH.

Surgical excision is the mainstay of therapy for MFH. Because this tumor can spread a considerable distance beyond the gross tumor margins, aggressive wide and deep local excision or even possible amputation has been recommended. Recurrence rates are directly related to the adequacy of the surgical treatment and establishment of tumor-free margins. One of the major problems in dealing with this soft tissue sarcoma is adequate local control of the primary tumor. MFH tumors with local recurrence do have a much worse prognosis, so complete excision of the primary tumor is important. Islands of tumor cells may extend well beyond what appears to be a well-encapsulated neoplasm. As with other aggressive cutaneous tumors, the MFH has a tendency to invade along fascial planes, muscle fibers, nerves, and blood vessels. Wide excisional margins of 3–5 cm may still result in recurrence rates of 30–40%, dependent somewhat on the previously described prognostic factors. Positive surgical resection margins will result in a local recurrence rate between 50 and 90%. Recurrence will usually recur within the first 2 years after surgery of the primary tumor. More radical surgical procedures such as complete muscle compartment excision or limb amputation will give higher cure rates but with greater patient morbidity. Less radical surgery in conjunction with radiation and/or chemotherapy is becoming more popular for soft tissue sarcomas. Even with adequate local control, metastatic disease will still occur. Only a minority of patients (less than 10%) will initially present with evidence of metastases. Because lymph node metastases are relatively infrequent, elective lymph node dissection of regional nodes is usually not recommended. Lymph node dissection should be reserved for those patients with clinically suspicious nodes and/or a positive nodal biopsy.

For the more superficially located MFH tumors, Mohs micrographic surgery appears to be an excellent surgical modality. Although a more time-consuming and meticulous procedure, Mohs surgery is capable of tracing out the deepest and widest extensions of the MFH tumor as it spreads along anatomic planes. The MFH tumor is easily visualized with frozen section technology. Brown et al. retrospectively looked at 17 patients with a total of 20 MFH tumors who underwent Mohs micrographic surgery. Half of these patients already had local recurrence of their MFH from a previous non-Mohs procedure. All patients were treated in an outpatient setting. Standard horizontal frozen sections were prepared in the usual manner after appropriate mapping and staining of the excised tissue. The location of these tumors were widespread with the average preoperative tumor size of 3 cm. The patients required an average of 2.5 stages and 16 tissue sections to achieve tumor-free margins. The average postoperative defect size was 4.8 cm. The average follow-up was approximately 4 years. There was local recurrence of only one tumor, and that patient subsequently underwent a second Mohs surgical procedure and remained tumor-free. One patient developed probable metastatic disease to the lungs, but an autopsy was not performed at the time of death. Thus, the overall success rate with Mohs surgery was excellent. These MFH tumors were primarily of the storiform-pleomorphic type with origin of the

Table 8 MFH: Evaluation

Size and anatomic location
Fixation to deep structures
Lymph nodes
Chest x-ray
MRI to assess depth and extent of local spread
CT of chest for high-risk patients
Consultation with radiation and medical oncology

tumor in the dermis and subcutis. However, a number of these tumors did extend into the muscle. The more superficial location and relatively smaller size may have contributed to the higher success rate. Nonetheless, for select MFH tumors, Mohs surgery offered a precise surgical approach with careful tracking of the tumor and clear definition of tumor-free margins. There was also the value of tissue sparing, which becomes extremely important for the approximately 10% of MFH tumors located in the head and neck region.

The preoperative evaluation of patients with MFH is outlined in Table 8. It is important to note the size of the tumor, its anatomic location, and possible fixation of the tumor to deeper structures such as muscle. Careful palpation of regional lymph nodes should be performed. Clinically suspicious nodes should be biopsied. Because the lungs are the most common site of metastatic disease, a chest x-ray should be performed for all MFH tumors. For the higher-risk deep and large MFH tumors, a CT of the chest should be undertaken. Evidence of metastatic disease may well alter the overall treatment plan. At times, resection of a solitary pulmonary metastasis can be performed, but only after a complete evaluation and staging of the metastatic disease. CT or MRI scans can also be helpful to assess the depth and extent of local spread of these MFH tumors.

Due to the high recurrence and metastatic rate of these soft tissue sarcomas, early consideration should be given to the use of adjuvant radiation and/or chemotherapy. Occult micrometastases may respond to adjuvant therapy, although this has not been well studied specifically for MFH tumors. Soft tissue sarcomas do appear to respond to radiation therapy. Radiation therapy is usually given postoperatively, but also has been used preoperatively. The value of adjuvant chemotherapy remains controversial. A prospective randomized study at the National Cancer Institute has shown improvement in disease-free and survival rates in patients with high-grade extremity sarcomas who underwent adjuvant chemotherapy. Other studies have not shown a distinct advantage. The drug that appears to be most efficacious is doxorubicin. Radiation and/or medical oncology should be consulted for the early aggressive management of these patients. Table 9 outlines the treatment options for fibrohistiocytic tumors.

Table 9 Treatment of Fibrohistiocytomas

Tumor	Excisional margins (cm)	Mohs surgery	Adjuvant radiation/chemo Rx
AFX	1	Tissue sparing for important cosmetic areas	No
MFH	3–5	Yes (except for deep skeletal and retroperitoneal tumors)	Yes, for high-risk tumors
DFSP	3	Yes	No

ANGIOSARCOMA

The angiosarcoma is a malignant tumor of endothelial cell origin. It is one of the rarest of soft tissue sarcomas, representing less than 10% of all sarcomas. Due to its marked predilection for skin and superficial soft tissue, it will be encountered by dermatologists. The angiosarcoma has a wide morphologic spectrum, ranging from low-grade tumors that resemble hemangiomas to highly anaplastic, poorly differentiated tumors. Unlike other STS that favor deeper locations, the angiosarcoma occurs frequently in the skin and superficial soft tissue. A review of 366 cases at the AFIP indicates one third of angiosarcomas to be located in the skin and one quarter in the subcutaneous soft tissue. Enzinger and Weiss divide angiosarcomas into four groups: (1) cutaneous angiosarcoma unassociated with lymphedema, (2) cutaneous angiosarcoma associated with lymphedema (Stewart-Treves lymphangiosarcoma), (3) angiosarcoma of the breast, and (4) angiosarcoma of deep soft tissue. This discussion will focus on the first group which is the most common form and the one most likely to be encountered by the dermatologic surgeon.

Chronic lymphedema is a clear etiologic factor in the development of angiosarcomas, yet it only accounts for 10% of the tumors. Radiation-induced angiosarcomas do occur, although they are rare. Despite an endothelial cell line of origin, malignant change in a preexisting benign vascular tumor is a rare occurrence. There is little information about the role of environmental carcinogens.

Angiosarcoma most commonly affects elderly persons but can occur in any age group. There is a 2:1 male predilection. The most common site of involvement is the scalp and forehead, with over 50% of angiosarcomas being on the head and neck. Less common anatomic sites include the extremities (20%) and trunk (13%). The angiosarcoma has an insidious onset, growing slowly and asymptomatically. Clinically, the tumor will initially present as an ill-defined, blue to purple, bruiselike indurated plaque. As it grows, the tumor will become elevated and nodular with soft compressible areas (Fig. 6). In more advanced lesions, there can be bleeding, ulceration, and tenderness. In up to 50% of cases, the tumor will be multifocal, with indistinct clinical margins. The tumor is typically large (6–12 cm). At the time of surgery, the angiosarcoma will spread horizontally in the dermis for considerable distances, well beyond apparent clinical margins. In more aggressive, poorly differentiated tumors, invasion into subcutis and fascia is seen.

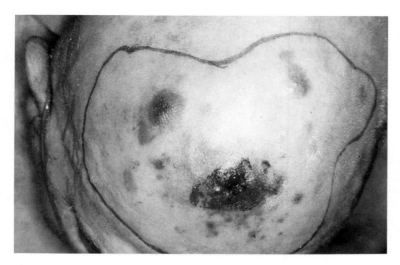

Figure 6   Ill-defined angiosarcoma on scalp of elderly male.

Histologically, the angiosarcoma develops irregular anastomosing sinusoids and dilated vascular spaces with endothelial-lined papillae infiltrating the dermis. These vascular channels appear to create their own tissue planes, dissecting through the dermal collagen. Although the cells may resemble normal endothelium, they typically show larger and more chromatic nuclei and create papillations along the lumina. Mitotic activity is variable. In high-grade tumors, there may be focal areas resembling fibrosarcoma.

Surgery is the primary method of treatment, although it is difficult due to extensive subclinical extensions and the multifocality of the tumor. Frozen section analysis is difficult due to vascular tissue distortion from frozen section processing, thus leading to a high rate of false negativity. Although Mohs surgery is able to track out subclinical extensions of cutaneous tumors, it is not well suited for angiosarcoma because of tumor multifocality (noncontiguous tumor foci) and problems with frozen section interpretation. One novel approach to the problem of margin control is the use of preoperative tumor mapping with multiple punch biopsies. Punch biopsies are performed circumferentially at increasing distances around the suspected edge of the tumor. The biopsies are read by standard permanent section technique. Connecting the negative biopsies closest to the neoplasm, a resection perimeter is established. The final resection margin is slightly more to account for any undetected tumor extending between the punch biopsy sites. Prophylactic lymph node dissection is not typically recommended, due in part to the overall poor prognosis and the usual hematogenous spread of the tumor. Of 72 patients with angiosarcoma, only 12% survived 5 years or longer, with 50% dying within 15 months. In a smaller study of 17 patients, 16 died from their disease. Common metastatic sites include cervical lymph nodes, lung, liver, and spleen. The size of the tumor appears to affect prognosis: tumors less than 5 cm at initial presentation do better than larger lesions. The role of adjuvant radiotherapy has not been clearly defined. Radiation alone (without surgery) does not appear adequate to achieve local control.

KAPOSI'S SARCOMA

Kaposi's sarcoma (KS) was first described in 1872 by Moricz Kaposi, who noted five cases of an unusual multifocal tumor, which he termed "idiopathic multiple pigmented sarcoma of the skin." There remains ongoing controversy about whether KS is a true neoplasm versus a diffuse, atypical hyperplasia of vascular tissue, likely in response to a viral infection. KS has a variable course, occurs in differing clinical settings, and is apparently influenced by genetic, geographic, and immunologic factors. There are four differing clinical settings: classic, endemic, AIDS-related, and immunosuppression-associated (e.g., organ transplantation). The exact etiology of KS is unknown, though most current investigation is aimed at identifying a viral association. Evidence that suggests that KS may be viral induced includes identification of viral DNA and viral antigens in KS tumor cells, association with AIDS and other immunosuppressive states, geographic distribution in equatorial Africa, a variable disease course with occasional regression, and the multifocality of the KS tumor. Although a causative agent has yet to be identified, CMV and retrovirus have been implicated. Based on immunohistochemical studies, the cell of origin of KS is probably the endothelial cell, or lymphatic and/or blood vessel derivation.

Histologically, KS has no difference in appearance related to its various clinical settings. However, the microscopic appearance does differ dependent upon the stage of the disease. In its earliest macule or patch stage, KS appears as a flat lesion with a proliferation of bland-appearing vessels surrounding larger ectatic vessels. There are irregular thin-walled vascular channels and dilated lumina lined by flattened endothelial cells. As the neoplasm evolves into the papule or plaque stage, there is proliferation of vascular channels and spindle-shaped cells involving the dermis and extending into the subcutis. Intertwining fascicles of spindle cells line well-defined vascular slits (Fig. 7). The spindle cell foci coalesce and give rise to nodular tumors, with a more clear-cut sarcomatous pattern. Solid cords and bundles of spindle cells intersect between jagged-shaped vascular channels. In the more aggressive KS tumors, there may be transitional areas that resemble a well-differentiated angiosarcoma. However, there is usually minimal pleomorphism and nuclear atypia. Mitotic figures are occasionally seen but not prominent. A mixed inflammatory infiltrate is present at the periphery.

In *classic KS,* the vascular neoplasm affects certain ethnic groups, such as Mediterranean Italians and central European Jews. This form of KS is relatively rare in the United States, accounting for only 0.02% of malignancies. It suggests genetic factors, yet familial occurrence is rare. The sarcoma begins as a bluish-red macule, typically on the lower leg or foot. It progresses slowly to form plaques and nodules. Although often beginning as a solitary lesion, it evolves into a bilateral, multifocal pattern (Fig. 8). As lesions age, they become a brownish color with a hyperkeratotic surface, which can eventually erode and ulcerate. Whereas early lesions are soft and compressible, later lesions are firm and hard to touch. The mean age is 60–70 years, with more than two thirds of patients over 50 years old. Earlier data suggested a male-to-female predominance of 10–15:1, but more recent studies show a 2–3:1 ratio. There is slow disease progression, with the average duration being 8–10 years. Overall mortality is 10–20%, but up to 25% die of a second malignancy, especially neoplasms of lymphoreticular origin. However, a more fulminant course can occur. Gastrointestinal lesions are common at autopsy, but usually are asymptomatic. KS can involve lymph nodes, spleen, heart, and lungs.

The *endemic form* of KS occurs in central Africa. It can occur in young children and steadily increases throughout adult years. Children may have minimal skin disease but often have extensive lymphatic tumor involvement and a fulminant course, with a greater tendency toward visceral involvement.

AIDS-related KS was first reported in 1981 and has become a well-established part of the AIDs epidemic. It is estimated that 30–40% of patients with AIDS develop KS lesions, but they are

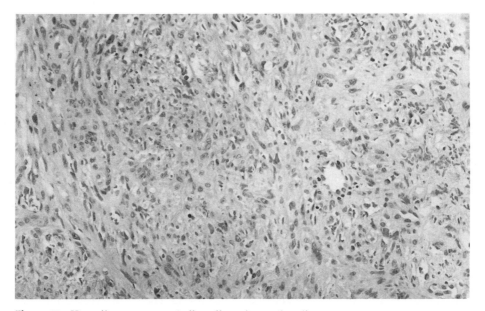

Figure 7   Kaposi's sarcoma: spindle cells and vascular slits.

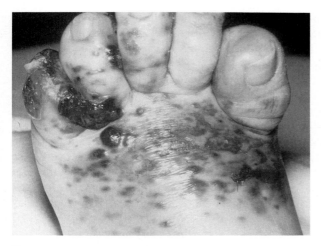

Figure 8 Classic Kaposi's sarcoma on lower leg of elderly Italian female.

most commonly seen in homosexual men. Recent trends have shown a decreasing incidence of KS in AIDS patients. Reasons for this decline are uncertain. KS lesions in AIDS patients are typically small in size, not confined to the lower extremities, multifocal, and common in the mouth and mucous membranes. Early lesions are flat, pink to red patches and progressively develop a blue-violet papular or nodular appearance.

Finally, KS can be associated with lymphoproliferative malignancies and organ transplantation. Treatment with cyclosporine appears to give a higher risk of involvement.

Treatment of KS is usually *not* surgical due to its multifocality and high rate of recurrence. KS is a very radiosensitive tumor; radiation is the treatment of choice for both solitary and disseminated cutaneous tumors. Different modes of delivery and dosages are used depending upon the severity of disease. For more rapidly progressive and visceral disease, chemotherapy is the mainstay of treatment; vinblastine and vincristine are commonly used. For smaller cutaneous lesions, cryotherapy is effective.

LEIOMYOSARCOMA

Leiomyosarcoma (LMS) is a malignant smooth muscle tumor. It comprises 7% of all soft tissue sarcomas. Superficial leiomyosarcomas, confined to the skin and subcutaneous tissue, account for 2–3% of all superficial STS. Classification and prognosis of LMS depends upon site of origin and anatomic location. Retroperitoneal and intraabdominal LMS are the most common group (50%) and have the worst prognosis. Rarely, LMS arise in large veins (e.g., vena cave) and have a similar poor prognosis. LMS of the cutaneous and subcutaneous tissue have a good prognosis, analogous to other STS restricted to the superficial soft tissue. Fortunately, this is the type encountered by dermatologists, and it is discussed in detail below.

Superficial LMS are most common in the 40- to 60-year-old age group, with males more commonly affected than females. The extremities are by far the most common site (85%), especially hair-bearing extensor surfaces. However, any anatomic area can be involved. The LMS is typically a solitary tumor, unlike the benign leiomyosarcoma, which commonly is multiple. If multiple lesions are seen, the possibility of cutaneous metastatic disease from a deeper retroperitoneal or intraabdominal location must be considered.

The etiology of the LMS is uncertain. Like other STS, trauma and previous radiation have been implicated. Development of a LMS from a preexisting benign leiomyosarcoma has been described but is a rare event. In the skin, LMS originates from the arrector pilorum muscle; those that develop in the subcutis are probably vascular in origin.

Superficial LMS can be divided into two groups: cutaneous (arising in the dermis) and subcutaneous (arising in the subcutis). It is important to distinguish between the two because of differing prognosis and treatment. Cutaneous leiomyosarcomas rarely develop metastatic disease, whereas those arising in the subcutis will metastasize in 30–40% of patients.

Clinically, the cutaneous LMS is relatively small at the time of diagnosis, usually less than 2 cm in size. Subcutaneous LMS will grow faster and achieve larger sizes (up to 6 cm). The correct diagnosis is rarely made preoperatively, and the duration from tumor appearance to eventual diagnosis and treatment is 2 years. The tumor is round to oval in shape. The overlying skin can show color change, umbilication, and rarely ulceration. Pain or tenderness may occur.

Histologically, LMS show poorly delineated, atypical, spindle-shaped myomatous cells with interlacing fascicles that weave and blend into a collagenous stroma. Most superficial LMS are well to moderately differentiated, and atpyical mitoses are common. The cells are spindle-shaped or ribbonlike with elongated nuclei and blunted ends. The tumor may be confined to the dermis, but extension into the subcutis is common. LMS arising in the subcutaneous soft tissue have a more circumscribed appearance with the creation of a pseudocapsule from a compressed rim of connective tissue. The subcutaneous LMS also shows a prominent vascular pattern, lacking in the cutaneous LMS.

Prognosis of superficial LMS is dependent upon location. In the largest series from the AFIP, 40% of cutaneous LMS recurred, but none metastasized. For subcutaneous LMS, 50% recurred, and one third developed metastases and/or died from their disease. The overall recurrence rate was 42%, apparently unrelated to tumor size or number of mitoses. Dahl and Angwell noted a similar recurrence rate of 40%, with 27% developing metastases; 10% of cutaneous tumors and 40% of subcutaneous tumors developed metastatic disease. Stout and Hill had the highest rate of recurrence (60%) and metastasis (50%), explained by the fact that most of their cases were subcutaneous and some penetrated deeper soft tissue. The primary site of metastasis is the lung.

The treatment of choice for LMS is complete surgical excision. Specific excision margins are not well documented, other than general statements such as "excised widely enough to require skin grafting for closure of the defect" or "a generous amount of uninvolved tissue surrounding the mass." At times, amputation has been recommended, usually for the larger, subcutaneous tumors. Radiotherapy has been tried but is of minimal value as a primary therapy. The role of radiation as adjunctive therapy is not well studied for LMS. Sporadic case reports of Mohs surgery for LMS have been documented, but at this time the numbers are too small to make definitive recommendations. The greatest utility for Mohs surgery may be for recurrent tumors or large tumors where tissue sparing is necessary for functional and/or cosmetic concerns. LMS of subcutaneous origin require aggressive surgical management due to the higher risk of metastasis.

BIBLIOGRAPHY

Antman K, Amato D, Lerner H, et al. Adjuvant doxorubicin for sarcoma. *Cancer Treat Symp* 1985;3: 109–115.

Bardwill JM, Moceza EE, Butler JJ, et al. Angiosarcomas of the head and neck regions. *Am J Surg* 1968; 116:548.

Barnes L, Coleman JA, Johnson JT. Dermatofibrosarcoma protuberans of the head and neck. *Arch Otolaryngol* 1984;110.

Barr RJ, Wuerker RB, Graham JH. Ultrastructure of atypical fibroxanthoma. *Cancer* 1977;30:736.

Bartlebort SW, Stahl R, Ariyan S. Cutaneous angiosarcoma of the face and scalp. *Plastic Reconstr Surg* 1989;84:55–59.

Bertoni F, Capanna R, Biagini R, et al. Malignant fibrous histiocytoma of soft tissue: An analysis of 78 cases located and deeply seated in the extremities. *Cancer* 1985;56:356.

Bramwell VHC, Rousse J, Santoro A, et al. European experience of adjuvant chemotherapy for soft tissue sarcoma. *Cancer Treat Symp* 1985;3:99–107.

Brown MD, Swanson NA. Treatment of malignant fibrous histiocytoma and atypical fibrous xanthomas with micrographic surgery. *J Dermatol Surg Oncol* 1989;15:1287–1292.

Chang AE, Rosenberg SA. Clinical evaluation and treatment of soft tissue tumors. In *Soft Tissue Tumors*. FM Enzinger, SW Weiss ed. St. Louis, CV Mosby Co., 1988, pp. 19–42.

Chen KTK, Huffman KD, Hendricks EJ. Angiosarcoma following therapeutic irradiation. *Cancer* 1979;44:2044.

Cutler SJ, Young IL. Third National Cancer Survey. Incidence Data. *NCI Monogr* 1975;41:1.

Dahl I, Angerval L. Cutaneous and subcutaneous leiomyosarcoma—a clinicopathologic study of 47 patients. *Pathol Eur* 1974;9:307.

Darier J, Ferrard M. Dermatofibromas professifs et recidivans on fibrosarcomes de la peau. *Ann Dermatol Venereol* 1924;5:545–562.

Ding JA, Hashimoto H, Sugimoto T, et al. Bednar tumor (pigmented DFSP). An analysis of six cases. *Acta Pathol Jpn* 1990;40:744–754.

Durach DT. Opportunistic infections and Kaposi's sarcoma in homosexual men. *N Engl J Med* 1981;305:1465.

Enzinger FM. Angiomatoid maglinant fibrous histiocytoma: a distinct fibrohistiocytic tumor of children and young adults simulating a vascular neoplasm. *Cancer* 1979;44:2147.

Enzinger FM, Weiss SW. *Soft Tissue Tumors*. St. Louis, CV Mosby Co., 1988.

Fields JP, Helwig EB. Leiomyosarcoma of the skin and subcutaneous tissue. *Cancer* 1981;47:156.

Fletcher CDM, McKee PH. Sarcomas—a clinicopathologic guide with particular reference to cutaneous manifestation. In *Clinical and Experimental Dermatology*. 1984, pp. 451–465.

Fretzin DF, Helwig EB. Atypical fibroxanthoma of the skin. *Cancer* 1973;31:1541.

Giraldo G, Beth E, Coeur P, et al. Kaposi's sarcoma: a new model in the search for viruses associated with human malignancies. *J Natl Cancer Inst* 1972;49:1495.

Guccion JG, Enzinger FM. Malignant giant cell tumor of soft parts. An analysis of 32 cases. *Cancer* 1972;29:1518.

Harcrood AR, Osoba D, Hofstader SL, et al. Kaposi's sarcoma in recipients of renal transplants. *Am J Med* 1979;67:759.

Headington JT, Niederhuber JE, Repola DA. Primary malignant fibrous histiocytoma of the skin. *J Cutan Pathol* 1978;5:329–338.

Helwig ED, May D. Atypical fibroxanthoma of the skin with metastases. *Cancer* 1986;57:368.

Hobbs ER. DFSP. In *Surgical Dermatology: Advances in Current Practice*. RK Roenigk, HH Roenigk, eds. Martin Dumitz, 1993, pp. 191–200.

Hobbs ER, Wheeland RG, Bailen PL, et al. Treatment of Dermatofibrosarcoma protuberans with Mohs micrographic surgery. *Ann Surg* 1988;207:102–107.

Holden CA, Spittle MJ, Jones EW. Angiosarcoma of the face and scalp. Prognosis and treatment. *Cancer* 1987;59:1046.

Huang ES. Cytomegalovirus: its oncogenes and Kaposi's sarcoma. *Antibiot Chemother* 1984;32:27.

Hudson AW, Winkelmann RK. Atypical fibroxanthomas of the skin. *Cancer* 1972;29:413.

Hymes KB. Kaposi's sarcoma in homosexual men—report of 8 cases. *Lancet* 1981;2:598.

Ivetzin DF, Helwig EB. Atypical fibrous xanthoma: a clinicopathologic study of 140 cases. *Cancer* 1973;31:1541–1552.

Jacobs, DS, Edwards WD, Ye RC. Metastatic atypical fibroxanthoma of the skin. *Cancer* 1975;35:457.

Kaposi M. Idiopathisches multiples Pigment sarkom der Haut. *Arch Derm Syph* 1872;4:265.

Karakousis CP, Perez RP. Soft tissue sarcomas in adults. *Ca Cancer J Clin* 1994;44:200–210.

Kearney MD, Soule EH, Ivins JC. Malignant fibrous histiocytoma: a retrospective study of 167 cases. *Cancer* 1980;45:167–178.

Lawrence W, Donegan WL, Natarajan N, et al. Adult soft tissue sarcomas: a pattern of care survey of the American College of Surgeons. *Ann Surg* 1987;205:349-359.

Lever WF, Schaumburg-Lever G. Tumors of fibrous tissue. In *Histopathology of the Skin*. New York, J.B. Lippincott Co., 1983, pp. 597-622.

Lo TCM, Salzman RA, Simedal MI, et al. Radiotherapy for Kaposi's sarcoma. *Cancer* 1980;45:684.

Maddox JC, Evans HL. Angiosarcoma of the skin and soft tissue. *Cancer* 1981;14:1186.

McNeer GP, Cantin J, Chu F, et al. Effectiveness of radiation therapy in the management of sarcoma of the soft somatic tissues. *Cancer* 1968;22:391-397.

McPeak CJ, Cruz T, Nicastri AD. Dermatofibrosarcoma proturberans: an analysis of 86 cases—five with metastases, *Ann Surg* 1967;166:803-816.

Panje WR, Moran WJ, Bostwick DG. Angiosarcoma of the head and neck: review of 11 cases. *Laryngoscope* 1986;96:1381-1384.

Penn. Cancer following cyclosporine therapy. *Transplantation* 1987;43:32.

Phelan JT, Shen W, Mesa P. Malignant smooth muscle tumors of soft tissue origin. *N Engl J Med* 1962; 266:1027.

Rappersberger K, Wolff K, Stingl G. Kaposi's sarcoma. In *Dermatology in General Medicine*. TB Fitzpatrick, ed. New York, McGraw-Hill, 1993, pp. 1244-1256.

Rieber E, et al. Vincristine and Kaposi's sarcoma in the acquired immunodeficiency syndrome. *Ann Intern Med* 1984;101:876.

Robinson JK. Dermatofibrosarcoma protuberans resected by Mohs surgery. *J Am Acad Dermatol* 1985; 12:1093-1098.

Rosenberg SA, Chang AE, Glatstein E. Adjuvant chemotherapy for treatment of extremity soft tissue sarcomas: review of National Cancer Institute experience. *Cancer Treat Symp* 1985;3:83-88.

Rowsell AR, Poole MD, Godfrey AM. Dermatofibrosarcoma protuberans: The problem of surgical management. *Br J Plast Surg* 1986;39:262-264.

Rutgers EJT, Kroon BBR, Albus-Lutter CE, et al. Dermatofibrosarcoma protuberans: treatment and prognosis. *Eur J Surg Oncol* 1992;18:241-248.

Safai B, Mike V, Giraldo G, et al. Association of Kaposi's sarcoma with second primary malignancies: possible etiopathogenic implications. *Cancer* 1980;45:1472.

Shiu MH, Brennan MF. Staging of soft tissue sarcoma: Surgical managment of soft tissue sarcoma. Philadelphia, Lea & Febiger, 1989.

Stout AP, Hill WT. Leiomyosarcoma of the superficial soft tissue. *Cancer* 1964;11:844.

Suit HD, Mankin JH, Schille AL, et al. Results of treatment of sarcoma of soft tissue by radiation and surgery at Massachusetts General Hospital. *Cancer Treat Symp* 1985;3:43-47.

Taylor HB, Helwig ED. Dermatofibrosarcoma protuberans: a study of 115 cases. *Cancer* 1962;15:717-725.

Vezeridis MP, Moore R, Karakousis CP. Metastatic patterns in soft tissue sarcomas. *Arch Surg* 1983; 118:915-918.

Volberding PA, et al. Vinblastive therapy for Kaposi's sarcoma in the acquired immunodeficiency syndrome. *Ann Intern Med* 1985;103:335.

Weedon D, Kerr JFR. Atypical fibroxanthoma of skin: an electron microscopic study. *Pathology* 1975;7:173.

Weiss SW, Enzinger FM. Malignant fibrous histiocytoma—an analysis of 200 cases. *Cancer* 1978;41: 2250-2266.

Weiss SW, Enzinger FM. Myxoid variant of malignant fibrous histiocytoma. *Cancer* 1977;39:1672.

35

Unusual Tumors

James E. Fitzpatrick
Fitzsimons Army Medical Center, Aurora, Colorado

Loren E. Golitz
University of Colorado School of Medicine, Denver, Colorado

The tumors discussed in this chapter arise from epithelial cells differentiating toward adnexal structures except for the Merkel cell tumor, which is considered to be a primary neuroendocrine carcinoma of the skin. The derivation, classification, and nomenclature of the adnexal tumors are controversial, and important disagreements will be discussed. This chapter is organized into subunits based on the differentiation toward hair, sebaceous glands, apocrine glands, and eccrine glands, with the final section discussing Merkel cell tumor.

Management of the majority of benign tumors involves surgical excision, although important alternatives do exist for some lesions. All the malignant tumors are capable of metastasis and their management is more controversial. Special emphasis will be placed on the clinical and histologic diagnosis of the malignant tumors.

TUMORS OF FOLLICULAR DIFFERENTIATION

Trichofolliculoma

Trichofolliculoma is an uncommon benign hair follicle tumor originally described by Miescher. It is one of the few adnexal tumors that may be recognized clinically. The typical lesion is a solitary, firm, dome-shaped, skin-colored papule measuring 3–5 mm in diameter with a dilated, centrally placed pore. Trichofolliculomas are characteristically located on the face or scalp (Fig. 1). Careful examination of some tumors may reveal a small wisp of fine white hairs originating from the follicular orifice. This has been described as a "wool-wisp" or "feather" hair.

Histologic examination reveals a centrally placed keratin-filled primary follicle surrounded by

The opinions or assertions contained herein are the views of the authors and are not to be considered as reflecting the views of the Department of the Army or the Department of Defense. This is a U.S. government publication and is in the public domain.

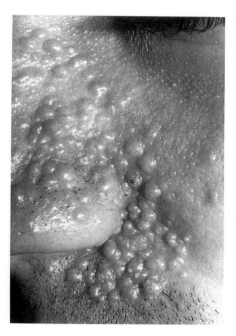

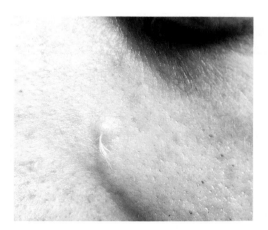

Figure 1   Trichofolliculoma: Small skin-colored papule with characteristic white feathery tuft composed of miniature hairs.

Figure 2   Multiple trichoepitheliomas: Small papules and nodules in characteristic distribution. Small white areas representing foci of keratinization can be seen in several of the papules.

multiple secondary hair follicles that radiate from the primary follicle. Epithelial strands may connect some of the secondary hair follicles. The primary follicle contains multiple small vellus hairs, and the secondary follicles demonstrate variable degrees of follicular differentiation ranging from immature basaloid islands with horned cysts to formed hair papillae with vellus hairs. The tumor is surrounded by a well-circumscribed fibrotic stroma. If mature sebaceous glands are present, some authorities use the term "sebaceous trichofolliculoma."

This tumor is not associated with other tumors or disorders, and surgical removal is curative. Exophytic lesions may be removed by shave biopsy, but the majority require either a punch biopsy or excision biopsy to remove the deep component.

Fibrofolliculoma

Fibrofolliculomas are typically multiple, associated with trichodiscomas and acrochordons, and inherited in an autosomal dominant fashion (Birt–Hogg–Dubé syndrome), although solitary lesions may occur. The primary lesion is a 1- to 4-mm white or yellow-white, dome-shaped papule with a central keratin plug in some cases. Fibrofolliculomas are most dense on the head and neck, although they may also be located on the trunk and arms.

Histologic examination reveals a dilated central follicle filled with keratin. Radiating from this follicle are thin strands of follicular epithelium that may anastomose with adjacent follicular strands. Surrounding this abortive follicle is a well-demarcated thick mantle of fibrous tissue composed of collagen, elastin, and dermal mucin. This is thought to represent a proliferation of the fibrous root sheath. The associated trichodiscomas are thought to represent a proliferation of the *Haarscheibe*, or hair disc. Histologically, they demonstrate a perifollicular proliferation of loose fibrous tissue associated with increased vascularity and occasional myelinated nerves.

Individual cosmetically unacceptable fibrofolliculomas may be removed by elliptical excisional biopsy or punch biopsy. Exophytic lesions are best removed by shave biopsy.

Trichoepithelioma

Trichoepitheliomas are poorly differentiated benign follicular tumors that are particularly important because they may be clinically and histologically confused with basal cell carcinomas. The recognized variants of trichoepithelioma include the solitary conventional trichoepithelioma, multiple conventional trichoepitheliomas, and desmoplastic trichoepithelioma. The solitary conventional trichoepithelioma is nonhereditary and most commonly occurs on the midface, although it may occur on the scalp, neck, trunk, or extremities. The primary lesion is a firm, flesh-colored or white papule usually measuring 0.2–2 cm. Multiple conventional trichoepitheliomas (epithelioma adenoides cysticum, Brooke's tumors) are inherited in an autosomal dominant fashion and may be associated with other adnexal tumors such as cylindromas or eccrine spiradenomas. The primary lesions are identical to the solitary form and are typically located on the nasolabial folds, nose, forehead, upper lips, and around the eyes (Fig. 2). A linear and dermatomal distribution of multiple trichoepitheliomas has also been described. The clinical differential diagnosis includes tuberous sclerosis, basal cell nevus syndrome, multiple perifollicular fibromas, and multiple syringomas. Desmoplastic trichoepithelioma is a clinical and histologic variant that is usually solitary. The primary lesion is a firm, white or yellow, often slightly annular papule measuring 3–8 mm. The most common location is the face, with almost one-half occurring on the cheek. The annular appearance is so characteristic that the diagnosis can be suspected clinically.

The solitary and multiple forms of trichoepithelioma have an identical histologic appearance. The dermis is filled with variably sized basaloid islands of epithelium with a characteristic "lacelike" pattern. The tumor, unlike basal cell carcinomas, is well demarcated and does not demonstrate an infiltrative growth pattern. Some epithelial islands are solid, while others have central keratinizing centers producing small cystic structures thought to be an abortive attempt at hair differentiation. Some lesions may demonstrate more differentiated areas, with the production of primitive hair bulbs or distinct fibroblastic aggregations that have been termed "papillary mesenchymal bodies," since they resemble normal follicular papillary mesenchyme. The surrounding stroma demonstrates a fibroblastic response. Desmoplastic trichoepithelioma is characterized by the presence of narrow basaloid epithelial strands, horn cysts, and desmoplastic stroma. Some lesions may demonstrate variable calcification and foreign body reaction. The relative absence of epidermal connections, deep invasion, prominent peripheral palisading, and retraction between the tumor and stroma help to differentiate it from morpheaform basal cell carcinoma.

Solitary conventional and desmoplastic trichoepitheliomas are best managed by simple excision of the tumor. Multiple trichoepitheliomas represent a significant cosmetic problem. They are not easily amenable to surgical excision because they are so numerous. Methods that aim to restore a normal contour to the facial surface, including dermabrasion, multiple shave excisions, and cryotherapy, usually produce a good cosmetic result. However, since these techniques usually do not remove the entire tumor, partial regrowth may occur over a period of years. Excellent results have also been reported with carbon dioxide laser vaporization. Other recommended treatment modalities, including electrocautery and irradiation, generally produce less satisfactory long-term results.

Pilomatricoma (Calcifying Epithelioma, Pilomatrixoma)

Pilomatricoma is a benign follicular tumor thought to arise from the cells of the hair matrix. The tumor is typically single but can be multiple. Multiple pilomatricomas may occur sporadically, be inherited as an autosomal dominant trait, or be associated with myotonic dystrophy. This tumor typically arises before the age of 20 years, with 40% occurring before the age of 10 years. The most common locations are the head and extremities, with more than three fourths of all pilomatricomas occurring at these sites. The tumors are characterized by slow growth, although a distinct subset demonstrates rapid growth. The primary lesion is a dermal or subcutaneous nodule that is frequently exophytic. The overlying skin is usually normal, although variants extruding granular calcified material have been described. The lesions may be skin-colored, erythematous, violaceous, or demonstrate focal yellow or white discoloration near the surface (Fig. 3). When the skin is stretched, multiple facets of the tumor may be appreciated, producing the "tent sign" associated with this neoplasm. The clinical differential diagnosis includes epidermoid cyst, trichilemmal cyst, and other adnexal neoplasms. The clinical presentation, positive tent sign, and hardness to palpation are features that clinically suggest the diagnosis.

Histologic examination of pilomatricomas reveals the tumor to be composed of three cell types. The first is a basophilic cell that tends to be present at the periphery of the tumor but may be absent in older tumors. Increased numbers of mitotic figures may be present. These cells typically differentiate into "shadow" cells that are eosinophilic and show a centrally unstained shadow at the former site of the nucleus. The basophilic cells may also differentiate into islands of squamous keratinocytes. Calcification, ossification, and foreign body reaction are also commonly observed.

This tumor is best managed by surgical excision, which is usually curative, although recurrences may develop if the entire tumor is not removed. Tumors that recur should be excised because of the rare occurrence of pilomatrix carcinoma.

Proliferating Trichilemmal Tumor (Pilar Tumor)

The nomenclature for this tumor is controversial. The consensus is that it arises from the outer root sheath of the hair follicle, but at least nine terms have been used in the literature to describe this tumor. This neoplasm usually affects the scalp of elderly women. The primary lesion is a slow-growing, firm, subcutaneous nodule.

The tumor is particularly important because it can be confused histologically with squamous cell carcinoma. Low-power examination reveals a large subcutaneous or dermal tumor that is well

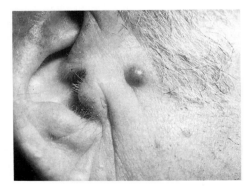

Figure 3   Pilomatricoma: Violaceous nodule that was hard to palpation.

demarcated and composed of interlacing lobules of squamous epithelium, demonstrating trichilemmal keratinization in the center of at least some islands. However, the presence of variable pleomorphism, cytologic atypia, dyskeratotic cells, mitotic figures, and squamous eddies are all features that might suggest a diagnosis of squamous cell carcinoma.

The tumor is best treated by surgical excision with clear surgical margins. While the tumor is generally regarded by most authorities as benign, others regard it as a low-grade squamous cell carcinoma. Because of this controversy, patients should have careful follow-up after removal. At least one tumor inadvertently treated as a squamous cell carcinoma with bleomycin and radiotherapy responded to the regimen, but this is not recommended.

SEBACEOUS GLAND TUMORS

Sebaceous Adenoma

Sebaceous adenoma is a rare benign adnexal tumor most commonly occurring as a solitary lesion on the face, scalp, or anterior trunk. Most patients report a history of slow growth, although rapid growth may occur. The primary lesion is not clinically distinctive and is usually described as a tan, pink, red, yellowish, skin-colored papule usually smaller than 5 mm, although larger lesions (up to 9 cm) have been described. Less commonly, the papules may be ulcerated or pedunculated.

Sebaceous adenomas are particularly important; they may be markers for Muir-Torre syndrome. Muir-Torre syndrome consists of the association of sebaceous neoplasms with colonic polyposis. In some cases there has been a family history suggesting an autosomal dominant pattern of inheritance, while other cases have appeared to be sporadic. In a large series of solitary sebaceous adenomas reviewed by the Armed Forces Institute of Pathology, 11 of 46 patients also gave a history of visceral malignancy. Although controlled studies are needed, this preliminary evidence suggests that even solitary sebaceous adenomas may be markers for visceral malignancies.

Histologic examination reveals a well-demarcated tumor composed of multiple lobules that connect to the overlying epidermis. The individual lobules are composed of two cell types: a germinative cell layer of smaller basophilic cells arranged around the periphery of the lobules and larger cells demonstrating variable sebaceous differentiation toward the center of the lobule. Those tumors demonstrating incomplete differentiation and increased numbers of mitotic figures may be difficult to separate from basal cell carcinoma with sebaceous differentiation (sebaceous epithelioma) and sebaceous carcinoma.

Sebaceous adenomas are best managed by ablative therapies including surgical excision, curettage, and shave excision. Cryosurgery may also give good cosmetic results. Short-term studies have demonstrated that multiple sebaceous adenomas will either decrease in size or disappear entirely following the administration of oral isotretinoin.

Sebaceoma

Sebaceomas are benign sebaceous neoplasms that clinically present as yellow to yellowish-orange papules on nodules in adults, most commonly women. Almost all the reported tumors have been on the face or scalp.

Histologically, sebaceomas are composed of smooth-bordered dermal aggregates of basaloid cells that demonstrate cystic spaces within the epitheloid islands. These cystic spaces frequently contain eosinophilic amorphous debris consistent with sebaceous holocrine secretion. Within the basaloid islands there are differentiated sebaceous cells, either singly or in small clusters. The surrounding stroma is often sclerotic. The histologic differential diagnosis includes basal cell carcinoma with sebaceous differentiation (sebaceous epithelioma).

These are benign sebaceous tumors, and complete removal is not required except for cosmesis. Their primary importance lies in the fact that they may be histologically confused with basal carcinoma and be treated with overly aggressive therapy. Ablation by desiccation and curettage, cryosurgery, shave biopsy, or excision biopsy are all curative.

Sebaceous Carcinoma

Sebaceous gland carcinoma may present as either an eyelid or cutaneous malignancy. The eyelid sebaceous carcinomas usually originate from the meibomian glands, although they may also arise from the glands of Zeis or caruncle. The pathogenesis is unknown, but occasional cases have been associated with a history of local radiation therapy. The tumor most commonly arises from the upper eyelid. Eyelid sebaceous gland carcinomas typically present as firm nodules (Fig. 4), although they may present as papillomatous growths or mimic chronic inflammatory conditions such as chalazions, blepharoconjunctivitis, or keratoconjunctivitis. This subset of sebaceous carcinoma is very important because it is regarded as one of the most lethal tumors of the eye. Large reviews have reported high local recurrence rates (32%), frequent lymph node metastasis (17%), and high mortality rates (6–25%).

Extraocular sebaceous gland carcinoma arising in the skin is less common. The most common location is the scalp or face (75%), followed by the trunk (15%), and extremities (10%). In the past this tumor has been regarded as a locally invasive tumor that rarely metastasizes. However, recent reports documenting metastatic disease suggest that this neoplasm is more aggressive than previously appreciated.

Histologically, this tumor is distinguished by irregular lobules of tumor that demonstrate an atypical growth pattern. In some cases the overlying epidermis may be ulcerated or the tumor may demonstrate invasion of lymphatics, vascular structures, or perineural spaces. An important histologic feature of the ocular variant is pagetoid spread across mucosal surfaces to include the cornea. The lobules of tumor are composed of variable numbers of basophilic germinative cells and larger cells undergoing sebaceous differentiation. The cells typically demonstrate increased numbers of atypical mitotic figures, pleomorphism, and hyperchromaticity, which suggest a malignant diagnosis; however, occasional well-differentiated tumors may demonstrate aggressive biologic behavior.

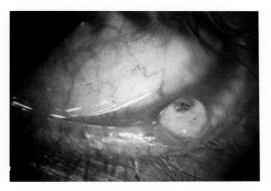

Figure 4 Ocular sebaceous carcinoma: Tumor was cleared by Mohs micrographic surgery and referred back to ophthalmology for reconstruction.

Treatments for primary lesions have included wide local excisions with histologic examination of clear margins and Mohs micrographic surgery. Microscopically controlled excision appears to be particularly well suited for the management of the ocular subset of sebaceous carcinoma, since cosmesis and preservation of the eyelid function are important. Recurrent sebaceous gland carcinomas have been managed by curettage and electrosurgery, wide local excision, Mohs micrographic surgery, and radiation therapy. Microscopically controlled excision is ideally suited for the management of recurrent lesions. Nonresectable tumors have been successfully managed by local radiation. Metastatic sebaceous carcinoma is best managed by surgical excision of resectable lesions and radiation of nonresectable tumors.

APOCRINE GLAND TUMORS

Syringocystadenoma Papilliferum

Syringocystadenoma papilliferum is a benign sweat gland tumor of debatable origin. Some authorities favor either an eccrine or apocrine origin. However, the association of this tumor with hair follicles, underlying normal apocrine glands, other apocrine gland tumors (apocrine cystadenoma), hamartomas that affect pilar structures (organoid nevus), and resemblance to other tumors (erosive adenomatosis or papillary adenoma of the nipple) of modified apocrine glands such as breast, suggests that this tumor arises from the apocrine gland duct. These tumors most commonly present as congenital lesions of the scalp, but they may not be noticed until puberty, when they may enlarge. Approximately one third of all lesions are associated with an organoid nevus (nevus sebaceus). Immature lesions tend to be smooth papules with developed lesions being papillomatous or verrucous. In some cases the papules are grouped, producing large plaques, while in other cases they may be arranged in a linear or segmental fashion. The surface may demonstrate variable scale, crust, and dried blood, with some lesions demonstrating a clear or mucoid secretion. While the literature reports that this tumor is associated with basal cell carcinomas, this usually only occurs when there is a coexistent organoid nevus.

Histologic examination at low power typically reveals a papillomatous appearance. The tumor itself is composed of ductal structures lined by two layers, with the outer cell layer being cuboidal and the luminal layer appearing somewhat columnar. The ductal structures are contiguous with the overlying epidermis or, less commonly, can be seen originating from the infundibular portion of a hair follicle. The surrounding collagenous stroma characteristically contains abundant plasma cells. Serial sections often demonstrate an underlying apocrine sweat gland.

Since basal cell carcinomas may develop in this tumor, it is best managed by surgical excision, although cautery and electrodesiccation have been used successfully.

Hidradenoma Papilliferum

Hidradenoma papilliferum is a benign apocrine gland tumor that occurs almost exclusively in women, on the vulva, although other sites such as eyelid, breast, or anus have been reported. The tumor is characteristically a solitary, dome-shaped nodule 0.5–1.5 cm in size. Rarely, it may be multiple. The overlying epidermis is normal, although occasional lesions may demonstrate a central red papular area if there is a large connection of the tumor to the overlying surface.

Histologic examination reveals a well-circumscribed dermal nodule that is often not connected to the overlying epidermis. The tumor is composed of intricate papillary structures lined by two cell layers. The peripheral layer is composed of small or cuboidal cells, while the luminal cells are composed of cuboidal to columnar cells that demonstrate variable decapitation secretion. Characteristically, plasma cells are absent, although occasional plasma cells may be seen near the surface if a connection to the overlying epidermis is present.

The lesion is best treated with simple surgical excision.

Apocrine Cystadenoma (Apocrine Hidrocystoma)

Apocrine cystadenoma is a relatively common, benign, cystic tumor that demonstrates both ductal and glandular differentiation. This tumor characteristically affects older patients and is rare in children. Apocrine cystadenomas are usually solitary, but multiple lesions may occur. The face is the most common location, with the majority of tumors being located around the eyes. Many of the periorbital lesions probably arise from the glands of Moll, which are modified apocrine glands. Apocrine cystadenomas arising in locations other than the head and neck are uncommon, but they have been documented. The primary lesion is a soft, translucent cyst varying in size from several millimeters to several centimeters. The lesions are typically skin-colored, although less commonly they appear blue or brown (Fig. 5).

Histologic examination at low power reveals that the tumor is composed of large, multi-loculated cystic spaces. The most superficial portions of the cyst are lined by ductal epithelium composed of two layers of cuboidal cells that do not demonstrate decapitation secretion. Examination of the epithelial lining of the deeper parts of the cystic spaces reveals the luminal layer to be composed of high columnar cells with eosinophilic cytoplasm and apical caps that project into the lumina. A peripheral layer of small cuboidal cells (myoepithelial cells) is typically present by may be difficult to appreciate. Areas of papillomatous hyperplasia projecting into the lumen are often, but not invariably, present.

Incision and drainage of the cyst provide temporary improvement, but the cyst lining must be destroyed or removed to prevent recurrence. The wall may be destroyed by electrodesiccation or cauterization, but better cosmetic results are usually obtained by surgical excision of the cyst. Recent success in the treatment of multiple apocrine cystadenomas with carbon dioxide laser has also been reported.

Apocrine Adenoma (Tubular Apocrine Adenoma)

Apocrine adenoma is a rare tumor that typically occurs on the scalp, face, axillae, or anogenital area. This tumor may occur alone or in association with an organoid nevus. The primary lesion is a skin-colored papule or nodule that may be pedunculated or lobular.

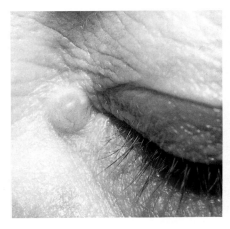

Figure 5 Apocrine cystadenoma: Characteristic solitary translucent cyst near the eye.

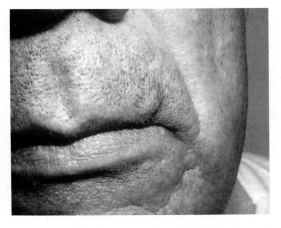

Figure 6 Mixed tumor of the skin: Firm dermal nodule of left upper lip.

Histologic examination reveals a dermal tumor that may be focally connected to the overlying epidermis by stratified squamous epithelial conduits. The tumor itself is composed of small to medium-sized tubules or cystic spaces lined by cuboidal to columnar epithelium that demonstrates variable papillary projections. Some portions of the tumor appear to be more ductal, and other areas are more glandular. The surrounding stroma may be fibrous. Focal areas may demonstrate pleomorphism or perineural invasion, which may make the differentiation from apocrine adenocarcinoma difficult.

This tumor is best managed by surgical excision. Lesions that demonstrate pleomorphism or an abnormal growth pattern should be excised with clear surgical margins since differentiation from apocrine adenocarcinoma may be difficult.

Apocrine Adenocarcinoma

Apocrine adenocarcinoma is a rare malignant neoplasm of the apocrine gland that most commonly arises in the axillae but may arise in other apocrine-bearing areas such as the eyelid (Moll's glands), external auditory canal (ceruminous glands), and anterior chest. This tumor may also arise in organoid nevi. The primary lesion is not distinctive and is usually described as a nodular or multinodular firm, rubbery, or cystic tumor measuring 1.0–8.0 cm. The tumor is red to violaceous in color with occasional ulceration. Regional lymph node metastases have occurred in approximately one half of all cases.

Histologic examination reveals a dermal tumor that often demonstrates an invasive growth pattern. This tumor demonstrates marked variation of the histologic pattern depending on the degree of differentiation. The tumor typically is composed of irregular cystic spaces lined by cuboidal or columnar cells with varying degrees of cytologic atypia and abundant eosinophilic cytoplasm. The number of mitotic figures varies from rare to more than four per high-power field. Careful examination will usually reveal diagnostic areas of eosinophilic apical caps projecting into the lumina. Less differentiated areas may demonstrate solid cellular sheets and cordlike infiltrations. The surrounding stroma may demonstrate variable fibrosis. Suspected apocrine gland carcinomas in women that arise in the axilla may be microscopically difficult to differentiate from breast gland carcinomas arising in the axillary tail of Spence.

This tumor is best managed by wide local excision with histologic examination to ensure that the margins are tumor-free. Mohs micrographic surgery may be useful in areas where preservation of normal tissue and function is important. Attempts to treat metastatic apocrine adenocarcinoma with radiotherapy have not been effective.

SWEAT GLAND TUMORS OF UNCERTAIN HISTOGENESIS

Mixed Tumor of the Skin (Chondroid Syringoma)

Mixed tumor of the skin is an uncommon benign sweat gland tumor of uncertain origin. The majority of authors have concluded that this is an apocrine tumor, while others have concluded that it is eccrine. Other authorities have suggested that there are both eccrine and apocrine variants or that this tumor arises from pleuripotential cells that may differentiate toward either eccrine or apocrine glands. Mixed tumor of the skin demonstrates histologic and ultrastructural similarities to the mixed tumor of the salivary gland and breast. Clinically, the tumor is typically solitary and located on the head, although truncal and extremity lesions have been described. The primary lesion is a firm dermal or subcutaneous nodule with a normal overlying dermis (Fig. 6). A correct clinical diagnosis is almost never made prior to biopsy.

Histologic examination reveals well-circumscribed dermal or subcutaneous nodules with both epithelial and stromal components. The epithelial component consists of nests of cuboidal or polygonal cells often arranged in a lacelike pattern with ductal structures. The ductal structures often demonstrate eosinophilic cytoplasmic protrusions into the lumina, suggesting apocrine differentiation; however, some tumors are composed of small ductal structures with a single row of cuboidal cells that do not demonstrate apocrine differentiation. Keratinous cysts may also be present. The matrix, like the epithelial component, is extremely variable. Some areas are sclerotic, myxoid, or demonstrate cartilaginous differentiation.

This tumor is easily managed surgically because of its distinct tendency to shell out during removal. Recurrences are rare unless some other form of therapy, such as electrodesiccation, is used.

Cylindroma (Turban Tumor)

Cylindroma is a benign sweat gland tumor of debatable origin. Histochemical and ultrastructural studies as well as the occasional association with tumors of follicular origin (trichoepithelioma) suggest an apocrine origin. However, other ultrastructural and immunoperoxidase studies, along with the rare finding of this tumor in association with a tumor of accepted eccrine origin (eccrine spiradenoma), suggest an eccrine differentiation. While this tumor is classically thought of as being multiple, in fact, it most commonly occurs as a solitary, firm, pink to violaceous nodule measuring 0.2–6.0 cm (Fig. 7). The most common locations are the scalp, hairline, or temple. Multiple cylindromas may present sporadically or be inherited in an autosomal fashion and be associated with multiple trichoepitheliomas. In some cases of multiple cylindromas the tumors of the scalp have been so numerous and large that the descriptive label "turban tumor" has been used. Rarely, malignant transformation has been described.

Histologic examination reveals a poorly circumscribed dermal tumor that rarely demonstrates connections to the overlying epidermis. The tumor is composed of numerous discrete, basaloid

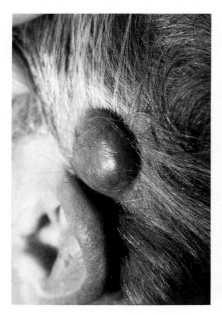

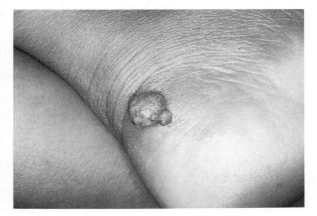

Figure 7   Cylindroma: Large violaceous nodule of the scalp. The patient had similar lesions elsewhere on the scalp.

Figure 8   Eccrine poroma: Large pedunculated nodule of heel with overlying erosion secondary to trauma. (Courtesy of Dr. Richard Gentry.)

islands of tumor that vaguely conform to adjacent islands of tumor, producing a characteristic "jigsaw puzzle" pattern. The lobules are composed of a smaller, more basophilic cell that tends to arrange around the periphery of the lobule and a larger, paler cell that tends to form the remainder of the tumor. Many lobules demonstrate characteristic droplet accumulations of an eosinophilic, hyaline material, and some areas may demonstrate ductal structures lined by cuboidal epithelium. The individual lobules are ensheathed by a thick, periodic acid-Schiff (PAS)–positive, diastase-resistant, hyalinized membrane.

Solitary cylindromas or multiple small cylindromas may be easily managed by simple excision. Recurrence is common if the entire tumor is not removed, and for this reason Mohs micrographic surgery has been advocated for cosmetically critical areas or when there is the histologic suggestion of malignant transformation. Multiple small cylindromas have also been successfully managed by electrocautery, cryotherapy, or radiation therapy, but these would appear to be less than optimal therapies. Multiple cylindromas severe enough to be designated as turban tumors may be so massive that simple excision with primary closure is not feasible. Extensive cases have been managed by total excision of the scalp under general anesthesia followed by split-thickness skin grafts. Dermabrasion may be palliative but not curative.

ECCRINE GLAND TUMORS

Eccrine Poroma

Eccrine poroma is a benign tumor arising from the intraepidermal portion of the eccrine sweat duct. The term "hidroacanthoma simplex" has been used to describe variants of this tumor confined to the epidermis. This tumor is closely related to eccrine acrospiroma, and in some cases both tumors may be present on the same histologic section. Some authorities regard this as a variant of eccrine acrospiroma. The tumor most commonly occurs as a solitary lesion, but linear variants and diffuse eccrine poromas in association with hidrotic ectodermal dysplasia have been reported. The tumors usually develop during adult life and are most commonly located on the plantar surface or lateral surface of the feet or, less commonly, on the hands. The primary lesion is a soft, skin-colored to red papule that may be pedunculated. The overlying epidermis is normal or may be ulcerated if located near a point of friction or pressure (Fig. 8).

Microscopic examination reveals a well-circumscribed tumor connected to the epidermis. The tumor is composed of lobules formed by small, uniform basaloid cells that clearly demarcate from the normal keratinocytes at the site of epidermal attachment. Palisading of nuclei at the periphery of the tumor is conspicuously absent. Focal accumulations of melanin or horn cyst formation may be present. Some cells may be clear due to increased glycogen. Occasional small eccrine ducts are often present within the lobules. The surrounding stroma usually demonstrates a loose stroma and increased vascularity.

Pedunculated lesions may be effectively removed by a deep shave biopsy, while more endophytic lesions require an excision biopsy to prevent recurrence.

Eccrine Acrospiroma (Nodular Hidradenoma, Cystic Hidradenoma, Clear Cell Hidradenoma, Dermal Duct Tumor)

Eccrine acrospiroma is a benign sweat gland tumor thought to demonstrate differentiation toward the eccrine duct. Within the spectrum of eccrine tumors, it has been postulated that eccrine acrospiroma fills the gap between the eccrine poroma and eccrine spiradenoma. The term "eccrine acrospiroma" is not universally accepted, and some authorities prefer other terms or use several different terms to describe histologic subsets. Clinically, the lesion is usually solitary and typically arises in adults. This tumor does not have a characteristic location. The primary lesion is a cyst or nodule that is skin-colored or violaceous (Fig. 9). The overlying epidermis is normal, thickened, or verrucous. The clinical features are not distinctive enough to suggest the correct diagnosis. Although this tumor is generally regarded as benign, a malignant counterpart that may be aggressive has been described.

Microscopic examination reveals the tumor to be composed of a well-circumscribed, multilobular tumor that may or may not appear to be connected to the overlying epidermis. The superficial portion may be histologically identical to an eccrine poroma. The deeper lobules of the tumor are composed of varying portions of larger clear cells that are rich in glycogen and smaller epidermal cells. In some areas the cells may be distinctly fusiform. Most tumors demonstrate ductal structures varying from small, round ducts lined by cuboidal epithelium to large cystic structures lined by flattened epithelium. The surrounding stroma varies from delicate to hyalinized.

Eccrine acrospiromas are managed by simple excisions. Occasional lesions may be so large (up to 6 cm) that surgical flaps or grafts are necessary to close the defect after removal.

Syringoma

Syringoma is a common benign sweat gland tumor with differentiation toward the eccrine sweat duct. It more common in women than men and usually appears after puberty. Syringomas may be familial, inherited as an autosomal dominant trait, or be associated with Down's syndrome. These tumors are usually multiple and characteristically located around the eyes, although scalp, genitalia, trunk, and extremities may also be involved. Linear or unilateral distributions have also been documented. The primary lesion is a small, 1- to 5-mm white-to-yellow papule that is firmer than the surrounding skin when palpated (Fig. 10). Rarely, some syringomas may present as plaques several centimeters in size.

Syringomas are composed of ductal structures placed in a dense sclerotic stroma in the upper dermis. The ducts are typically small and lined with two layers of flattened or cuboidal cells. Frequent epithelial extensions arise from the duct, producing a structure resembling a "tadpole" or "comma." The cells lining the duct have variable amounts of glycogen, and, in rare cases, the glycogen may be so abundant that the term "clear cell syringoma" has been used. Occasion-

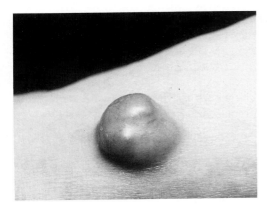

Figure 9 Eccrine acrospiroma: Large, multilocular, cystic nodule of anterior shin. Histologic examination revealed the cystic hidradenoma variant of eccrine acrospiroma.

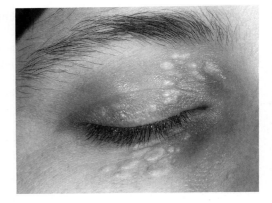

Figure 10 Multiple syringomas: Multiple, small, firm papules in characteristic periocular location in a woman. (Courtesy of Dr. Richard Gentry.)

ally, structures resembling small epidermoid cysts may be seen, most commonly at the most superficial portion of the tumor.

Management of multiple syringomas is complicated by the fact that they are typically multiple and may produce cosmetic disfigurement. Single lesions may be excised with excellent cosmetic results, but the large numbers of lesions preclude extensive use of this modality. Scissor excision using fine ophthalmologic spring-action scissors and secondary intention healing has been reported to be rapid and produce excellent cosmetic results. Electrodesiccation has been advocated, but this often results in incomplete destruction and may produce unattractive scars. In selected cases dermabrasion has been advocated and works well except in the thin skin just under the eye, which is a common location for syringomas. The carbon dioxide laser has been reported to be a fast, efficient method for removing extensive syringomas and produces good cosmetic results. Careful steps should be taken to prevent inadvertent laser-induced eye injury when using this modality around the orbit.

Eccrine Spiradenoma

Eccrine spiradenoma is a benign sweat gland tumor generally regarded as eccrine in origin, although arguments have also been made for an apocrine origin. It does not have a particular sex predilection and typically appears in adults. The majority of lesions are asymptomatic, although a significant percentage are associated with spontaneous pain or tenderness. Eccrine spiradenomas are usually solitary, although they rarely may be multiple or associated with multiple cylindromas and trichoepitheliomas. The primary lesion is a 0.2- to 2.5-cm papule or nodule. The majority are skin-colored or violaceous (Fig. 11). Malignant transformation has been reported rarely.

Histologic examination reveals one to several large, extremely basophilic, well-circumscribed dermal lobules without a connection to the overlying epidermis. The lobules are of two cell types: small, dark, basaloid cells, which tend to be arranged at the periphery, and larger cells with paler nuclei located in the center. Occasional ducts or hyaline droplets, as seen in cylindromas, may be present. The associated stroma is variably delicate or hyalinized. Occasional eccrine spiradenomas may demonstrate smaller lobules that are indistinguishable from cylindroma. The tumor is best removed by surgical excision. Characteristically, the tumor shells out easily during excision.

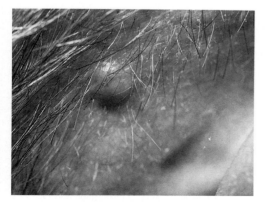

Figure 11 Eccrine spiradenoma: Small violaceous papule behind the ear that was spontaneously painful.

Papillary Eccrine Adenoma

Papillary eccrine adenoma is a rare, benign sweat gland tumor usually located on the extremities of black patients. The primary lesion is a nodule measuring 0.5–0.3 cm. The overlying skin is normal, although occasional lesions may be verrucous. The color is usually red, brown, or gray.

The tumor is composed of a fairly well-circumscribed dermal mass formed by ducts of varying sizes surrounded by a fibrous or sclerotic stroma. The ducts are lined by two cell layers that in some areas form complex intraluminal papillations. The cells are cytologically benign, and mitotic figures are rare or absent.

The treatment of papillary eccrine adenoma is surgical excision. Recognition of this sweat gland tumor variant is important because it has been confused with eccrine adenocarcinoma, which resulted in aggressive surgery.

Eccrine Carcinoma

Eccrine sweat gland carcinomas are an extremely rare group of malignant neoplasms that have been described by a bewildering array of different terms. The reason for this confusion is that this group of tumors is so rare that most descriptions involve a single case report and not large series. Some malignant sweat gland tumors are named by relating them to their benign counterpart (i.e., eccrine porocarcinoma, malignant eccrine spiradenoma, hidradenocarcinoma, malignant chondroid syringoma), while others are classified by their histologic patterns such as adenocystic carcinoma, mucinous carcinoma, ductal carcinoma, or microcystic adnexal carcinoma. Eccrine porocarcinoma, adenocystic eccrine adenocarcinoma (mucinous adenocarcinoma), adenoid cystic carcinoma, ductal eccrine carcinoma, and microcystic adnexal carcinomas are the most completely described and generally widely accepted and will be discussed here. Clinically, eccrine carcinomas tend to affect older patients and have no distinguishing clinical characteristics. Radiation therapy has been identified as an important predisposing factor in some cases. The primary lesions are typically painless, slow-growing papules or nodules. The most characteristic locations are the head, neck, and extremities (Fig. 12).

Histologic examination of eccrine porocarcinoma reveals a tumor connected to the epidermis by cellular cords of tumor. Since this tumor is thought to arise from the acrosyringium, it is often present intraepidermally. A benign eccrine poroma may be present. The dermal component is

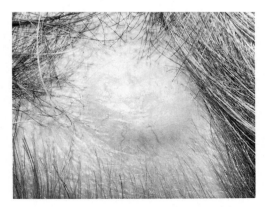

Figure 12 Eccrine carcinoma: Slow-growing firm nodule of frontal scalp line. The patient had received radiation therapy for tinea capitis as a child.

composed of an infiltrating pattern of growth by lobules of tumor that may demonstrate foci of necrosis and calcification. The individual cells demonstrate cytologic atypia. Adenocystic carcinoma is composed of islands of atypical epithelial cells that may form ductal structures and demonstrate perineural invasion. Some tumors may demonstrate foci of mucin or the mucin may be so abundant that the term "mucinous carcinoma" is used. Adenoid cystic carcinoma is characterized by basaloid islands of tumor that demonstrate a characteristic cribriform growth pattern. Eccrine ductal carcinomas are histologically similar to ductal carcinoma of the breast. Microcystic adnexal carcinoma demonstrates features of both follicular and sweat duct differentiation. The tumor is composed of cytologically benign-appearing cells but demonstrates an aggressive local growth pattern and may demonstrate invasion of perineural spaces of even deep muscle. The superficial portions of the tumor often demonstrate small keratinous cysts, and the deeper portion of the tumor is composed of round, oval, or tadpole-shaped islands of epithelium that demonstrate focal ductal differentiation. The surrounding stroma is typically fibrotic.

Optimal management of all forms of eccrine carcinomas has not been delineated. Microcystic adnexal carcinoma, mucinous carcinoma, and adenoid cystic carcinoma are low-grade sweat gland carcinomas that are locally invasive and rarely metastasize. They can be managed by excision with examination of the surgical margins. Recurrence is common if these tumors are not completely excised, and Mohs micrographic surgery is an ideal method. Eccrine ductal carcinoma and eccrine porocarcinomas are locally aggressive, more commonly metastasize, and may cause death. Wide excision is the treatment of choice in these histologic variants (Figs. 13,14). Regional lymph node dissection has been recommended for the eccrine ductal carcinoma variant, but it is not of proven benefit. Radiation therapy for recurrent or metastastic lesions does not appear to be effective, and the role of cytotoxic agents has not been determined conclusively.

MERKEL CELL TUMOR (TRABECULAR CELL TUMOR, TOKER TUMOR, PRIMARY NEUROENDOCRINE CARCINOMA OF THE SKIN)

Merkel cell tumor was originally thought to represent a poorly differentiated eccrine sweat gland carcinoma, but ultrastructural and histochemistry studies have identified it as a neuroendocrine tumor thought to arise from the Merkel cell. This tumor typically affects older patients, and it

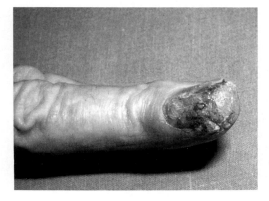

Figure 13 Eccrine porocarcinoma arising in an eccrine poroma: Lesion was initially mistaken for a verruca vulgaris and treated with liquid nitrogen.

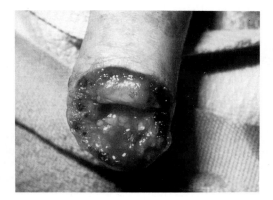

Figure 14 Eccrine porocarcinoma: Distal amputation of tumor depicted in Figure 13. This was done in the dermatology clinic following Mohs micrographic surgery.

arises as a rapidly growing nodule on sun-exposed skin, although other sites such as the sacrum or buttocks are not uncommonly affected. Regional lymph node metastasis occurs in approximately one half of all patients and death in almost 20% of the reported cases.

Histologic examination reveals a dermal tumor composed of uniform, small, densely packed basophilic cells with scanty cytoplasm. The cells are arranged in trabeculae or cords with some areas demonstrating a rosette pattern. Lymphatic invasion may be present. Decoration of tumor cells by neuron-specific enolase, cytokeratin, and epithelial membrane antigen by immunoperoxidase technique are useful diagnostic procedures. Electron microscopy is useful if electron-dense membrane-bound granules are found in the cytoplasm.

Merkel cell carcinoma is best managed by wide local excision of the tumor, although the optimal size of the surgical margin has not been established. Mohs micrographic surgery has been used if preservation of function is a prime concern. Due to noncontiguous spread of this tumor, Mohs micrographic surgery may be unsatisfactory and wide excision should be considered. The efficacy of regional lymphadenectomy when nodal metastasis is suspected has not been established, but it has been advocated on the basis of anecdotal cases. The tumor is also radiosensitive, but studies have not been done to determine if radiotherapy changes the overall mortality rates. Chemotherapy has been recommended as adjunctive therapy for metastatic disease, but it does not appear to be curative. More recently advanced cases have been treated by primary excision followed by induction chemotherapy and radiotherapy.

BIBLIOGRAPHY

Banse-Kupin L, Morales A, Barlow M. Torre's syndrome: report of two cases and review of the literature. *J Am Acad Dermatol* 1984;10:803–817.

Bickley LK, Goldberg DJ, Imaeda S, et al. Treatment of multiple apocrine hidrocystomas with the carbon dioxide (CO_2) laser. *J Dermatol Surg Oncol* 1989;15:599–602.

Birt AR, Hogg GR, Dube WJ. Hereditary multiple fibrofolliculomas with trichodiscomas and acrochordons. *Arch Dermatol* 1977;113:1674–1677.

Brooke JD, Fitzpatrick JE, Golitz LE. Papillary mesenchymal bodies: a histologic finding useful in differentiating trichoepitheliomas from basal cell carcinomas. *J Am Acad Dermatol* 1989;21:523–528.

Brownstein MH, Shapiro L. Desmoplastic trichoepithelioma. *Cancer* 1977;40:2979–2986.

Chesser RS, Bertler DE, Fitzpatrick JE, Mellette JR. Primary cutaneous adenoid cystic carcinoma treated with Mohs micrographic surgery toluidine blue technique. *J Dermatol Surg Oncol* 1992;18:175–176.

Crain RC, Helwig EB. Dermal cylindroma (dermal eccrine cylindroma). *Am J Clin Pathol* 1961;35:504–515.

Dixon RS, Mikhail GR, Slater HC. Sebaceous carcinoma of the eyelid. *J Am Acad Dermatol* 1980;3: 241–243.

Duhra P, Paul JC. Cryotherapy for multiple trichoepithelioma. *J Dermatol Surg Oncol* 1988;14:1413–1415.

Fenig E, Lurie H, Klein B, Sulkes A. The treatment of advanced Merkel cell carcinoma: a multimodality chemotherapy and radiation therapy treatment approach. *J Dermatol Surg Oncol* 1993;19:860–864.

Fleischmann HE, Roth RJ, Wood C, et al. Microcystic adnexal carcinoma treated by microscopically controlled excision. *J Dermatol Surg Oncol* 1984;10:873–875.

Forbis R, Helwig EB. Pilomatrixoma (calcifying epithelioma). *Arch Dermatol* 1961;83:606–618.

Goldman B. Total excision of the scalp and portions of face; restoration by skin grafting: The surgical management of massive cylindroma of the scalp and face. *Ann Surg* 1951;133:555–560.

Gray HR, Helwig EB. Trichofolliculoma. *Arch Dermatol* 1962;86:619–625.

Gray HR, Helwig EB. Epithelioma adenoides cysticum and solitary trichoepithelioma. *Arch Dermatol* 1963; 87:102–114.

Headington JT. Mixed tumors of skin: Eccrine and apocrine types. *Arch Dermatol* 1961:84:989–996.

Hirsch P, Helwig EB. Chrondroid syringoma. *Arch Dermatol* 1961;84:835–847.

Janitz J, Wiedersberg H. Trichilemmal pilar tumors. *Cancer* 1980;45:1594–1597.

Kersting DW, Helwig EB. Eccrine spiradenoma. *Arch Dermatol* 1956;73:199–227.

Lo JS, Snow SN, Mohs FE. Cylindroma treated by Mohs micrographic surgery. *J Dermatol Surg Oncol* 1991;17:871–874.

Maloney ME. An easy method for removal of syringoma. *J Dermatol Surg Oncol* 1982;8:973–975.

Mambo NC. Eccrine spiradenoma: clinical and pathologic study of 49 tumors. *J Cutan Pathol* 1983; 10:312–320.

Mammino JJ, Vidmar DA. Syringocystadenoma papilliferum. *Int J Dermatol* 1991;30:763–766.

Mellette JR Jr, Amonette RA, Gardner JH, et al. Carcinoma of sebaceous glands on the head and neck. *J Dermatol Surg Oncol* 1981;7:404–407.

Moehlenbeck FW. Pilomatrixoma (calcifying epithelioma). *Arch Dermatol* 1973;10:532–534.

Okun MR, Finn F, Blumental G. Apocrine adenoma versus apocrine carcinoma. *J Am Acad Dermatol* 1980; 2:322–326.

Pinkus H, Rogin JR, Goldman P. Eccrine poroma. *Arch Dermatol* 1956;74:511–521.

Roenigk HH Jr. Dermabrasion for miscellaneous cutaneous lesions (exclusive of scarring from acne). *J Dermatol Surg Oncol* 1977;3:322–328.

Roenigk RK, Goltz RW. Merkel cell carcinoma—a problem with microscopically controlled surgery. *J Dermatol Surg Oncol* 1986;12:332–336.

Rulon DB, Helwig EB. Cutaneous sebaceous neoplasms. *Cancer* 1974;33:82–102.

Rulon DB, Helwig EB. Papillary eccrine adenoma. *Arch Dermatol* 1977;113:596–598.

Smith JD, Chernosky ME. Apocrine hidrocystoma (cystadenoma). *Arch Dermatol* 1974;109:700–702.

Snow SN, Reizner GT: Eccrine porocarcinoma of the face. *J Am Acad Dermatol* 1992:27:306–311.

Troy JL, Ackerman AB. Sebaceoma: A distinctive benign neoplasm of adnexal epithelium differentiating toward sebaceous cells. *Am J Dermatopathol* 1984;6:7–13.

Warkel RL, Helwig EB. Apocrine gland adenoma and adenocarcinoma of the axilla. *Arch Dermatol* 1978; 114:198–203.

Wheeland RG, Bailin PL, Kronberg E. Carbon dioxide (CO_2) laser vaporization for the treatment of multiple trichoepithelioma. *J Dermatol Surg Oncol* 1984;10:470–475.

Wheeland RG, Bailin PL, Reynolds OD, et al. Carbon dioxide (CO_2) laser vaporization of multiple facial syringomas. *J Dermatol Surg Oncol* 1986;12:225–228.

Wick MR, Goellner JR, Wolfe JT III, et al. Adnexal carcinomas of the skin. I. Eccrine carcinomas. *Cancer* 1985;56:1147–1162.

Wick MR, Goellner JR, Wolfe JT III, et al. Adnexal carcinomas of the skin. II. Extraocular sebaceous carcinomas. *Cancer* 1985;56:1163–1172.

Woodworth H, Jr, Dockerty MB, Wilson RB, et al. Papillary hidradenoma of the vulva: a clinicopathologic study of 69 cases. *Am J Obstet Gynecol* 1971;110:501–508.

36

Keloids

Steven C. Bernstein
University of Montreal, Montreal, Quebec, Canada

Randall K. Roenigk
*Mayo Clinic/Foundation and Mayo Medical School,
Rochester, Minnesota*

HISTORY

The earliest recorded description of keloid scars is found in the Smith Papyrus dating back to approximately 3000 B.C. Reference is made to "the existence of swelling on his breast, large, spreading, and hard, touching them is like touching a ball of wrappings." The Yorubas, a tribe in West Nigeria, described many observations relating to the character and presentation of keloids as early as the tenth century A.D. The Yorubas practiced ritual facial markings and earlobe perforations. These acts were usually performed during the first week of life, as the Yorubas were aware that scarring during adolescence or adult life often became keloidal. They noted the tendency of the lesions to appear within the same family, but that not all family members were necessarily affected. Also, they described a time interval observed between a trauma and the appearance of a keloid. Finally, the Yorubas knew that once a lesion was present it had no remedy, except when "the Divine power is suitably appropriated to intervene in bringing about its resolution."

Jean Louis Alibert, a founder of the French School of Dermatology, is commonly credited with being the first to describe cicatricial tumors in the modern literature (1806) and to suggest the current name, keloid, in 1817. Retz in 1790 also described these tumors clinically, but he referred to them as "dartre de graisse" or "fatty hernias." Initially, Alibert was convinced that these lesions were cancerous in origin and consequently chose the term "cancroides." When the noncancerous nature of these tumors became apparent, he modified the term to "cheloide," *chele* being derived from the Greek for crab's claw and *oid* meaning like. This new term referred both to the clawlike extension of the lesions and to their tendency toward lateral growth.

Between 1825 and 1854, an artificial distinction was made between "true keloids" (spontaneously arising) and "false keloids" (arising secondary to trauma). In 1884, Addison described "true" keloids, which are now thought to be morphea or scleroderma.

It is now recognized that keloids are unique to humans. Keloidlike lesions have been reported in a few animals, but in all cases the excessive collagen that is deposited in animals is reabsorbed when the tissue insult ceases.

EPIDEMIOLOGY

The incidence of keloids in the general population varies with age, sex, race, anatomic location, and type of trauma. Additional confounding variables include difficulty in distinguishing keloids from hypertrophic scars and the broad time frame during which keloids form or reform. Accordingly, the reported incidence of keloids ranges from a high of 16% among adults in Zaire to a low of 0.09% in England. Keloids are more common among the darker-pigmented races. African Americans form keloids more often than Caucasians, with reported ratios ranging between 2 and 19:1. Arnold and Grauer found that in Hawaii, keloids are five times more common in Japanese and three times more common in Chinese than among Caucasians. There is also an increased incidence in people from East India, Aruba, and Polynesia. There are no known reports of keloids in Albinos.

Many theories have been espoused to explain the difference in keloid incidence between African Americans and Caucasians. Bohrod suggested that it was based on the principle of long-term social and religious mores for sacrification, which consequently determined genetic predisposition. Another theory implicates excessive secretion of melanocyte-stimulating hormone (MSH) and increased sensitivity of the melanocytes to this MSH in the pathogenesis of keloids, which may also account for the increased incidence in African Americans.

Keloids are uncommon at the extremes of life. They may occur at any age but develop most commonly between the ages of 10 and 30. The median age of onset is equal for both sexes. The incidence of keloids is usually reported to be equal among males and females, although some studies do report a higher incidence among females. This is most likely considered attributable to the greater frequency of ear piercing and the greater cosmetic concern in the female population.

These are regional predilections as well. The most susceptible anatomic locations are the presternal area, anterior chest, back, shoulder, and posterior neck. Moderately susceptible are the ears, beard areas, and the rest of the neck. Mildly susceptible areas include the abdomen, forearms, and the rest of the face. Keloids are rarely seen on the scalp, eyelids, genitalia, palms, soles, mucous membranes, tongue, and even the cornea (Table 1).

ETIOLOGY

Many factors are associated with keloid formations (Table 2). However, most lesions result from some form of trauma to a genetically susceptible individual. Keloids usually form within 2–4 weeks and up to 1 year following injury. Nevertheless, not all keloids result from trauma. Several authors have described spontaneous keloids. Notably, Kelly describes these keloids as appearing usually on the middle chest, without a history of antecedent trauma, in patients with a strong family history of keloid formation. Keloids have been reported to occur following numerous types of skin injury: surgery, ear piercing, lacerations, tattooing, abrasions, BCG and other vaccinations, insect bites, injections, specified or blunt trauma, and chemical and thermal burns. Many dermatologic diseases capable of inciting inflammation can also induce keloid formation: chicken pox, herpes zoster, vaccinia, folliculitis, perifolliculitis, and foreign body reactions (Figures 1, 2). Additionally, any process leading to follicular occlusion such as dissecting cellulitis of the scalp, acne vulgaris or conglobata, hidradenitis suppurativa and pilonidal cysts can all precede keloid scarring. Keloids have also been reported in several genodermatoses, including

Table 1 Regional
Susceptibility to Keloids

High risk
  presternal area
  anterior chest
  superior back
  shoulder
  posterior neck
Moderate Risk
  ear lobe
  beard
  anterior and lateral neck
  upper arms
Mild Risk
  abdomen
  forearms
  centrofacial area
  legs
Negligible Risk
  scalp
  eyelids
  genitalia
  palms
  soles
  mucous membranes

Ehlers-Danlos syndrome, Rubinstein-Taybi syndrome, pachydermioperiostosis, progeria, sclero-derma, osteogenesis imperfecta, and trichorhinophalangeal syndrome. Atypical keloids have been described following dermabrasion in patients having recently completed a course of isotretinoin. One case of congenital keloids has been reported (Fig. 3).

There is a tendency for keloids to occur within certain families. The inheritance pattern is still uncertain, although autosomal recessive and autosomal dominant patterns have been reported. Human leukocyte antigen (HLA) studies have been largely inconclusive, but one group has re-

Table 2 Etiological Factors in
Keloid Formation

1. Trauma
  genetic susceptibility
  nonspecific skin injury
  dermatologic disease
  follicular occlusion tetrad
  genodermatoses
2. Familial tendency
3. Anatomic sites
4. Wound tension
5. Sebum autoimmune mechanism
6. Foreign body reaction
7. Infection
8. Endocrine factors

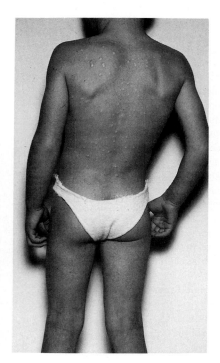

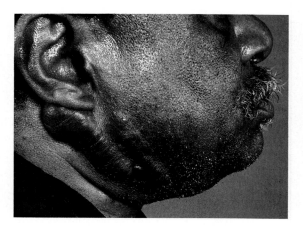

Figure 1   Keloids in pseudofolliculitis barbae.   **Figure 2**   Keloids postvaricella.

cently implicated HLA B14, BW16, and blood group A as being affiliated with a predisposition to keloid formation, and another group reports an increase of HLA DR5 and DQW3 in patients with keloids.

Although trauma is clearly a major provoking factor, not all trauma leads to keloid formation even in the predisposed individual. Many individuals with keloids will frequently have other scars with a normal behavior and appearance if they are located in areas free of tension. The anatomic sites with the highest predilection for keloid formation are those with the highest skin tension, such as the upper back, shoulders, anterior chest, and upper arms. Tension can occur from nonanatomic sources such as following the excision of a large skin tumor or a traumatic avulsion where there is loss of tissue. When an attempt is made to close the wound, there will be increased tension on the wound edges. There is also constant tension on skin from the underlying bony and cartilaginous structures. These tensions directed along certain paths are responsible for the "lines of relaxed skin tension." Many authors report a decreased risk of keloid formation with orientation of the wound along lines of relaxed skin tension. Studies have shown that scars crossing Langer's lines had twice the tensile strength of those running parallel. Increased skin tension is also responsible for the "coiffure keloid" that results from tight braiding of the scalp hair in Africa and increasingly in the United States. Interestingly, if a keloid is removed and grafted into an area of relatively little tension, it will undergo atrophic degeneration.

Osman and associates introduced the "sebum autoimmune mechanism" concept of keloid formation. According to this theory, sebaceous glands remaining in the skin following trauma secrete sebum intradermally, which acts to elicit an autoimmune granulomatous response with

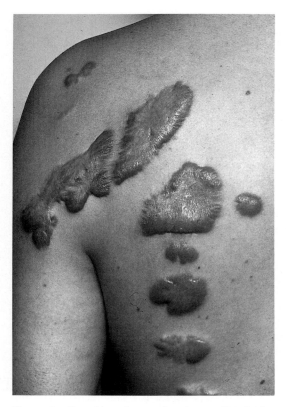

Figure 3 Broad-based posterior chest wall keloids.

progression to keloid formation. In support of this theory is the rarity of keloid scarring on areas lacking sebaceous glands such as the palms and soles. Other groups have suggested that it is the presence of an intralesional foreign body (e.g., ritual object, epidermal fragment, suture material) that leads to keloid formation.

Infection has also been proposed as an etiologic agent in the initiation of keloids. Wound infection constitutes an adverse healing scenario and as such can lead to keloid formation. Over the years, many organisms have been incriminated as being "keloidogenic" (e.g., tuberculosis, syphilis), but there is currently no evidence to support this.

Endocrine factors have also been implicated in the cause of keloids. The ages of the most keloids correlate with the periods of physical (puberty) and pituitary growth. The pituitary has long been incriminated due to the observations that acromegalics are particularly susceptible to keloid formation. Additionally, keloid growth is increased during puberty and pregnancy, periods with augmented pituitary activity. The predisposition for keloid formation has been associated with abnormal function of the hypothalamus, thyroid, and parathyroid. It has been proposed that increased MSH may be the unifying feature of the endocrinologic disorders. The hypothesis is supported by the increased incidence of keloids in dark-skinned races and more deeply pigmented individuals, the anatomic site of predisposition being parts of the body with the greatest melanocyte distribution, the increased incidence during puberty and pregnancy, and even the response to intralesional steroid injections.

CLINICAL MANIFESTATIONS

Keloids are benign fibrous growths that result from the excessive dermal connective tissue that forms in response to trauma in predisposed individuals. Clinically, their appearance is highly variable, reflecting the variation in antecedent trauma. Their location and configuration, but not their size, appear predetermined by the site of skin trauma. Characteristically, keloids generally appear within 1–2 months of trauma, but onset may be delayed up to 1 year or more. Classically, keloids are said to grow beyond the margins of the original injury progressively invading the surrounding normal skin. In contrast, the hypertrophic scar, with which the keloid is often confused, is confined to the tissue damaged by the original injury. Additionally, keloids never spontaneously regress, whereas regression is frequently seen in hypertrophic scars within 12–18 months (see Table 3 for comparison of keloids and hypertrophic scars).

Keloids vary in size from small papules to large pendulous tumors. Shape may vary from evenly contoured, symmetric protrusions with regular margins to irregular clawlike projections from an unevenly twisted mass (Fig. 4). The physical characteristics of the keloid are somewhat dependent on anatomic location. Keloids on the anterior chest tend to be broad-based, raised, and may have irregular clawlike projections (Fig. 5). Earlobe keloids are clinically diverse (Figs. 6, 7). Keloids range in consistency from soft and doughy to rubbery to rock hard. The color is variable, ranging from mildly erythematous in newer lesions to vivid purple in maturing lesions to hypo- or hyperpigmented in older lesions. The clinical course of keloids is also variable. Most keloids have a growth phase followed by a stable period of little or no growth. Often intense pruritus accompanies the growth phase. The epidermis commonly becomes thinned but only rarely ulcerates or drains necrotic material. Keloids rarely regress. Malignant transformation has been described, but such cases are rare and poorly documented. Patients consult physicians due to cosmetic concerns or symptomatology. Keloids following sternotomy or thoracotomy are notoriously painful (Figs. 8, 9). The clinical appearance is characteristic, and the differential diagnosis is limited. Aside from hypertrophic scar, lesions such as dermatofibrosarcoma protuberans, leiomyosarcoma, and other sarcomas may bear clinical resemblance. Infectious lesions such as lupus vulgaris and blastomycosis need to be eliminated by histopathology and culture. Sarcoidosis should be considered in the black population and superficial fascial fibromatoses in whites.

HISTOPATHOLOGY

Keloids are characterized histologically by the intradermal presence of highly compacted hyalinized collagen in nodular formations. The nodules gradually increase in size and ultimately show

Table 3 Clinical Features Distinguishing Keloids from Hypertrophic Scars

Keloid	Hypertrophic Scar
Not limited to site of trauma	Limited to site of trauma
No spontaneous regression	Spontaneous regression
Onset 1 month to 1 year or longer	Onset <3 months
High-risk anatomic areas	Anywhere
Familial tendency	? Familial tendency
Associated symptoms	No associated symptoms
May be worsened by surgery	Improved with appropriate surgery

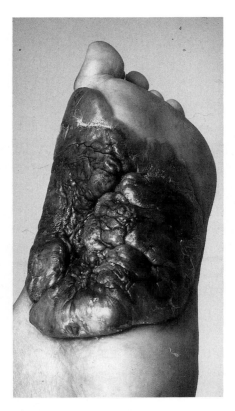

Figure 4 Unusual twisted mass on the dorsal and plantar foot.

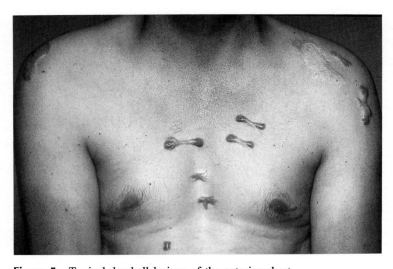

Figure 5 Typical dumbell lesions of the anterior chest.

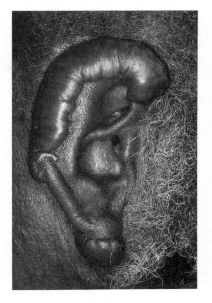

Figure 6 Unusual keloid of the helix and lobe of the ear. (Courtesy of Dr. John Ratz.)

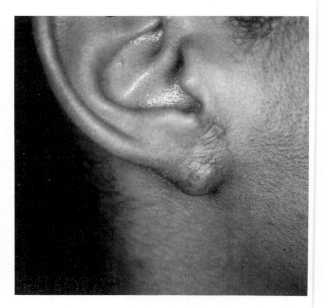

Figure 7 Earlobe keloid.

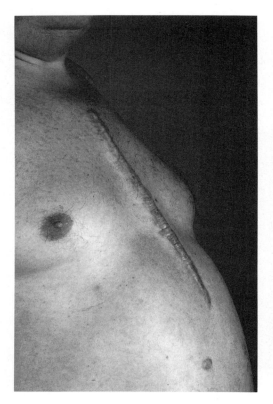

Figure 8 Postthoracotomy keloid.

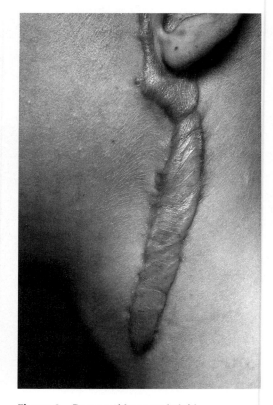

Figure 9 Postcarotidectomy keloid.

thick, highly compacted, hyalinized bands of collagen lying in a concentric arrangement. The collagen fibers are thickened, glassy, pale staining, and faintly refractile. Individual fibrils are large and irregular. Blood vessels, the number of fibroblasts, and ground substance are all increased. Depending upon whether the nodules of collagen encroach upon the papillary dermis, the epidermis appears either flattened or normal.

Craig and coworkers reported that mast cells are present only in the dermis and never in the epidermis, as in normal skin. However, the mast cells are more diffusely distributed than the normal periadnexal location. The actual number of mast cells in keloids is increased due to the presence of a much thicker dermis.

According to Lever and other authors, hypertrophic scars and keloids are indistinguishable from one another on histologic exam. However, with time, the thick and hyalinized collagen bundles that compose the hypertrophic scar gradually become thinner and straighten out so that the collagen bundles assume an orientation parallel to the epidermal surface. In keloids, the nodular condensation of collagen persists indefinitely.

PATHOGENESIS

Keloid scars are a result of an aberrant form of wound healing in which factors necessary for regulation of normal healing and remodeling are defective (Table 4). These keloid tumors ex-

Table 4 Biochemistry of Keloids

Abnormal Collagen Synthesis
    Increased collagen synthesis
    Increased immature soluble collagen
    Increased type I and type III collagen
    Abnormal cross-linking between collagen molecules
    Increased proline hydroxylase
Abnormal Collagen Catabolism
    Increased concentration of collagen
    Defective collagenase
    Collagenase inhibitors
        α_1-antitrypsin
        α_2-macroglobulins
        chondroitin-4-sulfate
    Increased collagenase
Increased Cellularity
    Increased concentration of DNA
    Increased fibroblast number
    Increased mastocyte number
Abnormal Proteoglycans
    Increased total proteoglycans (water retention)
    Major increase in chondroitin-r-sulfate
    (stimulates) fibroblast synthesis
Increased Metabolic Activity
    Increased glycolytic enzyme activity
    Increased glycoprotein synthesis
    Increased fibronectin deposition
Growth Factors
    Transforming growth factor B
    ? Increased

hibit abnormal collagen metabolism and overabundance of extracellular matrix components. Both the increased extracellular matrix and water account for the tissue bulk that forms a keloid.

Excessive collagen deposition is a hallmark of keloids. Collagen synthesis in keloids has been estimated at 20 times greater than in normal skin and 3 times greater than in a hypertrophic scar. It has been shown that the increased collagen synthesis falls to normal within 2–3 year following injury. Keloid scars are composed of both type I and type III collagen, although the actual proportion of each is a matter of controversy. Reports in the literature have demonstrated decreased, normal, and increased amounts of type III collagen ranging between 0 and 32% (normal being approximately 19%). Other studies state that the ratio of genetically distinct collagens type I/III is significantly increased, as compared to normal skin. This is paralleled by a specific increase in $\propto$ 1(I) procollagen mRNA. It is generally agreed upon, however, that collagen synthesis is increased as reflected by the increased level of the prolyl hydroxylase enzyme. Abergel et al. reported increased procollagen synthesis in tissue-cultured keloid fibroblasts, while procollagen peptidase activity was decreased. The collagen cross-linking in keloidal scars has been shown to be abnormal. This has been postulated to be due to a decrease in lysyl oxidase activity. This enzyme is copper dependent, and keloids have been shown to be copper deficient. Additionally, keloidal collagen is more acid soluble than normal dermal collagen. The collagen found in keloids is less mature and less stable than that found in normal skin.

Collagen deposition, however, represents only part of the pathogenesis. Collagen degradation has also been shown to be defective. Actual collagenase activity in keloids, hypertrophic scars, and mature scars is greater than in normal skin. Keloids demonstrate as much as 14 times the collagenase activity and hypertrophic and mature scars four times as much. Nevertheless, the increased degradation is overmatched by the increased deposition, and thus there is excess scar formation. The presence of plasma proteins known as α-globulins help explain this phenomenon. These proteins, such as α-1-antitrypsin and α-2-microglobulin, have been shown to be serum proteinase inhibitors and thus inhibit degradation of connective tissue. The proteoglycan chondroitin-4-sulfate has been shown to be extremely abundant in keloidal tissue. This proteoglycan provides a stimulus to collagen production while coating the collagen fibers and inhibiting their degradation by collagenase.

Keloids and hypertrophic scars are more cellular than normal dermis. This is reflected by an increased concentration of deoxyribonucleic acid. The collagen-producing fibroblasts are increased in number and metabolic activity. Mast cells are also prominent and may underlie the pruritus often associated with these tumors.

The role of growth factors has been the focus of some recent study. Transforming growth factor β (TGF-β) has been shown to stimulate collagen growth in keloids. TGF-β may be released from endothelial cells of small capillaries, making vascular damage a possible initiating event to keloid formation.

TREATMENT

It is dogma in clinical medicine that the more treatment modalities described for any one malady, the more refractory it is to cure. Nowhere is this more evident than in the treatment of keloids. Kelly states that the cardinal rule of keloid therapy is prevention. He advises that nonessential cosmetic surgery be withheld from patients prone to keloid formation. However, he considers patients with only earlobe keloids and a negative family history not to be at increased risk.

It is clear that there is no ideal, uniformly effective treatment for all keloids. Therapy must be tailored to the unique characteristics of the individual keloid such as the location, size, depth, age of the patient, and response to previous treatment. Also, the patient's goals and expectations must be considered. It is important to distinguish the keloid from the hypertrophic scar if appropriate treatment is to be instituted. Hypertrophic scars may spontaneously regress and can be treated effectively surgically or with less invasive measures such as intralesional corticosteroid injections, pressure devices, topical retinoid therapy, or flash lamp dye laser. Many diverse treatment modalities have been described for keloids, but the search for a uniformly effective therapy has proved elusive. For any regimen to be deemed effective, there must be symptomatic and cosmetic improvement as well as normal function. Most importantly, a minimum 2-year follow-up period is necessary to determine recurrence. Finally, one may have to accept the philosophy that treatments for keloids may last up to 2 years, but that it is the nature of the disease for regular retreatment to be required.

Surgery

Surgical excision of keloid tumors was described as early as 1844 by Druit. By 1903, DaCosta reported on the futility of surgical excision: "it is also useless to remove keloid by operation, as it will usually return and a study of the growth removed shows no reason for the inevitable return." Recent studies have shown that surgical excision alone has been associated with a 55% recurrence rate. Long-term follow-up studies have shown as many as 80% of keloids regrowing at 2 years and close to 100% over a lifetime. Although surgery alone is often ineffective, it remains the only method by which the larger, tumorous keloids can be effectively removed. This dilemma has led to the development of specialized surgical techniques to decrease wound tension and the implementation of adjuvant therapies such as intralesional corticosteroids, pressure devices, and radiation therapy.

Several surgical approaches are available. Very small lesions may be excised and closed primarily if the surrounding tissue is not under excessive tension. Such lesions must be removed atraumatically and closed precisely with a minimum amount of foreign material and without dead space or hematoma resulting. If a layered closure is necessary, sutures with low tissue reactivity such as polyglycolic acid should be chosen. Monofilament nylon may be used to close the epidermis, although monofilament polybutester sutures offer the advantage of greater elasticity and low tissue reactivity.

Larger lesions may be treated by excision and grafting or by various flap techniques to minimize tension. Unfortunately, excision followed by skin grafting has had a recurrence rate of 59%, and 50% develop a keloid at the donor site. One way to avoid this complication is to harvest the graft from the overlying epithelium of the keloid, thus creating no secondary wound. This technique is particularly useful for very large or flat pancakelike keloids. The surface epithelium is resected from the keloid using a scalpel or scissors, and the keloid is then resected or debulked. Finally, the harvested skin is sutured into the defect as a full-thickness skin graft. Excision of the keloid, while retaining a rim to which the graft is anchored, is thought to decrease recurrence. The scar rim serves as a splint and decreases the transmission of tensile forces to the rest of the graft. It is important to note that keloid remnants do not cause recurrence. Partial thickness skin grafts generally yield poor results, and the open donor site is at high risk for abnormal scar formation.

Skin flaps are useful for small- to medium-sized lesions or even larger pedunculated earlobe lesions. The skin overlying the keloid can be used to create a low-tension flap. A flap of epidermis may be gently folded down to create less skin tension than pulling surrounding skin over the defect. Additionally, the skin match is superior to that of a skin graft taken from another anatomic site. Earlobe keloids can also be managed by two other useful techniques. Dumbell-shaped keloids can be completed excised using the core-excision technique whereby elliptical incisions are made at the base of the lesion on the anterior and posterior sides of the pinna and the scalpel pushed through the earlobe, dissecting the core of the keloid from normal tissue. Thus, most of the lower earlobe tissue is spared. Shave excision of posterior earlobe keloids has been advocated as a fast, efficient technique. Healing by second intention with accompanying wound pressure is often adequate for treatment of keloids on skin that is not readily visible.

For all surgical techniques in which suture closure is performed, adjuvant therapy is strongly recommended to diminish recurrence. Most clinicians suggest infiltration of 0.1–1.0 ml of 40 mg/ml triamcinolone acetonide into the operative bed after the placement of sutures. Some clinicians suggest injecting the base of the wound with 10 mg of triamcinolone before closing the wound. The quantity of steroid injected should be sufficient to infiltrate the entire lesion. Steroids are generally reinjected at the time of suture removal and then at monthly intervals for 3–6 months. Thereafter, the interval between treatments can be progressively increased to 2, 3, and 4 months, and thereafter can be lengthened to a year. If there is any sign of recurrence, such as pruritus or skin thickening, the patient should be encouraged to return as needed.

Carbon dioxide (CO_2) laser removal of keloids as opposed to "cold steel" surgery was originally reported to have a lower recurrence rate (Figs. 10, 11). This method sterilizes tissue, seals blood vessels up to 0.5 mm as it cuts, and causes minimal necrosis to surrounding tissue. Unfortunately, once the initial enthusiasm subsided, there appeared to be no advantage if suture closure was subsequently performed. However, if the wound is left to heal by second intention and adjuvant therapy employed, the results are more encouraging. Intralesional triamcinolone acetonide at 40 mg/ml is injected after excision into the wound edges and then monthly for 6 months during healing. This time frame is arbitrary, and some clinicians have achieved better results by giving intralesional steroids at 2- to 3-week intervals.

Surgical removal of keloid tissue is appropriate for some lesions if proper technique is observed and adjuvant therapy employed. Excision is the only technique that provides debulking of the keloidal mass. Patients must understand the risk of recurrence and the consequent need for follow-up evaluation.

Pressure

Pressure therapy is useful both for therapy of established keloids and for prophylactic prevention. It is used for its proposed thinning effects. Bedridden patients resting on their sacrum or ischial tuberosities develop dermal thinning. In 1860, Herman Lawrence of Melbourne treated a keloid with multiple scarifications followed by compression for several months. After 1 year,

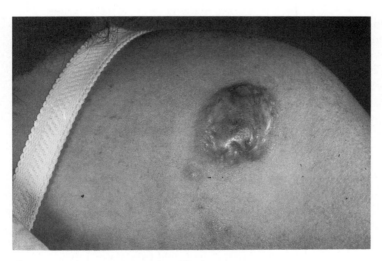

Figure 10 Keloid preoperative CO_2 laser.

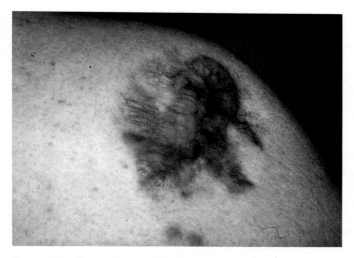

Figure 11 Six months post-CO_2 laser excision with healing by second intention and two intralesional steroid treatments. Note recurrence.

only a thin scar remained. Rayer in 1894 was the first to use pressure alone in keloid treatment. Larsen in 1971 showed that nodules did not develop under pressure treatment. Kishcher et al. proposed in 1978 that pressure produced hypoxia, resulting in fibroblast degeneration and altering the ratio of collagen metabolism so that catabolism became dominant. Another group suggested that the decreased blood flow to the scar resulted in the reduced delivery of α_2-macroglobulin, an α-protein known to inhibit collagenase function. Asboe-Hansen reported that mast cells degranulate under edematous conditions and that their products encourage the formation of increased ground substance. Pressure, therefore, would decrease the availability of water and diminish the degranulation of mast cells.

Pressure therapy following surgical excision is an effective method to help prevent recurrence of earlobe keloids. Both spring-pressure earring devices and acrylic ear splints have been reported to be beneficial. Large clip-on earrings may be used with flurandrenolide tape for greater preventative effect. Pressure devices for other locations include elastic garments tightly fitted to involved anatomic sites. The pressure exerted should be at least 24 mmHg to exceed the inherent capillary pressure. It must be maintained day and night for a minimum of 4–6 months to 1 year or more. Daily discontinuances of pressure for hygiene should not exceed 30 min. Kelly suggests that a pressure gradient elastic garment should be warn at least 12 hr a day for 4–6 months after cutaneous trauma in patients at high risk for the development of keloids.

Radiation

Radiation therapy is used either alone or as an adjunct to surgical excision. In 1906, DeBeurman and Gougerot were the first to describe x-ray treatment for keloids. Homans, in 1940, recommended radiation after excision or pressure therapy. In 1961, Cosmon et al. found that radiation treatment given in the early postoperative period was most advantageous in the prevention of recurrence. No advantage has been shown for preoperative radiation therapy alone or in combination with postoperative therapy.

The rationale for radiotherapy involves the destruction of fibroblasts by ionizing radiation. These fibroblasts are not replaced by bloodborne cells from distant tissues. Through the destruction of a sufficient quantity of cells, a balance may be reached between collagen synthesis and degradation.

Inalsingh reported a series of 501 patients given either superficial radiation alone or radiation following excisional therapy. Patients received 400 rads monthly and five or fewer treatments. Good cosmetic results and relief of symptoms were reported in 26.5% of patients. Over a 2-year follow-up, no adverse effects from radiation were observed. In 1989, Sällström et al. treated 124 patients with postoperative x-ray radiation begun within 24 hr of surgery. The treatment results were evaluated 6 and 24 months after treatment. Good or excellent results were observed in 92% of the patients. Side effects included slight hyperpigmentation in 31% and telangiectasia in 15%. Other reported side effects include pruritus, paresthesias, and pain. The results of radiation alone are cosmetically inferior to surgery and radiation combined.

Many clinicians remain concerned about the possible carcinogenic effects of radiation therapy. Radiation is known to increase the incidence of malignancy. However, Ketchum et al. claim to know of no case of carcinomas caused by radiation for keloids. It appears that although radiation therapy appears to be an effective adjuvant therapy, it should be used with caution, and then only in elderly patients with significant symptoms or loss of function from their keloids.

Intralesional Corticosteroids

A preferred initial approach to the treatment of keloids is the intralesional injection of steroids. Proper placement of the needle and medication within the lesion is important and often the reason this approach fails. Such injections may be used alone or in combination with other therapies such as surgery (as discussed above) or cryotherapy. Intralesional injections alone serve to diminish symptoms and soften and flatten the upraised scar. The patient must be informed that this treatment will not result in narrowing or disappearance of the scar. The response rate to intralesional steroid injections is variable. In 1970, Griffith et al. reported recurrence of only 5 of 56 treated keloids after 4 years of follow-up. However, Kiil in 1977 reported a 50% recurrence rate over 5 years.

Corticosteroids alter the balance between collagen synthesis and degradation. Collagen synthesis is diminished, and collagen breakdown is enhanced by decreasing levels of the known inhibitors α_2-macroglobulin and α_1-antitrypsin. It appears that early keloids are more responsive to treatment. This may be explained by the younger fibroblast's increased collagenase production in response to steroids.

Several preparations may be used for intralesional injection. Many clinicians routinely use triamcinolone acetoinde (Kenalog) 40 mg/ml for initial treatment. However, others suggest starting with a 10 mg/ml dose and monitoring response. Lack of response after two or three injections would dictate the need to increase the concentration or switch to a triamcinolone diacetate (Aristocort 25 mg/ml) preparation. Another approach is to vary the concentrations of triamcinolone acetonide in different lesions or within different areas of the same lesion. Corticosteroids can also be diluted with equal parts of 2% lidocaine. The lidocaine is most useful in decreasing the pain of multiple injections as well as the pain immediately following treatment.

The steroid preparation may be delivered in a number of fashions. Usually, a needle and syringe delivery system is used. A Luer-Lok needle and syringe are necessary to prevent separation of the syringe from the needle while injecting. A small-gauge needle is used; ideally, a 30- or 27-gauge needle is recommended. Occasionally, clogging and near impossible injection result, necessitating the use of a 25-gauge needle, especially while using triamcinolone acetonide at 40 mg/ml. Other delivery systems include mechanical injectors such as the spring or CO_2-powered device. Mechanical injectors are said to cause less pain on injection, but most clinicians feel that steroid placement is less efficient and there is greater wastage. Dental syringes are preferred by some as they are said to facilitate injection.

Intralesional injections are directed at the center or bulk of the keloid mass. Care must be taken to inject only the keloid itself or the base of the keloid. Superficial infiltration beneath the epidermis or deep deposition within the adipose will increase the risk of side effects such as atrophy and hypopigmentation. Occasionally, injection will be extremely difficult due to the fibrotic nature of the tumor. A technique for facilitating injection involves creating a needle tract by inserting the needle into the keloid and injection while slowly withdrawing. Another effective method is to use light cryosurgery prior to injection. Cryosurgery induces tissue edema and provides the additional advantage of subsequent cellular and collagen disruption. The liquid nitrogen is applied only briefly to establish a skin frost. An alternative used by the author (RKR) is to inject local anesthesia, followed by a freeze–thaw cycle with liquid nitrogen for 1½ min, which results in tissue necrosis plus the steroid effect. After 10 or 15 min, the lesion is injected. The technique also allows for better dispersal of the corticosteroid throughout the keloidal tissue and minimizes its deposition in the subcutaneous or surrounding tissue. Keloids become easier to inject with increasing treatment number. Treatment intervals are arbitrary, but most clinicians separate treatments by 3–4 weeks for maximal effect.

Intralesional steroid injections are not without potential risk. Hypopigmentation and atrophy are not uncommon side effects. Overenthusiastic use of steroids may result in telangiectases, necrosis, ulceration, and even cushingoid habitus. A rare complication results from the pooling of 40 mg/ml of triamcinolone acetonide in injected sites. This leads to the formation of subepidermal insoluble xanthomatous deposits, which must be removed for maximum cosmesis.

Cryotherapy

Cryotherapy has already been discussed for use in conjunction with intralesional corticosteroids. Two recent studies have reported excellent results using cryotherapy alone. Zouboulis et al. in 1993 performed a prospective trial on 93 white patients including 32 months of average follow-up. They reported excellent response in 32%, good response in 29%, poor response in 29%, and no response in 10%. Treatment was administered using the contact method for one freeze–thaw cycle of 30 sec per lesion. Treatment was repeated as needed every 20–30 days. Rusciani et al. treated 65 lesions with a hand-held liquid nitrogen spray unit. They reported complete flattening in 73% of the scars, most of which were less than 2 years old. No recurrence was seen during follow-up of 17–42 months.

The major side effect associated with cryotherapy is hypopigmentation due to enhanced melanocyte sensitivity to such cold temperatures. When cryotherapy is combined with intralesional steroid injection, hypopigmentation is almost inevitable.

Silastic Gel Sheeting

A newer approach to the treatment of keloid scars is with silastic gel sheeting. However, these authors are skeptical, not having much success with our patients. This is a semiocclusive scar cover made of cross-linked polydimethylsiloxane polymer. Silicon gel was shown to be of value in the treatment of hypertrophic scars, especially following thermal injury. Quinn proposed that it is the low molecular weight of the silicone oil continuously released from gel sheeting that is responsible for the clinical effect. Mercer described 18 patients with 22 keloid scars treated for 6 months with silicone gel. He reported improvement in texture and color in greater than 80% and height in 68%.

Sawada and Sone compared a silicone cream containing 20% silicone oil covered with an occlusive dressing to the cream formulation alone. They reported remarkable improvement in the cream/occlusive dressing group (82%) and only mild improvement (22%) in the cream alone group. The authors consequently suggested that occlusion and hydration are the principal modes of action of both the silicone gel sheeting method and the silicone cream/occlusive dressing method. They recently went on to compare the efficacy of an occlusive dressing technique using cream that did not contain silicone with an application of Vaseline as a control. Greater scar improvement was noted in the cream-tested areas, and the authors once again emphasized the importance of hydration and occlusion. Silastic gel sheeting is a new form of treatment, and consequently side effects are not well known at present. It appears that sensitization to silicone oil does not occur, nor does it cause irritation. There is no evidence to date of silicone absorption.

Lasers

Laser surgery using the carbon dioxide laser has already been discussed. Disappointing results have consistently been reported with the argon laser. Recently, however, some authors have reported softening and flattening of lesions with the neodynium-yttrium-garnet (Nd:YAG) laser. Abergel et al. reported initial success in two patients with 3 years of follow-up. They suggested that the mechanism of action was a specific bioinhibition of collagen production without altering viability or replication of cells. Collagen production was selectively inhibited after treatment with the Nd:YAG laser. Sherman et al. in 1990 also reported improvement with the Nd:YAG laser in 20 patients with keloid scars. Long-term follow-up and larger population sampling are necessary to judge the ultimate utility of this treatment modality.

Finally, in a recent article, Dierickx et al. reported the use of the flashlamp pulsed dye laser at 585 nm and 6.0–7.5 J/cm^2 fluence for the treatment of refractory hypertrophic scars. They reported that 47% of the patients had 100% improvement after one to three treatments. The authors had used the laser with the goal of improving scar color. An unexpected consequence was an improvement in the scar texture, with flattening and softening of the scar. Data suggest that patients with hypertrophic scars have an early increased microcirculatory perfusion. The authors suggest that selective photothermolysis of the increased vasculature by the flashlamp pulsed dye laser may reduce scar hypertrophy. The hypoxia induced by the laser treatment of the vessels has been proposed to alter the collagen metabolism, favoring catabolism by collagenase activity.

Systemic Therapy

Many keloids are associated with significant symptoms such as pain and pruritus. These symptoms are frequently ascribed to histamine release. Additionally, there is some evidence that the elevated histamine content in keloid tissue may be responsible for the development of the lesion. Antihistamines have been reported to inhibit the growth of fibroblasts derived from human keloids in addition to alleviating pruritus.

Other oral medications have also been suggested to have antifibrotic effects. Systemic D-penicillamine has been used with some success in the treatment of keloids. It is a prototypical thiol that inhibits the synthesis of collagen cross-links. In vitro D-penicillamine chelates copper which thereby reduces the activity of lysyl oxidase. Uncross-linked collagen is more susceptible to collagenase, and therefore conditions for collagen breakdown are more favorable.

Pentoxifylline, an analog of methyl xanthine theobromine, causes a dose-dependent inhibition of collagen, fibronectin, and glycoaminoglycan production from keloid-derived fibroblasts. Colchicine and beta-aminopropiontile fumarate (BAPN) are also effective antifibrotic agents. BAPN, like penicillamine, is a lysyl oxidase inhibitor, which interferes with collagen cross-linking. Colchicine increases tissue collagenase degradation. These treatments are still largely experimental and require further study.

Topical Therapy

Topical retinoic acid is thought to have an inhibitory effect on DNA synthesis in fibroblasts. It has been reported to reduce growth and soften keloid scars. Delimpens reported 28 patients treated with 0.025% solution of retinoic acid daily for up to 22 months. Favorable results were achieved in 77% and consisted of decreased symptomatology, improved coloration, and decreased tumor bulk. Zinc, in the form of zinc oxide, has also been used topically. One study reported scars reduced to the level of the surrounding skin within 6 months. No further studies followed.

Cytokines

Two types of cytokine, interferons (IFNα, β, and γ), and transforming growth factor β (TGF-β) have been investigated for their effects on collagen synthesis. The interferons and especially IFN-γ have been shown to inhibit collagen synthesis, while TGF-β is a cytokine that enhances extracellular matrix production by a variety of cells in vitro and in vivo. Further study will exploit methods to inhibit the effect of TGF-β on collagen production.

BIBLIOGRAPHY

Abdalla Osman AA, Gumma KA, Satir AA. Highlights on the etiology of keloid. *Int Surg* 1978;63(6):33–37.

Abergel RP, Pizzuro RD, Meeker CA, Lask G, et al. Biochemical composition of the connective tissue in keloids and analysis of collagen metabolism in keloid fibroblast cultures. *J Invest Dermatol* 1985; 84:284–290.

Abergel RP, Pizzurro D, Meeker CA, Lask G, Matsuoka LY, Minor RR, et al. Biochemical composition of the connective tissue in keloids and analysis of collagen metabolism in keloid fibroblast cultures. *J Invest Dermatol* 1985;84(5):384–390.

Addison T. On the keloid of Alibert and on true keloid. *Med-Chir Trans* 1854;37:27–47.

Alibert JLM. Description des maladies de la peau observees a l'hopital Saint-Louis et exposition des meilleures methodes suivies pour leur traitment. Paris, Banois L'Aine et Fils, 1806, p. 113.

Alibert JLM. Quelques recherches sur la cheloide. Mem Soc Medicale d'Emulation, 1817, p. 744.

Alibert JLM. Description des maladies de la peau observees a l'hopital Saint-Louis et exposition des meilleures methodes suivies pour leur traitment. Bruxelles, Auguste Whalen, 1825, vol. 2, p. 37.

Amar Inalsingh CHA. An experience in treating 501 patients with keloids. *Johns Hopkins Med J* 1974; 134:284–290.

Apfelberg DB, Maser MR, Lash H. The use of epidermis over a keloid as an autograft after resection on the keloid. *J Dermatol Surg* 1976;2(5):409–411.

Asboe-Hanson G. The mast cell in health and disease. *Acta Dermatol Venereol* (Suppl) 1973;23:139.

Babu M, Diegelmann R, Oliver N. Fibronectin is overproduced by keloid fibroblasts during abnormal wound healing. *Mol Cell Biol* 1989;9(4):1642–1650.

Bailly C, Dreze S, Asselineau D, Nusgens B, Lapiere C, et al. Retinoic acid inhibits the production of collagenase by human epidermal keratinocytes. *J Invest Dermatol* 1990;94:47–51.

Breasted JH. The Edwin Smith surgical papyrus. Vol. 1. Hieroglyphic text translation and commentary. Chicago, University of Chicago Press, 1930, pp. 403–406.

Brown LA Jr., Pierce HE. Keloids: scar revision. *J Dermatol Surg Oncol* 1986;12(1):51–56.

Ceilley RI, Babin RW. The combined use of cryosurgery and intralesional injection of suspension of fluorinated adrenocorticosteroids for reducing keloids and hypertrophic scars. *J Dermatol Surg Oncol* 1979; 5:54–56.

Chait LA, Kadwa MA. Hypertrophic scars and keloids. Cause and management—current concepts. *S Afr J Surg* 1988;26(3):95–98.

Cohen IK, McCoy BS. Keloid: biology and treatment. In *The Surgical Wound.* P Dineen, G Hildick-Smith, ed. Philadelphia, Lea & Febiger, 1981, pp. 123–131.

Combemale P, Cantaloube D. Traitement des cheloides. *Acta Dermatol Venereol* 1991;118(9):665–673.

Cosman B, Crikelair GF, Ju DM, Gaulin JC, et al. The surgical treatment of keloids. *Plast Reconstr Surg* 1961;27:335–358.

Craig RR, Schofield JD, Jackson DS. Collagen biosynthesis in normal and hyptertrophic scars and keloid as a function of the duration of the scar. *Br J Surg* 1975;62:741–744.

Daly TJ, Weston WL. Retinoid effects on fibroblast proliferation and collagen synthesis in vitro and on fibrotic disease in vitro. *J Am Acad Dermatol* 1986;15:900–902.

Datubo-Brown Department of Dermatology: Keloids: a review of literature. *Br J Plast Surg* 1990;43(1):70–77.

Delimpens AMPJ. The local treatment of hypertrophic scars and keloids with topical retinoic acid. *Br J Dermatol* 1980;103:319.

Di Cesare PE, Cheung DT, Perelman N, Libaw E, Peng L, et al. Alteration of collagen composition and cross-linking in keloid tissues. *Matrix* 1990;10(3):172–178.

Diegelmann RF, Cohen IK, McCoy BJ. Growth kinetics and collagen synthesis of normal scar and keloid fibroblasts in vitro. *J Cell Physiol* 1979;98(2):341–346.

Dierickx C, Goldman MP, Fitzpatrick RE. Laser treatment of erythematous/hypertrophic and pigmented scars in 26 patients. *Plast Reconstr Surg* 1995;95:84–92.

Dinehart SM, Herzberg AJ, Kerns BJ, Pollack SV. Acne keloidalis: a review. *J Dermatol Surg Oncol* 1989;15(6):642–647.

Doyle-Lloyd DJ, White JA. Keloids. *J La State Med Soc* 1991;143(12):9–12.

Edlich RF, Haines PC, Nichter LS, Silloway KA, Morgan RF. Psudofolliculitis barbae with keloids. *J Emerg Med* 1986;4(4):283–286.

Friedman DW, Boyd CD, Mackenzie JW, Norton P, et al. Regulation of collgen gene expression in keloids and hypertrophic scars. *J Surg Res* 1993;55(2):214–222.

Griffith BH. Treatment of keloids with triamcinolone acetonide. *Plast Reconstr Surg* 1966;30:202–208.

Inalsingh CHA. An experience in treating five hundred and one patients with keloids. *Johns Hopkins Med J* 1974;134:284–290.

Janssen de Limpens AM, Cormane RH. Keloids and hypertrophic scars—immunological aspects. *Aesthetic Plast Surg* 1982;6(3):149–152.

Janssen de Limpens AM, Cormane RH. Studies on the immunologic aspects of keloids and hypertrophic scars. *Arch Dermatol Res* 1982;274(3-4):259–266.

Jutley JK, Ng KY, Cunliffe WJ, Layton AM, Wood EJ. Analysis of collagen composition in acne keloids. *Biochem Soc Trans* 1993;21(3):303S.

Kelly AP. Keloids. *Derm CL* 1988;6(3):413–424.

Ketchum LD, Cohen IK, Masters FW. Hypertrophic scars and keloids. A collective review. *Plast Reconstr Surg* 1974;53(2):140–154.

Kiil J. Keloids treated with topical injections of triamcinolone acetonide (kenalog). Immediate and longterm results. *Scand J Plast Reconstr Surg* 1977;11:169–122.

Kischer CW, Shetlar MR, Chvapil M. Hypertrophic scars and keloids: a review and new concept concerning their origin. *Scanning Electron Microscopy* 1982;1699–1713.

Kischer CW. The microvessels in hypertrophic scars, keloids and related lesions: a review. *J Submicroscopic Cytol Pathol* 1992;24(2):281–296.

Larson DL, Abston S, Evans EB, et al. Techniques for decreasing scar formation and contractures in the burned patient. *J Trauma* 1971;11:807.

Layton AM, Yip J, Cunliffe WJ. A comparison of intralesional triamcinolone and cryosurgery in the treatment of acne keloids. *Br J Dermatol* 1994;130(4):498–501.

Lever WF. *Histopathology of the Skin.* 7th ed. Philadelphia, J.B. Lippincott, 1990, pp. 668–669.

Low SQ, Moy RL. Scar wars strategies. Target collagen. *J Dermatol Surg Oncol* 1992;18(11):981–986.

Mercer NS. Silicone gel in the treatment of keloid scars. *Br J Plast Surg* 1989;42(1):83–87.

Moulton-Levy P, Jackson CE, Levy HG, Fialkow PJ. Multiple cell origin of traumatically induced keloids. *J Am Acad Dermatol* 1984;10(6):986–988.

Muir IF. On the nature of keloid and hypertrophic scars. *Br J Plast Surg* 1990;4(1):61–69.

Murray JC. Keloids and hypertrophic scars. *Clin Derm* 1994;12(1)27–37.

Murray JC. Scars and keloids. *Dermatol Clin* 1993;11(4):697–708.

Murray JC, Pollack SV, Pinnell SR. Keloids: a review. *J Am Acad Dermatol* 1981;4(4):461–470.

Murray JC, Pollack SV, Pinnell SR: Keloids and hypertrophic scars. *Clin Dermatol* 1984;2(3):121–133.

Nemeth AJ. Keloids and hypertrophic scars. *J Dermatol Surg Oncol* 1993;l9(8):738–746.

Omo-Dare P. Yoruban contributions to the literature on keloids. *J Natl Med Assoc* 1973;65:367–372.

Peltonin J, Hsiao LL, Jaakkoic S, et al. Activation of collagen gene expression in keloids: colocalization of type I and VI collagen and transforming growth factor-B_1 MRNA. *J Invest Dermatol* 1991;97:240.

Placik OJ, Lewis VL, Jr. Immunologic associations of keloids. *Surg Gynecol Obstet* 1992;175(2):185–193.

Quinn KJ, Evans JH, Courtney JM, et al. Nonpressure treatment of hypertrophic scars. *Burns* 1988;12:102.

Retz N. Des maladies de la peau et de celles d l'esprit. 3. Paris, Mequinon, 1790, p. 155.

Rockwell WB, Cohen IK, Ehrlich HP. Keloids and hypertrophic scars: a comprehensive review. *Plast Reconstr Surg* 1989;84(5):827–837.

Rudolph R. Wide spread scars, hypertrophic scars, and keloids. *Clin Plast Surg* 14(2):253–60, 1987.

Rusciani L, Rossi G, Bono R. Use of cryotherapy in the treatment of keloids. *J. Dermatol Surg Oncol* 1993;19:529–534.

Sahl Jr., WJ, Clever H. Cutaneous scars. Part I. *Int J Dermatol* 1994;33(10):681–691.

Sallstrom KO, Larson O, Heden P, Eriksson G, Glas JE, et al. Treatment of keloids with surgical excision and postoperative x-ray radiation. *Scand J Plast Reconstr Surg Hand Surg* 1989;23(3):211–215.

Sawada Y, Sone K. Hydration and occlusion treatment for hypertrophic scars and keloids. *Br J Plast Surg* 1992;45(8):599–603.

Sawada Y, Sone K. Treatment of scars and keloids with a cream containing silicone oil. *Br J Plast Surg* 1990;43(6):683–688.

Selmanowitz VJ, Stiller MJ. Rubinstein-Taybi syndrome. Cutaneous manifestations and colossal keloids. *Arch Dermatol* 1981;117(8):504–506.

Sherman R, Rosenfeld H. Experience with the ND:YAG laser in the treatment of keloid scars. *Ann Plast Surg* 1988;21:231–235.

Sherman R, Rosenfeld H. Differential oxygen sensitivities in G6PDH activities of cultured keloid and normal skin dermis single cells. *J Dermatol* 1991;18(10):572–579.

Topol BM, Lewis VL Jr., Benveniste K. The use of antihistamine to retard the growth of fibroblasts derived from human skin, scar, and keloid. *Plast Reconstr Surg* 1981;68(2):227–232.

Zouboulis C, Blume V, et al. Outcomes of cryosurgery in keloids and hypertrophic scars. *Arch Dermatol* 1993;129:1146–1151.

Zubert TJ, DeWitt DE. Earlobe keloids. *Am Fam Phys* 1994;49(8):1835–1841.

Axillary Hyperhidrosis, Apocrine Bromhidrosis, Hidradenitis Suppurativa, and Familial Benign Pemphigus: Surgical Approach

Harry J. Hurley
*University of Pennsylvania School of Medicine,
Philadelphia, Pennsylvania*

Several axillary dermatoses for which medical or dermatologic treatment may be unsuccessful respond favorably to surgical management. They include axillary hyperhidrosis, apocrine bromhidrosis, hidradenitis suppurativa, and familial benign pemphigus (Hailey–Hailey disease). The essential pathogenetic and clinical features will be discussed here, followed by a description of the surgical therapy and its rationale.

AXILLARY HYPERHIDROSIS

Axillary hyperhidrosis is a genetic, autosomal dominant hyperactivity of the eccrine glands of the axilla. It results from increased sudomotor impulses from the cerebral cortex that are generated almost exclusively during waking hours by mental, emotional, and sensory stimuli. The disappearance of such stimuli during sleep coincides with virtual cessation of the excessive sweating at such times. Moreover, anatomic, histologic, histochemical, electron microscopic, and physiologic studies fail to reveal any abnormalities of the hyperactive glands that would explain their increased secretory activity. The glands cannot be distinguished from axillary eccrine sweat glands of the normhidrotic individual. Axillary hyperhidrosis is seen in whites, blacks, and Asians and has been reported in most, if not all, areas of the world.

The onset of axillary hyperhidrosis is typically postpubertal, usually occurring between the ages of 14 and 17. Axillary eccrine sweating normally begins just before or at puberty, unlike eccrine sweating on most other skin surfaces, including the palms and soles, which starts shortly after birth. Characteristically, typical of eccrine sweat, it is clear or watery (Fig. 1) and not turbid, opalescent, or occasionally colored as is apocrine sweat. Moreover, careful visualization defines the points of origin of individual droplets as nonfollicular, consistent with their eccrine origin.

The quantities of sweat in axillary hyperhidrosis can be dramatically excessive. In most patients, clothing is stained with the moisture after 15–30 min active sweating due to emotional

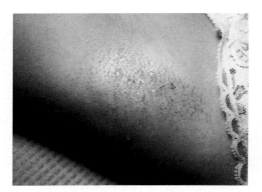

Figure 1 Axillary hyperhidrosis. Clear, watery sweat droplets appearing after mental activity.

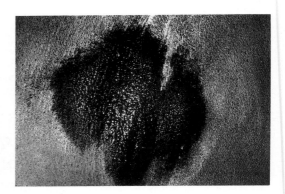

Figure 2 Axillary sweating pattern: starch-iodine colorimetric technique for demonstration of active sweating loci. Where sweating is most active, pooling of blue-black droplets is seen.

or mental excitation. As much as 2000 mg can be produced in a single axilla within 5 min. No mere cosmetic problem, it can alter a patient's life so that work is impaired or modified markedly, and social activities become difficult or are simply avoided. This problem can be costly, since clothes must be dry cleaned more frequently or discarded because of the stains. Axillary hyperhidrosis is defined as sweating in an axilla exceeding 125 mg/5 min measured gravimetrically. Not all patients with a rate of sweating this high complain of clinical wetness, since some simply tolerate the problem. Women are more likely to find this sweating distressing, and some with rates below 125 mg/5 min seek professional help for the problem. Because of the variance of concern among patients, the prevalence of axillary hyperhidrosis has never been precisely established. It is not uncommon, however, to which a billion dollar commercial antiperspirant industry readily attests. Moreover, surveys of dry cleaning establishments indicate that at least 25% of all garments cleaned are heavily stained in the underarm areas, typical of hyperhidrosis. The concurrence of axillary and volar (palmoplantar) hyperhidrosis is common, although each may exist separately.

Because it is an eccrine disorder, axillary hyperhidrosis does not normally coexist with axillary bromhidrosis. Excessive amounts of eccrine sweat wash away odor-producing apocrine sweat, preventing its accumulation on the axillary skin and hair. It is virtually axiomatic that patients complaining of axillary odor do not have axillary hyperhidrosis. Patients with axillary odor rarely have gravimetric sweating rates above 50 mg/5 min, and their sweating patterns are distinctively different.

Seasonal variation in axillary sweating rates is not marked, although, in general, eccrine glands are conditioned by heat. They secrete earlier and at higher rates under hot ambient conditions. Patients with axillary hyperhidrosis notice little or no difference in sweating rates in winter and summer, however, and many are less bothered in the summer when open or lighter-weight apparel permits more evaporative loss of sweat. Clearly this sweating is not induced by ambient or metabolic heat.

It should be emphasized that not only is the axillary sweating diurnal, beginning on awakening (coincident with the onset of mental activity), but it is also generally continuous, varying only moderately through the day. If a particularly intense emotional stimulation is experienced, however, sweating rates sharply increase and then recede as the stimulation subsides. During sleep, sweating decreases dramatically or ceases completely.

Commercial antiperspirants, with the exception of 20% aluminum chloride hexahydrate in anhydrous ethanol, applied under occlusion during sleep, are ineffective in these patients. Moreover, there is usually little or no relief from ataractic or anticholinergic medications.

Sweating Patterns

When one is examining patients with axillary hyperhidrosis, axillary sweating patterns can be evaluated by one of several colorimetric techniques to visualize eccrine sweat. The method used most commonly is the Minor technique, involving iodine and starch. This provides a topographic, semiquantitative determination of the axillary sweating response. It permits an estimate of the sweating rate and a delineation of the glandular loci from which the sweat derives. A solution of 3% iodine, 3% potassium iodide in 95% ethyl alcohol is painted on the shaved axillae and allowed to dry. Corn starch powder is dusted over the painted areas. Sweat droplets appear at ductal orifices and solubilize the iodine, which reacts with the starch to produce a blue-black color at each sweat pore. Where sweating is most active, the droplets become confluent (Fig. 2), and puddles of bluish sweat are noted at sites with high rates of sweating.

Studies of axillary sweating patterns in patients with hyperhidrosis as well as normal controls reveal that eccrine sweating is not diffuse and even across the axilla. Also, it is not necessarily most active in the center or dome of the vault. There is considerable variation from person to person to the point of being individually unique, much like a fingerprint. Furthermore, the pattern is consistently reproducible, varying only in degree with the intensity of stimulation. These constant, individual sweating patterns reflect the regular responsiveness of identifiable groups of glands to emotional, mental, or sensory stimuli. This forms the rationale for the Hurley–Shelley axillary resection technique and others to be discussed later that require preliminary mapping of the axillary sweating patterns. It should be noted that thermally induced sweating patterns differ from those of emotional induction in that the former involve more marginal glands, that is, those of thoracic or brachial areas outside the hairy axilla.

In most hyperhidrotic patients, one or two, and occasionally three, loci of high rates of sweating can be defined in the axilla (Fig. 3). The areas may vary in size, shape, and location, measuring from 2 to 6 cm in diameter. Smaller satellite loci of sweating may also be noted. The largest locus is most often in the center or dome of the axilla but may also be found at either end of the axilla. In exceptional cases a diffuse pattern of sweating over the entire axilla can be seen, but even in such patients, pooling of sweat on the blue-black background will delineate one or two areas that are the most active. Axillary sweating patterns are different qualitatively and quantitatively on opposite sides. While the right axilla usually exceeds the left in sweat secretion, this asymmetry is not based on right- or left-handedness. The cortical center for sweating is not necessarily in the dominant cerebral hemisphere. The difference quantitatively in sweating from opposing axillae is usually small but may at times be extreme. We have seen surgically treated patients with hyperhidrosis in one axilla and hypohidrosis or near anhidrosis in the other.

Patterns of sweating in axillary hyperhidrosis do not follow the distribution of apocrine glands in the axilla. Apocrine glands are characteristically densest in the center of the axilla and are smaller and less numerous peripherally and at the poles. This distribution is evidence against proposals identifying apocrine glands as the source of excessive secretion in axillary hyperhidrosis.

Medical Treatment

Some patients can accept greater sweating activity and its consequences psychologically as well as physically more readily than can others. It is regrettable that many patients with axillary hyperhidrosis do not consult dermatologists or other physicians for treatment. They live with the

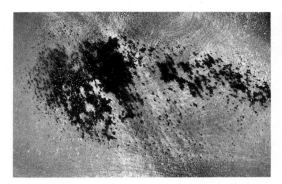

Figure 3 Axillary sweating patterns: starch-iodine colorimetric technique. Note demarcation of loci of most active sweating.

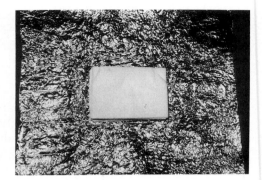

Figure 4 Tared collection pads used for gravimetric determination of eccrine sweating. Webril or gauze pads, preweighed, are placed in axilla for a 5-min period of mentally induced sweating and then weighed again to determine axillary sweating rate.

problem, convinced that the failure of modern commercial antiperspirants leaves them without any other recourse. Many physicians outside the field of dermatology do not realize that successful treatment is available.

Patients with axillary hyperhidrosis deserve a trial with one of several medical approaches before surgical management is recommended. The most effective and best-tolerated method is the topical application of 20% aluminum chloride hexahydrate in anhydrous ethanol (Drysol) under occlusion at bedtime. Some patients find this formulation irritating, but, if effective, it can be used indefinitely. There is little risk of allergic sensitization or toxicity.

The administration of systemic medications, such as anticholinergics or calcium channel blockers, is generally ill-advised for long periods of time. Some of these drugs, especially the anticholinergics, suppress sweating only at dosages that produce unpleasant side effects. A possible special use of systemic anticholinergics is in the initial phases of use of the topical aluminum chloride technique cited above, when 2–3 days' dosage of glycopyrrolate or its equivalent inhibits axillary sweating enough to prevent the aluminum chloride from being washed away from the sweat pores. While propoxyphene is reportedly suppressive in some patients with spinal sweating and clonidine is helpful in some patients with gustatory hyperhidrosis, neither drug has been evaluated in axillary hyperhidrosis and should not be used on a long-term basis.

Topical anticholinergics suppress axillary sweating in some normohidrotic individuals but are not similarly suppressive in hyperhidrotic patients. They also carry the risk of side effects, especially in patients with undiagnosed glaucoma or prostatic hypertrophy. Topical anesthetics have also been used to inhibit axillary eccrine sweating but are not as effective as aluminum chloride hexahydrate in anhydrous ethanol. Tap water iontophoresis and biofeedback or behavioral therapy should also be considered as alternatives to surgical treatment.

Surgical Treatment

Until the early 1960s, axillary hyperhidrosis was managed surgically by thoracic sympathectomy. While this is effective for palmar hyperhidrosis, it is not routinely helpful for axillary hyperhidrosis, usually because the fifth thoracic autonomic ganglion is not included or because anatomic variations preclude complete denervation of the axillary skin.

Side effects such as Horner's syndrome and a distressing compensatory hyperhidrosis (thermal, emotional, or gustatory) of other areas, notably the trunk, may occur after sympathectomy.

Therefore, sympathectomy is not recommended for axillary hyperhidrosis. Only in patients with combined palmar and axillary hyperhidrosis is it now indicated. An upper thoracic sympathectomy, which removes the second and third thoracic ganglia, controls the palmar hyperhidrosis of these patients, and local (axillary) ablative surgery is recommended for their axillary hyperhidrosis.

Local Axillary Surgical Treatment

Women who undergo radical mastectomy with extensive axillary dissection to remove lymph nodes and breast tissue in the axillary tail of Spence detect appreciable reduction or cessation of axillary sweating on that side. The effect is permanent and obviates the need for antiperspirants. While this effect has been known for years, these observations did not stimulate the development of local surgical techniques to control axillary hyperhidrosis until the early 1960s, when Skoog and Thyresson and Hurley and Shelley independently described the first two procedures for this condition.

The Skoog-Thyresson technique does not involve mapping of sweat patterns. The goal is to inactivate all glands across an axilla. Carefully placed incisions permit reflection of skin flaps for dissection of the sweat gland layer over the entire axilla. This results in marked reduction in sweating. Residual sweating can be eradicated by smaller localized procedures.

The Hurley-Shelley operation is based on identification of the most active sweating loci by mapping out sweating patterns, as described above. Surgery is tailored to fit the sweating pattern. Since the pattern of axillary sweating is constant and reproducible in a given axilla, this tissue can be selectively ablated.

Most patients can be treated satisfactorily with the Hurley-Shelley procedure. Those with extreme hyperhidrosis and axillary sweating rates greater than 2000 mg/5 min with diffuse sweating over the entire axilla may require the Skoog-Thyresson operation or total excision of the axilla, as in the Bretteville-Jensen procedure. Many modifications of these procedures have been described (Table 1). Cryosurgical removal of axillary sweat glands through a small incision has also been utilized. Some have advocated the use of subcutaneous tissue shavers, liposuction, or curettage removal of sweat glands through skin incisions, but the efficacy of these methods has been questioned.

In the Hurley-Shelley operation, the patient is informed that there should be 70–90% reduction in sweating following surgery. Details of the procedure, the postoperative period, and possible complications are discussed. The medical history should include questions about bleeding tendency, platelet disorder, hypofibrinogenemia, or other hematologic diatheses. Other pertinent information such as keloid formation and reactions to medications (specifically antibiotics) should be ascertained. An informed consent form should be signed and witnessed.

Examination of the patient preoperatively should include both gravimetric measurement of the axillary sweating, using tared sweat collection pads (Fig. 4), and axillary sweating patterns. The

Table 1 Surgical Treatment of Axillary Hyperhidrosis

Selective glandular removal based on sweating patterns
  Hurley–Shelley procedure
  Eldh–Fogdestam operation (M or W excision)
Broad glandular removal across axilla: no preliminary sweating patterns
  Skoog–Thyresson technique
  Bretteville–Jensen (Z-plasty)
  Total excision of axilla
  Subcutaneous tissue shavers
  Curettage removal through skin incisions
  Cryosurgical ablation

pattern should be drawn or photographed during the initial examinations and compared with a second pattern prepared just prior to the operation, when the patient should be anxious. This ensures adequate emotional stimulation and a marked sweating response. Mental stimulation or pain production may also be used to stimulate axillary sweating. The areas of greatest sweating are marked with a sterile dye.

The author recommends that this operation be performed in the hospital. Preoperative laboratory studies include a complete blood count, serum chemistry tests, a chest x-ray, and electrocardiogram done as an outpatient procedure within 7–10 days of the operation. The patient may be admitted in the morning on the day of surgery. Preoperative preparation includes shaving the axillary hair and two cleansings of the axillary skin, 6–12 hr apart, with a germicidal soap or detergent. Sedatives and anticholinergics are avoided until after the sweat patterns are obtained immediately before the operation because these drugs alter the sweat rate significantly. Local anesthesia is obtained with 1–2% lidocaine or mepivacaine without epinephrine infiltrated superficially into or just below the dermis along the marked excision lines. If necessary, sedation or light general anesthesia may be administered after the sweat patterns have been established. Most patients require, at most, a mild ataractic sedative such as hydroxyzine 100 mg intramuscularly.

The operation is performed with the patient in the supine position and the axilla exposed with the arm extended and flexed at the elbow and the hand placed under the head. This is also the position used to obtain the preoperative sweat patterns. Be aware of possible brachial plexus injury, particularly when general anesthesia or deep sedation is used and when both axillae are operated on simultaneously.

The Hurley–Shelley procedure involves a fusiform excision, transversely oriented, to remove the center of each sweating locus based on the starch-iodine test. This is followed by undermining on each side of each excision to reflect lateral flaps and permit resection of sweat glands on the undersurface of the dermis to the limits of each locus of sweating. The primary excision usually measures 5–6 cm in length and 1.5–2.5 cm in width at its midpoint (Fig. 5). Depending on the size and shape of the sweating loci, the excisions may occasionally be directed obliquely across the axilla. Transverse orientation is preferred, however, to minimize longitudinal contracture of the scar that could inhibit abduction of the limb. Undermining laterally is done just below the dermis for 2–4 cm on each side, depending on the sweating pattern.

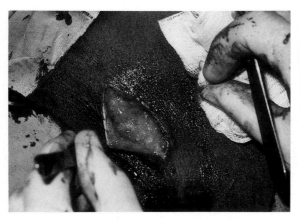

Figure 5   Hurley–Shelley operation for axillary hyperhidrosis. Elliptical excision of primary sweating locus.

In the subdermal glandular resection, the skin is reflected over the fingertip so that sweat gland lobules can be carefully resected with fine-curved scissors (Fig. 6a). While the eccrine glands are not grossly visible, apocrine gland lobules are, and these lobules must be visualized and resected. Since the eccrine glands are closely intermixed with or adjacent to the apocrine glands, this resection ensures removal of most of the eccrine glands. Trimming the undersurface too closely should be avoided so that as many hair follicles as possible are preserved. This contrasts with some techniques that stress close stripping of the dermal undersurface with a safety razor. Although hair follicle removal, especially in female patients, may be desirable, I believe that damage to hair follicles should be minimized to avoid damage to the deep dermal plexus, which may compromise flap survival.

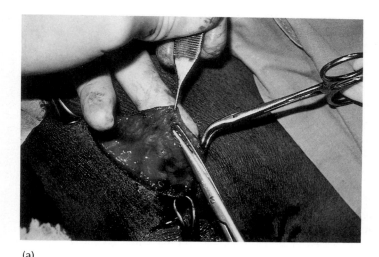

(a)

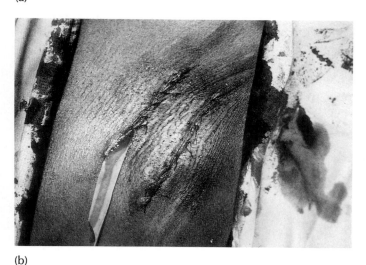

(b)

Figure 6 Hurley–Shelley operation for axillary hyperhidrosis. (a) Subdermal resection of sweat gland lobules on undersurface of flaps on each side of sweating locus. (b) Sutured wounds (with drain in one wound) at completion of operation.

Additional minor areas of sweating are treated with excisions that vary in size based on the sweating pattern, with proportionately less undermining and subdermal glandular resection. When more than one area is ablated, undermining should not overlap. This leaves some skin between the wounds not traumatized to ensure adequate blood supply for wound healing in the axilla.

Hemostasis is essential and must be established before closure. Electrocoagulation or suture ligature of clamped vessels will control major sources of bleeding. Moderate pressure may be applied for 5–10 min to arrest small vessel bleeding. Drains (1/4–3/8" wide) are placed if there is uncertainty about hemostasis, but these are usually unnecessary. Deep sutures to obliterate dead space are unnecessary since proper skin suturing and postoperative pressure dressings serve this purpose. This author prefers vertical mattress sutures with 5-0 nylon or silk for skin closure (Fig. 6b). Skin edges should be precisely approximated using skin hooks at each end of the wound.

Pressure dressings are applied directly over each wound, with the pressure directed upward toward the apex of the axilla. A gauze dressing may also be tied in place with retention sutures. Patients are advised to keep their arms at their sides for 48 hr postoperatively. Half of the skin sutures are removed in 6–7 days and the balance at 10–12 days. Normal activity can be resumed 2–3 days postoperatively except for work or exercise that involves raising the arms above the head. Abduction of the arms is avoided for 3 weeks, and then a graduated program of exercise is begun.

A side effect of this procedure is increased axillary odor, usually noticed within 2 days of the operation. The reduction in eccrine sweating permits retention of odorogenic apocrine sweat that is normally washed away by the excessive perspiration. Deodorants may be used as soon as the wounds are healed. Topical gentamicin can be used while sutures are in place for a deodorant effect.

The Hurley–Shelley operation results in sweat reduction of approximately 70–90%. The removal of skin and contained sweat glands by excision alone significantly reduces eccrine sweating. The additional reduction resulting from resection of glands from the dermal undersurface of the flaps usually brings the swelling rate down to acceptably low levels. Thus a preoperative sweating rate of 500 mg/5 min is normally decreased to between 50 and 100 mg/5 min or lower. Diminished sweating is also evident in postoperative sweating patterns (Fig. 7). Results of this degree have been achieved in 90–95% of patients in our series, but a few may require a second operation. Sweating patterns will reveal residual active loci of sweating, and they can be readily ablated using the same basic surgical approach on a smaller scale. It is not necessary to perform surgery beyond a second minor procedure.

Results from the operation are permanent. Examination 6–24 months later has shown no change from the postoperative sweating patterns. Results are best assessed at 6–8 weeks postoperatively, when edema and inflammation have subsided.

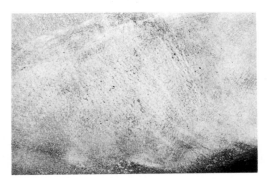

Figure 7   Postoperative sweating patterns (compare with Figs. 2,3).

Topical aluminum or zirconium antiperspirant preparations can be used to reduce axillary sweating after surgery. Aluminum chloride hexahydrate, 6.25% in anhydrous ethanol (Xerac AC) applied at bedtime without occlusion is the most satisfactory nonocclusive approach. Occlusion with polyvinylidine (Saran wrap) or polyethylene (Handiwrap) can be used for a greater antiperspirant effect. An axillary deodorant effect is also noted with this treatment along with the diminution of sweating.

Scars resulting from this operation are characteristically soft and pliable and do not inhibit mobility of the arms. Keloids may occur but must be rare in the axilla, and they have not developed in our series of patients. Infection or hematoma is uncommon, as for most dermatologic surgery, if care is given to operative details. One problem that occurs occasionally, 1–2 weeks after the operation, is a retrograde lymphangitis of a major brachial lymphatic vessel. A cordlike thickening is noted extending from the lower, brachial pole of the axilla down the arm. It may feel like a tendon or vein to the patient. This resolves without treatment in about 3 weeks and results in no permanent sequelae. Compensatory hyperhidrosis at another location, a common complication of sympathectomy, does not occur after this procedure.

A completely dry axilla is not expected and is probably undesirable because of frictional irritation that might occur with normal movement of the arms. The objective is a reduction of sweating to levels compatible with work and social activities without appreciable wetting of undergarments. Topical antiperspirants may still be necessary in some patients and are useful also for their deodorant effect.

APOCRINE BROMHIDROSIS

Bromhidrosis means excessive or abnormal body odor and includes both apocrine and eccrine varieties (Table 2). Apocrine bromhidrosis is far more common and is the only form for which local surgery may be indicated.

Table 2 Types of Bromhidrosis

Apocrine
Axillary
Eccrine
Keratinogenic
Plantar
Intertriginous
Metabolic
Heritable aminoacidurias
Phenylketonuria
Maple syrup urine disease
Oasthouse syndrome
Methionine malabsorption syndrome
Hypermethionemia
Isovaleric acidemia
n-Butyric/*n*-Hexanoic acidemia
Trimethylaminuria
Exogenous
Foods
Drugs
Chemicals

Reprinted with permission from Hurley HJ. Apocrine glands. In *Dermatology in General Medicine*. TB Fitzpatrick et al., eds. McGraw-Hill, New York, 1987, p. 705.

Epidemiology, Causes, and Clinical Features

Apocrine bromhidrosis occurs only in the axilla, since it is the only site where there are a large number of actively functioning apocrine glands. Like all apocrine disorders, apocrine bromhidrosis does not occur until puberty or thereafter when the apocrine glands begin secretion. Blacks have the largest and most active apocrine glands, while eastern Asians have the least active; these races represent the extremes in frequency of apocrine bromhidrosis.

Some apocrine odor is expected in all individuals with axillary apocrine glandular function. When the odor is excessive or qualitatively distinctive, the diagnosis of bromhidrosis can be made. Apocrine sweat is the only cutaneous secretion or breakdown product whose degradation yields the classic acrid axillary odor. This is the result of bacterial action on apocrine sweat, which is odorless and sterile when it first appears on the skin surface. Aerobic diphtheroids generate the most common odor, while micrococci produce a different, less offensive smell. Short-chain fatty acids and ammonia are the major odorogens resulting from bacterial breakdown. Certain androgenic steroidal compounds with odors similar to natural axillary odor may be important also. Unusual odors reflect individual variation in the composition of apocrine sweat. Thus, odors described as rancid, musty, pungent, fecal, sour, and sweet may be encountered. Factors that intensify axillary odor and apocrine bromhidrosis are poor bathing habits and the presence of axillary hair on which apocrine sweat can be retained. Concurrent axillary eccrine hyperhidrosis usually prevents significant apocrine bromhidrosis, because excessive quantities of eccrine sweat wash away odorogenic apocrine sweat.

The diagnosis of apocrine bromhidrosis is made clinically. It is essential to confirm its presence; however, bromhidrosiphobia, which is usually indicative of impending schizophrenia, should be excluded. Moreover, temporal lobe tumors may produce olfactory hallucinations. A neurologic examination is indicated in patients who complain of body odor but have none discernible by the examiner.

Treatment

In most patients, apocrine bromhidrosis is satisfactorily managed by nonsurgical methods to remove excessive apocrine sweat from the axilla or reduce axillary microflora. Thorough cleansing with an antibacterial soap, shaving of axillary hair, and application of a topical antibacterial agent are helpful. Commercial aluminum, zirconium, or zinc formulations and topical antibiotics such as neomycin, gentamicin, and clindamycin are effective deodorants. Absorption of odorogens with ion-exchange resins or powders or masking the odor with perfumes is less helpful. Systemic antibiotics generally do not suppress axillary odor.

The most effective topical deodorant is aluminum chloride hexahydrate in ethanol applied at bedtime, as described for the management of axillary hyperhidrosis. Its eccrine antiperspirant action is also helpful, but in apocrine bromhidrosis aluminum chloride is acting as an antibacterial. A weaker concentration (Xerac AC, 6.25%) may be tried first, but the stronger concentration (Drysol, 20%) is often necessary for more severe forms of apocrine bromhidrosis.

Surgical treatment of apocrine bromhidrosis is rarely necessary. When it is required, however, either of the two techniques described for axillary hyperhidrosis (the Skoog–Thyresson operation or the Hurley–Shelley operation and their variants) may be used. Rather than outline patterns of high-eccrine activity, an effort is made to remove as many apocrine sweat glands as possible through a fusiform excision in the center of the axilla and subdermal resection of glands. Smaller procedures may be done at the thoracic and brachial poles of the axilla to remove additional apocrine glands. Since the largest and most active apocrine glands are located in the center or dome of the axilla and glandular density, size, and activity decrease toward the axillary poles and the periphery, this surgery markedly decreases the amount of apocrine sweating and thus controls bromhidrosis.

HIDRADENITIS SUPPURATIVA

Hidradenitis suppurativa is a distinctive inflammatory disorder of apocrine gland–bearing skin. Inflammatory and pustular in its earliest stages, it is chronic and cicatrizing in its late recurrent forms. It is a painful, at times disabling, disease causing high morbidity. Moreover, it is misdiagnosed and mismanaged commonly and may involve several different medical specialists including the dermatologist, plastic surgeon, general surgeon, gynecologist, urologist, proctologist, and family practitioner. Hidradenitis suppurativa is a disease clearly made more troublesome and recalcitrant by delaying definitive surgical treatment when it is indicated. Although hidradenitis suppurativa was described and attributed to a disturbance of the apocrine glands in the early nineteenth century, clinical study of the disease did not take place until almost 100 years later.

Epidemiology

The prevalence of hidradenitis suppurativa has never been precisely established. It is not a common disorder, but it is by no means rare and is undoubtedly underdiagnosed. Axillary, mammary, and inguinal hidradenitis suppurativa is more common in women, but perianal disease occurs more frequently in men. Blacks and whites are both affected, while Asians do not appear to develop it as often.

Pathogenesis

The most striking evidence in favor of apocrine gland participation in hidradenitis suppurativa is its peculiar localization to apocrine gland–bearing skin areas. In order of frequency of involvement, these are the axillae, inguinal, perianal, mammary, buttock, abdominal, chest, scalp, and eyelid skin. End-stage hidradenitis suppurativa is difficult to distinguish from other cicatrizing, sinus tract–producing diseases, including acne.

The essential role of the apocrine glands in hidradenitis suppurativa has been disputed in recent years. Experimental reproduction of the disease by Shelley and Cahn in 1960 using adhesive tape occlusion of normal axillary skin suggested that the earliest pathologic event in hidradenitis suppurativa is apocrine sweat retention, secondary to keratinous ductal occlusion. Rupture of the apocrine glandular system at the tubular or proximal ductal level follows, with entrapped apocrine sweat and bacteria spilling into the surrounding dermis and subcutaneous tissue. However, careful histopathologic studies fail to confirm apocrine involvement in many specimens, and lesions typical of hidradenitis suppurativa may be found in skin areas devoid of apocrine glands. Additional microscopic analysis indicates that small cystic changes commonly arising from follicles are the most important early lesions in hidradenitis. Such cysts form and eventually become inflamed, probably secondary to a folliculitis, which is commonly induced by frictional trauma, as stressed below. If apocrine glands are present and are in the vicinity of the cystic lesions, they can be involved in the inflammatory process. It is well to recall that the apocrine ductal orifice is superficially located, immediately subjacent to the follicular pore, well above the sebaceous glands and ducts that lie along the midshaft of the hair. With follicular inflammation and cyst formation, which are probably the vital pathogenetic developments, apocrine gland involvement is inevitable if such glands are present. Spread of infection and inflammation to adjacent tissue and glands results in an expanding abscess and, eventually, fibrosis and sinus tract formation. With recurrent chronic disease, there is increased scarring and sinus tract formation and often persistent low-grade inflammation, with or without drainage. Clinical flares are marked by acute inflammation, infection, and suppurativa.

Thus, based on current information, hidradenitis suppurativa is best regarded as a follicular disorder with cyst formation, and not a primary alteration of the apocrine glands. A number of pathogenetic factors have been considered in the development or recrudesence of the disease and are worthy of discussion.

Local Frictional Trauma

A common, indeed the usual, incitant in hidradenitis suppurativa is local frictional trauma produced by the rubbing of opposing or redundant skin folds or tight-fitting clothing, such as brassieres or panty hose, or athletic equipment. The local edema and inflammation produced may result in portal and ductal occlusion, cystic change and rupture, and abscess formation typical of the disease. Epithelial encapsulation results in large cyst formation and eventually inflammation and rupture as the process repeats itself. If apocrine glands are present, they may become involved but can be spared. It is likely that a preliminary pustular folliculitis represents the primary lesion in the pathogenesis of hidradenitis (see below) with cysts, sinus tracts, and scarring sequential developments. Yu and Cook have identified these changes histologically, emphasizing that apocrine involvement is not essential in the genesis of hidradenitis suppurativa.

Folliculitis

Subtle or obvious bacterial folliculitis can be found in almost all areas of hidradenitis suppurativa (Fig. 8) at some time. The importance of folliculitis in pathogenesis has been stressed above. It is important to realize that most such folliculitic lesions usually regress without incident, but some persist and extend more deeply to result in the classical alterations of hidradenitis suppurativa.

Specific Bacteria

Various bacteria (notably staphylococci, streptococci, and *E. coli* in early lesions and *Proteus* species in chronic, recurrent hidradenitis suppurativa) have been isolated, but their relationship is unclear. They may be essential to ductal occlusion, as in eccrine miliaria, or simply part of concomitant bacterial folliculitis. Certainly bacteria produce most of the inflammation once the disease process has begun, as well as in its late stages. Anaerobes and unusual species, such as *Streptococcus milleri*, derived from the bowel and found in anogenital hidradenitis suppurativa may also be present. To state that hidradenitis suppurativa is caused by any bacterial species and thus suggest that antibacterial therapy is curative is not justified by our experience to date.

Associated Acne

Contrary to popular belief, acne is not a sine qua non of hidradenitis suppurativa. Over half of these patients, especially women and those with axillary involvement alone, have no acne, whether active or quiescent. Only a small percentage of patients, usually those with chronic multiple site disease, have had an active pilonidal sinus or cicatrizing folliculitis of the scalp.

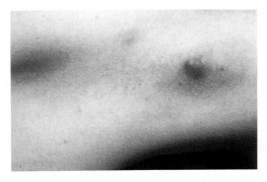

Figure 8   Hidradenitis suppurativa folliculitis in the axilla.

Associated Systemic Disease

These patients are usually healthy. No systemic disease has been associated with hidradenitis suppurativa. While obesity is common in patients with hidradenitis suppurativa, it is not found routinely. Diabetes mellitus is not seen more frequently in patients with hidradenitis suppurativa, but impaired glucose tolerance has been noted.

Hormonal Factors

Pubertal or postpubertal onset of hidradenitis suppurativa and premenstrual exacerbations suggest an endocrine influence that is as yet unidentified. Pregnancy may result in amelioration of hidradenitis suppurativa, but much less regularly than it does Fox-Fordyce disease. A recent study suggested a functional disturbance of the hypothalamopituitary axis in some patients with hidradenitis suppurativa, but this has not been confirmed.

Genetic Predisposition

Reports of familial cases suggest a genetic predisposition. HLA antigen frequencies do not differ from those in the normal population.

Defective Immune Response

Humoral and cell-mediated immunity appears to be normal, and there is no deficit in phagocytic function or any other known local defense mechanism. Some patients with severe hidradenitis suppurativa appear to have a significant reduction in circulating T lymphocytes.

Local Eccrine Sweating

In patients with hidradenitis suppurativa, increased eccrine sweating in affected skin tends to aggravate existing lesions and precipitate the development of new ones. Patients with axillary hyperhidrosis show no increased incidence of hidradenitis suppurativa, so increased eccrine sweating alone is not enough to induce hidradenitis suppurativa.

Antiperspirant-Deodorant Formulations and Depilatories

Antiperspirants and deodorants containing aluminum or zirconium salts do not promote or aggravate hidradenitis suppurativa, with the possible exception of those in a stick or ointment base. The use of an aluminum chloride hexahydrate in anhydrous ethanol may actually be helpful. No special pathogenic significance can be attached to depilatories, and very few patients give a history of their antecedent use in affected areas.

Clinical Course

Hidradenitis suppurativa develops after puberty, usually in the second or third decade of life. Classically, early lesions are solitary, painful, erythematous abscesses (Fig. 9) in an area rich in apocrine glands. Often described as blind boils or inflamed pilar cysts, they ultimately rupture, draining purulent material. Healing with fibrosis results and is usually followed by recurrences in or near the original site. Sinus tracts eventually form with dense bridges of scar tissue (Fig. 10). When it is severe, such scarring can decrease mobility of a limb and may rarely produce lymphatic obstruction and edema. The majority of patients with early or advanced hidradenitis suppurativa have small follicular lesions in the affected areas. Some are clearly pustular, others simply erythematous and macular (Figs. 8,11,12). Cysts and comedones are noted in chronic hidradenitis suppurativa, but they are absent in early disease.

The axillae are involved most commonly in hidradenitis suppurativa and often are affected similarly. Involvement of more than one site including the inguinal, perianal, and breast skin is not uncommon, however. With extensive hidradenitis across an axilla, diminished apocrine sweating and reduction in the usual axillary odor are noted. Regional adenopathy is usually in-

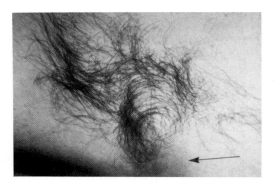

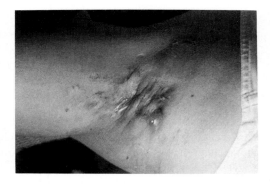

Figure 9 Stage I hidradenitis suppurativa. Solitary abscess in the axilla (arrow).

Figure 10 Recurrent hidradenitis suppurativa stage III, with dense scarring, sinus tracts, and acute abscess formation.

significant or absent. During the acute phase with abscess formation, there may be mild constitutional symptoms.

Untreated hidradenitis suppurativa is typically a relentlessly progressive disease. In the affected sites there is periodic abscess and sinus tract formation, marked scarring, interference with local lymphatic drainage, and decreased mobility of the affected limb. In the anal and inguinal regions, fistulous tracts may involve the rectum, urethra, and vagina. Anemia, interstitial keratitis, inflammatory arthritis, and secondary amyloidosis are also possible with severe chronic advanced disease. Occasionally the process may burn out but usually not until there is extensive fibrosis and tissue destruction and no remaining functional apocrine glands. Squamous cell carcinoma may develop in chronic lesions, especially those with ulceration.

Less than half of the patients with hidradenitis suppurativa also have acne of the face or trunk, while a smaller number have cicatrizing folliculitis of the scalp and a pilonidal sinus.

Histopathologic Findings and Laboratory Studies

Microscopic study of early lesions reveals keratinous obstruction of the distal apocrine duct with dilation and rupture of the subjacent apocrine tubule. Neutrophils are present within the tubule

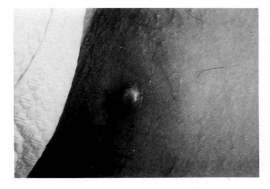

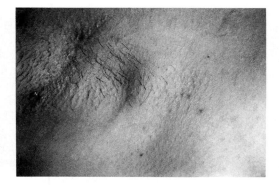

Figure 11 Prominent pustular folliculitis in hidradenitis suppurativa of axilla. Compare with Figure 8.

Figure 12 Stage II hidradenitis suppurativa. Multiple foci of activity, independent from one another and amenable to individual local surgical ablation.

before its rupture and afterwards in the surrounding dermis. Gram stain reveals bacteria within the neutrophils and extracellularly. A chronic lymphocytic infiltrate, granulation tissue, fibrosis, sinus tract formation, pseudoepitheliomatous hyperplasia, and obliteration of glandular elements occur as the disease progresses. While the early lesions of hidradenitis suppurativa are diagnostic, later the disease cannot be distinguished from severe acne or other disorders that cause chronic sinus tract formation.

Blood counts, blood chemistry tests, cell-mediated and immediate immune responsiveness, T-cell and B-cell levels, and routine endocrine assays are usually normal. Reports of abnormal hypothalamopituitary and T-cell response suggest the need for special study along these lines. Diabetes mellitus occurs with the same frequency as in the general population.

Smears and cultures from an acute abscess usually reveal coagulase-positive staphylococci, streptococci, and occasionally *E. coli. Streptococcus milleri* has been found in perianal lesions, but its significance is uncertain. Anaerobes are not commonly isolated. *Proteus* strains are regularly isolated from chronic recurrent disease, and with repeated courses of antibiotics more resistant strains emerge as the dominant organisms.

Treatment

Systemic antibiotics and topical therapy are ineffective once hidradenitis suppurativa shows evidence of progression or recurrence. Early solitary lesions may be treated by simple nonsurgical measures, but it is imperative to proceed surgically once reactivation or chronic recurrent hidradenitis suppurativa is recognized. This principle applies to patients with early unresponsive or recurrent hidradenitis suppurativa as well as those with more advanced disease.

In the axilla, it is convenient to approach treatment in a staged fashion (Table 3). Stage I, the initial manifestation of hidradenitis suppurativa, may be treated nonsurgically as follows. Intralesional triamcinolone (acetonide or diacetate suspension) is injected into the abscess. Distention of the inflamed abscess or tract with 5–10 mg triamcinolone suspension, diluted with saline, often results in involution within 12–24 hr. Incision and drainage of the abscess prior to the injection are avoided unless rupture is imminent.

Minocycline 100 mg twice daily should be given for 5–6 days or longer until the abscesses involute and should be maintained at 100 mg daily until all signs of inflammation are gone. This usually requires at least 2 weeks of antibiotic therapy but must be extended if necessary. Cephalosporins in the usual dosage for soft tissue infections are also effective. Drainage should be cultured and antibiotic sensitivities determined. Patients with slowly responsive or recalcitrant cases should be given antibiotics based on these findings.

Daily, gentle cleansing should be done with a germicidal soap. Warm compresses with saline or Burow's solution (1:40) are helpful during the acute stages. Topical antibiotics, such as

Table 3 Clinical Staging in Hidradenitis Suppurativa

Stage I
    Abscess formation, single or multiple, without sinus tracts and cicatrization
Stage II
    Recurrent abscesses with tract formation and cicatrization
    Single or multiple, widely separated lesions
Stage III
    Diffuse of near diffuse involvement, or multiple interconnected tracts and
        abscesses across entire area

2% clindamycin lotion, may be applied but are not very effective. They may be helpful for prophylaxis after surgical or adjunctive therapy.

Avoidance of tight-fitting garments that cause frictional trauma, such as T-shirts, body shirts, snug-fitting blouses or shirts, or straps from athletic equipment, is essential. In the groin, skin-tight blue jeans are a particular problem.

If a stage I lesion heals after conservative management with no recurrence, further therapy is not required. Careful, gentle cleansing and avoidance of tight-fitting clothing should be maintained. There is no restriction on the use of antiperspirants. Xerac AC (6.25% aluminum chloride hexahydrate) without occlusion may be used. It has a strong, local antibacterial and deodorant effect as well as an antiperspirant action. This provides prophylaxis against regional folliculitis and hidradenitis suppurativa.

At the first sign of recurrent hidradenitis suppurativa, surgical intervention is warranted. For unresponsive or recurrent stage I and stage II disease (Fig. 12), the following surgical approach is recommended.

Exteriorization

This technique is designed to destroy completely the hidradenitis tract and abscess and diseased epithelial tissue. Healing is by second intention, obliterating the defect with fibrosis. The scar may be depressed or irregular but is surprisingly smooth and insignificant in most instances. It has been called marsupialization by some observers, which is an inappropriate designation, since formation of a pouch is certainly to be avoided.

Preoperative preparation is routine, and local anesthesia is administered with lidocaine, 1–2%, or mepivacaine without epinephrine. Complete anesthesia may be difficult to obtain in larger fibrotic areas; therefore, supplemental analgesia, with meperidine 100 mg intramuscularly or general anesthesia, is sometimes necessary.

Where there is an opening in the tract, a soft probe can be inserted to guide the incision. Secondary tracts that emanate from the primary one should be probed as well. If tract openings are not detectable, an incision is made over the abscess and it is drained. The roof of the abscess or tract is then excised, exposing the interior of the lesion. In stage I lesions with little or no fibrosis and tract formation, palpation and visualization will reveal whether all the indurated disease tissue has been removed. Curettage is performed along the base of the entire lesion to remove granulation tissue and debris even from the smaller fibrotic pockets. Electrocoagulation of the sides and base of the wound is done both for hemostasis and to destroy residual necrotic epithelial and fibrotic tissue. In some instances, when the base of the wound is clean and free of deeply placed tracts, electrocoagulation is kept to a minimum. The wound may be quite large and irregularly shaped (Fig. 13). Upon completion of surgery, there is often an appreciable reduction or absence of pain. Pressure dressings are not required, but sterile petroleum jelly--impregnated gauze or Adaptic dressings are applied.

Postoperative care includes warm saline compresses applied twice daily for 15–20 min for 3–4 days, then decreased to alternate days. Antibiotic ointment can be applied under a light gauze dressing. The dressing can be omitted once the wound is dry and crusted. Healing takes 4–7 weeks, depending on the size and depth of the wound.

Exteriorization can be used on the axillary, inguinal, inframammary, suprapubic, and trunk skin, including the buttock. It is generally not used in the perianal region. While it should be applicable to that site as well, injury to the anal sphincter must be avoided. The scars produced are usually quite acceptable and become soft and increasingly pliable with time (Fig. 14).

Excision and Primary Closure

A sinus tract or fibrotic area may be sharply defined and limited in size, without irregular or poorly outlined tract extensions. In such instances, surgical excision of the entire area with pri-

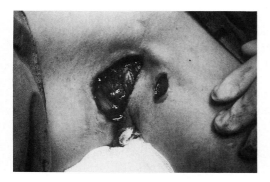

Figure 13 Exteriorization procedure for axillary hidradenitis suppurativa. After each tract is delineated with a soft probe or by visualization and palpation, it is incised. The tract roof is excised and curettage and electrocoagulation performed along the interior of the tract.

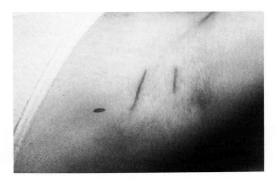

Figure 14 Postexteriorization scars of axilla. Patient had several tracts of hidradenitis suppurativa exteriorized surgically 6 months earlier.

mary closure may be used. If no residual disease has been missed, it produces a good result with minimal scarring. If there is any doubt about the complete removal of hidradenitis suppurativa, however, these areas are best left to heal by second intention. Generally, excision and closure is more likely to be complicated by recurrent disease than is exteriorization, and the former is only recommended for selected patients.

Total Excision

Eradication of stage III hidradenitis suppurativa usually requires total excision of the diseased region with closure utilizing flaps or grafts. In certain situations, such as involvement of the genital and perianal areas, closure or resurfacing may be best avoided, with healing by second intention aided by specialized dressings such as Silastic foam. In the axilla, total excision followed by transverse primary closure has been successful. Limited upward extension of the arm on the operated side is anticipated and at times is unacceptable. The use of flaps, including Z-plasty, balloon tissue expansion with flaps, and grafting techniques such as mesh grafts, split-thickness, and full-thickness grafts, are discussed elsewhere in this book. All these techniques may be useful in closing the remaining wound after removal of all the diseased tissue.

While results from total excision are very good and the disease is usually arrested, freedom from recurrence cannot be ensured. Moreover, proper skin care and avoidance of frictional trauma are important. Skin examination is recommended for several months before a cure can be assumed with certainty.

Other Modalities

Cryosurgery with liquid nitrogen for treatment of stage I lesions is an acceptable alternative and may result in minimal scarring.

Treatment with oral 13-*cis*-retinoic acid (Accutane) has been helpful in some patients but is normally used for recurrent or chronic disease rather than stage I hidradenitis suppurativa. The response is inconsistent (about 50% of cases respond) and not as dramatically effective as in cystic acne.

Spironolactone has been recommended for patients with chronic hidradenitis suppurativa. Its antiandrogen action may reduce the activity of hidradenitis suppurativa appreciably at times, but it is not regularly effective.

High-dosage corticosteroids (prednisone 60–80 mg daily) have been advocated to reduce inflammation in recurrent, extensive hidradenitis suppurativa. This is only adjunctive therapy to hasten involution of the acute changes. Other treatment, particularly surgery, must be undertaken.

Liposuction may also be helpful in certain obese patients in an effort to minimize the local frictional trauma produced by opposing skin surfaces or folds, especially in hidradenitis involving the upper medial thigh or lower abdominal fold. Although there are no reports of its efficacy, in principle it is worthy of consideration in the appropriate patient.

Radiation

The use of radiation for hidradenitis suppurativa has essentially been abandoned. Popular in the 1930s and 1940s, it has been supplanted by the treatments described above.

Conclusions

The management of hidradenitis suppurativa has improved but is far from perfect. Surgical eradication of lesions is necessary in all but the earliest forms of the disease. Clinical staging is useful to define and quantify appropriate treatment and response. Dermatologic care must be continued to avoid recurrences. The best chance for cure is by proper treatment of stage I or early stage II hidradenitis suppurativa. The need for early diagnosis and proper treatment cannot be overemphasized. Despite the best available treatment, hidradenitis suppurativa recurs in some patients.

FAMILIAL BENIGN PEMPHIGUS

Familial benign pemphigus or Hailey–Hailey disease was described by the Hailey brothers in 1939. It is an uncommon heritable eruption, primarily vesicular and often localized to crural areas. The pattern of inheritance is autosomal dominant, but the genetic mechanism is unknown. The histologic hallmark of familial benign pemphigus is acantholysis. It is distinguished from pemphigus and other acantholytic disorders by the presence of suprabasalar clefts, basal cell–lined villous projections into the blister space, and occasional dyskeratotic cells. Ultrastructurally, the defect is due to faulty cellular adhesion or an altered tonofilament–desmosome complex. (Although keratin profiles, as outlined by monoclonal antibody techniques, of uninvolved skin are normal, those of involved skin show a delayed suprabasal keratin expression probably secondary to acantholysis.) Sweat, various forms of local trauma, including patch testing for contact allergy, bacterial, candidal, and herpes simplex infections, are important in precipitating or aggravating the disease. Ultraviolet light induces acantholysis and can be used to diagnose the disease when it is in remission.

The consensus is that familial benign pemphigus is not a variant of Darier's disease, despite their histologic similarities. Differences in genetic profile, clinical presentation, and course justify a nosologic separation of the two diseases.

Clinical Features

Familial benign pemphigus usually appears in late adolescence or early adult years as clusters of crusted, erythematous, vesicular, or vesiculopustular lesions in crural areas, especially the neck, axillae, and groin (Fig. 15a). Perianal, inframammary, and antecubital skin may be involved less frequently. A recent clinical study suggested the diagnostic importance of asymptomatic longitudinal white bands in the fingernails, which were found in 38 of 50 patients examined. The disease is worse in summer months. Friction from clothing or opposing skinfolds, increased sweating and heat, or growth of microorganisms, notably staphylococci and *Candida* species, play major roles in exacerbating and prolonging the disease. Pruritus and burning pain are common. Large erosive areas become fissured with time. Unusual chronic variants may be hyperkeratotic, verrucous, neurodermatitic, and papular. Extension to portions of the trunk, especially the upper back and suprapubic area, may also occur. Remissions and exacerbations are the rule. Disease-free periods last from months to years; however, the disease tends to persist well into the later years of life. Mucosal lesions (mouth, larynx, esophagus, and vagina) occur rarely. In the anogenital area, verrucous papules must be distinguished histopathologically from viral verrucae.

Involvement of other organ systems has not been seen, and patients' general health is unaffected. During its active phase, familial benign pemphigus makes normal occupational and social activities difficult and causes considerable discomfort.

Diagnosis

The clinical features are usually characteristic. Histologic examination of skin with light and electron microscopy is diagnostic. There are no other laboratory abnormalities of importance. The differential diagnosis includes impetigo, pemphigus vulgaris, pemphigus foliaceus, pemphigus vegetans, keratosis follicularis (Darier's disease), and subcorneal pustular dermatosis.

Treatment

Nonsurgical

Systemic antibiotics are predictably effective therapy. Tetracycline, in daily dosages of 1–2 g initially and tapered to 250–500 mg for maintenance, is helpful during the first attack and early recurrences of the disease. Minocycline, erythromycin, and penicillin are also effective. Topical antibiotics such as clindamycin and erythromycin, in lotion or cream bases, are helpful less regularly, as are topical corticosteroids. The local application of cyclosporine has also been advocated. Systemic corticosteroids will suppress the disease if given in adequate doses but are not recommended for long-term use. Resistant cases may respond to dapsone 100–200 mg daily until clearing and then a maintenance dosage of 50–100 mg per day. Grenz radiation in weekly dosages of 300 rads for 3–4 weeks may also be helpful.

Surgical

When familial benign pemphigus is persistent locally in one area, and especially if it is resistant to other forms of treatment, surgical management should be considered. Dermabrasion is reportedly beneficial, as is carbon dioxide vaporization of lesions. However, the usual surgical approach is surgical excision of the affected area with skin grafting. Split-thickness grafts, usually of the thick type, are used to cover the defect (Fig. 15), although mesh grafts could be used in certain situations. Any affected area is amenable to this approach, and it has been used in the axillae, groin, scrotum, perineum, and perianal sites. Donor skin for the grafts is taken from normal, uninvolved sites such as the thigh. Generally there is no recurrence of the disease, although occasionally this has been observed within the grafted skin.

The success of surgical excision in familial benign pemphigus suggests that the areas typically involved have an intrinsic predisposition to the disease not shared by uninvolved skin of the graft donor sites. No pathogenetic role can as yet be assigned to the sweat glands, apocrine or eccrine, of the affected skin areas. The donor skin contains eccrine sweat glands, of course, and they will

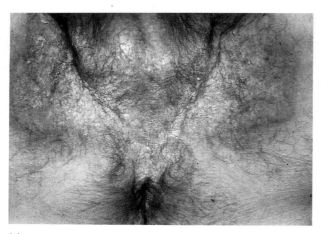

(a)

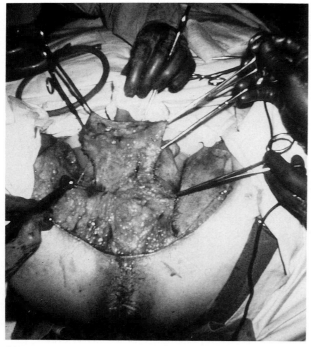

(b)

Figure 15   Familial benign pemphigus, inguinal: operative treatment. Sequential photographs showing (a) preoperative changes, (b) resection of diseased tissue, (c) placement of thick split-thickness grafts, and (d) healed postoperative state 6 months later showing no signs of recurrence. (Courtesy of Harold O. Perry, M.D.)

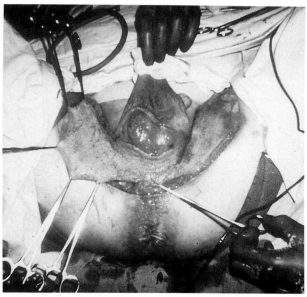

(c)

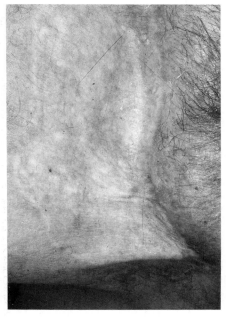

(d)

Figure 15 Continued

assume the functional responsiveness of sweat glands of the recipient site. Thus, eccrine sweat glands of the thigh transplanted in a graft to the axilla will then respond to emotional stimuli and probably also to thermal stimulation. Apparently such a functional change has not been responsible for recurrence of familial benign pemphigus in the graft.

BIBLIOGRAPHY

Ashby EC, William JL. Cryosurgery for axillary hyperhidrosis. *Br Med J* 1976;2:1173.

Bergman R, Levy R, Pam Z, Lichtig C, et al: A study of keratin expression in benign familial chronic pemphigus. *Am J Dermatopathol* 1992;14:32–36.

Bretteville-Jensen G, et al. Surgical treatment of axillary hyperhidrosis in 123 patients. *Acta Derm Venereol (Stockh)* 1975;55:73.

Burger SM. Hailey-Hailey disease: the clinical features, response to treatment and prognosis. *BJD* 1992;126:275–282.

Conway H, et al. Surgical treatment of chronic hidradenitis suppurativa. *Surg Gynecol Obstet* 1952;95:455–463.

Crotty CP, et al. Surgical treatment of familial benign chronic pemphigus. *Arch Dermatol* 1981;117:540.

Duller P, Gentry WD. Use of biofeedback in treating chronic hyperhidrosis. *Br J Dermatol* 1980;103:143.

Eldh J, Fogdestam I. The surgical treatment of hyperhidrosis axillae. *Scand J Plast Reconstr Surg* 1976;10:227.

Dvorak VC, et al. Host-defense mechanisms in hidradenitis suppurativa. *Arch Dermatol* 1977;113:450.

Fitzsimmons JS, et al. Evidence of genetic factors in hidradenitis suppurativa. *Br J Dermatol* 1985;113:1.

Harrison BJ, et al. Hidradenitis suppurativa: Evidence for an endocrine abnormality. *Br J Surg* 1985;72:1002.

Highet AS, et al. *Streptococcus milleri* causing treatable infection in perineal hidradenitis suppurativa. *Br J Dermatol* 1980;103:375.

Hurley HJ. Local surgical treatment of axillary hyperhidrosis. In *Skin Surgery*, 6th ed. E Epstein, E Epstein, Jr., eds. Philadelphia, WB Saunders, 1987, pp. 598–606.

Hurley HJ. Apocrine glands. In *Dermatology in General Medicine*, 3rd ed. Fitzpatrick, AZ Eisen, K Wolff, eds. New York, McGraw-Hill, 1987, pp. 704–717.

Hurley HJ, Shelley WB. A simple surgical approach to the management of axillary hyperhidrosis. *JAMA* 1963;186:109.

Hurley HJ, Shelley WB. Axillary hyperhidrosis. Clinical features and local surgical management. *Br J Dermatol* 1966;78:127.

Inaba M, et al. Radical operation to stop axillary odor and hyperhidrosis. *Past Reconstr Surg* 1978;62:355.

Jemec B. Abrasio axillae in hyperhidrosis. *Scand J Plast Reconstr Surg* 1975;9:44.

Jitsukuwa K, Ring J, Weyer U, et al. Topical cyclosporine in chronic benign familial pemphigus. *J Am Acad Dermatol* 1992;27:625–626.

Juhlin L, Rollman O. Vascular effects of a local anesthetic mixture in atopic dermatitis. *Acta Derm Venereol (Stockh)* 1984;64:439.

Kartamaa M, Reitamo S. Familial benign chronic pemphigus (Hailey-Hailey disease). Treatment with carbon dioxide laser vaporization. *Arch Drematol* 1992;128:646–648.

Kirtschig G, Gieler U, Happle R. Treatment of Hailey-Hailey disease by dermabrasion. *J Am Acad Dermatol* 1993;28:784–786.

Landes VE, Kapesser HJ. Zur operativen Behandlung der hyperhidrosis Axillaris. *Fortschr Med* 1979;97:2169.

Langenber A, Berger TG, Cardelli M, et al. Genital benign chronic pemphigus (Hailey-Hailey disease) presenting as condylomas *J Am Acad Dermatol* 1992;26:951–955.

Leach RD et al. Anaerobic axillary abscess. *Br Med J* 1979;2:5.

Levit F. Simple device for treatment of hyperhidrosis by iontophoresis. *Arch Dermatol* 1968;98:505.

Morgan WP, et al. A comparison of skin grafting and healing by granulation following axillary excision for hidradenitis suppurativa. *Ann R Coll Surg Engl* 1983;65:235.

O'Loughlin S, et al. Hidradenitis suppurativa: Glucose tolerance, clinical, microbiologic and immunologic features and HLA frequencies in 27 patients. *Arch Dermatol* 1988;124:1043.

Paletta FX. Hidradenitis suppurativa: Pathologic study and use of skin flaps. *Plast Reconstr Surg* 1963; 31:307.

Peppeatt T, Keefe M, White JE. Hailey-Hailey disease-exacerbation by herpes simplex virus and patch tests. *Clin Exp Dermatol* 1992;17:201.

Pollock WJ, et al. Axillary hidradenitis suppurativa. A simple and effective surgical technique. *Plast Reconstr Surg* 1972;49:22.

Rasmussen SS et al. Management of massive perianal hidradenitis suppurativa. *Ann Plast Surg* 1985;15:218.

Rosner IA, et al. Spondyloarthropathy associated with hidradenitis suppurativa and acne conglobata. *Ann Intern Med* 1982;97:520.

Shelley WB, Cahn MM. Pathogenesis of hidradenitis suppurativa in man. Experimental and histologic observations. *Arch Dermatol* 1955;72:562.

Skoog T, Thyresson N. Hyperhidrosis of the axillae. A method of surgical treament. *Acta Chir Scand* 1962;124:531.

Tashjian EA, Richter KJ. The value of proxyphene hydrochloride (Darvon) for the treatment of hyperhidrosis in the spinal cord injured patient. *Paraplegia* 1985;23:349.

Yu C C, Cook MG: Hidradenitis suppurativa: disease of follicular epithelium rather than apocrine glands. *Br J Dermatol* 1990;122:763–767.

38

Scarring Alopecia

Wilma F. Bergfeld
The Cleveland Clinic Foundation, Cleveland, Ohio

Dirk M. Elston
Brooke Army Medical Center, Fort Sam Houston, Houston, Texas

Any surgical approach to the treatment of alopecia must be based on a thorough understanding of the pathogenesis and natural history of the disorders that result in scarring alopecia. Accurate diagnosis and appropriate medical management are essential before surgery can be considered. Surgical correction of alopecic patches can be of great benefit in cases of quiescent or "burnt-out" scarring alopecia. Surgical management is seldom indicated in cases of active, progressive scarring alopecia. We will present an overview of the classification and appropriate diagnostic work-up as well as medical and cosmetic management of scarring alopecia.

The evaluation of alopecia can be frustrating. One source of frustration is the considerable degree of clinical and histological overlap that exists between various entities. Accurate diagnosis has therapeutic implications and is crucial. History, physical examination, serologic evaluation, and biopsy may all be important in establishing the diagnosis. A dermatopathologist skilled in the histological diagnosis of alopecia may be especially helpful.

The term "scarring alopecia" is archaic and would be more correctly termed permanent alopecia. A scar is the result of reparative fibrosis after destruction of connective tissue. Many causes of permanent alopecia, such as morphea, do not produce a histologic scar. Recent research suggests that hair follicles regenerate from the "bulge area" near the insertion of the erector pili muscle. Although the exact site of the germinative stem cell population has been debated, there is considerable evidence that the new anagen hair arises from the midportion of the follicle, near the erector pili insertion. Therefore, destruction of the midportion of the follicle appears to be the histologic hallmark of permanent alopecia.

A classification of scarring and nonscarring alopecia is offered in Figure 1. Causes of alopecia are classified based on their clinical and histological features. These include evidence of anagen arrest (tapered fracture), alterations in hair growth cycles (anagen:telogen ratio), and tricho-

---

The opinions expressed are those of the authors and are not to be construed as official or as representing those of the United States Army or the Department of Defense.

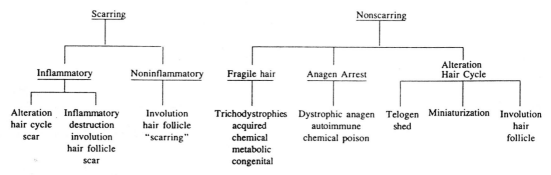

Figure 1 Classification of scarring and nonscarring alopecia.

Table 1 Scalp Alopecia, Nonscarring

Fragile hair	Alteration hair cycle	Anagen arrest
Structured abnormality (trichodystrophy)	Autoimmune	Complete
Congenital	Alopecia areata	Alopecia areata
Acquired	Early cicatricial alopecias	Chemotherapeutic drugs
	Pseudopelade (others)	Radiation
	Other	Burn 2–3°
	Androgenic alopecia	Incomplete arrest—telogen shed
	Inflammatory scalp disorders	Medical event
		Metabolic disorder
		Drugs
		Surgery
		Stress
		Nutrition
		Radiation
		Scalp inflammation

dystrophy (hair shaft abnormalities). Table 1 provides an overview of these mechanisms present in common types of alopecia. Anagen arrest is the result of an extreme insult to the hair follicle matrix, causing temporary cessation of DNA synthesis and keratinization. The result is a narrowed segment of hair shaft and tapered fractures. This manifests clinically as an acute shed of anagen hairs with tapered proximal cells. Shedding generally begins 1–2 weeks following the insult. Among the most frequent causes are antimetabolites and alkylating and cytotoxic drugs. Anagen effluvium may also herald the onset of the acute type of alopecia areata or a severe flare of lupus erythematosus.

Alterations in hair follicle growth cycles present clinically with increased shedding of telogen hairs, retarded rate of growth or miniaturization of the hair follicle. Telogen shedding most commonly results from an incomplete insult to the anagen matrix, causing premature transformation to telogen phase. Increased numbers of telogen hairs are reflected in alterations of the normal anagen:telogen ratio (telogen hairs > 25%). Premature transformation to telogen may occur with high fevers, crash diets, or major surgical procedures.

Other mechanisms for telogen effluvium include short cycling of anagen follicles (as occurs in androgenic pattern alopecia), delayed shedding of telogen hairs (as occurs in seasonal hair shedding), early release of telogen hairs (as occurs early in minoxidil therapy), and delayed transformation of large numbers of anagen hairs into telogen (as occurs with pregnancy). Headington recently published an excellent and comprehensive review of these mechanisms for telogen effluvium.

The mechanisms resulting in the various trichodystrophies are not yet totally understood. Fragile hair can be classified into congenital and acquired types. Acquired abnormalities may result from physical, chemical, and metabolic disorders. Congenital types may be markers for syndromes with metabolic or embryonic developmental abnormalities.

The remainder of this chapter is devoted to conditions that result in scarring alopecia (Table 2). Scarring results from inflammatory, physical, or chemical destruction of follicular epithelium and connective tissue, followed by reparative fibrosis. Scarring alopecia is divided clinically and histologically into inflammatory and noninflammatory types. Inflammatory scarring alopecia includes discoid lupus erythematosus, lichen planopilaris, mixed inflammatory destructive alopecia, erosive pustular dermatosis, and bacterial and fungal infections. Noninflammatory scarring alopecia includes physical trauma, some keratinizing disorders, and alopecia neoplastica. Table 3 summarizes the histological features of scarring alopecia.

True scarring is easily identified in biopsy specimens with the aid of an elastic tissue stain. True scars are devoid of elastic tissue. End-stage scarring alopecia is one form of permanent alopecia. Nonscarring conditions may also result in permanent alopecia. In these conditions, the follicular epithelium involutes, but no true scarring occurs. Linear scleroderma is one cause of permanent nonscarring alopecia. Elastic tissue stains reveal normal elastic fibers in cases of linear scleroderma.

Inflammatory and noninflammatory pseudopelade are other examples of permanent nonscarring alopecia. In pseudopelade, elastic tissue stains reveal apparent hyperplasia of all connective tissue elements. Collagen fibers appear sclerotic and mimic scarring in hematoxylin- and eosin-stained sections, but elastic tissue stains reveal normal or hypertrophic elastic fibers.

Table 2 Scalp Alopecia, "Scarring"

Inflammatory	Noninflammatory
Autoimmune alopecia	Autoimmune
Bullous (cicatricial) pemphigoid	Pseudopelade
Epidermolysis bullosa	Keratinizing defect
Erosive pustular dermatosis	Ichthyosis
Lichen planopilaris	Neoplasia
Lichen sclerosus et atrophicus	Benign:
Lupus erythematosus	keloid
Mixed inflammatory destructive alopecia	sarcoidosis
Necrobiosis lipoidica	Malignant:
Pseudopelade	angiosarcoma
Scleroderma	metastatic neoplasms
Infectious	mycosis fungoides
Folliculitis decalvans succedaneum	
Herpes and bacterial folliculitis	
Pyoderma	
Tinea capitis	
Chemical-Physical	
Burns, radiation, pressure	
Traction	
Trichotillomania	

Table 3 Scarring Alopecia, Histology

Noninflammatory		
Acute	Partial or complete absence of hair follicles	
	Widened fibrous tracts	
Chronic	Dermal fibrosis or sclerosis (lacks elastic fibers)	
	Absence of inflammation	
Inflammatory		
Acute	Inflammatory	
	Folliculitis: acute and chronic	
	Partial or complete absence of hair follicles	
Chronic	Frequent mucinous degeneration of fibrous tracts	
	Widened sclerotic fibrous tracts	
	Dermal fibrosis, scar (lacks elastic fibers)	

LUPUS ERYTHEMATOSUS

The most common form of inflammatory scarring alopecia is chronic cutaneous lupus erythematosus (Fig. 2), which occurs more frequently in females than in males and is observed more commonly during adulthood (30–60 yr). Systemic lupus may or may not be present. Occasionally, subacute cutaneous lupus produces a permanent alopecia. Histologically, in chronic lupus erythematosus, there is usually prominent vacuolar alteration of the basal cell layer of the epidermis and follicular epithelium (Fig. 3). A moderate to dense patchy perivascular and periadnexal lymphoid inflammatory infiltrate and basement membrane thickening are noted. A superficial lichenoid interface dermatitis resembling lichen planus may occasionally be seen. Direct immunofluorescent studies demonstrate granular deposition of IgG and C3 at the dermal-epidermal junction of the surface and follicular epithelium (Fig. 4). Dermal fibrosis (true scarring) occurs in the late stages with destruction of adnexal structures.

Lupus erythematosus can present clinically as an inflammatory patch or as a clinically noninflammatory patch resembling pseudopelade (Fig. 5). These cases lack changes at the dermalepidermal junction. However, perifollicular inflammation and follicular interface dermatitis will be present. Histologic examination with elastic tissue stains easily distinguishes lupus from pseudopelade. If a hair follicle is present, direct immunofluorescence may show a positive lupus band. Identification of other more typical lesions of lupus erythematosus aids in the clinical diagnosis of noninflammatory lesions of lupus.

The agents of greatest value in treating chronic cutaneous lupus are the corticosteroids (topical, intralesional, and systemic) and the antimalarials. Oral retinoids, dapsone, and thalidomide have also been used successfully. Labeled indications, the risk of teratogenesis, and appropriate contraceptive measures must always be discussed. Combination therapy with several agents may be necessary.

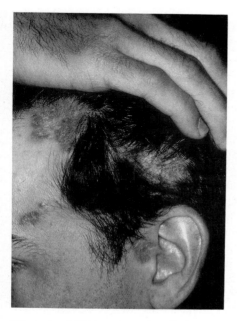

Figure 2 Middle-aged male with inflammatory discoid lupus erythematosus, active.

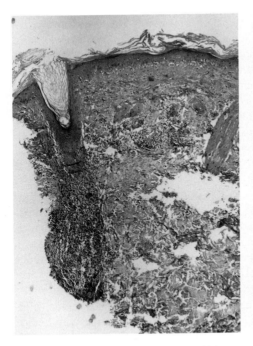

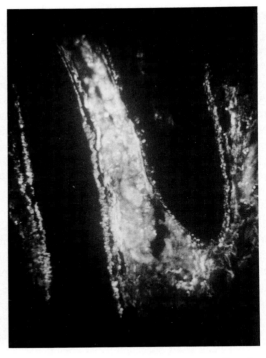

Figure 3   Scalp biopsy of acute discoid lupus erythematosus reveals follicular plugging with dense conical perifollicular and perivascular mononuclear infiltrates. Adjacent to the follicle, along the epidermis, there is notable basalar vacuolopathy. Diagnosis: discoid lupus erythematosus. (×10)

Figure 4   Direct immunofluorescence of scalp discoid lupus erythematosus reveals granular IgG, IgM, and C3 immunoreactants at the basement membrane zone. (×20)

LICHEN PLANOPILARIS

Lichen planopilaris presents as a patchy alopecia. It is seen more frequently in females and occurs most often in middle-aged adults. It may be seen on any hair-bearing area of skin and may be associated with more typical lesions of lichen planus. Individual lesions may present as erythematous follicular papules or as patches with follicular hyperkeratosis (Fig. 6). Lichen planopilaris runs a prolonged and slowly progressive but ultimately self-limited course. Small patches of 2–5 mm may expand and coalesce into larger areas, resembling lupus erythematosus. Clinically noninflammatory cases may resemble pseudopelade. Histological examination with elastic tissue stains will generally allow differentiation from pseudopelade. The degree of clinical and histological overlap with lupus erythematosus may pose more difficulty. They can be differentiated best by a combination of routine histology and immunofluorescence. Lichen planopilaris (LPP) demonstrates a lichenoid interface dermatitis involving follicular epithelium. This eventually results in true scarring. Epidermal interface dermatitis (lichenoid type) may also occur. Lichenoid dermatitis may occasionally be seen in cases of lupus erythematosus. Direct immunofluorescence in LPP reveals globules of IgM, IgA, IgG, and C3 within the adventitial dermis below the surface epithelium and adjacent to hair follicles. Linear heavy fibrin deposition may also be seen. In contrast, lupus erythematosus typically demonstrates a granular band of immunoglobulin. Occasionally globular immunofluorescence and linear fibrin below the surface epi-

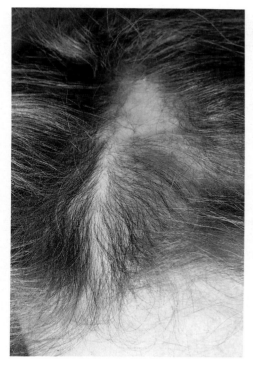

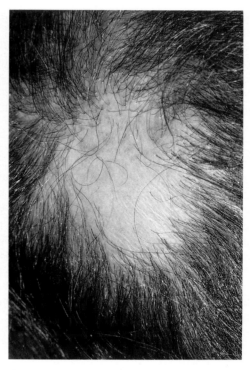

Figure 5 Discoid lupus erythematosus of scalp with flesh-colored discoid sclerotic patch. Consistent with scarring alopecia, end-stage.

Figure 6 Lichen planopilaris of the scalp: central sclerotic patch bordered by hair with perifollicular crusting.

thelium are noted in lupus. In our experience, the most reliable distinguishing feature in LPP is the presence of globular immunofluorescence *adjacent to follicular epithelium*. Serologic tests for lupus erythematosus are negative.

Topical, intralesional, and systemic corticosteroids are effective for the treatment of lichen planopilaris. Oral retinoids and griseofulvin have been tried with variable success. As stated previously, labeled indications, teratogenesis, and effective contraception must always be discussed.

MIXED INFLAMMATORY DESTRUCTIVE ALOPECIA

Mixed inflammatory destructive alopecia, a term coined by one of the authors (WFB), presents with clinical, histological, and immunofluorescent features of both lupus erythematosus and lichen planopilaris. Serologic testing for lupus is negative. Clinically, small alopecic patches coalesce to form larger patches. Lesions may appear inflammatory or noninflammatory clinically. No other more typical lesions of lupus or lichen planus are present. Histologically, a patchy lymphoid dermal infiltrate is seen within fibrous tracts of telogen follicles. In the late stage, widening of fibrous tracts and true scarring with absence of elastic fibers is seen. The epidermal and follicular epithelium demonstrates changes similar both to lichen planopilaris and chronic cutaneous lupus erythematosus. Direct immunofluorescence reveals a mixed pattern, with both globular and linear/granular immunoglobulin deposition. Please note that the linear pattern is one of *immunoglobulin* deposition, not linear fibrin deposition. Linear fibrin is more commonly seen in lichen planopilaris but may be seen in lupus. In our experience, mixed inflammatory destructive alopecia is extremely rare. The term should be reserved for those rare cases that demonstrate mixed clinical, histological, *and immunoglobulin* patterns. The term should not be used as a "wastebasket" for the many cases of lupus and lichen planopilaris that demonstrate some degree of clinical or histological overlap.

Mixed inflammatory destructive alopecia responds to corticosteroid therapy. In refractory cases, it is reasonable to consider agents used to treat lupus and lichen planopilaris.

PSEUDOPELADE OF BROCQ

Pseudopelade presents with clinically noninflammatory patches of alopecia, which may coalesce (Fig. 7). The clinical course is prolonged, but ultimately self-limited. Biopsy demonstrates involution of hair follicles, dermal sclerosis, and expanded fibrous tracts. In the late stages, widened fibrous tracts form broad columns, which extend from the subcutaneous tissue to the epidermis. Elastic fibers appear normal or hypertrophic. The only true scarring that occurs is a thin band of scar immediately below the epidermis. Lymphoid infiltrates are occasionally seen. Granulomatous inflammation, which represents a foreign body response to the exposed hair fibers is common. On direct immunofluorescence, IgM and C3 may be seen at the basement membrane zone of hair follicles. Pseudopelade, like linear scleroderma, is a permanent nonscarring alopecia.

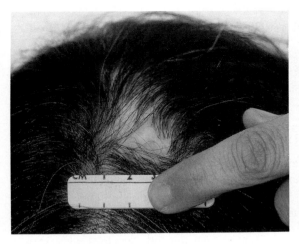

Figure 7 Pseudopelade: multiple flesh-colored alopecic patches, scalp. This presentation overlaps with end-stage scarring alopecia of DLE, LPP, and alopecia areata.

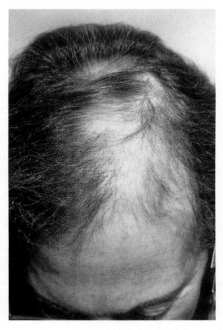

Figure 8 Scleroderma (linear scleroderma, scalp) associated with skin atrophy and alopecia (collagen hyperplasia without scarring).

It is unclear whether pseudopelade represents a single condition or a group of disorders with similar histological findings. We believe that as the pathophysiologic mechanisms of pseudopelade are uncovered, it will be subdivided into types by etiology and response to treatment.

The follicular degeneration syndrome, which includes many cases classified in the past as "hot comb alopecia" in black women, appears to represent the most common type of pseudopelade. Clinically, patients present with apical thinning or patches of alopecia, which clinically suggest scarring. Histologically, involuting follicles with asymmetrical thinning of the isthmus are seen. Collagen is sclerotic and elastic fibers are normal to hypertrophied. Therefore, these cases fit the histological pattern of pseudopelade. Patients with the follicular degeneration syndrome appear to run a prolonged but self-limited course. The value of specific treatments remains to be proved, but we would consider the use of antimalarials, as they have been reported to be of benefit in some cases of pseudopelade. Corticosteroids and tetracycline have also been reported as effective in some cases of pseudopelade.

SCARRING PEMPHIGOID

Scarring pemphigoid is a rare disorder that affects older individuals and may present as a scarring alopecia. Subtle bullous scalp lesions may be associated with bullae of mucous membranes, genitalia, and glabrous skin. Clinically, unless bullae are noted, the alopecic patches share clinical features with pseudopelade, scleroderma, and end-stage lupus and lichen planopilaris. Histology and immunofluorescent studies can be diagnostic. Subepidermal blistering with a variable polymorphous infiltrate and dermal fibrosis are noted. Direct immunofluorescence demonstrates linear immunoglobulin and C3 at the basement membrane zone. Treatment with corticosteroids or dapsone may be effective.

EPIDERMOLYSIS BULLOSA

Dermolytic types of epidermolysis bullosa may present in a fashion similar to scarring pemphigoid. Large cutaneous erosions and secondary infection may be seen. Electron microscopy, immunofluorescent studies, and immunoblotting may be necessary to distinguish epidermolysis bullosa acquisita and inherited epidermolysis bullosa types from each other and from scarring pemphigoid.

LINEAR SCLERODERMA

Linear scleroderma presents as a self-limiting permanent alopecia of the scalp. This disorder may affect any age and is equally distributed between the sexes. The slowly progressive linear alopecic patch presents as a clinically noninflammatory alopecia with occasional spared indeterminate hairs. In the late stages, an atrophic linear tract is present. The resemblance to a saber scar has given rise to the term "en coup de sabre morphea" (Fig. 8). Biopsy reveals the characteristic changes of scleroderma. Nodular lymphoplasmacytic perivascular infiltrates are noted in the deep dermis. Vasculitis and panniculitis may be present. Dermal sclerosis is present, but elastic tissue stains are normal. Like pseudopelade, this is a nonscarring permanent alopecia caused by involution of the hair follicle. Response to treatment is unpredictable, but corticosteroids and antimalarials have been tried. The relationship of scleroderma variants to *Borrelia* spirochetes and to ingested agents (tryptophan, toxins as in Spanish toxic oil syndrome) requires further investigation. The role of antibiotic therapy remains controversial.

EROSIVE PUSTULAR DERMATOSIS

Erosive pustular dermatosis is synonymous with or closely related to folliculitis decalvans (Fig. 9). These disorders present with suppurative folliculitis, which results in scarring alopecia. Recurrent bouts occur, with pustules or erosions occurring at the periphery of the scarred area. Gradually, the scarred area expands. The disorder occurs in both sexes, all races, and at all ages. *Staphylococcus aureus* is sometimes cultured from the pustules, but the disorder is not simply a staphylococcal folliculitis. The disorder may represent a hypersensitivity response, with staphylococci serving a triggering role. Immunologic studies have provided evidence of defective lymphocyte function, increased immunoglobulins, abnormal neutrophil chemotaxis, and hypocomplementemia. Skin biopsy in the acute phase demonstrates a suppurative folliculitis. In later stages, fibrosis and scarring are present. Residual hair fiber granulomas and a patchy polymorphous infiltrate may be seen. Patients sometimes respond to prolonged suppressive antibiotic therapy, such as erythromycin 500 mg BID. Rifampin has been used. It should be used in combination with a semisynthetic penicillin or cephalosporin. Similar regimens have been used to eradicate chronic staphylococcal carrier states. Zinc therapy has been reported as useful. Zinc therapy is not without complications and may be associated with decreased copper levels and anemia.

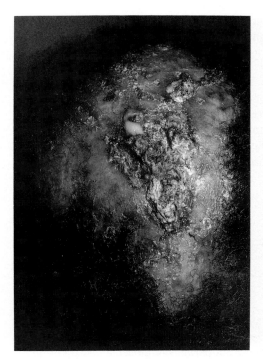

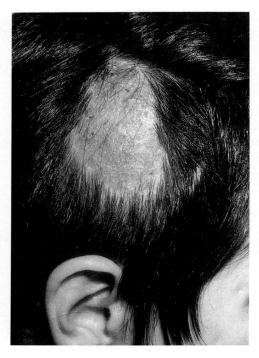

Figure 9 Erosive pustular dermatosis with secondary staphylococcal infection. Acute and chronic inflammation with evidence of scarring alopecia.

Figure 10 Chronic tinea capitis with kerion. Cultures demonstrated trichophyton tonsurans.

DISSECTING CELLULITIS OF THE SCALP

Dissecting cellulitis of the scalp (perifolliculitis capitis abscedens et suffodiens, Hoffman's disease) presents with boggy, tender alopecic plaques, which result in scarring. The lesions may be associated with acne conglobata or hidradenitis suppurativa. Hypersensitivity to infectious organisms may play a role. Long-term suppressive antibiotic therapy, combined antibiotic regimens, zinc therapy, and retinoid therapy have been tried with variable success.

INFECTIOUS DISORDERS

Tinea capitis with kerion (Fig. 10), hepetic folliculitis, and occasionally bacterial folliculitis can result in permanent scarring alopecia. Boggy inflammatory plaques, vesicles, pustules, or abscess formation may be seen. Therapy is dependent upon confirmation of the diagnosis by KOH examination, Tzanck preparation, Gram stain, and culture. Occasionally, these methods fail to identify the cause, and the diagnosis is made by histological examination.

LICHEN SCLEROSIS ET ATROPHICUS AND NECROBIOSIS LIPOIDICA

Lichen sclerosis and necrobiosis lipoidica have occasionally been reported to cause permanent alopecia. In necrobiosis lipoidica, true scarring is present. In lichen sclerosis, the pathophysiology of the alopecia is less well understood.

PHYSICAL AND CHEMICAL TRAUMA

Physical and chemical trauma can physically remove or destroy adnexal structures or cause an inflammatory response that results in scarring and alopecia. Chronic traction alopecia and trichotillomania (Fig. 11) represent special forms of physical trauma. Anagen hairs are extracted, causing the follicles to cycle into catagen phase. Repeated traction can result in pigment casts within the follicular infundibulum, trichomalacia, and follicular disruption. If traction or compulsive plucking are stopped early, all hairs will regenerate. Long-standing trichotillomania can result in a scarring alopecia with clinical characteristics similar to pseudopelade. Biopsy at this stage will demonstrate a true scarring alopecia. Some patients with trichotillomania will benefit from antidepressant therapy and behavior modification.

KERATINIZING DISORDERS

Permanent alopecia has been noted in keratinizing disorders such as ichthyosis and scarring keratosis pilaris. In patients with ichthyosis, alopecia may be the result of secondary bacterial or fungal infection. Appropriate stains and culture are often warranted in addition to treatment of the underlying keratinizing disorder.

NEOPLASMS

Alopecia neoplastica may mimic a scarring alopecia. Cutaneous adnexal neoplasms as well as metastatic carcinoma (especially breast and renal) may initially present as alopecic patches.

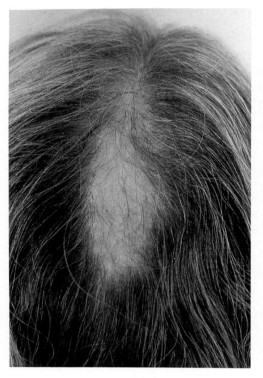

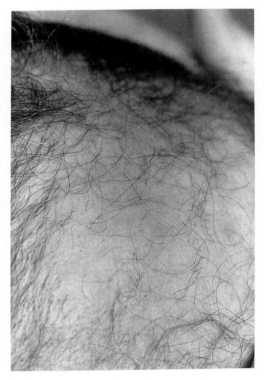

Figure 11 Chronic trichotillomania (traction alopecia). Chronic, slowly expanding alopecic patch of the vertex and parietal area, which contained a few hairs. Scalp biopsy was compatible with scarring alopecia. Differential diagnosis included pseudopelade.

Figure 12 "Scarring alopecia," end-stage. Etiology unclear; suspected autoimmune alopecia with involution of hair follicles without loss of elastic fibers.

Histology is diagnostic. Displacement and involution of follicles, follicular destruction, and inflammation may result in alopecia.

CAMOUFLAGE TECHNIQUE

Camouflage techniques can be extremely helpful for the patient with alopecia. In addition to hairpieces, hair coiffures, hair coloring, scalp crayons, and dyes can be of great benefit. Identification of a local cosmetologist who can assist the patient with these techniques (Table 4), in privacy and at reasonable cost, can be an important part of total patient management.

Approaches to surgical camouflage are covered in great depth in other chapters of this text. Hair transplantation, scalp reduction, flaps, and tissue-expansion techniques can play an important role in the management of stable quiescent permanent alopecia. Artificial fiber implantation should be avoided, since this procedure can produce great morbidity.

Table 4   Cosmetic Camouflage

Curl; style; hair coiffures
Lighter color
Scalp crayons
Hair prostheses
Combinations
Surgical therapies
    Hair transplantation (HT)
    Scalp reduction
    Combination HT and scalp reduction
    Tissue expansion–scalp reduction
    Juri flap

GLOBAL EVALUATION

Prior to considering surgical correction of an alopecic patch (Fig. 12), a global assessment of the patient is in order. This may include history, physical examination, serology, and biopsy. Biopsy may be particularly helpful in establishing a diagnosis, determining prognosis and differentiating a true scarring alopecia (Fig. 13) from conditions such as alopecia neoplastica. In addition to establishing a diagnosis, the stage and activity of the disorder must be determined.

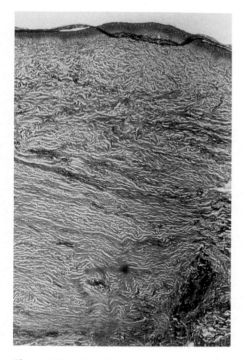

Figure 13   Skin biopsy demonstrating scarring alopecia, end-stage. Biopsy revealed absence of all adnexal structures and horizontal alignment of the collagen. Elastic fiber stains demonstrate absent elastic fibers. (×20)

Table 5 Medical Therapies

Anti-inflammatory/Immune modulators
  Antibiotics (tetracycline)
  Antifungals
  Antimalarials
  Antimetabolites
  Cimetidine
  Corticosteroids
  Isotretinoin
Anti-infectious
  Antibiotics (tetracycline, erythromycin)
  Antifungals (griseofulvin, ketoconazole)
  Antiviral (acyclovir)
  Other (minerals)
Biologic response modifiers
  Minoxidil
  Cyclosporin
  Doxepin
  Diazoxide
  Vitroprosal

Maximum benefit should be obtained from medical therapies when possible (Table 5). Surgical correction is seldom appropriate for an active case of alopecia, but can provide definitive therapy for "burnt-out" patches of alopecia.

BIBLIOGRAPHY

Bulge-Activation Hypothesis

Cotsarelis G, Sun TT, Lavker R. Label-retaining cells reside in the bulge area of pilosebaceous unit: implications for follicular stem cells, hair cycle and skin carcinogenesis. *Cell* 1990;61:1329–1337.
Holecek B, Ackerman AB. Bulge-activation hypothesis: is it valid? *Am J Dermatopathol* 1993;15(3):235–247.
Lavker RM, Fryer E, Margolis-Fryer J, Ostad M. Cells in the bulge region of mouse hair follicle undergo transient proliferation during onset of anagen and in response to physical and chemical stimuli. *J Invest Dermatol* 1992;98(4):581.
Sun T, Cotsarelis G, Lavker R. Hair follicle stem cells: the bulge activation hypothesis. *J Invest Dermatol* 1991;96(suppl):77–78.

Disease and Etiologic Agents

Bergfeld WF. Hair disease. In *Office Microbiology*. Roenigk HH, ed. Batltimore, Williams and Wilkins, 1981, pp. 335–347.
Bergner T, Braun-Falco O. Pseudopelade of Brocq. (letter) *J Am Acad Dermatol* 1991;25:865.
Binazzi M. In tema di folliculiti decalvanti. *Ann Ital Dermatol Sifiligr* 1954;9:325.
Birnbaum PS, Baden HP. Heritable disorders of hair. *Dermatol Clin* 1987;5(1):137–153.
Bogg A. Folliculitis decalvans. Acta Dermatovenereol 1963;43:14.
Braun-Falco O, Bergner T, Heilgemeir GP. Pseudopelade Brocq—Krankheitsbild oder Krankheitsentitat. *Hautarzt* 1989;40:77–83.

Brown AC, Crounse RG, Winkelmann RK. Generalized hair-follicle hamartoma associated with alopecia, aminoaciduria, and myasthenia gravis. *Arch Dermatol* 1969;99:478–493.

Bulengo-Ransby SM, Headington JT. Pseudopelade of Brocq (reply) (letter). *J Am Acad Dermatol* 1991; 25:865–866.

Dawber RPR, Ebling FJG, Wojnarowska FT. Disorders of Hair. In *Textbook of Dermatology*, 5th ed. Champion RH, Burton JL, Ebling FJG, eds., Oxford, Blackwell Scientific Publications, 1992, pp. 2533–2613.

Dupre A, Bonafe JL, Christol B. Syringomas as a causative factor for cicatricial alopecia (letter). *Arch Dermatol* 1981;117:315.

Ebling FJG, Dawber R, Rook A. The hair. In *Textbook of Dermatology*, 4th ed. Rook A, Wilkinson DS, Ebling FJ, Champion RH, Burton JL, eds. Oxford, Blackwell Scientific Publications, 1986, pp. 1937–2037.

Foulds IS. Lichen sclerosus et atrophicus of the scalp. *Br J Dermatol* 1980;103:197.

Frazer NG, Grant PW. Folliculitis decalvans with hypocomplementemia. *Br J Dermatol* 1982; 107(suppl 22):88.

Goerz G, Kind R, Lehmann P. Cicatricial alopecias. In *Hair and Hair Diseases*. Orfanos CE, Happle R, ed. Berlin, Springer-Verlag, 1990, pp. 611–639.

Hinter H, Wolff K. Generalized atrophic benign epidermolysis bullosa. *Arch Dermatol* 1982;118(6):375–384.

Kamalam A, Thambiah AS. Genetic ichthyosis and trichophyton infection in infants. *Mykosen* 1982; 25(5): 281–283.

Knight TE, Robinson HM, Jr, Sina B. Angiosarcoma (angioendothelioma) of the scalp. An unusual case of scarring alopecia. *Arch Dermatol* 1980;116(6):683–686.

Loewenthal LJA. A case of lupoid sycosis or ulerythema sycosiforme, beginning in infancy. *Br J Dermatol* 1957;69:443.

Mehregan AH, Baker S. Basaloid follicular hamartoma. *J Cutan Pathol* 1985;12:55–65.

Miller RF. Epilating folliculitis of the glabrous skin. *Arch Dermatol* 1961;83:115.

Moyer DG, Williams RM. Perifolliculitis capitis abscedens et suffodiens. *Arch Dermatol* 1962;85:378–384.

Navaratnam A, Hodgson GA. Necrobiosis lipoidica presenting on the face and scalp. *Br J Dermatol* 1973; 89(suppl 9):100.

Pye RJ, Peachey RD, Burton JL. Erosive pustular dermatosis of the scalp. *Br J Dermatol* 1979;100:559–566.

Ridley CM, Smith N. Generalized hair follicle hamartoma associated with alopecia and myasthenia gravis: report of a second case. *Clin Exp Dermatol* 1981;6:283–289.

Shelley WB, Wood MG. Occult syringomas of the scalp associated with progressive hair loss. *Arch Dermatol* 1980;116:843–844.

Shitara A, Igareshi R, Morohashi M. Folliculitis decalvans and cellular immunity—two brothers with oral candidiasis. *Jpn J Dermatol* 1974;28:113.

Slepyan AH, Burks JW, Fox J. Persistent denudation of the scalp in cicatricial pemphigoid. Treatment by skin grafting. *Arch Dermatol* 1961;84:444–451.

Sperling LC, Sau P. The follicular degeneration syndrome in black patients. *Arch Dermatol* 1992;128:68–74.

Stocker WW, Richtsmeier AJ, Rozycki AA, Baughman RD. Kerion caused by Trichophyton verrucosum. *Pediatrics* 1977;45:912–915.

Traupe H, Happle R. Alopecia ichthyotica. A characteristic feature of congenital ichthyosis. *Dermatologica* 1983;167:225–230.

Wagner W. Alopezia und Nagelveranderungen bei Epidermolysis bullosa hereditaria. *Zeitschr Haut Geshlechtskr* 1956;20:278–284.

Welton DG. Keratosis follicularis with unusual involvement of the scalp. *Arch Dermatol Syphilol* 1943;47:398–404.

Wheeland RG, Thurmond RD, Gilmore WA, Blackstock R. Chronic blepharitis and pyoderma of the scalp: an immune deficiency state in a father and son with hypercalcemia and decreased intracellular killing. *Pediatric Dermatol* 1983;1(2):134–142.

Histology and Immunology

Abell E. Immunofluorescent stain technic in the diagnosis of alopecia. *South Med J* 1977;70:1407–1410.

Bergfeld WF. Skin biopsy findings in androgenic alopecia. *Cutis* 1978;22:190–95.

Binkley W, Starsnic J, Valenzuela R, Bergfeld WF. A histochemical approach to differentiation of lichen planus from lupus erythematosus. *Am J Clin Pathol* 1983;79:486.

Braun-Falco O, Imai S, Schmoeckel C, Steger O, Bergner T. Pseudopelade of Brocq. *Dermatologica* 1986; 172:18–23.

Jordon RE. Subtle clues to diagnosis by immunopathology: scarring alopecia. *Am J Dermatopathol* 1980; 2:157–159.

Harrist TJ, Mihm MC. Cutaneous immunopathology: the diagnostic use of direct and indirect immunofluorescence techniques in dermatologic disease. *Human Pathol* 1979;10:625–653.

Lachapelle JM, Pierard GE. Traumatic alopecia in trichotillomania. *J Cutan Pathol* 1977;4:51–67.

Laymon CW. The cicatricial alopecias. *J Invest Dermatol* 1947;8:99.

Mehregan AH. Trichotillomania. *Arch Dermatol* 1970;102:129–133.

Mehregan AH. Histopathology of alopecias. *Cutis* 1978;21:249–253.

Messenger AG, Slater DN, Bleehen SS. Alopecia areata: alterations in the hair growth cycle and correlation with the follicular pathology. *Br J Dermatol* 1986;114:337–347.

Muller SA. Trichotillomania: a histologic study of sixty-six patients. *J Am Acad Dermatol* 1990;23:56–62.

Muller SA, Winkelmann RK. Trichotillomania. *Arch Dermatol* 1972;105:535–540.

Newton RC, Hebert AA, Freese TW, Solomon AR. Scarring alopecia. *Dermatol Clin* 1987;5:603–618.

Pierard-Franchimont C, Pierard GE. Massive lymphocyte-mediated apoptosis during the early stage of pseudopelade. *Dermatologica* 1986;172:254–257.

Pinkus H. Differential patterns of elastic fibers in scarring and non-scarring alopecias. *J Cutan Pathol* 1978;5:93–104.

Suter DE, Adams L. Scarring alopecia. *Arch Dermatol* 1972;106(6):915.

Tuffanelli DL. Cutaneous immunopathology: recent observations. *J Invest Dermatol* 1975;65(1):143–153.

Tuffanelli DL, Kay D, Fukuyama K. Dermal-epidermal junction in lupus erythematosus. *Arch Dermatol* 1969;99:652–662.

Waldorf DS. Lichen planopilaris. Histopathologic study of disease progression to scarring alopecia. *Arch Dermatol* 1966;93:684–691.

Valenzuela R, Bergfeld WF, Deodhar SD. Lupus erythematosus: immunohistopathology. In *Interpretation of Immunofluorescent Patterns in Skin Diseases*. Chicago, American Society of Clinical Pathologists Press, 1984, pp. 66–79.

Valenzuela R, Bergfeld WF, Deodhar SD. Lichen planus. In *Interpretation of Immunofluorescent Patterns in Skin Diseases*. Chicago, American Society of Clinical Pathologists Press, 1984, pp. 127–131.

Medical Treatment

Bazzano GS, Terezakis N, Galen W. Topical tretinoin for hair growth promotion. *J Am Acad Dermatol* 1986;15(4 pt 2):880–883.

Berne B, Venge P, Ohman S. Perifolliculitis capitis abscedens et suffodiens (Hoffman). Complete healing associated with oral zinc therapy. *Arch Dermatol* 1985;121:1028–1030.

Bjellerup M, Wallengren J. Familial perifolliculitis capitis abscedens et suffodiens in two brothers successfully treated with isotretinoin. *J Am Acad Dermatol* 1990;23:752–753.

Brozena SJ, Cohen LE, Fenske NA. Folliculitis decalvans—response to rifampin. *Cutis* 1988;42:512–515.

Coburn PR, Shuster S. Dapsone and discoid lupus erythematosus. *Br J Dermatol* 1982;106:105–106.

DeVillez RL. Androgenetic alopecia treated with topical minoxidil. *J Am Acad Dermatol* 1987;16 (3 pt 2):669–672.

Hasper MJ, Klokke AH. Thalidomide in the treatment of chronic discoid lupus erythematosus. *Acta Dermatovener* (Stockholm) 1982;62:321–324.

Holm AL, Bowers KE, McMeekin TO, Gaspari AA. Chronic cutaneous lupus erythematosus treated with thalidomide. *Arch Dermatol* 1993;129:1548–1550.

Ikeda M, Arata J, Isaka H. Erosive pustular dermatosis of the scalp successfully treated with oral zinc sulphate. *Br J Dermatol* 1982;106:742–743.

Mahrle G, Meyer-Hamme S, Ippen H. Oral treatment of keratinizing disorders of skin and mucous membranes with etretinate. *Arch Dermatol* 1982;118:97–100.

Norris D. Zinc and cutaneous inflammation. *Arch Dermatol* 1985;121:985–989.

Rubenstein DJ, Huntley AC. Keratotic lupus erythematosus: treatment with isotretinoin. *J Am Acad Dermatol* 1986;14:910–914.

Schewach-Millet M, Ziv R, Shapira D. Perifolliculitis capitis abscedens et suffodiens treated with isotretinoin (13-cis-retinoic acid) (letter). *J Am Acad Dermatol* 1986;15:1291–1292.

Shaffer N, Billick RC, Srolvitz H. Perifolliculitis capitis abscedens et suffodiens. Resolution with combination therapy. *Arch Dermatol* 1992;128:1329–1331.

Swedo SE, Lenane MC, Leonard HL. Long-term treatment of trichotillomania (hair pulling) (letter). *N Engl J Med* 1993;329:141–142.

Taylor AEM. Dissecting cellulitis of the scalp: response to isotretinoin (letter). *Lancet* 1987;2:225.

Tuffanelli DL. Lupus erythematosus. *J Am Acad Dermatol* 1981;4:127–142.

Verbov J. The place of intralesional steroid therapy in dermatology. *Br J Dermatol* 1976;94(suppl 12):51–58.

Sehgal VN, Abraham GJS, Malik GB. Griseovfulvin therapy in lichen planus. *Br J Dermatol* 1972;87:383–386.

Surgical Treatment

Hanke CW, Bergfeld WF. Fiber implantation for pattern baldness. *JAMA* 1979;241(2):146–148.

Hanke CW, Ceilley RI, Bergfeld WF. Complications of fiber implantation for baldness. *Am Fam Phys* 1981;24(1):115–118.

Hanke CW, Norins AL, Pantzer JG Jr, Bennett JE. Hair implant complications. *JAMA* 1981;245(13):1344–1345.

McCray MK, Roenigk HH, Jr. Cosmetic correction of alopecia. *Am Fam Phys* 1983;28(4):207–214.

Nordstrom RE. Hair transplantation. The use of hair bearing compound grafts for correction of alopecia due to chronic discoid lupus erythematosus, traumatic alopecia, and male pattern baldness. *Scand J Plast Reconstr Surg* 1976;(suppl 14):1–37.

Roenigk RK, Wheeland RG. Tissue expansion in cicatricial alopecia. *Arch Dermatol* 1987;123:641–646.

Savin RC. Hair transplants in burn scars and other alopecias. *Conn Med* 1973;37(10):501–503.

Schultz BC, Roenigk HH. Scalp reduction for alopecia. *J Dermatol Surg Oncol* 1979;5:808–811.

Stegman SJ, Tromovitch TA. Cosmetic dermatologic surgery. *Arch Dermatol* 1982;118:1013–1016.

39

Evaluation and Management of Leg Ulcers

Gregory J. Wilmoth and Thom W. Rooke
Mayo Clinic/Foundation, Rochester, Minnesota

INTRODUCTION

Lower extremity ulcers are a common and troublesome problem affecting up to 1% of the adult population. They occur more frequently in the elderly, and their prevalence is likely to increase with the changing demographics of an older population. While the differential diagnosis of leg ulcerations is broad (see Table 1), the majority are caused by venous insufficiency, arterial insufficiency, or neuropathy (in patients with diabetes mellitus). Fortunately, with a careful history, good physical examination, and select laboratory evaluations, a prompt diagnosis can usually be reached. Ulcers that elude initial investigations, are of unusual location or morphology, or are unresponsive to treatment may need further evaluations (see Table 2), such as biopsy and culture.

DIAGNOSIS

History

Directed questions can be extremely helpful in establishing the cause of a leg ulcer.

1. How did the ulcer develop? Injury, infection, cold, or thrombophlebitis can be factors precipitating ulcerations. Neuropathic ulcers are often unnoticed.

2. Did it develop rapidly or slowly? Rapidly developing ulcers suggest venous insufficiency, acute thrombosis, embolic causes, or pyoderma gangrenosum. Slowly developing ulcers may reflect chronic arterial insufficiency or malignancy.

3. How painful is the ulcer? Ulcers from arterial insufficiency, livedoid vasculitis, sickle cell anemia, and cutaneous polyarteritis nodosa are typically very painful. Pain is not a prominent feature of venous ulcers. Neuropathic ulcers are often painless; however, there may be associated paresthesias or burning pain generalized to the leg. These neuropathic pains can also be seen in systemic vasculitis or cutaneous polyarteritis nodosa.

Table 1 Classification of Leg Ulcers

I. Vascular diseases
   A. Venous
   B. Arterial
      Atherosclerosis obliterans
      Thromboangiitis obliterans
      Arteriovenous malformations
      Cholesterol embolism
      Hypertension
   C. Lymphatics
      Lymphedema

II. Vasculitis
   A. Small vessel
      Hypersensitivity vasculitis
        Drugs
        Cryoglobulinemia
        Infection
        Henoch-Schönlein purpura
        Malignancy
      Autoimmune associated
        Rheumatoid arthritis
        Lupus erythematosus
        Scleroderma
        Sjogrens syndrome
        Behcets disease
        Livedoid vasculitis
   B. Medium and large vessel
      Polyarteritis nodosa
      Cutaneous polyarteritis nodosa
      Wegener's granulomatosis
      Churg-Strauss granulomatosis
      Giant cell arteritis

III. Neuropathic
   Diabetes
   Tabes dorsalis
   Poliomyelitis
   Leprosy
   Traumatic and toxic neuropathies
   Inherited sensory deficiency

IV. Metabolic
   Diabetes
   Gout
   Prolidase deficiency
   Vitamin C deficiency

V. Hematologic diseases
   A. Red blood cell disorders
      Sickle cell anemia
      Thalassemia
      Polycythemia rubra vera
   B. Leukemia
   C. Thrombocythemia
   D. Dysproteinemias
      Cryoglobulinemia

V. Hematologic diseases (continued)
      Cryofibrinogenemia
      Macroglobulinemia
   E. Coagulation defects
      Protein S and C deficiencies
      Antithrombin III deficiency
      Antiphospholipid antibody syndromes

VI. Drugs
   Halogens
   Ergotism
   Methotrexate
   Illicit drugs (injected)
   Vasopressors
   Hydroxyurea
   Coumadin

VII. Trauma
   Pressure
   Cold injury (frostbite, pernio)
   Radiation
   Burns (chemical, thermal)
   Factitial

VIII. Neoplastic
   Squamous cell carcinoma
   Basal cell carcinoma
   Melanoma
   Sarcoma (Kaposi's)
   Lymphoma
   Cutaneous T-cell lymphoma

IX. Infection
   A. Bacterial
      Furuncle
      Ecthyma gangrenosum
      Septic emboli
      Anthrax
      Diphtheria
      Synergistic anaerobic infections
      Gas gangrene
      Necrotizing fascitis
      Tuberculosis (lupus vulgaris)
      Leprosy
      Atypical mycobacteria
      Syphilis
   B. Fungal
      Blastomycosis
      Coccidiomycosis
      Histoplasmosis
      Sporotrichosis
      Majocchi's granuloma (dermatophyte)
   C. Actinomycosis (Madura foot)
   D. Leishmania
   E. Infestations and bites

Table 1 Continued

X. Dermatosis	XI. Panniculitis
Pyoderma gangrenosum	Pancreatic fat necrosis
Necrobiosis lipoidica diabeticorum	Lupus panniculitis
Lichen planus	α_1-Antitrypsin deficiency
Sarcoidosis	
Necrobiotic xanthogranuloma	
Papulonecrotic tuberculid	

4. Are there exacerbating or relieving factors? Pain from arterial ulcers worsens with elevation or exercise and may be relieved with dependency and rest. The discomfort of venous ulcers may improve with elevation.

5. Are there predisposing factors? Is there a history of claudication (arterial) or edema and blood clots (venous)?

6. What is current treatment? Topical agents may impair healing or promote contact dermatitis. Compression therapy in a patient with arterial insufficiency may lead to new ischemic ulcerations.

7. What are current medications? Systemic corticosteroids, methotrexate, and immunosuppressive or chemotherapeutic agents can inhibit wound healing. Coumadin and hydroxyurea can cause ulcers. There may be a drug-induced vasculitis or lupus erythematosus.

Table 2 Laboratory Tests

I. Routine	III. Skin biopsy
Complete blood count	Routine histopathology
Differential blood count	Immunohistochemical stains
Peripheral smear	Cultures
Urinalysis	bacterial
Serum chemistry group	fungal
Bacterial culture	mycobacterial
Syphilis serology	Molecular genetic analysis lymphomatous
	infiltrates
II. Special laboratory tests	
Antinuclear antibodies	IV. Vascular
Lupus antibodies (ENA, anti-DNA)	A. Arterial
Total complement, C3, C4	Ankle brachial pressure ratio
Rheumatoid factor	Segmental pressures
Antineutrophilic cytoplasmic	Cutaneous temperature
antibodies	Doppler waveforms
Sickle cell preparation	Pulse volume recordings
Hemoglobin electrophoresis	Duplex ultrasound
Serum protein electrophoresis	B. Venous
Immunoelectrophoresis	Volume plethysmography
Cryoglobulins	Photoplethysmography
Routine and special coagulation	Doppler directional analysis
Chest radiograph	Duplex ultrasound
Limb radiographs	C. Cutaneous flow correlates
CT and MRI for malignancy detection	Laser Doppler flowometry
Colonoscopy (ulcerative colitis)	Transcutaneous oxygen tension
Vitamins C and A, iron, zinc	D. Angiography

8. *What is past medical history?* Systemic diseases contributing to ulcers can be identified. These include diabetes mellitus, rheumatoid arthritis, systemic lupus erythematosus, hematologic disorders, thrombosis or pregnancy loss (suggesting antiphospholipid antibodies), inflammatory bowel disease (suggesting pyoderma gangrenosum), and ischemic heart disease or stroke (suggesting atherosclerosis).

9. *How is general health?* Weight loss and fever may signal infection or malignancy. Smoking can impair wound healing and is an important aggravating factor in atherosclerosis and thromboangiitis obliterans.

10. *What is social history?* Does the patient have proper housing and nutrition? Is there anyone available to help with wound care?

11. *What is family history?* Are there inherited diseases present such as diabetes mellitus, hemoglobinopathies, connective tissue diseases, or atherosclerosis?

Physical Exam

The physical examination can help differentiate causes of leg ulcers. Questions to ask include the following.

1. *What is the location?* Venous ulcers tend to develop on the distal third of the leg. They may occur anywhere at this level, but commonly the medial malleolar area is involved. Ischemic ulcers affect the toes and distal foot. Embolic processes usually involve the toes. Neuropathic ulcers predominate under pressure points on the sole of the foot or at sites of trauma from shoes.

2. *What is the appearance?* Venous ulcers tend to be shallow and exudative, with ample granulation tissue. Arterial ulcers are usually dry and deep, with necrotic tissue or eschar at the base. Vasculitic ulcers are commonly well demarcated with necrotic base, giving a "punched-out" appearance, or they may have irregular serpiginous borders. Pyoderma gangrenosum has an exudative necrotic center to the ulcer with a ragged undermined violaceous border bounded by a halo of erythema. Ulcers of livedoid vasculitis tend to be shallow and sharply demarcated with linear and angled configurations.

3. *Are the foot and leg pulses present, adequate, and symmetrical?* Pulse changes or asymmetry indicate large vessel arterial occlusive disease.

4. *What is the appearance of the surrounding skin?* Is there evidence of venous insufficiency with edema, varicosities, and hemosiderin pigmentation? Is there pallor or reactive dependent hyperemia from ischemic disease? Evidence of livedo reticularis suggests systemic lupus erythematosus, livedoid vasculitis, cutaneous polyarteritis nodosa, cholesterol emboli, or antiphospholipid disease. The scarring of atrophie blanche is seen in livedoid vasculitis and venous disease. Is there infection with signs of lymphangitis or cellulitis? Subcutaneous nodules suggest panniculitis or cutaneous polyarteritis nodosa. An elevated "heaped-up" border suggests squamous cell carcinoma.

5. *Are there associated signs?* Arthritis may indicate rheumatoid disease or systemic lupus. Are there signs of scleroderma? Are there sensory losses or other signs of neuropathy such as altered gate? Are there heart or lung findings indicating endocarditis, tuberculosis, or systemic fungal disease? Does the patient's general appearance suggest malnutrition or malignancy?

LABORATORY STUDIES

Routine laboratory screening is helpful for any ulceration of the leg and includes complete blood count, serum chemistries, urinalysis, and syphilis serology. Testing may demonstrate evidence of hematologic disorders, infection, diabetes mellitus, nutritional deficiency, and systemic diseases such as vasculitis or systemic lupus erythematosus. Local radiographs are useful to rule out osteomyelitis.

Swab cultures of the wound should be obtained even without evidence of infection since they may reveal occult fungal or mycobacterial disease, identify candida yeast overgrowth that can slow wound healing, and guide empiric antibiotic coverage pending definitive culture and sensitivity if infection should occur.

Any ulceration that is not felt to be from venous, arterial, or neuropathic causes should probably have a biopsy. Biopsy is essential in the diagnosis of malignancy, vasculitis, infection, panniculitis, and small-vessel occlusive diseases such as those associated with antiphospholipid syndromes or cryoglobulinemia. Tissue should be taken from skin at the ulcer edge, not the healing tissue or necrotic debris of the base. Ideally, it should be deep enough to contain ample pannicular tissue. The wound should be closed unless obvious necrosis and infection are encountered. Tissue should be submitted for bacterial, fungal, and mycobacterial culture. Of note, several ulcer-causing atypical mycobacteria have temperature requirements in culture of 30–33°C instead of the routine 37°C. The laboratory should therefore be notified so that they may set up appropriate cultures. It is also wise to freeze a portion in liquid nitrogen and set it aside in the event that special immunohistochemical stains or molecular genetic studies are required. Specialized testing can be useful and should be directed by clinical suspicion. Helpful tests are summarized in Table 2.

NONINVASIVE VASCULAR STUDIES

Differentiation between venous and arterial ulcers is important in planning appropriate therapy and avoiding iatrogenic complications. A useful office procedure to evaluate arterial insufficiency is the ankle-to-brachial systolic blood pressure ratio, or ankle-brachial index (ABI). With the patient supine, a blood pressure cuff is placed over the calf while arterial flow is monitored over the dorsalis pedis or posterior tibial arteries with a hand-held doppler instrument. The cuff is inflated until no flow is detected, then the cuff is slowly released until the pressure at which return of flow occurs is identified. This is the systolic blood pressure. A similar reading is obtained over the brachial artery. Normally the ankle systolic pressure is equal to or greater than the brachial systolic pressure. Thus a normal ABI is between 0.8 and 1.1, but may be greater on occasion. An ABI of less than 0.8 indicates significant arterial obstructive disease. It is important to note that leg systolic pressure can be falsely elevated in patients with noncompressable arteries caused by medial calcification or severe atherosclerosis. Thus, in diabetic patients, a normal ABI may overlook significant ischemic disease. Other noninvasive techniques can be used to identify arterial insufficiency in diabetic patients.

If arterial insufficiency alone, arterial and venous insufficiency combined, or diabetes mellitus is identified, then the noninvasive vascular laboratory can be extremely helpful in reaching a diagnosis. The laboratory can determine if underlying arterial or venous disease is complicating other causes of ulcers. Localization of disease to certain segments or locations can be helpful. Vasculitis and thromboangitis obliterans typically involve more peripherally located vessels than atherosclerosis. Venous studies are useful in detecting thrombosis, obstruction, or incompetent valves. Disease can be localized to the superficial system, the perforators, or the deep system. These distinctions have prognostic and therapeutic implications regarding surgical options and anticoagulation. Techniques such as transcutaneous partial pressures of oxygen ($TcPO_2$) may be able to yield prognostic and therapeutic information. Several reports have associated threshold $TcPO_2$ levels (20–40 mmHg) below which healing is severely impaired.

SPECIFIC CLINICAL TYPES

Venous Insufficiency Ulcers

The primary pathologic event leading to venous ulceration is failure of the calf muscle pump, which is responsible for venous return against gravity. The venous systems of the leg consist of the superficial system (short and long saphenous veins with their tributaries), the perforating veins, which connect the superficial to the deep system, and the deep veins within the musculature. One-way valves, which are present throughout the system, direct flow from the superficial to deep system via the perforators, then cephalad to the pelvic veins. The calf muscle group is invested in a tough fibrous fascia, preventing distension and providing support. During ambulation and muscle contraction, pressure increases in the deep venous system, forcing blood cephalad. Backflow and high pressures in the superficial system are prevented by valves in the perforators. During muscle relaxation the cephalad blood is held in check by valves, deep venous pressure falls, and filling of the deep veins occurs from the muscular tributaries and the superficial system. The siphoning effect of the pump is extremely effective in draining the superficial system and skin, maintaining a low superficial venous pressure during exercise.

Obstruction or valve incompetence in the deep system and perforators prevents the fall in pressure normally seen with ambulation and exposes the venous system to hydrostatic pressures. This persistent venous hypertension leads to chronic venous changes and ulcerations. Previous deep thrombosis with valve damage, primary valve incompetence, obstruction, or pump failure secondary to neuropathies, arthropathies, or inflammatory diseases all may find a common endpoint leading to persistent venous hypertension.

Several theories exist on how venous hypertension leads to ulcerations. One idea is that venous hypertension is transmitted to the capillary system leading to microvascular distension, fluid migration, and widened endothelial pores. This allows leakage of macromolecules and fibrin into the interstitial space, where the fibrin forms pericapillary cuffs. The fibrin cuffs then become a barrier to oxygen and metabolites, leading to ulceration. Fibrin deposition has not been well documented in other causes of leg ulcers. Of interest, defects in fibrinolysis and decreased protein C levels have been documented in some patients with venous disease. Another theory proposes that leukocytes are attracted to pressure-altered endothelial cells and trigger the release of inflammatory mediators, leading to subsequent capillary damage, increased permeability, and fibrin accumulation. Again, diffusion barriers are created. A recently formulated hypothesis unrelated to barrier effects is the "trap" hypothesis, in which macromolecules and fibrin leak into the dermis because of pressure or inflammation. They then bind up essential growth factors, rendering them unavailable for routine tissue homeostasis and repair.

Venous ulcers can be located anywhere on the distal third of the leg (Fig. 1). They are relatively shallow with granulation tissue and exudation. Pain is not a prominent symptom. The pulses are typically intact. Pigment changes are common with "cayenne pepper" purpura and hemosiderin deposition leading to a red-brown color. Edema is often a prominent sign but may be absent. Varices are commonly present. In long-standing cases the dermis and panniculus become fibrotic and woody hard, a change known as lipodermatosclerosis. In severe cases the fibrotic area on the distal third of the leg excludes edema, which persist cephalad, giving the leg an inverted "champagne bottle" appearance. Repeated episodes of cellulitis may damage lymphatics, producing a component of lymphedema.

Often there is an associated dermatitis with erythema, scaling, pruritus, and excoriation. This may be a direct consequence of venous disease or secondary to contact allergy. Common sensitizers include adhesives, neomycin, bacitracin, balsam of Peru, lanolins, benzocaine, parabens, and ethylenediamine.

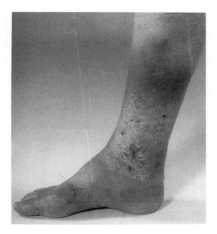

Figure 1   Venous ulcer.

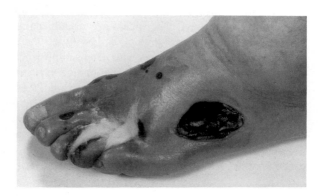

Figure 2   Ischemic ulcer.

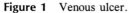

The diagnosis of venous ulceration is usually made based on clinical impression supported by noninvasive vascular labs.

Ischemic Ulcers

Leg ulcers caused by arterial insufficiency may be associated with ischemic heart disease, cerebrovascular disease, diabetes mellitus, and hypertension. Atherosclerosis is the leading cause, usually occurring in patients 45 years of age or greater. In younger patients who smoke, thromboangiitis obliterans should be considered.

Ischemic ulcerations are usually painful and exhibit increased pain with elevation and exercise, while pain is relived with dependency and rest. Rest pain is a sign of more severe disease. These ulcerations usually appear sharply demarcated and occasionally punched out (Fig. 2). They are dry with a necrotic base and poor granulation response. Typically, they occur on distal points such as the toes or the distal foot and at sites of pressure or trauma such as bony prominences. The peripheral pulses are usually diminished, asymmetric, or absent. They are rarely normal. Capillary refill time is prolonged. Elevation of the leg leads to pallor, and subsequent leg lowering leads to a reactive hyperemia and erythema. Upon lowering there will also be a delay in venous filling beyond 15–20 sec. This is valid only in the absence of venous incompetence, because if present, it would lead to erroneously normal findings.

The diagnosis can be confirmed with noninvasive vascular testing, and subsequent referral should be made to a vascular specialist to plan medical, interventional, or surgical management.

Neuropathic Ulcers

Sensory neuropathic ulcers arise from frequent trauma or persistent pressure leading to tissue ischemia, necrosis, and ulceration. Concurrent autonomic neuropathy may lead to the absence of vasodilator reflexes, which can contribute to ischemia. Traumatic tissue damage of this magnitude would not be tolerated in a sensate limb because of the pain. Diabetes mellitus is the most common cause, but neuropathic ulcers may be seen in leprosy, tabes dorsalis, traumatic neuropathy, or in children with inherited sensory neuropathies.

Neuropathic ulcers are usually located over points of pressure, especially on the plantar foot surfaces under the metatarsal heads or heel (Fig. 3). Footwear may also cause enough trauma for ulceration. Motor neuropathies may lead to altered weight bearing and gate, creating preferred areas of trauma. The ulcers are usually painless, with a necrotic or purulent base, and are surrounded by a rim of thick callus. Often the extent of the ulcer is not appreciated upon surface inspection. Deep ulcers with extension to tendon or bone are common. Many of the ulcers will show signs of infection with surrounding erythema, cellulitis, or purulent drainage. Wounds that appear trivial at first inspection can rapidly expand and necrose secondary to infection. Baseline immune deficiencies in diabetes mellitus combined with ischemia and neglect often lead to gangrene and amputation.

Radiographic evaluation is required to evaluate osteomyelitis. Special studies such as plain films of the involved bones, nuclear medicine scans, computed tomography, and magnetic resonance imaging may help in distinguishing osteomyelitis from noninfected osteopathy in a diabetic foot.

Noninvasive vascular studies can identify underlying ischemia and diagnose major vessel obstructive disease that can benefit from revascularization procedures. In contrast, a subset of patients will not have ischemia, but only pure neuropathic ulcerations, and may heal with conservative measures.

Simple neurologic evaluation with soft touch and vibration testing will reveal sensory neuropathy. Special nylon filaments of a uniform diameter are available to aide clinical evaluation. Inability to sense 10 g of pressure (normal sensation senses 1–2 g) indicates a high risk of ulceration.

Autoimmune and Vasculitic Ulcerations

The incidence of leg ulcers attributed to autoimmune and vasculitic causes is around 7%. Many, but not all, of these ulcers will reveal vasculitis upon biopsy of skin at the lesion's edge. A finding

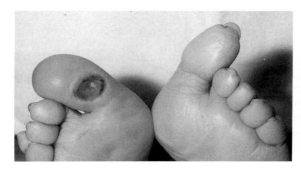

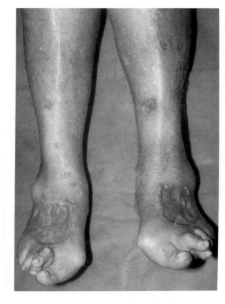

Figure 3   Neuropathic ulcer.   **Figure 4**   Rheumatoid vasculitis ulcer.

of vasculitis directly under the ulcer base is nonspecific and can be seen with any ulceration. Excisional biopsy of suspected lesions, including panniculus, is important because it provides enough tissue that the pathologic architecture is preserved, it increases sampling of the process, and it provides information on the location and type of vessel involved in the process. Findings of vasculitis on biopsy may reflect a primary vasculitic syndrome or a vasculitis associated with infection, drug, autoimmune disease, or neoplasm. If vasculitis is noted on biopsy, then historical, physical, and laboratory evidence of other organ system involvement should be sought with attention to vasculitic syndromes and associated causes. Lower extremity pulses are usually intact if autoimmune disease or vasculitis is the only cause of the ulceration.

Leg ulcers may affect up to 10% of patients with rheumatoid arthritis. The etiology is multifactorial. Necrotizing vasculitis is seen in the majority of biopsies; however, other factors may contribute to poor healing and ulceration. These factors include corticosteroid therapy (which leads to thin, fragile, poorly healing skin), peripheral neuropathies (causing neuropathic ulcerations), and venous insufficiency due to poor calf muscle pump function (resulting from neuropathy, deformity, and immobility). Rheumatoid ulcerations may have multiple appearances related to the underlying causes: ulcerative infarction and necrosis, deep punched-out dry ulcers of the feet, or shallow geographic exudative ulcers of the legs (Fig. 4).

Systemic lupus erythematosus can cause leg ulcerations, which are usually due to vascular occlusion associated with vasculitis or thrombosis. Patients with the lupus anticoagulant and antiphospholipid antibodies are at a greater risk of ulceration, and the ulcers are usually of the thrombotic occlusive nature. Vasculitic ulcers are usually seen in patients with active systemic disease (Fig. 5). Livedo reticularis, periungual erythema, a malar rash, oral ulcerations, and photosensitivity may be important differential clues. Systemic disease is often found with testing. Antiphospholipid antibodies may be seen primarily without evidence of systemic lupus erythematosus. These patients have a similar risk of ulceration. Ulcers related to antiphospholipids usually have a similar appearance to the ulceration of livedoid vasculitis.

Scleroderma may ulcerate, particularly long-standing severely involved lower limbs. Smaller ulcerations are common on the tips of involved digits. The etiology is multifactorial relating to functional (vasospasm) and structural (intimal proliferation and occlusion) vascular abnormalities supplying sclerotic and easily traumatized skin.

Livedoid vasculitis is a chronic relapsing segmental hyalinizing occlusive process of the dermal vessels accompanied by lymphocytic perivascular inflammation. Clinically the ulcers are small, extremely painful, and have stellate or linear configurations associated with livedo reticularis of the involved limb. The ulcers often heal with the white scars of atrophie blanche (Fig. 6). The process is often idiopathic but has been associated with autoimmune disease such as systemic lupus erythematosus or antiphospholipid antibodies.

Necrotizing venulitis or leukocytoclastic vasculitis causes palpable purpuric lesions, vesicles, pustules, or necrotic papules. Occasionally these lesions will progress to ulcerations. This vasculitis is usually a reactive process, but in the proper clinical setting may be a primary finding, as occurs, for example, in Henoch-Schönlein purpura. Inciting events include infection, autoimmune disease, drug reactions,cryoglobulinemia, malignancy, or systemic vasculitis.

Cutaneous polyarteritis nodosa and systemic polyarteritis nodosa can both cause leg ulcerations. In the cutaneous group, findings are limited to the skin and tend to have a chronic, recurrent course. Both diseases present with punched-out painful ulcerations on the legs associated with tender, erythematous, deep dermal, and subcutaneous nodules (Fig. 7). Often there is a "starburst" or linear irregular "lightning bolt" livedo pattern radiating from the ulcerated areas. Biopsy of a nodule (including panniculus) will often reveal necrotizing vasculitis of a small- to medium-sized artery at the dermal-pannicular junction.

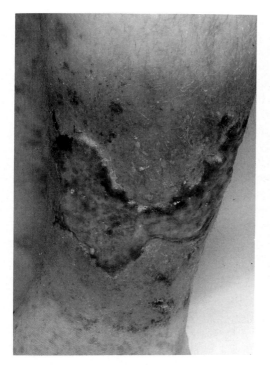

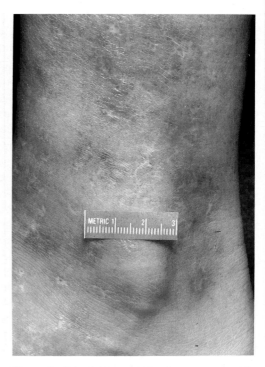

Figure 5   Lupus erythematosus ulcer.   **Figure 6**   Livedoid vasculitis ulcers and atrophie blanche scarring.

Leg ulcer biopsies revealing vasculitis can be seen in Wegener's granulomatosis or Churg-Strauss vasculitis. Other common findings include erythematous papules and nodules. Systemic associations are necessary for diagnosis. In Wegener's granulomatosis a necrotizing granulomatous vasculitis is noted in the upper respiratory tract and lung. Glomerulonephritis is seen in the kidney, and antineutrophil cytoplasmic antibodies are detected in the plasma. In Churg-Strauss granulomatosis patients have a history of asthma, peripheral blood and tissue eosinophil, necrotizing granulomatous vasculitis (affecting the lung and other organs), and extravascular granulomas in the lung and the skin.

Miscellaneous Causes

Pyoderma gangrenosum is a well-recognized clinical entity. The lesions commonly begin as a purple nodule or pustule that rapidly spreads to produce necrosis and ulceration (Fig. 8). The border is characteristically undermined with a violaceous color and a surrounding erythematous halo. Central healing often leads to cribriform scarring. The lesions frequently begin at sites of minor trauma or after skin incision, ulcerating to a larger size than initially damaged. This process is known as pathergy. The most common systemic associations are inflammatory bowel disease and the presence of a monoclonal gammopathy. Biopsies are not specific and reveal neutrophilic central inflammation surrounded by intense perivascular lymphocytic inflammation at the periphery. The diagnosis is based on characteristic clinical findings and the exclusion of other causes by history, exam, vascular evaluation, biopsy, and cultures. Case reports exist where necrotizing fasciitis has been mistaken for pyoderma gangrenosum, resulting in inappropriate steroid treatment with severe consequences.

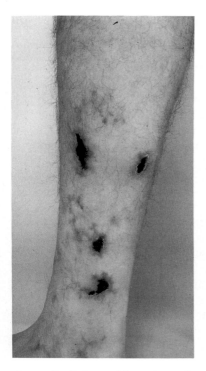

Figure 7 Polyarteritis nodosa ulcers.

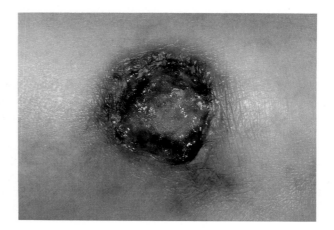

Figure 8 Pyoderma gangrenosum.

Necrobiosis lipoidica diabeticorum may ulcerate. Diagnosis is established by the characteristic yellow-brown, atrophic, telangiectatic plaques on the pretibial leg in a patient who often has diabetes mellitus. Biopsy reveals palisading necrobiotic granulomas in the dermis.

Hematologic causes are an important consideration. The ulcers typically involve the ankle area and are often painful, shallow, and small. Upon biopsy the majority of these processes reveal thrombotic occlusive phenomena. Red blood cell disorders such as sickle cell anemia, thalassemia, and polycythemia vera are common causes. Other disorders such as thrombocytosis and dysproteinemias (cryoglobulins, cryofibrinogenemia) may produce thrombotic or vasculitic ulcers. Fibrinolytic defects are a recently recognized cause of ulcers; they include protein C and S deficiencies and antithrombin III deficiency.

Emboli from atheroma, aneurysms, or endocarditis usually cause ulcerations in the distal extremities and the digits. There may be a preceding history of intravascular manipulations such as angiography. Initiation of coumadin therapy can sometimes cause showers of emboli from atheromatous plaques.

Infection is an important cause of leg ulcers, particularly in the immunocompromised patient. Causes that should be considered include deep fungal infections, tuberculosis, atypical mycobacteria, leprosy, syphilis, actinomycosis, septic emboli, and synergistic bacterial infections such as necrotizing fasciitis. Appropriate tissue must be submitted for culture and the biopsy examined with special stains.

Malignancy should be excluded with biopsy. Common malignant causes include squamous cell carcinoma (particularly in old burn scars and indolent ulcers of any cause), basal cell carcinoma,

Kaposi's sarcoma, classic cutaneous T-cell lymphoma (mycosis fungoides), and peripheral T-cell lymphomas (Fig. 9).

Several drugs may contribute to leg ulceration, including hydroxyurea, methotrexate, halogen ingestion, coumadin, infiltrated vasopressors, and intravenous or subcutaneous illicit drugs, particularly amphetamines.

Factitial ulcers are not a rare problem, and diagnosis can be difficult. The location, pattern, size, and shape of the ulcers can provide clues (Fig. 10). History of "physician shopping" or an indifferent attitude and obvious secondary gain may also help in diagnosis.

Panniculitis can ulcerate. The most likely causes of ulcerating panniculitis include pancreatic fat necrosis, α_1-antitrypsin deficiency, and lupus.

GENERAL TREATMENT MEASURES

Impairments to wound healing should be recognized and corrected. Nutritional deficiencies of protein, vitamin C, magnesium, iron, and zinc are important considerations. Glucocorticoids and cytotoxic agents will impair healing, although in autoimmune or malignant ulcers these agents can also promote healing.

If any evidence of active infection such as cellulitis, lymphangitis, leukocytosis, fever, or persistent drainage is encountered, then treatment with systemic antibiotics is essential. This should be based upon culture and sensitivities. Empiric coverage of common skin organisms such as *Staphylococcus* and *Streptococcus* species should be started pending culture data. If deep or necrotic wounds are present, empiric coverage for anaerobic species should also be provided.

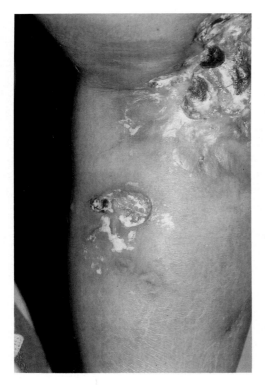

Figure 9   Angiocentric T-cell lymphoma ulcer.

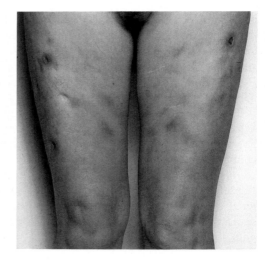

Figure 10   Factitial ulcers.

Candida overgrowth under occlusive dressings or in topically treated wounds can be a cause of delayed wound healing. If cultures indicate *Candida* in high numbers, the addition of several days of topical antifungal therapy can be extremely helpful.

Treatment of dermatitis from venous disease or contact allergy will speed healing and decrease portals of entry for infection. A few days of topical steroids and nonirritating wet dressings (saline, water, or mild antiseptics such as aluminum subacetate or dilute acetic acid) will provide rapid control. The steroids may then be discontinued and the liberal use of lubricating creams begun as a protective measure.

Wound Care

Standard wound care consists of infection control, removal of necrotic debris (a sanctuary and media for bacteria and fungi), and provision of a moist wound environment promoting granulation tissue and epithelialization.

Mild antiseptic wet dressings are a historic and effective method of microbial control and gentle debridement. Wetting agents include aluminum subacetate and acetic acid. Povidone iodine inhibits wound healing in concentrations above 0.001% solution, as does Dakin's sodium hypochlorite solution above 0.005% solution and hexachlorophene at any concentration. Because of inhibition of wound healing, these last three should probably be avoided. All five of these compounds have shown in vitro fibroblast toxicity, therefore it seems prudent to use normal saline once debridement has been accomplished.

Wet-to-dry dressing changes can be very effective in debridement of necrotic wounds. The original moist wound surface dries as the wetting agent evaporates, binding wound exudate and debris to the gauze dressing material. When the dressing is removed, the necrotic debris is mechanically pulled away. Unfortunately, it may also pull away new epithelium and granulation tissue, so it should be stopped once debridement has been achieved. Newer occlusive dressings have the capacity to provide painless debridement by holding autolytic wound exudates against the ulcer bed. This process may lead to an erroneously perceived worsening and increase in size when actually it reflects loss of necrotic tissue.

Surgical debridement may be necessary for thick eschars, infectious ulcers, and deep ulcers extending to tendon and bone. Caution must be used to limit the debridement to devitalized tissues only, particularly in ischemic and neurotrophic ulcers. For superficial ulcers, topical 2% lidocaine gel followed by sharp curettage may be sufficient debridement.

Once granulation tissue is forming and the wound is clean, maintenance of a moist non-traumatic environment is desired for the fragile new tissues. This can be done with continuous wet dressings of saline or water, being careful not to macerate or overly dry the wound through evaporative losses. Gauze- and bandage-covered bland ointments and creams can be effective, including erythromycin ointment, silver sulfadiazine cream, or petrolatum-impregnated gauze. Harsh antiseptics and sensitizing chemicals are to be avoided. Care should be taken to remove cream buildup with occasional wet dressings or soaks. Occlusive dressings are helpful at this stage of healing as well.

Wound Dressings

There are a variety of new dressing materials available (see the chapter on wound dressings in this text). In general these dressings provide painless debridement, stimulate granulation tissue, encourage epithelialization, reduce wound pain, provide protection, and decrease dressing change needs. Initial concerns that increased bacterial counts in the trapped wound fluid would lead to greater incidence of infection have proved unfounded. Indeed, wounds treated with these dressings have a decreased infection rate. Infected draining wounds should not be occluded. Disadvantages are expense, availability, adhesives that rip away new epithelium if dressings are changed too frequently, malodorous leakage of wound fluid, and induction of an exudative wound phase in a previously dry wound. For chronic wounds several types of occlusive dressings seem to have an advantage. The hydrocolloids are useful in all stages of wound healing since they have some ability to debride, absorb exudate, provide protection, and maintain moisture. These dressings are self-adhesive and may be used under compression therapy. Hydrogels will absorb and allow the passage of exudate to overlying gauze while maintaining a moist wound environment. They must be held in place with bandages. For exudative wounds the alginates have the unique ability to absorb abundant exudate into a gel-like matrix. These dressings promote exudative wounds into dry wounds, so it is recommended that a moisture-maintaining regime be used once the exudation ceases.

Skin Grafting

Any ulcer that is clean and granulating may benefit from skin grafting. Well-granulating but poorly epithelialized ulcers from venous insufficiency or previous occlusion therapy may show particular benefit. Often the graft will stimulate epithelial healing even at sites not covered by the graft. This may relate to growth factor release or production of matrix materials for epithelial migration.

Given the compromised healing in chronic wounds, the most successful grafting methods have been pinch grafts and split-thickness skin grafts. Both of these grafts have fewer metabolic requirements than full-thickness grafts. Advantages of pinch grafts include the fact that they can be harvested in the office and will allow passage of wound exudate. Split-thickness grafts generally cover greater areas, leave better-appearing donor and recipient sites, and may heal faster. Fenestrations should be provided to allow passage of exudate. Meshing of split-thickness grafts offers wider coverage from a given size donor site and allows passage of exudate. Routine procedures for these grafting techniques should be followed (described elsewhere in this text). For small areas, all may be done in the office under local anesthesia.

Any large ulcer or ulcer with exposed bone and poorly vascularized deep structures, such as tendon, should have full-thickness skin and soft tissue coverage via flaps or free microvascular reconstructed flaps.

Systemic Agents

Systemic agents are sometimes used as primary or supportive treatment in leg ulcer management. Platelet-inhibiting drugs like aspirin and dipyridamole have proven beneficial adjuncts to routine wound care. Processes where they are used include livedoid vasculitis, necrobiosis lipoidica diabeticorum, atheromatous and cholesterol emboli, and antiphospholipid antibody disease. Anticoagulation with heparin and coumadin has been useful in patients with livedoid vasculitis, coagulopathies, and antiphospholipid antibody disease.

Fibrinolytic agents such as phenformin and the anabolic steroid stanazolol are used to treat antiphospholipid antibody disease, livedoid vasculitis, and cryofibrinogenemia. Controversy remains whether stanazolol provides benefit in venous ulcerations. Low-dose tissue plasminogen activator has been successful in healing ulcerations of livedoid vasculitis and antiphospholipid antibody disease.

Ketanserin, a serotonergic blocker, has direct vasodilating effects and indirect effects via blocking serotonin-mediated platelet degranulation and the inflammatory and vasoconstricting sequelae. This also inhibits the serotonin-driven platelet degranulation-amplification loop. It has shown benefit in treating ischemic ulcers, venous ulcers, livedoid vasculitis and systemic scleroderma.

Pentoxifylline produces hemorrheologic effects by increasing red blood cell deformity, thereby allowing easier passage through the microvasculature and preventing sludging. Recent support on fibrinolytic effects, platelet aggregation effects, and changes in prostacyclin synthesis have been published. Studies support its use in a wide variety of ulcerations including ischemic ulcers, venous ulcers, necrobiosis lipoidica diabeticorum, sickle cell anemia, and thalassemia.

Corticosteroids and immunosuppressive agents are the mainstay of treatment for vasculitis, pyoderma gangrenosum, and autoimmune diseases. Antibiotics, antifungals, and antimycobacterials are essential in the treatment of infectious ulcerations.

TREATMENT OF SPECIFIC ULCERATIONS

Venous Ulcers

Specific measures to reduce ambulatory venous hypertension are essential in the treatment of venous ulcers. While hospitalization (for bed rest and wound care) has been a standard and effective treatment for venous and other ulcers, cost-control measures are quickly making this impossible. Benefits from an outpatient approach to ulcer management include less deconditioning and lower risks of falls, decreased risk of deep venous thrombosis, and patients who can remain active and at work.

One method to decrease venous hypertension is by using support hose that provide 30–40 mmHg of pressure. They should be put on first thing in morning and worn until retiring for the night, and in most cases they need to be worn indefinitely. Hose will lose elasticity over time and should be replaced on a regular basis. Routine wound care can usually be done with dressings underneath the stockings. Ischemic disease should always be sought and ruled out, because with any compression therapy, ischemia can be exacerbated.

Several problems make the use of compression hose difficult; for example, exudative wounds require frequent dressing changes, resolution of initial edema causes poor stocking fit, and mobility limitations make it hard to treat the disabled and elderly. One method that addresses some of these problems is the Unna boot. This impregnated bandage consists of a mixture of zinc oxide, calamine lotion, and glycerin. It is used to wrap the extremity from forefoot to knee, creating a semirigid cast that provides compression, occlusion, and protection. During the initial treatment of exudative or edematous wounds, the dressing must be changed every 2–4 days. After the edema and exudation resolve, the dressing can be changed every 7–10 days. Experience in application is required to provide adequate compression without inducing ischemia or creating pressure points. The Unna boot is particularly suited to disabled and noncompliant patients since the only requirements on the wearer are to come for office visits and keep the boot dry. Once the ulcer is healed, use of Unna boots or compression hose may continue. Continued boot use can provide prophylactic compression for patients unwilling or unable to use support hose. Problems with continued boot use include maceration and sensitization to the boot compounds. Intermittent pneumatic compression devices are helpful for rapidly reducing edema in a day or two, allowing support hose or Unna boots to be fit.

Elastic wraps are another compression method for treating venous ulcers, especially when they are exudative wounds, alternative limb shapes, changing states of limb edema, or in disabled patients. By nature they adapt to changing limb size and shape and are easily applied by health care providers. Some patients may also find them easier to use. They are inexpensive and can easily be replaced when soiled or when elasticity is lost. While wrapping a limb requires some degree of skill, it can usually be learned without difficulty. The wrap is started at the malleolar area for the first turn, then down over the ankle and forefoot. It is then reversed back up over the ankle to the knee. Wrapping direction should be from medial to lateral on the way up the leg. The overlap should be one-half to one-third of the width. Since the elastic recoil can be quite significant, care should be used not to wrap the limb too tightly. Underlying gauze pads can be used to absorb exudate and supply additional pressure over concave areas such as ulcers and the perimalleolar areas. Once healing occurs, the wraps may be continued or compression hose may be used.

The role of venous surgery in healing and preventing leg ulceration remains controversial. Procedure choices include sclerotherapy of superficial system and perforators, superficial system ligation, stripping with perforator ligation, bypass techniques, and deep venous valve reconstruction or brachial vein segment transplants. Proper patient selection appears to be important to outcome. In general, if deep venous system disease is present (as it is in the majority of the cases), then neither superficial nor perforator surgery is likely to help healing or prevent recurrence. Deep venous procedures combined with superficial procedures may play a role, but this remains to be proven conclusively. Isolated superficial system disease and ulceration will likely respond to surgical therapy, although this is a small portion of venous ulcer patients.

Arterial Disease

Simple measures can be done to benefit patients with ischemic ulcers. Smoking should be prohibited. Diabetes mellitus and hypertension should be controlled. The limbs should be protected from trauma (going barefoot, ill-fitting shoes) and protected from direct heat and cold environments. Surgical debridement should be undertaken cautiously. In general, despite theoretical advantages, vasodilator drugs such as calcium channel blockers have not been beneficial in ischemic ulcers. This may be due to a "shunting" effect into the muscle vasculature, resulting from the muscle's ability to increase blood flow beyond that of damaged skin. Invasive interventions that are beneficial in selected patients include angioplasty, atherectomy, reconstruction, and bypass procedures.

Neuropathic Ulcerations

Prevention of trauma to the healing ulcer or surrounding tissues is the main therapeutic goal. Patients should inspect their feet daily for any evidence of trauma, fissuring, persistent erythema, or nonhealing wounds, no matter how minor. A similar examination should be done at each physician visit. Before dressing, shoes should be inspected by the patient to avoid walking on unnoticed foreign objects. Inspection may also reveal pressure points on the shoes. The shoes should fit, support, and distribute weight well. Consultation with orthopedics and podiatry can be extremely helpful in providing orthotics and special shoes for these patients. Tinea pedis should be sought and treated to decrease portals of entry for infection. Extreme care should be undertaken during nail trimming and corn or callus management. In many patients this is best done by a physician or podiatrist. Patients must not go barefoot, wear pressure-inducing sandals or thongs, or apply heat or hot water to the feet. Bath water should always be tested before stepping into the tub. Patients should quit smoking and control their diabetes and hypertension.

Once ulceration develops, the severity of tissue destruction may not be apparent. It is important to inspect the wound for undermined areas that might extend to deep structures. Adequate debridement is important and should be done by a physician experienced in these wounds. Relief of pressure over the ulcer and non–weight bearing are essential until full healing has occurred. If this cannot be done adequately with crutches or a wheelchair, then total contact casting is recommended so that the patient can ambulate without placing pressure on the ulcer. Frequent inspections of the ulcer are needed to avoid overlooking complications.

Evaluation of infection is essential, and studies to rule out underlying osteomyelitis must be done. Treatment of ulcer-associated infection may require intravenous antibiotics, and 6–8 weeks of antibiotics may be needed to eradicate osteomyelitis. Necrotic tissue, including bone, should be debrided. Antibiotic therapy should be guided by culture and sensitivity. Once healing occurs, preventive measures remain essential to prevent recurrence.

Autoimmune and Vasculitic Ulcers

Identification of the cause is the most important aspect in proper treatment of these ulcers. Once a diagnosis is reached, treatment of specific autoimmune or vasculitic disorders is the goal. General wound care measures are important. The main therapeutic agents for the vasculitic syndromes are systemic corticosteroids. Dosing depends upon the specific syndrome and response to therapy. Other useful agents include azathioprine and cyclophosphamide. The ulcers will often heal when the vasculitic syndrome is treated. In other cases, once the underlying process is controlled, the immunosuppressive medications may need tapering to a minimal beneficial level, so that wound healing may progress.

The treatment for autoimmune diseases is specific according to the disease process and ulcer cause. Vasculitic ulcers associated with rheumatoid arthritis usually require systemic corticosteroids. If associated with systemic vasculitis as well, cyclophosphamide or chlorambucil has been used. Vasculitis limited to the skin may respond to methotrexate or dapsone. Nonvasculitic rheumatoid leg ulcers may benefit from routine agents used in rheumatoid arthritis, including hydroxychloroquine, methotrexate, azathioprine, and penicillamine.

Systemic lupus erythematosus ulcerations are treated according to the cause. In cases revealing vasculitis, corticosteroids and immunosuppressants are used. If they are thrombotic in nature (usually associated with antiphospholipid antibodies), they are treated with antiplatelet agents, fibrinolytics, and anticoagulants (as in livedoid vasculitis).

Livedoid vasculitis has been treated successfully as a thrombotic occlusive disease without the need for immunosuppression. Methods that have been used include anticoagulation with heparin and coumadin, aspirin, low-dose tissue plasminogen activator, pentoxifylline, nicotinic acid, phenformin, and ketanserin.

Necrotizing venulitis (hypersensitivity vasculitis) is treated by removal of inciting agents and treatment of any stimulating disease processes. In idiopathic cases dapsone and colchicine have been used.

Scleroderma ulcers have been treated with vasodilating agents such as nifedipine, nitrates, prazosin, hydralazine, and methyldopa. Other approaches have used antiplatelet therapy with aspirin, dipyridamole, and ketanserin. Pentoxifylline and immunosuppressives have also been reported as beneficial.

Miscellaneous Conditions

Pyoderma gangrenosum is generally treated with corticosteroids. For small superficial lesions, intralesional triamcinolone may be effective. For larger and multiple lesions, systemic prednisone is required. In refractory cases other agents are used, including rifampin, minocycline, dapsone, azathioprine, cyclosporin, and cyclophosphamide. Standard wound care measures support systemic therapy.

Necrobiosis lipoidica diabeticorum may respond to aspirin, dipyridamole, and pentoxifylline when combined with wound care.

Hemoglobinopathy-associated ulcers often respond to transfusion therapy, antiplatelet therapies, and pentoxifylline. Coagulation disorders and dysproteinemias may respond to antiplatelet therapies, anticoagulation, or fibrinolytics. Thrombocythemia-related ulcers often respond to therapy directed at lowering the platelet count.

Malignant lesions are treated according to type, location, extent, size, and distribution. Methods include local excision, Mohs micrographic surgery, amputation, radiation therapy, and systemic chemotherapy.

FUTURE DIRECTIONS IN LEG ULCER TREATMENT

Cultured Epidermal Grafting

Keratinocytes can now be propagated in tissue culture to produce sheets of cells. If grown on a collagen matrix, these sheets resemble normal epidermis. This allows coverage of large defects with minimal donor skin and has been used successfully in patients with widespread severe burns. These grafts are now being tested on chronic wounds including leg ulcers. Autografts are created from a sample of the patient's own skin. These grafts have been used on leg ulcers to speed healing of large or refractory ulcers. The main disadvantages are the patient-specific costs of individual preparation, time waiting for cultures to grow, and increased risks of fungal and bacterial contamination of the tissue culture due to harvesting from patients with colonized wounds.

Allografts provide improved efficiency through economies of time and scale, which has led to experiments using allograft keratinocyte cultures from unrelated donor. Neonatal foreskin cultures may have added benefits through increased response to growth factors and more rapid wound coverage. Allografts may also be frozen, allowing long-term storage and banking benefits as well as easing transportation pressures. Allografts have also been shown to speed healing in chronic leg ulcerations from a variety of causes. While originally thought to be immune tolerant (since no detectable signs of rejection were originally noted), this theory has been disproven using chromosomal analysis of wound-covering keratinocytes. It appears that the allografts serve as temporary dressings that stimulate wound healing and growth of host keratinocytes. No donor keratinocytes are noted in the wound after about day 14. One hypothesis to explain these findings is that the allograft provides growth factors or manufactures matrix protein structures that stimulate wound healing.

Growth Factors

The basic science literature on wound healing and growth factors has expanded exponentially over the last several years. Clinical applications of growth factor research are now being tested in a variety of settings. The most successful approach reported thus far utilizes an extract of autologous platelets isolated by apheresis. The platelets are then stimulated to release their storage granules, producing a variety of peptide growth factors including platelet-derived growth factor, transforming growth factors alpha and beta, and epidermal growth factor. This growth factor–rich extract is then applied to the wound surface, where it can speed healing of refractory leg ulcers from a variety of causes. This platelet-derived wound healing extract can also be prepared from donor platelets. Trials of individual and combined growth factor treatment in chronic wounds are currently underway.

Electrical Stimulation

Numerous human and animal studies have demonstrated that direct galvanic electrical stimulation can dramatically improve healing of skin wounds. The majority of the clinical studies have been in the treatment of pressure ulcers in bedridden patients or in patients with diabetic neuropathy. Even when compared to routine therapies, electrical stimulation showed improved healing. Several theoretical benefits exist which are supported by experimental data. They include attraction of macrophages, stimulation of fibroblast activity, induction of keratinocyte migration, bacteriostasis, improving edema, liquefaction of necrotic debris, expression of growth factor receptors, and stimulation of neurite growth and associated trophic factors. Devices manufactured for other uses are available, but none have Federal Drug Administration approval for use in wound healing.

Topical Hyperbaric Oxygen Therapy

Total body hyperbaric oxygen chambers have proven useful in the healing of chronic wounds. The main disadvantage has been oxygen toxicity affecting multiple organs. A simple method of local topical hyperbaric oxygen therapy has been described using routinely available oxygen delivery systems and disposable polyethylene bags. It has been used with success in the treatment of chronic wounds including leg ulcers secondary to venous disease, arterial disease, diabetes mellitus, vasculitis, and pyoderma gangrenosum.

BIBLIOGRAPHY

Venous Ulcers

Bishop JB, Phillips LD, Musto TA, et al. A perspective randomized evaluator-blinded trial of 2 potential wound healing agents for the treatment of venous stasis ulcers. *J Vasc Surg* 1992;16:251–257.

Blair SD, Wright DD, Blackhouse CM, et al. Sustained compression and healing of chronic venous ulcers. *Br Med J* 1988;297:1159–1161.

Burnand KG, Clemenson G, Morland M, et al. Venous lipodermatosclerosis: treatment by fibrinolytic enhancement and elastic compression. *Br Med J* 1980;280:7–11.

Burnand KG, Whimster I, Naidoo A, et al. Pericapillary fibrin disposition in the ulcer-bearing skin of the lower limb: the cause of lipodermatosis sclerosis in venous ulceration. *Br Med J* 1982;285:1071–1072.

Cikrit DF, Nichols WK, Silver D. Surgical management of refractory venous stasis ulceration. *J Vasc Surg* 1988;7:473–477.

Colgan MP, Dormandy JA, Jones PW, et al. Oxpentifylline treatment of venous ulcers of the leg. *Br Med J* 1990;300;972–975.

Comp PC, Esman CT. Recurrent venous thromboembolism in patients with partial deficiency of protein S. *N Engl J Med* 1984;311:1526–1528.

Falanga V. Venous ulceration. *J Dermatol Surg Oncol* 1993;19:764–771.

Falanga V, Bontempo FA, Eaglstein WH. Protein C and protein S plasma levels in patients with lipodermatosclerosis and venous ulceration. *Arch Dermatol* 1990;126:1195–1197.

Falanga V, Eaglstein WH. The "trap" hypothesis of venous ulceration. *Lancet* 1993;341:1006–1008.

Falanga V, Moosa HH, Nemeth AJ, et al. Dermal pericapillary fibrin in venous disease and venous ulceration. *Arch Dermatol* 1987;123:620–623.

Gaylarde PM, Dodd HJ, Sarkany I. Venous leg ulcers and arthropathy. *Br J Rheum* 1990;29:142–144.

Goodfield MJD. A relative thrombocytosis and elevated mean platelet volume are features of gravitational disease. *Br J Dermatol* 1986;115:521–528.

Herrick SE, Sloan P, McGurk M, et al. Sequential changes in histologic pattern and extracellular matrix deposition during the healing of chronic venous ulcers. *Am J Pathol* 1992;141:1085–1095.

Hopkins NFG, Spinks TJ, Rodes CG, et al. Positron emission tomography in venous ulceration and lipodermatosclerosis: study of regional tissue function. *Br Med J* 1983;286:333–336.

Jarrett F. Leg ulcers of vascular etiology. *Clin Dermatol* 1990;8:40–48.

Kirsner RS, Pardes JB, Eaglstein WH, et al. The clinical spectrum of lipodermatosclerosis. *J Am Acad Dermatol* 1993;28:623–627.

Layton AM, Ibbotson SH, Davies JA, et al. Randomized trial of oral aspirin for chronic venous leg ulcers. *Lancet* 1994;344:164–165.

Luetolf O, Bull RH, Bates DO, et al. Capillary under perfusion in chronic venous insufficiency: a cause for leg ulceration? *Br J Dermatol* 1993;128:249–254.

O'Donnell TF. Chronic venous insufficiency and varicose veins. In *Peripheral Vascular Diseases*. JR Young, RA Graor, JW Olin, and JR Bartholomew, eds. St. Louis, Mosby-Year Book, 1991, pp. 443–480.

O'Donnell TF, MacKay WC, Shepherd AD, et al. Clinical, hemodynamic, and anatomic follow-up of direct venous reconstruction. *Arch Surg* 1987;122:474–482.

Phillips TJ, Dover JS. Leg ulcers. *J Am Acad Dermatol* 1991;25:965–987.

Sarkany I, Dodd HJ, Gaylarde PM. Surgical correction of venous incompetence restores normal skin blood flow and abolishes skin hypoxia during exercise. *Arch Dermatol* 1989;125:223–226.

Wolfe JHN, Morland M, Browse NL. The fibrinolytic activity of varicose veins. *Br J Surg* 1979;66:185–187.

Ischemic Ulcers

Christensen JH, Freundlich M, Jacobsen BA, et al. Clinical relevance of pedal pulse palpation in patients suspected of peripheral arterial insufficiency. *J Int Med* 1989;226:95–99.

Duncan HJ, Faris IB. Martorell's hypertensive ischemic leg ulcers are secondary to an increase in the local vascular resistance. *J Vasc Surg* 1985;2:581–584.

Friedman SA. The diagnosis and medical management of vascular ulcers. *Clin Dermatol* 1990;8:30–39.

Joyce JW. Thromboangiitis obliterans (Buerger's disease). In *Peripheral Vascular Diseases*. JR Young, RA Graor, JW Olin, JR Bartholomew, eds. St. Louis, Mosby-Year Book, 1991, pp. 331–337.

Krajewski LP, Olin JW. Atherosclerosis of the aorta and lower extremity arteries. In *Peripheral Vascular Diseases*. JR Young, RA Graor, JW Olin, JR Bartholomew, eds. St. Louis, Mosby-Year Book, 1991, pp. 179–200.

Neuropathic Ulcers

Bockers M, Benes P, Bork K. Persistent skin ulcers, mutilations, and acro-osteolysis in hereditary sensory and autonomic neuropathy with phospholipid excretion. *J Am Acad Dermatol* 1989;21:736–739.

Flynn MD, Tooke JE. Microcirculation in the diabetic foot. *Vasc Med Rev* 1990;1:121–138.

Huntley AC. The cutaneous manifestations of diabetes mellitus. *J Am Acad Dermatol* 1982;6:427–455.

Levin ME. Diabetic foot lesions. In *Peripheral Vascular Diseases*. JR Young, RA Graor, JW Olin, JR Bartholomew, eds. St. Louis, Mosby-Year Book, 1991, pp. 669–711.

Logerfo FW, Coffman JD. Vascular and microvascular diseases of the foot in diabetes: Implications for foot care. *N Engl J Med* 1984;311:1615–1619.

McGoey JW. Metabolic causes of leg ulcers. *Clin Dermatol* 1990;8:86–91.

Miller OF. Essentials of pressure ulcer treatment: the diabetic experience. *J Dermatol Surg Oncol* 1993;19:759–763.

White RR, Lynch DJ, Verheyden CN, et al. Management of wounds in the diabetic foot. *Surg Clin North Am* 1984;64:735–42.

Autoimmune and Vasculitic Ulcers

Alegre VA, Gastineau DA, Winkelmann RK. Skin lesions associated with circulating lupus anticoagulant. *Br J Dermatol* 1989;120:419–429.

Bard JW, Winkelmann RK. Livedoid vasculitis: segmental hyalinizing vasculitis of the dermis. *Arch Dermatol* 1967;96:489–499.

Cawley M. Vasculitis and ulceration in rheumatic diseases of the foot. *Clin Rheumatol* 1987;1:315–333.

Diaz-Perez JL, Winkelmann RK. Cutaneous periarteritis nodosa. *Arch Dermatol* 1974;110:407–414.

Goslen JB. Autoimmune ulceration of the leg. *Clin Dermatol* 1990;8:92–117.

Grattan CEH, Burton JL. Antiphospholipid syndrome and cutaneous vasoocclusive disorders. *Semin Dermatol* 1991;10:152–159.

Kerdel FA. Inflammatory ulcers. *J Dermatol Surg Oncol* 1993;19:772–778.

Lawley TJ, Kubota Y. Vasculitis. *Dermatol Clin* 1990;8:681–687.

Petry M. Antiphospholipid antibodies: lupus anticoagulant and anticardiolipin antibody. *Curr Probl Dermatol* 1992;4:171–201.

Roenigk HH, Young JR. Leg ulcers. In *Peripheral Vascular Diseases*. JR Young, RA Graor, JW Olin, JR Bartholomew, eds. St. Louis, Mosby-Year Book, 1991, pp. 605–638.

Tuffanelli DL, Winkelmann RK. Systemic scleroderma: a clinical study of 727 cases. *Arch Dermatol* 1961;84:359–371.

Wallace DJ, Dubois EL. Dubois-Lupus Erythematosus. 3rd ed. Philadelphia, Lea & Febiger, 1987.

Miscellaneous Causes

Callen JP. Pyoderma gangrenosum and related disorders. *Adv Dermatol* 1989;4:51–70.

Fellner MJ, Ledesma GN. Leg ulcers secondary to drug reactions. *Clin Dermatol* 1990;8:144–149.

Galinberti RL, Flores V, Gonzalez Ramos MC, et al. Cutaneous ulcers due to *Candida albicans* in an immunocompromised patient: Response to therapy with itraconazole. *Clin Exp Dermatol* 1989;14:295–297.

Geller JD, Peters MS, Su WPD. Cutaneous mucormycosis resembling superficial granulomatous pyoderma in an immunocompetent host. *J Am Acad Dermatol* 1993;29:462–465.

Hansson C, Jekler J, Swanbeck G. *Candida albicans* infections in leg ulcers and surrounding skin after the use of ointment impregnated stockings. *Acta Dermato-Vener* 1985;65:424–427.

Harahap M. Leg ulcers caused by bacterial infections. *Clin Dermatol* 1990;8:49–64.

Helm KF, Su WPD, Muller SA, Kurtin PJ. Malignant lymphoma and leukemia with prominent ulceration: clinicopathologic correlation of 33 cases. *J Am Acad Dermatol* 1992;27:553–559.

Jemic GBE, Konradsen L. Pyoderma gangrenosum complicated by a necrotizing fasciitis. *Cutis* 1994;53:139–141.

Koshy M, Entsuah R, Koranda A, et al. Leg ulcers in patients with sickle cell disease. *Blood* 1989;74:1403–1408.

Leoni A, Cetta G, Tenni R, et al. Prolidase deficiency in two siblings with chronic leg ulcerations. Clinical, biochemical, and morphologic aspects. *Arch Dermatol* 1987;123:493–499.

Milligan A, Graham-Brown RA, Burns DA, et al. Prolidase deficiency: a case report and literature review. *Br J Dermatol* 1989;121:405–409.

Parish LC, Witkowski JA. Leg ulcers due to miscellaneous causes. *Clin Dermatol* 1990;8:150–156.

Peters MS, Su WPD. Panniculitis. *Dermatol Clin* 1992;10:37–57.

Piette WW. Hematologic associations of leg ulcers. *Clin Dermatol* 1990;8:66–85.

Sedgwick-O'Donnell SK, Kaplan RP. Primary and secondary skin cancers affecting the lower extremities: tumorous leg ulcers. *Clin Dermatol* 1990;8:118–143.

Sehgal VN. Leg ulcers caused by deep mycotic infection. *Clin Dermatol* 1990;8:157–165.

Sehgal VN. Leg ulcers caused by yaws and endemic syphilis. *Clin Dermatol* 1990;8:166–175.

Additional Therapies

Angelides NS, Angastiniotis C, Pavlides N. Effect of pentoxifylline on treatment of lower limb ulcers in patients with thalassemia major. *Angiology* 1992;43:549–554.

Callen JP, Case JD, Sager D. Chlorambucil—an effective corticosteroid sparing therapy for pyoderma gangrenosum. *J Am Acad Dermatol* 1989;21:514–519.

Callen JP, Spencer LV, Bhatnagar Burruss J, Holtman J. Azathioprine. An effective corticosteroid sparing therapy for patients with recalcitrant cutaneous lupus erythematosus or with recalcitrant cutaneous leukocytoclastic vasculitis. *Arch Dermatol* 1991;127:515–522.

Ely H, Bard JW. Therapy of livedo vasculitis with pentoxifylline. *Cutis* 1988;42:448–453.

Falanga V, Kirsner RS, Eaglstein WH, et al. Stanozolol in the treatment of leg ulcers due to cryofibrinogenemia. *Lancet* 1991;338:347–348.

Fredenberg MF, Malkinson FD. Sulphonamide on therapy in the treatment of leukocytoclastic vasculitis. *J Am Acad Dermatol* 1987;17:355–359.

Gilliam JN, Herndon JH, Prystowski SD. Fibrinolytic therapy for vasculitis of atrophie blanche. *Arch Dermatol* 1974;109:664–667.

Gupta A, Ellis C, Nickoloff B, et al. Oral cyclosporine in the treatment of inflammatory and noninflammatory dermatoses. *Arch Dermatol* 1990;126:339–350.

Heng MCY, Song MK, Heng MK. Healing of necrobiotic ulcers with antiplatelet therapy: correlation with plasma thromboxane levels. *Int J Dermatol* 1989;28:195–197.

Janssen PAJ, Janssen H, Cauwenbergh G, et al. Use of topical ketanserin in the treatment of skin ulcers: a double-blind study. *J Am Acad Dermatol* 1989;21:85–90.

Johnson RB, Lazarus GS. Pulse therapy: therapeutic efficacy in the treatment of pyoderma gangrenosum. *Arch Dermatol* 1982;118:76–84.

Klein KL, Pittekow MR. Tissue plasminogen activator for treatment of livedoid vasculitis. *Mayo Clin Proc* 1992;67:923–933.

Rustin MAJ, Bunker CB, Dowd PM. Chronic leg ulceration with livedoid vasculitis, and response to oral ketanserin. *Br J Dermatol* 1989;120:101–105.

Samlaska CP, Winfield EA. Pentoxifylline. *J Am Acad Dermatol* 1994;30:603–621.

Sawada K, Segal AM, Malchesky PS, et al. Rapid improvement in patient with leukocytoclastic vasculitis with secondary mixed cryoglobulinemia treatment with cryofiltration. *J Rheumatol* 1991;18:91–94.

Yamamoto M, Danno K, Shio H, Imanura S. Antithrombotic treatment in livedoid vasculitis. *J Am Acad Dermatol* 1988;18:57–62.

Noninvasive Vascular Studies

Bernstein EF. *Vascular Diagnosis*. 4th ed. St. Louis, Mosby-Year Book, 1993.

Mani R, Gorman FW, White JE. Transcutaneous measurment of oxygen tension at edges of leg ulcers: preliminary communication. *J R Soc Med* 1986;79:650–654.

Nemeth AJ, Falanga V, Alstadt SP, Eaglstein WH. Ulcerated edematous limbs: effect of edema removal on transcutaneous oxygen measurements. *J Am Acad Dermatol* 1989;20:191–197.

Schabauer AMA, Rooke TW. Cutaneous laser doppler flowmetry: applications and findings. *Mayo Clin Proc* 1994;69:564–574.

Wound Healing and Future Directions

Beck SL, DeGuzman L, Lee WP, et al. One systemic administration of transforming growth factor-$\beta1$ reverses age- or glucocorticoid-impaired wound healing. *J Clin Invest* 1993;92:2841–2849.

Bennett NT, Schultz GS. Growth factors and wound healing: Part II. Role in normal and chronic wound healing. *Am J Surg* 1993;166:74–81.

Brain A, Purkis P, Coates P, et al. Survival of cultured allogeneic keratinocytes transplanted to deep dermal bed assessed with probes specific for Y chromosome. *Br Med J* 1989;298:917–919.

Brennan SS, Leper DJ. The effect of antiseptics on the healing wound: a study using the rabbit ear chamber. *Br J Surg* 1985;72:780–782.

Brown CD, Zitelli JA. A review of topical agents for wounds and methods of wounding: Guidelines for wound management. *J Dermatol Surg Oncol* 1993;19:732–737.

Brown GL, Naney LB, Griffin J, et al. Enhancement of healing by topical treatment with epidermal growth factor. *N Engl J Med* 1989;321:76–79.

Carley PJ, Wainapel SF. Electrotherapy for acceleration of wound healing: low intensity direct current. *Arch Phys Med Rehabil* 1985;66:443–446.

Chen WYJ, Lydon MJ. Identification of growth factor activities of wound fluid collected under hydrocolloid dressings. *J Invest Dermatol* 1990;94:513.

Davis SC, Ovington LG. Electrical stimulation and ultrasound in wound healing. *Derm Clin* 1993;11:775–782.

De Luca M, Albanese E, Cancedda R, et al. Treatment of leg ulcers with crypreserved allogeneic cultured epithelium. *Arch Dermatol* 1992;128:633–638.

Eaglstein WH. Occlusive dressings. *J Dermatol Surg Oncol* 1993;19:716–722.

Falanga V. Growth factors in chronic wounds: the need to understand the microenvironment. *J Dermatol* 1992;19:667–672.

Falanga V. Growth factors in wound healing. *J Dermatol Surg Oncol* 1993;19:711–715.

Gentzkow GD. Electrical stimulation to heal dermal wounds. *J Dermatol Surg Oncol* 1993;19:753–758.

Geronemus RG, Mertz PM, Eaglstein W. Wound healing: the effects of topical antimicrobial agents. *Arch Dermatol* 1979;115:1311–1314.

Gilchrist T, Martin AM. Wound treatment with Sorbsan: an alginate fiber dressing. *Biomaterials* 1983;4:317–320.

Harris IR, Bottomley W, Wood EJ, Cunliffe WJ. Use of autografts for the treatment of leg ulcers in elderly patients. *Clin Exp Dermatol* 1993;18:417–420.

Hefton JM, Caldwell D, Biozes DG, et al. Grafting of skin ulcers with cultured autologous epidermal cells. *J Am Acad Dermatol* 1986;14:399–405.

Heng MCY. Topical hyperbaric therapy for problem skin wounds. J Dermatol Surg Oncol 1993;19:784–793.

Hutchinson JJ. Prevalence of wound infection under occlusive dressings, a collective survey of reported research. *Wounds* 1990;1:123–133.

Katz MH, Alvarez AH, Eaglstein WH, et al. Human wound fluid from acute wound stimulates cellular proliferation. *J Invest Dermatol* 1990;94:541A.

Kirsner RS, Falanga V. Techniques of split-thickness skin grafting for lower extremity ulcerations. *J Dermatol Surg Oncol* 1993;19:779–783.

Knighton DF, Ciresi K, Fiegel VD, et al. Stimulation of repair in chronic nonhealing cutaneous ulcers using platelet-derived wound-healing formula. *Surg Gynecol Obstet* 1990;170:56–60.

Lundeberg TC, Eriksson SV, Malm M. Electrical nerve stimulation improves healing of diabetic ulcers. *Ann Plast Surg* 1992;29:328–331.

Lydon MJ, Hutchinson JJ, Rippon M, et al. Dissolution of wound coagulum and promotion of granulation tissue under DuoDerm. *Wounds* 1990;1:95–106.

Mertz PM, Eaglstein WH. The effect of semiocclusive dressing on the microbial population in superficial wounds. *Arch Surg* 1984;119:287–289.

Mertz PM, Ovington LG. Wound healing microbiology. *Derm Clin* 1993;11:739–748.

Phillips TJ. Biologic skin substitutes. *J Dermatol Surg Oncol* 1993;19:794–800.

Phillips TJ. Cultured skin grafts: past, present, and future. *Arch Dermatol* 1988;124:1035–1038.

Phillips TJ, Bhawan J, Leigh IM, et al. Cultured epidermal allografts: a study of differentiation and allograft survival. *J Am Acad Dermatol* 1990;23:189–198.

Phillips TJ, Kehinde O, Green H, et al. Treatment of skin ulcers with cultured epidermal allografts. *J Am Acad Dermatol* 1989;21:191–199.

Pittelkow MR. Growth factors in cutaneous biology and disease. *Adv Dermatol* 1991;7:55–81.

Rothe M, Falanga V. Growth factors: their biology and promise in dermatologic diseases and tissue repair. *Arch Dermatol* 1989;125:1390–1398.

Sporn MB, Roberts AB. A major advance in the use of growth factors to enhance wound healing (editorial). *J Clin Invest* 1993;92:2565–2566.

Steed DL, Goslen JB, Holloway GA, et al. Randomized prospective double-blind trial in healing chronic diabetic foot ulcers. *Diabetes Care* 1992;15:1598–1604.

Telfer NR, Moi RL. Drug and nutrient aspects of wound healing. *Derm Clin* 1993;11:729–738.

Teepe RGC, Roseeuw DI, Hermans J, et al. Randomized trial comparing cryopreserved cultured epidermal allografts with hydrocolloid dressings in healing chronic venous ulcers. *J Am Acad Dermatol* 1993; 29:982–988.

Weiss DS, Kirsner R, Eaglstein WH. Electrical stimulation in wound healing. *Arch Dermatol* 1990;126:222–225.

Winter GD. Formation of scab and the rate of epithelialization of superficial wounds in the skin of the young domestic pig. *Nature* 1962;193:293–294.

Review Articles and Special Issue Periodicals

Falanga V, ed. Wound healing. *J Dermatol Surg Oncol* 1993;19:677–812.

Harahap M, ed. Leg ulcers. *Clin Dermatol* 1990;8:1–175.

Nemeth AJ, ed. Wound healing. *Dermatol Clin* 1993;11:629–809.

Phillips TJ, Dover JS, eds. Leg ulcers. *J Am Acad Dermatol* 1991;25:965–987.

Roenigk HH, Young JR. Leg ulcers. In *Peripheral Vascular Diseases*. JR Young, RA Graor, JW Olin, JR Bartholomew, eds. St. Louis, Mosby-Year Book, 1991, pp. 605–638.

40

Tattoos

John Louis Ratz
*Tulane University, Louisiana State University, and
The Ochsner Clinic, New Orleans, Louisiana*

Those who remove decorative tattoos know that these patients, on the whole, are a unique group. Often characterized as unusual, eccentric, and unreliable, not all tattoo patients warrant these distinctions. Nevertheless, a physician can never be sure that a person requesting removal of a tattoo will keep the scheduled appointment, return for subsequent stages of tattoo removal, or return for simple follow-up appointments. Their expectations regarding removal are often unrealistic, especially since the tattoo was applied so easily, quickly, and inexpensively.

The word tattoo is derived from the Tahitian word "tatau" and, according to Webster's *New Collegiate Dictionary,* is "an *indelible* mark or figure fixed upon the body by insertion of pigment under the skin or by the production of scars." In fact, tattoo pigments are actually placed into the skin, rather than under it, but they are, without question, indelible.

Dermatologic surgeons are principally interested in the various methods of tattoo removal. Before I discuss this, several other aspects of tattooing deserve attention.

TATTOO APPLICATION

Reasons patients give for getting tattoos range from the fraternity prank to "I was drunk" to "everybody else did, so I did." In some culture or religious groups, particularly in the Far East and the South Seas, tattooing is an accepted method of body adornment and symbolizes attainment of maturity, fertility, and other cultural or social identification or distinction. In these societies, it is not only accepted but expected.

In our culture, most tattoos are considered provocative. They may allude to sexual or antisocial rebellion (Fig. 1). Sexually oriented tattoos are often quite explicit (Fig. 2) and can have both heterosexual and homosexual implications (Fig. 3). Tattoos can reflect a myriad of antisocial messages: antireligion, antiparents, antigovernment, anti–law-enforcement, etc. (Fig. 4). Often such tattoos are required for membership in a particular club or organization and may be of an identifying nature (Fig. 5).

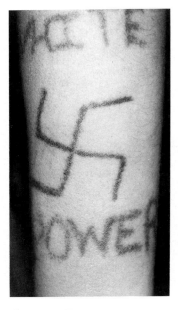

Figure 1 Tattoos are provocative and often carry a message of antisocial rebellion.

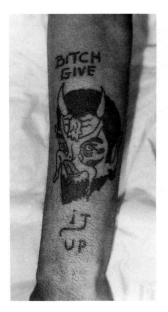

Figure 2 Sexually oriented tattoos are frequently quite explicit.

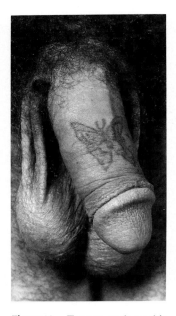

Figure 3 Tattoos such as this butterfly, by virtue of its location, may have homosexual or heterosexual implications.

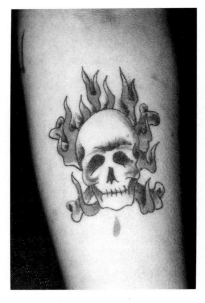

Figure 4 This tattoo is one of a dozen on one young lady representing her rebellion against parental restrictions.

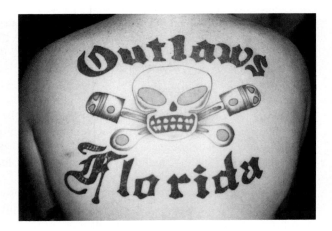

Figure 5 Tattoos may represent membership in gangs.

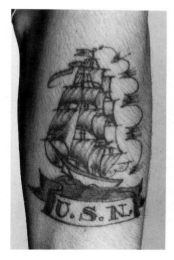

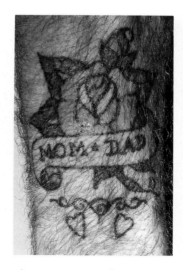

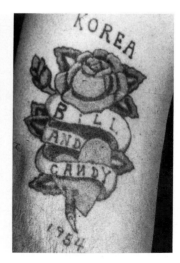

Figure 6 This tattoo reflects love of country.

Figure 7 Tattoos may reflect love of family.

Figure 8 Tattoos frequently reflect affection for a loved one.

Many people have tattoos applied while in the armed forces. Such tattoos reflect love of country (Fig. 6), family (Fig. 7), or lover (Fig. 8) but probably are applied most often because of intoxication, group behavior, or "macho" designation. Tattoos have also been used to identify prisoners or undesirables, especially in Nazi concentration camps.

Occasionally tattoos occur accidentally secondary to injury. Traumatic tattoos (Fig. 9) are often difficult to remove because of their depth and variability. Other tattoos are basically unintentional since their application may have been a consequence of psychological disease or may have occurred while the patient was under the influence of intoxicating drugs (Fig. 10).

Tattoos are sometimes applied in an acceptable fashion in our culture. A tattoo may be applied to cover up another, less acceptable tattoo (Fig. 11), to mask a birthmark or injury (Fig. 12), to mark boundaries for radiation therapy, or to camouflage missing appendages such as nipples, hair, or other structures. One highly fashionable type is eyeliner tattooing, which enhances dull eyes and eliminates the need for daily application of eyeliner makeup (Fig. 13).

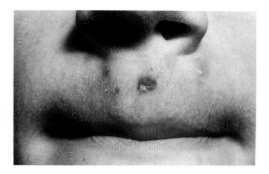

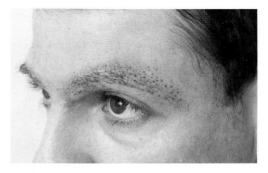

Figure 9 Traumatic tattoos, such as this one caused by gunpowder, can be difficult to remove because of their depth and distribution. (Courtesy of Randall K. Roenigk, M.D.)

Figure 10 Extremely unusual tattoos may occur as a consequence of psychological disease or indiscriminate drug use. This patient was mimicking Groucho Marx while under the influence of cocaine.

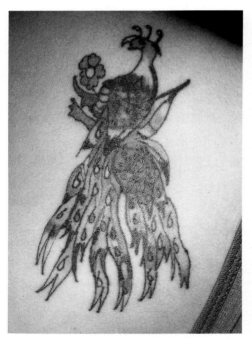

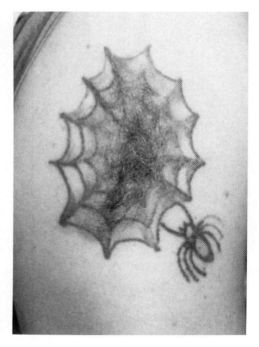

Figure 11 This bird of paradise tattoo covers a less acceptable *pair of dice* which can be seen on careful examination.

Figure 12 A tattoo may be used to cover an unwanted birthmark, such as the hairy nevus here.

TECHNIQUE

Though much has been written about tattoo psychology and tattoo removal, very little is available regarding tattoo application. Although details of the procedure may vary, the procedure for professional tattoos is essentially the same. Unlike amateur tattoos done with India ink and a needle, by which the tattoo pigment can be deposited at various depths, professionally applied tattoos are applied so that the pigment is at a uniform depth. The exact depth of pigment depo-

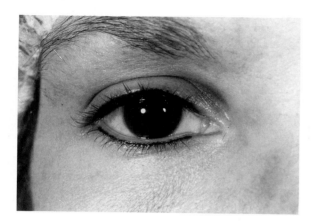

Figure 13 Eyeliner tattoo.

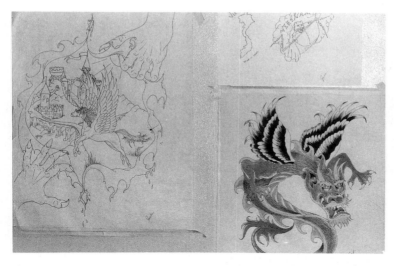

Figure 14 Thousands of patterns can be applied by a creative tattoo artist.

sition depends on the downward pressure applied to the tattooing instrument. Depth of penetration is generally set at a constant 1/32 inch (roughly 1 mm). However, it is likely that the pigment is actually deposited much deeper because of downward pressure.

A professionally applied tattoo can be done either freehand or from a stencil. The first step is to complete the tattoo outline. If a stencil is used, the pattern can be done freehand or can be taken from one of thousands of available patterns (Fig. 14). The stencil is produced on a flexible plastic mat with a simple engraving instrument (Fig. 15). This results in a rough undersurface that serves as a template for the tattoo. This roughened surface is covered with graphite and imprinted on the tattoo site (Fig. 16). The site is prepared by shaving, cleansing the skin, and, in some tattoo salons, application of antibiotic ointment.

Outlining is completed with a liner. This instrument has only one needle and is dipped into the tattoo pigment as needed (Figs. 17,18). Once the outline has been completed (Fig. 19), the detail lines are applied with the same instrument. Shading is done with an instrument similar to the liner, but containing more needles and called a shader. The shader routinely contains 5 needles

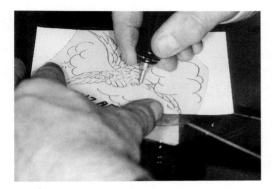

Figure 15 A tattoo stencil is made with an engraving tool.

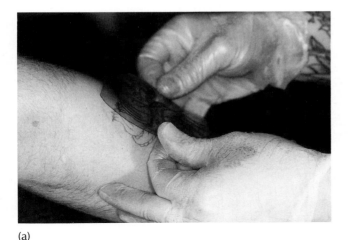

(a)

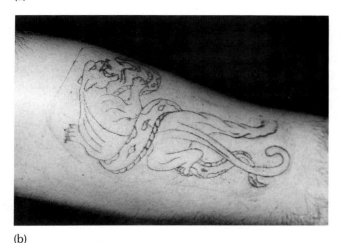

(b)

Figure 16   The stencil is imprinted and serves as a pattern for the tattoo artist.

but can have up to 21 for working on larger areas. Shading is done to give pictoral depth and intricacy (Fig. 20). Once shading is completed, the tattoo is then colored with the darker colors first, then the next darkest, and so on, until white or yellow is applied last (Fig. 21). The dressings for the tattoo site are variable but can include antibiotic ointment.

Sterile technique is not used, so there is considerable concern regarding transmission of disease. The same instruments are often used on consecutive customers without sterilization. A particular fear is possible transmission of HIV and hepatitis virus from this procedure. Despite this danger, the art of tattooing continues to flourish.

COMPLICATIONS

The transmission of disease is only one complication of tattoo application. Wound infection is possible, but it is difficult to know how often this occurs. Dermatologists sometimes see post-application allergic contact dermatitis (Fig. 22). This allergy can be mediated by ultraviolet light, depending on the pigment employed. One local tattoo artist described reaction to a certain lav-

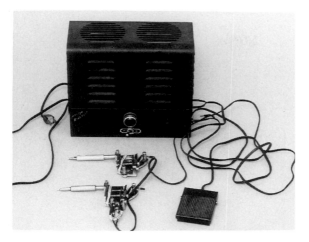

Figure 17 Tattoo guns are electrically operated and controlled by a foot switch.

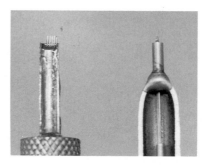

Figure 18 Liners have a single needle and are used for the outline. The shader usually has 5 needles but may have as many as 21.

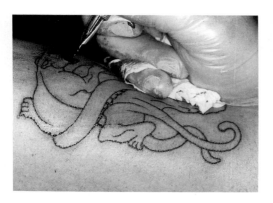

Figure 19 The outline is done first.

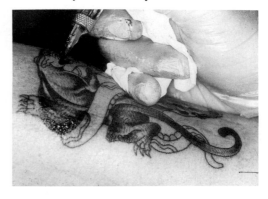

Figure 20 Shading is done to give the work depth and intricacy.

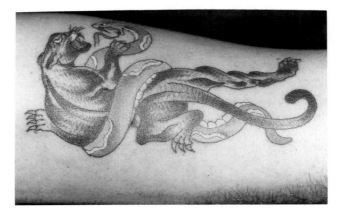

Figure 21 Darkest colors are applied first, followed by successively lighter colors.

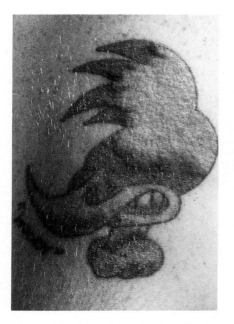

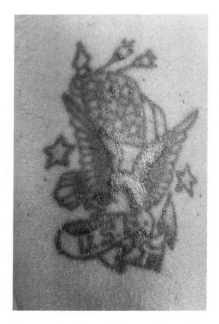

Figure 22 Allergic and photoallergic contact dermatitis can occur, depending on the pigment used.

Figure 23 Sarcoid in a decorative tattoo.

ender dye in customers using cocaine or "crack." No scientific data exist for such an unusual relationship, however.

Keratinization or activation of a preexisting condition such as psoriasis, lichen planus, or sarcoid can also occur as a consequence of tattoo application (Fig. 23). Hypertrophic scar or keloid formation is also theoretically possible, but this has not been reported with significant frequency. Perhaps the most significant complication, though not often considered as such, is the social impact the presence of a tattoo can have.

REMOVAL

The presence of a tattoo may be considered highly inappropriate in certain situations and may affect interpersonal relationships and employment opportunities. Such social pressure can serve as the rationale for tattoo removal. The need to remedy one of the complications mentioned above may also be the reason for having a tattoo removed.

Whether a broken relationship or social impact, the reason for removal is usually a strong motivating force. However, expectations usually exceed possible outcomes. Most people want the tattoo removed simply, quickly, completely, and as painlessly as possible. They do not want the tattoo duplicated by a scar bearing the same subject matter, nor do they expect a cosmetically unacceptable scar. They prefer one-step procedures and may not return for subsequent stages. They often expect removal to cost no more than application. A tattoo may cost $50–$60 to apply; removal may cost 10 times as much or more.

Technique

There are many methods for tattoo removal. They vary from topical chemical applications to complex excision and reconstruction. The discussion here will be limited to surgical modalities, since most topical methods are strikingly unimpressive.

As with most procedures, the simplest method is usually the best. It is wise to use a single-stage procedure whenever possible, although this is not always practical. Duplication of tattoo by a scar in the same image does little service to the patient. It is better to include some un-involved tissue to avoid duplication. The patient should have reasonable knowledge about the procedure, pain, cost, and final outcome. Surgical removal of a tattoo invariably results in a scar. The physician must make certain that the patient understands this. Patients should know that there are ways to minimize the size of the scar and to maximize its quality.

Professionally applied tattoos are easier to remove than amateur tattoos because of the uniform depth of deposition of the pigment. The longer a tattoo has been present, however, the more difficult is its removal. This is because the pigment migrates horizontally and longitudinally with time. It is not unusual to remove an old professional tattoo and find pigment present at the bottom of the dermis and in the subcutaneous tissue.

When tattoos are small, simple excision should be used. In some locations larger tattoos can be effectively excised and closed primarily or with the use of a local flap (Fig. 24). The linear or semilinear scars are much more preferable than scars produced by other procedures. Because of this, excision remains the procedure of choice for tattoo removal.

Often the tattoo is present in an anatomic location that makes excision impossible or the size of the tattoo is such that excision could only be carried out in a multiple-staged procedure. Total excision or dermatomal removal followed by skin grafting can be used for larger tattoos. In the majority of cases, however, grafting gives an unacceptable final cosmetic result distinctly inferior to that achieved with other methods of removal.

Cryosurgery can be used but is quite imprecise. It is difficult to estimate the level of freeze to remove all of the pigment since the depth is uncertain. It is not particularly useful for large tattoos but may be reasonable for small tattoos, particularly those that appear to be shallow.

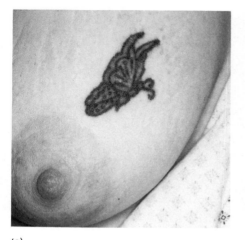

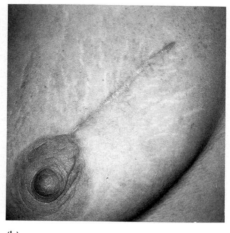

(a)   (b)

Figure 24 Excision is the removal method of choice when possible. The resulting scar in the A to T closure seen here is more acceptable than either a dermabrasion or laser scar would have been.

Abrasive removal is a common, effective technique for tattoo removal. Several abrasives have been used both with and without the application of chemicals afterward. Results following use of these postoperative chemicals have been less than impressive, and they will not be discussed further.

Salabrasion

The most common abrasion methods for tattoo removal are salabrasion and dermabrasion. Salabrasion uses simple table salt or a variety with coarser texture. Salt is placed on the field and is rubbed with an applicator. The applicator can be made with several tongue depressors on which are fixed gauze pads that serve as the abrading surface. Considerable downward force is required with this technique. Salabrasion should be terminated when the surface is bright red (Fig. 25). The tattoo will still be present, but wound healing and inflammatory reaction should result in removal of a considerable amount of the pigment. Salabrasion is often repeated several times before all the pigment is completely removed. Results can be satisfactory, but other removal methods are less laborious. Although effective, salabrasion has the drawbacks of being a multi-staged procedure and causing some discomfort to the patient. Postabrasion care is not uniform. Some suggest leaving the salt in place, while others support removing the salt and dressing the wound.

Dermabrasion

Dermabrasion is a standard procedure used for tattoo removal. The biggest controversies are whether a wire brush or diamond fraise should be used, and whether all or part of the pigment should be removed. The brush has the advantage of faster, deeper abrasion but is perhaps less

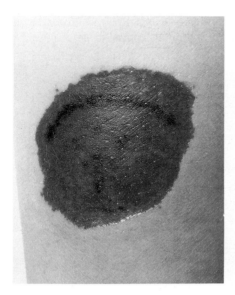

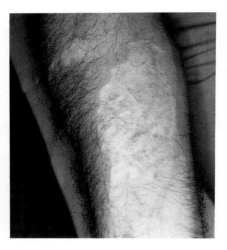

Figure 25   The end point of a salabrasion; the treatment field is entirely bright red. The pigment will still be visible and may not be completely removed after healing.

Figure 26   A tattoo "ghost" may remain after argon laser photocoagulation.

precise than the diamond fraise. The question of residual pigmentation in the wound site will be addressed later. Cosmetic results following dermabrasion are reasonable and, as with any other modality, are dependent on depth of pigment deposition and anatomic location.

Laser

Laser removal of tattoos is a new, popular method. Results are subject to the same restrictions as other techniques: depth of pigmentation and anatomic location. The essentials of laser surgery are described adequately in other chapters, and the theoretical and practical considerations of laser removal will be discussed only briefly here. Laser removal of tattoo pigmentation can be done with color-specific lasers or those not color-specific.

Color-Specific Removal

Lasers producing colored light are capable of color-specific absorption of their energy by complementary pigments. Thus blue-green argon laser energy can be selectively absorbed by black, brown, or red. A yellow dye laser would have much the same absorption, and a red laser, such as the ruby laser, would have just the opposite affinity. In theory, such specific absorption would be ideal, but several problems exist. Destruction is limited to complementary colored pigments as well as by depth of light penetration. The argon laser, for example, penetrates to a maximum depth of 1.6 mm. Use of such a laser, therefore, often leaves residual pigmentation (Fig. 26) in the treated site. There is also potential for burn scarring because of the tremendous heat that can be absorbed by surrounding tissues. More recently, several Q-switched lasers have shown the ability to remove tattoos with minimal risks for scarring or textural change. These include the Q-switched ruby, Q-switched Nd-YAG, and Alexandrite lasers. These lasers are more color-specific and each has pigments that it cannot remove. Additionally, multiple treatments are usually necessary for complete pigment removal. A detailed description of their use can be found elsewhere in this book. At this point in time, they have become a significant development in the treatment of decorative tattoos.

Lasers Not Color-Specific

Infrared lasers, such as the Nd-YAG and CO_2 lasers, are tissue destroyers. The Nd-YAG laser does so by tissue coagulation, the CO_2 laser by vaporization. The idea is similar to that of dermabrasion: to remove all overlying, involved tissue. The Nd-YAG laser has been used only sparingly for tattoo removal because of its tremendous energy scatter and deep penetration, which are conducive to burn scar formation.

The CO_2 laser is capable of removing large, professional (superficial) tattoos. Its precise action and limited energy spread result in minimal damage to the wound, bloodless surgery, diminished postoperative pain, and high-quality, soft, supple scar formation. However, the final result, as with dermabrasion, depends on the depth of pigment deposition and anatomic location of the tattoo (Fig. 27).

Complications

The most common complications of tattoo removal are hypertrophic scarring (Fig. 28) and the presence of residual pigment in the healed wound (Fig. 29). Scarring is usually unavoidable, but the quality of the scar can be improved by removing the least amount of tissue and inflicting the least amount of damage to surrounding tissue. Residual pigmentation can only be avoided by ensuring that all pigment is removed at the time of removal. However, this may create more damage than is desirable and result in an unacceptable scar. Another complication is duplication of the original tattoo by scar (Fig. 30). This can be avoided by removing normal tissue in a

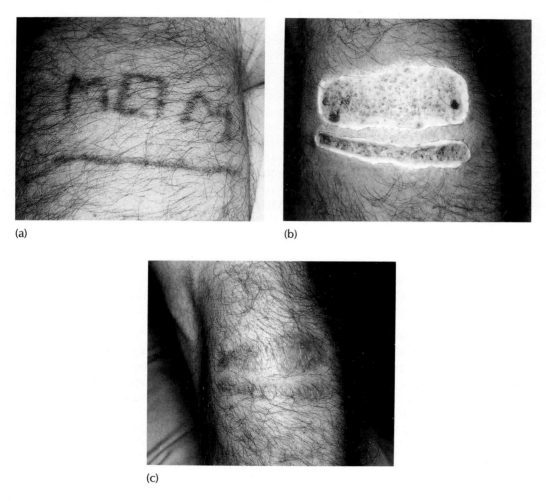

(a)   (b)

(c)

Figure 27   Tattoo (a) before, (b) immediately postoperative, and (c) 2 months after CO_2 laser vaporization.

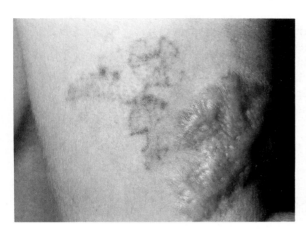

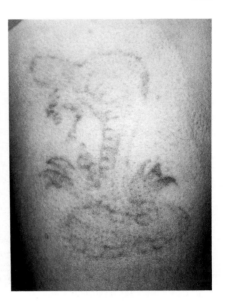

Figure 28 The most common complication of tattoo removal is hypertrophic scarring. This example resulted from dermabrasion.

Figure 29 Residual pigmentation can be a complication of any technique.

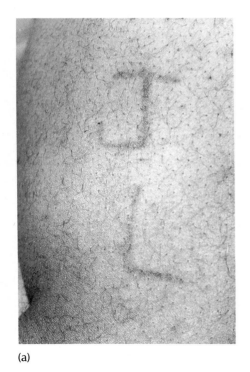

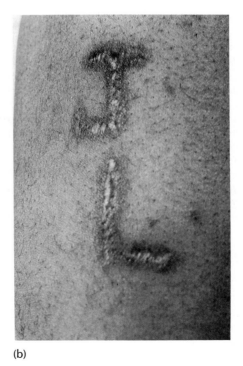

(a)   (b)

Figure 30 The scar should not duplicate the original tattoo. It is better to sacrifice a small amount of uninvolved tissue to produce a geometric scar.

geometric or random pattern around the tattoo. Other complications are not unique to tattoo removal but can occur in any surgical situation. These include wound infection and allergic reaction to dressing materials.

Some problems can be avoided or minimized. Removal of tattoos from the shoulder, midchest, or deltoid often leads to hypertrophic scars or keloid formation. Recognizing this fact and discussing it with the patient is important. Written informed consent outlining the possible complications is advisable. The patient should be told that a scar is to be expected and that it may require treatment, such as intralesional corticosteroid injection. When dermabrasion or CO_2 laser is used, it is usually appropriate to remove all of the pigment unless the subcutaneous fat is involved. Patients are generally more tolerant of hypertrophic scar formation than they are of residual pigmentation and the possibility of additional procedures.

BIBLIOGRAPHY

Angres GG. Blepharopigmentation and eyebrow enhancement techniques for maximum cosmetic results. *Ann Ophthalmol* 1985;17:605–611.

Bailin PL, Ratz JL, Wheeland RG. Laser therapy of the skin: A review of principles and applications. In *Dermatologic Clinics*. PL Bailin, JL Ratz, RG Wheeland, eds. Philadelphia, W.B. Saunders, 1987.

Bailin PL, Ratz JL. Use of the carbon dioxide laser in dermatologic surgery. In *Lasers in Cutaneous Medicine and Surgery*. JL Ratz, ed. Chicago, Yearbook Medical Publishers, 1986, pp. 73–104.

Bailin PL, Ratz JL, Levine HL. Removal of tattoos by CO_2 laser. *J Dermatol Surg Oncol* 1980;6:997–1001.

Dvir E, Hirshowitz B. Tattoo removal by cryosurgery. *Plast Reconstr Surg* 1980;66(3):373–379.

Fitzpatrick PE, Goldman MP, Ruiz-Esparza J. Use of the alexandrite laser (755 nm, 100 nsec) for tattoo pigment removal in an animal model. *J Am Acad Dermatol* 1993;(May 28):745–750.

Goldstein N. Tattoo removal. In *Dermatologic Clinics*. PL Bailin, JL Ratz, RG Wheeland, eds. Philadelphia, W.B. Saunders, 1987.

Goldstein N. (Guest Editor). Special issue: tattoos. *J Dermatol Surg Oncol* 1979.

Johannesson A. A simplified method of focal salabrasion for removal of linear tattoos. *J Dermatol Surg Oncol* 1985;11(10):1004–1005.

Kilmer SL, Lee MS, Grevelink JM, Flotte TJ, Anderson RR: The Q-switched Nd:YAG laser effectively treats tattoos. A controlled, dose-response study. *Arch Dermatol* 1993;(Aug 129):971–978.

Kilmer SL, Anderson RR. Clinical use of the Q-switched ruby and the Q-switched Nd:YAG (1064 nm and 532 nm) lasers for treatment of tattoos. *J Dermatol Surg Oncol* 1993;(Apr 19):330–338.

Ratz JL. Laser applications in dermatology and plastic surgery. In *Surgical Application of Lasers*. J Dixon, ed. Chicago, Yearbook Medical Publishers, 1987, pp. 160–182.

Reid PJ. McLeod A, Ritchie A, et al. Q-switched ruby laser treatment of black tattoos. *Br J Plast Surg* 1983;36(4):455–459.

Shelley WB, Shelley ED. Focal salabrasion for removal of linear tattoos. *J Dermatol Surg Oncol* 1984;19(3):216–218.

Thomson W, McDonald JC. Self-tattooing by schoolchildren. *Lancet* 1983;2:1243–1244.

41

Indications for Mohs Micrographic Surgery

Henry W. Randle
Mayo Clinic/Foundation, Jacksonville, Florida

Randall K. Roenigk
*Mayo Clinic/Foundation and Mayo Medical School,
Rochester, Minnesota*

The definitive treatment for cutaneous malignant disease that spreads contiguously is micrographic surgery as described by Mohs (Fig. 1). Basically, Mohs micrographic surgery is an excision modified to obtain accurate histologic tumor-free margins. This method allows precise visualization of all peripheral margins, a distinct advantage over traditional vertical sections that allow the pathologist to evaluate only a minute sample of the margin (Fig. 2). This procedure requires a specially trained surgeon and technician and an on-site laboratory that processes frozen sections on demand. It is tedious but cost-effective and is not indicated for all cutaneous malignant lesions. Standard therapies such as electrodesiccation and curettage, cryosurgery, excision, and radiation are excellent options in many cases. The cutaneous oncologic surgeon must evaluate each tumor preoperatively to determine its risk for recurrence and subsequent morbidity or mortality. The surgeon can then decide if a standard therapy will suffice or if Mohs micrographic surgery might be indicated. Cure rates after Mohs micrographic surgery are well documented in the literature. Robins and Reyes summarized Dr. Robins' 20 years of experience, which is surpassed only by that of Dr. Mohs.

Cutaneous malignant disease is the most common form of cancer, with 1,000,000 cases treated annually. Within that group, basal cell carcinoma is by far the most common, followed by squamous cell carcinoma. Mohs micrographic surgery has had its greatest use and success in the treatment of difficult forms of these two malignancies. When the diagnosis of either of these tumors is made, it is important to evaluate several characteristics, including histologic subtype, size, location, and previous therapy, to determine whether Mohs micrographic surgery is indicated (Fig. 3). Less common cutaneous malignant lesions can also be treated by Mohs technique. These are keratoacanthoma, verrucous carcinoma, and dermatofibrosarcoma protuberans, among others. Specific areas where Mohs surgery may be indicated are the eyes, ears, and nose, but the technique can be applied to any area on the skin. Some patients elect to have Mohs micrographic surgery as their primary treatment because of its very high cure rates and conservation of normal tissue.

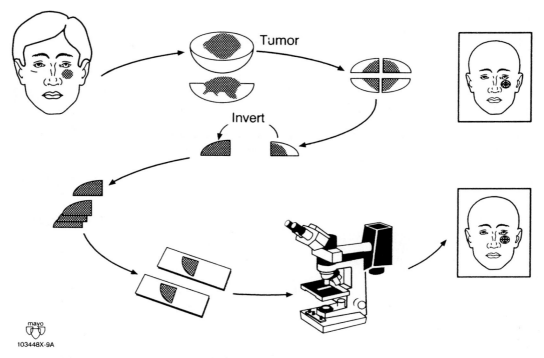

Figure 1 General procedure for micrographic surgery.

BASAL CELL CARCINOMA

Basal cell carcinoma is so common and so clinically benign in many cases that it would be unreasonable to apply Mohs micrographic surgery to each tumor. Accurate cure rates of 95–99% are obtained by standard therapies, especially when used for small tumors in uncomplicated areas. Use of the Mohs procedure is limited to tumors that are more likely to recur. It must be remembered, however, that guidelines for treating high-risk tumors must include an evaluation of the general health of the patient. Often, other operations are more reasonable in light of the total clinical picture.

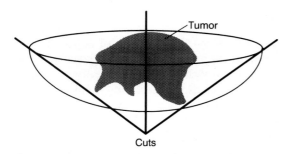

Figure 2 Mohs micrographic surgery provides histologic sections of the peripheral margins only. These sections include both the superficial and the deep margins.

Tumor

Tumor remains localized or metastasizes late
Significant subclinical spread, clinically ill-defined
High recurrence rate if treated by traditional methods
Continguous growth

Indications
  Location:
      High recurrence rate if treated by traditional methods
      Embryonic fusion planes--site of least resistance:
         - nasolabial fold
         - philtrum
         - ala
         - mid lower lip
         -chin
         - preauricular
         - retroauricular sulcus
         - temple
         - periocular
      Tissue conservation important:
         - penis
         - digits
         - nose
         - eyelids
  Histology (Subtype, aggressive):
      BCC--morpheaform, metatypical, micronodular BCC
      SCC--grade II, III, IV; Clark level IV, V
      Perineural
      Marjolin
      Recurrent
      Large, invasive (> 2 cm)
      Immunosuppressed patient
      Patient preference

Figure 3   Indications for Mohs micrographic surgery.

When a patient with basal cell carcinoma is evaluated, Mohs micrographic surgery might be indicated for five general reasons.

Large Tumors

Tumor size is directly related to recurrence rate of basal cell carcinoma following any method of treatment. The recurrence rate following surgical excision for primary basal cell carcinomas less than 6 mm was 3.2% vs. 8% for basal cell carcinomas of 6–10 mm and 9% for basal cell carcinomas greater than 1 cm. Generally speaking, tumors greater than 2 cm in diameter have been present for a long time and have a greater likelihood of recurring if treated by standard methods. The 5-year cure rate for basal cell carcinoma less than 3 cm in diameter treated by Mohs micrographic surgery is greater than 99%. For tumors greater than 3 cm, the cure rate is 93%. When large lesions occur in areas of vital importance or in cosmetically important sites, not only must the tumor be cured with the initial therapy, but sparing normal tissue also makes the reconstruction easier.

Generally speaking, tumors greater than 2 cm in diameter have been present for a long time and have a greater likelihood of recurring if treated by standard methods. When large lesions occur in areas of vital importance or in cosmetically important sites, not only must the tumor be cured with the initial therapy but sparing normal tissue makes the reconstruction easier.

Indistinct Clinical Margins

Some basal cell carcinomas, especially those with histologic patterns that are morpheaform or infiltrating, have indistinct clinical margins. The tumor seems to blend in with the normal skin at its periphery, especially in areas like the temple (Fig. 4) or when extending into an embryonic fusion plane (Fig. 5). When the extent of clinical disease is difficult to determine, Mohs micrographic surgery is a good option, since the distinction between normal and abnormal tissue is much more clear histologically.

Recurrent Tumor

If a lesion has already been treated by a standard therapy and has recurred, Mohs micrographic surgery is strongly indicated. Retreatment with standard therapy is complicated by the fact that tumor now has been interspersed with scar tissue from previous treatment. There may be several foci of tumor, both at the periphery of the old site and at the deeper margins (Fig. 6). One must assume that the tumor was never completely eradicated and has had time to invade more deeply into the subcutaneous tissues.

It was once thought that if tumor-free margins were not obtained after removal of basal cell carcinoma, most of these lesions would not recur—somehow wound healing would obliterate residual tumor cells. Although this may happen in a small percentage of cases, clearly many lesions recur, especially when patients are followed closely. The 5-year recurrence rate for treatment of recurrent basal cell carcinoma using Mohs micrographic surgery is 5.6% compared to 19.9% for all non-Mohs modalities and 40% for electrodesiccation and curettage.

Another consideration is that Mohs micrographic surgery is tissue sparing. Since most basal cell carcinomas occur on the face and neck, the cosmetic appearance after reconstruction is important (Fig. 7). If tissue can be spared for reconstruction while a high cure rate is assured, a satisfying functional and cosmetic result is likely (Fig. 8).

Incompletely Excised Basal Cell Carcinoma

Basal cell carcinoma that has been excised with margins involved with tumor should be reexcised. Mohs micrographic surgery is an effective way to remove the remaining tumor cells.

Site

Most basal cell carcinomas occur on the face and neck, most commonly on the nose. Common sites of recurrence are the nose, eyes, and ears. There are many reasons why lesions in these areas may be more difficult to eradicate. Because the skin in these areas is close to vital structures, standard therapy may be less effective when the therapist is trying to avoid damage to the vital structure. There are many embryologic fusion planes in these areas, such as along the nasolabial fold, that provide a path of least resistance for the extension of tumor. This probably accounts for the high recurrence rate for basal cell carcinoma in these high-risk locations. Therefore, the "midfacial triangle," which includes the eyes, nose, and upper lip, or the "H" zone, which includes the ears, temple, and midcentral portion of the face, are areas considered at high risk for recurrence, and tumors in these sites should be considered for Mohs micrographic surgery because of its ability to follow these "silent" extensions. Artificial fusion planes created by grafts or flaps also allow paths for tumor growth (Fig. 9).

An exception is tumors that have invaded a vital organ at presentation (Fig. 10). Extension of basal cell carcinoma into the cranium, orbit, or the deeper tissues is a difficult problem.

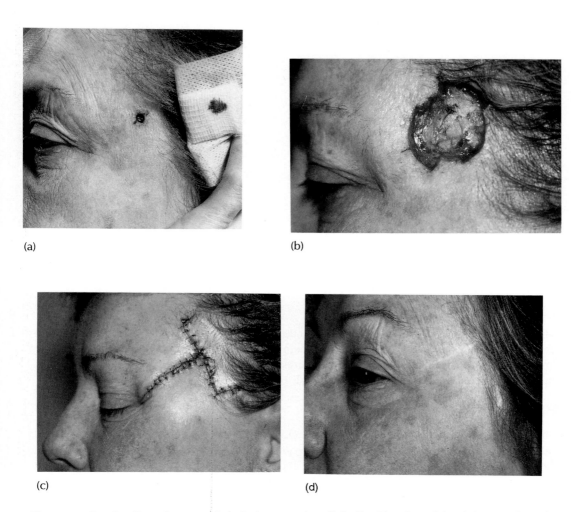

(a)

(b)

(c)

(d)

Figure 4 Basal cell carcinoma with indistinct margins clinically. The size of the defect can be quite alarming to the patient; however, creative reconstruction provides a cosmetically acceptable closure. (a) Preoperative view. (b) Micrographic tumor-free margins. (c) A to T closure. (d) Result 3½ years postoperatively.

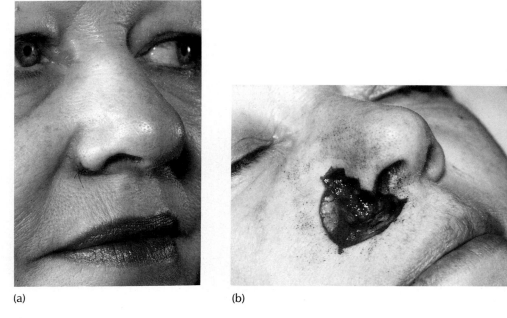

(a)   (b)

Figure 5 Basal cell carcinoma with indistinct margins clinically. The nasolabial fold and its embryologic fusion planes are notorious for allowing tumor to dissect well beyond what might be suspected clinically. (a) Preoperative view. (b) Micrographic tumor-free margins.

Maintaining accurate margins by Mohs technique becomes difficult. In these instances, the operation must be performed in an operating room rather than in the outpatient setting. Deeply invasive basal cell carcinoma is rare and requires the support of our colleagues in other surgical subspecialties, possibly in combination with radiation therapy or chemotherapy.

Histologic Subtype

There are at least 26 subtypes of basal cell carcinoma. The most common is nodular basal cell carcinoma, and because the cells in this tumor are closely compacted and well circumscribed, the histologic extensions correlate well with the clinical disease, usually being well circumscribed. The prognosis for cure for primary tumors of most subtypes of basal cell carcinoma is as good as that for the nodular type. The major exceptions are morpheaform, metatypical, and micronodular basal cell carcinomas.

Morpheaform basal cell carcinoma contains anaplastic strands with nests of small numbers of cells. This tumor has the propensity for dissecting along embryologic fusion planes, perineural spaces, and perivascular spaces, and can have extensions well beyond the clinical margins of the lesion (Fig. 11). An average of 7.2 mm of subclinical tumor extension was found in morpheaform basal cell carcinomas compared with 2.1 mm of extension in well-circumscribed nodular lesions. If left unchecked, these tumors can be quite invasive, involving vital organs such as the eye, parotid gland, and ethmoid sinus.

Metatypical basal cell carcinoma has features of squamous differentiation and keratinization within a tumor that is predominantly basal cell carcinoma. Some dermatopathologists call this basosquamous cell carcinoma. There is some controversy about the existence of this tumor, most

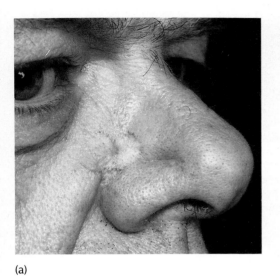

(a)

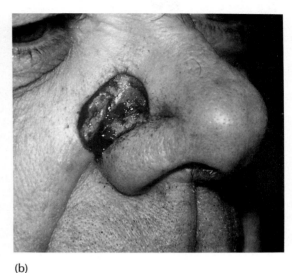

(b)

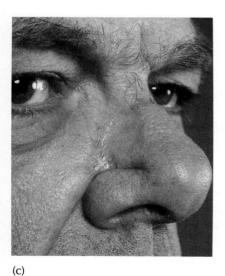

(c)

Figure 6   Recurrent basal cell carcinoma along the ala-nasolabial fold, an area where embryologic fusion planes allow invasion of the tumor. (a) Preoperative view. (b) Micrographic tumor-free margins. (c) Good cosmetic result after second intention healing 6 weeks postoperatively.

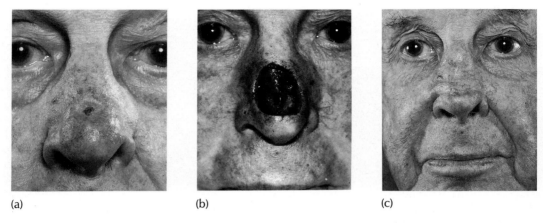

(a)   (b)   (c)

Figure 7   Residual basal cell carcinoma that was treated several months earlier by electrodesiccation and curettage and healed poorly. (a) Preoperative view. (b) Micrographic tumor-free margins. Note exposure of septal and alar cartilages. (c) Five weeks after reconstruction with bilateral nasolabial transposition flaps by an otolaryngologist.

recognizing that this may be a form of malignant degeneration that occurs in basal cell carcinoma that has been present for a long time. Metatypical basal cell carcinoma occurring as a small primary lesion is less common. Tumors with these histologic subtypes statistically have a higher risk of recurrence (12–30% vs. 1–6% for nodular lesions) and therefore should be considered for treatment by Mohs micrographic surgery.

SQUAMOUS CELL CARCINOMA

Squamous cell carcinoma has a greater propensity for metastasis and lymphatic or hematogenous spread. In the skin, this risk is still small enough that most regard this tumor as one that spreads contiguously as its main form of invasion, and therefore can appropriately be treated by Mohs micrographic surgery. Squamous cell carcinoma should be divided into three groups: sun-induced cutaneous, sun-induced mucocutaneous, and chronic inflammation or injury related.

Squamous cell carcinoma that occurs in actinically damaged skin, such as that on the dorsum of the hand, accounts for the greatest percentage of these tumors. The tumors act benignly, as reflected in low rates of metastasis. When small, most of these tumors can easily be treated by standard therapy, such as excision or electrodesiccation and curettage. Mohs micrographic surgery is generally indicated for larger lesions in difficult locations (Fig. 12). The rate of recurrence correlates with preoperative size. Incidence of metastasis correlates with the thickness; lesions thicker than 4 mm may warrant Mohs surgery. Other indicators of Mohs surgery would be signs of poor differentiation, perineural invasion, or a patient who is immunosuppressed.

Mucocutaneous squamous cell carcinoma may also be actinically related, but other risk factors are chronic trauma and smoking. This tumor most commonly occurs on the lower lip, and the incidence of metastatic disease is approximately 10%. Squamous cell carcinoma of the lower lip may be treated by Mohs micrographic surgery and the resulting defect may be small enough to allow a simple primary closure rather than a larger wedge resection. In the presence of lymph node involvement, Mohs surgery may be appropriate for removal of the primary tumor.

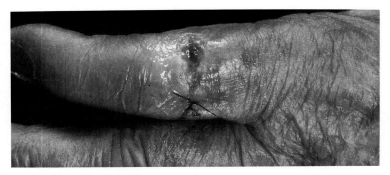

(a)

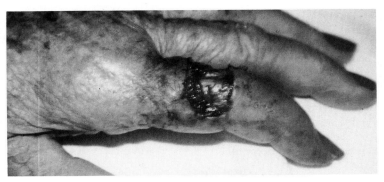

(b)

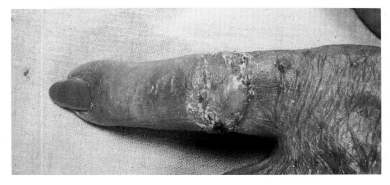

(c)

Figure 8 Morpheaform basal cell carcinoma in a site of previous burn injury. (a) Preoperative view. (b) Micrographic tumor-free margins. Tumor extended down to but did not include the extensor tendon. Use of Mohs micrographic surgery probably prevented amputation of the digit. (c) One month after placement of graft by a plastic surgeon.

Cutaneous squamous cell carcinoma secondary to inflammation, scar, and degenerative processes has an incidence of metastasis ranging from 10 to 30%. Mohs micrographic surgery is indicated for these lesions, although on occasion they become quite large (Fig. 13). Squamous cell carcinoma extending into deeper musculature and other vital organs requires aggressive excision and occasionally amputation, with consideration of adjunctive therapies.

(b)

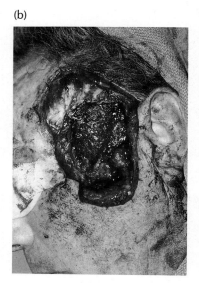

(a)

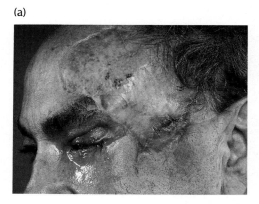

Figure 9   Aggressive basal cell carcinoma treated by excision and grafting on five previous occasions. Tumor extended beneath the old graft superiorly and down to the superficial lobe of the parotid gland inferiorly, involving the temporalis muscle fascia. By micrographic techniques, histologic tumor-free margins could be obtained without removing the eye or involving the trunk of the facial nerve. (a) Preoperative view. (b) Micrographic tumor-free margins.

When squamous cell carcinoma occurs in locations where tissue sparing is an important consideration, Mohs surgery may be a reasonable option (Fig. 14). An example is radiation-induced squamous cell carcinoma on the digits in dentists or papillomavirus-induced tumors on the penis. Traditional approaches might include amputation, whereas Mohs surgery would maximally spare residual normal tissue and increase the likelihood that normal function would be preserved.

Recurrent squamous cell carcinoma is also an indication for Mohs micrographic surgery. As with basal cell carcinoma, recurrences may be multifocal; therefore, even the Mohs technique may miss peripheral foci of tumor. This consequence is reflected in cure rates that are slightly lower for all recurrent tumors. A special subgroup of squamous cell carcinoma consists of tumors previously treated by radiation. In some patients, radiotherapy causes the tumor to become quite biologically aggressive. Often, despite histologic tumor-free margins and excision of normal tissue beyond the tumor, recurrences occur. A combination of therapies may be a consideration, along with a wide block dissection.

MELANOMA

The use of Mohs micrographic surgery for melanoma has been advocated by Dr. Mohs because the lesion can be accurately excised with clear margins while tissue is spared. He has observed that malignant melanomas spread either locally in cohesive contiguity or more or less by "embolism" of discontinuous melanomatous cells to adjacent and more distant tissues (lymph node metastasis). Clinical stage I, thin melanomas (Breslow thickness less than 0.75 mm) statistically have cure rates approaching 100% when treated with wide excision. It may be that tumors this thin have not begun to spread hematogenously and therefore it would be reasonable to believe that histologic tumor-free margins would be curative. Cure rates published by Dr. Mohs are similar to those published by others performing wide excision (up to 3 cm margins) for the same tumors.

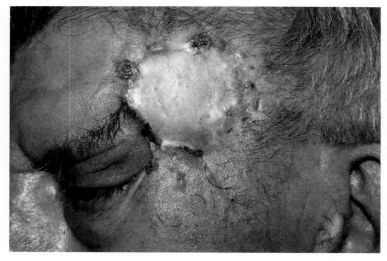

(a)

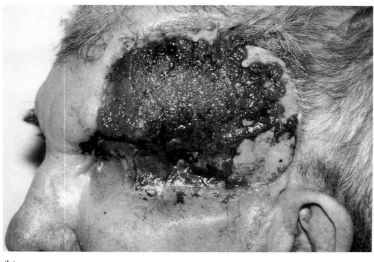

(b)

Figure 10 Recurrent morpheaform basal cell carcinoma after several excisions and grafting. Note ulcers and nodules at the periphery of the graft. This tumor extended down to bone and into the retro-orbital space, requiring enucleation of the orbit. Invasive tumor such as this requires the expertise of other surgical specialists and is beyond the capabilities of Mohs surgery done in an outpatient setting. (a) Preoperative view. (b) Two months postoperatively, granulation tissue is regenerating in preparation for graft placement.

Mohs' impression is that the spread of melanomas, in the form of satellites, in-transit metastasis, and lymph node metastasis, is almost always by embolism. He believes that clumps of cells break off and travel to other sties rather than that there is continuous permeation through lymphatic vessels. They spread in the direction of regional lymph nodes, but a few extend in the retrograde direction. There is no sharp distinction between in-transit metastasis and satellites, and Mohs considers outbreaks within 5 cm of the primary lesion to be satellites and those beyond to be in-transit metastatic lesions. The latter have a less favorable prognosis.

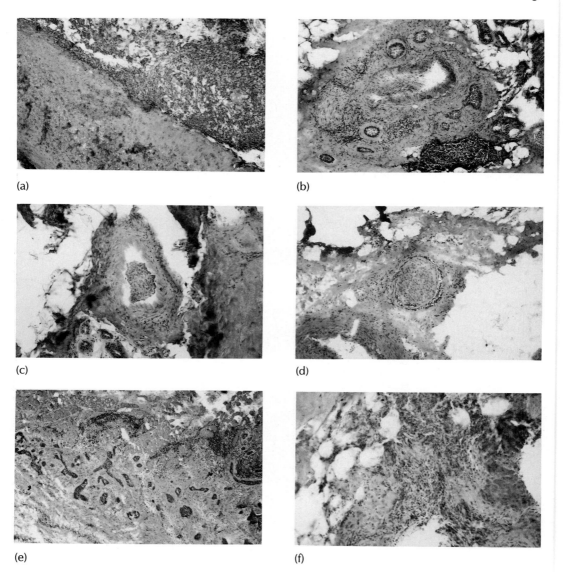

(a)

(b)

(c)

(d)

(e)

(f)

Figure 11 Basal cell carcinoma has the capacity to dissect into embryologic cleavage planes: (a) perichondrial (b) perivascular; (c) intravascular; (d) perineural; (e) intramuscular. recurrent tumor underneath a myocutaneous flap; (f) parotid gland involvement. Note normal parotid gland mixed superficially with subcutaneous fat and squamous cell carcinoma invading (right of figure).

The approach advocated by Mohs is that the primary tumor be excised using the older fixed technique, applying the zinc chloride paste. Presumably, this prevents hematogenous dissemination of living tumor cells intraoperatively when cutting through tumor. He then excises an extra margin of skin and subcutaneous tissue (5–15 mm); if the neoplasm appears highly aggressive, he removes a wider margin (15–30 mm) in order to remove invisible satellites and the lymphatics around the neoplasm.

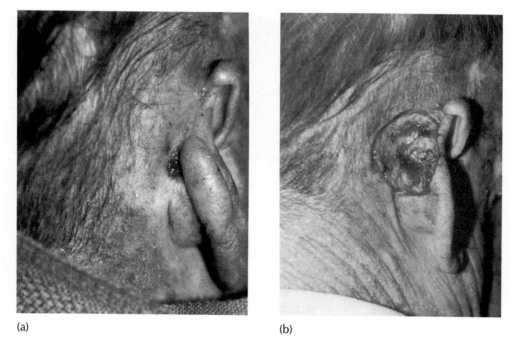

(a)   (b)

Figure 12 Squamous cell carcinoma recurrent after previous excision and irradiation. Clinically, a small erosion in the retroauricular sulcus resulted in a large postauricular defect. (a) Preoperative view. (b) Micrographic tumor-free margins.

Wide margin excision of clinical stage I disease in melanoma is itself controversial. Recommendations for wide excision range from margins of as little as 1 cm up to 3 cm (most recommended 2–3 cm). The essential point may be that whether Mohs surgery or wide excision is done, both therapies are intended to prevent local recurrences. There is probably no significant relationship between the recurrence of melanoma within a 5 cm area of the primary site and subsequent mortality. Clearly, tumors greater than 1.69 mm in thickness have a greater incidence of lymphatic spread, lymph node involvement, metastatic dissemination, and death. Lymph node dissections may be warranted for thicker lesions, but the efficacy of this procedure remains controversial as well.

KERATOACANTHOMA

Keratoacanthoma is a neoplasm of uncertain origin that may resolve spontaneously if left untreated. The neoplasm is unpredictable and in its growth phase may cause massive tissue destruction before involution. There is an overlap with squamous cell carcinoma, and metastatic disease has developed in patients with keratoacanthoma.

There are many methods for treating keratoacanthoma, including excision, electrodesiccation and curettage, cryosurgery, radiation, intralesional steroids, topical or intralesional 5-fluorouracil, intralesional bleomycin, topical podophyllin, methotrexate, systemic isotretinoin or etretinate, interferon, and observation. Larson reported a cure of 42 out of 43 keratoacanthomas using Mohs micrographic surgery. The one recurrence was a central facial lesion. Central facial keratoacanthomas have a propensity to be more aggressive (Fig. 15). Mohs micrographic surgery

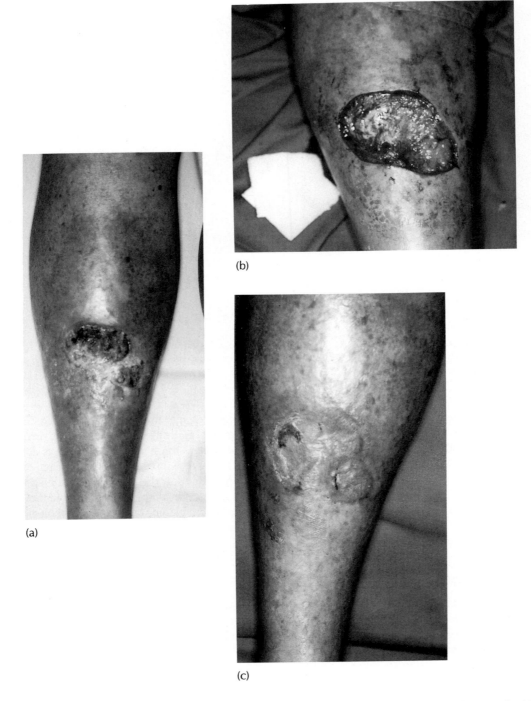

(a)

(b)

(c)

Figure 13 Squamous cell carcinoma on the lower extremity in a patient with psoriasis treated with methotrexate and psoralen with ong wave ultraviolet light. (a) Preoperative view. (b) Micrographic tumor-free margins. (c) One month postoperatively, after placement of a graft by a plastic surgeon. (Photo courtesy of Ronald G. Wheeland, M.D.)

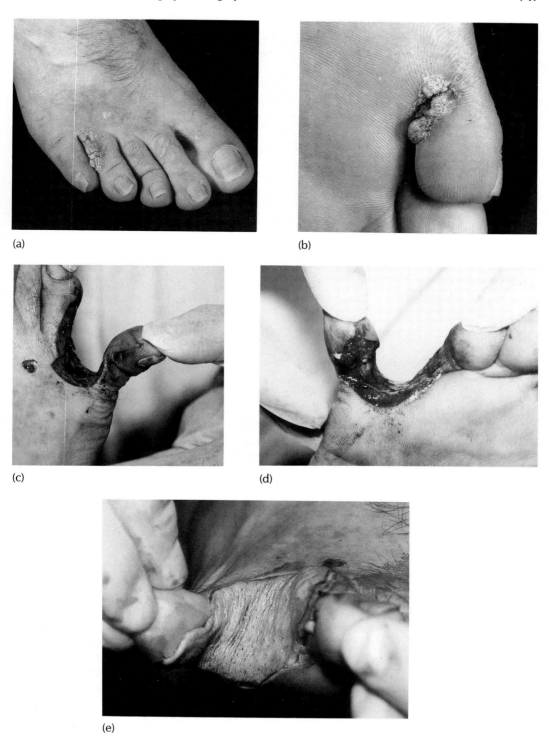

(a)

(b)

(c)

(d)

(e)

Figure 14 Verrucous squamous cell carcinoma in the interdigital space between the fourth and fifth toes. Micrographic surgery probably spared amputation of one or both digits. (a) Preoperative dorsal view. (b) Preoperative ventral view. (c) Micrographic tumor-free margins, dorsal view. (d) Micrographic tumor-free margins, ventral view. (e) Intraoperative placement of skin graft by a plastic surgeon.

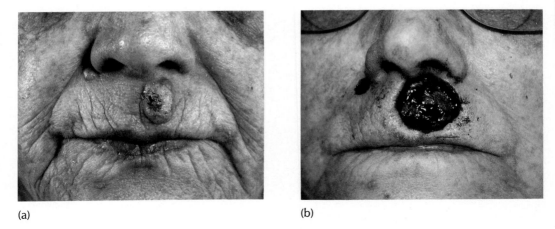

(a)   (b)

Figure 15 Keratoacanthoma enlarging rapidly. (a) Preoperative view. (b) Micrographic tumor-free margins. Tumor involved part of the orbicularis oris muscle.

may be indicated for large, more aggressive keratoacanthomas but should not be considered the treatment of choice for the routine tumor.

VERRUCOUS CARCINOMA

Verrucous carcinoma is a variant of squamous cell carcinoma that may be induced by human papillomavirus. It has been reported in the oral cavity, penis, foot, and larynx, usually under a variety of confusing terms, including giant condyloma acuminatum, Buschke-Löwenstein tumor, papillomatous cutis carcinoides, and epithelioma cuniculatum. The tumor is characterized by sheets of well-differentiated, pale-staining keratinocytes with infrequent mitoses. Although considered a low-grade carcinoma, well-documented cases of recurrence and metastasis have been described. The recurrence rate after local excision is approximately 20%. Metastasis may occur at a similar rate. Since it is clear that this tumor may extend well into the subcutaneous tissues, treatment by Mohs micrographic surgery, especially for large primary lesions, is warranted (Fig. 16).

BOWEN'S DISEASE

Bowen's disease is squamous cell carcinoma in situ. The lesion occurs most commonly on the face, hands, and trunk and rarely in the perianal region and on the vulva and penis (erythroplasia of Queyrat). There are several destructive ways in which this tumor can be treated, but Mohs micrographic surgery may be indicated when tissue sparing is important, particularly on the digits, penis, and vulva (Fig. 17). Histologic tumor-free margins are important for accurate excision and for sparing normal tissue to minimize reconstruction or allow for second intention healing.

ATYPICAL FIBROXANTHOMA

This is typically a rapidly growing red nodule, often ulcerated, on the sun-damaged skin of the head and neck of elderly males, which has an ominous histology but a good prognosis. The

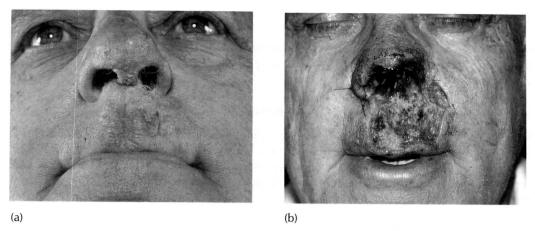

(a)   (b)

Figure 16 Verrucous carcinoma is considered a low-grade malignant lesion but has the potential to metastasize. (a) Preoperative view. (b) Micrographic tumor-free margins.

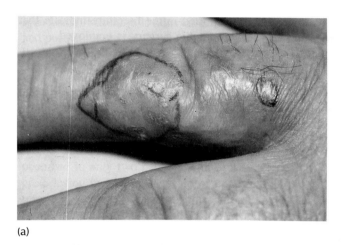

(a)

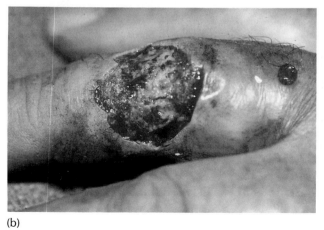

(b)

Figure 17 Bowen's disease that has recurred after treatment with the CO_2 laser. The lesion is characteristically superficial; therefore an excision that risks the viability of the digit would not be warranted. (a) Preoperative view. (b) Micrographic tumor-free margins.

Ears

Malignant tumors of the auricle and periauricular structure constitute only 6% of all skin cancers. However, the recurrence rate for tumors in this area is higher than that for most other areas. Tumors of the ear have a predictable pattern of growth and spread. Tumors arising in the periauricular or postauricular area tend to spread to the ear. Tumors in the preauricular area spread toward the tragus and the anterosuperior aspect of the helix. Once at the tragus, tumor can spread down the external part of the tragus between tragal cartilage and the parotid gland to involve deeper structures. Once the superior helix is reached, spread is along the superior helix and down the helix itself. Tumors arising in the preauricular or postauricular region do not involve the ear canal itself until very late in their course. The spread of these tumors is probably related to the embryologic development of the auricle.

Eyes

It was in the eyelid region that Mohs first used micrographic surgery with the fresh tissue technique in 1953. In 1969, Mohs had reported a 100% 5-year cure rate for 66 basal cell carcinomas and 4 squamous cell carcinomas treated in this way. Others, notably Tromovitch and Stegman, applied the fresh frozen tissue technique, which is now used almost exclusively by most dermatologic surgeons performing micrographic surgery.

Lesions on the eyelids can present some special problems. On the upper lid, excess skin often allows small lesions to be treated by surgical excision and primary closure, with good results. However, if the tumor extends to the tarsal plate and levator muscle, repair by an ophthalmoplastic specialist is indicated. Electrodesiccation and curettage is not recommended for treatment of eyelid lesions or those on the inner canthi, because these areas are of vital functional importance and assurance of the highest possible cure rate is essential (Fig. 19). As with Mohs micrographic surgery, cryosurgery or radiation therapy in these areas requires special training and experience.

Of all basal cell carcinomas on the head and neck, 5–10% involve the eyelids. Approximately 90% of malignant tumors around the eyes are basal cell carcinoma. Squamous cell carcinoma, sebaceous carcinoma, malignant melanoma, malignant lymphoma, Bowen's disease, and adenocarcinoma of the glands of Moll make up the rest. Mohs micrographic surgery has resulted in the highest cure rates for cutaneous carcinoma. Mohs micrographic surgery is especially beneficial for recurrent tumors, for which standard forms of therapy often fail. This may be followed by immediate reconstruction by the dermatologic surgeon in small, uncomplicated cases. Healing by second intention is especially effective in the medial canthal region. For larger defects, eyelid reconstruction can be performed by an ophthalmoplastic surgeon, providing optimal function and cosmesis with minimal morbidity. This type of tumor removal followed by reconstruction combines the best the two specialties have to offer in managing these difficult tumors.

Lips

In the perioral region, tumors of the keratinizing skin of the upper lip are most frequently basal cell carcinomas (Fig. 20). On the lower lip, the most common tumor is squamous cell carcinoma. These lesions generally arise in the mucosal epithelium posterior to the vermilion border. This tumor is notable for its capacity to metastasize regionally, becoming life-threatening.

Mohs micrographic surgery has been effective in treating squamous cell carcinoma of the lower lip. Mohs experience has been the most extensive, showing that expected cure rates are very high, but that certain subgroups can be identified preoperatively as having a higher risk for recurrence.

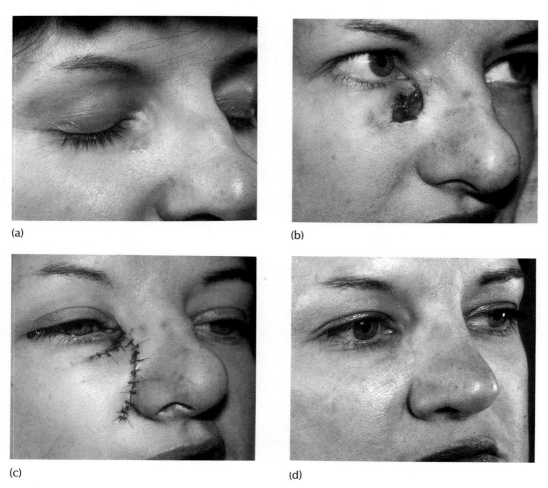

Figure 19 Primary nodular basal cell carcinoma on the medial lower eyelid. Aside from cosmetic importance, the function of the lacrimal duct and the ability to close the eyelid once the tumor has been removed must be considered. Tissue sparing is important in this location so that reconstruction may be done on the smallest defect possible, sparing as much adjacent normal tissue as can be made available. (a) Preoperative view. (b) Micrographic tumor-free margins. (c) Reconstruction with an inferiorly based rotation flap. (d) Six months postoperative.

The overall cure rate for squamous cell carcinoma of the lower lip in Mohs series is 94.2%. Lesions less than 2 cm in diameter had a cure rate of 96.6%, whereas those greater than 2 cm in diameter had a cure rate of only 59.6%. If tumors are categorized by degree of cellular differentiation based on Broders' classification (grades I–IV), a cure rate of 96.3% can be expected for tumors of grade I or II. This contrasts with a cure rate of 66.7% for tumors with grade III or IV differentiation.

Use of Mohs micrographic surgery for tumors that had recurred from previous therapy results in a highly respectable cure rate of 88.2%. However, evidence of metastatic disease either before treatment or shortly thereafter lower the expected cure rate to only 27.3%. Mohs surgery accurately controls the primary tumor.

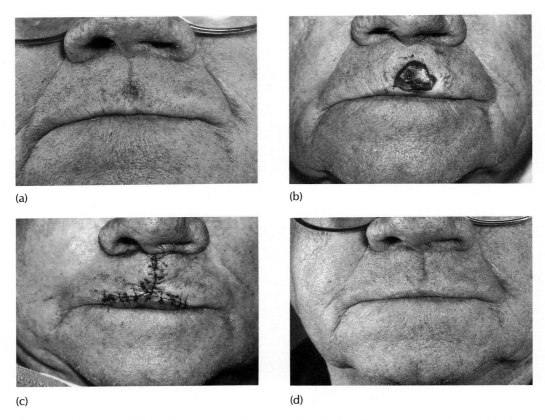

(a) (b)

(c) (d)

Figure 20 Recurrent basal cell carcinoma of the upper lip. Basal cell carcinoma characteristically occurs on the upper lip, whereas squamous cell carcinoma characteristically occurs on the lower lip. (a) Preoperative view. (b) Micrographic tumor-free margins. (c) Closure in an A to T fashion. (d) Four months postoperative.

If these statistics are used as a guide during the preoperative management of patients with squamous cell carcinoma of the lower lip, it seems reasonable that smaller (less than 2 cm), well-differentiated tumors unassociated with metastatic disease can be treated effectively by Mohs micrographic surgery to obtain high cure rates and also to spare normal tissue for immediate cosmetic and functional reconstruction. Larger and more aggressive tumors may require wider excision, node dissection, and adjunctive therapy, with the cooperation of the otolaryngologist and other specialists.

Nails

Subungual epidermal carcinomas, such as Bowen's disease or squamous cell carcinoma, are not uncommon, and the course of the disease is often prolonged, since the clinical diagnosis can be confused with onychomycosis, paronychia, verruca, and other common disorders of the nail. Once a tumor has been established histologically, local excision with histologic tumor-free margins is optimal, because these are low-grade malignancies with a low incidence of metastasis. The use of Mohs micrographic surgery often avoids amputation of the digit, so that function is maintained.

Nose

The nasal area is the single most common site for presentation of basal cell carcinoma and also the most common site for recurrence. Approximately 40% of all recalcitrant basal cell carcinomas of the head and neck involve the nasal skin. This occurrence is in part related to the many embryologic fusion planes in this region that offer decreased resistance to the spread of neoplasm. Standard forms of treatment in this area are acceptable for tumors less than 0.5 cm in diameter. For larger tumors, however, Mohs micrographic surgery may be indicated, especially if the tumor has recurred after previous treatment or has an aggressive histologic growth pattern (morpheaform or metatypical basal cell carcinoma). In areas such as the junction between the ala and the nasolabial fold, the tumor can be deceivingly extensive. In addition, the alar rim and nasal tip are areas where tissue conservation is critical for reconstruction. A cooperative effort between the Mohs micrographic surgeon and the reconstructive surgeon is critical for treatment of tumors in this location (Fig. 21).

Penis

Conventional excision of squamous cell carcinoma of the glans penis has been reported to result in recurrence at the primary site in approximately 40% of patients. This high recurrence rate may result from an inability to assess the tumor margins accurately by clinical evaluation. Therefore, many urologists have recommended penectomy at a level of 1.5–2 cm proximal to the tumor unless the lesion is on the distal prepuce, in which case circumcision may suffice. The location of tumor on the penis with or without metastasis strongly affects the prognosis. Cure rates of 80% can be expected when tumors are localized to the glans or prepuce, but this cure rate decreases to 57% when the shaft is involved. Size of the primary lesion also affects cure rates, as in other locations, with a 100% cure rate expected for lesions less than 1 cm, but no better than 50% for lesions greater than 3 cm. Grading malignancies histologically also predicts the success

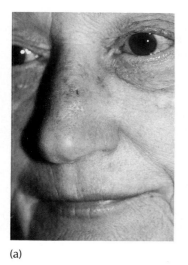 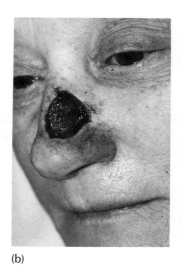 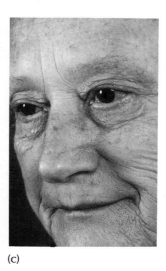

(a) (b) (c)

Figure 21 Recurrent basal cell carcinoma on the nasal sidewall. Despite extensive involvement in this cosmetically important area, reconstruction can yield a very acceptable result. (a) Preoperative view. (b) Micrographic tumor-free margins. (c) Eight months after a nasolabial transposition flap was placed by an otolaryngologist.

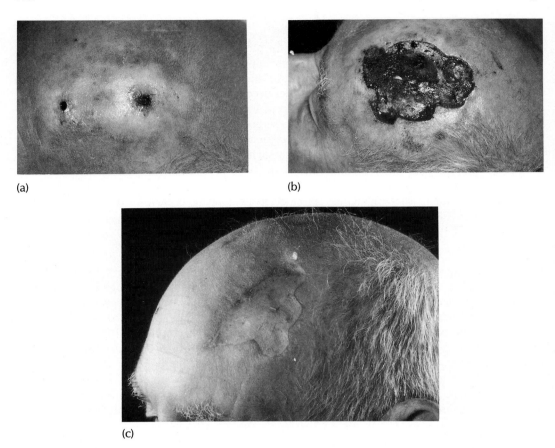

(a)   (b)

(c)

Figure 22 Basal cell carcinoma on the scalp can be quite extensive and have indistinct clinical margins. (a) Preoperative view. It was anticipated that two separate small tumors would be present (blanching due to local anesthesia). (b) Micrographic tumor-free margins. (c) Six weeks postoperatively after placement of a split-thickness skin graft by a plastic surgeon.

of treatment with more well-differentiated tumors being treated more successfully. Mohs micrographic surgery is useful for patients with genital tumors to control the local disease. However, patients with squamous cell carcinoma should be considered for regional lymph node biopsy or dissection in conjunction with excision of the primary tumor.

Scalp

Carcinomas of the scalp have a tendency to spread peripherally in several tissue planes, including the dermis, fascia above and below the galea, periosteum, and, occasionally, the lymphatics (Fig. 22). The bone generally acts as a barrier to vertical growth, but eventually the tumor may follow paths of least resistance into foramina or osseous suture lines, reaching the bony cortex and breaking through the inner table to involve the dura, vascular sinuses, and brain. Basal cell carcinoma invasive to this extent has been reported several times in the literature.

The cure rate with traditional therapy for tumors on the scalp is very high. This location is not considered a high risk for recurrence. However, as in other locations, treatment with Mohs micrographic surgery also allows a 99% cure rate. Preoperative evaluation of the size and histologic subtypes of tumors in this location helps determine whether basal cell carcinoma or squamous cell carcinoma of the scalp should be treated by Mohs micrographic surgery.

BIBLIOGRAPHY

Albright SD III. Treatment of skin cancer using multiple modalities. *J Am Acad Dermatol* 1982;7:143–171.

Anderson RL, Ceilley RI. A multispecialty approach to the excision and reconstruction of eyelid tumors. *Ophthalmology* 1978;85:1150–1163.

Bailin PL, Levine HL, Wood BG, Tucker HM. Cutaneous carcinoma of the auricular and periauricular region. *Arch Otolaryngol* 1980;106:692–696.

Baker SR, Swanson NA, Grekin RC. An interdisciplinary approach to the management of basal cell carcinoma of the head and neck. *J Dermatol Surg Oncol* 1978;13(10):1095–1106.

Baker SR, Swanson NA. Management of nasal cutaneous malignant neoplasms: An interdisciplinary approach. *Arch Otolaryngol* 1983;109:473–479.

Baran RL, Gormley DE. Polydactylous Bowen's disease of the nail. *J Am Acad Dermatol* 1987;17:201–204.

Brown M, Swanson N. Treatment of malignant fibrohystiocytoma and atypical fibroxanthoma with micrographic surgery. *J Derm Surg Oncol* 1989;15:1287–1292

Brown MD, Zachary CB, Grekin RC, Swanson NA. Genital tumors: Their management by micrographic surgery. *J Am Acad Dermatol* 1988;18:115–122.

Bumstead RM, Ceilley RI. Auricular malignant neoplasms: Identification of high-risk lesions and selection of method of reconstruction. *Arch Otolaryngol* 1982;108:225–231.

Ceilley RI, Anderson RL. Microscopically controlled excision of malignant neoplasms on and around eyelids followed by immediate surgical reconstruction. *J Dermatol Surg Oncol* 1978;4(1):55–62.

Davidson TM, Haghighi P, Astarita R, Baird S, Seagren S. Microscopically oriented histologic surgery for head and neck mucosal cancer. *Cancer* 1987;60:1856–1861.

Dickson RS, Mikhail GR, Slater HC. Sebaceous carcinoma of the eyelid. *J Am Acad Dermatol* 1980;3:241–243.

Dzubow LM, Grossman DJ, Johnson B. Chemosurgical report: Eccrine adenocarcinoma—report of a case, treatment with Mohs' surgery. *J Dermatol Surg Oncol* 1986;12(10):1049–1053.

Dzubow LM, Rigel DS, Robins P. Risk factors for local recurrence of primary cutaneous squamous cell carcinomas: Treatment by microscopically controlled excision. *Arch Dermatol* 1982;118:900–902.

Friedman HI, Cooper PH, Wanebo HJ. Prognostic and therapeutic use of microstaging of cutaneous squamous cell carcinoma of the trunk and extremities. *Cancer* 1985;56:1099–1105.

Folber R, Whitaker DC, Tse DT, Nerad JA. Recurrent and residual sebaceous carcinoma after Mohs' excision of the primary lesion. *Am J Ophthalmol* 1987;103:817–823.

Goldstein DJ, Barr RJ, Santa Cruz DJ. Microcystic adnexal carcinoma: A distinct clinicopathologic entity. *Cancer* 1982;50:566–572.

Hobbs E. Dermatofibrosarcoma protuberans. In: Roenigk R, Roenigk H, eds. *Surgical Dermatology*. St. Louis: Mosby, 1993.

Hobbs ER, Wheeland RG, Bailin PL, Ratz JL, Yetman RJ, Zins JE. Treatment of dermatofibrosarcoma protuberans with Mohs' micrographic surgery. *Ann Surg* 1988;207(1):102–107.

Howell JB, Caro MR. Morphea-like epithelioma. *Arch Dermatol* 1957;75:517–524.

Koplin L, Zarem HA. Recurrent basal cell carcinoma: A review concerning the incidence, behavior, and management of recurrent basal cell carcinoma, with emphasis on the incompletely excised lesion. *Plast Reconstr Surg* 1980;65:656–664.

Lang PG Jr, Maize JC. Histologic evolution of recurrent basal cell carcinoma and treatment implications. *J Am Acad Dermatol* 1986;14:186–196.

Larson PO. Keratoacanthomas treated with Mohs' micrographic surgery (chemosurgery): A review of forty-three cases. *J Am Acad Dermatol* 1987;16:1040–1044.

Levine HL, Bailin PL. Basal cell carcinoma of the head and neck: Identification of the high risk patient. *Laryngoscope* 1980;90(6):955–961.

Levine H, Bailin P, Wood B, Tucker H. Tissue conservation in treatment of cutaneous neoplasms of the head and neck: Combined use of Mohs' chemosurgical and conventional surgical techniques. *Arch Otolaryngol* 1979;105:140–144.

Mehregan AH, Hashimoto K, Rahbari H. Eccrine adenocarcinoma: A clinicopathologic study of 35 cases. *Arch Dermatol* 1983;119:104–114.

Mehregan D, Roenigk R. Management of superficial squamous cell carcinoma of the lip with Mohs micrographic surgery. *Cancer* 1990;66:463–468.

Mikhail GR. Subungual epidermoid carcinoma. *J Am Acad Dermatol* 1984;11:291–298.

Mohs FE. *Chemosurgery: Microscopically Controlled Surgery for Skin Cancer*. Springfield, IL: Charles C Thomas, 1978.

Mohs FE. Micrographic surgery for the microscopically controlled excision of eyelid cancers. *Arch Ophthalmol* 1986;104:901–909.

Mohs FE. Micrographic surgery for the microscopically controlled excision of eyelid cancer: History and development. *Adv Ophthalmol Plast Reconstr Surg* 1986;5:381–408.

Mohs FE. Micrographic surgery for satellites and intransit metastases of malignant melanomas. *J Dermatol Surg Oncol* 1986;12(5):471–476.

Mohs FE. The width and depth of the spread of malignant melanomas as observed by a chemosurgeon. *Am J Dermatopathol* 1984;6 (Suppl 1):123–126.

Mohs FE, Blume RF, Sahl WJ. Chemosurgery for familial malignant melanoma. *J Dermatol Surg Oncol* 1979;5(2):127–131.

Mohs FE, Snow SN. Microscopically controlled surgical treatment for squamous cell carcinoma of the lower lip. *Surg Gynecol Obstet* 1985;160:37–41.

Mohs FE, Snow SN, Messing ME, Kuglitsch ME. Microscopically controlled surgery in the treatment of carcinoma of the penis. *J Urol* 1985;133:961–966.

Mohs FE, Zitelli JA. Microscopically controlled surgery in the treatment of carcinoma of the scalp. *Arch Dermatol* 1981;117:764–769.

Moller R, Reymann F, Hou-Jensen K. Metastases in dermatological patients with squamous cell carcinoma. *Arch Dermatol* 1979;115:703–705.

Nickoloff BJ, Fleishmann HE, Carmel J, Wood CC, Roth RJ. Micrycystic adnexal carcinoma: Immunologic observations suggesting dual (pilar and eccrine) differentiation. *Arch Dermatol* 1986;122:290–294.

Padilla RS, Bailin PL, Howard WR, Dinner MI. Verrucous carcinoma of the scalp and its management by Mohs' surgery. *Plast Reconstr Surg* 1984;73(3):442–447.

Peters CR, Dinner MI, Dolsky RL, Bailin PL, Hardy RW Jr. The combined multidisciplinary approach to invasive basal cell tumors of the scalp. *Ann Plast Surg* 1980;4(3):199–204.

Preston D, Stern R. Nonmelanoma cancers of the skin. *N Engl J Med* 1992;327:1649–1662.

Randle H, Roenigk R, Brodland D. Giant basal cell carcinoma (T3). Who is at risk? *Cancer* 1993;72:1624–1630.

Ratz JL, Luu-Duong S, Kulwin DR. Sebaceous carcinoma of the eyelid treated with Mohs' surgery. *J Am Acad Dermatol* 1986;14:668–673.

Rigel DS, Robins P, Friedman PJ. Predicting recurrence of basal-cell carcinomas treated by microscopically controlled excision: A recurrence index score. *J Dermatol Surg Oncol* 1981;7(10):807–810.

Robins P, Nix M. Analysis of persistent disease of the ear following Mohs surgery. *Head Neck Surg* 1984;6:998–1006.

Robins P, Dzubow LM, Rigel DS. Squamous cell carcinoma treated by Mohs' surgery: An experience with 414 cases in a period of 15 years. *J Dermatol Surg Oncol* 1981;7(10):800–801.

Robins P, Rodriguez-Sains R, Rabinovitz H, Rigel D. Mohs' surgery for periocular basal cell carinomas. *J Dermatol Surg Oncol* 1985;11(12):1203–1207.

Robinson JK. Dermatofibrosarcoma protuberans resected by Mohs' surgery (chemosurgery): A 5-year prospective study. *J Am Acad Dermatol* 1985;12:1093–1098.

Roenigk RK. Mohs' micrographic surgery. *Mayo Clinic Proc* 1988;63:175–183.

Roenigk RK, Ratz JL, Bailin PL, Wheeland RG. Trends in the presentation and treatment of basal cell carcinomas. *J Dermatol Surg Oncol* 1986;12(8):860–865.

Rowe D, Carroll R, Day C. Mohs surgery is the treatment of choice for recurrent (previously treated) basal cell carcinoma. *J Dermatol Surg Oncol* 1989;15:524–531.

Rowe D, Carroll R, Day C. Prognostic factors for local recurrence, metasteses, and survival rates in squamous cell carcinoma of the skin, ear, and lip. *J Am Acad Dermatol* 1992;26:976–990.

Salashe S, Amonette R. Morpheaform basal cell epitheliomas, a study of subclinical extension in a series of 51 cases. *J Dermatol Surg Oncol* 1981;7:387–394.

Silverman M, et al. Recurrence rate of treated basal cell carcinoma. *J Dermatol Surg Oncol* 1992; 18:471–476.

Swanson NA. Mohs surgery: Technique, identification, applications, and the future. *Arch Dermatol* 1983; 119:761–773.

Swanson NA, Taylor WB. Plantar verrucous carcinoma: Literature review and treatment by the Mohs' chemotherapy technique. *Arch Dermatol* 1980;116:794–797.

Tromovitch TA, Stegman SA. Microscopically controlled excision of cutaneous tumors—chemosurgery, fresh tissue technique. *Cancer* 1978;41:653–658.

Wade T, Ackerman A. The many faces of basal cell carcinoma. *J Dermatol Surg Oncol* 1978;4:23–28.

42

Mohs Micrographic Surgery Technique

Ronald G. Wheeland
University of New Mexico, Albuquerque, New Mexico

John Louis Ratz
*Tulane University, Louisiana State University, and
The Oschner Clinic, New Orleans, Louisiana*

Philip L. Bailin
The Cleveland Clinic Foundation, Cleveland, Ohio

Mohs micrographic surgery is a technique first described by Dr. Frederic Mohs, and subsequently modified, which permits the complete removal of contiguously spreading skin cancers. When properly performed, this procedure allows for immediate and total microscopic evaluation of all surgical margins and precise identification and localization of any residual tumor through the use of fresh frozen section. The location of residual tumor cells can be accurately identified on a detailed anatomic diagram or map, and those positive areas can be selectively removed. This serial or staged excision technique is repeated until no microscopic evidence of tumor remains, permitting all contiguous extensions of the tumor to be mapped and removed. This can be completed on an outpatient basis over several hours, using local anesthesia. The resulting defect can be repaired immediately or allowed to heal by second intention.

PREOPERATIVE EVALUATION

At the initial consultation with the candidate for Mohs surgery, a complete history should be taken and a complete physical examination performed. A history of previous treatment affects the prognosis of this tumor as well as the repair to be considered. Previous radiation exposure, intake of arsenic, or significant exposure to ultraviolet light should be noted to evaluate the potential for new tumors. The consultation may also be used to educate the patient about these risk factors. After the lesion has been examined, it is measured and photographed. The nature of the problem, pathogenesis, prognosis, treatment options, risks, benefits, complications, and anticipated extent of the postoperative defect are discussed in detail with the patient. If there is a history of cardiac disease, bleeding disorder, or any other internal disease that may influence the procedure or the postoperative course, appropriate laboratory, electrocardiographic, and radiologic examinations are also performed at the initial consultation.

Work represents a combined effort from the Section of Mohs micrographic surgery at the Cleveland Clinic.

To minimize potential bleeding during the operation or postoperatively, the patient should discontinue use of all nonsteroidal antiinflammatory agents or aspirin for 2 weeks preoperatively and use of any alcoholic beverage for 72 hr prior to the procedure. If the patient is required to take medications regularly for preexisting internal disease, he or she should take the usual dose on the day of surgery. Also, it is recommended that the patient eat a light breakfast the morning of surgery. Most patients are advised to come to the office with a family member or friend. Since the patient usually does not remain in the Mohs operating suite during tissue processing, it is often helpful to have someone present to lessen the anxiety of waiting for results of the microscopic analysis. Additionally, if the lesion is located in the periorbital area, where a dressing may interfere with vision, a family member or friend can accompany the patient home.

PROCEDURE

The extent of the tumor is first determined as accurately as possible (Fig. 1) and the apparent peripheral border is outlined with a surgical skin marker such as brilliant green or gentian violet (Fig. 2). The outlined tumor is measured, and the size is recorded on an anatomic diagram from which the surgical map will be generated. The affected area is then prepped with surgical scrub such as Hibiclens or Betadine. Local anesthesia, typically 1% lidocaine with epinephrine (1:100,000 or 1:200,000), is administered by intradermal injection. The operative field is covered with sterile towels or drapes.

If the tumor is large or particularly thick, debulking may be useful. This is accomplished by simple curettage with or without the use of electrodesiccation. It may be beneficial to determine

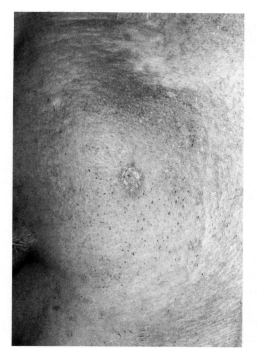

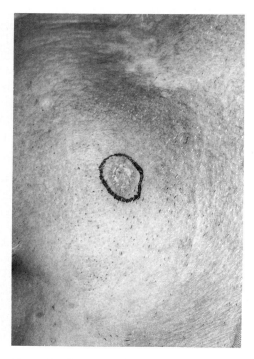

Figure 1   Preoperative clinical appearance of a primary basal cell carcinoma of the cheek.

Figure 2   Apparent clinical extent of the tumor is outlined with brilliant green ink.

the extent of primary tumors by performing curettage and electrodesiccation prior to taking the first Mohs layer. This modification may help to reduce the number of layers necessary to eradicate the tumor.

The first micrographic specimen should include all clinically evident tumor plus a very small peripheral margin of normal-appearing tissue. Before the specimen is removed, the margin is marked with several small incisions (Figs. 3,4) to orient the removed tissue properly. These marks are made in both the specimen and adjacent normal tissue. An incision is then made along the outlined margin with the scalpel angled in the traditional perpendicular position. Then the blade is beveled slightly inward and the incision is repeated along the margin. Subsequent cuts, each increasingly beveled inward (Fig. 5), are made until the plane of the incision is horizontal (Fig. 6). This is the plane of dissection along which the entire specimen is removed. This yields a thin disc of tissue (Fig. 7). The tissue is held at only one edge with forceps to preserve the proper orientation of the specimen. Once the specimen has been removed, orientation must be verified. This is accomplished by aligning the specimen in its original position using the scored incisions made previously. The specimen is then placed with proper orientation on an anatomically marked transfer card (Fig. 8).

Although epinephrine will aid hemostasis, additional measures for limiting blood loss may be necessary. In most cases, this is achieved with standard electrosurgery, either direct as electrofulguration or indirect as electrocoagulation, with the aid of forceps or a hemostat. Larger transected blood vessels may require suture ligation. If the operative field is large and there is significant capillary bleeding from the skin edges, chemical cautery, bovine thrombin, or hemostatic gauze (Oxycel, Gelfoam) may be helpful. Between layers, a pressure dressing is applied.

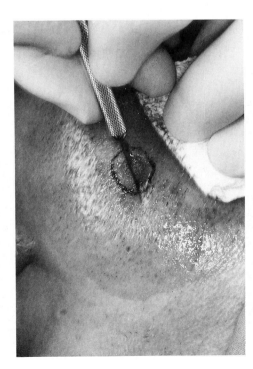

Figure 3 One small superficial score mark is made at the inferior edge of the planned excision to facilitate orientation.

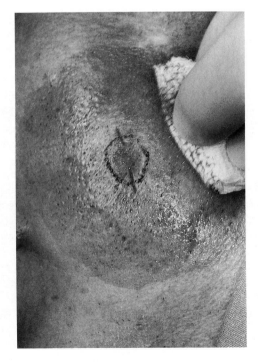

Figure 4 A second superficial score mark has been added to the superior edge of the planned excision.

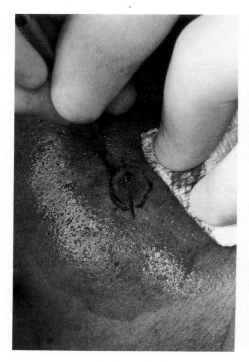

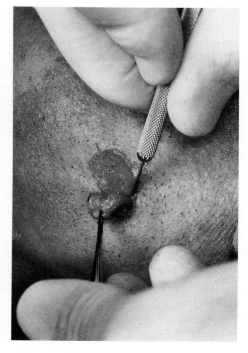

Figure 5 With the scalpel held in nearly horizontal fashion, a flat specimen can be harvested.

Figure 6 As the specimen is removed, the scalpel bevels the edge of the incision line.

If immediate repair is anticipated, Gelfoam is placed in the wound as a temporary hemostatic aid. However, if the wound is allowed to heal by second intention, oxidized cellulose cotton (Oxycel) can be used instead. An antibiotic ointment is applied topically followed by a non-adherent gauze (Telfa). A simple bulk dressing is placed on the surface and, when appropriate, a pressure dressing applied.

To ensure proper orientation of the specimen, an accurate schematic representation of the surgical defect is drawn on an appropriate anatomic diagram. The alignment is aided by the "scored" incisions made for orientation, which are also marked on the diagram. For small specimens the entire disk of tissue can be processed in its entirety as a single piece. However, in most cases, the original disk of tissue is subdivided into several smaller pieces (Fig. 9) to fit on a standard glass microscope slide to be processed. These pieces are drawn on the map to maintain proper orientation. Relatively straight lateral epidermal margins must be obtained when the specimen is being divided in order to facilitate histologic sectioning and ensure that the entire peripheral margin is represented on each section. Specimens having acutely curved epidermal margins are difficult to evaluate after processing since the skin edge is often only found deeply embedded in the frozen block.

After the specimen has been divided, each piece is lifted from the transfer card, and all margins not at the periphery are marked with colored dyes (Fig. 10). After being marked, the

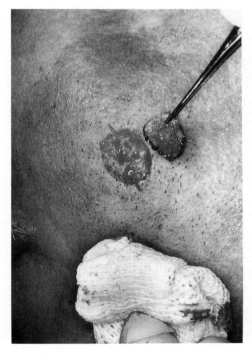

Figure 7 The thin piece of tissue is held next to the defect.

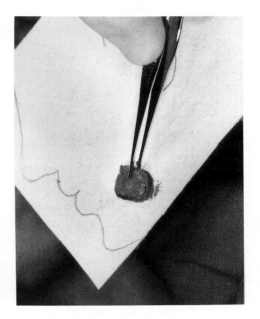

Figure 8 The specimen is placed on a card on which anatomic features are sketched to preserve orientation.

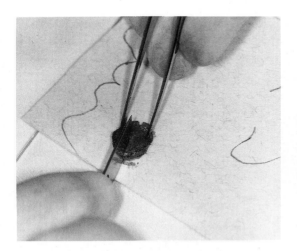

Figure 9 The harvested tissue is divided in half to fit on a standard microscope slide.

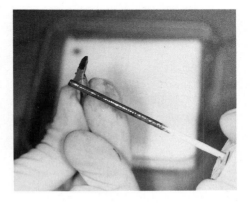

Figure 10 The cut edge of the specimen is color-coded with special dyes to orient the sectioned tissue under the microscope.

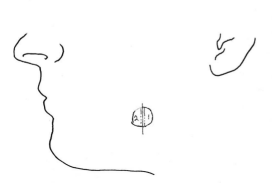

Figure 11 Color-coding is used to mark each half of the specimen.

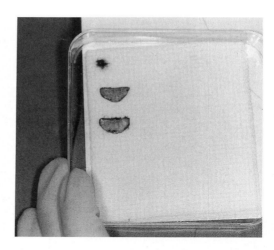

Figure 12 The color-coded specimens are placed on a saline-moistened gauze within a plastic container for transportation to the laboratory.

pieces are numbered consecutively, and the colored margins are recorded on the map. For diagrammatic purposes, a straight line on the map represents a red-colored margin, a dotted line on the map represents a blue one (Fig. 11), and a jagged line on the map represents a black one. Each piece of the specimen is placed on a saline-moistened gauze pad in ordered sequence in a Petri dish (Fig. 12) so that the peripheral skin edge margin is pointed down. This routine simplifies handling by the technician.

The technician begins the processing with piece number one and proceeds consecutively. Optimal cutting temperature (OCT) medium is placed on the cryostat chuck (Fig. 13); the specimen is inverted and placed horizontally on the chuck (Fig. 14) so that the deepest margin now faces up. If the specimen is quick-frozen in liquid nitrogen (Fig. 15), the OCT partially solidifies, and the specimen can be molded. This may be done by using the flat portion of a Bard-

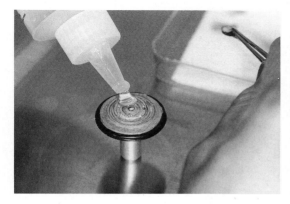

Figure 13 A small quantity of OCT medium is placed on the top of the cryostat chuck.

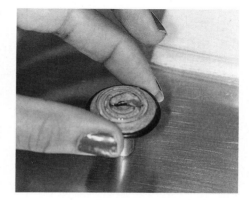

Figure 14 The specimen is turned over and placed horizontally on top of the OCT medium so that its deepest margin now faces upward.

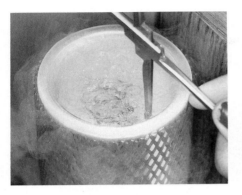

Figure 15 The specimen is frozen quickly in liquid nitrogen.

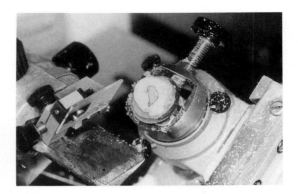

Figure 16 The chuck is mounted in the cryostat.

Parker scalpel handle, a spatula, or similar instrument. After the instrument is warmed over an alcohol flame, it is used to compress the semirigid specimen into a flat plane. The peripheral skin margin is elevated until it is in the same plane as the rest of the specimen. Once this has been accomplished, the entire specimen is covered with OCT medium and frozen in liquid nitrogen.

The chuck with the attached specimen is then placed in the cryostat for storage until all specimens have been mounted. The specimens are stored in consecutive order to maintain proper identification. The tissue is then sectioned (Fig. 16) at a thickness of 4–8 μm. The first sections processed represent the deepest and most lateral margins of that piece and are the most important. These sections are placed on a standard glass slide beginning at the end away from its frosted portion. Deeper sections into the block are actually closer to the epidermal surface and are placed on the slide in sequence progressing toward the frosted end of the slide. Once all sections have been positioned on the slide, it is dried on a slide warmer and stained with hematoxylin and eosin.

After staining, a coverslip is applied (Fig. 17) and each slide is carefully examined microscopically. Residual tumor can then be identified (Fig. 18) and its exact location determined, since precise orientation is revealed by the colors on the dyed margins. If residual tumor is identified,

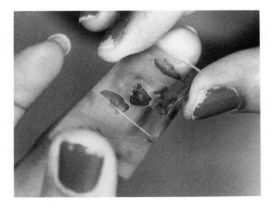

Figure 17 After the sections are stained, a coverslip is applied to the slide.

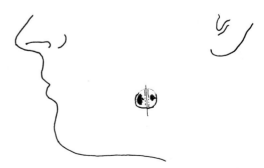

Figure 18 Residual tumor is identified microscopically and marked on the anatomic diagram.

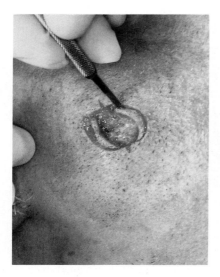

Figure 19   Residual tumor is removed in the next layer.

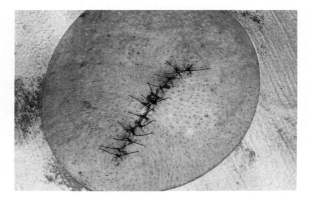

Figure 20   The defect is repaired in simple primary fashion.

the patient is returned to the operating room for removal of any areas with persistent tumor. Those areas positive for tumor are removed (Fig. 19) in a similar manner as in the first stage of the procedure. Each specimen encompasses the area of residual tumor and a small amount (1–2 mm) of surrounding clinically normal tissue. The mapping, marking, and processing of specimens from the second stage of the procedure are carried out exactly as in the initial stage.

If any areas still contain residual tumor, they are treated in a third stage. This process continues until there is no further evidence of tumor. Once a tumor-free plane has been reached, the final defect is measured and recorded. The resulting defect is evaluated to consider whether immediate repair (Fig. 20) should be undertaken or if the wound should be allowed to heal by second intention.

INDICATIONS

Mohs micrographic surgery has proven to be the most effective form of treatment for cutaneous neoplasms that spread by contiguous growth. These include basal cell carcinoma, squamous cell carcinoma, sebaceous carcinoma, verrucous carcinoma, keratoacanthoma, squamous cell carcinoma in situ, and dermatofibrosarcoma. In addition, it has also been used effectively in the management of other, less common, malignancies, including extramammary Paget's disease, atypical fibroxanthoma, malignant fibrous histiocytoma, eccrine adenocarcinoma, adenocystic carcinoma, leiomyosarcoma, granular cell tumor, angiosarcoma, apocrine adenocarcinoma, and melanoma. Although Mohs micrographic surgery is an extremely effective form of therapy, it is not necessary to utilize it for the treatment of all of these tumors. This is especially true in the management of melanoma, where significant controversy exists around the country as to the questionable benefits offered by this technique. However, Mohs micrographic surgery is considered the treatment of choice for recurrent epithelial cancers, cancers greater than 2 cm in size, and those found in known high-risk locations for recurrence. These include the midfacial triangle and ear and periauricular areas. Mohs micrographic surgery should also be considered for the treatment of clinically or histologically aggressive basal cell carcinomas, such as the metatypical and morpheaform subtypes.

CONTRAINDICATIONS

Mohs micrographic surgery is not indicated for patients who are considered poor surgical candidates. Several factors to be considered include poor general health and the presence of metastatic disease. Patients with an allergy to local anesthetic agents or who do not tolerate injected field blocks may require general anesthesia. Patients with bleeding disorders, hypertension, diabetes, and other cardiovascular conditions must be evaluated individually.

COMPLICATIONS

Fortunately, complications of Mohs micrographic surgery are infrequent. Patient anxiety is a common problem and may be due to uncertainty about the extent of the neoplasm and the potential for poor cosmetic results following complete removal of the tumor. Occasionally, as a consequence of this anxiety, a patient may hyperventilate and become syncopal. This is treated by placing the patient in reverse Trendelenburg position. On rare occasions, use of oxygen supplementation via nasal cannula or facial mask may be necessary.

Many patients are afraid of needles and fear that the administration of local anesthesia will be painful. Slow injections of anesthesia through a small bore needle and advancing the needle through previously anesthetized sites can minimize the discomfort in virtually all cases.

If anxiety is excessive, sedation may be administered orally. Diazepam, at doses of 5–10 mg, may be administered 1–2 hr preoperatively. If anxiety is not manifest until just prior to the surgical procedure, sublingual diazepam tablets in a similar dose can provide more rapid relief. On occasion, an intramuscular injection of hydroxyzine 25–50 mg can be used as a sedative in the elderly patient who might react adversely to the use of other agents.

An adverse or allergic reaction to lidocaine, the most commonly used local anesthetic agent, is rare. This agent does not cross-react with other anesthetics that are commonly responsible for allergic reactions. If allergic reactions or anaphylaxis should occur, the surgeon must be prepared for emergency medical care.

Epinephrine is frequently added to standard formulations of local anesthetic agents in a concentration of 1:100,000. In the elderly patient, or in a patient with labile hypertension, this concentration of epinephrine may be sufficient to elevate the blood pressure significantly. Since a much lower concentration of epinephrine can provide sufficient hemostasis, diluting the standard mixture with plain 1% lidocaine solution can provide a lower concentration for use that is safe and still effective. The standard concentration is 1:200,000, although, on occasion, a dilution of 1:400,000 is used with good results.

Hemorrhage is always a potential complication of skin surgery. While this risk is minimized by epinephrine in the local anesthetic, which acts as a vasoconstrictor, bleeding from small arterioles or capillary beds can still occur. The most common site for significant arterial damage is the temple in the area of the superficial temporal artery. If this artery is transected, suture ligation is usually required. Smaller bleeding points from the capillary plexus can be treated with electrocoagulation.

For tumors that are either deeply invasive or have recurred after previous therapy, injury to cutaneous sensory and motor nerves can be a complication of the Mohs surgery. Since the normal location of the common sensory and motor nerves of the face and extremities is well known, the Mohs surgeon should anticipate when injury to nerve structures is possible and inform the patient in advance of this potential complication. The surgeon can minimize the risk of inadvertent nerve injury by injecting additional local anesthetic or normal saline into the treatment site immediately prior to excision of the next layer. This causes the soft tissues to balloon out, providing a safe distance between the level of excision and the deeper vital nerve structure.

Tumors treated with Mohs micrographic surgery commonly occur in the midfacial triangle and periauricular areas. Mohs surgery is tissue-sparing, but if a significant amount of tissue must be removed in order to reach a tumor-free plane, there may be considerable anatomic disfigurement, including distortion of the eyelids, nose, lips, and ears.

One potential complication of Mohs surgery performed in the periorbital region is inadvertent injury to the eye. If the tumor is not present on the eyelid margin, the eyes can be protected by taping cotton gauze pads over the eyelids during the surgical procedure. This also blocks the bright operating room lights from the patient's eyes. However, if the tumor is present on the eyelid margin, a plastic methylmethacrylate eye shield can be placed directly on the cornea after topical anesthesia is applied.

Once the tumor has been completely removed, a decision is made as to whether the wound should be primarily repaired or if healing by second intention is preferable. This decision is based on the nature, location, and extent of the tumor. Most tumors that have recurred after previous therapy have a slightly lower chance of cure with the Mohs technique than do primary tumors (96% versus 99% cure). Because of this risk many Mohs surgeons recommend that defects from recurrent tumors be allowed to heal by second intention. This permits the surgeon to identify sites of subsequent recurrence earlier in the course of the disease.

A period of at least 3–6 weeks is required before complete second intention healing can be expected. The rate of healing is largely dependent on the physical condition of the patient and the size and depth of the wound. Anatomic location also accounts for variation in the time required for complete healing: extremities heal more slowly than the face. Diligent wound care by the patient consists of twice daily cleansing with hydrogen peroxide followed by application of an antibacterial ointment. Frequently, this is all that is required to ensure satisfactory healing.

Postoperative bleeding is only a rare complication when the Mohs defect is allowed to heal by second intention. If meticulous hemostasis is obtained at the completion of surgery, the risk of postoperative bleeding is minimal. When bleeding does occur, it is seen most commonly in the patient who does not keep the wound covered with an antibacterial ointment, resulting in desiccation, fissuring, and subsequent bleeding. Patients who show a tendency to bleed excessively during the procedure, or have deep invasive tumors in highly vascular areas, are instructed to apply firm pressure externally for 10 min should bleeding occur at home or work. The patient may apply a small quantity of oxidized cellulose cotton (Oxycel) at home to the wound if bleeding cannot be controlled by firm external pressure.

Pain is uncommon following surgery. In most situations, acetaminophen is sufficient analgesia for any postoperative discomfort. Oral narcotic analgesics may rarely be required in patients with a low pain threshold, large tumors, or tumors located on dependent areas of the body. Anatomic areas that are frequently moved or stretched, such as the lips, shoulders, and waist, may also be uncomfortable postoperatively.

The most common psychological concern following Mohs micrographic surgery is the effectiveness of the treatment and the final cosmetic result. If the defect is on a concave surface of the face and postoperative care is good, the final cosmetic result from second intention healing can be exceptional. Patients who have an ill-defined tumor or one that has recurred after prior therapy should have reconstruction delayed for a minimum of 1 year. If this is discussed prior to surgery, the patient usually accepts the temporary deformity that may result. While the primary concern must be eradication of the tumor, the cosmetic result is important also. Retraction of the eyelid or lip may occur when tumors are removed close to these free margins of tissue.

Repair may be considered immediately to prevent this complication. The poor results following second intention healing in these areas probably outweigh the risk of recurrent tumor.

Chondritis may result when the tumor is on the ear or nasal alae. If removal of all overlying soft tissue structures, including perichondrium, is required, chondritis may develop during healing by second intention. Chondritis may also result if electrocoagulation is used adjacent to cartilaginous structures. This complication can be minimized with a short course of oral antibiotics, such as erythromycin. The benefit of this medication relates more to its effect on lysosomes and decrease in inflammation than to its antibacterial properties.

When deeply infiltrating tumors of the nasal alae result in removal of the cartilaginous support for the nose, the ball-valve effect may occur with deep inspiration. The unsupported side of the ala retracts slightly, restricting air flow through the affected naris. Most patients' respiration functions adequately during the day but they may become short of breath when asleep. Reconstruction of the nasal ala would be recommended.

When Mohs surgical wounds are closed primarily, the same complications that may occur with any surgical excision may develop, including hematoma or seroma formation, bleeding, and secondary infection. These risks can be kept to a minimum with meticulous surgical technique, application of sterile compression dressings, and diligent postoperative care by the patient. Appropriate precautions should be taken in the patient with a known predisposition to bleeding or secondary infection.

Necrosis of a repaired wound is no more common following Mohs micrographic surgery than any other comparable soft tissue repair. Necrosis usually occurs when wounds are closed under tension. Necrosis of a poorly designed flap from vascular compromise or the shedding of a full-thickness or split-thickness graft is not more likely to occur following Mohs surgery than the repair of any other similar surgical defect.

SPECIAL CONSIDERATIONS

For exceedingly apprehensive individuals, patients with massive tumors, or tumors occurring in difficult anatomic areas, the use of general anesthesia may be indicated. No absolute criteria can be established for these situations, so these cases may be evaluated individually. General anesthesia may be required for several hours due to laboratory processing time, especially for larger tumors. The risks of prolonged general anesthesia must be considered in these cases.

Extensive tumor involvement may be anticipated by preoperative evaluation with computed axial tomography or other diagnostic aids. When an extensive procedure is likely, the comfort of the patient must be considered. In these circumstances, it may be advantageous to perform this technique using a team. Colleagues from otolaryngology, plastic surgery, oculoplastic surgery, and neurosurgery should be consulted freely. In these cases, the dissection may be done by the appropriate surgical specialist and margin control of the specimen performed by the Mohs surgeon. This approach allows the patient to be treated by the individual physician with the greatest expertise in a given area of specialization. It also serves to maximize the chance for a successful outcome. This team approach has proven especially useful in patients with large tumors of the eyelids, periorbital area, external auditory canal, and for dermatofibrosarcoma regardless of its anatomic location.

Described more than 40 years ago, the original Mohs technique began by topical application by a zinc chloride fixative. This fixative was applied to the surface of the tumor, resulting in localized tissue necrosis. Twenty-four hours after the application of this agent, layers of tissue could be removed and examined histologically for evidence of residual tumor. This technique was painful and slow. Consequently, it has been replaced by most Mohs surgeons with what is known as the fresh tissue technique. On occasion, the traditional fixed tissue technique may be used. The indications include tumors that are deeply invasive or involve highly vascular tissue. In these cases, the zinc chloride fixative permits bloodless removal of tissue layers with minimal risk of significant hemorrhage. In addition, when deep excision has occurred on the scalp with bone involvement, the outer table of bone can be removed with the fixed tissue technique without the need for bone chisels or other similar instruments. Some Mohs surgeons use the fixed technique when treating tumors that are capable of hematogenous spread, such as squamous cell carcinoma and malignant melanoma. The advantage of using the fixed tissue technique is that the vascular channels adjacent to the tumor will be sealed by the fixative, limiting the potential for dissemination of tumor cells as a consequence of incision through the tumor.

The carbon dioxide laser can be used in similar situations, because of its hemostatic properties when focused as a cutting instrument. As a consequence, carbon dioxide laser-assisted Mohs micrographic surgery is used frequently for patients taking anticoagulants or for those with tumors at risk for hematogenous spread. The laser permits treatment of these tumors without blood loss or significant risk of dissemination of tumor cells.

In hypertensive patients, special consideration must be given to the amount of epinephrine used in the local anesthetic. A concentration of epinephrine as low as 1:400,000 can provide effective vasoconstriction without elevating blood pressure significantly. If epinephrine cannot be used, the carbon dioxide laser can provide necessary hemostasis.

POSTOPERATIVE MANAGEMENT

Initially, Dr. Mohs allowed virtually all wounds to heal by second intention. Three to 6 weeks may be required for complete healing of the wound, depending on the size of the lesion and its location. Management of a wound that is healing by second intention is relatively simple. Patients leave the initial dressing in place for 24 hr. This dressing is then removed, and the base is cleansed with 3% hydrogen peroxide solution; a fine film of antibiotic ointment is applied, and the wound is covered with a nonadherent dressing. This procedure is repeated twice daily. The hydrogen peroxide acts as an excellent debriding agent and helps remove necrotic material. A topical antibiotic ointment is used since moist, petrolatum-coated wounds heals more quickly than wounds that have been allowed to dry. The antibiotic used in the ointment may decrease surface bacteria, but this function probably is less important that the occlusive properties of petrolatum.

Second intention healing is chosen for recurrent tumors, large wounds for which primary closure or closure with grafts and flaps would be exceedingly difficult, and for lesions on concave surfaces of the face. Wounds on concave surfaces heal with more satisfactory cosmetic results than those on convex surfaces. Second intention wounds appear slightly red and edematous after complete reepithelialization. This improves with time, and sites often attain fairly normal texture, sensation, and color 6 months after surgery. If healing by second intention does not yield acceptable results, consideration can be given to reconstructive surgery.

Immediate repair of defects following Mohs surgery is performed most frequently when a primary tumor has been treated. Closure is especially useful when the defect is on a convex surface or in the periorbital or perioral area. Primary closure is most common, but local skin flaps or skin grafts can be created when necessary.

BIBLIOGRAPHY

Anderson RL, Ceilley RI. A multispecialty approach to the excision and reconstruction of eyelid tumors. *Ophthalmology* 1978;85:1150–1163.

Bailin PL, Ratz JL, Lutz-Nagey L. CO_2 laser modification of Mohs' surgery. *J Dermatol Surg Oncol* 1981; 7:621–623.

Baker SR, Swanson NA. Management of nasal cutaneous malignant neoplasms. An interdisciplinary approach. *Arch Otolaryngol* 1983;109:473–479.

Braun M. The case for MOHS surgery by the fixed-tissue technique. *J Dermatol Surg Oncol* 1981; 7:634–640.

Bumsted RM, Ceilley RI, Panje WR, Crumley RL. Auricular malignant neoplasms. When is chemotherapy (MOHS technique) necessary? *Arch Otolaryngol* 1981;107:721–724.

Bumsted RM, Ceilley RI. Auricular malignant neoplasms. Identification of high-risk lesions and selection of method of reconstruction. *Arch Otolaryngol* 1982;108:225–231.

Casson PR, Baker DC. Reconstruction of defects following MOHS surgery. *J Dermatol Surg Oncol* 1981; 7:811–817.

Cottel WI, Bailin PL, Albom MJ, et al. Essentials of Mohs micrographic surgery. *J Dermatol Surg Oncol* 1988;14:11–13.

Dzubow LM. False-negative tumor-free margins following Mohs surgery. *J Dermatol Surg Oncol* 1988; 14:600–602.

Goldberg DJ, Kim YA. Angiosarcoma of the scalp treated with Mohs micrographic surgery. *J Dermatol Surg Oncol* 1993;19:156–158.

Grabski WJ, Salasche SJ, McCollough ML, et al. Interpretation of Mohs micrographic frozen sections: A peer review comparison study. *J Am Acad Dermatol* 1989;20:670–674.

Hanke CW, Lee MW. Cryostat use and tissue processing in Mohs micrographic surgery. *J Dermatol Surg Oncol* 1989;15:29–32.

Harris DWS, Kist DA, Bloom K, Zachary CB. Rapid staining with carcinoembryonic antigen aids limited excision of extramammary Paget's disease treated by Mohs surgery. *J Dermatol Surg Oncol* 1994; 20: 260–264.

Hobbs ER, Wheeland RG, Bailin PL, et al. Treatment of dermatofibrosarcoma protuberans with Mohs micrographic surgery. *Ann Surg* 1988;207:102–107.

Hruza GJ, Snow SN. Basal cell carcinoma in a patient with acquired immunodeficiency syndrome: Treatment with Mohs micrographic surgery fixed-tissue technique. *J Dermatol Surg Oncol* 1989;15:545–551.

Kirsner RS, Garland LD. Squamous cell carcinoma arising from chronic osteomyelitis treated by Mohs micrographic surgery. *J Dermatol Surg Oncol* 1994;20:141–143.

Lang PG. Mohs micrographic surgery: Fresh tissue technique. *Dermatol Clin* 1989;7:613–626.

Levine HL, Bailin PL. Basal cell carcinoma of the head and neck: Identification of the high-risk patient. *Laryngoscope* 1980;90:955–961.

Miller LJ, Argeny ZB, Whitaker DC. The preparation of frozen sections for micrographic surgery: A review of current methodology. *J Dermatol Surg Oncol* 1993;19:1023–1029.

Mohs FE. Chemosurgery: Microscopically controlled methods of cancer excision. *Arch Surg* 1941; 42: 279–295.

Mohs FE. Mohs micrographic surgery: A historical perspective. *Dermatol Clin* 1989;7:609–611.

Mohs FE, Zitelli JA, Larson P, Snow S. Mohs micrographic surgery for melanoma. *Dermatol Clin* 1989; 7:833–843.

Mora RG, Robins P. Basal cell carcinomas in the center of the face: Special diagnostic, prognostic, and therapeutic considerations. *J Dermatol Surg Oncol* 1978;4:315–321.

Peters CR, Dinner MI, Dolsky RL, Bailin PL, Hardy RW Jr. The combined multidisciplinary approach to invasive basal cell tumors of the scalp. *Ann Plast Surg* 1980;4:199–204.

Rapini RP. Pitfalls of Mohs micrographic surgery. *J Am Acad Dermatol* 1990;22:681–686.

Robins P, Pollack SV, Robinson JK. Immediate repair of wounds following operations by Mohs fresh-tissue technique. *J Dermatol Surg Oncol* 1979;5:329–336.

Roenigk RK, Ratz JL, Bailin PL, Wheeland RG. Trends in the presentation and treatment of basal cell carcinomas. *J Dermatol Surg Oncol* 1986;12:860–865.

Rustad OJ, Kaye V, Cerio R, Zachary CB. Postfixation of cryostat sections improves tumor definition in Mohs surgery. *J Dermatol Surg Oncol* 1989;15:1262–1267.

Sato K, Kennard CD. Phase contrast microscopy for identifying epidermal margins in unstained cryosections for Mohs micrographic surgery. *J Dermatol Surg Oncol* 1993;19:869–874.

Stanley RB Jr, Burres SA, Jacobs JR, Mathog RH. Hazards encountered in management of basal cell carcinomas of the mid-face. *Laryngoscope* 1984;94:378–385.

Swanson NA. MOHS surgery. Technique, indications, applications, and the future. *Arch Dermatol* 1983; 119:761–773.

Tromovitch TA, Stegman SJ. Microscopic-controlled excision of cutaneous tumors: Chemosurgery, fresh-tissue technique. *Cancer* 1978;41:653–658.

43

Cure Rates for Cancer of the Skin: Basal Cell Carcinoma, Squamous Cell Carcinoma, Melanoma, and Soft Tissue Sarcoma

Clark C. Otley and Katherine K. Lim
Mayo Clinic/Foundation, Rochester, Minnesota

Randall K. Roenigk
Mayo Clinic/Foundation and Mayo Medical School,
Rochester, Minnesota

GENERAL CONSIDERATIONS

The goal of this chapter is to present an overview of the cure rates for local, regional, and distant metastatic involvement with malignant cutaneous neoplasms. Because the neoplasms discussed range from locally invasive basal cell carcinomas to highly lethal soft tissue sarcomas, discussion will focus on either recurrence rates or survival rates as indicated by the biologic tendencies of specific neoplasms. The quality of the literature with regard to consistency and depth is less than optimal in many areas, and attempts will be made to highlight controversial points. Finally, it is important to realize that the majority of therapies have not been subjected to head-to-head comparison, and the inevitable selection bias between study populations has a major impact on the cure rates cited. Therefore, direct comparisons of cure rates for different modalities should be viewed in the context of these inherent biases.

BASAL CELL CARCINOMA

Basal cell carcinoma (BCC) is the most common malignant cutaneous neoplasm in the United States. BCC is a low-grade epithelial neoplasm, which grows in a contiguous manner with rare metastasis, making local control the primary therapeutic objective. Because of the locally invasive nature of BCC, cure rates are generally presented in terms of absence of local recurrence, rather than survival. Because BCC can recur 5 yr or longer after treatment, the cure rates cited in this chapter are derived from those studies with follow-up of 5 yr or greater. Cure rates will also be analyzed according to a variety of clinical and histologic variables, including location, size, histologic subtype, and patient characteristics. Discussion will focus on cure rates for primary BCC, with additional discussion of recurrent BCC.

Cure Rates: Summary for Primary Basal Cell Carcinoma

Rowe et al. systematically reviewed the literature between 1947 and 1987 regarding recurrence rates after treatment of BCC. Recurrence rates based on studies with 5-yr follow-up were generally 2–3.5 times higher than in studies with less than 5-yr follow-up, emphasizing the inadequacy of studies with less than 5-yr follow-up. In fact, 18% of recurrences occurred between the fifth and tenth year after treatment. The authors conclude that recurrence rates should be standardized using 5-yr life-table analysis as outlined by Cutler, which compensates for patients lost to follow-up.

Overall, 5-yr recurrence rates divided by treatment modality as presented in Figure 1 are as follows: Mohs micrographic surgery, 1.0%; surgical excision, 10.1%; curettage and electrodesiccation, 7.7%; radiation therapy, 8.7%; and cryosurgery, 7.5%. Clearly the highest cure rate is obtained by Mohs micrographic surgery, which relies on immediate and complete histologic confirmation of tumor-free margins. However, for well-defined tumors with favorable histology in low-risk areas, the cost:benefit ratio may favor other modalities when applied to a large population.

Cure Rates: Summary for Recurrent Basal Cell Carcinoma

Recurrent tumors are often embedded in a cicatricial stroma and have prolonged opportunity to infiltrate into deeper levels of dermis and subcutaneous tissue. It is intuitively obvious that recurrent tumors would be associated with higher rates of recurrence regardless of retreatment modality, a notion supported by the literature. Recurrent BCC treated with non-Mohs modali-

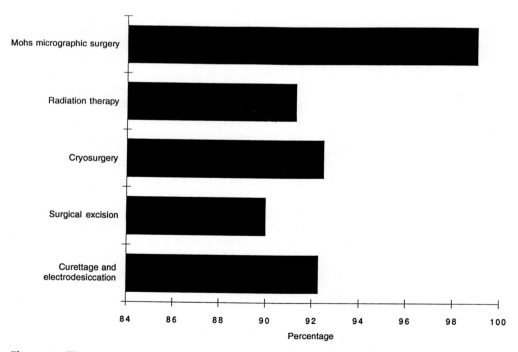

Figure 1 Five-year cure rates for primary basal cell carcinoma by treatment modality. (Modified from Rowe et al. Long-term recurrence rates in previously untreated (primary) basal cell carcinoma: implications for patient follow-up. *J Dermatol Surg Oncol* 1989; 15:315–328.)

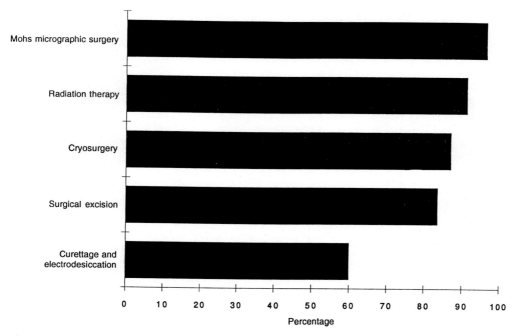

Figure 2   Five-year cure rates for recurrent basal cell carcinoma. (Modified from Rowe et al. Mohs surgery is the treatment of choice for recurrent (previously treated) basal cell carcinoma. *J Dermatol Surg Oncol* 1989;15:424–431.)

ties is associated with an average 19.9% 5-yr recurrence rate, while the precision offered by Mohs micrographic surgery reduces this rate to 5.6%. By modality, 5-yr recurrence rates for recurrent BCC are 17.4% for surgical excision, 40.0% for curettage and electrodesiccation, 13% for cryotherapy, and 9.8% for radiation therapy, as demonstrated in Figure 2. Given the high rates of local recurrence when non-Mohs modalities are applied to recurrent BCCs, caution should be used when considering such therapy.

Cure Rates for Primary Basal Cell Carcinoma by Treatment Modality

Curettage and Electrodesiccation

Curettage and electrodesiccation (C & E) is a simple, rapid method for the eradication of primary BCC, which results in acceptable cosmesis and avoids the need for sutures. Silverman et al. reviewed 2314 primary BCCs treated by C &E between 1955 and 1982 at the Skin and Cancer Unit of New York University Medical Center. The overall 5-yr recurrence rate for low-risk sites (neck, trunk, extremities) was 3.3% as determined by the life-table method, which is lower than the recurrence rate reported by Rowe et al. Silverman et al. analyzed recurrences by anatomic site and found that low-risk areas (neck, trunk, extremities) were associated with an 8.6% recurrence rate, while middle-risk (scalp, forehead, malar, and pre- and postauricular) and high-risk (nose, paranasal, nasolabial groove, ear, chin, mandibular, perioral, and periocular) areas had recurrence rates of 12.9 and 17.5%, respectively. Figure 3 graphically displays recurrence rates for BCCs treated with C & E in low-, middle-, and high-risk anatomic sites.

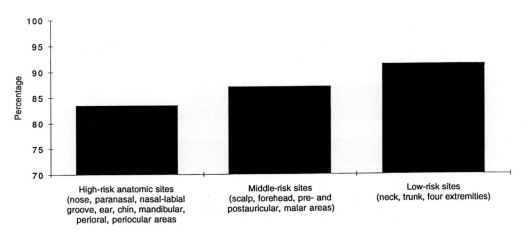

Figure 3 Five-year cure rates for primary basal cell carcinomas treated with curettage and electrodesiccation according to anatomic location. (Modified from Silverman et al. Recurrence rates of treated basal cell carcinomas. Part 2: Curettage-electrodesiccation. *J Dermatol Surg Oncol* 1991;17:720–726.)

Anatomic location and size of the primary BCC were key determinants of recurrence with electrodesiccation and curettage, whereas gender, age, and duration of the BCC prior to treatment had no effect on recurrence rate. Differences in recurrence rates according to size of the BCC were most evident at middle- and high-risk sites, as noted in Figure 4. Recurrence rates for BCCs of greater than 10 mm in middle-risk sites have an unacceptably high 5-yr rate of recurrence of 22.7%, while BCCs of greater than 6 mm in high-risk sites have a poor 5-yr recurrence rate of 17.6%. Therefore, electrodesiccation and curettage remains an excellent modality for BCCs of any size in low-risk areas but is not recommended for treatment of BCCs greater than 6 mm on high-risk sites or BCCs greater than 10 mm on middle-risk sites.

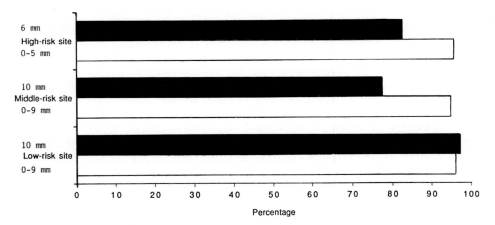

Figure 4 Five-year cure rates of primary basal cell carcinomas treated with curettage and electrodesiccation according to size. (Modified from Silverman et al. Recurrence rates of treated basal cell carcinomas. Part 2: Curettage-electrodesiccation. *J Dermatol Surg Oncol* 1991;17:720–726.)

Surgical Excision

Surgical excision is associated with a 10.1% 5-yr recurrence rate according to Rowe et al. This relatively high rate may be partially explained by a bias toward referral of more complicated tumors for excision as opposed to other, non-Mohs modalities. In a review of 588 primary BCCs treated with surgical excision between 1955 and 1982 at New York University, the cumulative 5-yr recurrence rate was 4.8%. Independent, statistically significant risk factors for recurrence included male gender and location on the head, whereas age, size, and duration of the BCC prior to treatment were not predictive of recurrence. As shown in Figure 5a, the 5-yr recurrence rate for BCC on the head was 6.6% in contrast to 0.7% at all other sites. Men had a 6.6% recurrence rate as opposed to a 3.1% rate for women. The same sites categorized as low-risk (neck, trunk, extremities) in Silverman's study of C & E were low-risk for surgical excision. However, the middle- and high-risk sites noted in Silverman's study of C & E were indistinguishable when analyzed for excision. Although size was not statistically predictive of recurrence for BCCs as a group, when only BCCs on the head were analyzed, recurrence rate increased with diameter (Fig. 5b). Because BCCs of less than 6 mm diameter have a 3.2% recurrence rate, while larger tumors have greater than 8% recurrence rate, surgical excision without margin control is most effective for small BCCs on the head.

With regard to the impact of surgical margins on recurrence rates for basal cell carcinomas, Wolf and Zitelli's study demonstrated an inverse correlation between width of margins and rate of recurrence with BCC. The margins necessary for the eradication of 117 BCCs were determined by obtaining serial 2-mm margins beginning at the clinically apparent border until eradication of all tumor was confirmed by frozen histology via Mohs micrographic surgery. A surgical margin of 4 mm resulted in the eradication of 98% of tumors less than 2 cm, whereas margins of 3 mm and 2 mm resulted in eradication of only 85 and 75% of tumors, respectively.

Curettage and Excision

Preoperative curettage of basal cell carcinomas may enhance delineation of tumor margins and was associated with a 2.4% recurrence rate with mean follow-up of 3.1 yr in a study by Johnson et al. The results of this study are comparable to those cited by Rowe et al. The authors conclude that preexcision curettage may be beneficial in the treatment of BCCs with indistinct clinical borders.

Cryosurgery

The 7.5% recurrence rate for cryotherapy of BCCs cited above was based on a retrospective study of 164 eyelid tumors by Fraunfelder et al. This study, with 5-yr follow-up, demonstrated that nodular and infiltrative BCCs less than 10 mm had cure rates of 97 and 94%, respectively. Nodular and infiltrative BCCs greater than 10 mm had cure rates of 85 and 82%, respectively, while recurrent BCCs had a 93% cure rate. The largest experience in the treatment of BCCs with cryotherapy is presented in a study of 3450 skin cancers, the majority of which were BCCs, by Kuflik and Gage. Primary BCCs treated between 1980 and 1984 were associated with a 99% 5-yr cure rate, while those treated between 1971 and 1989 had a 98.4% overall 5-yr cure rate. Cryosurgery is an effective therapeutic modality for the management of BCCs in a variety of clinical settings, but does not permit histologic verification of tumor eradication. Data regarding the relative risk of recurrence over 5-yr follow-up with BCCs in high-risk areas other than the eyelid are scant.

Radiation Therapy

Radiation therapy is an effective modality for managing BCCs with a unique set of advantages and disadvantages. Silverman et al. reported a 5-yr recurrence rate of 7.4% for 862 primary

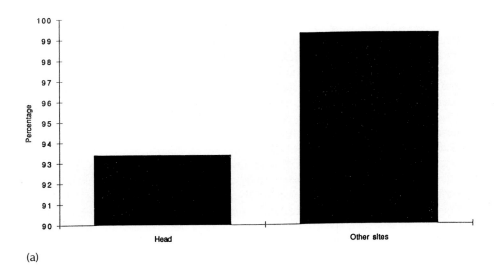

(a)

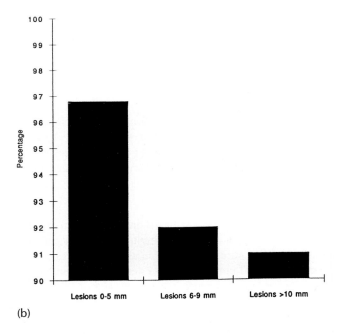

(b)

Figure 5 (a) Five-year cure rates for primary basal cell carcinomas treated with surgical excision according to anatomic site. (b) Five-year cure rates for primary basal cell carcinomas on the head treated with surgical excision according to diameter of the lesion. (Modified from Silverman et al. Recurrence rates of treated basal cell carcinomas. Part 3: Surgical excision.

BCCs treated with radiation between 1955 and 1982. Increased diameter of tumor correlated with increased recurrence, with 4.4% of BCCs 9 mm or less on the head recurring over 5 yr in contrast to 9.5% of tumors 10 mm or greater. Other variables, such as age, gender, anatomic location, duration of treatment, and duration of BCC prior to treatment, did not significantly affect recurrence rates. Cosmetic outcome was felt to diminish with time, and the authors concluded that radiation therapy is an effective modality if cosmesis is not a primary consideration. A recent long-term study by Childers et al. found a similar 96% local control rate with good to excellent cosmetic outcome. The adverse effect of tumor size on recurrence rates was demonstrated with 61 recurrent BCCs by Wilder, who found 5-yr remission rates of 96% for tumors 0.5–1.0 cm but 81% for tumors greater than 1.0 cm.

Mohs Micrographic Surgery

Because it offers the ability to confirm complete tumor-free margins prior to reconstruction or healing by second intention, Mohs micrographic surgery is associated with superior cure rates in the management of BCC. Impressive cure rates of approximately 99% as reported by Rowe et al. and Miller et al. can be achieved with the additional advantage of significant tissue conservation. Although a comparison of published studies by Lawrence revealed comparable 98.3 and 98% cure rates for Mohs micrographic surgery and surgical excision, respectively, this recurrence rate for surgical excision is significantly below the 10.1% recurrence rate cited by Rowe et al. and the 4.8% recurrence rate found in the New York University study. Furthermore, when data was analyzed for recurrent BCCs, Mohs micrographic surgery was associated with a superior 3.5% recurrence rate compared with 13% for excision. Based on significant experience and supported by extensive data, Mohs micrographic surgery is associated with the highest cure rates of any modality for the treatment of BCCs. It is the treatment of choice for many recurrent or large BCCs as well as those arising in high-risk sites, with ill-defined margins, or with aggressive histologic subtype.

As with any treatment modality, tumors with unfavorable characteristics, such as large size and recurrence, are associated with increased rates of recurrence even with Mohs micrographic surgery, albeit at lower rates than with other modalities. Recurrent and primary BCCs smaller than 1 cm have a cure rate of 99.6% with Mohs micrographic surgery in contrast to a 92.2% cure rate for tumors greater than 5 cm. Similarly, primary BCCs have been associated with a 98.2% cure rate compared with a 96.6% cure rate with recurrent BCCs. Younger patients, who may have more aggressive BCCs, have slightly higher recurrence rates than older patients. Treatment failures with Mohs micrographic surgery, which theoretically should have a 100% cure rate, have been traced to technical or interpretive difficulties or rare instances of discontiguous growth in studies by Hruza et al. and Madsen et al.

Cure Rates: Anatomic Location

An analysis by Roenigk et al. utilized odds ratios to demonstrate the increased risk of recurrence of BCC at certain anatomic units, such as the nose, ears, and periorbital region. Odd ratios of greater than 1.00 connote higher risk of recurrence for a particular site, and values less than 1.00 indicate a lower risk. Table 1 reveals that BCCs of the nose are associated with a high risk of 2.38, while other sites such as the ears (1.43), periorbital region (1.17), and remaining face (1.04) have slight to moderate increased risk.

Managed by non-Mohs techniques, nasal BCCs have a 24% recurrence rate, compared with recurrence rates of 0.9–2.6% for a combination of primary and recurrent BCCs treated with Mohs micrographic surgery in studies by Robins et al. and Mohs. Recurrence rates for primary BCCs of the periorbital area, inner canthus, retroauricular area, and scalp managed by Mohs micrographic surgery were 1.9, 4.7, 14, and 1.3%, respectively, in the study by Robins et al. Re-

Table 1   Odds Ratio (Risk of Recurrence)

Location	Odds ratio
Lips	0.96
Eyes	1.17
Ears	1.43
Nose	2.38
Other/Face	1.04
Neck/Scalp	0.55
Trunk	0.22

Source: Modified from Roenigk RK, Ratz JL, Bailin PL, Wheeland RG. Trends in the presentation and treatment of basal cell carcinomas. *J Dermatol Surg Oncol* 1986; 12(8):860–865.

current BCCs of the periorbital area and inner canthus managed by Mohs micrographic surgery have 6.4 and 9.5% recurrence rates, respectively. Because of a higher propensity for perichondral spread, BCCs and squamous cell carcinomas of the ear have a 6.8% recurrence rate in the study by Robins et al.

Cure Rates: Histologic Subtype

BCCs with histologic evidence of infiltration, sclerosis, or multifocality are associated with increased rates of recurrence, estimated at 12–30%. In a histopathologic study of 156 BCCs by Sloane, infiltrative and multifocal types had recurrence rates of 20–30% as compared to 6–12% for nodular BCCs with or without infiltrative marginal features. A review of 51 recurrent BCCs by Lang and Maize revealed that 65% were characterized by poor palisading and a micronodular or infiltrative growth pattern. A multivariate analysis of prognostic histologic features for recurrent BCCs revealed that infiltrative, multicentric, or morpheaform growth patterns within 0.38 mm of the surgical margin were predictive of 82% probability of recurrence. Salasche et al. found that morpheaform BCCs had, on average, 7.2 mm of subclinical extension beyond clinical borders. Roenigk et al. found statistically significant odds ratios for recurrence with multicentric and morpheaform BCCs of 5.80 and 3.62, respectively. The effect of histologic subtypes on recurrence rates makes pretherapy biopsy and knowledge of the prognostic significance of histologic features essential. BCCs evidencing aggressive histologic subtypes may best be managed with Mohs micrographic surgery.

Cure Rates for Alternative Therapeutic Modalities

A variety of nonsurgical, innovative modalities have been utilized in the treatment of BCCs. Brenner et al. demonstrated that twice-daily 0.05% tretinoin was ineffective in treating arsenic-induced BCCs. Treatment of BCC with isotretinoin and etretinate results in complete and partial remission rates of less than 20 and 70%, respectively, far inferior to conventional therapies. In a study of 12 patients with multiple BCCs, including patients with nevoid basal cell carcinoma syndrome, Peck et al. showed that isotretinoin in a mean dose of 3.1 mg/kg/day resulted in only 8% complete clinical and histologic remission after a mean of 8 months. However, low-dose isotretinoin (0.25–1.5 mg/kg/day) has demonstrated a chemopreventive effect in three patients for 3–8 yrs.

   In a large trial by Cornell et al. of intralesional interferon alpha-2b (1.5 million IU three times weekly for 3 weeks) versus placebo in the treatment of 172 patients with noduloulcerative or superficial BCCs, 86% of interferon-treated BCCs and 29% of placebo-treated BCCs were histologically negative after 16–20 weeks. Due to the high cost and need for repeated administration of interferon, the indications for intralesional interferon are as yet unclear.

Photodynamic therapy is a promising new modality for the treatment of BCCs, but it has been associated with high recurrence rates in the literature. Wilson et al. treated 37 patients with 151 tumors with intravenous Photofrin II^R and visible light with complete response in 88% of lesions but with an 18% recurrence rate. Retreatment of the recurrent BCCs resulted in 100% complete response, but with an eventual 26% recurrence rate. Treatment of superficial BCCs with topical PDT with 5-aminolevulinic acid resulted in a 50% complete response rate. Another investigative modality, intralesional 5-fluorouracil implants, have been associated with 25–50% cure rates depending on the dosage.

Locally advanced BCCs unsuitable for salvage therapy with either surgery or radiation therapy have been treated with cisplatin-based chemotherapy, with a durable (>5 yr) complete response rate of 14% according to a study by Guthrie et al. Neoadjuvant, cisplatin-based chemotherapy has also been utilized with 12% complete and 62% partial response rates to shrink locally advanced BCCs in order to make definitive surgical resection or radiation therapy technically feasible. Systemic chemotherapy is best viewed as primarily a palliative modality in the management of advanced BCC.

Survival Rates for Metastatic Basal Cell Carcinoma

Although very uncommon, metastasis from large, neglected, or highly aggressive BCC does occur. As reviewed by von Domarus and Stevens, 50% of patients with metastatic BCC are deceased within 8 months after metastasis. Patients with isolated lymph node metastases survive for an average of 3.6 years, whereas prognosis after distant, visceral metastasis is extremely poor. Once distant spread occurs, response to chemotherapy with methotrexate, 5-fluorouracil, bleomycin, and cisplatin is marginal and survival rarely exceeds 1.5 yr.

SQUAMOUS CELL CARCINOMA

Squamous cell carcinoma (SCC) is the second most common skin cancer in the United States. The majority of SCCs are small, low-risk tumors associated with high cure rates with standard treatment modalities. Unlike basal cell carcinoma, SCC is associated with a measurable risk of nodal and disseminated metastasis and even death. Therefore discussion will include not only cure rates for local SCC, but also for regional and distant metastasis. Factors significant in the selection of treatment modality include tumor size, location, and histologic differentiation as well as patient characteristics.

Local Cure Rates for Cutaneous Squamous Cell Carcinoma

Local Cure Rates for Conventional Modalities

Conventional modalities for the treatment of primary cutaneous SCC include surgical excision, radiation therapy, curettage and electrodesiccation, cryosurgery, and Mohs micrographic surgery. In a systematic review of the literature between 1947 and 1987 on recurrence rates for SCC of the lip, ear, and skin, Rowe et al. found that Mohs micrographic surgery provided the highest cure rates for primary tumors in all locations. As shown in Figure 6, management of SCC of skin other than lip or ear by Mohs micrographic surgery affords a 5-yr local cure rate of 96.9% versus 92.1% for non-Mohs modalities. Similarly, primary SCC of the lip and ear had higher local cure rates with Mohs micrographic surgery than non-Mohs modalities as seen in Figures 7 and 8. With regard to local cure rates of specific non-Mohs modalities, Rowe et al. cite 5-yr

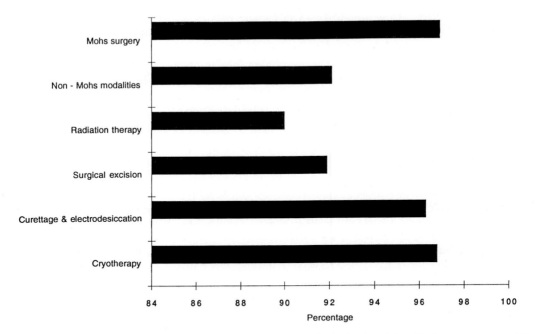

Figure 6 Five-year local cure rates for primary squamous cell carcinoma of the skin by treatment modality. (Modified from Rowe et al. Prognostic factors for local recurrence, metastasis, and survival rates in squamous cell carcinoma of the skin, ear, and lip. *J Am Acad Dermatol* 1992;26:976–990.)

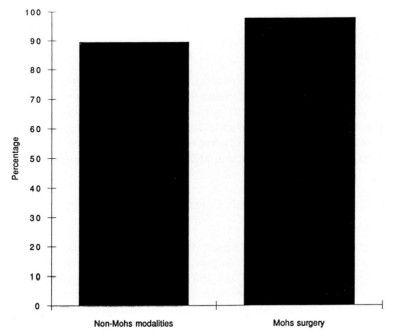

Figure 7 Five-year local cure rates for primary squamous cell carcinoma of the lip according to treatment modality. (Modified from Rowe et al. Prognostic factors for local recurrence, metastasis, and survival rates in squamous cell carcinoma of the skin, ear, and lip. *J Am Acad Dermatol* 1992;26:976–990.)

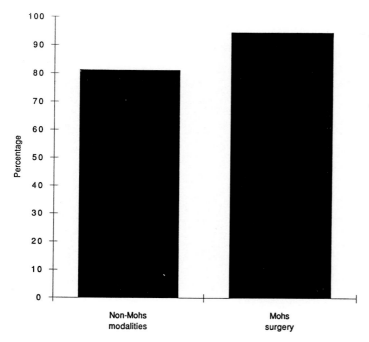

Figure 8 Five-year local cure rate for primary squamous cell carcinoma of the ear by treatment modality. (Modified from Rowe et al. Prognostic factors for local recurrence, metastasis, and survival rates in squamous cell carcinoma of the skin, ear, and lip. *J Am Acad Dermatol* 1992;26:976–990.)

cure rates of 90.0, 91.9, 96.3, and 96.8% for primary SCC treated with radiation therapy, surgical excision, C & E, and cryosurgery, respectively (Fig. 6). It is important to note, however, that the majority of tumors treated by C & E and cryosurgery were smaller than 1 cm and that the follow-up for cryosurgery was less than 5 yr. A study of cryosurgery of SCC less than 2 cm by Kuflik et al. reported a 5-yr local cure rate of 96.1%. As noted in the introduction, the presence of selection bias between studies of different treatment modalities is inevitable, rendering direct comparison of cure rates imprecise. In general, high-risk tumors are more frequently managed by Mohs micrographic surgery than by non-Mohs modalities, resulting in lower cure rates for Mohs micrographic surgery than might occur with a random selection of tumors.

Recurrent SCC is associated with an increased risk of recurrence and metastasis regardless of treatment modality. As with primary SCC, Mohs micrographic surgery is associated with superior 5-yr local cure rates of 90–93.3% in studies by Rowe et al. and Dzubow et al. as shown in Figure 9. Recurrence rates were higher with tumors on the lower extremities, in male patients younger than 60 years of age, and in male patients requiring five or more Mohs stages. A study of Mohs micrographic surgery for recurrent SCC by Hruza with 4-yr follow-up had a 98.6% local cure rate. Surgical excision was associated with recurrence rates of 23.3% for recurrent SCC in the study by Rowe et al.

Clinical Predictors of Local Recurrence and Metastasis

Because SCC has a definite potential for metastasis and death, factors predictive of increased risk of dissemination have been extensively investigated. Clinical features predictive of increased metastatic risk include size greater than 2 cm, history of recurrence, high-risk location (ear, lip), rapid growth, association with a preexisting scarring process (burn, ulcer, scar), and immunosuppression of the patient. Figure 10 presents the prognostic significance of various factors in

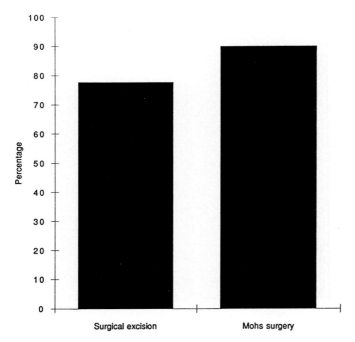

Figure 9 Five-year local cure rates for locally recurrent squamous cell carcinoma of the skin. (Modified from Rowe et al. Prognostic factors for local recurrence, metastasis, and survival rates in squamous cell carcinoma of the skin, ear, and lip. *J Am Acad Dermatol* 1992;26:976–990.)

local recurrence and metastasis of SCC based on more than 30 studies summarized by Rowe et al. For SCCs greater than 2 cm, the local recurrence rates are more than double and metastatic rates triple those of SCCs less than 2 cm. A study by Breuninger et al. found rates of metastasis of 1.4, 9.2, and 14.3% for 500 primary cutaneous SCCs of less than 2 cm, 2–5 cm, and greater than 5 cm, respectively. Five-year local cure rates after Mohs micrographic surgery are 98.1% for tumors less than 2 cm versus 74.8% for SCCs greater than 2 cm.

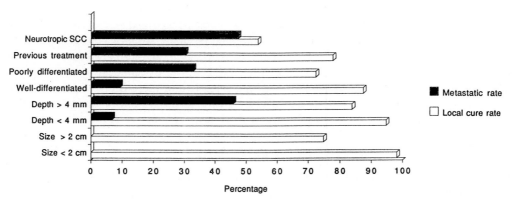

Figure 10 Local cure rates and metastatic rates associated with prognostic variables. (Modified from Rowe et al. Prognostic factors for local recurrence, metastasis, and survival rates in squamous cell carcinoma of the skin, ear, and lip. *J Am Acad Dermatol* 1992;26:976–990.)

As mentioned before, recurrent SCCs have high local recurrence rates of 23.3% and metastatic rates of 30.3% with excision and a 10% local recurrence rate with Mohs micrographic surgery according to Rowe et al. Recurrent SCCs of the lip and ear are associated with high metastatic rates of 31.5 and 45%, respectively, according to Salasche et al. SCCs arising in association with a chronic ulcer or sinus tract have an 18–30% metastatic rate, while those arising in radiation dermatitis or scar have 20–26 and 26.2–37.9% metastatic rates, respectively. A report of SCCs in immunosuppressed patients noted a 12.9% metastatic rate.

SCCs in particular anatomic locations, especially ear and lip, have an increased risk of recurrence and distant metastasis. According to Rowe et al., SCC of the lip has local recurrence and metastatic rates of 10.5 and 13.7%, respectively, compared to 7.9 and 5.2%, respectively, for tumors at other sites. The relatively high recurrence rates may be related to horizontal spread of SCC on the mucosa not adequately treated by wedge excision, as suggested by Mehregan and Roenigk. SCC of the ear has more than double the rate of local recurrence and metastasis at 18.7 and 11%, respectively, compared with other sites. Mohs et al. reported a 5-yr local cure rate of 92.3% for SCC of the ear managed by Mohs micrographic surgery. Experience at the Mayo Clinic as studied by Daoud et al. revealed a 3.75% recurrence rate with a mean follow-up of 41 months for auricular SCCs in 74 patients.

Mohs and Zitelli reported a 5-yr local cure rate of 98.8% for SCC of the scalp treated by Mohs micrographic surgery. However, because of unpredictable peripheral tumor extension with SCC on the scalp, modalities lacking histologic confirmation of tumor-free margins suffer from inferior cure rates, with a 66% 5-yr local cure rate for radiation therapy. In a review of SCC of the trunk and limbs, Joseph et al. reported a 4.9% metastatic rate, 3.4% overall mortality rate, and a 70.6% mortality rate among patients with metastatic disease. Risk factors associated with metastasis include delayed presentation, large neglected tumors, misdiagnosis, and recurrence.

Histologic Predictors of Local Recurrence and Metastasis

Histologic features correlating with worse prognosis include depth greater than 4 mm, poor histologic differentiation, and neurotropism. Several studies have suggested that the risk of recurrence and metastasis increases with invasion of SCC into or through the reticular dermis (Clark level IV/V). Rowe et al. found that SCCs less than 4 mm in depth have rates of local recurrence and metastasis of 5.3 and 6.7%, respectively, whereas tumors 4 mm or greater carry rates of 17.2 and 45.7%, respectively. Seemingly more reasonable estimates were derived from a study by Breuninger in which 0, 4.5, and 15% rates of metastasis were found with SCCs less than 2, 2–6, and greater than 6 mm in depth.

Poorly differentiated (Broders grades 3 and 4) SCCs are twice as likely to recur locally (28.6% vs. 13.6%) and three times more likely to metastasize (32.8% vs. 9.2%) than well-differentiated SCCs according to Rowe et al. Mohs micrographic surgery offers significant advantages when managing both well- and poorly differentiated SCC. Well-differentiated SCCs treated with non-Mohs modalities or Mohs micrographic surgery have local cure rates of 81.0 and 97.0%, respectively, while poorly differentiated SCCs have local cure rates of 46.4 and 67.4%, respectively.

The presence of tumor within the perineural space, known as neurotropism, has been associated with poor prognosis in several studies. SCCs with histologic evidence of perineural invasion managed with excision have local recurrence and metastatic rates of 47.2 and 47.3%, respectively, according to Rowe et al. Mohs micrographic surgery offers improved outcome for neurotropic SCC compared with excision, with local recurrence and metastatic rates of 0 and 8.3%, respectively. Lawrence and Cottel reported a survival probability of 88.7% for SCC with perineural invasion managed with Mohs micrographic surgery. Adjuvant radiation therapy has been employed in the management of neurotropic SCCs with 100 and 50% local cure rates for primary and recurrent tumors, respectively, as reported by Barrett et al.

Local Cure Rates with Alternative Modalities

Photodynamic therapy (PDT) is a promising therapeutic modality in which a systemic or topical photosensitizer is preferentially absorbed by neoplastic cells with resultant selective killing of tumor cells after exposure to photons. In a study by McCaughan et al. 27 patients with cutaneous and subcutaneous malignancies (7 BCC, 3 SCC, 3 melanoma, 1 liposarcoma, 12 breast cancer) were treated with photodynamic therapy with a 67% complete response and 26% partial response rate. After one year, 48% of patients initially experiencing complete response remained free of disease. A phase I trial of PDT with topical 5-aminolevulinic acid in the treatment of Bowen's disease had a 97% complete response rate at 2 months, falling to 89% at a median of 18 months follow-up.

Interferon has been utilized in the treatment of cutaneous SCC as well as BCC. Edwards et al. treated 36 SCCs ranging from 0.5 to 2.0 cm with 1.5 million units of intralesional interferon alpha-2a three times weekly for 3 weeks with an 88.2% complete response, histologically confirmed. Combination subcutaneous interferon alpha-2a with oral isotretinoin has been utilized in a study by Lippman et al. in 28 patients with inoperable SCC, with 25% complete remission and 43% partial remission. As with BCC, treatment of SCC with isotretinoin or etretinate alone has been disappointing, with 3 of 13 patients experiencing complete remission in one study.

As with BCC, cisplatin-based chemotherapy has resulted in 40% complete response rates in patients with locally advanced SCC unsuitable for salvage therapy with either surgery or radiation according to a study by Guthrie et al. When used neoadjuvantly to shrink SCCs to allow for easier surgical or radiation therapy, cisplatin-based chemotherapy has resulted in 25% complete and 25–50% partial response rates in the studies of Guthrie et al. and Sadek et al. Systemic chemotherapy may have a palliative or neoadjuvant role in the management of advanced SCC.

Survival Rates: Regional Lymph Node Metastasis

Salasche et al. estimated that 2–6% of actinically derived SCCs will metastasize to regional lymph nodes, contrary to earlier estimates of 0.5%. Once histologically confirmed lymph node metastases are present, therapeutic options include lymphadenectomy, radiation therapy, or combination therapy. Overall, survival rates after lymph node metastasis are poor, with 34.4% of patients alive after 5 yr. Therapeutic lymphadenectomy results in 5-yr survival rates of 26.8, 25.6, and 47.5% for SCC of the skin, ear, and lip, respectively, according to Rowe et al. Radiation therapy is associated with 5-yr survival rates of 28.6 and 26.5% for ear and lip SCCs metastatic to regional nodes, respectively. Combination therapy with lymphadenectomy and radiation therapy results in improved 5-yr survival rates of 45.5 and 58.6% for ear and lip SCCs with nodal metastases, respectively, as shown in Figure 11. To date, systemic chemotherapy has not been shown to improve survival significantly beyond that achieved with surgery and radiation in patients with metastatic nodal involvement of the neck.

Survival Rates: Distant Metastasis

Fifteen to twenty percent of metastatic SCC will bypass the regional lymph nodes and directly affect other organs according to Salasche et al. Additionally, patients with regional nodal metastases in whom the SCC is not cured by therapeutic lymphadenectomy may develop distant metastases. Once extranodal SCC is present, prognosis is grim. However, unlike melanoma, there are few data regarding survival rates once SCC is distantly disseminated.

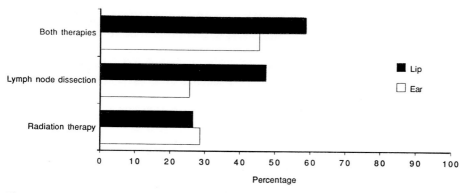

Figure 11 Five-year survival rates after nodal metastasis of squamous cell carcinoma. (Modified from Rowe et al. Prognostic factors for local recurrence, metastasis, and survival rates in squamous cell carcinoma of the skin, ear, and lip. *J Am Acad Dermatol* 1992;26:976–990.)

SURVIVAL RATES FOR MELANOMA

Unlike basal cell carcinoma, in which cure rates are defined in terms of local recurrence, cure with a potentially lethal melanoma is best defined by prolonged disease-free survival. Sophisticated prognostic models based on well-defined clinical and histologic variables have been developed for melanoma. Thus, discussion of cure rates for melanoma centers on the predictive value of various prognostic factors for survival. The utility of carefully defining prognostic factors in melanoma relates to the potential to target aggressive surgical or systemic, adjuvant or neo-adjuvant therapy to those patients at highest risk of metastasis. Although an updated American Joint Committee on Cancer (AJCC) staging system was issued in 1992, most available data are based on the 1983 American Joint Committee on Cancer (AJCC) Staging System, which will be referred to in this section (Table 2). Survival rates in general are calculated with the exclusion of level I, in situ melanoma, as these are considered to have no metastatic potential.

Historical Considerations

Advances in the early diagnosis of melanoma, independent of changes in therapeutic modalities, have had a major impact on the cure rate for melanoma over the past few decades. As aware-

Table 2 1983 AJCC Staging System for Melanoma

Stage	Criteria
Stage IA	Localized melanoma ≤ 0.75 mm thick or level II (T1,N0,M0)
Stage IB	Localized melanoma 0.76–1.50 mm thick or level III (T2,N0,M0)
Stage IIA	Localized melanoma 1.51–4.00 mm thick or level IV (T3,N0,M0)
Stage IIB	Localized melanoma ≥ 4.00 mm thick or level V (T4,N0,M0)
Stage III	Limited nodal metastasis involving only one regional lymph node basin or <5 in-transit metastases but without nodal disease (any T,N1,M0)
Stage IV	Advanced regional metastases (any T, N2, M0) or any patient with distant metastases (any T, any N, M1, or M2)

Source: Modified from American Joint Committee on Cancer. *Manual for Staging of Cancer*. 2nd ed. Philadelphia, J.B. Lippincott, 1983.

ness of melanoma increases among both the public and medical professionals, there has been a trend toward clinical presentation with lower stage, less ulceration, and decreased thickness and level as outlined by Little et al. As a result of earlier diagnosis, cumulative 5-yr survival rates for stage I and II malignant melanoma exclusive of in situ disease improved from 78 to 86% between 1970 and 1980 in a series from the Sydney Melanoma Unit, likely independent of any therapeutic innovations. For this reason, comparison of new survival data with historical controls not stratified by other variables is inappropriate.

Breslow Thickness

Currently, the most reliable predictor of survival in melanoma is the measured, histologic thickness of the tumor from the top of the granular cell layer to the deepest malignant cell, known as the Breslow thickness. As shown in Figure 12, increased thickness correlates with worsening prognosis. Five-year survival data for stage I and II (localized) melanoma stratified by thickness are presented in Table 3. It is important to note that, of patients with melanomas 4 mm thick or greater, approximately 30% survive long term. Predictions of inevitable metastasis in patients with thick melanomas should thus be avoided. When compared with other prognostic factors in melanoma, Breslow thickness is the most sensitive, with most other factors deriving significance from their secondary relation to thickness.

Clark's Level

As melanoma cells penetrate to deeper levels within the dermis, known as Clark's levels, survival decreases according to univariate analysis. However, when level is compared to thickness as a prognostic indicator, Breslow thickness is a more accurate predictor of metastasis and survival as demonstrated in the studies of Balch et al., Cascinelli et al., and Day et al., among others. Thus, a 0.6-mm, level IV tumor extending into the midreticular dermis is associated with a favorable prognosis, while a 4-mm, level IV melanoma carries a poor prognosis. In the majority of cases, increased thickness correlates with deeper levels, resulting in fair correlation

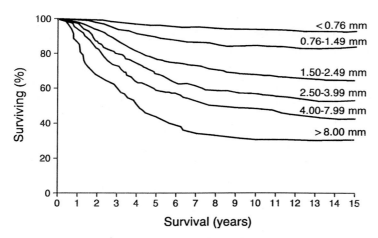

Figure 12 Survival for stage I and II (localized) melanoma by tumor thickness. (Modified from Balch CM, Soong S-J, Shaw HM, et al. An analysis of prognostic factors in 8500 patients with cutaneous melanoma. In: *Cutaneous Melanoma*, 2nd ed. CM Balch, AN Houghton, GW Milton, et al., eds. Philadelphia, J.B. Lippincott Co, 1992, p. 170.)

Table 3 3 Five-Year Survival Rates for
Stage I and II (Localized) Melanoma

Thickness (mm)	Survival (%)
<0.76	96
0.76–1.49	87
1.50–2.49	75
2.50–3.99	66
≥4.00	47

Source: Modified from Balch CM, Cascinelli N,
Drzewiecki KT, et al. A comparison of prog-
nostic factors worldwide. In: *Cutaneous Mela-
noma*. 2nd ed. Balch CM, Houghton AN,
Milton GW, et al., eds. Philadelphia, J.B.
Lippincott Co, 1992, p. 194.

between the two prognostic indicators. However, when thickness and level are discordant, prognosis is more accurately predicted by measurement of thickness. The prognostic significance of
Clark's level may be greater for melanomas arising from regions with thin skin, such as eyelid
or ear.

Additional Histologic Factors

Nodular and acral lentiginous melanomas tend to be thicker at presentation and are thus associated with a worse prognosis. However, when tumor thickness is controlled for, nodular and
superficial spreading melanomas have similar 10-yr survival rates. Lentigo maligna melanoma
may be associated with a slightly better 10-yr survival rate and acral lentiginous melanoma with
a slightly worse survival rate than either superficial spreading or nodular melanoma, even after
controlling for thickness according to McGovern et al. Ulceration is associated with slight negative
prognostic significance when thickness is controlled for whereas the prognostic value of both host
response and regression is controversial.

Gender and Anatomic Location

Although melanoma in women is associated with a more favorable prognosis than in men, the
survival difference is due to the decreased thickness of melanoma at presentation in women. The
better prognosis for acral, other than hands and feet, than axial melanomas, however, is only
partially accounted for by decreased thickness of acral melanomas at presentation. Melanoma of
the scalp is associated with a worse prognosis than other sites on the head.

Lymph Node Metastases

Approximately 21% of patients with stage I or II melanoma (localized) eventually develop local recurrence or metastases. For patients with occult metastatic nodal melanoma detected by
elective lymph node dissection, the 10-yr survival rate is 48%. The 5-yr survival rate for all stage
III (nodal metastases) patients is approximately 27–42%, with 15-yr survival rates of 20–25%.
Prognosis worsens with an increase in the number of involved nodes and a primary melanoma
with axial location and ulceration.

Distant Metastases

Once distant metastases are present, median survival is 6 months, with 1-yr survival rates of 8% in the study by Balch et al. Patients with a greater number of metastatic sites, shorter duration of remission after primary treatment, and metastases to visceral organs tend to have significantly worse prognoses. Occasionally, patients with metastatic melanoma survive more than 5 yr. Also intriguing is the fact that 2–3% of patients with melanoma will develop recurrences 10 yr or more after treatment of their primary tumor, with rare relapses more than 30 yr after initial diagnosis.

Surgical Margin

Many studies support the concept that the width of surgical margin has no effect on survival in cutaneous melanoma. Two prospective, randomized, controlled trials on patients with thin- to intermediate-thickness (<4 mm) melanomas by Veronesi et al. and Balch et al. recently demonstrated no statistically significant difference in survival rates between those receiving narrow (1–2 cm) versus wide (3–4 cm) margins. Based on these studies, recommended resection margins have decreased to 1 cm for thin melanomas (≤1 mm), 1–2 cm for melanomas 1–2 mm thick, and 2 cm for melanomas 2–4 mm thick. Thick (>4 mm) melanomas still warrant 3-cm surgical margins. Several studies, including Veronesi's, have demonstrated that narrow surgical margins may be associated with increased local recurrence rates. The discordance between the negative effect of narrow surgical margins on local recurrence but not on survival challenges the concept that melanoma spreads via localized lymphatics prior to nodal or hematogenous dissemination.

Mohs Micrographic Surgery

Mohs micrographic surgery ideally offers the possibility of decreased surgical margins without increased risk of local recurrence, distant metastasis, or death. Although not universally accepted, the use of Mohs micrographic surgery for the removal of cutaneous melanoma is supported by clinical experience as outlined by Zitelli. According to the most complete reports, survival and local recurrence rates obtained with Mohs micrographic surgery are comparable to those of standard wide excision. Of 20 patients with invasive melanoma, Zitelli reported only one death at 5 yr for a 95% 5-yr survival, comparable to that expected from life-table analysis from other studies involving standard excisions. Mohs micrographic surgery for melanoma can be regarded as an extension of the general trend toward narrower margins for melanoma with the additional security of immediate and complete histologic verification of tumor-free margins. Prospective, randomized comparison with standard excision would clarify the role of Mohs micrographic surgery in the management of melanoma.

Lymph Node Dissection

Results of studies regarding the impact of elective lymph node dissection in clinical stage I melanoma are conflicting, with some studies demonstrating improved survival while others reveal no impact on ultimate outcome. The two prospective, randomized studies from the WHO Melanoma Group and the Mayo clinic failed to demonstrate a statistically significant increase in survival rates for patients with localized melanoma of the limbs undergoing elective lymph node dissection. These trials have been criticized for enrolling disproportionately large numbers of patients with thin melanomas and excluding patients with melanoma of the head, neck, and trunk, who may have increased risk of metastatic disease. The ongoing Intergroup Melanoma Committee and WHO Melanoma Group studies will hopefully provide more definitive data regarding the efficacy of elective lymph node dissection in the not too distant future. For patients with metastatic melanoma localized to regional lymph nodes, therapeutic nodal dissection has been associated with a 20% 10-yr survival rate. Thus, therapeutic lymph node resection can result in long-term survival in patients with metastatic melanoma of the lymph nodes.

Treatment of Disseminated Metastatic Disease

At the present time, no nonsurgical modality has been shown in randomized, blinded trials to consistently and significantly improve survival in patients with metastatic melanoma. As shown in the study by Wong et al., 5–20% of patients with solitary visceral metastasis amenable to resection will survive more than 5 yr. However, chemotherapy, radiotherapy, and biologic therapies have shown poor efficacy with regard to curative intent in metastatic melanoma and are best regarded as palliative. Chemotherapy with dacarbazine (DTIC) or paclitaxel (Taxol) is associated with objective response rates of 20%, while combination DTIC, carmustine, cisplastin, and tamoxifen has been associated with response rates of 46%. Neither regimen has demonstrated the ability to improve survival rates. Autologous bone marrow transplantation after high-dose combination chemotherapy has been attempted, with overall response rates of 65%. For patients with extremity-based in-transit metastases, isolated limb perfusion with combination melphalan, tumor necrosis factor, and interferon-alpha was recently associated with a 90% response rate and is currently being evaluated in controlled trials. None of the above regimens has been shown to improve disease-free or overall survival significantly and consistently. Ongoing investigations of isolated limb perfusion, adjuvant radiotherapy, megestrol acetate, and levamisole will hopefully identify treatments with more significant impact on metastatic melanoma than current regimens.

Biologic therapy with interferon-alpha in patients with metastatic melanoma is associated with a 15% objective response rate. Although preliminary, interim analysis of the Eastern Cooperative Oncology Group EST 1684 trial with interferon-alpha revealed a significant increase in disease-free survival. Recently, high-dose interleukin-2 has been associated with occasional long-term remissions in an uncontrolled trial in patients with metastatic melanoma. Such promising results must be viewed with caution, however, until interleukin-2 can be evaluated in a controlled trial. Trials of adjuvant interferon-alpha and vaccines in high-risk stage II patients are ongoing.

SOFT TISSUE SARCOMA

With only 5700 new cases reported in 1990, soft tissue sarcomas are relatively uncommon, and extensive prognostic data on specific sarcoma histologic types is not readily available. Because histologic type is not the most sensitive prognostic factor for soft tissue sarcomas, the majority of prognostic data regarding cure rates and survival are derived from grading and staging systems based on collective series of all types of soft tissue sarcomas. In many systems, the histologic characteristics of specific tumors are integrated into the overall grade of the tumor. Analogous to melanoma, "cure" rates for high-grade soft tissue sarcomas are more appropriately defined in terms of long-term survival, given the potentially lethal nature of these neoplasms. Conversely, for low-grade sarcomas local recurrence is a more relevant concept given their indolent, locally invasive nature. As with melanoma, current therapy of soft tissue sarcomas centers on surgical resection, with adjuvant modalities essential but inadequately curative themselves. Most available data are based on the 1992 American Joint Committee on Cancer Staging System (Table 4) which will be referred to in this section. Table 5 outlines the most common soft tissue sarcomas.

Table 4   1992 AJCC Staging System for Soft Tissue Sarcomas

Stage	Criteria
Stage I	
Stage 1a($G_1T_1N_0M_0$)	Grade 1 tumor less than 5 cm in diameter with no regional lymph node or distant metastasis
Stage 1b($G_1T_2N_0M_0$)	Grade 1 tumor 5 cm or greater in diameter with no regional lymph node or distant metastasis
Stage II	
Stage IIa($G_2T_1N_0M_0$)	Grade 2 tumor less than 5 cm in diameter with no regional lymph node or distant metastasis
Stage IIb($G_2T_2N_0M_0$)	Grade 2 tumor 5 cm or greater in diameter with no regional lymph node or distant metastasis
Stage III	
Stage IIIa($G_{3,4}T_1N_0M_0$)	Grade 3 tumor less than 5 cm in diameter with no regional lymph node or distant metastasis
Stage IIIb($G_{3,4}T_2N_0M_0$)	Grade 3 tumor 5 cm or greater in diameter with no regional lymph node or distant metastasis
Stage IV	
Stage IVa($G_{1-4}T_{1-2}N_1M_0$)	Tumor of any grade or any size with regional lymph node metastasis but without distant metastasis
Stage IVb($G_{1-4}T_{1-2}N_{0-1}M_1$)	Tumor with distant metastasis

Source: Modified from American Joint Committee on Cancer, *Manual for Staging of Cancer*, 3rd ed. J.B. Lippincott, Philadelphia, 1992.

Survival Rates

Grade and Histologic Type

Grading systems attempt to objectify the degree of malignancy of a particular tumor. The grade of a soft tissue sarcoma is the most reliable predictor of survival. A variety of grading systems for soft tissue sarcomas have been proposed based on factors including cellularity, cellular pleomorphism, growth pattern, tumor necrosis, specific tumor type, vascular invasion, and mitotic rate. Of these prognostic factors, mitotic rate, vascular invasion, and necrosis are the most reliable. Depth of tumor penetration has also been shown to predict decreased survival. Because pathologists are concordant on histologic type, mitotic rate, and tumor necrosis in only 61, 73, and 81% of cases, respectively, examination by a pathologist experienced with soft tissue sarcomas is paramount for prognostic and therapeutic information.

Table 5   Common Soft Tissue Sarcomas

Malignant fibrous histiocytoma (25.1%)
Liposarcoma (11.6%)
Rhabdomyosarcoma (9.7%)
Leiomyosarcoma (9.1%)
Synovial sarcoma (6.5%)
Malignant schwannoma (5.9%)
Fibrosarcoma (5.2%)

% = Percent of total soft tissue sarcomas.

Table 6 5-Year Survival Rates for Grade 1–3 Soft Tissue Sarcomas

Grading system	Grade 1	Grade 2	Grade 3	Grade 4
Markhede	100	100	68	47
Myhre Jensen	97	67	38	
Costa	100	73	46	

In general, increasing grade correlates with decreased survival. There are notable exceptions as in malignant granular cell tumors, which display only moderate pleomorphism and little mitotic activity yet behave aggressively. Intermediate- and high-grade sarcomas are associated with a poor prognosis in general, with 50% of patients dying within 5 yr according to Myhre Jensen et al. Table 6 outlines the differences in trends toward decreased survival in various grading systems. Figure 13 demonstrates typical corrected survival curves for grade 1, 2, and 3 sarcomas based on the grading system of Myhre Jensen et al. As can be seen in the curves, death from soft tissue sarcomas can occur as much as 10 yr after initial presentation, although 80% of local or distant recurrences occur within 5 yr.

Five-year survival rates for specific histologic types of intermediate- and high-grade sarcomas are compiled in Table 7. As many of these sarcomas arise in the deep soft tissues and retroperitoneum, dermatologic surgeons have infrequent exposure to many of these tumors. A notable exception is cutaneous leiomyosarcoma, which rarely metastasizes, in contrast to the highly aggressive deep leiomyosarcoma, as shown by Fields and Helwig. Leiomyosarcomas localized to the dermis are associated with a 32% local recurrence rate after standard excision and have been successfully managed with Mohs micrographic surgery, as reported by Davidson et al.

Low-grade or locally invasive soft tissue sarcomas rarely metastasize but frequently recur, which makes complete surgical resection imperative. Dermatologic surgeons have made significant contributions to the therapeutic options available for these tumors. Table 8 outlines recurrence rates for low-grade, locally invasive soft tissue sarcomas.

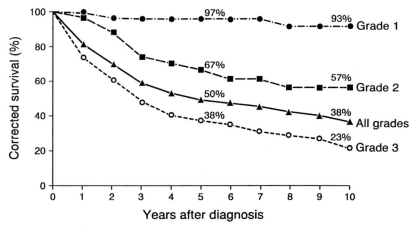

Figure 13 Survival rates by grade for soft tissue sarcomas. (Modified from Myhre Jensen O, Kaae S, Hjollund Madsen E, et al. Histopathological grading in soft-tissue tumors. *Acta Pathol Microbiol Immunol Scand* 1983;91A:145–150.)

Table 7 5-Year Survival Rates for Aggressive Soft Tissue Sarcomas

Tumor type	Survival (%)
Fibrosarcoma	39–54
Malignant fibrous histiocytoma	36–69
Liposarcoma	59–73
Leiomyosarcoma	
Retroperitoneal	0–29
Extremity	64
Rhabdomyosarcoma	26–88
Hemangioendothelioma	87 (4 yr)
Angiosarcoma	12
Synovial sarcoma	36–82
Malignant peripheral nerve sheath tumor	20–44
Neuroblastoma	60 (2 yr)
Extraskeletal Ewing's sarcoma	66
Extraskeletal myxoid chondrosarcoma	73 (10 yr)
Extraskeletal mesenchymal chondrosarcoma	55
Epitheliod sarcoma	60

Tumor Size, Depth, and Anatomic Location

Although tumor grade is the most important prognostic indicator in soft tissue sarcomas, the size of the primary tumor is the clinical variable most predictive of disease-free survival. Tumor size and duration of survival are inversely related, as shown in Table 9. Although soft tissue sarcomas arising in the subcutaneous tissue are associated with a better prognosis than deeper sarcomas, the difference is attributable to the smaller size of subcutaneous tumors when subjected to multivariate analysis, according to a study by Peabody et al.

Due to modification of surgical margins at locations adjacent to vital structures, the risks of local recurrence and death are increased in sarcomas on the head and neck. According to the large study by Gustafson, the increased rate of local recurrence and decreased survival associated with proximal as opposed to distal sarcomas is secondary to the larger size of proximal tumors when analyzed by multivariate analysis. Treatment of distal extremity sarcomas with radical excision or amputation results in local control rates near 100% according to Owens et al. Sarcomas arising in the abdomen, retroperitoneum, and body wall are all associated with worse prognosis than extremity sarcomas, largely due to advanced local and distant disease by the time of presentation.

Table 8 Recurrence Rates for Locally Invasive Soft Tissue Sarcomas[a]

Tumor type	Recurrence rate (%)
Dermatofibrosarcoma protuberans	18
Giant cell fibroblastoma	50
Angiomatoid fibrous histiocytoma	20
Plexiform fibrohistiocytic tumor	40
Atypical fibroxanthoma	6.4
Granular cell tumor	6.5

[a]Length of follow-up varied.

Table 9 5-Year Survival by Tumor Size for Intermediate- and High-Grade Sarcomas in Patients Treated with Surgery and Radiation

Tumor size (cm)	No. of patients	Percentage disease-free at 5 yr
<2.5	17	94
2.6-4.9	48	77
5.9-10.0	55	62
10.1-15.0	24	51
15.1-20.0	9	42
>20.0	6	17
Total	159	65

Source: Modified from Suit HD, Mankin HJ, Wood WC, et al. Treatment of the patient with stage M_0 soft tissue sarcoma. *J Clin Oncol* 1988;6:854–862.

Extent of Surgery and Local Recurrence

Soft tissue sarcomas grow in an expansile and microscopically infiltrative manner, which results in a 60–80% local recurrence rate if excisions are performed at the periphery of the pseudocapsule. En bloc wide excisions, which encompass a 1- to 3-cm margin of clinically normal tissue around the entire periphery of the tumor but remain within the muscular compartment of origin, result in an overall 30% recurrence rate. Wide excision alone is considered adequate therapy for small, superficial, or low-grade sarcomas, as supported by the study of Rydholm et al. Wide excision or lesser procedures can be utilized for higher grade sarcomas only with the addition of adjuvant radiation or chemotherapy, as demonstrated by Rosenberg et al. Radical excision involves extirpation of the entire compartment from which the sarcoma arose, either by radical muscle compartment excision or radical amputation. Eighty percent of patients treated with radical excision or amputation achieve local control; of the 20% with local recurrences, 69% will be alive 3 yr after reexcision.

Stage

Staging systems attempt to define the extent of tumor involvement at presentation. The American Joint Committee on Cancer staging system for soft tissue sarcomas is based on the TNM staging system, with the addition of histologic grade as an additional feature (GTNM) (Table 4). Survival decreases with increased stage at presentation, as shown in Figure 14.

Lymph Node Metastases

Whereas lymph node metastasis commonly occurs in metastatic melanoma and squamous cell carcinoma, regional lymph nodes are involved in <4% of patients at presentation and only 5% overall with soft tissue sarcomas. Because of this, elective lymph node dissection is not recommended. The histologic type rather than grade of the tumor is the most important factor predicting lymph node metastasis. Nodal metastasis carries the same prognosis as distant metastasis, uniformly poor, with a 2–3% 10 yr survival. Radical lymphadenectomy for sarcoma metastatic to lymph nodes alone can be curative, with 5-yr survival rates of 34–46%, as reported by Fong et al.

Distant Metastases

At presentation, 10–23% of patients with soft tissue sarcomas will have distant metastases, most commonly to the lung, liver, bone, and central nervous system, according to Lawrence et al. Metastatic soft tissue sarcomas are associated with a dismal prognosis, with 10-yr survival rates of 2–3%. A report by Verazin et al. documented a 21% overall 5-yr survival and an 11% disease-

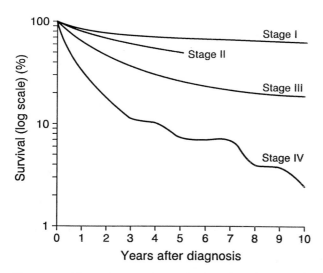

Figure 15 Survival rates by stage for soft tissue sarcomas. (Modified from Enzinger FM, Weiss SW. General consideration. In: *Soft Tissue Tumors*. FM Enzinger, SW Weiss, eds. St. Louis, Mosby, 1995, p. 13.)

free survival after complete resection of lung metastases from soft tissue sarcomas of various types. Whereas isolated distant metastases can be surgically resected, chemotherapy would be appropriate palliative therapy for disseminated metastases. Novel therapeutic modalities such as cytokines and monoclonal antibodies have not shown efficacy in metastatic sarcoma.

Adjuvant Radiation Therapy

Radical excision and amputation can be associated with considerable functional morbidity, which has stimulated therapeutic approaches based on less radical surgical therapy. Other than small, superficial, and low-grade sarcomas, most surgically excised sarcomas are treated with adjuvant radiation therapy to optimize cure rates, as reviewed by Suit et al. Radiation can be administered pre- or postoperatively, either externally or via implanted brachytherapy. Radiation therapy alone as discussed by Tepper and Suit is associated with a 28% 5-yr survival, inadequate for monotherapy when compared with adequate surgical resection. When used in conjunction with surgical excision, control rates are superior to either approach alone, with decreased surgical morbidity.

Adjuvant Chemotherapy

Intermediate- and high-grade sarcomas are associated with a 50% 5-yr survival rate despite aggressive local therapy. The high propensity of sarcomas toward early microscopic metastasis has prompted trials of adjuvant systemic chemotherapy in an attempt to achieve cure while tumor burden is low. However, to date, randomized, controlled trials of postoperative adjuvant chemotherapy have not revealed definitive evidence of improved survival. Randomized trials utilizing adjuvant doxorubicin failed to demonstrate improved survival compared with surgery alone, according to Elias and Antman. The findings of randomized trials utilizing multiagent chemotherapy postoperatively are conflicting, but a recent meta-analysis by Zalupski et al. suggests that aggressive, adjuvant, multiagent chemotherapy may increase survival in patients with high-grade extremity sarcomas.

Recurrence Rates for Soft Tissue Sarcomas Managed with Mohs Micrographic Surgery

Although many types of soft tissue sarcoma have been managed with Mohs micrographic surgery, the paucity of reported cases prevents reasonable estimates of recurrence rates for most tumors. However, reports of dermatofibrosarcoma protuberans (DFSP) treated with Mohs micrographic surgery now exist in larger numbers, as reviewed and expanded in the work by Gloster et al. They reported a cumulative recurrence rate of only 0.6% for DFSP treated by Mohs micrographic surgery, which compares favorably to an average 18% recurrence rate after wide (>2 cm) surgical excision. This relates to the well-known capability of peripheral strands of DFSP to extend into fat and fascia well beyond the clinical margins of tumor in a haphazard fashion. Because of the impressive cure rates and opportunity for significant normal tissue sparing associated with Mohs micrographic surgery, it is considered the treatment of choice for DFSP by many authors.

In a series of 25 superficial primary and recurrent malignant fibrous histiocytomas and atypical fibroxanthomas treated with Mohs micrographic surgery, Brown and Swanson noted a 94% tumor-free survival after an average 3-yr follow-up. When compared with the higher recurrence rates associated with standard excisional surgery, Mohs micrographic surgery may offer a uniquely precise and controlled method for the removal of superficial malignant fibrohistiocytic neoplasms.

BIBLIOGRAPHY

Basal Cell Carcinoma

Amonette RA, Salasche SJ, Chesney TM, Clarendon CCD, Dilawari RA. Metastatic basal-cell carcinoma. *J Dermatol Surg Oncol* 1981;7:397–400.

Bollag W, Holdener EE. Retinoids in cancer prevention and therapy. *Ann Oncol* 1992;3:513–526.

Brenner S, Wolf R, Dascalu DI. Topical tretinoin treatment in basal cel carcinoma. *J Dermatol Surg Oncol* 1993;19:264–266.

Cairnduff F, Stringer MR, Hudson EJ, Ash DV, Brown SB. Superficial photodynamic therapy with topical 5-aminolaevulinic acid for superficial primary and secondary skin cancer. *Br J Cancer* 1994;69:605–608.

Childers BJ, Goldwyn RM, Ramos D, Chaffey J, Harris JR. Long-term results of irradiation for basal cell carcinoma of the skin of the nose. *Plast Reconstr Surg* 1994;93:1169–1173.

Cornell RC, Greenway HT, Tucker SB, Edwards L, Ashworth S, Vance JC, Tanner DJ, Taylor EL, Smiles KA, Peets EA. Intralesional interferon therapy for basal cell carcinoma. *J Am Acad Dermatol* 1990;23:694–700.

Cutler S, Ederer F. Maximum utilization of the life table method in analyzing survival. *J Chron Dis* 1958;8:699–712.

Dixon AY, Lee SH, McGregor DH. Histologic features predictive of basal cell carcinoma recurrence: results of a multivariate analysis. *J Cutan Pathol* 1993;20:137–142.

Edwards L, Tucker SB, Perdnia D, Smiles KA, Taylor EL, Tanner DJ, Peets E. The effect of intralesional sustained-release formulation of interferon alfa-2b on basal cell carcinomas. *Arch Dermatol* 1990;126:1029–1032.

Fraunfelder FT, Zacarian SA, Wingfield DL, Limmer BL. Results of cryotherapy for eyelid malignancies. *Am J Ophthalmol* 1984;97:184–188.

Graham GF. Cryosurgery. *Clin Plast Surg* 1993;20:131–147.

Guthrie TJ, Porubsky ES, Luxenberg MN, Shah KJ, Wurtz KL, Watson PR. Cisplatin-based chemotherapy in advanced basal and squamous cell carcinomas of the skin: results in 28 patients including 13 patients receiving multimodality therapy. *J Clin Oncol* 1990;8:342–346.

Hruza GJ. Mohs micrographic surgery local recurrences. *J Dermatol Surg Oncol* 1994;20:573–577.

Johnson TM, Tromovitch TA, Swanson NA. Combined curettage and excision: a treatment for primary basal cell carcinoma. *J Am Acad Dermatol* 1991;24:613–617.

Kuflik EG. Cryosurgery updated. *J Am Acad Dermatol* 1994;31:925–944.

Kuflik EG, Gage AA. *Cryosurgical Treatment for Skin Cancer.* New York: Igaku-Shoin, 1990.

Kuflik EG, Gage AA. The five-year cure rate achieved by cryosurgery for skin cancer. *J Am Acad Dermatol* 1991;24:1002–1004.

Lang PG, Maize JC. Histologic evolution of recurrent basal cell carcinoma and treatment implications. *J Am Acad Dermatol* 1986;14:186–196.

Lawrence CM. Mohs surgery of basal cell carcinoma—a critical review. *Br J Plast Surg* 1993;46:599–606.

Levine H. Cutaneous carcinoma of the head and neck: management of massive and previously uncontrolled lesions. *Laryngoscope* 1983;93:87–105.

Madsen A. Studies on basal cell epithelioma of the skin. *Acta Pathol Microbiol Scand* 1965; 177(suppl):1047–1049.

Miller PK, Roenigk RK, Brodland DG, Randle HW. Cutaneous micrographic surgery: Mohs procedure. *Mayo Clin Proc* 1992;67:971–980.

Mohs FE. Chemosurgery. A microscopically controlled method of cancer excision. *Arch Surg* 1941; 44:279–295.

Orenberg EK, Miller BH, Greenway HT, Koperski JA, Lowe N, Rosen T, Brown DM, Inui M, Korey AG, Luck EE. The effect of intralesional 5-fluorouracil therapeutic implant (MPI 5003) for treatment of basal cell carcinoma. *J Am Acad Dermatol* 1992;27:723–728.

Peck GL, DiGiovanna JJ, Sarnoff DS, Gross EG, Butkus D, Olsen TG, Yoder FW. Treatment and prevention of basal cell carcinoma with oral isotretinoin. *J Am Acad Dermatol* 1988;19:176–185.

Preston DS, Stern RS. Nonmelanoma cancers of the skin. *N Engl J Med* 1992;23:1649–1662.

Raszewski RL, Guyuron B. Long-term survival following nodal metastases from basal cell carcinoma. *Ann Plast Surg* 1990;24:170–175.

Riefkohl R, Wittels B, McCarty K. Metastatic basal cell carcinoma. *Ann Plast Surg* 1984;13:525–528.

Rigel DS, Robins P, Friedman RJ. Predicting recurrence of basal-cell carcinomas treated by microscopically controlled excision. *J Dermatol Surg Oncol* 1981;7:807–810.

Robins P. Chemosurgery: my 15 years of experience. *J Dermatol Surg Oncol* 1981;7:779–789.

Roenigk RK. Mohs' micrographic surgery. *Mayo Clin Proc* 1988;63:175–183.

Roenigk RK, Ratz JL, Bailin PL, Wheeland RG. Trends in the presentation and treatment of basal cell carcinomas. *J Dermatol Surg Oncol* 1986;12:860–865.

Roenigk RK, Roenigk HH, Jr., *Dermatologic Surgery: Principles and Practice.* New York, Marcel Dekker, Inc., 1989.

Roenigk RK, Roenigk HH, Jr., eds. *Surgical Dermatology.* St. Louis, Mosby Year Book, 1993.

Rowe DE, Carroll RJ, Day CL, Jr. Long-term recurrence rates in previously untreated (primary) basal cell carcinoma: implications for patient follow-up. *J Dermatol Surg Oncol* 1989;15:315–328.

Rowe DE, Carroll RJ, Day CL, Jr. Mohs surgery is the treatment of choice for recurrent (previously treated) basal cell carcinoma. *J Dermatol Surg Oncol* 1989;15:424–431.

Sahl W, Yessenow R, Brou J, Levine N. Mohs' micrographic surgery and prompt reconstruction for basal cell carcinoma: report of 62 cases using the combined method. *J Okla State Med Assoc* 1994;87:10–15.

Salasche SJ, Amonette RA. Morpheaform basal-cell epitheliomas. *J Dermatol Surg Oncol* 1981;7:387–394.

Scanlon EF, Volkmer DD, Oviedo MA, Khandekar JD, Victor TA. Metastatic basal cell carcinoma. *J Surg Oncol* 1980;15:171–180.

Silverman MK, Kopf AW, Grin CM, Bart RS, Levenstein MJ. Recurrence rates of treated basal cell carcinomas. Part 1: overview. *J Dermatol Surg Oncol* 1991;17:713–718.

Silverman MK, Kopf AW, Grin CM, Bart RS, Levenstein MJ. Recurrence rates of treated basal cell carcinomas. Part 2: curettage-electrodessication. *J Dermatol Surg Oncol* 1991;17:720–726.

Silverman MK, Kopf AW, Bart RS, Grin CM, Levenstein MJ. Recurrence rates of treated basal cell carcinomas. Part 3: surgical excision. *J Dermatol Surg Oncol* 1992;18:471–476.

Silverman MK, Kopf AW, Gladstein AH, Bart RS, Grin CM, Levenstein MJ. Recurrence rates of treated basal cell carcinomas. Part 4: x-ray therapy. *J Dermatol Surg Oncol* 1992;18:549–554.

Sloane JP. The value of typing basal cell carcinomas in predicting recurrence after surgical excision. *Br J Dermatol* 1977;96:127–132.

Stenquist B, Wennberg AM, Gisslen H, Larko O. Treatment of aggressive basal cell carcinoma with intralesional interferon: evaluation of efficacy by Mohs surgery. *J Am Acad Dermatol* 1992;27:65–69.

Torre D. Cryosurgery of basal cell carcinoma. *J Am Acad Dermatol* 1986;15:917–929.

Tromovitch TA, Allende M. Curette-excision techniques for skin cancer. *Cutis* 1970;6:1349–1352.

von Domarus H, Stevens PJ. Metastatic basal cell carcinoma. *J Am Acad Dermatol* 1984;10:1043–1060.

Wilder RB, Kittelson JM, Shimm DS. Basal cell carcinoma treated with radiation therapy. *Cancer* 1991;68:2134–2137.

Wilder RB, Shimm DS, Kittelson JM, Rogoff EE, Cassady JR. Recurrent basal cell carcinoma treated with radiation therapy. *Arch Dermatol* 1991;127:1668–1672.

Wilson BD, Mang TS, Stoll H, Jones C, Cooper M, Dougherty TJ. Photodynamic therapy for the treatment of basal cell carcinoma. *Arch Dermatol* 1992;128;1597–1601.

Wolf DJ, Zitelli JA. Surgical margins for basal cell carcinoma. *Arch Dermatol* 1987;123:340–344.

Zacarian SA, ed. *Cryosurgery for Skin Cancer and Cutaneous Disorders*. St. Louis, CV Mosby, 1985.

Squamous Cell Carcinoma

Barrett TL, Greenway HTJ, Massullo V, Carlson C. Treatment of basal cell carcinoma and squamous cell carcinoma with perineural invasion. *Adv Dermatol* 1993;8:277–304.

Bollag W, Holdener EE. Retinoids in cancer prevention and therapy. *Ann Oncol* 1992;3:513–526.

Breuninger H, Black B, Rassner G. Microstaging of squamous cell carcinoma. *Am J Clin Pathol* 1990;94:624–627.

Cairnduff F, Stringer MR, Hudson EJ, Ash DV, Brown SB. Superficial photodynamic therapy with topical 5-aminolaevulinic acid for superficial primary and secondary skin cancer. *Br J Cancer* 1994;69:605–608.

Daoud MS, Fett DL, Gloster HM, Roenigk RK. Micrographic surgery for the removal of squamous cell carcinoma of the ear. In: *American College of Mohs Micrographic Surgery and Cutaneous Oncology*. Hilton Head, SC, 1995.

Dinehart SM, Pollack SV. Metastases from squamous cell carcinoma of the skin and lip. *J Am Acad Dermatol* 1989;21:241–248.

Dzubow LM, Rigel DS, Robins P. Risk factors for local recurrence of primary cutaneous squamous cell carcinoma. *Arch Dermatol* 1982;118:900–902.

Edwards L, Berman B, Rapini RP, Whiting DA, Tyring S, Greenway HJ, Eyre SP, Tanner DJ, Taylor EL, Peets E., et al. Treatment of cutaneous squamous cell carcinomas by intralesional interferon alpha-2b therapy. *Arch Dermatol* 1992;128:1486–1489.

Frankel DH, Hanusa BH, Zitelli JA. New primary nonmelanoma skin cancer in patients with a history of squamous cell carcinoma of the skin. Implications and recommendations for follow-up. *J Am Acad Dermatol* 1992;26:720–726.

Guthrie TJ, Porubsky ES, Luxenberg MN, Shah KJ, Wurtz KL, Watson PR. Cisplatin-based chemotherapy in advanced basal and squamous cell carcinomas of the skin: results in 28 patients including 13 patients receiving multimodality therapy. *J Clin Oncol* 1990;8:342–346.

Hruza GJ. Mohs micrographic surgery local recurrences. *J Dermatol Surg Oncol* 1994;20:573–577.

Johnson TM, Rowe DE, Nelson BR, Swanson NA. Squamous cell carcinoma of the skin (excluding lip and oral mucosa). *J Am Acad Dermatol* 1992;26:467–484.

Joseph MG, Zulueta WP, Kennedy PJ. Squamous cell carcinoma of the skin of the trunk and limbs: the incidence of metastases and their outcome. *Aust NZ J Surg* 1992;62:697–701.

Kuflik EG, Gage AA. The five-year cure rate achieved by cryosurgery for skin cancer. *J Am Acad Dermatol* 1991;24:1002–1004.

Lippman SM, Parkinson DR, Itri LM, Weber RS, Schantz SP, Ota DM, Schusterman MA, Krakoff IH, Gutterman JU, Hong WK. 13-cis-Retinoic acid and interferon alpha-2a: effective combination therapy for advanced squamous cell carcinoma of the skin. *J Natl Cancer Inst* 1992;84:235–241.

McCaughan JJ. Photodynamic therapy of skin and esophageal cancers. *Cancer Invest* 1990;8:407–416.

Mehregan DA, Roenigk RK. Management of superficial squamous cell carcinoma of the lip with Mohs micrographic surgery. *Cancer* 1990;66:463–468.

Miller PK, Roenigk RK, Brodland DG, Randle HW. Cutaneous micrographic surgery: Mohs procedure. *Mayo Clin Proc* 1992;67:971–980.

Mohs F, Larson P, Iriondo M. Micrographic surgery for the microscopically controlled excision of carcinoma of the external ear. *J Am Acad Dermatol* 1988;19:729–737.

Mohs FE, Zitelli JA. Microscopically controlled surgery in the treatment of carcinoma of the scalp. *Arch Dermatol* 1981;117:764–769.

Preston DS, Stern RS. Nonmelanoma cancers of the skin. *N Engl J Med* 1992;23:1649–1662.

Robins P, Dzubow LM, Rigel DS. Squamous-cell carcinoma treated by Mohs' surgery: an experience with 414 cases in a period of 15 years. *J Dermatol Surg Oncol* 1981;7:800–801.

Roenigk RK, Ratz JL, Bailin PL, Wheeland RG. Trends in the presentation and treatment of basal cell carcinomas. *J Dermatol Surg Oncol* 1986;12:860–865.

Roenigk RK, Roenigk HH, Jr., eds. *Dermatologic Surgery: Principles and Practice*. New York, Marcel Dekker, Inc., 1989.

Rowe DE, Carroll RJ, Day CL. Prognostic factors for local recurrence, metastasis, and survival rates in squamous cell carcinoma of the skin, ear, and lip. *J Am Acad Dermatol* 1992;26:976–990.

Sadek H, Azli N, Wendling JL, et al. Treatment of advanced squamous cell carcinoma of the skin with cisplatin, 5-fluorouracil, and bleomycin. *Cancer* 1990;66:1692–1696.

Salasche SJ, Cheney ML, Varvares MA. Recognition and management of the high-risk cutaneous squamous cell carcinoma. *Curr Probl Dermatol* 1993;5:141–192.

Melanoma

Aebersold P, Hyatt C, Johnson S, et al. Lysis of autologous melanoma cells by tumor-infiltrating lymphocytes: association with clinical response. *J Natl Cancer Inst* 1993;85:622–632.

American Joint Committee on Cancer. *Manual for Staging of Cancer*. 2nd ed. Philadelphia, JB Lippincott, 1983.

Balch CM. The role of elective lymph node dissection in melanoma: rationale, results, and controversies. *J Clin Oncol* 1988;6:163–172.

Balch CM, Houghton AN, Peters LJ. Cutaneous melanoma. In: *Cancer: Principles and Practice of Oncology*. DeVita VT, Hellman S, Rosenberg SA, eds. Philadelphia, J.B. Lippincott Co., 1993, pp. 1612–1661.

Balch CM, Murad TM, Soong S-J, et al. A multifactorial analysis of melanoma. Prognostic histopathological features comparing Clark's and Breslow's staging methods. *Ann Surg* 1978;188:732–742.

Balch CM, Murad TM, Soong S-J, et al. Tumor thickness as a guide to surgical management of clinical stage I melanoma patients. *Cancer* 1979;43:883–888.

Balch CM, Soong S-J, Milton GW, et al. A comparison of prognostic factors and surgical results in 1,786 patients with localized (stage I) melanoma treated in Alabama, USA, and New South Wales, Australia. *Ann Surg* 1982;196:677–684.

Balch CM, Soong S-J, Murad TM, et al. A multifactorial analysis of melanoma.II. Prognostic factors in patients with stage I (localized) melanoma. *Surgery* 1979;86:343–351.

Balch CM, Soong S-J, Murad TM, et al. A multifactorial analysis of melanoma. IV. Prognostic factors in 200 melanoma patients with distant metastases (Stage III). *J Clin Oncol* 1983;1:126–134.

Balch CM, Soong S-J, Shaw HM, et al. An analysis of prognostic factors in 8500 patients with cutaneous melanoma. In: *Cutaneous Melanoma*. 2nd ed. Balch CM, Houghton AN, Milton GW, et al., eds. Philadelphia, J.B. Lippincott Co., 1992, pp. 165–187.

Balch CM, Soong S-J, Shaw HM, et al. Changing trends in the clinical and pathologic features of melanoma. In: *Cutaneous Melanoma*. 2nd ed. Balch CM, Houghton AN, Milton GW, et al., eds. Philadelphia, J.B. Lippincott Co., 1992, pp. 40–45.

Balch CM, Urist MM, Karakousis CP, et al. The efficacy of 2-cm margins for intermediate-thickness melanomas (1–4mm): results of a multi-institutional randomized surgical trial. *Ann Surg* 1993;218:262–267.

Barth A, Morton DL. The role of adjuvant therapy in melanoma management. *Cancer* 1995;75:726–734.

Breslow A. Thickness, cross-sectional areas and depth of invasion in the prognosis of cutaneous melanoma. *Ann Surg* 1970;172:902–908.

Breslow A, Macht SD. Optimal size of resection margin for thin cutaneous melanoma. *Surg Gynecol Obstet* 1977;145:691–692.

Callaway MP, Briggs JC. The incidence of late recurrence (greater than 10 years); an analysis of 536 consecutive cases of cutaneous melanoma. *Br J Plastic Surg* 1989;42:46–49.

Carmichael VE, Robins RE, Wilson KS. Elective and therapeutic regional lymph node dissection for cutaneous malignant melanoma: experience of the British Columbia cancer agency. *Can J Surg* 1992;35:600–604.

Cascinelli N, Van der Esch EP, Breslow A, et al. Stage I melanoma of the skin: the problem of resection margins. *Eur J Cancer* 1980;16:1079–1085.

Clark WH, Elder DE, Guerry D, et al. Model predicting survival in stage I melanoma based on tumor progression. *J Natl Cancer Inst* 1989;81:1893–1904.

Crowley NJ, Seigler HF. Late recurrence of malignant melanoma. Analysis of 168 patients. *Ann Surg* 1990;212:173–177.

Day CL, Jr, Lew RA. Malignant melanoma prognostic factors 3: surgical margins. *J Dermatol Surg Oncol* 1983;9:797–801.

Day CL, Jr, Mihm MC, Jr, Lew RA, et al. Cutaneous malignant melanoma: prognostic guidelines for physicians and patients. *CA* 1982;32:113–122.

Day CL, Jr, Mihm MC, Jr, Lew RA, et al. Prognostic factors for patients with clinical stage I melanoma of intermediate thickness (1.51-3.99 mm). A conceptual model for tumor growth and metastasis. *Ann Surg* 1982;195:35–43.

Day CL, Jr, Mihm MC, Jr, Sober AJ, et al. Narrower margins for clinical stage I malignant melanoma. *N Engl J Med* 1982;306:479–482.

Day Cl, Jr, Sober AJ, Kopf AW, et al. A prognostic model for clinical stage I melanoma of the upper extremity. The importance of anatomic subsites in predicting recurrent disease. *Ann Surg* 1981;193:436–440.

Day CL, Jr, Sober AJ, Kopf AW, et al. A prognostic model for clinical stage I melanoma of the lower extremity. Location on foot as independent risk factor for recurrent disease. *Surgery* 1981;89:599–603.

Day CL, Jr, Sober AJ, Kopf AW, et al. A prognostic model for clinical stage I melanoma of the trunk: location near midline is not an independent risk factor for recurrent disease. *Am J Surg* 1981;142:247–251.

Drzewiecki KT, Anderson PK. Survival with malignant melanoma. A regression analysis of prognostic factors. *Cancer* 1982;49:2414–2419.

Einzig AI, Hochster H, Wiernik PH, et al. A phase II study of taxol in patients with malignant melanoma. *Invest New Drugs* 1991;9:59–64.

Elder DE, Gverry D, Heiberger RM, et al. Optimal resection margin for cutaneous malignant melanoma. *Plast Reconstr Surg* 1983;71:66–72.

Eldh J, Boeryd B, Peterson LE. Prognostic factors in cutaneous malignant melanoma in stage I. A clinical, morphological and multivariate analysis. *Scand J Plast Reconstr Surg* 1978;12:243–255.

Falkson CI, Falkson G, Falkson HC. Improved results with the addition of interferon alpha-2b to decarbazine in the treatment of patients with metastatic malignant melanoma. *J Clin Oncol* 1991;9:1403–1408.

Fewkes J, Mohs FE. Microscopically controlled surgical excision (the Mohs technique). In: *Dermatology in General Medicine*. 3rd ed. Fitzpatrick TB, Eisen AZ, Wolff K, et al., eds. New York, McGraw-Hill, 1987, pp. 2557–2563.

Gajetta E, Di Leo A, Zampino MG, et al. Multicenter randomized trial of dacarbazine alone or in combination with two different doses and schedules of interferon alpha-2a in the treatment of advanced melanoma. *J Clin Oncol* 1994;12:806–811.

Hafstrom L, Rudenstam CM, Blomquist E, et al. Regional hyperthermic perfusion with melphalan after surgery for recurrent malignant melanoma of the extremities. *J Clin Oncol* 1991;9:2091–2094.

Hill GJ II, Moss SE, Golomb FM, et al. DTIC and combination therapy for melanoma. DTIC [NSC 45388] surgical adjuvant study COG protocol 7040. *Cancer* 1981;47:2557–2562.

Johnson TM, Smith JW II, Nelson BR, Chang A. Current therapy for cutaneous melanoma. *J Am Acad Dermatol* 1995;32:689–707.

Karakousis CP, Velez A, Driscoll DL, et al. Metastasectomy in malignant melanoma. *Surgery* 1994;115:295–302.

Kaspar TA, Wagner RF, Jr. Mohs micrographic surgery for thin stage I malignant melanoma: rationale for a modern management strategy. *Cutis* 1991;50:350–351.

Koh KH. Cutaneous melanoma. *N Engl J Med* 1991;325:171–182.

Koh K, Michalik E, Sober AJ, et al. Lentigo maligna melanoma has no better prognosis than other types of melanoma. *J Clin Oncol* 1984;2:994–1001.

Legha SS, Ring S, Papadopoulos N, et al. A phase II trial of taxol in patients with malignant melanoma. *Cancer* 1990;65:2478–2481.

Little JH, Holt J, Davis N. Changing epidemiology of malignant melanoma in Queensland. *Med J Aust* 1980;1:66–69.

Mansson-Brahme E, Carstensen J, Erhardt K, et al. Prognostic factors in thin cutaneous melanoma. *Cancer* 1994;73:2324–2332.

McCarthy WH, Shaw HM, Thompson JF, et al. Time and frequency of recurrence of cutaneous stage I malignant melanoma with guidelines for follow-up study. *Surg Gynecol Obstet* 1988;166:497–502.

McClay EF, Mastrangelo MJ, Spradnio JD, et al. The importance of tamoxifen to a cisplatin-containing regimen in the treatment of metastatic melanoma. *Cancer* 1989;63:1292–1295.

McGovern VJ, Shaw HM, Milton GW, et al. Is malignant melanoma arising in a Hutchinson's melanotic freckle a separate disease entity? *Histopathology* 1980;4:235–242.

Mohs FE. *Chemosurgery: Microscopically Controlled Surgery for Skin Cancer*. Springfield, IL, Charles C Thomas, 1978.

Mohs FE. Fixed-tissue micrographic surgery for melanoma of the ear. *Arch Otolaryngol Head Neck Surg* 1988;114:625–631.

Mohs FE, Bloom RF, Sahl WL. Chemosurgery for familial malignant melanoma. *J Dermatol Surg Oncol* 1979;5:127–131.

Myerskens FL, Jr, Berdeaux DH, Parks B, et al. Cutaneous malignant melanoma (Arizona Cancer Center experience).I. Natural history and prognostic factors influencing survival in patients with stage I disease. *Cancer* 1988;62:1207–1214.

National Institutes of Health Consensus Development Panel on Early Melanoma. Diagnosis and treatment of early melanoma. *JAMA* 1992;286:1314–1319.

Pontikes LA, Temple WJ, Cassar SL, et al. Influence of the level and depth on recurrence rates in thin melanomas. *Am J Surg* 1993;165:225–228.

Prade M, Bognel C, Charpentier P, et al. Malignant melanoma of the skin: prognostic factors derived from a multifactorial analysis of 239 cases. *Am J Dermatopathol* 1982;4:411–412.

Pyrhonen S, Hahka-Kemppinen M, Muhonen T. A promising interferon plus four-drug chemotherapy regimen for metastatic melanoma. *J Clin Oncol* 1992;10:1919–1926.

Reintgen DS, Vollmer R, Tso CY, et al. Prognosis for recurrent stage I malignant melanoma. *Arch Surg* 1987;122:1338–1342.

Rosenberg SA, Yang JC, Topalian SL, et al. Treatment of 283 consecutive patients with metastatic melanoma or renal cell cancer using high-dose bolus interleukin 2. *JAMA* 1994;271:907–913.

Schmoeckel C, Bockelbrink A, Bockelbrink H, et al. Low- and high-risk malignant melanoma—I. Evaluation of clinical and histological prognosticators in 585 cases. *Eur J Cancer Clin Oncol* 1983;19:227–235.

Schmoeckel C, Bockelbrink A, Bockelbrink H, et al. Low- and high-risk malignant melanoma—II. Multivariate analyses for a prognostic classification. *Eur J Cancer Clin Oncol* 1983;19:237–243.

Schmoeckel C, Bockelbrink A, Bockelbrink H, et al. Low- and high-risk malignant melanoma—III. Prognostic significance of resection margin. *Eur J Cancer Clin Oncol* 1983;19:245–249.

Shea TC, Antman KH, Elder JP, et al. Malignant melanoma. Treatment with high-dose combination alkylating agent chemotherapy and autologous bone marrow transplantation. *Arch Dermatol* 1988;52:1792–1802.

Shumate CR, Carlson GW, Giacco GG, et al. The prognostic implications of location for scalp melanoma. *Am J Surg* 1991;162:315–319.

Sim FH, Taylor WF, et al. A prospective randomized study of the efficacy of routine elective lymphadenectomy in management of malignant melanoma. Preliminary results. *Cancer* 1978;41:948–956.

Sim FH, Taylor WF, Pritchard DJ, et al. Lymphadenectomy in the management of stage I malignant melanoma: a prospective randomized trial. *Mayo Clin Proc* 1986;61:697–705.

Slingluff CL Jr, Dodge RK, Stanley WE, et al. The annual risk of melanoma progression: implications for the concept of cure. *Cancer* 1992;70:1917–1927.

Thompson DB, Adena M, McLeod GR. Interferon alpha-2a does not improve response or survival when compared with dacarbazine in metastatic malignant melanoma: results of a multiinstitutional Australian randomized trial. *Melanoma Res* 1993;3:133–138.

Thorn M, Ponten F, Berstrome, et al. Clinical and histopathologic predictors of survival in patients with malignant melanoma: a population-based study in Sweden. *J Natl Cancer Inst* 1994;86:761–769.

van der Esch EP, Cascinelli N, Preda F, et al. Stage I melanoma of the skin: evaluation of prognosis according to histologic characteristics. *Cancer* 1981;48:1668–1673.

Veronesi U, Adamus J, Aubert C, et al. A randomized trial of adjuvant chemotherapy and immunotherapy in cutaneous melanoma. *N Engl J Med* 1982;307:913–916.

Veronesi U, Adamus J, Bandiera DC, et al. Delayed regional lymph node dissection in stage I melanoma of the skin of the lower extremities. *Cancer* 1982;49:2420–2430.

Veronesi U, Adamus J, Bandiera DC, et al. Inefficacy of immediate node dissection in stage I melanoma of the limbs. *N Engl J Med* 1977;297:627–630.

Veronesi U, Adamus J, Bandiera DC, et al. Stage I melanoma of the limbs: immediate versus delayed node dissection. *Tumori* 1980;66:373–396.

Veronesi U, Cascinelli N. Narrow excision (1-cm margin): a safe procedure for thin cutaneous melanoma. *Arch Surg* 1991;126:438–441.

Veronesi U, Cascinelli N, Adamus J, et al. Thin stage I primary cutaneous malignant melanoma. Comparison of excision with margins of 1 or 3 cm. *N Engl J Med* 1988;318:1159–1162.

Vollmer RT. A multivariate analysis of prognostic factors. *Pathol Ann* 1989;24:383–407.

Wong JH, Skinner KA, Kin KA, et al. The role of surgery in the treatment of nonregionally recurrent melanoma. *Surgery* 1993;113:389–394.

Zeitels J, LaRossa D, Hamilton R, et al. A comparison of local recurrence and resection margins for stage I primary cutaneous malignant melanomas. *Plast Reconstr Surg* 1988;81:688–693.

Zitelli JA. Mohs surgery for melanoma. In: *Mohs Micrographic Surgery*. Mikhail GR, ed. Philadelphia, W.B. Saunders, 1991, pp. 275–288.

Zitelli JA, Mohs FE, Snow S. Mohs micrographic surgery for melanoma. *Dermatol Clin* 1989;7:833–843.

Soft Tissue Sarcomas

Broders AC, Hargrave R, Meyerding HW. Pathologic features of soft tissue fibrosarcoma with special reference to the grading of its malignancy. *Surg Gynecol Obstet* 1939;69:267–280.

Brown MD, Swanson NA. Treatment of malignant fibrous histiocytoma and atypical fibrous xanthomas with micrographic surgery. *J Dermatol Surg Oncol* 1989;15:1287–1292.

Brown MD, Zachary CB, Grekin RC, et al. Genital tumors: their management by micrographic surgery. *J Am Acad Dermatol* 1988;18:115–122.

Cantin J, McNeer GP, Chu FC, et al. The problem of local recurrence after treatment of soft tissue sarcoma. *Ann Surg* 1968;168:47–53.

Chang AE, Sondak VK. Clinical evaluation and treatment of soft tissue tumors. In: *Soft Tissue Tumors*. Enzinger FM, Weiss SW, eds. St. Louis, Mosby, 1995, pp. 17–38.

Costa J, Wesley RA, Glatstein E, et al. The grading of soft tissue sarcomas. Results of a clinicohistopathologic correlation in a series of 163 cases. *Cancer* 1984;53:530–541.

Davidson LL, Frost ML, Hanke CW, et al. Primary leiomyosarcoma of the skin. *J Am Acad Dermatol* 1989;21:1156–1160.

Elias AD, Antman KH. Adjuvant chemotherapy for soft-tissue sarcoma: a critical appraisal. *Semin Surg Oncol* 1988;4:59–65.

Enneking WF. *Musculoskeletal Tumor Surgery*. New York, Churchill Livingstone, 1983.

Enneking WF, Spanier SS, Malawer MM. The effect of the anatomic setting on the results of surgical procedures for soft parts sarcoma of the thigh. *Cancer* 1981;47:1005–1022.

Enzinger FM. Clinicopathological correlation in soft tissue sarcomas. In: *Management of Soft Tissue and Bone Sarcomas*. New York, Raven Press, 1986.

Enzinger FM, Weiss SW. General consideration. In: *Soft Tissue Tumors*. Enzinger FM, Weiss SW, eds. St. Louis, Mosby, 1995, pp. 1–16.

Fields JP, Helwig EB. Leiomyosarcoma of the skin and subcutaneous tissue. *Cancer* 1981;47:156–169.

Fong Y, Coit DG, Woodruff JM, et al. Lymph node metastasis from soft tissue sarcoma in adults. Analysis of data from a prospective database of 1772 sarcoma patients. *Ann Surg* 1993;217:72–77.

Geer RJ, Woodruff J, Caspar ES, et al. Management of small soft-tissue sarcoma of the extremity in adults. *Arch Surg* 1992;127:1285–1289.

Gloster HM, Harris KR, Roenigk RK. A comparison between Mohs' micrographic surgery and wide surgical excision for the treatment of dermatofibrosarcoma protuberans. *J Am Acad Dermatol* (in press).

Gustafson P. Soft tissue sarcoma. Epidemiology and prognosis in 508 patients. *Acta Otrhop Scand* 1994;259(suppl):1–31.

Hanke CW, Lee MW. Treatment of rare malignancies. In: *Mohs Micrographic Surgery*. Mikhail GR, ed. Philadelphia, W.B. Saunders, 1991, pp. 265–267.

Hashimoto H, Diamaru Y, Takeshita S, et al. Prognostic significance of histologic parameters of soft tissue sarcomas. *Cancer* 1992;70:2816–2822.

Hess KA, Hanke CW, Estes NC, et al. Chemosurgical reports: myxoid dermatofibrosarcoma protuberans. *J Dermatol Surg Oncol* 1985;11:268–271.

Hobbs ER, Wheeland RG, Bailin PL, et al. Treatment of dermatofibrosarcoma protuberans with Mohs micrographic surgery. *Ann Surg* 1988;207:102–107.

Huth JF, Eilber FR. Patterns of metastatic spread following resection of extremity soft-tissue sarcomas and strategies for treatment. *Semin Surg Oncol* 1988;4:20–26.

Iacobucci JJ, Stevenson TR, Swanson NA, et al. Cutaneous leiomyosarcoma. *Ann Plast Surg* 1987;19:552–554.

Lawrence W Jr, Donegan WL, Natarajan N, et al. Adult soft tissue sarcomas. A pattern of care survey of the American College of Surgeons. *Ann Surg* 1987;205:349–359.

Mandard AM, Chasle JC, Mandard JC, et al. The pathologist's role in a multidisciplinary approach for soft part tissue sarcoma: a reappraisal (39 cases). *J Surg Oncol* 1981;17:69–81.

Marcus SG, Merino MJ, Glatstein E, et al. Long-term outcome in 87 patients with low-grade soft tissue sarcoma. *Arch Surg* 1993;128:1336–1343.

Markhede G, Angervall L, Stener B. A multivariate analysis of the prognosis after surgical treatment of malignant soft-tissue tumors. *Cancer* 1982;49:1721–1733.

Mikhail GR, Kelly AP Jr. Malignant angioendothelioma of the face. *J Dermatol Surg Oncol* 1977;3:181–183.

Mikhail GR, Lynn BH. Dermatofibrosarcoma protuberans. *J Dermatol Surg Oncol* 1978;4:81–84.

Myhre Jensen O, Kaae S, Hjollund Madsen E, et al. Histopathological grading in soft-tissue tumors. *Acta Pathol Microbiol Immunol Scand* 1983;91A:145–150.

Owens JC, Shiu MH, Smith R, et al. Soft tissue sarcomas of the hand and foot. *Cancer* 1985;55:2010–2018.

Padilla RS, Shimazu C. Malignant Schwannoma treated by Mohs surgical excision. *J Dermatol Surg Oncol* 1991;17:793–796.

Peabody TD, Monson D, Montag A, et al. A comparison of the prognosis for deep and subcutaneous sarcomas of the extremities. *J Bone Joint Surg* 1994;76A:1167–1173.

Peters CW, Hanke CW, Pasarell HA, et al. Chemosurgical reports. Dermatofibrosarcoma protuberans of the face. *J Dermatol Surg Oncol* 1982;8:823–826.

Potter DA, Glenn J, Kinsella T, et al. Patterns of recurrence in patients with high-grade soft-tissue sarcomas. *J Clin Oncol* 1985;3:353–366.

Potter DA, Kinsella T, Glatstein E, et al. High-grade soft tissue sarcomas of the extremities. *Cancer* 1986;58:190–205.

Robinson JK. Dermatofibrosarcoma protuberans resected by Mohs' surgery (chemosurgery). *J Am Acad Dermatol* 1985;12:1093–1098.

Rosenberg SA, Suit HD, Baker LH. Sarcomas of soft tissues. In: *Cancer: Principles and Practice of Oncology*. DeVita VT, Hellman S, Rosenberg SA, eds. Philadelphia, J.B. Lippincott, 1985, pp 1243–1291.

Rosenberg SA, Tepper J, et al. The treatment of soft-tissue sarcomas of the extremities. Prospective randomized evaluations of (1) limb-sparing surgery plus radiation therapy compared with amputation and (2) the role of adjuvant chemotherapy. *Ann Surg* 1982;196:305–315.

Rydholm A, Gustafson P, Rooser B, et al. Limb-sparing surgery without radiotherapy based on the anatomic location of soft tissue sarcoma. *J Clin Oncol* 1991;9:1757–1765.

Simon MA, Enneking WF. The management of soft-tissue sarcomas of the extremities. *J Bone Joint Surg* 1976;58A:317–327.

Suit HD, Mankin HJ, Wood WC, et al. Treatment of the patient with stage M_0 soft tissue sarcoma. *J Clin Oncol* 1988;6:854–862.

Tepper JE, Suit HD. Radiation therapy of soft tissue sarcomas. *Cancer* 1985;55:2273–2277.

Verazin GT, Warneke JA, Driscoll DL, et al. Resection of lung metastases from soft-tissue sarcomas. *Arch Surg* 1992;127:1407–1411.

44

Random Pattern Flaps

Ronald G. Wheeland
University of New Mexico, Albuquerque, New Mexico

A skilled dermatologic surgeon quickly learns that the simplest and easiest repair for a cutaneous wound frequently results in fewer complications, faster healing, and minimal scarring. Yet there are many cases in which simple primary closure would fail to yield a desirable result because of the size of the wound or its anatomic location. In these circumstances more complex repairs with the use of local flaps may be required to obtain the most satisfactory functional and cosmetic result. It is important to understand the appropriate applications of several local random pattern cutaneous flaps. This greatly expands the number of surgical therapeutic options available to repair a cutaneous defect best. The basic concepts and principles of local flap repair and various clinical applications will be discussed.

A flap is defined as skin and its subcutaneous tissue with its own intact vascular supply moved from its original location to another. Movement of this type is possible due to the elasticity or redundancy of the skin. The terminology used to describe different types of flaps is confusing since many different names have been used to describe the same type of flap.

In general, flaps are named according to their proximity to the defect: local or distant (Table 1). Most local flaps are random pattern flaps since the vascularity is not based on a single blood vessel but arises from the deep dermal plexus. Local random pattern flaps are named according to the prevailing motion it makes to fill the adjacent defect (sliding, stretching, or pivoting). All local flaps present some combinatin of these basic types of movement. Typically, these flaps are divided into advancement or sliding flaps, rotational flaps that pivot in an arc about a point, or transpositional flaps.

A second major type of flap is known as the regional flap. It is moved into the wound from the same general anatomic area as a defect; however, this flap is based on a specific artery. This may also be called an axial pattern flap. The name of the blood vessel that supplies the flap is typically used to name the flap. The temporal artery flap is an example of a regional flap that allows tissue from the temple to be mobilized to fill a defect on the forehead. These flaps are also known as interpolation or pedicle flaps since the intact pedicle that contains the arterial supply

Table 1 Types of Flaps

Local: Random pattern flaps
    Advancement (sliding) flap
    Rotational (pivotal) flap
    Transpositional flap
Regional: Axial pattern flaps
    Temporal artery flap
    Deltopectoral flap
Distant flaps
    Bridging flap
    Tubed flap
Simple flaps
    Epidermis
    Dermis
    Subcutaneous tissue
Compound flaps
    Skin
    Subcutaneous tissue
    Bone (or) cartilage (or) muscle

crosses normal skin. Once circulation has been established from tissue surrounding the defect, the pedicle is divided and the wound revised.

A third major group of flaps includes distant flaps. These flaps are located at a significant distance from the anatomic location of the defect. Most distant flaps require a series of staged procedures to improve flap survival by augmenting circulation through the newly created pedicle. These flaps are typically tubed to bridge normal skin surrounding the defect.

A different classification of flaps divides them into simple or compound. The simple flap is composed of epidermis, dermis, and its attached subcutaneous tissue. The compound flap used for major reconstructive surgery is composed of skin, subcutaneous fat, and either bone, muscle, or cartilage. Flaps used by dermatologic surgeons are almost exclusively the local random pattern type, and this discussion will be limited to these.

REPAIR OF WOUNDS WITH UNEQUAL LENGTH

In order to use flaps, special suturing and wound closure techniques must be understood, because flaps often result in a wound of unequal sides. The first special technique is closure for wounds of unequal length. The simplest method for repairing a wound of this type is by the rule of halves (Fig. 1a). The incision on the longer side is spread out evenly over the entire length of the wound. This is done by placing the first stitch at the center of the excision. Then, the remaining halves are sutured half again to help spread out the excess tissue on the longer side over the remaining length of the wound. This process is repeated until the wound has been closed and all excess tissue has been distributed evenly over the length of the incision.

Burow's Triangle

A second way to close a wound of unequal sides is remove a small triangular piece of tissue, a Burow's triangle, from the longer side, thus decreasing its length (Fig. 1b). This triangular excision can be done anywhere along the longer side of the excision (Fig. 1c). If one recognizes

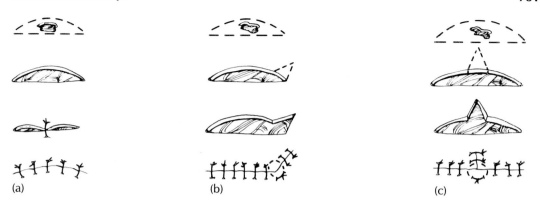

Figure 1 (a) Closing a wound of unequal sides by halves. (b) Closing a wound of unequal sides with a Burow's triangle. (c) Placement of Burow's triangle at any position on long side.

this, the linear closure that results from this triangular excision can frequently be hidden in an adjacent anatomic line, crease, fold, or hairline and does not add to the cosmetic deformity.

Dog Ear Repair

Another technique to remove excess tissue from one side of an unequal wound that puckers is dog ear repair. Dog ears generally result when a wound is closed primarily but the angles at the ends of the incision are greater than 30 degrees. Repair may be done in a number of ways, all of which yield an excellent cosmetic result. The simplest technique (Fig. 2) is to use a skin hook placed in the tip of the dog ear and to pull the tissue to one side. This side is incised with a scalpel extending the original incision. The partially transected piece of tissue is pulled to the opposite side of the suture line and completely incised in the same fashion. The triangular piece of tissue is discarded and the wound closed in a linear fashion.

Another technique is simply to excise the redundant tissue as a new ellipse (Fig. 3). This further extends the length of the original incision line but keeps it oriented in the same direction.

Dog ears can also be removed by creating two small triangles, dividing the apex of the dog ear in half with a scalpel. The redundant tissue from each side is then pulled over the incision line and cut off. Two small triangular pieces of tissue are removed, and the wound is repaired by simple linear closure (Fig. 4).

A recently described technique is the M-plasty (Fig. 5) for repair of dog ears. Curvilinear incisions are made on each side of the redundant tissue. The tissue is then unfolded and allowed to lie flat on top of the wound edge. The excess tissue is excised with a scalpel or sharp scissors as two small triangular pieces. This results in the creation of an M at the end of the incision line. The advantage of this technique is that normal tissue is spared. This results in a shorter incision. It also redirects the incision's orientation at the end and has particular advantages when one is excising close to natural free margins such as the lips or eye.

The Z-plasty may be used to equalize wound margins of different lengths as well. This technique will be discussed in greater detail later in this chapter. One (Fig. 6a) or two Z-plasties (Fig. 6b) can be done at the ends of the long margin of an excision to shorten its effective length.

M-Plasty

The M-plasty is used to shorten the overall length of an incision and is used most typically when one is performing a fusiform excision to a vital anatomic structure, natural body fold, or crease.

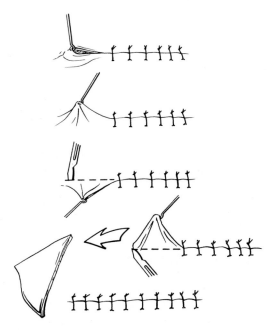

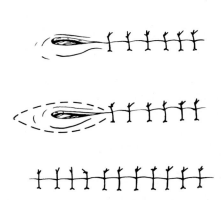

Figure 2 Repair of dog ear deformity by pulling excess tissue to each side of the incision line and removing a single triangular piece of excess tissue.

Figure 3 Correction of dog ear deformity by simple excision.

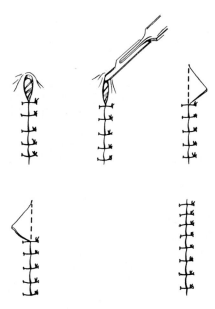

Figure 4 Correction of dog ear deformity by division of dog ear in half and excision of two small triangular pieces of tissue.

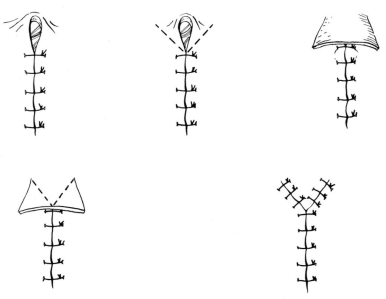

Figure 5 Correction of dog ear deformity with M-plasty.

It is also known as a crown closure because of the shape at the end of the wound. The M-plasty may be performed at one (Fig. 7a) or both ends (Fig. 7b) of an excision. Typically, a standard fusiform excision with 30 degree angles is drawn on the skin. Then two smaller 30 degree angles are drawn within the angle to form an M. These two lines at 30 degree angles are inset into the

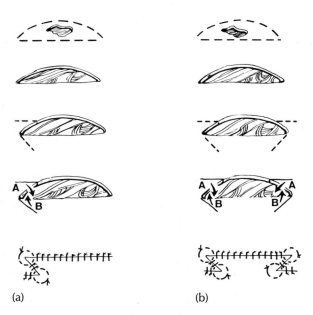

(a)   (b)

Figure 6 (a) Repair of anticipated dog ear from a wound of unequal sides by a single Z-plasty. (b) Repair of a wound of unequal sides with anticipated dog ear deformity with two Z-plasties.

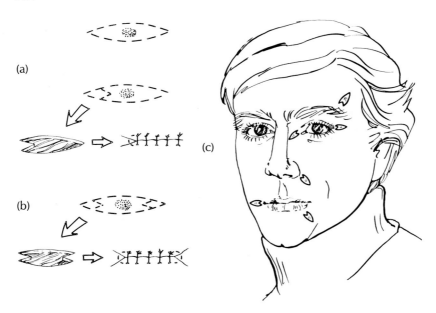

Figure 7 (a) Single M-plasty to shorten a fusiform excision. (b) M-plasty at both ends of excision. (c) M-plasty used at anatomic borders.

apex of the excision to form a rhomboid of equal sides with alternating 30 and 150 degree angles. The M-plasty may be used to remove a dog ear, as previously discussed, but is more typically used to shorten an excision. This is desirable when the excision is near areas such as the ocular canthi or the oral commissures (Fig. 7c). This helps to preserve the symmetry of anatomic structures by creating lines that fit into the natural folds.

Corner Stitch

The technique used most often to suture triangular defects is a half-buried horizontal mattress suture. This is also known as a corner stitch or three-point tie. This stitch is crucial for many of the flaps that will be discussed later. If standard closures are performed, impairment of vascular flow to the tip of the flap may result in necrosis. In addition, if standard simple interrupted suturing techniques are used to close a triangular defect, this may result in depression or elevation of the flap tip that may need to be revised later.

The corner stitch begins as the needle is inserted in the surrounding skin and exits at the middermis (Fig. 8a). The tip of the flap is then punctured with the needle oriented horizontally entirely within the middermis. This is carried across the tip in buried fashion and emerges from the tip at the same depth as its point of entrance. The needle is then rotated back to the traditional position and inserted in the middermis of the adjacent side. It exits on the skin surface and is tied. This stitch results in minimal vascular impairment of the tip and maintains the proper alignment with the surrounding skin. A four-corner stitch is typically used with double advancement flaps, where two rectangles of tissue meet in the middle of the wound. The procedure (Fig. 8b) is similar to that of the three-point stitch except that the additional flap tip is included in the buried horizontal segment.

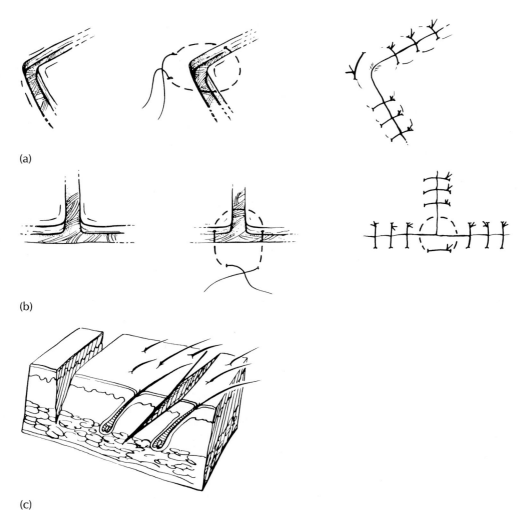

(a)

(b)

(c)

Figure 8 (a) Half-buried mattress suture as corner stitch. (b) Half-buried mattress suture as two-corner stitch. (c) Proper alignment of incision with direction of hair growth.

Undermining

Proper undermining of flaps is important in order to move tissue appropriately. The vascular supply for random pattern flaps is based on the deep dermal plexus. Consequently, the risk of injury to this vascular supply must be minimized. Blunt undermining with scissors and a skin hook is best done at the level of the upper subcutaneous tissue, especially when the location is the face. On the scalp undermining is in the subgaleal plane, and for the extremities undermining is performed within the subcutaneous tissue or fascial plane.

PLANNING WOUND CLOSURE

The next preliminary consideration that must be paramount to the surgeon considering use of a flap for repair of a defect is the relationship of the size and shape of the wound and adjacent donor tissue. Careful planning should begin with an evaluation of the vascular supply for a proposed flap. Vascular supply on the head and neck is usually good, but the length-to-width ratio of the proposed flap must always be considered. Also, elasticity of the adjacent donor tissue must be evaluated for its ability to tolerate tension. In addition, the effect tension from the flap will have on adjacent anatomic structures must be considered. It is important to remember that in addition to the primary defect from removal of the lesion, a secondary defect is also created as the flap is moved. Also, tissue surrounding both the flap and the defect moves in the opposite direction. This movement is known as the secondary motion.

Skin chosen for the flap should be evaluated for color, texture, and the presence or absence of hair. To obtain the best cosmetic result, tissue that closely matches the original tissue should be used.

In order to obtain the best cosmetic and functional result when considering wound closure options in the reconstruction of facial defects, several general aesthetic concepts must not be overlooked. It is always important to first carefully examine the patient's skin to identify the existing tension lines, creases, and natural folds. This will allow the surgeon to make incisions so the resulting scars can be effectively camouflaged by normal facial lines. These lines, also known as Langer's lines, vary from one patient to another but are typically perpendicular to underlying muscles of facial expression. The skin tension lines, which may be present at rest or with motion, can also be utilized to help properly orient the planned repair of the wound or defect. However, if the potential donor reservoir of tissue is of insufficient quantity to permit tensionless wound closure, then all of the preliminary planning will prove to be inadequate and the cosmetic and functional result impaired. The potential reservoirs of donor tissue for local flap reconstructive surgery vary from patient to patient and also with age and the amount of solar damage. However, common donor sites include the glabella, temple, cheek, nasolabial folds, neck, and preauricular area.

Children and teenagers may not have obvious skin tension lines. In this case, remove the lesion as clinically appropriate (usually in a circle). Then undermine the margins; by checking for tension in various directions with skin hooks, the most appropriate direction of closure can be chosen. Ask the patient to smile, frown, or purse the lips, and the natural creases may become more pronounced.

When incisions are to be made in or adjacent to hair-bearing skin, avoid advancing hair-bearing tissue into non-hair-bearing skin. It is also important, especially around the eyebrows or sideburns, that the incision be angled parallel to the hair shafts and not perpendicular to the surface as is typically performed (Fig. 8c). This will minimize transection or injury to hair follicle structures that may result in a permanent patch of alopecia.

TYPES OF RANDOM PATTERN FLAPS

In order to understand local random pattern flaps, remember that while each flap is named for a primary motion used to position it into the defect, there is always secondary motion. In fact, most flaps involve combinations of various types of motion. Illustrations used to represent flap closure use idealized squares, circles, triangles, or other geometric shapes. In fact, many flaps can be modified to fill a defect without converting it into a stylized geometric pattern. In general, flaps can be characterized by their primary motion as advancement, rotation, or transposition.

Advancement Flap

The advancement flap is one with which most dermatologic surgeons are familiar. The simplest fusiform excision can be viewed as a double advancement flap when undermining is necessary to permit tensionless closure. Since tissue from both sides of the excision is advanced to fill the defect, this can be considered a simple type of advancement flap.

Advancement flaps traditionally move in a straight line. This type of movement is possible due to the elasticity of the flap and the adjacent tissue. When one is creating an advancement flap, the tissue is stretched over the defect and the unequal sides of the wound are closed using techniques previously described. Flaps included in this category are the H-flap, U-flap, O–T flap, V–Y flap, and the Burow's triangle flap.

U-Flap

The U-flap, also known as the O–U repair, trapdoor flap, or single advancement flap, is one of the simplest flaps to use since the geometric pattern (Fig. 9) and incision lines can easily be oriented to fit natural folds. In general, this flap should have a length-to-width ratio of no more than 3:1 in order to maintain sufficient vascular supply to nourish the tip of the flap. There are several ways to modify this flap so that even moderate-sized defects can be repaired.

One U-flap that is useful for defects of the nasal tip is the Rintala flap (Fig. 10). This flap, also known as the median glabellar flap, is used to advance glabellar skin in a straight line down the nasal bridge to cover defects of the nasal bridge and tip. The dog ears are excised just above the medial ends of the eyebrows.

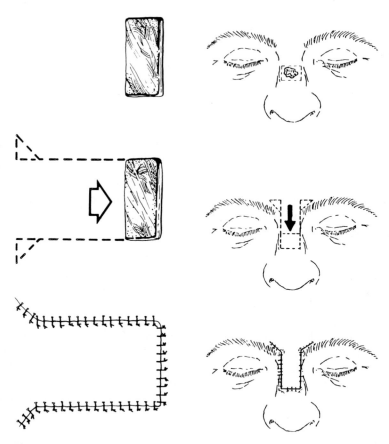

Figure 9   Single advancement, U-flap.

Figure 10   Advancement of Rintala flap along bridge of nose.

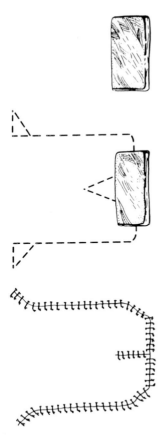

Figure 11 Peng variant of single advancement flap to increase base of pedicle.

A modified U-flap proposed by Peng (Fig. 11) increases the pedicle size to improve flap survival. This flap is designed to advance into and around a defect, and the dog ear is repaired centrally. The large flap pedicle with improved vascular supply has a greater chance of survival.

H-Flap

Synonyms for the H-flap include the double-U, double tab, or double advancement flap (Fig. 12a). This flap is commonly used to repair defects on the forehead (Fig. 12b), within the eyebrow (Fig. 12c), since it permits the remaining hair-bearing portion of the brow to be approximated to avoid alopecia, and on the upper lip (Fig. 12c). Burow's triangles are removed wherever excess tissue is present along the edge of the incision. This incision should be hidden as inconspicuously as possible. Redundant tissue may be distributed evenly along the closure, with suturing by the rule of halves, previously described, to avoid the Burow's triangle.

For a defect in the midline of the upper lip, tissue can be advanced from both lip margins. The Burow's triangles are removed within the nasolabial line (Fig. 12c). The forehead lends itself well to this closure since the incision lines can be placed within the natural folds (Fig. 13). Relatively large amounts of tissue can be mobilized with this flap.

Another location successfully repaired with an advancement flap is the helical rim of the ear (Fig. 14a–c). The helical sulcus is incised to the superior edge of the lobule. Since the lobe of

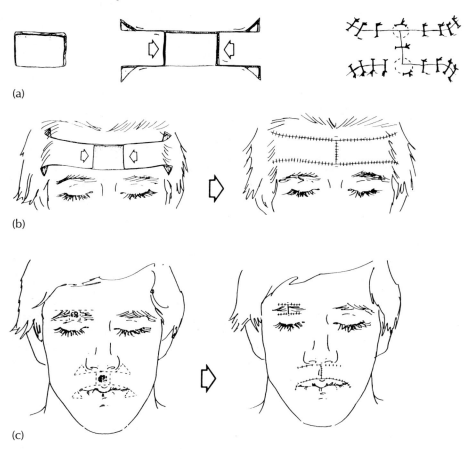

Figure 12 (a) Double advancement, H-flap. (b) H-flap to repair forehead defect. (c) H-flap to repair midbrow defect and upper lip defect.

the ear is mobile, it allows the helix to be advanced upward (Fig. 14d). Removal of a Burow's triangle permits advancement without significant distortion of the ear. The Burow's triangle may include full-thickness cartilage to permit the helical rim to advance without difficulty. A second advancement flap can be created using the superior pole of the helical rim if needed (Fig. 14e).

Defects around the nose or upper lip can frequently be closed with a crescent-shaped advancement flap. Redundant tissue from the cheek is advanced medially and closed along the nasolabial fold (Fig. 15). Large defects may be closed without deforming the base of the ala or the lip. Redundant tissue is removed at the junction of the nose and face at the nasofacial sulcus. A dog ear is excised, tissue from the medial portion of the cheek is undermined, and the triangular flap is advanced.

Burow's Triangle Flap

The Burow's triangle flap can be used to close a defect with tissue mobilized from areas some distance from the wound (Fig. 16). This flap can be visualized as a simple elliptical closure; however, part of the ellipse is separated from the remainder of the ellipse by a distance. This permits redundant tissue from nearby to be moved into the defect. The size of the defect dictates the size of the Burow's triangle and whether or not two triangles are used (Fig. 17). The distance between the defect and where the Burow's triangle is removed is a function of the

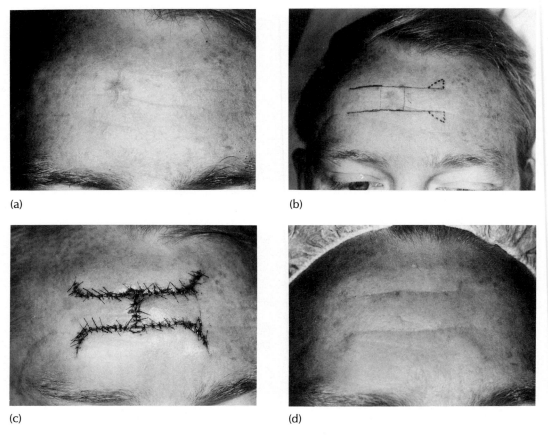

(a)

(b)

(c)

(d)

Figure 13 (a) Scar following curettage and electrodesiccation. (b) Double advancement flap planned. (c) Immediately after closure. (d) Double advancement flap 2 months postoperative.

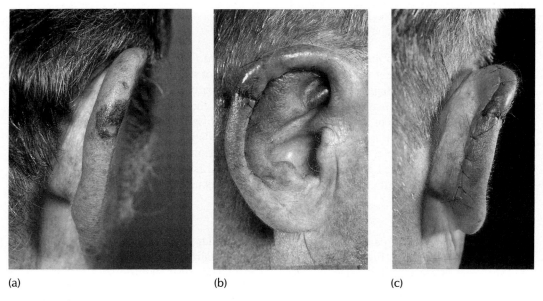

(a)

(b)

(c)

Figure 14 (a) Lentigo maligna melanoma. (b,c) Wide excision and closure with a double advancement flap. (d) Advancement flap of helix. (e) Burow's triangles to reduce ear distortion. (Figure 14a–c courtesy Randall K. Roenigk.)

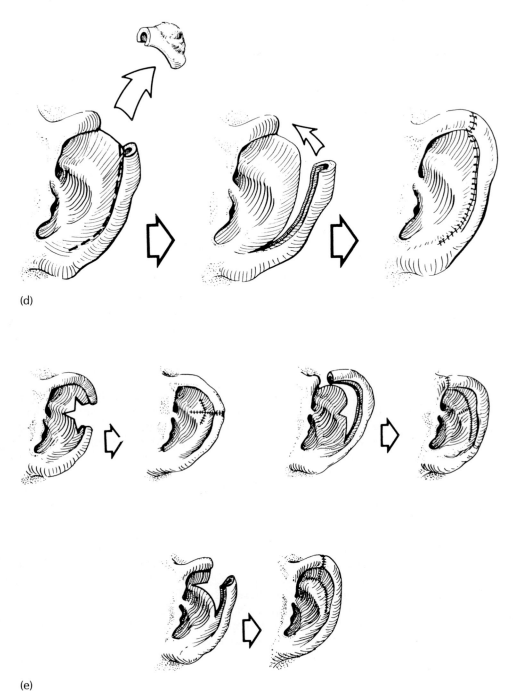

(d)

(e)

Figure 14 Continued

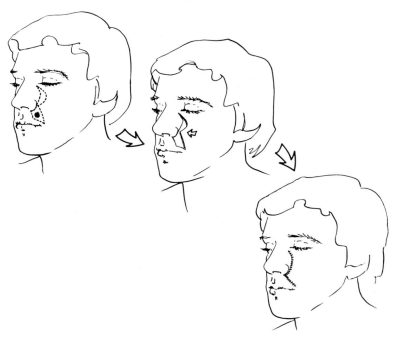

Figure 15 Perialar crescent-shaped advancement flap schematic.

anatomic location and degree of skin laxity. This versatile flap can be used in a number of areas but is especially useful when natural folds can be incorporated into the motion of the flap.

The flap can be modified by increasing or decreasing the distance between the defect and the Burow's triangle to take advantage of excess skin. By placing the Burow's triangle some distance from the defect, distortion of an important structure such as the upper lip or eyebrow is minimized. The secondary defect can be repaired in a less conspicuous tension line (Fig. 18). When two lesions are immediately adjacent to one another and are to be removed in one session, the Burow's triangle flap may be used to close both defects at once by advancing the tissue between them.

O–T or A–T Flap

The O–T or A–T flap is a bilateral advancement flap with incisions made at one end of the defect (Fig. 19). By extending the incision from the base of a triangular defect or the top of a circular defect, the adjacent tissue can be advanced and sutured in a straight line (Fig. 20). Burow's triangles are often necessary to accommodate secondary movement. The two pedicles advanced are broad-based, and there is little risk of vascular impairment. Furthermore, this closure is especially useful to shorten the final length of an ellipse that might otherwise extend across a

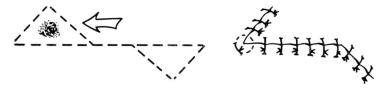

Figure 16 Burow's triangle flap.

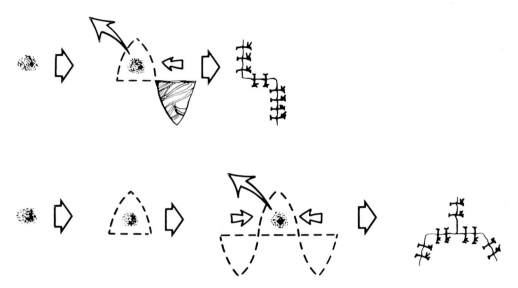

Figure 17 Variants of Burow's triangle flap.

vital anatomic structure such as vermilion border of the lip, eyebrow, or natural crease or fold such as the chin crease or nasolabial fold (Fig. 21). Placing the limbs of the T within a natural fold makes them inconspicuous (Fig. 22). Closure requires use of a four-corner stitch or the half-buried mattress suture previously discussed.

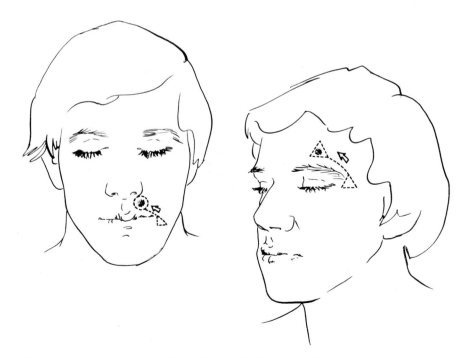

Figure 18 Locations where Burow's triangle flap is useful.

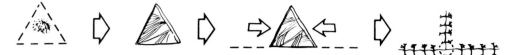

Figure 19   A–T flap used to close a wound.

V–Y or Y–V Advancement Flap

The V–Y advancement flap (Fig. 23) is created by initially making a V-shaped incision and advancing the triangular portion of the flap in a straight line toward its base. The wound is closed in the shape of a Y. This technique increases the overall length of the wound and is beneficial for the correction of wounds that have contracted around the eye or mouth. The lengthening of the scar depends on the size of the V. As a consequence, this may be limited by a desire to keep the incision as short as possible. The flap is closed with a three-point suture to avoid tip necrosis.

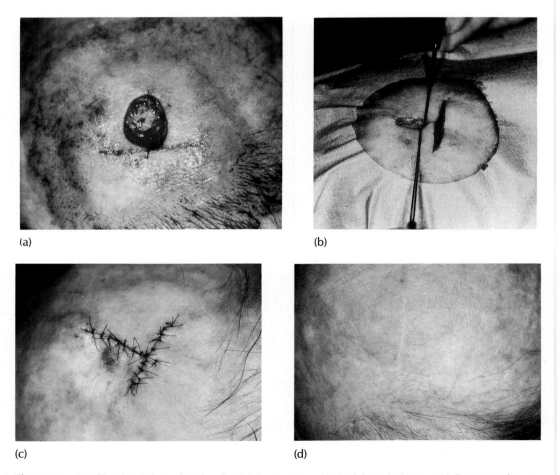

Figure 20   (a) Circular defect of scalp after Mohs surgery. (b) Anticipated closure. (c) Postoperative appearance. (d) Two months postoperative.

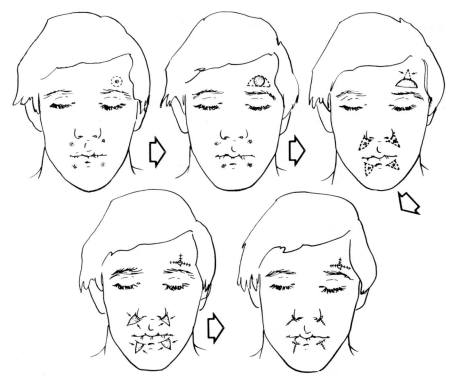

Figure 21 Clinical uses of O–T and A–T advancement flaps.

The Y–V incision is made in a Y-shape, and the tip of the triangular flap is advanced. This variation of the V–Y flap is used to move the oral commissures laterally when some defect has pulled the commissure toward the midline (Fig. 24).

Rotation Flap

The rotation flap is one of the simpler types of random pattern flaps. It uses lateral movement of tissue while at the same time rotating about a pivot point (Figs. 25,26). This flap exploits the elasticity of adjacent skin along the curved portion of the incision line to permit advancement of rather large flaps (Fig. 27). Safety is one major advantage of the rotation flap since it has a broad base, and thus a good vascular supply. Another advantage is that large amounts of tissue from virtually any side of a wound may be moved to close even large defects (Fig. 28). In general, the curved incision lines inherent with the rotation flap are easier to disguise and yield a better cosmetic result than the straight lines that result from repairs with some other flaps. This flap is typically used on the cheek and based inferiorly with advancement and rotation in a forward, medial direction (Fig. 29). By placing the curved incision within relaxed skin tension lines, this flap is relatively easy to camouflage.

The rotation flap is classically shown as a way to close triangular defects (Fig. 30), but it can be used successfully to close round and square defects as well (Fig. 31). Conversion of a round wound into a triangular defect is often not required.

To plan the rotation flap properly, the broad base pedicle should be inferior whenever possible. This maximizes gravitational assistance for both venous and lymphatic drainage. The pivot

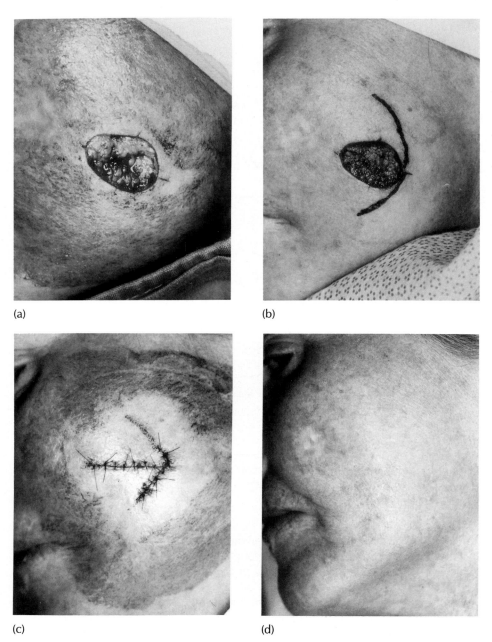

(a)   (b)

(c)   (d)

Figure 22   (a) Oval defect following Mohs surgery. (b) Curvilinear incisions to create the O–T flap. (c) Immediately postoperative. (d) Two months postoperative.

point, through which lies the line of maximum tension, determines the length of the advancing edge. The leading edge should be slightly longer than the length of the distal edge of the defect (Fig. 26). This is especially important for locations where tissue is thick, inelastic, or immobile. If the wound is closed with excess tension, the flap may become ischemic.

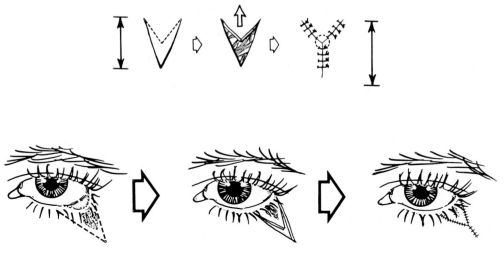

Figure 23 The V–Y flap used to lengthen a scar.

Back Cut

In some circumstances when closing a defect in inelastic tissue, a small back cut is made into the pedicle. This will release tissue for easier closure. The back cut is a relaxing incision (Fig. 32) that helps facilitate rotation. However, this incision may compromise vascularity of the flap since the pedicle has been made narrower.

Secondary movement adjacent to the flap may result in a dog ear. This redundant tissue can be excised at any point along the arc of the flap. Placement of this triangular excision should be planned so that it can be hidden in a natural hairline or skin tension line.

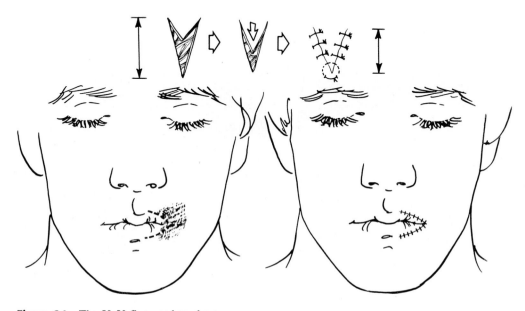

Figure 24 The Y–V flap used to shorten a scar.

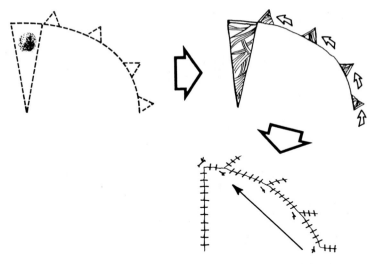

Figure 25   Classic rotation flap with various dog ear correction options. The line of maximal tension is shown.

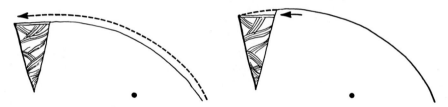

Figure 26   The step-up technique.

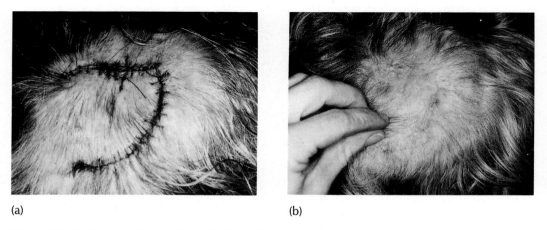

(a)   (b)

Figure 27   (a) Rotation flap of the scalp, immediately postoperative. (b) Six weeks postoperative.

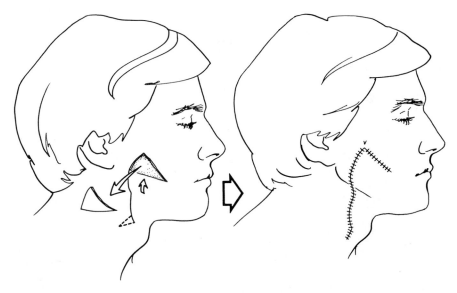

Figure 28   Large rotation flap of inferior cheek.

O–Z Closure

Many variations on the simple rotation flap can be used for wound closure. One of the more common variants is the O–Z closure. This consists of two rotation flaps, one on each side of the defect. Both flaps are rotated into the defect and closed side to side (Fig. 33a). Burow's triangles may be placed anywhere along the incision (Fig. 33b). The O–Z flap is traditionally used to decrease distortion of the anatomy at sites where loose tissue is limited (Fig. 34) on the face or trunk (Fig. 35). Because it does not excise the complete ellipse, the O–Z flap is a method

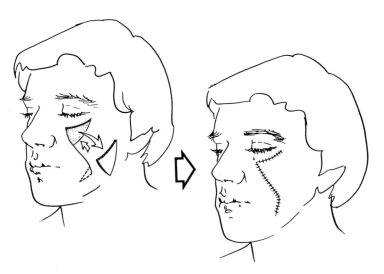

Figure 29   Large inferiorly based rotation flap for superior cheek defect.

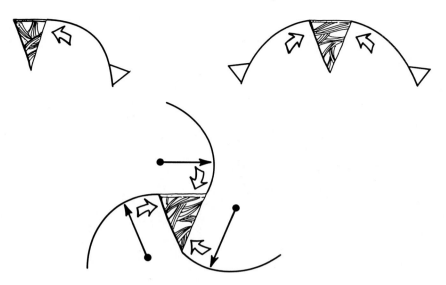

Figure 30   Rotation flaps used for closure of a triangular defect.

for conserving tissue since approximately one-half of the ellipse is not removed. Furthermore, the tension on this closure is parallel to the limbs of the Z. Therefore, this flap can be used when a traditional fusiform excision would distort the adjacent structure. It is commonly used adjacent to the eyebrow where one limb of the Z can be hidden within the hairline. It can also be used along the nasal bridge, adjacent to the free eyelid margin or near the outer canthus.

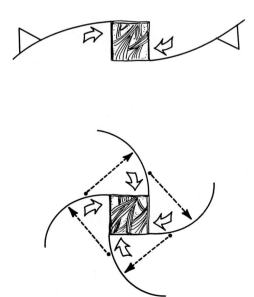

Figure 31   Closure of a square defect with rotation flaps.

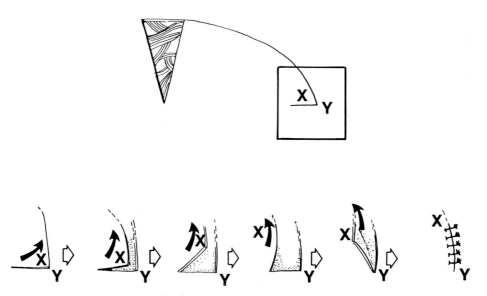

Figure 32   Lengthen the arc of a rotation flap with a back cut.

Glabellar, Anvil, or Banner Flap

This variant of the rotation flap is known as a glabellar flap. Synonyms are the anvil flap, dorsal nasal flap, or Banner flap. Movement of tissue uses excess skin in the glabellar area of the forehead. It is a rotation flap with a prominent back cut (Fig. 36). Tissue from the glabella can be rotated to fill defects of the inner canthus or the nasal root.

Transposition Flap

The transposition flap combines advancement and rotation to pivot about a given point (Fig. 37) without stretching the flap. An advantage of this flap is that the secondary defect can be placed away from the primary wound. The flap can be lifted over a zone of normal skin and moved

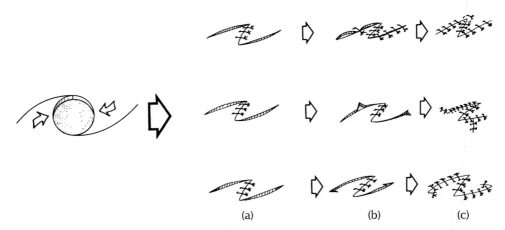

(a)   (b)   (c)

Figure 33   (a) O–Z closure of a circular defect: unequal edges are closed with the halving technique. (b) O–Z flap with Burow's triangles used to close uneven edges. (c) O–Z flap with Z-plasties to close unequal sides.

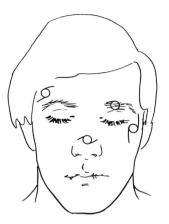

Figure 34   Various uses of O–Z flaps at different anatomic sites.

into a new position (Fig. 38). The main disadvantage of this flap is that it may be difficult to turn a transposition flap more than 90 degrees. Many different transposition flaps will be discussed separately, including the rhomboid or Limberg flap, the nasolabial flap, the labial-ala flap, the bilobed flap, and the Z-plasty.

Rhomboid Flap

The rhomboid flap is one of the most popular transposition flaps because of its versatility, since with proper planning, any one of eight individual flaps can be devised for closure of a given defect (Fig. 39). To design these flaps to allow proper closure, a precise geometric pattern is created. The defect is made into a rhombus, or equilateral parallelogram, with angles of 60 and 120 degrees. An incision is extended perpendicularly, usually from the point of the 120 degree angle. The length of this line is equal to the length of the other sides of the rhombus. Another incision of similar length is made at 60 degrees, parallel to one side of the rhombus. The flap and adjacent tissue are undermined and the flap is then transposed into the primary defect (Fig. 40). This closes not only the original defect but also the secondary defect (Fig. 41) created to develop this flap. The line of maximum tension occurs at the closure point of the secondary defect, so this is where the first stitch is placed.

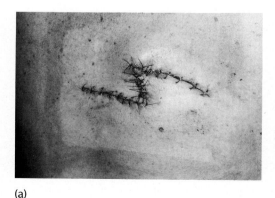

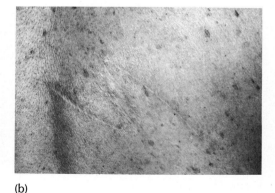

(a)   (b)

Figure 35   (a) Repair of defect on the back with O–Z flap. (b) Six months postoperative.

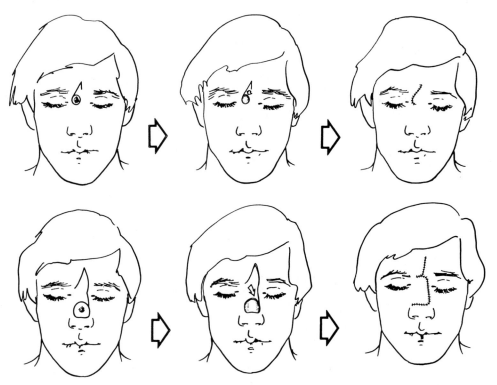

Figure 36 Banner flap variants of rotation flap used to repair a nasal defect: small (top), large (bottom).

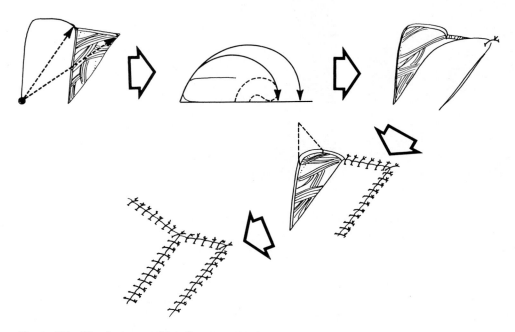

Figure 37 Classic transposition flap movement.

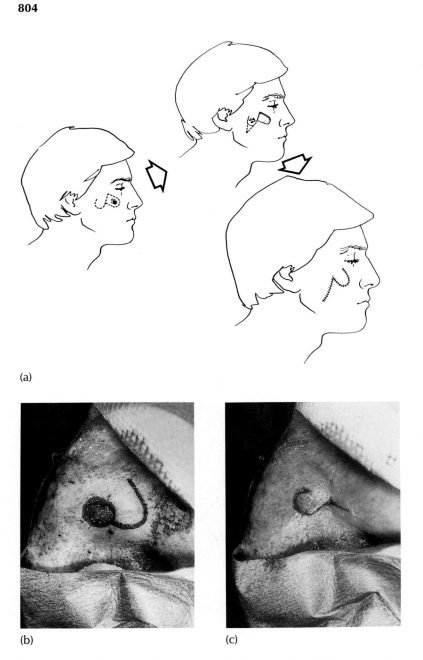

(a)

(b)   (c)

Figure 38 (a) Transposition flap on cheek. (b) Markings indicate planned transposition flap on the nose. (c) Transposed flap after single subcuticular suture. (d) Immediate postoperative appearance. (e) One month postoperative; compare appearance with alar rim defect that healed by second intention.

This flap can actually be used to transpose tissue in any direction (Fig. 42). This allows unlimited possibilities, so excess skin and the tension lines can be maximally considered. Rather than change the defect into a rhombus, a circular defect is maintained. The first incision is made perpendicular to the defect at an appropriate point for closure based on the location of the de-

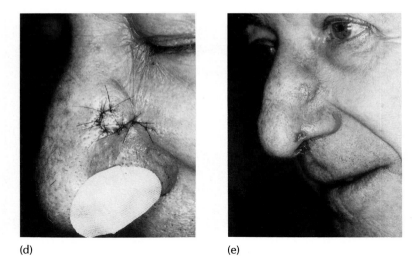

(d) (e)

Figure 38 Continued

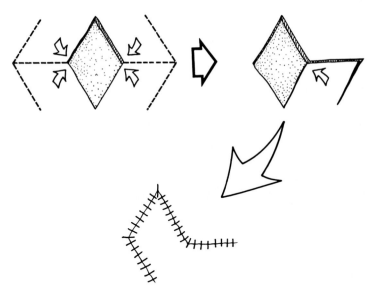

Figure 39 Schematic diagram shows four options available for repair of a rhomboid defect. Four more can be created with incisions from the other two points in the rhomboid.

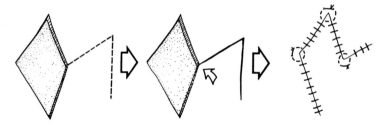

Figure 40 Closure of rhomboid flap.

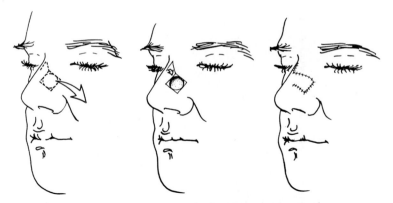

Figure 41   Rhomboid flap for closure of defect on side of nose.

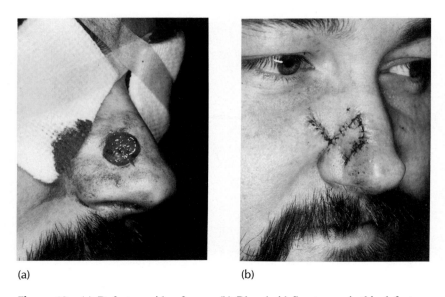

(a)   (b)

Figure 42   (a) Defect on side of nose. (b) Rhomboid flap to repair this defect.

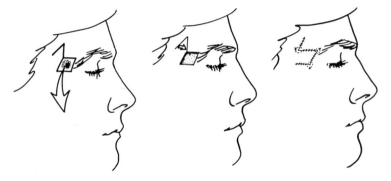

Figure 43   Rhomboid flap for temple defect.

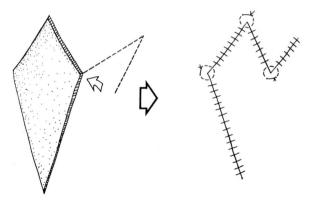

Figure 44 DuFourmental flap.

fect. The length of the incision is approximately equal to the radius of the circle. The second incision is the same length and at a 60 degree angle. After appropriate undermining, the flap is transposed and the circle trimmed and molded to fit the flap. In this way, this transposition flap can be very versatile and valuable (Fig. 43).

DuFourmental Flap. A modification of the rhomboid flap is the DuFourmental variation (Fig. 44). This flap is constructed by decreasing the angle of the first incision from the defect. This facilitates both transposition of the flap and closure of the secondary defect.

Webster 30 Degree Transposition Flap. Another variation on the rhomboid flap is the Webster 30 degree transposition flap (Fig. 45). The incision is made at a very narrow angle from the 120 degree angle of the defect. The normal 60 degree angle of the rhomboid defect is elongated into a 30 degree angle. This creates an uneven rhomboid that is closed with the transposed flap and an M-plasty.

W-Plasty or Double Rhomboid Flap. Another variant uses two rhomboid flaps to close one wound. This may be useful for closure of long defects. Two rhomboid flaps (Fig. 46) are placed end to end. This can be applied to circular defects that may be closed with three rhomboid flaps. The defect is converted into a hexagon that can be repaired using flaps planned from the 120 degree angles (Fig. 47).

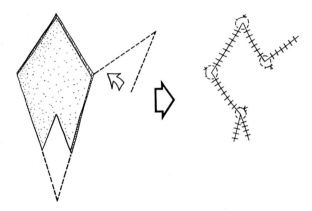

Figure 45 Webster 30 degree flap.

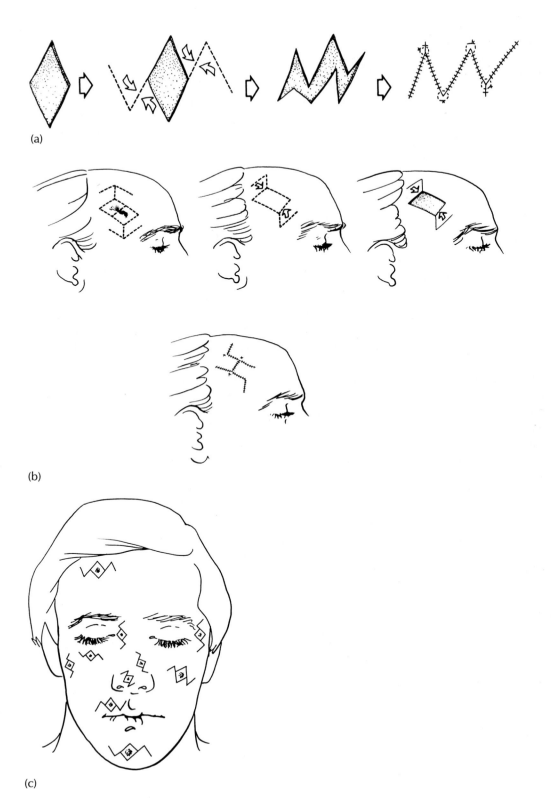

Figure 46 (a) Double rhomboid or W-plasty. (b) Double rhomboid for temple defect. (c) Clinical uses for W-plasties.

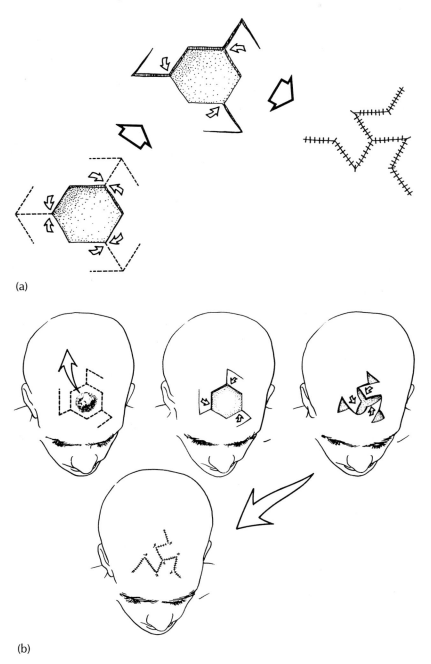

Figure 47 (a) Rhomboids used to close hexagonal defect. (b) Scalp closure.

The temple is an area where closure of a defect with a rhomboid flap is common. The area between the eyebrow and the anterior hairline is easily narrowed and distorted by many closure techniques. To minimize distortion, it is essential to maintain the distance between these two hair-bearing points. A rhomboid flap moved into such an area can maintain the relationship between these two hair-bearing structures and close the defect without significant tension. Excess tissue is utilized from the preauricular area. Closure of small defects on the bridge or side of the nose can also be done with a small rhomboid flap. Excess tissue comes from the glabella or lateral to the nasofacial sulcus.

Nasolabial Flap

The nasolabial flap is a transposition flap used to repair defects on the side of the nose or upper lip (Fig. 48). This flap utilizes excess tissue typically available from the nasolabial area. The pedicle of this flap can be based either superiorly or inferiorly. The vascular supply in this location is excellent.

The nasolabial flap is traditionally based in a superior fashion and extended down the nasolabial fold (Fig. 49). The secondary defect is primarily closed along the nasolabial fold. A narrow bridge of normal skin may separate the defect from the base of the flap. It is beneficial to excise this tissue and close it along with the original defect since this will avoid the need for a second procedure later to revise the wound. Once the flap is mobilized, the distal end is trimmed to fit the defect. The wound is then sutured in place.

While color and texture match are good, the main disadvantage of this flap is that the skin of the ala is thicker than skin from the medial cheek. This may result in irregularities in the margins of the flap. There also may be some blunting of the nasofacial sulcus at the side of the nose. If this blunting is unacceptable and shows no tendency to resolve with time, a revision may be done after the vascular supply has been established from the surrounding skin. A trapdoor deformity may occur with contraction around the distal end of the flap (Fig. 50). This deformity may resolve with time. Use of intralesional steroids (Fig. 51a,b) or correction with small Z-plasties (Fig. 51c) may help. When using this flap, remember not to transfer hair-bearing tissue onto the nose.

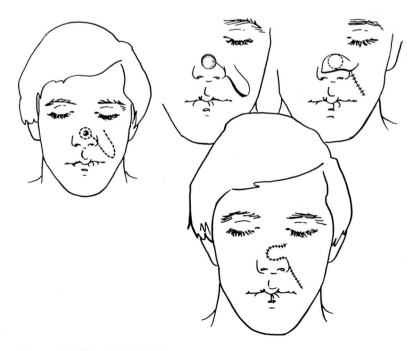

Figure 48   Nasolabial fold flap.

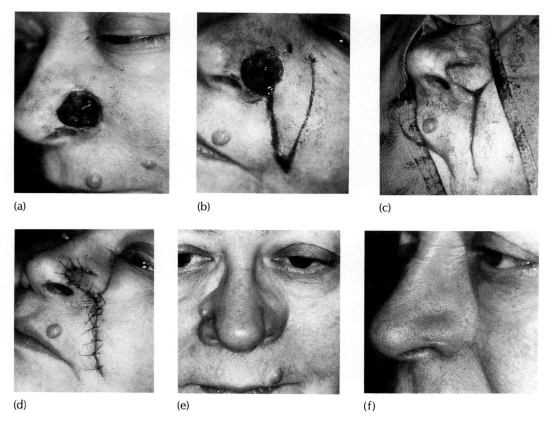

Figure 49 (a) Defect of nasal ala. (b) Planned nasolabial transposition flap. (c) The flap is trimmed and sutured in the defect. (d) Immediately after surgery. (e) Frontal view demonstrates blunting of the left nasofacial sulcus. (f) Three months following surgery the flap is thinner, conforming with the nasofacial sulcus.

When the nasolabial flap is used to repair defects on the lip, it can be based either superiorly or inferiorly (Fig. 52). The greater the angle the flap turns, the more likely is distortion of an inferiorly based flap. Nevertheless, this flap is useful for closure of defects in this area.

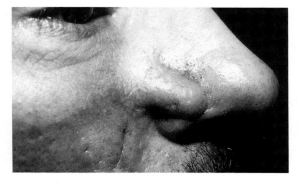

Figure 50 Six weeks postoperative; trapdoor deformity.

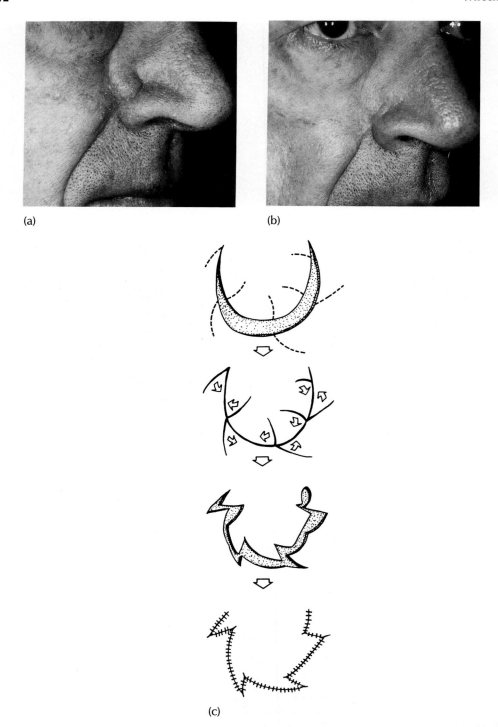

(a)   (b)

(c)

Figure 51   (a) Trapdoor defect after nasolabial flap repair for the alar defect. (b) Improvement 6 weeks after injection of intralesional steroids. (c) Correction of trapdoor with multiple Z-plasties.

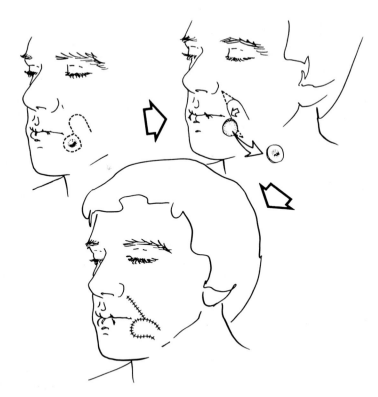

Figure 52 Inferiorly based nasolabial flap to repair defect on lip.

Labial-Ala Flap

Another transposition flap, the labial-ala flap, can also be used to repair small defects (<1 cm) on the nasal ala. This superiorly based flap has an advantage over the traditional nasolabial flap as the donor tissue is developed inferior to the nasal rim and does not cross or otherwise distort the nasofacial sulcus. In addition, the healed incision scars are easily hidden under the nasal sill rather that being present in the more visible melolabial fold. Pincushioning may occur as with any transposition flap, but this can be easily corrected using standard techniques.

Traditional Transposition Flaps

Another use of the transposition flaps is for correction of defects of the lower eyelids. This is known as the Tripier flap and is constructed with excess tissue from the upper eyelid (Fig. 53). The flap is elevated with its pedicle based laterally. The defect on the lower lid is closed when the flap is transposed. The secondary defect is closed in a primary fashion. Often a small amount of orbicularis oculi muscle is transposed with the flap to ensure vascularity.

Glabellar Transposition Flap

This flap is used to repair defects (Fig. 54) of the nasal root and inner canthus. Tissue from the glabella is transposed approximately 90 degrees. The secondary defect is closed primarily and the flap trimmed to fit the defect exactly. Glabellar skin is thicker than that of the nasal root or

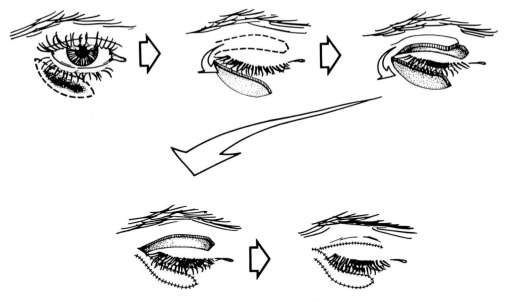

Figure 53 Tripier transposition flap for repair of a lower lid defect.

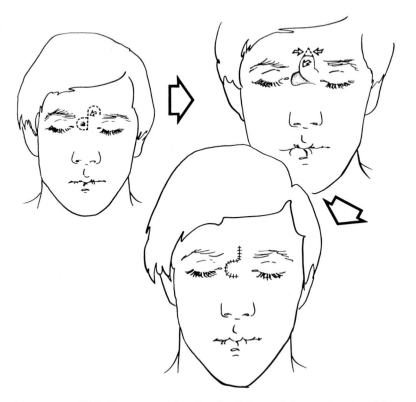

Figure 54 Glabellar transposition flap for defects of the nasal root and inner canthus.

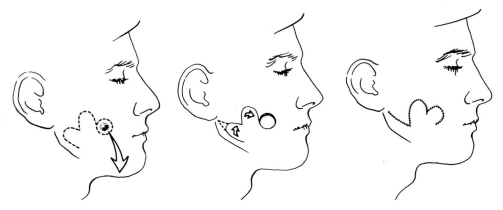

Figure 55   Bilobed flap for midcheek defect.

inner canthus, so all subcutaneous fat must be removed to prevent bulging. Care must be taken to minimize transposition of hair-bearing tissue into this area.

Bilobed Flap

The bilobed flap, also known as a double rotation flap, is used when a defect is in thick or inelastic tissue but adjacent to relatively loose tissue. This flap permits tissue transfer 180 degrees away from the donor area. The first lobe of the flap is constructed slightly smaller than the primary defect, and the second lobe is slightly smaller than the secondary defect (Fig. 55). This permits a gradual decrease in the donor defect so tension on the adjacent tissue is spread between both lobes of the flap. The bilobed flap is used to repair defects of the nose with tissue from the glabella (Fig. 56). Because these flaps are round, there is some potential for the development of a trapdoor deformity. Correction with Z-plasties or other modifications frequently leaves a good result but will require a delayed second procedure. Despite being useful for wounds with little adjacent donor skin, the role of this flap is relatively limited.

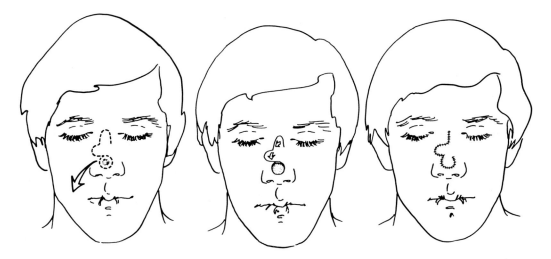

Figure 56   Bilobed flap repair on the nose.

Z-Plasty

The Z-plasty is another transposition flap used to lengthen scars, decrease tension, change direction, or reorient a preexisting scar (Fig. 57) to improve the cosmetic appearance. It is also used to prevent contraction of a straight line scar in a site of frequent motion.

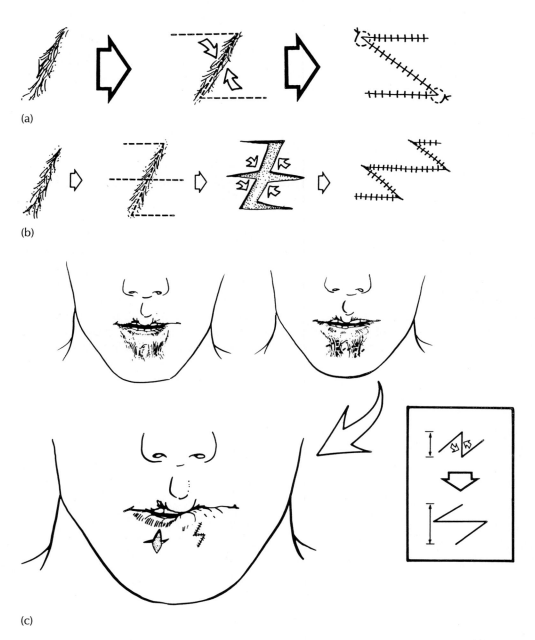

(a)

(b)

(c)

Figure 57 (a) Z-plasty changes the direction of a scar. (b) Z-plasty reorients a scar. (c) Z-plasty lengthens a scar to release a contracture.

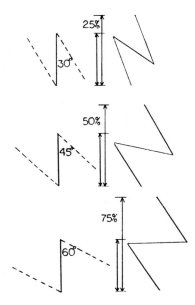

Figure 58 Different angles used in Z-plasty to adjust the final length of the scar.

The Z-plasty is usually designed at 60 degree angles with limbs of sufficient length to move tissue on either side of the central arm of the incision. The two flaps are transposed and sutured together in a new position. At 60 degree angles this will result in a 75% increase in length. If more acute angles are utilized, the net increase in length will be less (Fig. 58). For practical purposes, angles greater than 60 degrees are not used since the tension created would be unacceptable for flap closure.

Subcutaneous Island Pedicle Flap

The most elastic component of a skin flap is the subcutaneous tissue. The most inelastic component is the dermis. The subcutaneous pedicle flap or kite flap permits advancement of tissue from the ends of a fusiform excision without wasting normal tissue to close a wound and minimize tension. One or two island pedicle flaps may be advanced from the ends of an excision or from one end of a square defect (Figs. 59–61). Since the subcutaneous fat is left intact, there is sufficient vascular supply for the flap. The dermis is incised to the subcutaneous fat but is left attached. This permits skin to be shifted in the direction of the defect (Fig. 62). Sometimes the defect must be made deeper to accommodate the advancing pedicle, otherwise the flap meets resistance when advanced or will bulge.

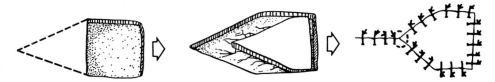

Figure 59 Single subcutaneous pedicle flap.

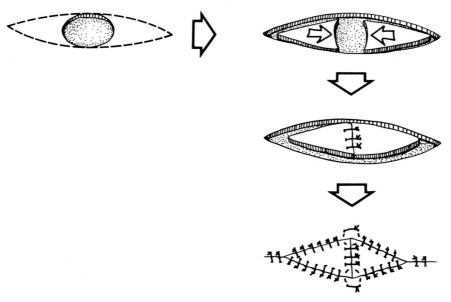

Figure 60 Double subcutaneous pedicle flap to repair a fusiform excision.

EVALUATING THE FLAP

Once a flap has been created, the vascular supply should be evaluated prior to final closure and application of the dressing. Typically, flaps should be either pink or slightly cyanotic. They tend to blanch slightly with light pressure and rapidly return to normal color. If the distal tip appears white, the flap should be released and an alternative closure considered.

Maximizing Flap Survival

To minimize interference with the circulation, close the flap with as few sutures as possible. The flap tissue should be handled with as much care as possible. Prior to suturing, complete hemostasis must be obtained. Hematoma formation will separate the flap from its base and predispose it to secondary infection. Secondary infection, although rare, may occur after flap surgery since at least some diminution of the normal vascular supply exists. As a consequence, a strict aseptic technique should be utilized during flap surgery, and any deadspace created should be closed. Tension on the flap must be avoided since this also impairs circulation and decreases survival.

   The postoperative dressing should lightly compress and immobilize the wound to permit rapid healing. External pressure should not be excessive since this will further impair the circulation to the flap. Epidermal blistering is a sign of impaired vascularity and occurs within several days after surgery.

Revising the Flap

All patients who undergo flap repair of a cutaneous wound or defect should be advised in advance that secondary procedures are often necessary to improve the small imperfections that may result from the flap. This may be a debulking or defatting procedure, dog ear repair at the point

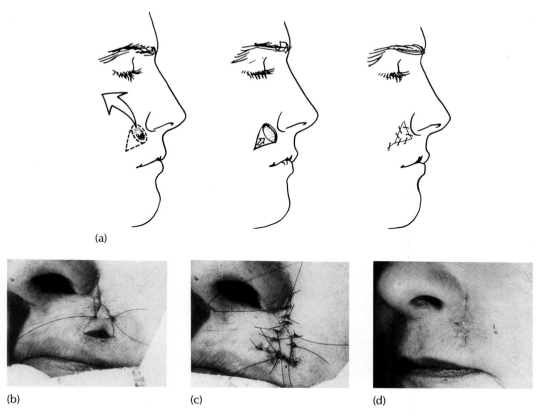

(a)

(b) (c) (d)

Figure 61 (a) Subcutaneous pedicle flap on upper lip. (b) Subcutaneous pedicle flap mobilized from nasofacial sulcus into defect of the upper lip; primary closure of the superior portion has been performed. (c) Postoperatively, closure obtained without crossing the vermilion border. (d) One month postoperative; no upward pull or distortion of the vermilion border.

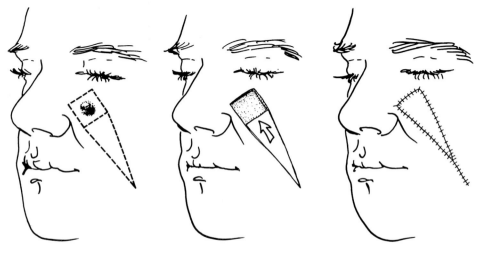

Figure 62 Large subcutaneous pedicle flap for medial cheek defect.

of pivot, dermabrasion of suture lines, or possibly injection of collagen to build up a depressed wound.

ADVANTAGES OF FLAP SURGERY

The advantages of flap surgery include a better chance of survival compared to skin grafting. This, of course, is due to the uninterrupted blood supply of the flap. In addition, the aesthetic appearance is usually better than a graft since tissue of similar color, texture, and thickness is used. The functional result of flap surgery compared to skin graft surgery is substantially better as well, since flaps tend to show greater durability than grafts and generally undergo less scar contracture. Normal function of sweat glands, oil glands, and hair growth function can be expected with flaps, especially if care is taken not to transect hair follicles. There may be a delay, however, of several months before normal sensation returns within flap tissue.

DISADVANTAGES OF FLAP SURGERY

One of the disadvantages of flap surgery is that while success rates are usually very high, failure can occur. If this happens, all of the adjacent donor skin is usually gone so repeated procedures are difficult to perform. Flap failure often requires coverage of the defect with a skin graft. Flap surgery is more difficult to perform in children since their skin is tight and does not lend itself well to stretching, and their scars tend to hypertrophy. Also, proper planning of a flap in a child may be difficult since natural creases and body lines may not have formed. Flap surgery may be associated with some anatomic distortion or asymmetry between sides of the face. Careful planning is the key to success.

COMPLICATIONS

Most complications with local random pattern flaps are due to an error in planning or execution of the flap. One main cause is poor design. When an incorrect method of closure is utilized, tension may result in necrosis. Flaps designed with insufficient length for closure may require a back cut that may impair the vascular supply, which will result in flap failure. A hematoma or seroma after flap surgery can disrupt vascular supply, predispose to infection (Fig. 63), and subsequently result in loss of the flap. The flap must be handled delicately since inadvertent injury to the vascular supply may result in necrosis.

Failure to use an inferiorly based flap, when possible, to improve venous return and limit lymphatic congestion can result in flap necrosis. This is a more common cause of flap failure than deficient arterial supply. Disruption of blood flow can result from seroma formation as well; if a seroma should develop beneath a flap it should be evacuated as soon as possible. The trapdoor defect typically occurs with U- or V-shaped flaps. This is secondary to scar contracture around the distal end of the flap. Much of this deformity improves spontaneously in about 6 months. Intralesional steroids injected into the base of the wound may improve this. Alternatively, this flap can be incised and excess fibrotic material or subcutaneous tissue removed. If this is not satisfactory, a series of small Z-plasties can be performed (see Fig. 51c).

Systemic Diseases and Flap Failure

Internal disease may also predispose to flap failure. Individuals with a bleeding diathesis or on anticoagulant medication are more likely to develop postoperative hematoma and associated

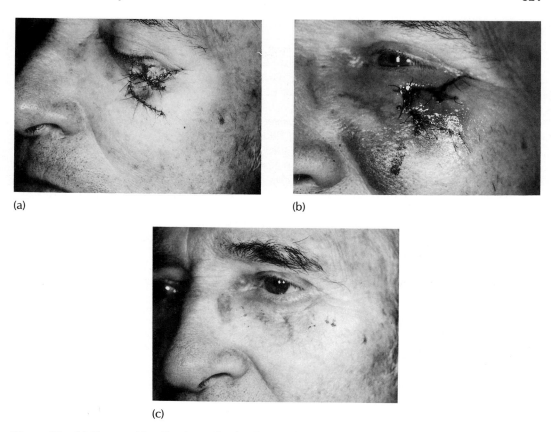

(a)

(b)

(c)

Figure 63 (a) Transposition flap immediately after repair. (b) Hematoma 48 hr postoperative and ecchymosis of the cheek. (c) Six weeks after evacuation of the hematoma.

complications. Diabetes, neoplasia, immunosuppressive therapy, and a variety of connective tissue diseases increase the risk of secondary infection and also result in slowed wound healing. Systemic or topical corticosteroid therapy may result in thinning of the skin such that poor wound healing or a flap failure may occur.

Infection

Infection is relatively uncommon with local random pattern flaps. Use of strict aseptic technique is important, however. Meticulous preparation with preoperative antiseptic scrubs, sterile instruments, and a sterile operating field are required. Prophylactic systemic antibiotics may be indicated if a large, complicated flap is performed. If infection should develop, appropriate measures include obtaining cultures and sensitivities to guide antibiotic therapy, draining any abscess formation, and debridement of necrotic tissue.

DRESSINGS

Immobilizing dressings that do not exert excess pressure to limit blood flow are beneficial. Instruction to the patient in proper postoperative care to minimize injury that might otherwise occur is also very important. Frequent follow-up visits are worthwhile.

BIBLIOGRAPHY

Asken S. A modified M-plasty. *J Dermatol Surg Oncol* 1986;12:369–373.

Becker FF. Local tissue flaps in reconstructive facial plastic surgery. *South Med J* 1977;70:677–680.

Becker FF. Rhomboid flap in facial reconstruction. *Arch Otolaryngol* 1979;105:569–573.

Becker H. The rhomboid-to-W technique for excision of some skin lesions and closure. *Plast Reconstr Surg* 1979;64:444–447.

Bennett RG. Local skin flaps on the cheeks. *J Dermatol Surg Oncol* 1991;17:161–165.

Borges AF. The rhombic flap. *Plast Reconstr Surg* 1981;67:458–466.

Borges AF. Pitfalls in flap design. *Ann Plast Surg* 1982;9:201–209.

Borges AF. Relaxed skin tension lines (RSTL) versus other skin lines. *Plast Reconstr Surg* 1984;73:144–150.

Bray DA, Eichel BS, Kaplan HJ. The dorsal nasal flap. *Arch Otolaryngol* 1981;107:765–766.

Cameron RR, Latham WD, Dowling JA. Reconstructions of the nose and upper lip with nasolabial flaps. *Plast Reconstr Surg* 1973;52:145–150.

Dzubow LM. Subcutaneous island pedicle flaps. *J Dermatol Surg Oncol* 1986;12:591–596.

Dzubow LM, Zack L. The principle of cosmetic junctions as applied to reconstruction of defects following Mohs surgery. *J Dermatol Surg Oncol* 1990;16:353–355.

Field LM. Design concepts for the nasolabial flap (letter). *Plast Reconstr Surg* 1983;71:283–285.

Gormley DE. A brief analysis of the Burow's wedge/triangle principle. *J Dermatol Surg Oncol* 1985;11:121–123.

Hallock GG, Trevaskis AE. Refinements of the subcutaneous pedicle flap for closure of forehead and scalp defects. *Plast Reconstr Surg* 1985;75:903–905.

Johnson TM, Baker S, Brown MD, Nelson BR. Utility of the subcutaneous hinge flap in nasal reconstruction. *J Am Acad Dermatol* 1994;30:459–466.

Katz AE, Grande DJ. Cheek-neck advancement-rotation flaps following Mohs excision of skin malignancies. *J Dermatol Surg Oncol* 1986;12:949–955.

Kolbusz RV, Goldberg LH. The labial-ala transposition flap. *Arch Dermatol* 1994;130:162–164.

Koranda FC, Webster RC. Trapdoor effect in nasolabial flaps. *Arch Otolaryngol* 1985;111:421–424.

Kraissl CJ. The selection of appropriate lines for elective surgical incisions. *Plast Reconstr Surg* 1951;8:1–28.

Mandy SH. The practical use of Z-plasty. *J Dermatol Surg* 1975;1:57–60.

McGregor IA. Local skin flaps in facial reconstruction. *Otolaryngol Clin North Am* 1982;15:77–98.

Mellette JR. Ear reconstruction with local flaps. *J Dermatol Surg Oncol* 1991;17:176–182.

Monheit GD. The rhomboid transposition flap reevaluated. *J Dermatol Surg Oncol* 1980;6:464–471.

Rubin LR. Langers lines and facial scars. *Plast Reconstr Surg* 1948;3:147–155.

Salasche SJ, Grabski WJ. Complications of flaps. *J Dermatol Surg Oncol* 1991;17:132–140.

Salasche SJ, Roberts LC. Dog-ear correction by M-plasty. *J Dermatol Surg Oncol* 1984;10:478–482.

Siegle RJ. Forehead reconstruction. *J Dermatol Surg Oncol* 1991;17:200–204.

Simmonds WL. Reflections on dermatologic surgery and the management of perioral and labial lesions. *J Dermatol Surg Oncol* 1978;4:383–389.

Spicer TE. Techniques of facial lesion excision and closure. *J Dermatol Surg Oncol* 1982;8:551–556.

Stegman SJ. Fifteen ways to close surgical wounds. *J Dermatol Surg* 1975;1:25–31.

Stegman SJ. Planning closure of a surgical wound. *J Dermatol Surg Oncol* 1978;4:390–393.

Summers BK, Siegle RJ. Facial cutaneous reconstructive surgery: General aesthetic principles. *J Am Acad Dermatol* 1993;29:669–681.

Summers BK, Siegle RJ. Facial cutaneous reconstructive surgery: Facial flaps. *J Am Acad Dermatol* 1993;29:917–941.

Walkinshaw MD, Chaffee HH. The nasolabial flap: a problem and its correction. *Plast Reconstr Surg* 1982;69:30–34.

Webster RC, Davidson TM, Smith RC. The thirty degree transposition flap. *Laryngoscope* 1978;88:85–94.

Wheeland RG. Reconstruction of the lower lip and chin using local and random-pattern flaps. *J Dermatol Surg Oncol* 1991;17:605–615.

Winton GB, Salasche SJ. Use of rotation flaps to repair small surgical defects on the ala nasi. *J Dermatol Surg Oncol* 1986;12:154–158.

Yanai A, Nagata S, Okabe K. The Z in Z-plasty must have a long trunk. *Br J Plast Surg* 1986;39:390–394.

Zimany A. The bi-lobed flap. *Plast Reconstr Surg* 1952;11:424–434.

Zitelli JA. The nasolabial flap as a single stage procedure. *Arch Dermatol* 1990;126:1445–1448.

Zitelli JA. A regional approach to reconstruction of the upper lip. *J Dermatol Surg Oncol* 1991;17:143–148.

Zitelli JA, Fazio MJ. Reconstruction of the nose with local flaps. *J Dermatol Surg Oncol* 1991;17:184–189.

45

Advancement Flaps

David G. Brodland
Mayo Clinic/Foundation, Rochester, Minnesota

INTRODUCTION

There are three reasons to close a defect with a flap. First, flaps can facilitate closure of defects that, due to size, are not otherwise closable by simple wound edge apposition. Second, flaps may be used to optimize aesthetic outcome. Finally, flaps can help maintain the function of adjacent structures by avoiding impingement of those structures in the process of reconstruction. An advancement flap can be defined as a unidirectional flap that moves tissue in a straight line. In a general sense, a simple fusiform closure is a type of advancement flap, since the majority of tissue movement is unidirectional and usually in a straight line. Traditional advancement flaps, however, are created when incisions are made tangential to the defect in the same plane as the planned tissue movement (Figs. 1,2). These incisions release the flap from tension in all directions except in the direction opposite to the planned tissue movement. As such, the utility of advancement flaps is primarily for improving the aesthetics of the closure and for maintaining the function of adjacent structures and of the tissue being closed. However, they are not as useful if the reason for considering a flap is that the defect is large and difficult to close. The very design of a traditional advancement flap focuses wound tension on the relatively narrow pedicle of the advancement flap rather than dispersing or displacing wound tension. Since the blood supply is dependent on this same pedicle, any tension potentially compromises the viability of the flap. Advancement of the flap into the defect relies on the inherent elasticity of the flap tissue, the inherent mobility of the tissue at the base of the pedicle, and secondary movement of the surrounding tissue in a direction opposite to the flap movement (Fig. 3). Therefore, the set of circumstances that would typically favor the choice of an advancement flap is when there is a wound that, when closed primarily or with another type of flap, would give a suboptimal aesthetic or functional outcome and that has adequate tissue laxity and mobility available in the desirable direction.

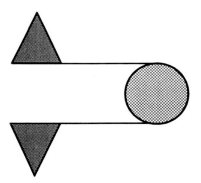

Figure 1 Traditional single-advancement flap characterized by two parallel, tangential incisions and displacement of the Burow's triangles laterally along the tangents.

Occasionally, there are situations in which a double advancement flap can be used to close a wound under tension since a sum total of the wound tension is divided between two flaps (Figs. 4,5). In this situation, other options should be considered first, since double advancement flaps have a total of seven incision lines and most other closures have fewer sutured wound edges.

PREOPERATIVE CONSIDERATIONS

Classically designed advancement flaps are not particularly good at closing high-tension defects. Defects under a great deal of tension necessitate careful preoperative planning. Preoperatively, it is very important to determine how much tension the closure will be under based on the tissue mobility and elasticity in the direction of the flap. This can be determined by the finger pinch test or by wound edge approximation using skin hooks. The finger pinch test requires attempted approximation of the wound edges in the direction of the planned flap between two fingers. Routine use of this method enables the surgeon to gain a sense of how much tissue can be

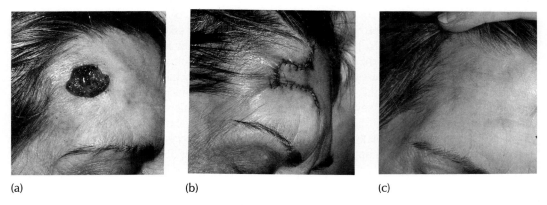

(a)   (b)   (c)

Figure 2 (a) Surgical defect. (b) Reconstruction with single-advancement flap. (c) Three months postoperative.

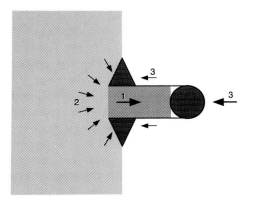

Figure 3 Tissue mobility of advancement flap comes from (1) inherent elasticity of flap tissue, (2) the inherent mobility of the tissue at the base of the pedicle, and (3) secondary movement of the surrounding tissue in a direction opposite to the flap.

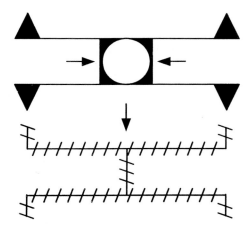

Figure 4 Diagram of classic double-advancement flap.

mobilized once the flaps are incised and the tissue is undermined. With experience, one can very accurately anticipate whether or not a particular flap closure is possible. Another way to test the tissue mobility and elasticity is with skin hooks. Approximating the wound edges using skin hooks gives a better idea of whether a wound can be closed under some tension without significantly injuring the viable wound edges.

Another consideration in planning closure with advancement flaps is blood supply. Factors that affect blood supply to the distal portion of a flap include flap length-to-width ratio, vascu-

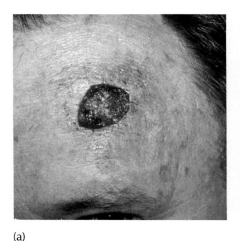

(a)

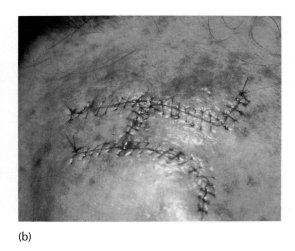

(b)

Figure 5 (a) Large defect, left forehead. (b) Closure with double-advancement flap. Note that Burow's triangles were taken at the less conspicuous lateral aspect of the flap.

lar supply at the pedicle base, anticipated wound tension, and anatomic disruption of local blood supply such as old scars from previous trauma or surgery. The traditional rule of thumb in designing advancement flaps is not to let the length-to-width ratio exceed 3 or 4:1. In practice, this rule is not inviolate, however, ratios greater than this should be considered risky and avoided when possible.

The very nature of the design of the advancement flap makes it risky with regard to blood supply. A classical advancement flap has had its blood supply severed in four of five directions (including the subcutaneous blood supply). The blood supply of the pedicle is often far removed from the distal aspect of the flap. When planning these flaps, in addition to considering the length-to-width ratio, other factors that can affect the blood supply need to be taken into account. For example, the blood supply may be compromised if there has been previous excisional surgery at or near the pedicle such that the normal vasculature may have been disrupted. Likewise, a pedicle based on retrograde blood supply, such as a distally based advancement flap on an extremity, should be avoided.

Philosophically, there are two main indications for the use of classical advancement flaps. The first reason has already been briefly discussed. When a defect exists in which displacement of the Burow's triangles to a position distant from the defect is desirable, an advancement flap is an ideal choice. It may be that the Burow's triangle in a standard fusiform closure would impinge upon a vital cosmetic structure, such as the eyebrow, eyelid, lip, or nose. Or it may be aesthetically advantageous to displace the Burow's triangles to a more imperceptible site along parallel expression lines in order to achieve the least noticeable final scar. The other major reason for using an advancement flap is if there is only one source of donor skin and adjacent distortable structures dictate a tangential unidirectional movement of skin. An example of this would be in repair of the upper lip, where the only adjacent donor skin exists laterally and there are distortable structures above (the nose) and below (the vermilion) (Fig. 6).

Another subtle feature of this flap is that the Burow's triangles can be made somewhat smaller when they are displaced toward the base of the flap since the redundant skin for which Burow's triangles are removed can be partially distributed along the length of the flap. The diminution of the triangle should be done with caution since it can lead to a taut-appearing flap and somewhat bulky skin on either side of the flap.

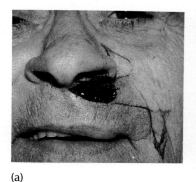
(a)

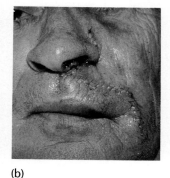
(b)

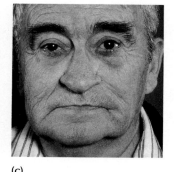
(c)

Figure 6 (a) Large, deep defect of the upper lip just below the nose. (b) Immediately after closure with advancement flap. (c) Seven months postoperative.

VARIATIONS ON ADVANCEMENT FLAPS

Single Tangent Advancement Flaps

Geometrically, a classical advancement flap is characterized by a defect with two parallel tangent lines extending in the same direction. Therefore, the classical advancement flap may be better described as a double-tangent advancement flap. A double advancement flap is simply two pairs of tangents extending in opposite directions. Another variation of the classical double tangent advancement flap is the single-tangent advancement flap. This flap is also known as the Burow's wedge advancement flap (Fig. 7a). Its bilateral form is the symmetric Burow's wedge advancement flap, also known as the A-to-T flap (Fig. 7b). The Burow's wedge advancement flap is characterized by a single tangential incision at the end of which is a Burow's triangle. A Burow's triangle is taken from the side of the tangent opposite the defect. After undermining, the flap is advanced along the tangent into the defect (Fig. 8). This flap, in contrast to the standard double-tangent advancement flap, is very broadly based and generally has a robust blood supply. Recruitment of skin in this flap is not unidirectional as with the double-tangent advancement flap. Therefore, if the flaps are carefully designed, more tissue mobilization can be anticipated and larger defects closed. These flaps are excellent in situations where only one of the two obligatory Burow's triangles of a simple fusiform closure must be displaced laterally to avoid undesirable functional or aesthetic disruption of adjacent structures. Single-tangent advancement flaps may also be used in defects that are difficult to close due to the wound tension.

A symmetric Burow's wedge flap, also known as the A-T flap is created by incising two tangents extending in opposite directions but in the same plane from the defect (Fig. 7b). At the end of both of these incisions, the Burow's triangle is excised. The flap is elevated, and wound edges undermined so the flaps can be advanced medially into the defect. Another Burow's triangle is taken at the pole (opposite of the defect) from the tangents. As with the single Burow's wedge flap, the A-T is very broad based and even better suited for closure of large wounds. This flap has the same advantage of laterally displacing one of the Burow's triangles that would be

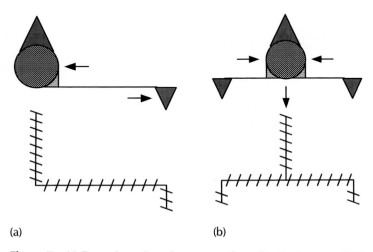

(a)   (b)

Figure 7 (a) Burow's wedge advancement flap with single tangential incision and lateral displacement of a single Burow's triangle. Stairstep-shaped sutured wound after closure. (b) Double Burow's wedge advancement flap, also known as A-to-T flap.

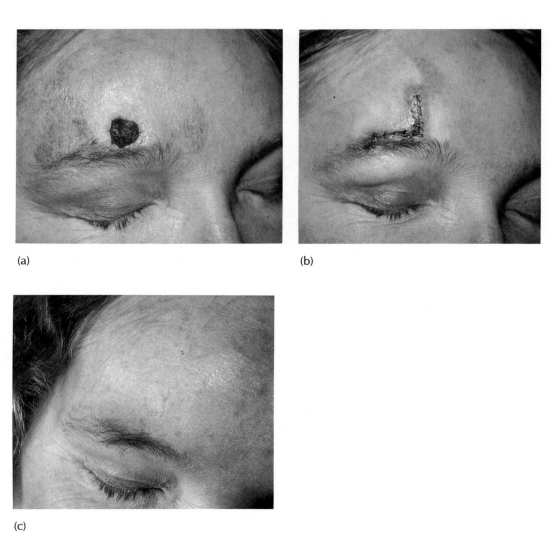

(a)

(b)

(c)

Figure 8 (a) Surgical defect prior to closure. (b) Immediately after reconstruction with single-tangent advancement flap. Note displacement of inferior Burow's triangle laterally to minimize loss of brow. (c) Three months postoperative.

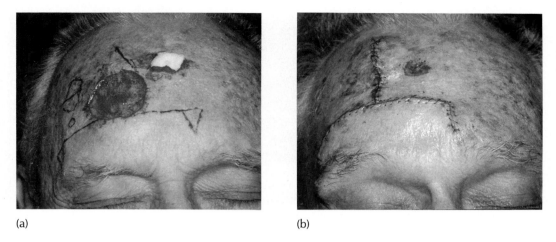

(a)   (b)

Figure 9   (a) Large defect of the right forehead. (b) Immediately following reconstruction with A-to-T flap.

taken if the defect was closed by simple fusiform closure. Therefore, these flaps are helpful in areas such as superior to the eyebrow where it is desirable to leave the eyebrow undisturbed and displace the Burow's triangles medially and laterally (Fig. 9).

Specialized Variations of Advancement Flaps

Over the years several variations of the advancement flap have been described. These flaps tend to be site and situation dependent in their use for reconstruction. Three variants commonly considered in discussions of advancement flaps include the crescentic advancement flap, the Peng flap, and the helical advancement flap.

The crescentic advancement flap is most useful for closure of defects near the nose and upper lip (Fig. 10). This flap is useful when a standard fusiform closure is not possible but there is an adjacent reservoir of donor skin. A crescentic equivalent of a Burow's triangle is excised in the donor area and is usually placed conveniently in the border of a cosmetic unit, such as the nasolabial fold. The crescentic skin that is excised not only serves the purpose of removing the redundant skin that would result from advancement of the flap into a defect but also creates

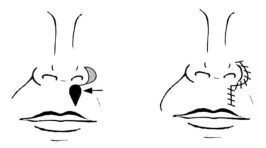

Figure 10   Typical crescentic advancement flap. Lateral displacement of the superior Burow's triangle in the form of a crescent avoids distortion of the nostril (see also Fig. 6).

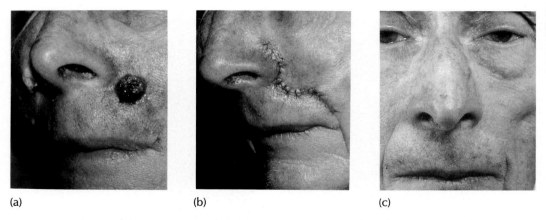

(a)   (b)   (c)

Figure 11   (a) Defect situated on both the upper lip and left cheek in which simple primary closure would impinge upon the ala and possibly cause mild eclabion laterally. (b) Immediately after reconstruction. (c) One year and 7 months postoperative.

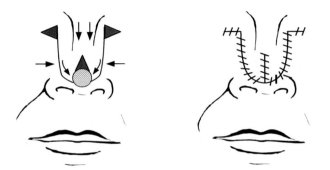

Figure 12   Typical design of Peng flap with tissue movement by combination of advancement and inward rotation of flap tips.

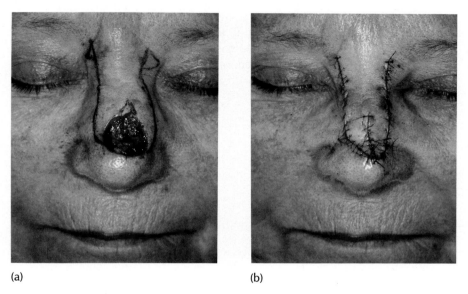

(a)   (b)

Figure 13   (a) Large and deep defect overlying the nasal tip and distal nasal dorsum. (b) Immediately after closure using Peng variation of advancement flap.

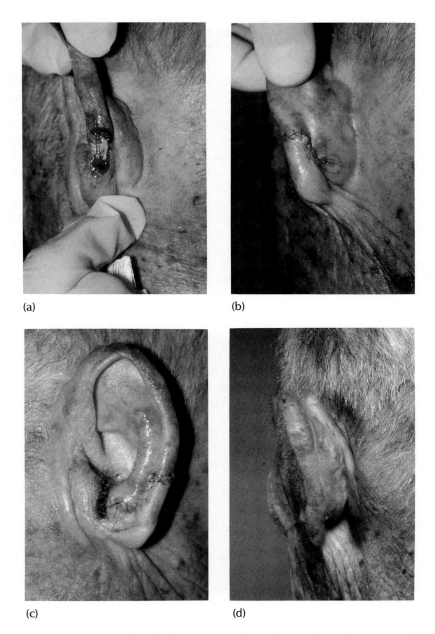

(a)   (b)

(c)   (d)

Figure 14 (a) Defect on lower helix. (b) Posterior view immediately after reconstruction. (c) Lateral view after reconstruction. (d) Six months postoperative.

edges of unequal length and allows the sliding of additional skin towards the defect from the donor site. Another consequence of the crescentic skin removal is a broadening of the flap pedicle and hence a more robust and well-vascularized flap. An ideal place to utilize the crescentic flap is in repairing defects on the superior and lateral portion of the upper lip (Fig. 11). In this situation, the crescentic triangle can be excised directly adjacent to the curved structure of the alar base, which results in a nicely hidden scar.

The Peng flap is a variation on the standard double-tangent advancement flap (Fig. 12). The curvilinear lines make this a combination advancement and rotation flap. While the overall flap advances into the defect, there is rotation from the adjacent skin into the defect.

This flap works nicely in situations where there may not be adequate unidirectional tissue laxity for an advancement flap but in which there is some laxity lateral to the defects. With advancement and inward rotational movement, the defect can be closed with minimal distortion of the surrounding structures. An area where this flap is commonly used is in defects on the distal third of the nose in which the skin is advanced down the length of the nose and rotated in from the nasal side wall (Fig. 13). The scalp is another area in which there is often not enough laxity to utilize a standard advancement flap, and the combination of advancement and rotation enable closure of the wound.

The helical advancement flap takes advantage of the laxity of the tissue along the margin of the helix. This principle is used in a similar fashion along other free margins, such as the eyelid and lips. The same principles of standard advancement flap design hold true in these flaps. The length-to-width ratio should not exceed 3 or 4:1, and the tissue laxity must be assessed. If a defect includes loss of the cartilage of the helical rim, then a chondrocutaneous helical advancement flap can be designed. In both cases, the incisions are made along the helical rim or in the scaphoid fossa below the rim (Fig. 14). Burow's triangles are taken at a point along the flap from the skin adjacent to the flap, and the adjacent skin is undermined enough to untether the advancing flap. It is then advanced along the curvature of the helical rim into the defect. Blood supply in this area is generally excellent. The size of the ear may be diminished but is usually less noticeable than with wedge resections of the ear. Often, the donor tissue is the earlobe and serves as an abundant supply of redundant skin, especially in defects of the mid- or inferior helix. Even large wounds of the helix can be repaired with minimal aesthetic consequence.

BIBLIOGRAPHY

Cavanaugh EB. Management of lesions of the helical rim using the chondrocutaneous advancement flap. *J Dermatol Surg Oncol* 1982;(Aug.):691–696.

Dzubow LM. *Facial Flaps. Biomechanics and Regional Application*. Norwalk, CT, Appleton and Lange, 1989.

Moy RL. *Atlas of Cutaneous Facial Flaps and Grafts: A Different Diagnosis of Wound Closures*. Philadelphia, Lee and Febiger, 1990, pp. 1–2.

Wheeland RG. Random pattern flaps. In *Dermatologic Surgery: Principles and Practice*. Roenigk RK, Roenigk HH Jr., eds. New York, Marcel Dekker, 1989, pp. 265–322.

Whitaker DC. Random-pattern flaps. In *Cutaneous Surgery*. Wheeland RG, ed. Philadelphia, W.B. Saunders Co., 1994, pp. 332–337.

46

Rotation Flaps

William J. Grabski
Brooke Army Medical Center, Fort Sam Houston, Houston, Texas

Stuart J. Salasche
University of Arizona Health Sciences Center, Tucson, Arizona

THE CLASSIC ROTATION FLAP

A rotation flap, one of the three main types of random-pattern flaps, is named after the method of tissue movement. The classic rotation flap can be conceptualized as a triangular defect closed by the rotation of skin around a pivot point (Fig. 1A). In actuality, as the primary defect is closed by the rotation of tissue, a secondary defect is created along the curvilinear arc of the flap (Fig. 1B). This longer and narrower secondary defect contains the same surface area as the primary defect but can often be closed by a combination of simple advancement of the curvilinear arc as well as secondary advancement of the surrounding skin (Fig. 1C). As will be discussed later, a dog ear usually forms along the outer curvilinear arc.

FLAP DESIGN

The design of the rotation flap is not complex in conception or execution. It consists of incising along the curvilinear arc drawn away from the defect, usually in a relaxed skin tension line or a junction line between cosmetic units. If possible, it is best to base the flap inferiorly and laterally to help with drainage and cosmesis as the new scar line will be displaced away from the midline (Fig. 2).

Unfortunately, the rotation flap is a relatively inefficient method of recruiting tissue as a long incision is often required. The arc may need to be three to four times the length of the primary defect. In selected situations a rotation flap with a short curvilinear arc can be utilized as a method of either changing the closure tension vector or moving redundant skin (dog ears) to a more advantageous location around a defect than could otherwise be accomplished by a side-to-side closure. The maneuver of creating a rotation flap also effectively shortens the scar line. This not only allows for closure without extension into an adjoining cosmetic unit, it also breaks up the scar line. Two short incision lines have a cosmetic advantage over a single long one.

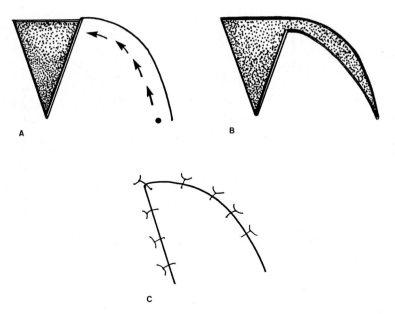

Figure 1 (A) Triangular defect and rotation flap design. (B) Creation of secondary defect after incision of flap. (C) Idealized closure of primary and secondary defects.

When required, there are two methods of increasing flap mobility. Each has the advantage of allowing less tension on the distal flap; however, both confer viability disadvantages. First, the curvilinear arc is successively lengthened until mobility is sufficiently increased to allow tension-free closure of the flap tip (Fig. 3A). In addition, a longer, narrower secondary defect is created, which also closes under less tension (Fig. 3B). The disadvantage of this lengthening maneuver is that a longer scar is created and vascular pedicle width decreases relative to the length of the flap. In a random-pattern flap, blood must reach the most distal portion of the flap via the subdermal plexus. Lengthening the distance blood must travel may put this area at risk of insufficient perfusion.

The second method of increasing flap mobility is to perform a back-cut incision into the vascular pedicle at the far end of the curvilinear arc (Fig. 4). A back-cut is an efficient maneuver to change the pivot point with a short incision and hence increase mobility. This contrasts with the much longer continuation of the curvilinear arc required to produce the same increase in flap movement. Unfortunately, the back-cut also decreases the pedicle width just as the lengthening of the curvilinear arc decreases the pedicle width relative to the length of the flap. In general, rotation flaps are designed with wide, thick vascular pedicles which can tolerate either a back-cut or lengthening of the arc. The gain in tissue mobility and decrease in tension from these maneuvers often more than compensate for the decrease in blood supply to the flap tip. Only clinical experience will help the surgeon decide how wide a vascular pedicle must be in order to supply the flap tip and how much tension can be tolerated.

There are two common errors in the design of a rotation flap. Both involve selection of the beginning point of the curvilinear arc. The first consists of starting this point too low around the defect. This does not compensate for the inevitable loss of height that occurs during the actual rotation of the flap. Tension is required to pull the flap tip into place, and the surgeon must often

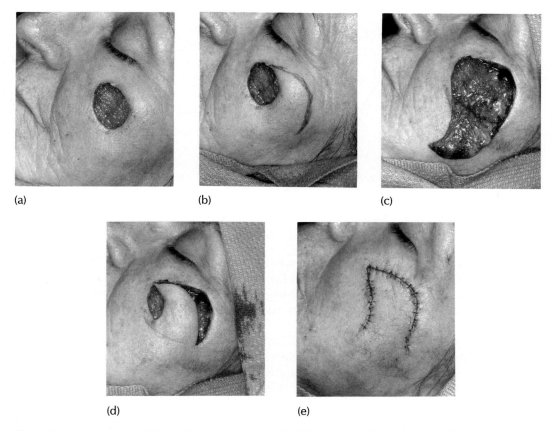

Figure 2 (a) A surgical defect of the malar cheek. (b) Inferior/lateral based rotation flap. The proposed incision is in the curvilinear RSTLs of the cheek. (c) The body of the flap is draped back. Undermining around primary and secondary defect already accomplished. (d) The key stitch is placed, partially closing the primary defect and creating a longer, narrower secondary defect. (e) After closure, both incision lines parallel the RSTLs of the cheek.

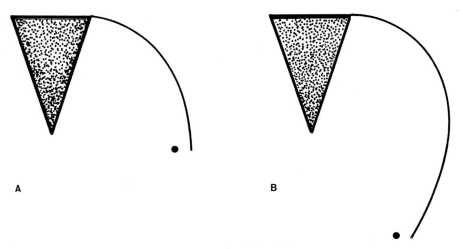

Figure 3 (A) Initial rotation flap design. (B) Flap lengthened to increase mobility. Area of secondary defect also increased.

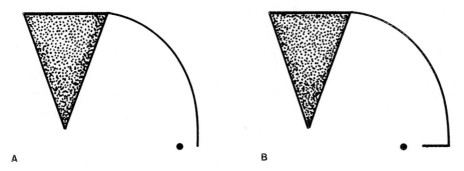

Figure 4 (A) Initial rotation flap design. (B) Back-cut changes pivot point and increases flap mobility.

resort to either lengthening the arc or back-cutting the pedicle. It is easier to account for the expected loss of height and raise the leading edge of the flap beforehand (Fig. 5). The flap then drapes into place with little or no vertical tension on the flap tip. The blood supply to the tip is not compromised, and vertical tension on important anatomic structures (i.e., eyelid or lip) is avoided.

The second error involves round or oval defects where the tip designed is too narrow. When pulled into place, it is obvious this small triangle will not fit in or survive. This, in effect, shortens the flap and the same problems as above are created. A better design would be to widen and raise the take-off point of the curvilinear arc (Fig. 6).

CLINICAL FLAP DESIGN

Although the classic rotation flap is conceptualized as beginning as a triangular defect, most cutaneous surgical defects tend to be circular or oval. Triangulating the defect is unnecessary and only creates a larger defect. The rotation flap should be designed and executed utilizing the original shape of the defect, with redundant tissue eliminated only as necessary. As stated earlier, the curvilinear arc of the flap should be designed so that it can be hidden in a junction line

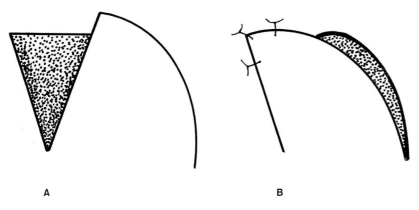

Figure 5 (A) Step-up design raises the lead edge of the flap. (B) The flap falls easily into place without tension.

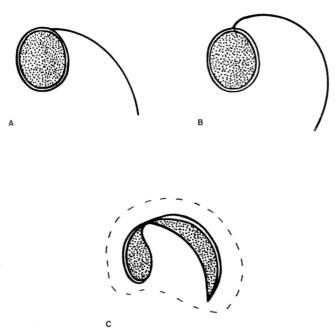

Figure 6 (A) Initial flap design. (B) Improved flap design. (C) Flap incised. Extent of undermining indicated.

or a relaxed skin tension line (RSTL) for best cosmesis. The length of the flap can initially be incised to a conservative length (one or two times the diameter of the primary defect) and then widely undermined. Undermining should include the tissue surrounding the flap to ensure good secondary movement, but should not extend too far under the pedicle to prevent compromising blood flow to the tip (Fig. 6C). The flap is undermined at the deepest safe level possible for that given anatomic site, but must always include at least some subcutaneous fat in order to include the subdermal plexus. The thicker the flap can be designed, the better the blood supply to the flap tip.

Once elevated, the flap can be pulled into place with a skin hook to test for the ease of flap mobility and the degree of closure tension. If an increase in flap mobility is required to fill the primary defect, an appropriate adjustment of arc lengthening or back-cutting can be made at this time. Once an adequate amount of flap tissue has been recruited to fill the defect, the flap tip can be tacked into place with a temporary suture. Placement of the tip is the key stitch in a rotation flap as the tension vector of closure runs through this point (Fig. 7). Placement of the tip stitch defines how much of the primary defect will be filled with the flap and how much by secondary movement of the surrounding skin. If there is an important anatomic structure adjacent to the primary defect that should not be distorted, the flap should be draped in to fill the whole defect. This creates a larger secondary defect and produces more pronounced dog ears. More often it is advantageous to partially close the primary defect, which creates two similar wounds that are easier to close and have less pronounced dog ears.

The actual closure consists of placing buried dermal absorbable sutures along the curvilinear arc (secondary defect) to relieve the tension on the tip stitch. They are arranged in a tangential

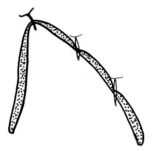

Figure 7   Placement of key stitch and tension reducing subcuticular stitches along secondary defect.

manner across the defect so that they pull the flap into place and distribute the tension to several points away from the tip (Fig. 7). Buried sutures are also placed in the primary defect not so much to decrease tension but to spread out and arrange the flap placement. If the flap tip forms a narrow angle, it is often best to trim a small amount off to create a better fit and avoid tip necrosis.

Two areas of tissue redundancy can be expected whenever a rotation flap is done to close a circular or oval defect (Fig. 8A). A symmetrical dog ear develops as the primary defect closes because it contains an angle greater than 30 degrees. The tissue redundancy should be resected in a direction that does not narrow the vascular pedicle of the flap (Fig. 8B). An asymmetric dog ear occurs along the closure of the secondary defect because of the difference in length of the two sides of the curvilinear arc. This dog ear can be removed anywhere along the arc, but classically it is resected at the distal end in a "hockey stick" manner. Nonabsorbable surface sutures are then placed to approximate the epidermal edges in a slightly everted manner. A simple running suture is often a quick and efficient way to complete the closure.

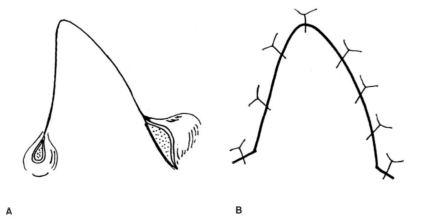

A   B

Figure 8   (A) Dog ears form predictably in rotations flaps. (B) After excision of dog ears.

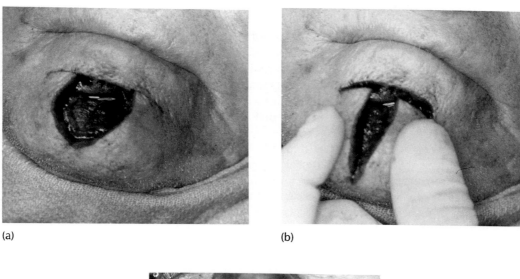

(a)　　　　　　　　　　　　　　　　　　(b)

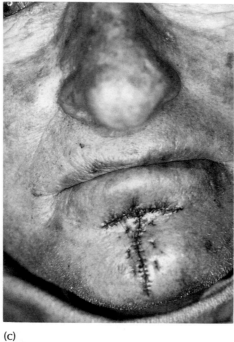

(c)

Figure 9 (a) Bilateral rotation flap created by paired incisions along mentolabial crease. (b) The two flaps rotate to meet each other in the midline. (c) The final closure is confined to the chin. Scar lines confined to the mentolabial crease and midline chin.

SPECIAL DESIGN MODIFICATIONS

Bilateral rotation flaps can be designed in selected situations to recruit tissue from both sides of a defect, thus creating two smaller secondary defects rather than one large one (Fig. 9). This becomes cosmetically advantageous when curvilinear junction lines or RSTLs are available on both sides of the primary defect. Bilateral rotation flaps may allow closure of a defect within a single cosmetic unit and obviate the need to cross over into the next cosmetic unit. The flap design is actually a rotational modification of an A-to-T or an O-to-T closure. The latter are considered advancement rather than rotation flaps.

Another variation is the O-to-Z flap (Fig. 10). This flap also borrows skin bilaterally. However, in this instance, the two curvilinear incisions are designed on opposite sides of the wound and arc away from each other rather than toward each other as in the standard bilateral rotation flap. This flap has limited application because of the resultant Z-shaped scar, which is not easily camouflaged, especially in one area where it is often attempted—the forehead. The vertex of the scalp is one area where this modification has proven useful.

REGIONAL APPLICATIONS

The rotation flap is one of the simpler random-pattern flaps, but one that requires careful planning and design as well as good surgical technique to obtain the best cosmetic results. This flap exploits the adjacent tissue elasticity along the curvilinear arc of the incision and has the potential to mobilize large volumes of tissue. One major advantage of the rotation flap is that it has a broad base. Thus it contains a good vascular supply and has a low incidence of necrosis. It is usually designed as an inferiorly based flap, which results in better venous and lymphatic drainage (Fig. 2). The rotation flap is best utilized in areas where the incision lines can be camouflaged in a curvilinear junction line or RSTL.

The cheek and temple are particularly receptive to repairs by rotation flap (Fig. 11). Temple and lateral cheek rotation flaps can be designed with the curvilinear incisions placed along the temporal hairline or the preauricular junction. The lateral dog ear repair can be hidden in the hairline or just inferior to the earlobe. These flaps take advantage of the lax tissue of the cheek, preauricular area, jowls, and neck.

Defects of the central cheek can be repaired effectively with inferolaterally based flaps. This is probably the "cleanest" indication for this flap. Wounds can be closed away from the central portion of the face. The superior dog ear that would form with a side-to-side closure and run onto the convex malar eminence is avoided. Finally, a long scar is broken up and camouflaged in the lateral cheek RSTL or preauricular folds.

Similarly, infraorbital cheek defects are especially challenging because of the need to avoid pull on the lower eyelid. The flap incision should arc superiorly along the infraorbital crease to compensate for the loss of flap height during rotation (Fig. 12). This allows the flap to drape across rather than having to be pulled up into place. Downward tension on the eyelid is avoided and ectropion prevented. A long flap is frequently required to mobilize sufficient tissue to minimize vertical tension upon closure of the secondary defect.

If small defects of the infraorbital cheek are closed in a side-to-side fashion, removal of the superior dog ear would carry the scar line onto the lower eyelid. This can be avoided by performing an inferolaterally based rotation flap. The tissue redundancy is repositioned to the inferior poles of the closure and the repair can be completed within the cheek cosmetic unit.

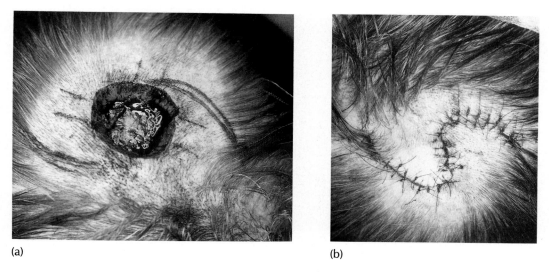

(a)   (b)

Figure 10   (a) An O-to-Z flap is created by two curvilinear incisions on opposite sides of a scalp defect. (b) The final closure after rotation toward the center.

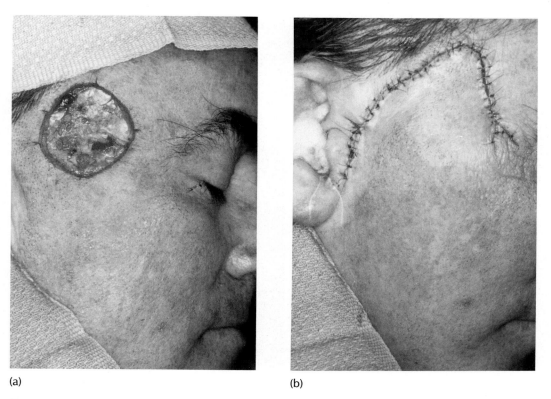

(a)   (b)

Figure 11   (a) A surgical defect of the temple. (b) Repair utilizing a lateral/inferior-based rotation flap. Arc incised along the hairline and the preauricular junction.

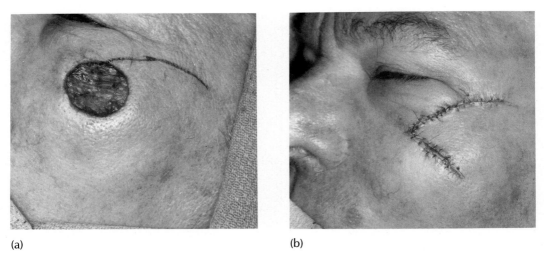

(a)   (b)

Figure 12   (a) The proposed flap arcs superiorly to compensate for loss of height during rotation. (b) The final closure without downward tension on the eyelid.

Medially displaced cheek wounds can also be repaired with a rotation flap. In these instances the flap is incised in the melolabial fold to tap into the lax, excessive skin of the inferior portion of the fold (Fig. 13). Often more efficient or more cosmetic flaps such as the subcutaneous pedicle flaps or the perialar advancement flaps are chosen for repair of defects in this region.

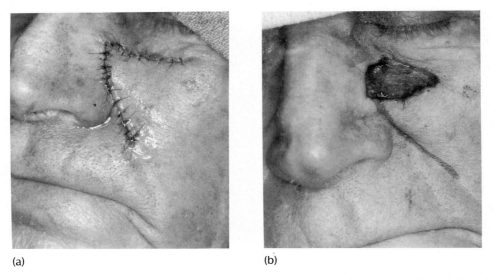

(a)   (b)

Figure 13   (a) Inferior based rotation flap designed in melolabial fold. (b) The key stitch tacks the flap tip to the medial aspect of the defect to avoid downward pull on the eyelid.

Surgical defects of the middle to upper portion of the cutaneous upper lip can also be repaired by designing a rotation flap with the curvilinear arc incised along the melolabial fold (Fig. 14). There must be sufficient lax skin to fill the wound but not pull up the labial commissure.

Rotation flaps have proven useful in the repair of small defects of the distal nose only in special situations where recruitment of only a few millimeters of tissue is required and there is sufficient lax skin in the nasal sidewall to allow it. The arc is designed superiorly into the RSTL, radiating down from the medial canthus. Unfortunately, if the defect is large or near the nostril rim, the tension vector will be directed to pull up on this free margin. In these situations, a transposition flap that changes the tension vector transversely would be a better choice to avoid unsightly elevation of the nostril.

Another useful repair for small to moderately sized defects of the distal nose is the dorsal nasal flap (Fig. 15). This is essentially a rotation flap with a back-cut built into the design. A curvilinear design is initiated from the lateral portion of the defect superiorly into the nasofacial sulcus and continuing into the ipsilateral glabellar frown line. The back-cut is continued into the contralateral frown line. The flap is widely undermined below the muscle plane at the level of the periosteum and the perichondrium. The flap is then draped into place to fill the defect. The secondary defect of the glabella is closed in a V-to-Y manner, which tends to push the flap further into place. The remaining closure lines are in junction lines and normal creases.

Bilateral rotation flaps are useful for larger repairs of the chin (Fig. 9). Curvilinear arcs fit nicely into the curved mentolabial crease. Tissue is recruited bilaterally and closure of the defect is completed within one cosmetic unit without extension onto the cutaneous lower lip. The glabella is another location that may be amenable to repair by a superiorly based bilateral rotation flap.

The O-to-Z bilateral rotation flap is a very useful flap for repairs on the hair-bearing scalp (Fig. 10). In this region the Z-shaped scar is well camouflaged. It may be the ideal repair for

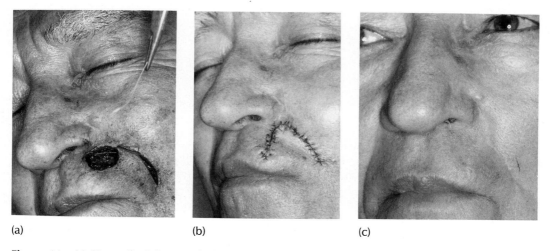

(a) (b) (c)

Figure 14 (a) Upper lip defect repaired with rotation flaps placed in melolabial fold. (b) Final closure. Incisions confirmed to RSTL of lip and melolabial fold. (c) At 2-month follow-up.

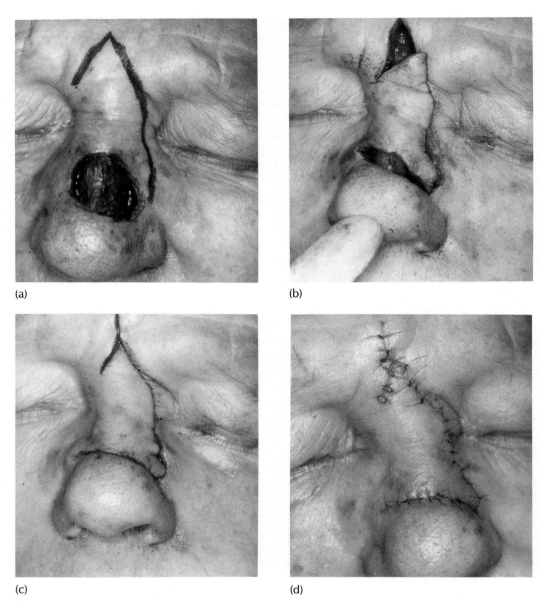

(a)

(b)

(c)

(d)

Figure 15   (a) Defect of nasal dorsum with back-cut rotation flap design. (b) Incisions confined to nasofacial junction and glabellar frown lines. (c) Flap rotated and advanced to fill primary defect. Secondary defect closed in a V-to-Y manner. (d) The final closure at 5 days.

defects of the vertex of the scalp because it results in a normal whorled configuration of the hair in this region.

BIBLIOGRAPHY

Albom MJ. Repair of large scalp defect by bilateral rotation flaps. *J Dermatol Surg Oncol* 1978;4:906–907.

Baron JL, Reynaud JP, et al. Specificity of hatchet flaps in the laterofacial region. *Ann Plast Esthet* 1990;35:47–52.

Cook TA, Israel JM, et al. Cervical rotation flaps for midface resurfacing. *Arch Otolaryngol Head Neck Surg* 1991;117:77–82.

Crow ML, Crow FJ. Resurfacing large cheek defects with rotation flaps from the cheek. *Plast Reconstr Surg* 1976;58:196–199.

Dzubow LM. The dynamics of flap movement: The effect of pivotal restraint on flap rotation and transposition. *J Dermatol Surg Oncol* 1987;13:1348–1353.

Golomb FM. Closure of the circular defect with double rotation flaps and Z-plasties. *Plast Reconstr Surg* 1984;74:813–816.

Hardaway RM. The useful rotation flaps. *Am J Surg* 1955;90:1013–1019.

Larrabee WR Jr, Sutton D. The biomechanics of advancement in rotation flaps. *Laryngoscope* 1981;91:726–734.

Snow SN, Mohs FE, Olansky DC. Nasal tip reconstruction: The horizontal "J" rotation flap using skin from the lower lateral bridge and cheek. *J Dermatol Surg Oncol* 1990;16:727–732.

Stark RB, Kaplan JM. Rotation flaps, neck to cheek. *Plast Reconstr Surg* 1972;50:230–235.

Winton GB, Salasche SJ. Use of rotation flaps to repair small surgical defects on the ala nasi. *J Dermatol Surg Oncol* 1986;12:154–158.

47

Transposition Flaps

Holly L. F. Christman and Roy C. Grekin
University of California, San Francisco, California

In the preceding chapters, the principles of flap surgery have been well covered. These serve as a good basis for understanding transposition flaps, which are conceptually the most difficult flaps to design and execute. In this chapter, we will present some general concepts about transposition flaps and then discuss specific examples. Finally, we will cover anatomic sites where they are most commonly used.

CLASSIFICATION

Flaps may be classified by a number of systems. Most flaps used in dermatologic surgery are *local*, indicating that they come from the same or adjacent cosmetic units. They usually have a blood supply, which is random pattern, i.e., not based on a specific artery but nourished by the network of the deep dermal plexus. They are most successful therefore in richly vascularized areas, such as the head and neck, or in other areas if they are small in size.

These principles apply to the transposition flaps most commonly used by dermatologic surgeons and the ones we will be considering in this chapter. There are transposition flaps that are harvested from more than one cosmetic unit away and performed as *staged* or *pedicle* flap, and they will be covered in the next chapter. There are also transposition flaps based on specific arteries, such as the many variations on the temperoparietal-occipital flap used in hair-replacement surgery, but we shall not discuss these specialized examples.

Flaps are also classified according to their type of movement. Advancement and rotation flaps are *sliding* flaps, but transposition flaps are not. Rather, they are cut, lifted, and rotated over *intervening tissue* into the primary defect.

DEFINITION OF TRANSPOSITION

To transpose means to change the place of without destroying the basic structure. The key concept in transposition flap design is that the vectors of the wound closure are transposed by 45–120 degrees. Often a primary defect cannot be closed along a certain axis, either because there is not enough tissue or because in so doing it will distort some adjacent structure. If there is tissue available 45–120 degrees from the defect, the surgeon can make use of this excess skin to create a transposition flap (Fig. 1).

The basic structure of the flap that is moved into place is maintained in transposition flaps, which are generally cut to fit the size and shape of the defect. In contrast, for sliding flaps (e.g., advancement and rotation flaps) the skin is stretched (pulled) into place.

ADVANTAGES OF TRANSPOSITION FLAPS

Efficient Use of Tissue

Because the flap is essentially the same size as the defect, transposition flaps are small compared to advancement and rotation flaps. The latter have 3:1 to 4:1 flap-to-defect size ratios, making transposition flaps economical in their tissue use.

Transferring Tension

The key suture in a flap is generally the first suture placed when moving a flap into position. It both aligns the flap over the primary defect and redirects the tension of the closure toward the

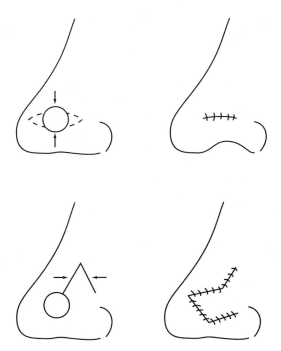

Figure 1 Schematic representation of transposition flap. Note direction of closure of secondary defect as compared to a side-to-side repair of this defect. Size of flap is approximately the same as the size of the defect.

secondary defect. In sliding flaps, such as rotation and advancement flaps, the key suture closes the primary defect and the tension is maintained across that primary site.

Transposition flaps are unique in that the key suture is the one that closes the secondary defect, i.e., the defect is 45–120 degrees away from the primary defect. In so doing, all of the tension is transferred to the secondary defect, allowing the flap to be "pushed" into place, rather than pulled, so that it drapes over the primary defect without any tension. Thus, transposition flaps are very useful for the closure of defects near free margins, such as the nasal alae or lower eyelids, where transfer of the tension can prevent distortion of those structures (Figs. 1,2).

Broken-Line Appearance

Long-term camouflage of scars is an important goal in dermatologic surgery. Our specialty teaches that hiding scars in skin tension lines or at the junction of cosmetic units aids in camouflage.

Another cosmetic principle is that a viewer's eye follows the lines of a linear scar more easily than the irregular pattern of a geometric design. Therefore, in certain areas, the geometric, broken-line scars that a transposition flap creates are preferred (Fig. 2).

SECONDARY DEFECT

In determining from where to elevate a transposition flap, several factors must be considered. First, in dealing with noncircular wounds, the flaps should always be designed off the short axis of the defect. Harvesting a transposition flap off the long axis results in a long, narrow-pedicled flap. This configuration also requires excessive rotation of the flap, placing increased tension on the pedicle and further limiting blood supply.

The next factor, and possibly the most important, is placement of the secondary defect in relation to surrounding anatomy. Since the tension of this repair is across the secondary defect, the donor site must be situated such that the tensions of its closure parallel free margins (Figs. 1,2).

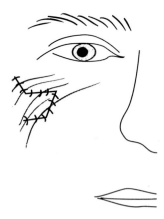

Figure 2 Transposition flaps have utility near free anatomic margins as the tension of the closure is directed across closure of the secondary defect, allowing the flap to "drape" into the primary defect in a tension-free manner. Proper flap design and placement of the secondary defect is essential to achieve this effect. Note that due to the rotation of a transposition flap, at least one incision line will traverse relaxed skin tension lines.

The third factor is camouflage. The multiple geometric broken lines and the small flap size facilitate camouflage. However, this can be maximized by using cosmetic borders and aligning these flaps as much as possible within skin tension lines (STLs). It is inherent in transposition flaps due to their 45–120 degree rotations that at least one closure line will cross rather than parallel STLs (Fig. 2).

TYPES OF TRANSPOSITION FLAPS

Banner Flap

The classic transposition flap is the banner flap, a finger-shaped flap that rotates from 45–120 degrees over intervening tissue into the primary defect (Fig. 3A). The flap width is the same size as the primary defect. Its length should be designed by determining the rotation point at the base of the flap and measuring from there to the most distal point of the primary defect. The novice surgeon will often be surprised by just how long the flap must be made. This is because of the effective shortening that occurs with rotation of the flap, and it is always prudent to add yet a few more millimeters to the measured length. These can always be trimmed if not needed, but it is difficult to salvage the situation if a flap is cut too short.

Once the flap is cut and elevated, the tissue surrounding the secondary defect is undermined to facilitate its closure. Undermining around the primary defect is controversial, but some believe it may lessen the chance of the flap becoming bulky or "pincushioning." The key suture is then placed to close the secondary defect. With this one suture, the genius of the transposition flap is evident—the tension is transferred from the primary defect to the secondary defect and the flap, without tension, drapes into place. The flap is then sutured into place, trimmed as

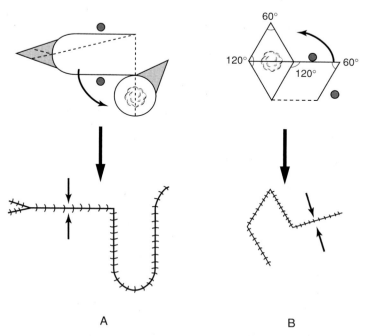

Figure 3   (A) Classic banner transposition flap. (B) Rhombic transposition flap. ● = Key suture placement; → ← = secondary tension.

required, and the rest of the secondary defect is closed. All transposition flaps will follow this basic pattern.

Dog ears are constant in all transposition flaps (Fig. 3A). One occurs at the point of rotation at the base of the primary defect. This redundant tissue, created by rotation of the flap into the primary defect, can be removed by excision of a triangle of tissue, called removal by "triangulation." Some surgeons design the removal of this as a part of the flap. We prefer to remove it once the flap is in place to better determine the exact location and amount of excess skin to be removed. There are situations where removing this would decrease the size of the base of the flap and compromise its blood supply, so it can be left. In several weeks to months, it may disappear or a small second procedure to remove it can be performed once the flap's blood supply is firmly established.

The second dog ear occurs at the superior aspect of the closure of the secondary defect and is dependent on the shape of the flap. If the flap has a rounded appearance or an angle of 60 degrees or greater, there will be a dog ear. Often the flap can be redesigned with a 30 degree angle or an M-plasty to prevent this. The M-plasty not only shortens the length of this secondary defect but confers upon the scar even more of a broken-line appearance (Fig. 3A).

Rhombic Flap

In contrast to the banner flap, the rhombic flap is designed with sharp angles. (*Note*: Due to technical definitions in geometry, these flaps are properly referred to as rhombic, but rhomboid is also in common use.) This design capitalizes on the concept presented earlier that sharp angles and zigzagging lines are less perceptible to the viewer's eye.

The first step in designing a rhombic flap is to draw a rhombus around the outer edges of the defect. Note that this is a parallelogram. It is not necessary to cut the defect into this shape. The flap is usually designed off the short axis of the rhombus so it extends out from one of the obtuse angles (Fig. 3B). One side of the rhombus is measured and a diameter extended through one of the obtuse angles for a distance equal to the rhombus side length. At the end of this length, a 60 degree angle is made and another line of the same length, which parallels the near side of the rhombic defect, is drawn (Fig. 3B).

At first glance, it seems that only a triangle has been drawn, and novice surgeons see only that shape. If one uses the mind's eye to extend yet another line parallel to the initial line drawn out from the obtuse angle to the near acute angle, it is clear that actually a parallelogram, specifically a rhombus, has been formed, of exactly the same measurement as the defect (Fig. 3B).

The flap is cut as designed and undermined, and as with the classic banner flap, the secondary defect will be closed first, allowing the flap to rotate into place without tension. Note that this transposes the vector of closure approximately 90 degrees from the primary defect. Again there will be dog ears to repair. This could be predicted because 60 degree angles are not favorable closure angles, and these exist at the base of the rhombic primary defect and at the superior tip of the rhombic secondary defect. The dog ear at the base of the rhombic primary defect can sometimes be designed out of the flap by extending the base to create a 30 degree angle. This sacrifices a lot of normal skin; therefore some surgeons prefer to design it as a M-plasty, but this can diminish the base of the flap. As discussed with the banner flap, one can wait until the flap is rotated into place and remove the dog ear by triangulation or leave the protrusion for correction at a later date.

When the rhombic flap is rotated into the primary defect, either it can be trimmed to fit the shape of the defect or the defect enlarged to accommodate the flap. Both options maintain the broken-line appearance, although the former does spare more normal tissue.

30 Degree Angle Flap

The 30 degree angle flap is a refinement of the rhombic flap designed to provide more favorable closure angles and thus eliminate the dog ear repairs. It does so by converting the 60 degree angles of the rhombic flap into 30 degree angles. The design, however, is predicated on the ability to close some of the primary defect by side-to-side motion; thus it loses the advantage of being able to transfer all the tension of the closure away from the primary defect. It follows that it is not a good choice for a primary defect located near a free margin. Since the tension of the closure is shared between the primary and secondary defect, it has the advantage of distributing tension over a larger area. Additionally, a smaller flap is required, since not all of the closure of the primary defect has to come from the flap.

This flap is designed by creating a rhombus out of the primary defect, with 60 degree angles top and bottom and 120 degree obtuse side angles. In the classic rhombic flap, the flap was designed by extending a line out that bisected the obtuse angle. Here, in contrast, a "plumb line" is drawn extending one side of the rhombus (Fig. 4A). This line serves as a base for design of the flap. The primary defect is measured across its short axis and one half of this width is taken to draw out the base of the flap along the plumb line starting from the obtuse angle. Then, using the measure of one side of the diamond, an isosceles triangle is created with the plumb line as its base. Thus, the isosceles triangle has its two long legs equal to a side of the primary defect, and its base is half the width. Because the flap is half the width of the primary defect, it closes half the defect, and the remaining closure is side to side (Fig. 4A).

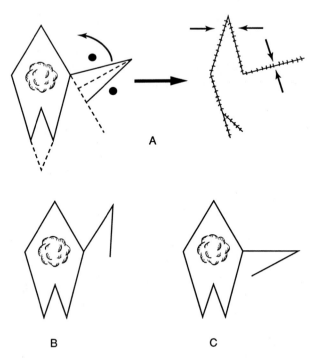

Figure 4 (A) Design and movement of a 30 degree angle flap. Note that the flap is one half the width of the defect and drawn off a "plumb line" created by extending one side of the defect downward. Tension is shared equally across both the primary and secondary defects. ● = Key suture; → ← = secondary tension. (B,C) Inappropriate designs fo 30 degree angle flap.

This flap can be hard to visualize, and two mistakes are commonly made in its design. One is to have the flap arise at too acute an angle from the plumb line (Fig. 4B). When this flap is closed, its vectors of closure are oriented in the same direction as those of the primary defect, so there is no sharing of the tension and thus no advantage to the flap. If the angle is too obtuse, i.e., greater than 90 degrees because of the 30 degree angle at the tip of the flap and its small size, the flap base will be narrowed and its blood supply compromised (Fig. 4C). This flap can be modified by converting the angle at the bottom of the rhombus into an M-plasty, thereby shortening the wound (Fig. 4A).

It is important with both the classic rhombic and the 30 degree angle flap to understand the appearance of the final incision lines. Because of the geometric pattern of this flap, clearly all lines will not be in relaxed skin tension lines. In fact, some lines will go against the RSTLs. The flap, however, can be pivoted to maximize its conformation to the RSTLs and thus its final cosmetic appearance (Fig. 2).

Bilobed Flap

The bilobed flap is another variation on the basic transposition flap (Fig. 5). It is considered when a transposition flap with all its advantages is desired but there is insufficient tissue movement immediately adjacent to the primary defect to close a secondary defect. By adding a second lobe to the flap, one "walks" the excess tissue from the more distant site so that the defect immediately adjacent to the primary defect can be closed. In this case, the key suture is placed to close the tertiary defect, which is the harvest site of the secondary lobe. As with all transposition flaps, the tension is transferred to this site at closure so that the flap drapes into place.

The actual size of the two lobes of the flap are dependent on how much secondary movement one can rely on from the surrounding skin. The first lobe is designed to be 75–100% of the size of the primary defect. For instance, if the flap is to be used to repair a nasal alar defect, and no closure is wanted to derive from the primary defect so as not to pull up the alar rim, one designs the lobe at 100%. If some closure of the primary defect is acceptable, then the size of the lobe can be closer to 75%. The second lobe is usually one-half the size of the first, relying on movement of the surrounding tissue to facilitate closure.

The two lobes may be designed with 30 degree angle tips to obviate dog ear repair. The primary lobe is generally rounded, as it is often closing a circular defect, and it will be closed by transfer of the secondary lobe into it. Some surgeons feel, however, that there is less pincushioning and better geometric line appearance if the primary lobe is designed with a 30 de-

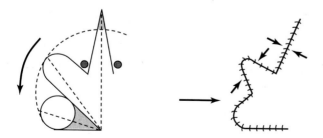

Figure 5 Schematic of the bilobed flap. Note the similarity to a rotation flap in its movement as well as its broad base. However, less tissue is moved than with a rotation flap, the geometric broken lines aid in camouflage, and tension is directed away from the primary defect. ● = Key suture; → ← = secondary tension.

gree angle. It has also been stated that undermining of the area around the primary defect will help prevent pincushioning.

The overall rotation of the flap may vary from 90 to 180 degrees depending on the location of excess tissue. The greater the angle of rotation, the more tissue protrusion there will be at the point of rotation. It is very important that each lobe rotate the same number of degrees or there will be "buckling" at the base of the lobe that has rotated to a greater degree.

Determining the length of the lobes is critical, and perhaps the trickiest task involved with transposition flaps. As with the classic banner flap, one must determine the point of rotation of the flap and remember that the length of the lobes will be effectively shortened in their rotation. If the lobe is made too short, it will not fit the primary defect and so the use of a flap will have been for naught; it is better to err by making the lobe several millimeters too long.

Once the tertiary defect is closed, allowing the flap to drape into place, and the flap is anchored, the dog ear created by the rotation may be excised by triangulation. As stated earlier, some surgeons prefer to design this into the flap, but we believe it is important to remove excess tissue only once the flap is in place. It can always be removed later, after the flap's blood supply is established.

Postoperatively, the appearance of the bilobed transposition flap is often compromised by the pincushioning discussed above. This can occur in both the primary and secondary lobes. Pincushioning can often be treated by the injection of steroids intralesionally beginning at 4–8 weeks postoperatively. We usually use triamcinalone acetonide 5–10 mg/cc, depending on the amount of bulkiness, and inject at 3- to 4-week intervals for a total of one to three injections. This will often result in a surprising reduction in bulkiness. Occasionally, we need to go back and revise the flap by incising the lobes, lifting them up, and paring down their undersurface. We would wait several months postoperatively before doing this, as time may result in a reduction in bulkiness. Dermabrasion 6–10 weeks postoperative aids in both camouflaging incision lines and debulking the flap.

AREAS OF UTILITY FOR TRANSPOSITION FLAPS

Because of their economy of size and the nature of their movement, transposition flaps can be used almost anywhere, particularly for facial defects. The main limitations relate to the ability

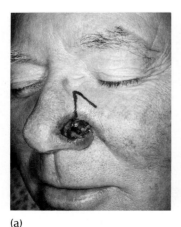 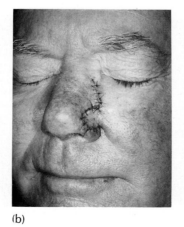 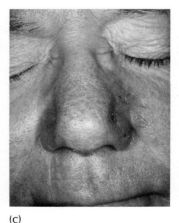

(a)   (b)   (c)

Figure 6   Rhombic flap on nasal ala: (a) defect; (b) closure; (c) long-term follow-up.

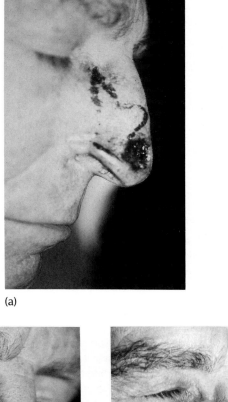

(a)

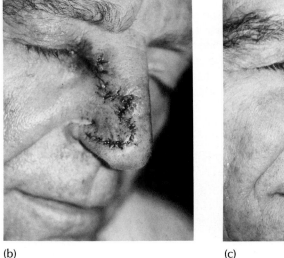

(b)

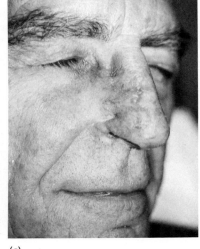

(c)

Figure 7 Bilobed flap on nasal ala: (a) defect; (b) closure; (c) long-term follow-up.

to close secondary defects primarily without compromising local anatomy and obtaining optimum camouflage within RSTLs and cosmetic borders.

Because transposition flaps are pushed into the primary defect, creating little or no tension at that site, they are ideally suited for closures near free margins. In these areas the secondary motion of an advancement or rotation flap may pull down on an eyelid or elevate a nasal ala. Flaps particularly useful on the nasal ala include the rhombic, bilobed, or nasolabial fold (Figs. 6,7,8). The decision to use one or the other of these depends on the size of the defect, the amount

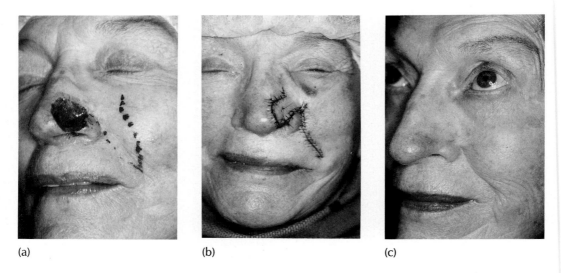

(a)   (b)   (c)

Figure 8   Nasolabial fold flap on nasal ala: (a) defect; (b) closure; (c) long-term follow-up.

and location of donor tissue, and the precise location of the defect in respect to the alar rim, nasal tip, or alar groove. On the lower eyelid defects can be repaired by a rhombic flap harvested from lateral canthal skin (Fig. 9) or a banner-type flap transposing upper eyelid skin to the lower lid. While cheek skin may be transposed superiorly to close a lower lid defect, this skin is much thicker than eyelid skin, and its weight may cause an ectropion.

Transposition flaps may be used around the free margins of the lips, but the nature of the incision lines and tissue movement inherent in these flaps will usually result in at least one scar cutting across rather than paralleling RSTL. Advancement and rotation flaps generally work better on the lips.

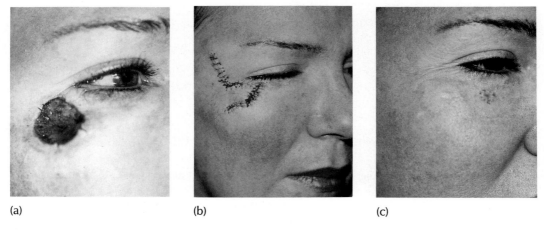

(a)   (b)   (c)

Figure 9   Rhombic flap repairing lower eyelid defect: (a) defect; (b) closure; (c) long-term follow-up.

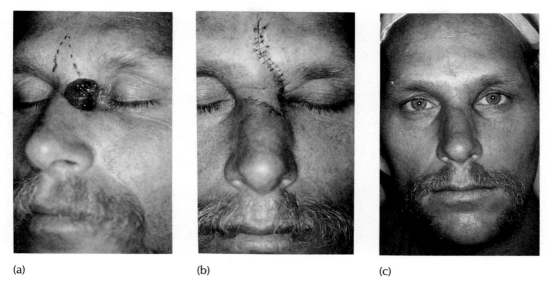

(a) (b) (c)

Figure 10 Banner transposition flap used to close a medial canthal-lateral nasal root defect: (a) defect, (b) closure; (c) one-month follow-up.

A banner-type flap may be raised from the glabella to repair nasal root or medial canthal defects. The surgeon must be sure that the closure of the secondary defect does not draw the eyebrows too close together. Also, the glabellar skin is considerably thicker than that of the lateral nasal root and may create a bulky appearance (Fig. 10). Another use for the banner flap is in repair of superior helical defects. A superiorly based flap may be raised from preauricular skin with secondary defect closure hiding well within the preauricular crease. The flap is then transposed onto the superior helix providing excellent coverage, cosmetic appearance, and more reliable take than a graft.

Transposition flaps have utility for repair of cheek defects. They are most useful for lateral and midcheek repairs where ample and extensible skin is available. They are less useful for medial cheek repairs where closure of the secondary defect may distort the eyelids or position of the melolabial fold. Also, camouflage with RSTLs is more difficult in the medial cheek. For lateral and midcheek repairs, a medially or inferiorly based rhombic flap should be designed to facilitate outflow drainage and lessen edema and flap thickening (i.e., pincushioning). A 30 degree angle flap is useful in this region because of good skin extensibility and the lack of nearby important anatomic structures. Bilobed flaps are neither necessary nor cosmetically advantageous on the cheek.

Rhombic flaps can be used for closure of wounds on the temple. However, they must usually be superiorly based, which may affect drainage of blood and lymph from the flap and in men may remove hairbearing cheek skin into this nonglabrous area.

The forehead skin is considered an extension of the scalp. As such is it thick and inelastic, making closure of the secondary defect created by a transposition flap difficult. This, combined with the well-defined horizontal skin tension lines, makes the region less amenable for use of transposition flaps. However, in patients with lax forehead skin, a rhombic or banner-type flap may be useful for closure of lateral or superolateral forehead defects.

BIBLIOGRAPHY

Arnold AT, Bennett RG. The bilateral dog-ear transposition flap. J Dermatol Surg Oncol 1990;16:667–672.

Borges AF. The rhombic flap. Plast Reconstr Surg 1981;67:458–66.

Davidson TM, Webster R, Gordon BR. The Principles and Dynamics of Local Skin Flaps. Alexandria: American Academy of Otolaryngology–Head and Neck Surgery Foundation Inc., 1988.

Dzubow LM. Design of an appropriate rhombic flap for a circular defect created by Mohs microscopically controlled surgery. J Dermatol Surg Oncol 1988;14:126–28.

Field LM. Design concepts for the nasolabial fold flap (letter). Plast Reconstr Surg 1983;71:283–85.

Field LM. Peripheral tissue undermining is not the final answer to prevent trapdooring in transposition flaps (letter). J Dermatol Surg Oncol 1993;1993:191131-2.

Holt PJA, Motley RJ. A modified rhombic transposition and its application in dermatology. J Dermatol Surg Oncol 1991;17:287–92.

Gormley DE. A brief analysis of the Burrow's wedge/triangular principle. J Dermatol Surg Oncol 1985;11:121–23.

Jackson IT. Local flaps in head and neck reconstruction. St. Louis, C. V. Mosby Co., 1985.

Kaufman AJ, Kiene KL, Moy RL. Role of tissue underminng in the trapdoor effect of transposition flaps. J Dermatol Surg Oncol 1993;19:128–32.

Kolbusz RV, Goldberg LH. The labial-ala transposition flap. Arch Dermatol 1994;130:162–64.

Larrabee WFJ, Trachy R, Sutton D, Cox K. Rhomboid flap dynamics. Arch Otolaryngol 1981;107:755–7.

Masson JK, Mendelsohn BC. The banner flap. Am J Surg 1977;134:419–23.

McGregor JC, Soutar DS. A critical assessment of the bilobed flap. Br J Plast Surg 1981;34:197–205.

Monheit GD. The rhomboid flap. In: Dermatologic Surgery. St. Louis, C. V. Mosby Co., 1988.

Moy RL. Atlas of cutaneous facial flaps and grafts— A differential diagnosis of wound closures. Philadelphia, Lea & Febiger, 1990.

Robinson JK, Horan DB. Modified nasolabial transposition flap provides vestibular lining and cover of alar defect with intact rim. Arch Dermatol 1990;126:1425–27.

Salasche SJ, Bernstein G, Senkarik M. Surgical Anatomy of the Skin. Norwalk, CT, 1988.

Salasche SJ, Grabski WJ. In: Grekin RC, ed., Flaps for the Central Face. New York, Churchill Livingstone, 1990.

Summers BK, Siegle RJ. Facial cutaneous reconstructive surgery: General aesthetic principles. J Am Acad Dermatol 1993;29:669–81.

Summers BK, Siegle, RJ. Facial cutaneous reconstructive surgery: Facial flaps. J Am Acad Dermatol 1993;29:917–41.

Swanson NA. Atlas of Cutaneous Surgery. Boston, Little, Brown, and Co., 1987:1–177.

Tromovitch TA, Stegmen SJ, Glogau RG. Flaps and Grafts in Dermatologic Surgery. Chicago, Mosby Year Book, 1989.

Walkinshaw M, Caffee HH. The Nasolabial Flap: A Problem and Its Correction. Plast Reconstr Surg 1982;69:30–34.

Webster RC, Davidson TM, Smith TC. The thirty degree transposition flap. Laryngoscope 1978;88:85–94.

Zitelli JA. The bilobed flap for nasal reconstruction. Arch Dermatol 1989;125:957–59.

Zitelli JA. The nasolabial fold flap as a single-stage procedure. Arch Dermatol 1990;126:1445–48.

Zitelli JA, ed. Special Issue: Local Flaps. J Dermatol Surg Oncol 1991;17:112–204.

48

Pedicle Flaps

J. Ramsey Mellette, Jr.
University of Colorado Health Sciences Center, Denver, Colorado

THE PARAMEDIAN FOREHEAD PEDICLE FLAP FOR NASAL RECONSTRUCTION

In the 27th edition of *Dorland's Illustrated Medical Dictionary*, a pedicle flap is defined as "a flap consisting of full thickness of skin and the subcutaneous tissue attached by tissue through which it achieves its blood supply." In practice most pedicle flaps remain attached to their source for a period of several days to a few weeks. Viability is thus assured by establishment of a blood supply in the recipient bed. In dermatologic surgery the three most common pedicle flaps utilized are the paramedian forehead flap for nasal reconstruction, the superiorly based naso-labial pedicle flap for extensive defects of the ear. This chapter will present applications of the forehead pedicle flap for nasal reconstruction. (*Editor's Note*. RKR also commonly prefers the subcutaneous island pedicle flap, especially for upper lip defects, as discussed in Chap. 44.)

HISTORICAL NOTES

The forehead flap for nasal reconstruction was known to have been performed by the Kanghiara family of India as early as A.D. 1440 and may well have been performed as early as 1000 B.C. The more modern reports on the forehead flaps extend back at least 150 years. In the last 40 years most practitioners have utilized either "the precise midline" forehead flap or the "paramedian" forehead flap. Both of these variations have been employed successfully with excellent aesthetic results; however, the paramedian version will be emphasized here.

GENERAL

The vascular supply for the pedicle forehead flap is provided primarily by the supratrochlear vessel system, which eminates from the supratrochlear foramen inferior to the medial orbital rim.

When based on both supratrochlear vessels, this flap is usually described as "midline"; when based on one of the paired supratrochlear vessels, it is described as "paramedian."

Although the paramedian flap appears to be have been utilized by Labat in the 1830s, Millard is generally credited with revealing it in the current reconstructive literature beginning in the 1960s. Burget and Menick, along with Millard, have provided much of the literature detailing the technique and its applications.

It is clear that the paramedian flap with its single-vessel system is equal in reliability to the two-vessel midline flap and offers significant advantages, which include:

1. A narrow pedicle of approximately 1 cm at its origin, with the result that there is less possibility of strangulation of the pedicle. This narrow pedicle can be amputated at its origin in the glabella with the defect closed simply side to side.
2. A longer flap is possible, since the incisions at its origins can be extended below the level of the brow in the area of the medial canthus and into the nasal bridge medially.
3. The opposite side can be utilized as a backup should there be a recurrence of skin cancer or other indications for forehead flap reconstruction.

The paramedian flap is unusually versatile. It can be used to reconstruct the entire surface of the nose and, when properly lined, can be used to repair full-thickness defects. Two procedures are necessary. The first requires insertion of the pedicle into the defect. The second involves division of the pedicle once its blood supply in the recipient area is assured, usually within 14–21 days. In many cases it can be done in the outpatient operatory under local anesthesia or local combined with regional block anesthesia.

ANATOMIC CONSIDERATIONS

McCarthy et al. have demonstrated that the forehead has a rich blood supply from the supraorbital, supratrochlear, infratrochlear, dorsal nasal, and angular branches of the facial artery (Fig. 1). Anastomoses among these vessels ensure more than adequate profusion of forehead flaps, but the supratrochlear vessel is the branch most important to the paramedian flap. It originates from the supratrochlear foramen medially beneath the orbital rim, where it lies between the corrugator and frontalis muscle. The corrugator frontal crease (the glabellar crease) serves as a landmark of the location of the supratrochlear vessel in this area. One can dissect over the orbital rim beneath the muscle without injury to the vessel. The flap origin can therefore be inferior to the level of the brow, which, as previously stated, provides extra length.

Consideration must be given to the length of tissue available from the forehead. The height from the glabella to the hairline varies significantly. One would see as ideal a male with a receded hairline with unlimited vertical height, but is not infrequently faced with a patient whose eyebrows seem to join his or her hairline (Fig. 2). In the case of short vertical height, there are two possible solutions. One is to extend the flap into the hairline. This soon-to-be-distal portion of the flap can be thinned extensively with an attended attempt to transect the hair bulbs. Another solution is to arch the flap horizontally along the forehead. This may present problems with healing of the forehead defect. However, due at least in part to the extensive anastomotic connections previously mentioned, even lengthy horizontal extensions have not compromised flap viability (Figs. 3–9).

The patient pictured presented an extreme case of an unusually short vertical forehead and the need for a long and wide forehead flap. The defect included the surface of the nose, the full thickness of the nasal ala and a portion of adjacent cheek (Fig. 3). The cheek was advanced to the nasal side wall, and the forehead flap was utilized to resurface the nasal defect (Fig. 4). The

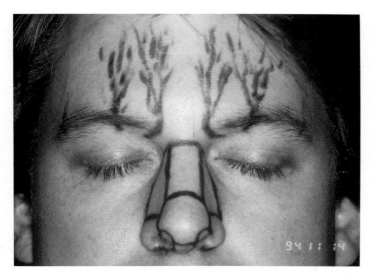

Figure 1 Extensive anastomoses of supratrochlear (medial brow) and supraorbital (midbrow) vessels.

aforementioned technique of extending the incision inferior to the orbital rim would have provided additional length and has been routinely employed in subsequent cases. There was minimal ecchymoses at the tip (Fig. 5), but no significant impedement to flap viability. After 2 weeks the pedicle was divided, the stump of the pedicle returned to the forehead, and the remainder of the forehead defect repaired with a full-thickness graft (Figs. 5,8). A superiorly based nasolabial flap was utilized to reconstruct the nasal ala (Figs. 6,7) with the long-term result as seen in Figure 9. An auricular composite graft to further reconstruct the inferior lateral alar was offered but refused by the patient.

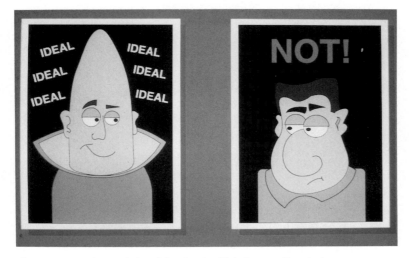

Figure 2 Vertical height of forehead will influence flap design.

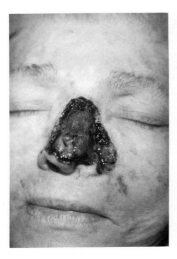

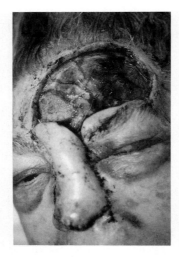

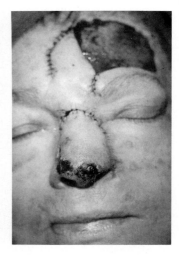

Figure 3 Extensive nasal and cheek defect following Mohs micrographic surgery. Note short vertical height of forehead.

Figure 4 Forehead flap arched to provide necessary length.

Figure 5 Stump of pedicle returned to forehead. Remainder of defect to receive full-thickness graft.

THE TECHNIQUE

The technique for the usual case is developed as follows: The forehead and nasal defect area are injected with 1% lidocaine 1:100,000 epinephrine buffered with 1:10 sodium bicarbonate. A template of the defect (Figs. 10–12) is made utilizing nonadherent pads (alternatively, aluminum foil or the metal wrapping of sutures may suffice).

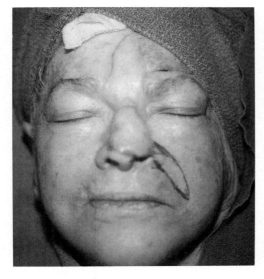

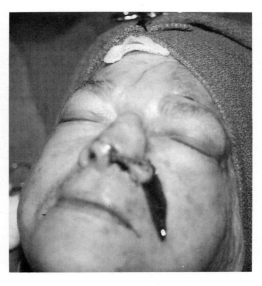

Figure 6 Design of superiorly based nasolabial fold flap to recreate nasal ala.

Figure 7 Nasolabial fold flap attached. Flap division planned in 2 weeks.

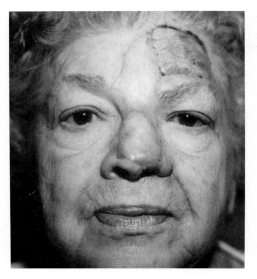

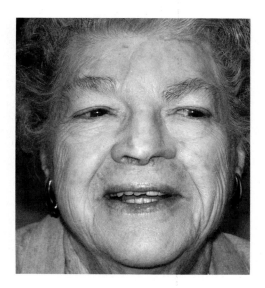

Figure 8 Six-week follow-up of full-thickness graft to forehead and nasolabial fold flap to alar rim.

Figure 9 Result at 1 year.

The length of the flap is carefully measured from the area of the chosen supratrochlear vessels to the lower limits of the defect (Fig. 12). A Doppler may be used to precisely identify the supratrochlear blood flow; however, no complications have been encountered in identifying the vessel location by anatomic landmarks. The template is applied to the forehead and outlined with a sterile marking pen (Fig. 13,14). The length and fit are verified. An incision (Fig. 15) is begun in the midglabella between the eyebrows. This incision is taken deep through the subcutaneous tissues down to the periosteum and is extended upward in the forehead precisely along the inked

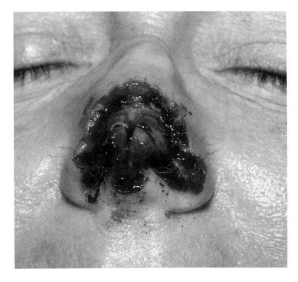

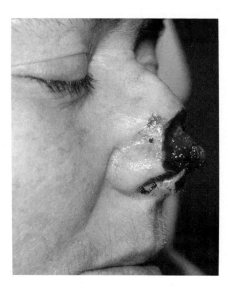

Figure 10 Extensive nasal tip and alar defect.

Figure 11 Right lateral view of defect.

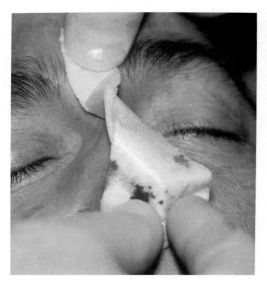

Figure 12 Dressing pad template including excess to allow for enfolding to reconstruct alar rims.

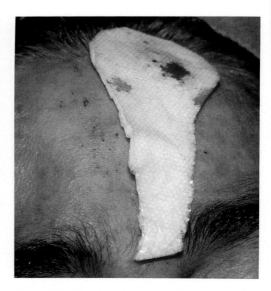

Figure 13 Precise placement of template.

margins. The incision is then continued downward toward the area of the medial eyebrow (Fig. 16). At a point just superior to the medial brow, the incision is made shallow through the epidermis and dermis until the flap can be fully elevated. At this point the flap is retracted away from the forehead, the incision is extended slightly inferior to the brow, and with good visualization the remaining attachment of the flap is bluntly dissected (Fig. 17). This dissection can

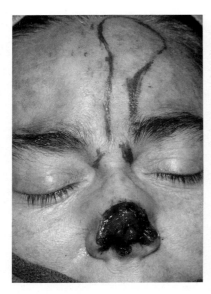

Figure 14 Inked outline of template and approximate location.

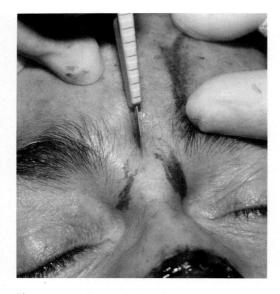

Figure 15 Midglabella incision. Note accurately estimated location of supratrochlear vessels.

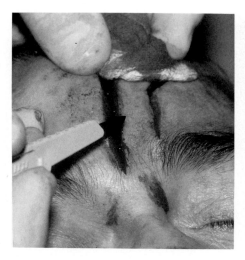

Figure 16 Incision to medial eyebrow.

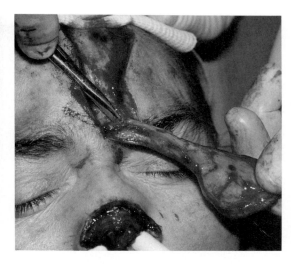

Figure 17 Scissor dissection of flap. For added length the incision can be extended below the brow.

be carried along and below the orbital rim. The raised flap is held in the hand and the tip of the flap is thinned of fascia and muscle with serrated iris scissors (Fig. 18). It is advisable to leave enough fat for additional vascularity (presumably provided in the fat by the subdermal plexus) but not so much as to compromise good wound apposition. The flap is then rotated inward on its axis and the tip placed in the defect (Figs. 19,20). Exceptionally, due to eccentric location of the defect an outward rotation of the flap may be desirable. In Figures 21 and 22 the

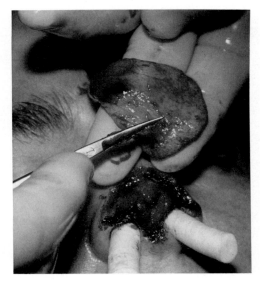

Figure 18 Scissor removal of fascia and muscle from the distal flap.

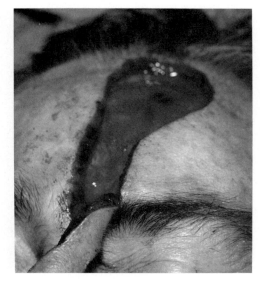

Figure 19 Inward 180° rotation of flap.

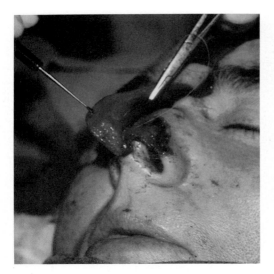

Figure 20 Tip of flap attached to columella.

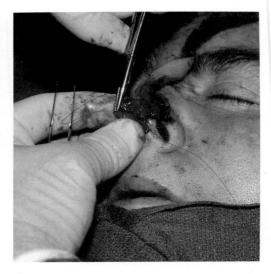

Figure 21 The suture needle is placed near the distal rim and exited 5 mm proximal.

flap is infolded with absorbable suture to recreate the alar rims. The wound edges are approximated with 5–0 nylon or other suitable suture material (23). Due partly to wound contracture, there is a tendency for wound inversion at the point of attachment. Vertical mattress sutures to evert the wound edge may be helpful in preventing this tendency.

With a properly designed flap, the pedicle width at its origin in the medial brow area generally need not be more than 1 cm wide; therefore, the lower part of the forehead defect can usually be closed side to side (Figs. 24,25). The undermining plane for the forehead closure lies above

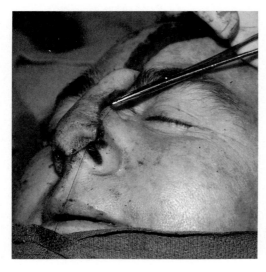

Figure 22 With the suture tied, the alar rim is recreated. This was repeated on the opposite side.

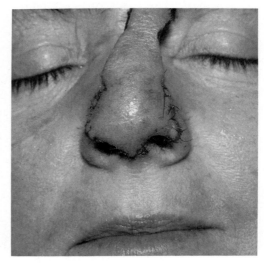

Figure 23 Flap is sutured with simple and vertical mattress suture.

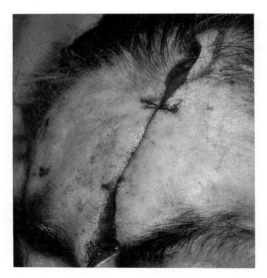

Figure 24 Partial closure of defect. Dog ear was rotated into defect to close widest part in hairline.

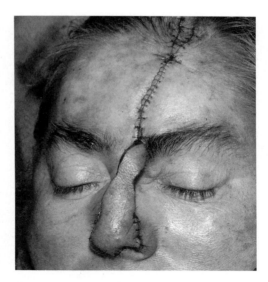

Figure 25 Complete closure of forehead defect.

the periostium in a manner similar to that employed for scalp reductions. The upper part of the forehead defect may be broad enough to require repair by flap (Fig. 24) or graft or to provide for healing by second intention.

The flap will be left attached to its pedicle for a period of 2–3 weeks. The stump is dressed with a moist dressing usually consisting of vaseline-impregnated gauze, antibiotic or a moisturizing ointment, nonadherent pads, and gauze. Within the first 24 h the wound is inspected in the office and is usually cleaned with saline or diluted hydrogen peroxide (1/2 hydrogen peroxide diluted with water) and redressed. The dressing is generally changed once or twice a week. If necessary, the dressing can be changed at home by family members or home care assistants.

After 2 weeks (rarely 3), the pedicle is ready to be divided (Fig. 26). Viability may be confirmed by compressing the stump with a penrose drain. There will be a slight blanching since there tends to be some hyperemia at the tip, but failure to adequately vascularize at this point has not been encountered. With sterile technique and under local anesthesia, the flap is divided at the superior point of insertion in the defect (Fig. 27). The proposed division should offer generous excess of tissue, which will be trimmed to assure appropriate wound apposition. It is again helpful to apply eversion techniques to decrease the tendency for a crease to form along the line of closure. The pedicle is then amputated in the glabella area (Fig. 28). Electrocautery is generally sufficient to seal the remaining supratrochlear vessels. There is usually sufficient tissue laxity to allow for simple side-to-side closure of the defect left by the amputated stump (Fig. 29). At 6 months the outstanding bulk and color match of the forehead flap can be appreciated (Figs. 30–33).

CONSIDERATION OF REGIONAL OR TOPOGRAPHIC SUBUNITS

Gonzales-Ulloa is generally credited with advancing the concept of reconstruction of regional or topographic subunits. This has been expanded and emphasized in recent articles by various re-

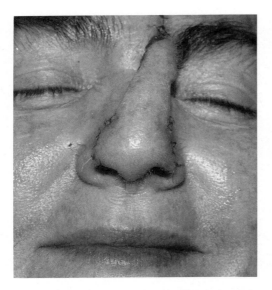

Figure 26 At 2 weeks flap viability is assured.

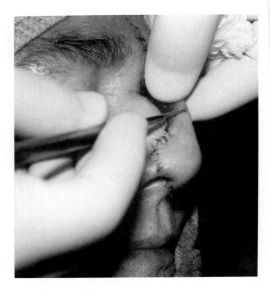

Figure 27 Division of pedicle.

constructive surgeons, most notably Burget and Menick, and is covered in detail elsewhere in this text (see Chap. 22). The concept is that the nose is considered an aesthetic unit of the face. The smaller parts of the nose are then designated topographic subunits (Fig. 34). When a significant part of a subunit or subunits has been lost, it is often advisable to replace the entire subunit or units. This is a valid consideration, and attempts are always made to adhere to its

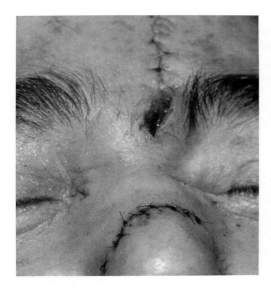

Figure 28 Amputated pedicle stump.

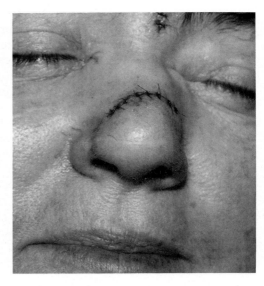

Figure 29 Completed closure of flap insertion and stump.

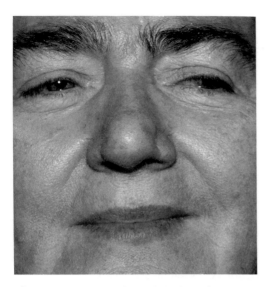

Figure 30 Frontal view of result at 6 months.

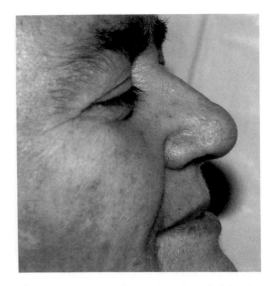

Figure 31 Result of reconstruction of right alar rim.

principals. On occasion, the potential size of the forehead defect—which should always be secondary in consideration of the nasal reconstruction—will require that the surgeon not follow these principals absolutely. Particularly in the case of some males, a less than perfect nasal reconstruction may be preferable to a very undesirable forehead scar.

A middle-aged male patient had a defect that was full-thickness beneath the alar rim (Fig. 35). His life-long style was to comb his hair backward away from the forehead. In consideration of

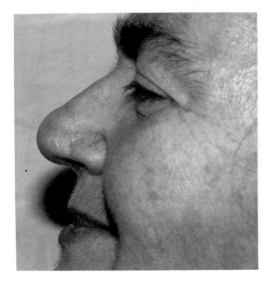

Figure 32 Result of reconstruct of left alar rim.

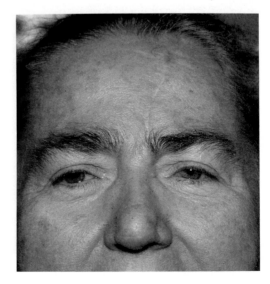

Figure 33 Acceptable forehead scar.

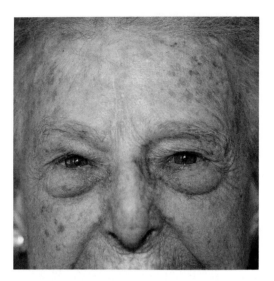

Figure 42   Six-month result of defects in Figures 41 and 42.

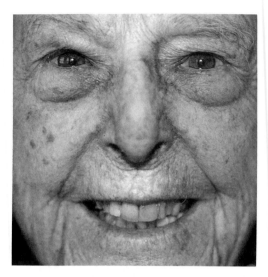

Figure 43   Close-up of forehead flap repair of defect in Figure 40.

An attractive middle-aged female patient had a full-thickness defect of the alar rim following Mohs micrographic surgery for a recurrent basal cell carcinoma (Fig. 44). Consideration was given to extending the defect to replace the lateral nasal tip and ala with a composite cartilage graft. Ultimately it was decided that a less complicated approach involving infolding of the fore-

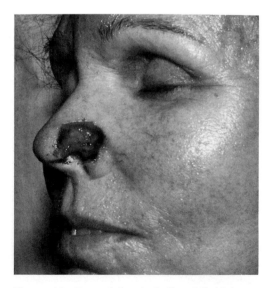

Figure 44   Deep defect including full thickness loss of mid-alar rim.

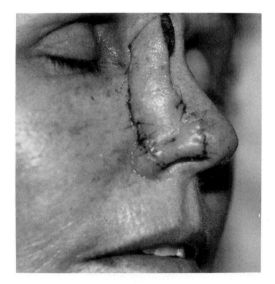

Figure 45   Alar rim recreated by enfolding flap. Note pexing suture.

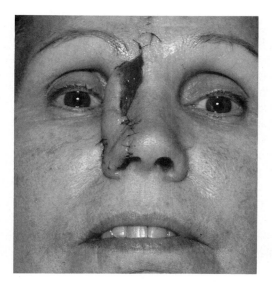

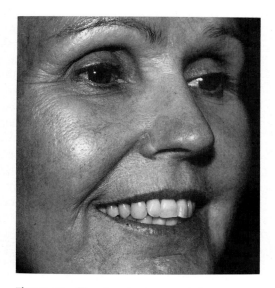

Figure 46 Frontal view of attached flap. Note pedicle origin inferior to brow.

Figure 47 The alar rim is recreated.

head flap to recreate the alar rim would provide an acceptable aesthetic result (Figs. 45,46). A pexing suture (Fig. 45) was utilized to assist in recreating the superior alar crease. Approximately 1.5 cm of added length for the flap was achieved by extending the incisions below the brow (Figs. 46). The long-term result is seen in Figures 47 and 48. The forehead defect was closed side to side. The resulting scar was minimally visible (Fig. 48).

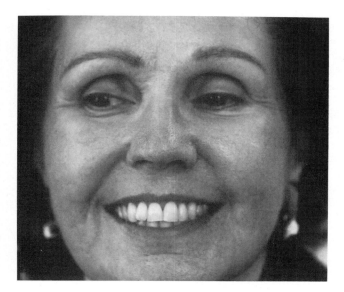

Figure 48 Acceptable long-term result with minimal forehead scar.

CONSIDERATIONS

The richly vascularized paramedian forehead flap is exceptionally suited for nasal reconstruction and can be done safely and reliably in the outpatient setting under local anesthesia. In bulk and color it more closely resembles normal nasal tissue than any other flap or graft. This technique may be used to reconstruct the entire surface of the nose and provides especially elegant tissue for replacement of the nasal tip and ala. Even if the vertical height of the forehead is short, a flap of sufficient length will be possible. Added length is obtained by incising over the orbital rim to a point just inferior to the medial brow. In exceptional circumstances the flap may extend vertically into the hairline, or it may be arched horizontally. With added flap length, the full-thickness defects, especially along the alar rim, tip, and columella, can be repaired by inward folding of the distal edge. More extensive full-thickness defects will require lining and support with various combinations of skin and cartilage grafts and adjacent tissue flap.

Difficulties and complications in utilizing these flaps have been minimal. Bleeding from the pedicle has occurred in 3 of 35 cases, developing in each case within the first 24 h. One episode was the result of direct trauma 4 h post operative. The patient stumbled and fell against the bedpost! The other two cases were detected at the time of initial dressing change 24 h postoperative and were controlled by electrocautery under local anesthesia. There have been no flap failures.

Prophylactic antibiotics are not routinely prescribed. In cases of long duration and/or if a break in sterile technique is known or suspected, antibiotics are given for 7–10 days. Infection has not been encountered. The forehead scar, especially the upper part, may rarely be significant. Intralesional steroids prove useful in softening these scars and hairstyling techniques may provide camouflage. Not uncommonly the flaps may have too much bulk. Revision, especially thinning, may be necessary to achieve optimal results.

BIBLIOGRAPHY

Antia NH, Daver BM. Reconstructive surgery for nasal defects. *Clin Plast Surg* 1981;8(3):535–563.
Burget GC. Aesthetic reconstruction of the nose. *Clin Plast Surg* 1985;12(3):463–480.
Burget GC, Menick FJ. *Aesthetic Reconstruction of the Nose.* St. Louis, Mosby, 1994.
Burget GC, Menick FJ. The subunit principal in nasal reconstruction. *Plast Reconstr Surg* 1985;76(2):239–247.
Dorland's Illustrated Medical Dictionary. 27th ed. Philadelphia, WB Saunders Co, 1988.
Gaze NR. Reconstructing the nasal tip with a midline forehead flap. *Br J Plast Surg* 1980;33:122–126.
Gonzales-Ulloa M. Restoration of the face covering by means of selected skin in regional aesthetic units. *Br J Plast Surg* 1957;9(3):212.
Gonzalez-Ulloa M. Reconstruction of the nose and forehead by means of regional aesthetic units. *Br J Plast Surg* 1961;13(4):305.
Kotler R. The midline forehead flap for resurfacing the nose. *J Dermatol Surg Oncol* 1981;7(1):57–66.
McCarthy JG, Lorene ZD, et al. The median forehead flap revisited: The blood supply. *Plast Reconstr Surg* 1985;76:866.
Menick FJ. Aesthetic refinements in use of forehead for nasal reconstruction: The paramedian forehead flap. *Clin Plast Surg* 1990;17(4):607–622.
Millard DR Jr. Hemirrhinoplasty. *Plast Reconstr Surg* 1967;40:440.
Millard DR Jr. Reconstructive rhinoplasty for the lower half of a nose. *Plast Reconstr Surg* 1974;53:133–139.
Millard DR Jr. Reconstructive rhinoplasty for the lower two-thirds of the nose. *Plast Reconstr Surg* 1978;57:722–728.

Shumrick, K. Arterial circulation of the forehead. Its importance in nasal reconstruction. In: Burgett CG, Menick FJ eds. *Aesthetic Reconstruction of the Nose*. St. Louis, Mosby, 1994:62.

Tardy ME Jr, Sykes S, Kron T. The precise midline forehead flap in reconstruction of the nose. *Clin Plast Surg* 1985;12(3):481–494.

Thomas R, Griner N, Cook TA. The precise midline forehead flap as a musculocutaneous flap. *Arch Otolaryngol Head Neck Surg* 1988;114:79–84.

49

Skin Grafts

Ronald G. Wheeland
University of New Mexico, Albuquerque, New Mexico

HISTORY

The first skin graft was performed in India nearly 3000 years ago. The Hindus reconstructed nasal defects with full-thickness skin grafts. It was not until 1869 that Reverdin published his experience with small pinch grafts in the treatment of a variety of cutaneous defects. In 1870, Lawson used full-thickness skin grafts to repair defects of the eyelid, and von Esmarck later used full-thickness skin grafts in other areas of the body. Thiersch reported the first use of split-thickness skin grafts in 1886. Since that time, the technique has improved. The dermatologic surgeon should be able to place several different types of skin grafts in order to treat most satisfactorily the patient with a cutaneous defect.

USE

Skin grafts are used when primary repair is impossible due to size, location, or tension on the wound. They are also indicated when repair with a flap would result in significant disfigurement or morbidity. Skin grafts are typically used to protect deeper vital structures such as bone or cartilage and keep them from becoming desiccated. Skin grafts prevent contraction of soft tissue. This is helpful when the defect is around the facial orifices such as the eyelids or lips. Skin grafts speed healing time compared to that required for second intention. Lastly, skin grafts may provide temporary coverage for a defect after oncologic surgery. This permits careful evaluation of the wound for evidence of recurrent tumor.

TYPES

There are essentially three types of skin grafts (Table 1). The split-thickness skin graft (Fig. 1) consists of full-thickness epidermis and partial thickness dermis. One type of split-thickness skin

Table 1 Comparison of Skin Grafts

	Full-thickness	Split-thickness	Composite
Nutritional requirements	High	Low	High
Color	Good	Poor	Good
Contraction	Low	High	Low
Durability	Fair	Poor	Fair
Sensation	Good	Fair	Fair
Appendageal functions (hair, eccrine, sebaceous)	Excellent	Poor	Good

graft is the pinch graft, which was described more than a century ago. The full-thickness skin graft consists of epidermis and a complete thickness of dermis. One type of full-thickness skin graft is the dog-ear graft. The composite graft is composed of skin and some other appendage such as hair or cartilage. Hair transplant autografts consist of both skin and hair follicle structures used for hair replacement.

SPLIT-THICKNESS SKIN GRAFTS

Pinch Graft

The pinch graft is the simplest type of split-thickness skin graft. It is used in the treatment of stasis ulceration, decubitus ulcers, slowly healing traumatic or burn wounds, or ulcers of chronic radiodermatitis. The benefit of this technique is largely its safety and simplicity. Pinch grafting can be performed by surgeons with little experience with skin grafting. It can be used for patients who have significant medical problems or who are on medication that might typically interfere with normal wound healing. No special instrumentation is required.

This procedure can be performed on an outpatient basis in most situations. The grafts are highly successful, because they have exceedingly low metabolic demands. For this reason, this type of graft is often successful when other grafts fail. Pinch grafts are capable of surviving in

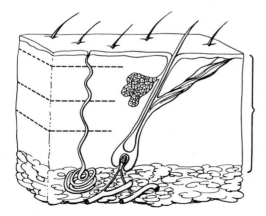

Figure 1 Various thickness of skin grafts: split-thickness (thin, medium, and thick) on left, full-thickness on right.

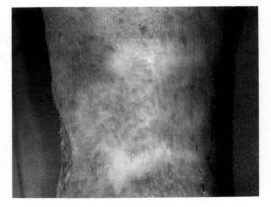

Figure 2 The irregular cobblestone appearance of a healed pinch-grafted site is obvious long after the wound has healed.

areas of decreased blood flow or in the presence of bacterial colonization. Functional results can be expected and grafting can be repeated as needed since the donor site is not permanently damaged.

A major disadvantage is that pinch grafting can be time-consuming. In addition, the small donor scars are obvious and may be difficult to hide. Most importantly, however, the ulcers that are treated have a typical cobblestone appearance (Fig. 2). This may be cosmetically unacceptable in spite of the fact they are functionally acceptable.

The ulcer bed must be clean, well vascularized, and devoid of necrotic debris. This can be done in several ways, the most expeditious being blunt surgical debridement. Other approaches include enzymatic debridement, application of synthetic membrane dressings, topical benzoyl peroxide, dextranomer granules, whirlpool baths, and antibacterial ointments. If the patient is to be treated at home, an effective way to obtain a clean ulcer bed is to use an oral hygiene device, such as WaterPik.

Once the ulcer bed is ready for grafting, wheals approximately 1 cm in diameter are raised on the donor site (Fig. 3a), which is typically the anterior thigh, by the intradermal injection of lidocaine 1%. The grafts are taken by shaving the top off each wheal using a #11 Bard-Parker blade (Fig. 3b) or sterile razor blade (Fig. 3c) at the level of the papillary dermis. These grafts are then placed in the ulcer bed spaced 1–2 mm apart (Fig. 3d). The grafted ulcer is then covered with a sheet of sterile transparent polyurethane (Fig. 3e) (Op-Site, Tegaderm, Bioclusive, or Ensure It). This membrane should overlap the ulcer bed by 2–3 cm onto the adjacent normal skin. A cotton-ball stent is placed on top of the polyurethane membrane to compress the grafts into the base of the ulcer. The grafted site is then immobilized and dressed with an elastic wrap, which is left in place for 7–8 days.

The donor site is treated in a similar fashion. This permits rapid wound healing by second intention. The polyurethane membrane is allowed to separate within 12–14 days after reepithelialization is complete (Fig. 3f). Pooling of blood or exudative fluids can be drained by puncturing the membrane with an 18-gauge needle. This puncture site can be repaired with a small piece of polyurethane membrane so that desiccation will not occur. If incomplete wound healing of the ulcer bed has not occurred in 6 weeks, these portions can be regrafted (Fig. 3g). While the patient may ambulate somewhat, walking should be kept to a minimum to avoid dislodging the grafts.

Classification

A split-thickness skin graft is the free transfer of epidermis and a portion of the dermis from one site to another. Split-thickness skin grafts are classified according to the thickness and are typically classified as thin (0.0006–0.0012"), intermediate (0.0012–0.0018"), or thick (0.0018–0.0024") (Fig. 1).

Split-thickness skin grafts are used to cover large defects. After tumor surgery, they permit observation of the wound for evidence of tumor recurrence, while a more definitive repair is planned at a later date. Split-thickness skin grafts can also be used to cover the second defect from a flap or to line composite grafts.

The benefit of split-thickness skin grafts is that there is almost no limitation to the size of the defect that can be treated, and virtually no part of the body cannot be used as a donor site (Fig. 4). The success rate is relatively high, especially with thinner split-thickness grafts. While these skin grafts do not prevent wound contraction, they will reduce what would normally occur. At the same time, split-thickness skin grafts will speed wound healing compared to healing by second intention.

To apply properly, a split-thickness skin graft requires more meticulous technique than pinch grafts. In addition, special equipment and assistance are necessary. While the appearance of

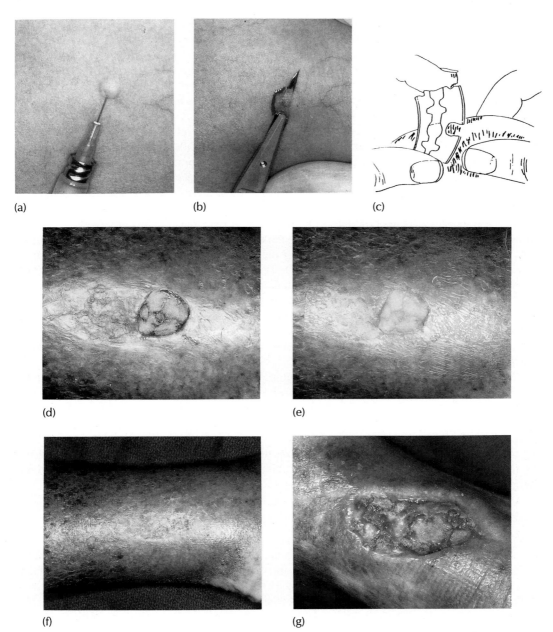

Figure 3 (a) Creation of a wheal by the intradermal injection of 1% plain lidocaine. (b) Harvesting a thin pinch graft with a sawing motion and a #11 Bard-Parker scalpel blade. (c) Alternative method for harvesting pinch grafts using a razor blade. (d) Immediate postoperative appearance of a small stasis ulcer with pinch grafts placed in the ulcer bed. (e) Stasis ulcer with translucent polyurethane membrane in place to assist healing and protect grafts. (f) Healed stasis ulcer 6 weeks postoperatively. (g) Large stasis ulcer with partial take of pinch grafts; complete healing can still occur by second intention after pinch-graft procedure.

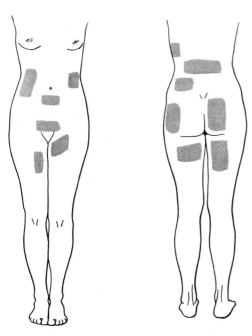

Figure 4 Typical split-thickness skin graft donor sites.

wound following split-thickness skin grafting is acceptable, it is not excellent, since in most cases there are both alopecia and differences in texture and color of the skin (Fig. 5a,b). In addition, split-thickness skin grafts may not recover normal sensation. The donor site heals by second intention and may be the source of postoperative pain as well as permanent disfigurement.

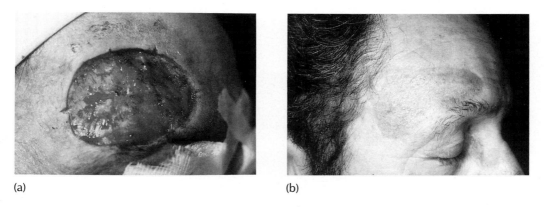

(a)   (b)

Figure 5 (a) Large defect on the forehead immediately following Mohs micrographic surgery. (b) Final appearance of treatment site 6 months after repair of wound with a split-thickness skin graft; note hyperpigmentation of grafted tissue compared to surrounding noral tissue.

Instrumentation

Several devices are available to harvest grafts of split thickness. The oldest are hand-operated knives, which are inexpensive but limited in the quality of grafts obtained. With the surgeon's increased experience these instruments are capable of providing split-thickness skin grafts of sufficient length and width to cover most wounds (Fig. 6a).

More popular today are the power dermatomes such as the Brown, Padgett, and Castroviejo types (Fig. 6b,c). These instruments are capable of providing minute variability in the thickness and width of split-thickness skin grafts. They are expensive but relatively easy to operate. The Simon-Davol battery-powered dermatome (Fig. 6d,e) is less expensive. It has only one setting—1-5/16" wide and 0.015" thick—but it is light, convenient, and the head is disposable.

Technique

The typical donor sites used include the anterior thigh, buttocks, abdomen, and back. The scalp can be used since the donor site will be hidden by the hair once it has regrown. For young patients who like to wear swimsuits, the pubic area has also been used as a donor site.

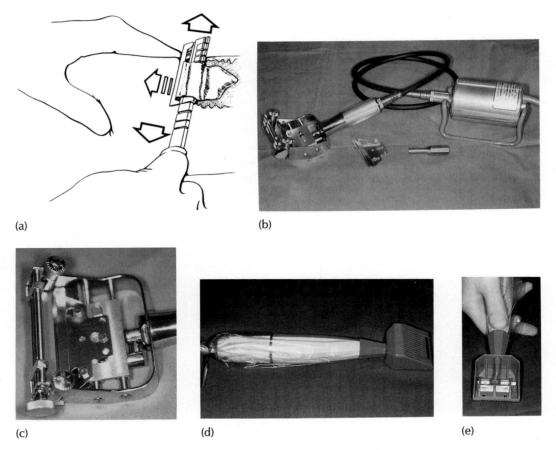

(a)   (b)

(c)   (d)   (e)

Figure 6 (a) Weck: free-hand blade harvesting split-thickness skin graft. (b) Brown dermatome with its electric motor. (c) Close-up shows head of Brown dermatome. (d) Profile view of Simon-Davol dermatome with disposable sterile head in place and handle containing battery pack within sterile plastic bag, ready for use. (e) Frontal appearance of Simon-Davol dermatome.

On the day of surgery, the donor site is shaved and prepped. The tissue to be harvested is marked at least 10–25% larger than the defect since contraction of the graft can be expected. Local anesthesia is obtained with lidocaine 1%. Hyaluronidase may be added to this solution to decrease the number of injections required.

A liberal amount of sterile lubricant is applied to the surface of the donor site. With the donor skin pulled taut, the dermatome is pushed with even pressure over the skin. To make harvesting easier, apply a sheet of sterile polyurethane to the donor site prior to cutting the graft. This makes the skin more rigid and allows the dermatome to harvest the graft uniformly. These membranes are all approximately 0.002" thick, so this must be considered when setting thickness on the dermatome. The polyurethane membrane remains adherent to the harvested graft. The graft is then lifted off the dermatome and draped loosely into the wound. Precise placement of the graft is not important since excess at the edges of the wound will undergo necrosis and shed (Fig. 7a). The edges are then sutured or stapled into place. A basting stitch may be required for larger wounds to ensure attachment to the base. If excessive exudate is expected, fenestrations are made in the graft to permit drainage (Fig. 7b,c). The defect is then irrigated under the graft with chilled saline and an immobilizing pressure dressing is applied.

After bleeding has stopped at the donor site, it is covered with a sheet of sterile polyurethane or hydrocolloid synthetic dressing material. If fluid accumulates beneath these membranes, it may be drained by puncturing the membrane with an 18-gauge needle.

Both graft and donor sites are reexamined at 24–48 hr to be sure no excess fluid has accumulated beneath the graft or the membrane at the donor site. If so, this is drained by puncturing the membrane with an 18-gauge needle and patching the puncture site with a small piece of the adhesive membrane. Graft adhesion is satisfactory within 2–3 weeks. Maturation may take many months. Dermabrasion may be considered at 6–12 weeks to even out the edges of the grafted site.

Meshed Split-Thickness Skin Grafts

Meshing a split-thickness skin graft is done when donor tissue is limited or the wound is relatively large (Fig. 8). Meshing allows the graft to expand like an accordion due to slits made by a mechanical mesher. A standard split-thickness skin graft placed through this meshing device can increase the area of coverage from 100 to 900%. The mesh graft is particularly beneficial for anatomic areas that are highly mobile such as the knee, scrotum, or axillae, since it easily fits irregular body folds.

The meshed graft allows drainage of exudate and blood without disruption of the healing process. The meshed spaces heal by second intention, which results in a slightly more irregular surface. However, the wound maintains its durability, and healing time is not substantially different from that of the traditional split-thickness skin graft.

FULL-THICKNESS SKIN GRAFTS

A full-thickness skin graft involves the free transfer of epidermis and the complete thickness of dermis from one site and its removal to another with disruption of the vascular supply. This type of graft is used for small to medium-sized defects where primary closure is not possible or where local skin flap surgery would create an undesirable effect and maximal cosmetic results are desired.

The primary benefit of this graft is that it prevents wound contraction in up to 80% of cases. At the same time, the cosmetic appearance is maximized because the tissue color, texture, and thickness match better. This graft allows excellent wound durability and is typically associated

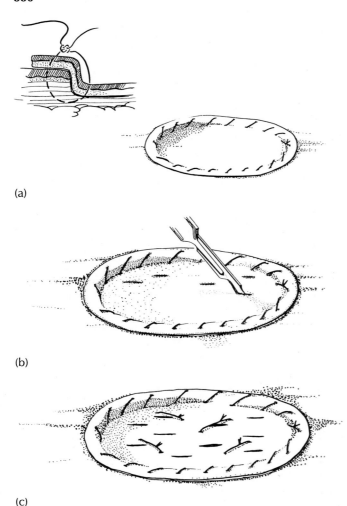

(a)

(b)

(c)

Figure 7 (a) Suturing technique for split-thickness skin graft. (b) Fenestrations made in split-thickness skin graft to permit egress of exudate. (c) Basting sutures in center of graft to provide maximum attachment of graft to base.

with less morbidity than local flaps. An additional advantage is that this procedure can be performed with standard surgical instruments, without the need for new or expensive instrumentation.

A disadvantage of full-thickness skin grafts is that there are only a limited number of donor sites available, and the donor site must match closely the tissue surrounding the defect. For example, for facial defects, the donor site must be superior to the blush line, which is typically the clavicle or nipple, so that the vessels in the graft will dilate when appropriate. The metabolic demands of this graft are relatively high and failure is not uncommon. As a consequence, grafts of this type are limited in size.

The recipient site for full-thickness grafts must be clean and well vascularized. Full-thickness skin grafts should not be placed directly on exposed bone, cartilage, tendon, or fat, which lack

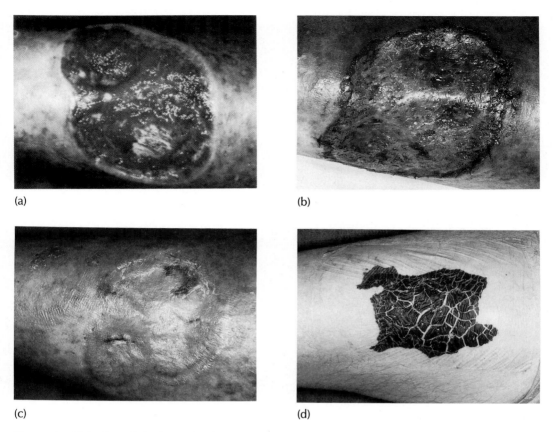

(a)   (b)

(c)   (d)

Figure 8 (a) Defect of the lower leg following removal of squamous cell carcinoma with Mohs micrographic surgery. (b) Meshed split-thickness skin graft in place. (c) One month postoperatively: irregular texture and color. (d) Donor site on anterior thigh with translucent polyurethane membrane placed; dried serosanguinous fluid is present beneath.

sufficient vascular supply. In spite of this, failure of the graft may be due to either hematoma or seroma formation and meticulous hemostasis is important.

Donor Site

Several areas of facial tissue excess are more likely to provide a graft that has good color and texture, matching the tissue adjacent to the defect. Typical donor areas (Fig. 9a) are the superior retroauricular area or upper eyelid used for the lower eyelid; lower retroauricular area used for defects on the cheek and temple; the preauricular area and lower lateral neck for the midcheek and chin; the supraclavicular area for both the medial canthus and lower eyelid; the upper lateral neck for the helix; and the glabella for the chin, forehead, and nose. The upper back in the area of the trapezius muscle (Fig. 9b) is good for defects on the nasal tip since the thickness of this tissue allows it to be sculptured to fit properly around the alar cartilages. The nasolabial fold may be sufficiently redundant to harvest a small graft for the nose as well (Fig. 9a). The inguinal fold and the antecubital fossa are used for defects on the hand (Fig. 9b).

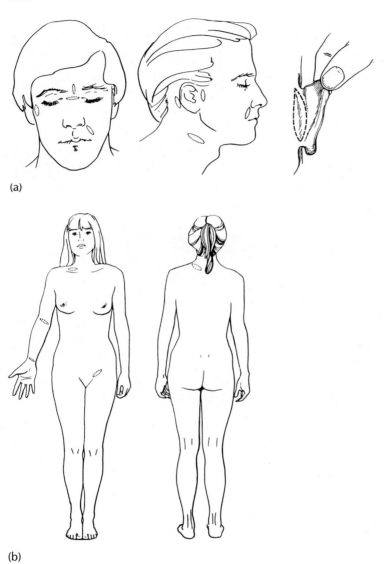

(a)

(b)

Figure 9 (a) Donor sites available for full-thickness skin grafts on the face and neck. (b) Donor sites for full-thickness skin graft on trunk and extremities.

Technique

First, the recipient site must be healthy, clean, well vascularized, and not contaminated with necrotic debris or microorganisms. There should be little subcutaneous fat on the base of the graft. A template that matches the defect can be made to harvest a graft of appropriate size and shape. This is only a rough approximation since the graft contracts 20–40% after harvesting. Once the size of the graft has been determined, the best donor site is selected according to color, texture, thickness, and presence or absence of appendageal structures such as hair follicles. The graft is harvested and all fat is stripped from the base (Fig. 10a). It is then cut to fit the defect, so it may be placed without tension or excess tissue at any margin.

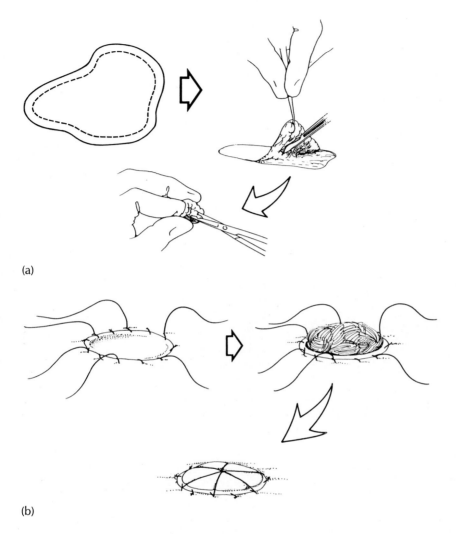

(a)

(b)

Figure 10 (a) Graft harvesting is planned 10–20% larger than defect (upper left); graft harvested in the subcutaneous plane (upper right); removal of subcutaneous fat prior to graft placement (bottom). (b) Graft sutured into place. Alternate sutures left long (upper left), cotton stent, or bolus applied on top of full-thickness skin graft (upper right), with tie-over suture (bottom).

The graft is sutured into position. Alternate sutures are left long to support a tie-over dressing (Fig. 10b). For larger grafts, a basting stitch may be placed through the graft to the wound bed. The space under the graft is then irrigated with chilled saline to flush our residual blood or debris.

Many different dressings have been used successfully to immobilize and support a skin graft. An interpositional membrane, such as N-terface, is placed between the graft and the dressing. This membrane permits easy removal of the dressing by preventing crust from adhering to the gauze stent. A nonadherent gauze pad is cut slightly larger than the graft so that the compression is outward and downward and not directly on the sutures themselves. A bulky cotton stent is placed over the gauze to absorb exudate and act as a buffer from external trauma. A button-foam dressing may be used instead of the cotton stent.

After the cotton stent is applied, the long sutures used to anchor the graft into position are tied over the stent (Fig. 10b). A bulky protective dressing is then placed over this. While not required, antibiotics are given to most patients for 1 week.

To minimize interference with wound healing, the graft is not examined for 5–7 days. At that time, the dressing is soaked with either sterile saline or hydrogen peroxide. The graft is typically cyanotic, and there may be epidermal blistering (Fig. 11a–c). This tissue should be left in place. An antibiotic ointment is applied to the surface of the graft, and a smaller protective dressing is applied to be changed daily for an additional week. Within several days, depending on the location, the epidermal crusting will disappear and revascularization of the graft can be expected (Fig. 11d). Dermabrasion can be considered in 6–12 weeks to smooth the edges and help blend the graft in with the surrounding skin.

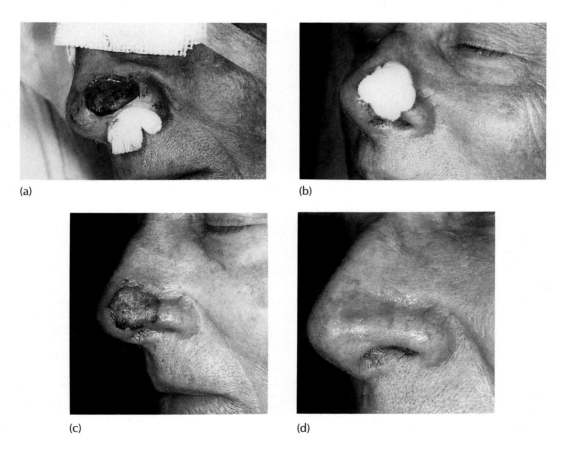

(a)

(b)

(c)

(d)

Figure 11   (a) Wound on the ala after removal of a basal cell carcinoma by Mohs micrographic surgery. (b) Tie-over stent dressing holding full-thickness skin graft compressed and immobile. (c) Full-thickness graft 1 week postoperatively shows epidermal crust and cyanosis. (d) Full-thickness skin graft 2 months postoperatively. Preservation of normal contours and good color match.

Dog-Ear (Burow's Triangle) Grafts

When full-thickness defects are created on the inelastic, thick skin, such as the forehead, sometimes only partial linear closure is possible. In these situations, the superfluous tissue that forms at one or both ends of the closure, commonly called "dog-ear" deformities, can sometimes be utilized advantageously as free full-thickness skin grafts to provide wound closure without the need to create a second donor defect elsewhere. These dog-ear or Burow's triangle grafts provide excellent color and texture match since they are obtained from the immediately adjacent area. The technique used for placement of these grafts is identical to that employed for more traditional full-thickness grafts, and either one or both of the excised Burow's triangles can be placed in the central defect and sutured in place (Fig 12a). A stent dressing is applied (Fig. 12b), and standard wound care is followed. If the defect is not entirely covered by the combined use of primary closure and Burow's triangle grafts, the remaining portion can be allowed to heal by second intention (Fig. 12c) with anticipated good cosmetic results. Since these grafts contribute a substantial amount of tissue to the overall repair of the wound, the time required for complete healing is reduced over that normally necessary for total healing by second intention.

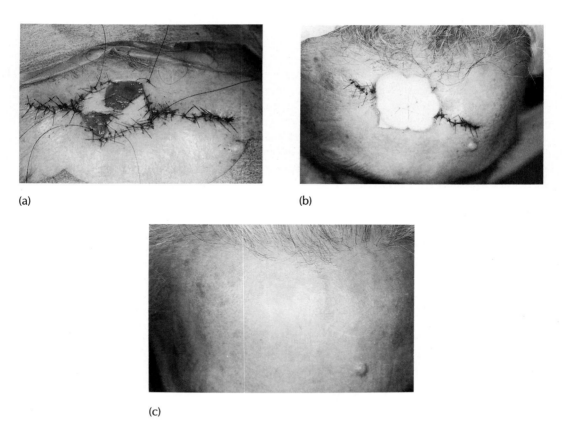

(a)

(b)

(c)

Figure 12 (a) Partial primary closure of a Mohs micrographic surgery defect. The dog ears have been used as full-thickness skin grafts. A portion of the defect is allowed to heal by second intention. (b) Stent dressing is placed over the dog-ear grafts for stability. (c) Postoperative result at 1 year.

Composite Grafts

Composite grafts are composed of more than one tissue type. These are typically used for defects on the alae, auricles, or eyelids (Fig. 13) that have no base. Hair transplants are a type of composite graft since they are composed of both skin and hair.

The main disadvantage of composite grafts is the higher failure rate due to their increased metabolic demands. This is especially true if the graft is greater than 1 cm in diameter. The ear is the typical donor site for many composite grafts, so there may be some distortion of the donor area. The technique varies significantly from one surgeon to another. Some allow the initial wound to heal by second intention before proceeding with the graft. Others will proceed with immediate repair.

The size of the defect is determined and marked on the anterior crus of the helix of the ear (Fig. 13). This zone is chosen because it is the right contour for defects of the nasal alae and has similar texture, color, and thickness. The donor area is harvested as an excision, and the graft is lined with either a mucosal flap from the nose or a split-thickness skin graft. This is then sutured into place, with great care taken to prevent injury to the vascular structures. Survival of the composite graft depends on circulation from the periphery and perfusing centrally. The donor site on the ear is then repaired, typically with an inferiorly based preauricular advancement flap.

Cultured Epithelial Autografts

Nearly 25 years ago initial laboratory techniques were developed for the cultivation of animal and human keratinocytes. Within a few years the technique had been sufficiently perfected to allow the growth of cultured keratinocytes in large enough quantities to permit their use as a type of skin graft known as a cultured epithelial autograft (CEA). This type of skin graft has now proven useful as a functional skin replacement and has been used experimentally at split-thickness skin graft donor sites as well as to treat wounds produced by Mohs micrographic surgery, carbon dioxide laser vaporization, or electrosurgery. CEAs are also routinely used in the management of patients with severe burns and to speed the healing of certain chronic wounds, like stasis and decubitus ulcers.

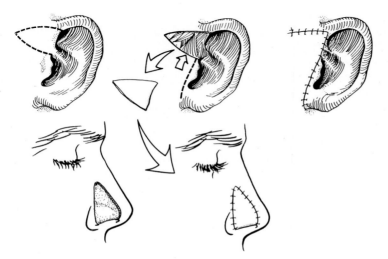

Figure 13   Composite graft from the ear is transferred to a full-thickness defect of the ala.

CEAs have been used for skin replacement after the excision of giant congenital nevi, but because these grafts are typically applied without any fibrous dermal component, they often appear atrophic. For that reason, when used as a sheet of epithelium, they are of only limited usefulness for most cosmetic problems. However, in order to improve the cosmetic results, a number of artificial tissues known as living skin equivalents have been developed, which employ autologous cultured keratinocytes suspended on a dermal substitute composed of an acellular, synthetic, porous membrane of cross-linked collagen, glycosaminoglycans, and autologous cultured fibroblasts or a bovine collagen gel to provide both dermal and epidermal components to the graft. Although additional clinical experience is required to substantiate the benefits these skin equivalents may provide, their promise seems substantial.

Dermal Graft

A dermal graft is a free graft of dermis without epidermis. This graft is infrequently used to correct nonrigid, shallow, depressed scars. Sometimes this type of graft is used to line flaps in order to give additional thickness to a depressed wound. This type of graft is well vascularized, but hematoma and small cysts sometimes occur due to the transection of pilosebaceous structures. This technique has largely been replaced by injectable tissue augmenting implants.

Overgrafting

Overgrafting is the serial application of split-thickness skin grafts applied to increase thickness. A split-thickness skin graft is placed into a wound and allowed to heal. Then the epidermis is removed by dermabrasion down to the papillary dermis. Another split-thickness graft is applied to the surface. This may be repeated two or three times to increase the thickness of a defect. This technique is also not commonly performed today since a variety of alternative flaps may be more appropriate. Also, since full-thickness skin grafts can be harvested from donor sites with a thicker dermis, there is little use for overgrafting. The occurrence of small cysts is typical since appendageal structures may be left intact and buried beneath the layers of grafted skin.

Delayed Grafting

Ceilley has reported that defects need not be repaired immediately. Instead, the wound is managed as if allowed to heal by second intention. This is done for 10–14 days, which allows removal of necrotic debris and the development of sufficient vascular supply and granulation tissue to support a graft. Since contraction of the wound may occur during this time, the small rim of advancing epithelium should be excised prior to performing the final closure. The main advantage of this technique, in addition to improving circulation, is that the depth of the wound may fill in significantly with granulation tissue during this delay period, which decreases the required thickness of grafted tissue. This will also improve the final cosmetic appearance by eliminating some of the irregular contours.

Substitutes for Human Skin

Several products are now available for use in place of the autologous skin graft. While they are traditionally used for larger wounds such as severe thermal injuries, a knowledge of these materials is important. One of the original grafts used for burn wounds is the porcine xenograft. This material is used as a temporary dressing until sufficient donor tissue can be harvested or cultured from the patient. In this same fashion, chorioamnion biologic membrane can be used as a temporary covering. A new product composed of polyurethane foam and polypropylene film may also be used to provide temporary coverage for a large wound. It also serves to demonstrate the ability of the body to accept a permanent graft according to the quantity and quality of the vascular supply generated.

CAUSES OF GRAFT FAILURE AND THEIR TREATMENT

General Causes

While there are many reasons (Table 2) for a graft to fail, the most common cause is disruption of the newly formed blood vessels by movement or shearing forces. For this reason a variety of different dressing, suturing patterns, and basting stitches have been used to minimize disruption of the healing wound. Another reason grafts are lost is secondary infection, especially due to *Staphylococcus, Streptococcus*, and *Pseudomonas*. The temporary impairment of circulation after injury or surgery predisposes to contamination, colonization, and necrosis.

Both hematoma and seroma are also causes of graft failure. Hematomas interfere with neovascularization to the graft, and it appears that breakdown products of the blood clot are toxic. In a similar fashion, seromas may predispose to inoculation and wound infection. For this reason, the wound must be meticulously examined for hemostasis prior to application of the graft and then be sufficiently compressed into the defect by sutures or dressings to minimize the collection of serum or blood beneath the graft.

Another common reason that grafts fail is that they are placed on an inappropriate recipient site. Exposed bone, cartilage, and tendons do not provide enough vascularity to support a graft. In these circumstances, if primary closure is possible, it is preferred. If a flap is not possible and yet, because of the size or location of the defect, wound closure is desirable, sufficient time

Table 2   Causes of Graft Failure

Technical errors
  Improper size or thickness
  Tension
  Incomplete hemostasis resulting in hematoma
  Error in timing of surgical repair
  Improper dressing
    Too tight
    Not immobilizing
Improper patient care
  Dependent position
  Motion
Insufficient bed vascularity
  Improper bed (fat, bone, cartilage, tendon)
  Necrotic debris
  Hematoma
  Seroma
Infection
  Staphylococcus
  Streptococcus
  Pseudomonas
Trauma
Motion
Systemic disease
  Diabetes
  Immunologic dysfunction

should be allowed for development of a well-vascularized wound bed to ensure graft survival. Many find that subcutaneous fat is not adequately vascularized for grafting and recommend that the fat be removed and the graft applied to the underlying fascia or muscle to improve graft survival. If a full-thickness graft is being used to repair a defect, all fat on the base of the graft should be removed. This serves to minimize the chance of secondary infection and maximize the chance for graft survival.

Excessive tension on a graft further impairs vascular supply since the caliber of the vessels within the graft is decreased by tension across the surface caused by wound closure. In this way, tension not only decreases the chance for survival but also predisposes to graft failure by increasing the risk of secondary intention.

Treatment of Failed Grafts or Grafts with Poor Cosmetic Results

It is important to be patient with performing graft surgery. Epidermal necrosis and cyanosis almost always occur with full-thickness skin grafts. The surgeon should expect these and warn the patient that they are not a sign of graft failure and provide sufficient emotional support for the patient during the healing process. Wound care, such as mild debridement during the postoperative period done at the office, is helpful. In many cases even when the graft appears to be nonviable, complete and satisfactory wound healing will still occur.

For the pinch graft, it appears that sufficient numbers of epidermal cells are transferred with this technique to allow the wound to heal despite apparent total graft failure. In a similar fashion, a split-thickness skin graft may provide a stimulus for wound healing in spite of the fact that the graft may have been lost entirely. Thus, if a graft fails, it does not necessarily represent an intrinsic problem with the procedure, anatomic location, or patient. Instead, once a new vascularized base has developed, regrafting should be attempted if necessary.

Spontaneous improvement in the texture or color of grafted tissue can be expected over a period of 6–12 weeks. Since improvement may be substantial over this period of time, patience is a necessity. If after 6–12 weeks the results have been less than optimal, dermabrasion may be performed to help blend the color with the surrounding tissue and improve the texture of the grafted site.

BIBLIOGRAPHY

Bell E, Erlich HP, Sher S, et al. Development and use of a living skin equivalent. *Plast Reconstr Surg* 1981;67:386–392.

Boyce ST, Hansbrough JF. Biologic attachment, growth, and differentiation of cultured human epidermal keratinocytes on a graftable collagen and chondroitin-6-sulfate substrate. *Surgery* 1987;103:421–431.

Ceilley RI, Bumsted RM, Panje WR. Delayed skin grafting. *J Dermatol Surg Oncol* 1983;9:288–293.

Fatah MF, Ward CM. The morbidity of split-skin graft donor sites in the elderly: The case for mesh-grafting the donor site. *Br J Plast Surg* 1984;37:184–190.

Field LM. Nasal alar rim reconstruction utilizing the crus of the helix, with several alternatives for donor site closure. *J Dermatol Surg Oncol* 1986;12:253–258.

Gallico III GG, O'Connor NE, Compton CC, et al. Permanent coverage of large burn wounds with autologous cultured human epithelium. *N Engl J Med* 1984;311:448–451.

Gallico III GG, O'Connor NE, Compton CC, et al. Cultured epithelial autografts for giant congenital nevi. *Plast Reconstr Surg* 1989;84:1–9.

Hansbrough JF, Boyce ST, Cooper ML, Foreman TJ. Burn wound closure with cultured autologous keratinocytes and fibroblasts attached to a collagen-glycosaminoglycan substrate. *J Am Med Assoc* 1989;262:2125–2130.

Gilmore WA, Wheeland RG. Treatment of ulcers on legs by pinch grafts and a supportive dressing of polyurethane. *J Dermatol Surg Oncol* 1982;8:177–183.

Harris DR. Healing of the surgical wound. *J Am Acad Dermatol* 1979;1:208–215.

Hefton JM, Caldwell D, Biozes DG, et al. Grafting of skin ulcers with cultured autologous epidermal cells. *J Am Acad Dermatol* 1986;14:399–405.

Hill TG. A simplified method for closure of full-thickness skin grafts. *J Dermatol Surg Oncol* 1980;6:892–893.

Hill TG. Reconstruction of nasal defects using full-thickness skin grafts: A personal reappraisal. *J Dermatol Surg Oncol* 1983;9:995–1001.

Hill TG. Enhancing the survival of full-thickness grafts. *J Dermatol Surg Oncol* 1984;10:639–642.

Hull BE, Finley RK, Miller SF. Coverage of full-thickness burns with bilayered skin equivalents: A preliminary clinical trial. *Surgery* 1989;107:496–502.

Igel HJ, Freeman AE, Boeckman CR, Kleinfeld KL. A new method for covering large surface area wounds with autografts. II. Surgical application of tissue culture and expanded rabbit skin autografts. *Arch Surg* 1974;108:724–729.

James JH, Watson ACH. The use of Op-site, a vapour permeable dressing, on skin graft donor sites. *Br J Plast Surg* 1975;28:107–110.

Johnson TM, Ratner D, Nelson BR. Soft tissue reconstruction with skin grafting. *J Am Acad Dermatol* 1992;27:151–165.

Leigh IM, Purkis PE. Culture grafted leg ulcers. *Clin Exp Dermatol* 1986;11:650–652.

Mareclo CL, Kim YG, Kaine JL, Voorhees JJ. Stratification, specialization and proliferation of primary keratinocyte cultures. *J Cell Biol* 1978;79:356–370.

Petry JJ, Wortham KA. Contraction and growth of wounds covered by meshed and non-meshed split-thickness skin grafts. *Br J Plast Surg* 1986;39:478–482.

Phillips TJ, Gilchrest BA. Cultured allogenic keratinocyte graft in the management of wound healing: Prognostic factors. *J Dermatol Surg Oncol* 1989;15:1169–1176.

Phillips TJ, Kehinde O, Green H, Gilchrest BA. Treatment of skin ulcers with cultured epidermal allografts. *J Am Acad Dermatol* 1989;21:191–199.

Porter JM, Griffiths RW, McNeill DC. The surgical management of intractable venous ulceration in the lower limbs: Excision, decompression of the limb, and split-skin grafting. *Br J Plast Surg* 1984;37:179–183.

Robinson JK. Improvement of the appearance of full-thickness skin grafts with dermabrasion. *Arch Dermatol* 1987;123:1340–1345.

Silfverskiold KL. A new pressure device for securing skin grafts. *Br J Plast Surg* 1986;39:567–569.

Stal S, Spira M. Mons pubis as a donor site for split-thickness skin grafts. *Plast Reconstr Surg* 1985;75:906–910.

Swanson NA, Tromovitch TA, Stegman SJ, Glogau RG. Skin grafting: The split-thickness graft in 1980. *J Dermatol Surg Oncol* 1980;6:524–526.

Wright JK, Brawer MK. Survival of full-thickness skin grafts over avascular defects. *Plast Reconstr Surg* 1980;66:428–431.

Yuspa SH, Morgan DL, Walker RJ, Bates RR. The growth of fetal mouse skin in cell culture and transplantation to F1 mice. *J Invest Dermatol* 1970;55:379–389.

Zitelli JA. Burow's grafts. *J Am Acad Dermatol* 1987;17:271–279.

50

Tissue Expansion in Head and Neck Reconstruction

Tom D. Wang
Oregon Health Sciences University, Portland, Oregon

Stephen S. Park
University of Virginia Medical Center, Charlottesville, Virginia

INTRODUCTION

The goal in any reconstructive endeavor is to recreate, as closely as possible, normal tissue appearance and function. Toward this end, a number of options have been described for reconstruction of soft tissue defects in the head and neck area. In general, repair of soft tissue defects in this region is best accomplished by means of a flap obtained from adjacent skin and subcutaneous tissues. These flaps provide the best skin color and texture match and also the potential to retain sensory and motor function. When the surrounding tissue is inadequate or particularly inextensible, one is forced to utilize less optimal coverage such as skin grafts or distant flaps, usually at the expense of cosmesis. The advent of tissue expansion as a reconstructive technique has significantly increased the role of local tissue flaps in soft tissue reconstruction of the head and neck.

Tissue expansion is a natural and ancient phenomenon as evidenced by normal pregnancy. The first description of therapeutic tissue expansion was made in 1957 by Neumann, who reported expanding postauricular skin with a rubber balloon for auricular reconstruction. In spite of his success, tissue expansion did not meet with wide acceptance for another 20 years. In 1976, Radovan described his clinical experience with the precursor to contemporary tissue expander implants. He also introduced the concept of breast reconstruction with a temporary expander following mastectomy.

HISTOLOGY

Understanding tissue expansion at the cellular level supports many of the physiologic changes known to occur, such as increased vascularity and dependability. It also directs us in experimentation and the potential future applications of selective expansion. Most of what we know about the histology of expansion comes from the pig model.

Epidermis

The epidermis of expanded tissue is unique from other layers of tissue in that it remains a constant thickness. It may even be slightly thicker during the actual expansion process. This suggests that this layer is not merely stretched but rather that there is an increase in cellular production and metabolic rate. The number of epidermal cells per unit surface area remains constant. The initial increase in the intercellular space and in the number of intracellular bridges probably stimulates the mitotic rate. All components of the epidermis can be identified and are in their appropriate proportions. More rapid expansion may flatten the rete ridges and basal membrane.

Dermis

A number of histologic changes are found at the dermal level. The thickness decreases by roughly 20% and does not fully recover after expansion. More rapid rates of expansion result in more dramatic thinning. The metabolically active basal layer, however, increases proportionally from comprising 10% of the dermal height to 40%.

The reticular dermis contains irregular, dense collagen bundles and is responsible for the lines of tension. These collagen fibers become more aligned in a parallel arrangement following expansion. There is increased fibroblast activity with more collagen deposition but not greater collagen concentration. Tensile strength is proportionally diminished.

Melanin production is also accelerated and accounts for the hyperpigmentation often found in expanded skin. This pigmentation usually fades over several months. Hair follicles and sebaceous glands do not change in number or morphology. Accordingly, there is a decrease in hair density. Sebaceous glands are, on occasion, occluded by the expansion process.

Subcutaneous Tissue

Subcutaneous tissue tolerates the expansion process poorly. The thickness decreases by as much as 50%, with a loss in the overall number and size of adipocytes. One also finds small areas of fat necrosis, especially with more rapid expansion. The recuperation of adipocytes is slow, taking longer than a year. The final thickness may ultimately surpass the preoperative thickness.

Muscle

Muscle is moderately sensitive to expansion. One finds decreased thickness and occasional muscle atrophy with expansion. There may be focal necrosis or calcification. Permanent sequelae and functional deficit, however, are not common.

Bone

Bone generally withstands expansive forces and does not undergo cortical erosion. During conservative expansion and when on relatively thin bone, such as the forehead, mild "bathtub" depression may be encountered. *Distraction osteogenesis* is a form of tissue expansion whereby new bone is deposited between two segments as they are gradually distracted. Instead of stretching skin, native bone is "stretched" in order to fill a defect or to lengthen a deficit segment. Adequate osteogenic potential for bone regeneration is dependent upon the presence of vascularized periosteum.

Vasculature

Vessels respond to expansion in two important ways. Although some small vessels probably do rupture, a majority will stretch in length without compromise to the integrity of the vessel wall.

Moreover, there is a proliferation of new vessels giving rise to an exceptionally robust vascular pattern and dependable tissue. Arterioles and venules respond similarly. The clinical effect of this vascular response is increased flap viability by roughly 120%. An analogy has been made with the phenomenon of delayed flaps.

Nerves

Neural tissue tolerates expansion well by stretching without necrosis, demyelination, or functional loss.

Capsule

A capsule forms around the expander and is composed of a dense outer layer of collagen and fibroblasts and an inner layer of macrophages. Its formation can be detected within 7 days and eventually resorbs upon removal of the expander. Microscopic evidence of the capsule may be present for up to a year.

The relationship between the capsule and tissue vascularity is unclear, but it probably makes little, if any, contribution to tissue viability. It may have a role in the "stretch-back" that occurs shortly following expander removal.

The term *biologic creep* refers to all of the metabolic and histologic events that occur during the course of tissue expansion. It is a dynamic cellular response to an external stimulus, i.e., expansion. The epidermis and neurovascular structures respond with proliferation and the other layers with extensibility.

GROSS CHANGES

Expanded skin develops a discoloration that originates at the cellular level. There is hyperemia from the increased neovascularization and at times a brownish hue from increased melanin production. Both changes are transient after expander removal. The texture does not change appreciably, as the normal stratum corneum persists following expansion.

Following expander removal all tissues probably undergo some degree of "shrink back." Certainly the more acutely stretched tissue will shrink more, but even conventionally expanded tissue will shrink if left alone. Clinically, the degree of shrinkage is minimal and held to the appropriate size by the peripheral tissues and underlying structural support.

INDICATIONS

Identifying the appropriate defect and patient is pivotal for tissue expansion. The defect should be of sufficient size such that the extensibility of surrounding tissues will not permit primary closure. Alternative means of resurfacing such as grafts and distant flaps should be considered. Ideally, the tissue to be expanded overlies a flap and solid buttress, such as the calvarium.

Large scalp defects are particularly suited for reconstruction with expansion because of the inextensibility of the scalp and the need to resurface with hair-bearing tissue. Nasal reconstruction with forehead flaps on occasion warrant preoperative expansion in order to increase the length of the nonhair-bearing portion of the flap. This is applicable to patients with nasal defects that involve the columella and ala yet also have a low frontal hairline. Preoperative expansion also facilitates donor site closure, however, secondary healing at this site contracts nicely and, alone, is not an indication for expansion.

The patient should have sufficient psychologic stability to understand and accept the slow process and temporary disfigurement of expansion. Patient dependability is paramount in order to maintain regular visits throughout the treatment. Finally, manual dexterity is needed if the patient elects to self inflate the expander.

TECHNIQUE

Devices

Most conventional expanders consist of a silicone bag attached to an inflation port. These may be attached by a narrow connecting tube, or the inflation port may actually be on the side of the main reservoir. The inflation reservoir consists of a self-sealing injection port, which allows penetration of a needle but prevents egress of fluid. Although small amounts of antibiotic solution may be recommended for initial inflation, sterile saline is used for the majority of expansion. Implants of different sizes and shapes are available commercially. In general, prostheses used in the head and neck are no greater than 250 ml in volume and rectangular in shape. Rectangular expanders yield the most efficient increase in surface area per unit volume, more so than dome or crescent-shaped expanders. As a general rule, the base of the expander should be roughly 2.5 times the surface area of the defect to be reconstructed. The devices are consistently of high quality and can be overexpanded 100%.

Variations of the conventional Radovan-type expander exist, such as permanent devices for breast augmentation and differential expanders for the treatment of male pattern baldness. In 1979, Austad and Rose described a self-inflating expander that did not depend upon external saline injections. The implant would extend by a net influx of water from the body tissues through a semipermeable membrane and across an osmotic gradient. These devices are not widely used due to the relatively long inflation period as well as the risk of implant rupture when compared to the Radovan-type implant. Other devices have the injection port immediately attached to the expander rather than connected through a silastic connecting tubing.

Incision Planning

Planning the reconstruction and the appropriate incisions are critical prior to placement of the expander. The incisions for expander placement should be made through preexisting incisions or at the advancing edge of the planned flap to minimize the resultant scar. Otherwise, the incision should be camouflaged in as distant a location from the expander as feasible to minimize direct tension on the wound edge during the expansion phase. Consideration must be given to the direction of the blood supply for the expanded tissue.

Insertion

A pocket is created to house the expander. Care must be taken to make a pocket of appropriate size. Too large a pocket may allow migration and an inadequate pocket may create folds and contour irregularities in the expander. These may lead to pressure necrosis in the skin during inflation. Flap elevation is done in a deliberate plane and is site specific. Excessive thinning will compromise the overlying tissue and increase the chance of tissue breakdown. The pocket for scalp expansion is in the subgaleal plane; for the forehead it is below the frontalis muscle. In the cheek and face the pocket is created in the usual face-lift plane. In the neck the expander may be placed either above or deep to the platysma muscle, depending on the area to be resurfaced.

The expander is inserted in the pocket and laid as flat as possible. A small amount of fluid is injected into the expander at the time of insertion to minimize the folds and irregularities. It also serves to maintain hemostasis and eliminate deadspace.

The injection port is tunneled through a subcutaneous pocket and placed at a site distant from the expander in order to avoid inadvertent puncture. Others leave the injection port exteriorized to facilitate home inflation by the patient, but this remains controversial because of the risk of infection.

The incision site for placement of expanders is closed in at least two layers. The subcutaneous layer is closed with either a long-lasting absorbable suture or a permanent one to withstand the tension during expansion. The skin is closed with a rapidly absorbing suture. Drainage is generally not needed, and a pressure dressing is applied for 24 hr. Postoperatively any hematomas must be promptly evacuated.

Expansion

Initial inflation is delayed 1–2 weeks to allow some wound healing to occur. Thereafter, in the head and neck area, inflation can be performed on a weekly basis. The amount of saline injected is dependent upon the appearance of the flap, patient discomfort during injection, and the anticipated amount of total inflation. Usually, 10–15% of the total volume may be injected each time, with the amount increasing as expansion progresses. The injection should be promptly terminated when blanching of the expanded skin flap occurs, indicating pressure vasoconstriction within the expanded skin. Some fluid may be withdrawn to allow capillary refill in the flap.

Measurements of transcutaneous oxygen saturation and implant pressure have been done in an effort to lower the risk of ischemic necrosis during expansion. These techniques are helpful in complicated situations but are cumbersome and not necessary for routine use. Aseptic technique is essential during each saline injection. This involves a sterile cleansing of the area over the injection port and the use of sterile gloves. A 23-gauge needle is used for the injection, since it minimizes the risk of subsequent leakage from the injection port while allowing adequate passage of the saline into the reservoir. Complete expansion generally takes between 6 and 8 weeks (Fig. 3).

Reconstruction

Immediately prior to removal of the expander, at the time of the definitive reconstruction, approximately twenty percent of the total expander volume is further added. This serves to stretch the capsule and minimize flap shrinkage.

For most locoregional flaps, the prosthesis is simply removed and the expanded tissue mobilized over the defect with the capsule intact. This is thought to enhance strength and dependability. Some flaps must be thinner in order to show underlying definition, such as forehead flaps in nasal reconstruction. These flaps are elevated in the subdermal plane, superficial to the capsule, with the expander in place to provide countertraction. Following flap elevation and rotation, the expander and capsule are removed.

COMPLICATIONS

Complications from tissue expansion are infrequent but may be a significant setback. *Infection* of the expander site is an uncompromising problem; once it develops, the expander is best promptly removed and the wound vigorously irrigated. The prosthesis has become a foreign body and nidus of infection. On rare occasion and in mild, superficial cases, systemic antibiotic therapy may suffice. Further expansion in the setting of infection is contraindicated, but it can be replaced to the same area once the infection has cleared. Meticulous sterile technique during insertion and expansion will minimize this occurrence.

Exposure also dictates prompt action. If it is early during the course of expansion, one is adviced to abort the expansion, remove the prosthesis, and try again at a future date. If it occurs late in the course, one may attempt to complete the reconstruction with the amount of expansion obtained at that point. Again, continued expansion is not recommended in the face of prosthesis exposure. With minimal exposure of the inflation port, however, continued expansion may be conservatively attempted. Wound dihiscence is usually the result of premature inflation and insufficient closure.

Skin slough/necrosis can be a devastating problem because not only is it a setback in timing, but the first-line tissue is destroyed. Prevention is critical and involves careful attention during expansion, avoiding persistent blanching or congestion.

Leakage from the prosthesis is rare with the current high-quality implants. If it does occur it does not necessitate immediate removal. Slow, guarded expansion can be continued. Puncture of the inflation port should be with a clean stick and perpendicular to the face of the port.

Migration may occur with excessively large pockets. This can be minimized with accurate dissection and suture fixation of the prosthesis to the underlying tissues.

Pain is an occasional problem for some patients. It immediately follows expansion and usually resolves upon withdrawing a small amount of fluid. At times it may be persistent for several hours and require mild analgesics.

Psychological instability and "second thoughts" are not infrequent during the disfiguring phase. Persistent support and optimism are helpful and necessary.

INTRAOPERATIVE "RAPID" EXPANSION

In 1987, Sasaki reported the use of rapid tissue expansion performed intraoperatively at the time of primary reconstruction. Roughly 2–3 cm of extra tissue can be obtained from intraoperative expansion. The disadvantage is that these tissues quickly shrink back and therefore must be mobilized and utilized for reconstruction in an expeditious manner. This procedure should not be used for delicate contour because the size is so unreliable. It is indicated for relieving some of the tension that arises from resurfacing larger defects of the scalp and forehead. It distributes the tension more evenly over the entire flap rather than concentrating it at the wound edges as would occur from vigorous suturing alone.

The biologic creep discussed earlier is not found because there is not sufficient time for increased mitosis and collagen synthesis. There is a *mechanical creep*, however, which is thought to be the mechanism of rapid expansion. It consists of four parts at the cellular level: (1) displacement of fluids (water and mucopolysaccharide ground substance) from the dermis, (2) parallel realignment of collagen bundles in the dermis, (3) micofragmentation of elastic fibers, and (4) recruitment from neighboring tissues as a result of effective undermining. The last part probably makes a significant, but not exclusive, contribution to rapid expansion.

The technique of rapid, intraoperative expansion is a cyclic loading and unloading of tension on the tissue. Several expanders (often 30 cc foley catheters) are inserted in the usual plane. They are inflated for 3 min, then deflated for 3 min. Each injection is with progressively larger amounts of saline. Four or five cycles are performed to a total of 60 cc per catheter. We have not found many situations where intraoperative expansion has provided clear advantages over extensive undermining, and thus it is rarely utilized.

THE FUTURE

Since its introduction, the role of tissue expansion in reconstructive surgery has blossomed proportionately with the experience and ingenuity of the surgeons utilizing this technique. Local tissue offers optimal color and texture for facial reconstruction. The practice of expanding this adjacent tissue is simple, elegant, and satisfying. Appropriate and knowledgeable use of expanders in the head and neck area can maximize reconstructive options and minimize complications.

Enhancement of tissue expansion through pharmacologic manipulation may be a standard for the future. Selective expansion of neurovascular pedicles or of bone segments will have great implications for future head and neck reconstruction. Expansion of visceral structures such as ureters and the esophagus will also have a tremendous impact. Currently, tissue expansion has a well-accepted place in facial reconstructive surgery.

REPRESENTATIVE CASES

Case 1

A 25-year-old man was involved in a motor vehicle accident and dragged down the road for several hundred feet. He presented 9 months later interested in improving his facial deformity (Figs. 1,2). He has contracture of the upper lip, scarring of the left cheek, lower eyelid defi-

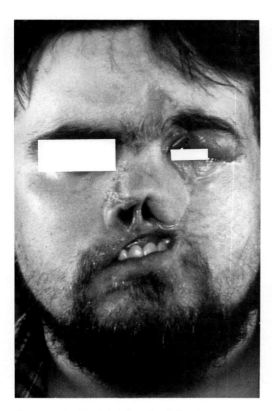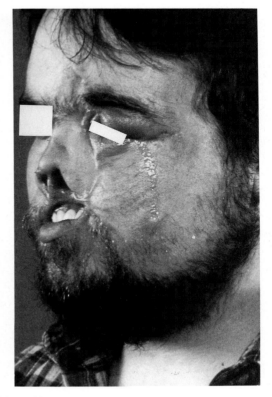

Figure 1,2 Facial deformity following a motor vehicle accident.

ciency, and a partially avulsed nose. The reconstruction involved a Karapandzic flap for the lip, scar revision to the cheek and lower eyelid, and a rebuilding of a nose. Internal lining of the nose was established with an epithelial "turn-in" flap from the dorsum. Structural support provided with split calvarial bone grafts cantalevered for a dorsum and conchal cartilage grafts for the ala, sidewalls, and onlay tip graft. The entire nose needed resurfacing from a midline forehead flap. There were concerns over the length of the flap needed to reach to the base of the columella. Options include shanking the flap in an oblique fashion, extending the flap into hair-bearing tissues, or designing the flap as an "up-and-down" flap. Another solution for this tissue deficiency is preoperative tissue expansion. This not only provides increase flap length, but also facilitates donor site closure.

A 250 cc rectangular tissue expander is placed in the forehead via an incision in the scalp (Fig. 3). The expander is positioned between the frontalis muscle and the pericranium, and inflated twice weekly for 5 weeks. A midline forehead flap is designed using a template and based on the right supratrochlear vessels (Fig. 4). The flap is then turned for nasal resurfacing and the donor site closed primarily with a transverse incision at the pretrichial line (Fig. 5). At 1 year he has an acceptable and functional nose (Fig. 6,7).

Case 2

A 50-year-old woman had a congenital hemangioma of the right cheek that was partially excised many years ago. She was interested in removing the obvious bulge and discoloration from the

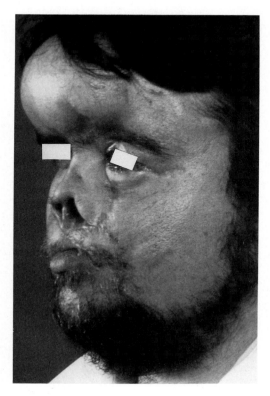

Figure 3   250-cc rectangular tissue expander in position.

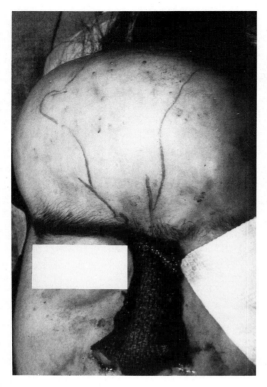

Figure 4 Incision planning for a midline forehead flap based on the right supratrochlear vessels.

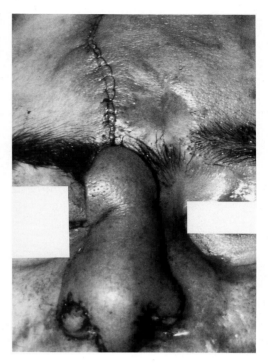

Figure 5 Forehead flap in position and donor site closed primarily.

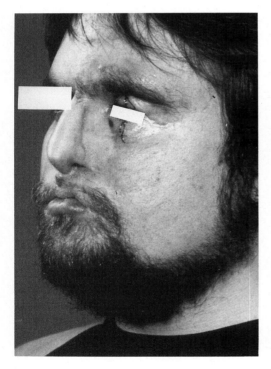

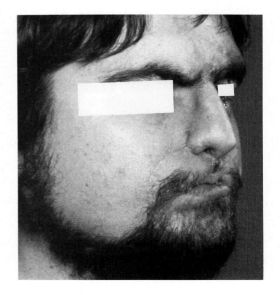

Figure 6,7 One year postoperative results.

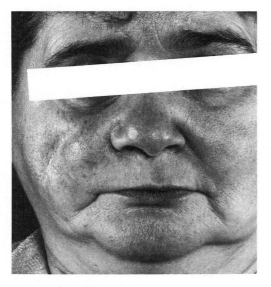

Figure 8 Residual hemangioma of right cheek.

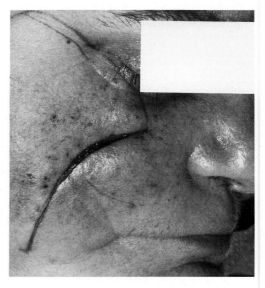

Figure 9 Incision for expander placement.

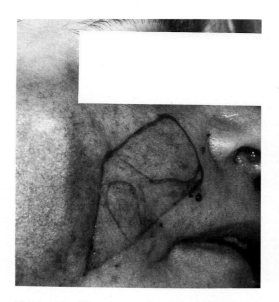

Figure 10 Tissue expander fully inflated with anticipated defect.

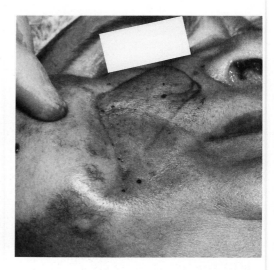

Figure 11 Additional expansion at time of repair.

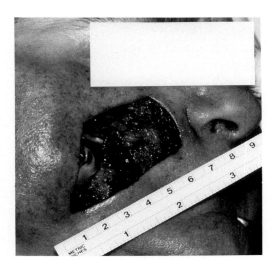

Figure 12 Skin defect defined.

residual hemangioma (Fig. 8). The entire lesion involved roughly the anterior half of her right cheek, and a sizable defect was expected. An incision is made at the leading edge of the anticipated flap, through which the tissue expander is inserted (Fig. 9). The lesion is located anterior to the incision. The expander is fully inflated and the hemangioma and probable defect outlined (Fig. 10). Immediately prior to reconstruction the expander is inflated one final time with about 15 cc (Fig. 11). The hemangioma is excised and the final defect measured 4½ cm in width (Fig.

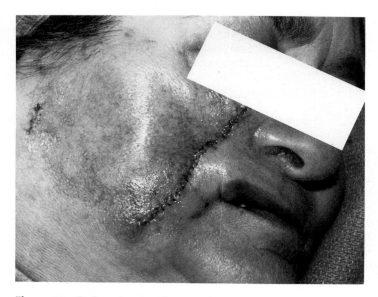

Figure 13 Defect closed without tension.

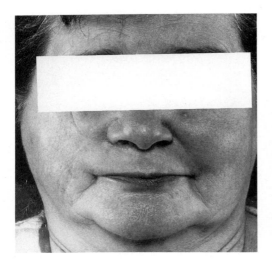 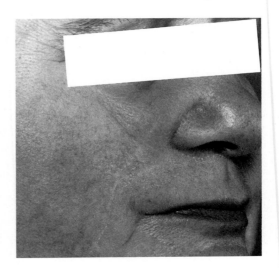

Figure 14,15   Nine months postoperative.

12). The flap is advanced medially and the wound closed without tension (Fig. 13). At 9 months she has healed nicely (Figs. 14,15).

BIBLIOGRAPHY

Austad E, Rose GL. A self-inflating tissue expander. *Plast Reconst Surg* 1982; 70:588–593.

Austad ED. Complications in tissue expansion. *Clin Plast Surg* 1987; 14:549–550.

Cherry GW, Austad E, Pasyk K, et al. Increased survival and vascularity of random-pattern skin flaps elevated in controlled, expanded skin. *Plast Reconstr Surg* 1983; 72:680–685.

Converse JM. Corrective and reconstructive surgery of the nose: Full-thickness loss of nasal tissue, in Converse JM (ed): *Reconstructive Plastic Surgery*, vol. 2. Philadelphia, WB Saunders Co. 1977, pp. 1209–1287.

Hallock GG, Rice DC. Objective monitoring for soft tissue expansion. *Plast Reconstr Surg* 1986;77:416–420.

Hong C, Stark GB, Futrell JW. Elongation of axial blood vessels with a tissue expander. *Clin Plast Surg* 1987;14:465–467.

Manders EK, Schenden MJ, Furrey JA, et al. Soft tissue expansion; concepts and complications. *Plast Reconst Surg* 1984;74:493–507.

Manders EK. Reconstruction by expansion in the patient with cancer of the head and neck. *Surg Clin North Am* 1986;66:201–212.

Manders EK, Saggers GC, Diaz-Alonso P, et al. Elongation of peripheral nerve and viscera containing smooth muscle. *Clin Plast Surg* 1987;14:551–562.

Maves MD, Lusk RP. Tissue expansion in the treatment of giant congenital melanocytic nevi. *Arch Otolaryngol Head Neck Surg* 1987;113:987–991.

Neumann CG. The expansion of an area of skin by progressive distention of a subcutaneous balloon. *Plast Reconstr Surg* 1957;19:124–130.

Oneal RM, Rohrich RJ, Izenberg PH. Skin expansion as an adjunct to reconstruction of the external ear. *Br J Plast Surg* 1984;37:517–519.

Pasyk K, Argenta LC, Austad ED. Histopathology of human expanded tissue. *Clin Plast Surg* 1987;14:435–445.

Radovan C. Breast reconstruction after mastectomy using the temporary expander. *Plast Reconst Surg* 1982;69:195–206.

Radovan C. Tissue expansion in soft tissue reconstruction. *Plast Reconst Surg* 1984;74:482–490.

Roenigk RK, Wheeland RG. Tissue expansion in dermatologic surgery. *Derm Clin* 1987; 5:429–436.

Sasaki GH. Intraoperative sustained limited expansion (ISLE) as an immediate reconstructive technique. *Clin Plast Surg* 1987;14:563–573.

Tardy ME, Sykes JM, Kron T. The precise midline forehead flap in reconstruction of the nose. *Clin Plast Surg* 1985;12:481–494.

Thornton JW, Marks MW, Izenberg PH, et al. Expanded myocutaneous flaps; their clinical use. *Clin Plast Surg* 1987;14:529–534.

51

Scar Revision by Dermabrasion

Christopher Barry Harmon
Keesler Medical Center, Keesler Air Force Base, Biloxi, Mississippi

John M. Yarborough, Jr.
Tulane University School of Medicine, New Orleans, Louisiana

The process by which wounds heal ranks among nature's wonders. It represents more than regeneration of cells and matrix; it is an awakening of primordial cellular states. Mitosis, formation of intercellular substance, and cellular migration occur during embryologic development just as during formation of tissue after injury. While our comprehension of the biologic mechanisms of wound repair is advancing, our understanding is incomplete. However, wounds heal by scar formation, some of which require surgical revision for functional or cosmetic improvement.

Dermabrasion gained its notoriety for treatment of acne scars. It was criticized because of its partial, rather than complete, effectiveness, despite the fact that other approaches to scar revision, generally postponed until 1 year after healing, also resulted in partial improvement. Scars of long duration, whether formed primarily or by second intention, are nearly always improved, though rarely eradicated, by dermabrasion (Figs. 1–3).

One of the most significant advances was derived from John Yarborough's observations that scars from facial lacerations—either surgical or accidental—planed 4–8 weeks after injury usually healed without visible evidence of residual cicatrization (Figs. 4–17). While the mechanisms by which this phenomenon occurs have not yet been completely defined, our understanding of the cellular and extracellular interactions has recently been expanded.

When planed earlier than 4 weeks after injury, most wounds lack sufficient tensile strength to prevent spread. Those abraded much after 8 weeks only are improved. Theoretically, obliteration of residual scar during the revised deposition of collagen may be achieved by upward and horizontal migration of epithelial cells from viable adnexal appendages prior to their atrophy during the early maturation phase of wound repair.

WOUND HEALING

Wounds that heal without apposition of their edges are said to heal by second intention, while sutured wounds heal by first intention. Second intention wounds may be classified according to

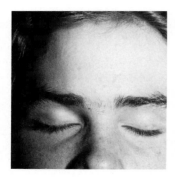

Figure 1 Stellate scar on forehead of 16-year-old boy from injury 13 years previously.

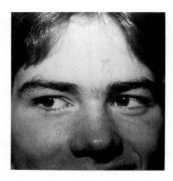

Figure 2 Appearance of scar 1 month after abrasion with coarse fraise.

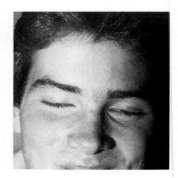

Figure 3 After 11 months, scar is improved but apparent.

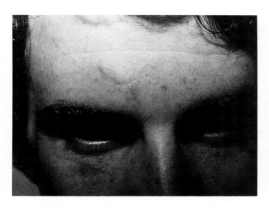

Figure 4 Traumatic scar above eyebrow 4 weeks after injury.

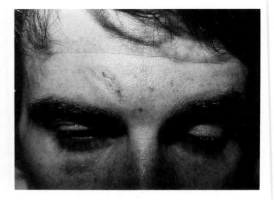

Figure 5 Appearance of scar 9 days after abrasion with brush, 5 weeks postinjury.

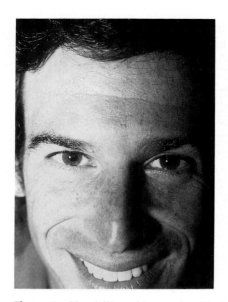

Figure 6 No visible evidence of residual scar.

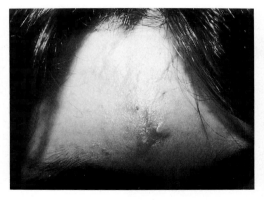

Figure 7 Fifteen-year-old with scars from multiple lacerations sustained in automobile accident 4 weeks earlier.

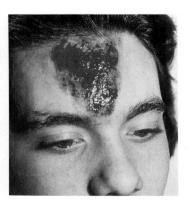

Figure 8 After wire-brush abrasion.

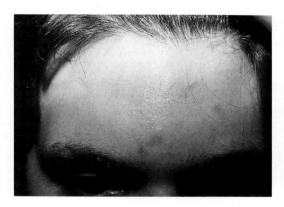

Figure 9 Modest evidence of residual scars 3 months after planing.

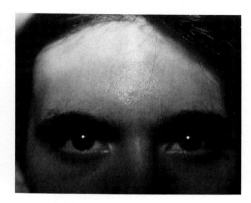

Figure 10 No evidence of residual scars 6 months after surgery.

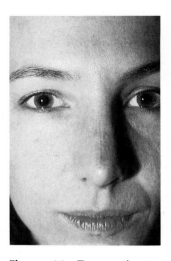

Figure 11 Four-centimeter surgical scar on nose of 28-year-old woman 6 weeks after debridement of scar tissue.

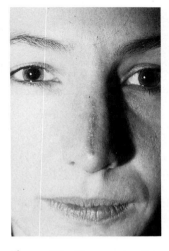

Figure 12 One week after planing, mild crusting and residual scar were apparent.

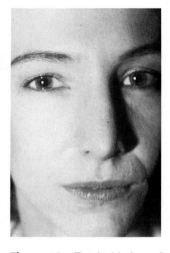

Figure 13 Total ablation of scar 6 months later.

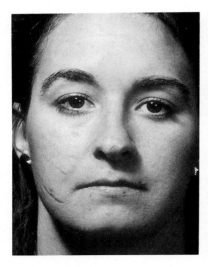 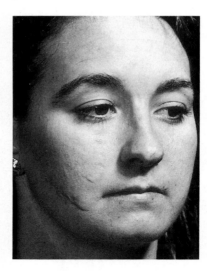

Figures 14, 15   Scars after injury due to broken glass sustained 3 weeks earlier.

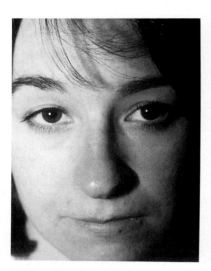 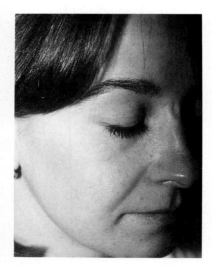

Figures 16, 17   Although faint residual evidence of scarification was apparent after 10 weeks, none was evident at 7 months.

width, depth, and degree of tissue loss into three types: (1) superficial (type I), whose injuries encompass epidermis and papillary dermis but not epidermal appendages; (2) deep (type IIA) wounds that penetrate deeply into or beneath the dermis without loss of tissue (i.e., traumatic laceration); and (3) deep (type IIB) penetrating wounds that incorporate substantial loss of tissue. Superficial (type I) lesions heal with little or no visible scars by epithelialization, a process by which the epidermis resurfaces an injury by horizontal epidermal migration from wound margins and vertical migration from adnexal appendages. Natural epidermis is formed. Deeper wounds heal by granulation, contraction, and ultimately epidermization, a process by which the epidermis resurfaces an injury without reforming epidermal appendages. Type IIA wounds heal without significant contraction, because the edges are closely apposed by the nature of the injury, whereas type IIB wounds are dependent upon contracture to close. Granulation tissue becomes contractile, after which epidermization bridges the residual gap.

Conventional dermabrasion causes superficial second intention wound healing. In describing the histopathologic events of the process, Burks observed that an eosinophilic exudate containing neutrophils and lymphocytes forms over the dermis immediately following dermabrasion. Within 48 hr, fibroplasia and capillary proliferation can be seen beneath the coagulum, and by 72 hr epidermal cells begin to migrate from the epithelial buds of pilosebaceous units onto the dermabraded surface. Epithelialization is complete in most patients within 8 days of abrasion. The epidermis is four to six cells thick with poorly developed rete ridges. The subepidermal collagen becomes more dense than nonabraded skin and by 30–90 days develops into a zone of mature fibrocytes with collagen bundle arrangements in a linear pattern.

The repair of deep wounds by second intention parallels to a degree the cellular and extracellular events of wounds that heal by first intention and can be divided into four phases: (1) inflammatory, (2) proliferative, (3) early maturation, and (4) late maturation. While staging is conceptually convenient, there is considerable overlap and interaction between these phases of repair.

The inflammatory phase, characterized initially by vasoconstriction and then vasodilatation and lasting about 5 days, begins immediately after injury when blood vessels are transected and serum, plasma proteins, and blood cells fill the wound, forming a coagulum. Fibroblasts, the architects of wound repair, appear during the first 48 hr to begin synthesis of collagen. The platelet clot develops complement, coagulation cascades are activated, and a fibrin-fibronectin matrix is laid down, thereby forming a scaffold upon which the subsequent cellular phases of neovascularization, reepithelialization, and fibroplasia occur. Concomitantly, polymorphonuclear leukocytes and macrophages improve the wound environment by phagocytizing bacteria and foreign body debris. Additionally, the macrophages serve to stimulate formulation of granulation tissue, fibroplasia, and further collagen deposition through the release of macrophage-derived growth factor, interleukin-1, other growth factors, and cytokines. New blood vessels are formed and the thickened epidermis migrates into the clot and across the defect.

During the early proliferative phase, there is multiplication of capillaries and fibroblasts that migrate along vertically oriented strands of fibrin. Within 24 hr of injury, epithelial cells begin to migrate from the wound edges and adnexal structure. Epithelialization is stimulated and guided by cell-matrix interactions via cell surface proteins and their receptors. As part of the adhesion molecule complex, bullous pemphigoid antigen, collagen type IV, laminin (a 125×103 MW polypeptide), and the integrins play important roles in the establishment and maintenance of cell-substratum adherence. In addition to serving as molecules for structural integrity, they also enhance keratinocyte migration and mitosis.

The integrins are a family of transmembrane adhesion receptors consisting of noncovalently associated alpha and beta subunits, which are involved in cell-matrix and cell-cell interactions. The alpha 6/beta 4 integrin heterodimer has been shown to be a component of the hemidesmosome, typically expressed along the dermal pole of the basal keratinocyte. With wounding the hemidesmosomes are dissassembled while keratinocytes migrate over the wound defect. Following migration the hemidesmosomes are reestablished at the basal pole of the basal cell keratinocyte.

Tenascin is also an extracellular matrix glycoprotein known to be associated with epithelial-mesenchymal interfaces during embryogenesis. The appearance of tenascin prior to keratinocyte and fibroblast migration has been demonstrated in fetal wounds. Furthermore it has been shown to interfere with integrin-mediated fibroblast attachment to fibronectin.

Three to four days after wounding, fibroblasts begin migrating and proliferating along the fibronectin matrix to form granulation tissue and synthesize collagen (primarily types I and III).

Fibroblast migration appears to occur preferentially in regions rich in fibronectin and poor in collagen, such that as the wound matures and more collagen is deposited fewer fibroblasts migrate into the area. The vertical deposition of soluble collagen by fibroblasts modestly increases tensile strength. Subsequently, the collagen assumes a more horizontal orientation, but the fibers lack extensive linkage. This *quantitative* phase of collagen production, usually of 1–2 weeks' duration, may represent the body's attempt to buy time so that collagen fibers may be arranged into a more functional pattern before becoming irretrievably fixed during the next phase.

The early maturation phase lasts 1–3 months, sometimes indefinitely. The wound matures as connective tissue remodeling proceeds with the sequential deposition of fibronectin, type III collagen, then type I collagen. Stromal reorganization occurs as more collagen is produced and fibronectin disappears. Type III collagen fibers are replaced by type I fibers. The reorganization of collagen fibers parallel to the direction of the scar coincides with an increase in intermolecular cross-linkages that serve to reinforce the tensile strength of the wound.

The late maturation phase may last a lifetime. With decline of the vascular network over the next 6–12 months, redness gradually fades. Collagen is continually synthesized and metabolized, and there is gradual appearance of elastic and nerve fibers. In spite of its perennial remodeling, collagen within a scar is always different from that in uninjured skin.

Dermabrasive scar revision superimposes the mechanisms of second intention wound healing on the remodeling phase of the primary scar. The process by which this method of scar revision (performed during the 4- to 8-week interval following injury) causes most facial lacerations to heal without visible evidence of cicatrization is not proven. A restructuring and layering of collagen parallel to lines of tension before completion of cross linking may afford smoother surface textures. Ultrastructural studies of biopsy specimens taken 24 hr to 6 weeks following dermabrasive revision of primary scars shows an increase in collagen density and bundle size with a tendency toward a more unidirectional orientation of fibers parallel to the epidermal surface. Furthermore, the reestablishment of a normal-appearing epidermis across initial scar boundaries may be influenced by changes in the extracellular formation of integrin and tenascin. Immunocytochemical staining of postabrasion specimens demonstrates a change in the staining of alpha 6/beta 4 integrin subunits from a linear basement membrane zone pattern to dispersed nonpolarized staining throughout the stratum spinosum. This postabrasive alteration in integrin expression coincides with more active cell migration and may regulate reepithelialization across the initial scar boundaries, ultimately yielding a less perceptible epidermal defect. The extracellular matrix glycoprotein tenascin is known to be associated with epithelial-mesenchymal interfaces during embryogenesis and wound healing. Prior to dermabrasive scar revision, tenascin staining is confined along either side of primary scars, whereas after dermabrasion tenascin is expressed throughout the papillary dermis. The dermabrasive procedure appears to upregulate tenascin expression from a localized event to a more dispersed one. Concordant with changes in integrin ligand expression, this alteration in tenascin expression may promote epithelial cell migration along the basement membrane zone and fibroblast movement across scar boundaries. In summary, these ultrastructural and immunocytochemical findings suggest that dermabrasion alters epithelial cell-cell interaction, epithelial cell-mesenchymal interaction, and fibroblast-mesenchymal interaction.

PREMATURE REABRASION

The healing process of the abraded site must not be interrupted by premature reabrasion, as illustrated in Figures 18–22. Although clinically the severe facial lacerations sustained in a windshield injury had not healed entirely by 6 weeks (Fig. 18), dermabrasion was performed, after which there was dramatic improvement in contour 4 weeks later (Fig. 19). Reabrasion of the

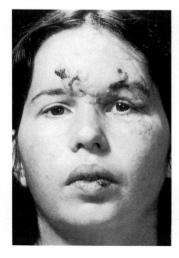

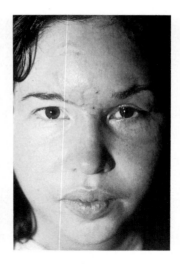

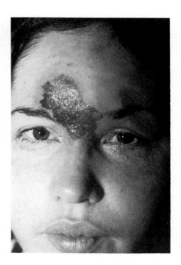

Figure 18 Facial lacerations incompletely healed 6 weeks after injury during an automobile accident.

Figure 19 Dramatic improvement of facial contour 1 month after abrasion with wire brush, but residual scars are apparent on the nasal bridge, medial aspect of the right eyebrow, and transecting the left eyebrow onto the upper eyelid.

Figure 20 Reabrasion of residual deformities 4 weeks after initial planing.

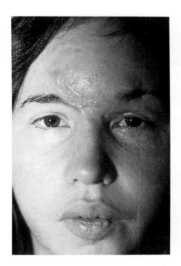

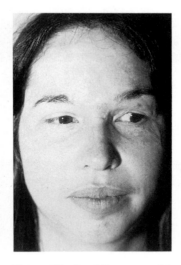

Figure 21 Four weeks after reabrasion, areas healed with atrophy and hypertrophic ridging.

Figure 22 Partially successful correction after implantation of bovine collagen.

residual scar at that time (Fig. 20) healed with atrophy and hypertrophic ridges (Fig. 21). Subsequently, partial correction was achieved by implantation of bovine collagen (Fig. 22). The recently synthesized soluble collagen could have been digested enzymatically by collagenase released in the tissue at the time of surgery.

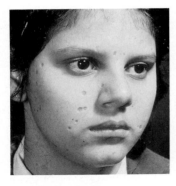
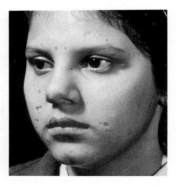

Figures 23, 24   Sharply marginated punched-out scars in 15-year-old child from type IIB wounds secondary to varicella at age 9 months.

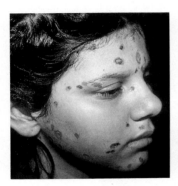
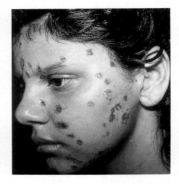

Figures 25, 26   Bases of scars elevated to improve cutaneous contour.

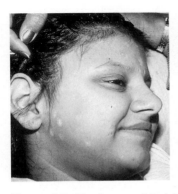
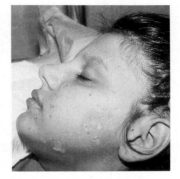

Figures 27, 28   Improved facial contour 18 days after punch elevation.

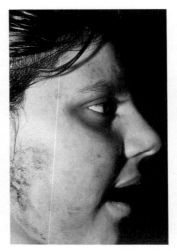

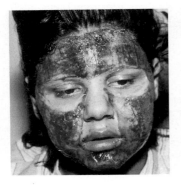

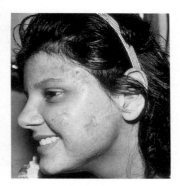

Figure 29 One day after wire-brush dermabrasion.

Figures 30, 31 Five days after dermabrasion, reepithelialization is almost complete and scars are less apparent.

SURGICAL ADJUNCTS TO DERMABRASION

Until recently, wide, deep, sharply marginated facial scars encompassing significant loss of tissue (type IIB) (i.e., "icepick" or "punched-out" scars such as those secondary to acne or varicella) were unimproved by dermabrasion alone. Adjunctive techniques such as punch elevation and punch replacement have made these deformities more amenable to improvement (Figs. 23–34). Punch elevation, which is ideal for larger pox scars, is accomplished by denuding the bases and vertical walls of the scars with a cone-shaped fraise, and then freeing the fibrotic bases

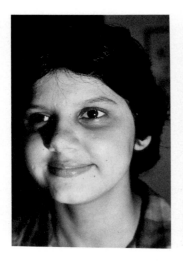

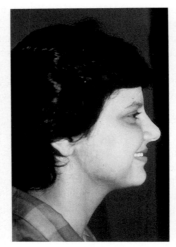

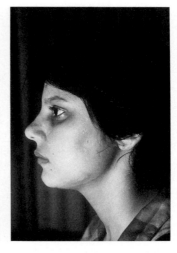

Figures 32–34 Several months after dermabrasion, defects are much improved although not totally obliterated.

with scalpel or dermal punches rotated into subcutaneous fat. Bases of these scars, whose function becomes analogous to cylindrical, full-thickness autografts, are then elevated to the surface for improved contour. Wide scars, 8 mm or larger, may require stabilization by one or two sutures to reduce retraction. "Ice-pick" scars may be excised by the punch technique and replaced with postauricular grafts 0.5 mm larger than the surgical defect. Healing after punch elevation or transfer of full-thickness autografts usually is sufficient for dermabrasion in 2 or 3 weeks, since cylindrical scars are not likely to spread.

BIBLIOGRAPHY

Bazin S, LeLous M Delaunary A. Collagen in granulation tissues. *Agents Actions* 1976;6:272.

Bennett RG, Robins P. Repair of tissue defects resulting from removal of cutaneous neoplasms. *J Dermatol Surg Oncol* 1977;3:512.

Billingham RE, Russell PS. Studies on wound healing, with special reference to the phenomenon of contracture of experimental wounds in rabbits skin. *Ann Surg* 1956;144:961.

Burks JW. *Dermabrasion and Chemical Peeling in the Treatment of Certain Cosmetic Defects and Diseases of the Skin.* Springfield, IL, Charles C Thomas, 1979.

Carrel A. The treatment of wounds. *JAMA* 1964;55:2148.

Chiquet-Erismann R, Kalla P, Pearson, CA, et al. Tenascin interferes with fibronectin action. *Cell* 1988;53:383–390.

Dann L, Glucksmann A, Tansley K. The healing of untreated experimental wounds. *Br J Exp Pathol* 1941;22:1.

Demarchez M, Harmann DJ, Herbage D, Ville G, Drunieras M. Wound healing of human skin transplanted onto the nude mouse. An immunohistological and ultrastructural study of the epidermal basment membrane zone reconstruction and connective tissue reorganization. *Dev Biol* 1987;121(1):119–129.

Dunphy JE, Udupa KN. Chemical and histochemical sequences in the normal healing of wounds. *N Engl J Med* 1955;253:847.

Eisen AZ, Jeffrey JJ, Gross J. Human skin collagenase: Isolation and mechanism of attack on the collagen molecule. *Biochim Biophys Acta* 1968;151:637.

Gabbiana G, Lelous M, Bailey AJ, et al. Collagen and myofibroblasts of granulation tissue: A chemical, ultrastructural and immunologic study. *Virchow's Arch (Cell Pathol)* 1976;21:133–145.

Gillman T, et al. Reactions of healing wounds and granulation tissue in man to auto-Thiersch, autodermal, and homodermal grafts. *Br J Plast Surg* 1953;6:153.

Harmon CB, Zelickson BD, Roenigk RK, Pittelkow MR, et al. Immuno-ultrastructural evaluation of dermabrasive scar revision. American Society of Dermatologic Surgery 20th Annual Meeting, Charleston, SC, March 25–28, 1993.

Kurpakus MS, Stock EL, Jones JC. Analysis of wound healing in an in vitro model: early appearance of laminin and a 125 × 103 WM polypeptide during adhesion complex formation. *J Cell Sci* 1990;96:651–660.

Lundberg C, et al. Quantification of the inflammatory reaction and collagen accumulation in an experimental model of open wounds in the rat: A methodological study. *Scand J Plast Reconstr Surg* 1982;16:123.

MacDonald RA. Origin of fibroblasts in experimental healing wounds. Autoradiographic studies using tritiated thymidine. *Surgery* 1959;46:376.

Mackie EJ, Tucker RP, Halfter W, Chiquet-Ehrismann R. The distribution of tenascin coincides with pathways of neural crest cell migration. *Development* 1988;102:237–250.

Majno G, et al. Contraction of granulation tissue in vitro: similarity to smooth muscle. *Science* 1971;173:548.

O'Hare RP, et al. Isolation of collagen-stimulating factors from healing wounds. *J Clin Pathol* 1983;36:707.

Olsen C, Forscher BK. Soluble collagen in acute inflammation. *Proc Soc Exp Biol Med* 1962;111:126.

Ordman LJ, Gillman T. Studies in the healing of cutaneous wounds. I. The healing of excisions through the skin of pigs. *Arch Surg* 1966;93:857.

Rigal C, Pieraggi MT, Vincent C, Prost C, et al. Healing of full-thickness cutaneous wounds in the pig. *J Invest Dermatol* 1991;96:777–85.

Ross R, Odland G. Human wound repair: Inflammatory cells, epithelial-mesenchymal interrelations, and fibrogenesis. *J Cell Biol* 1968;39:152.

Rovee DT, Miller CA. Epidermal role in the breaking strength of wounds. *Arch Surg* 1968;96:43.

Ryan GB,et al. Myofibroblasts in human granulation tissue. *Hum Pathol* 1974;5:55.

Silbert JE. Structure and metabolism of proteoglycans and glycosaminoglycans. *J Invest Dermatol* 1982;79 (suppl):31–37.

Snowden JM, Kennedy DF, Cliff WJ. The contractile properties of wound granulation tissue. *J Surg Res* 1984;36:108.

Sonnenberg A, Calafat J, Janssen J, et al. Integrin alpha 6/beta 4 complex is located in hemidesmosomes, suggesting a major role in epidermal cell-basement membrane adhesion. *J Cell Biol* 1991;113:907–917.

Stepp MA, Spurr-Michaud S, Tisdale S, et al. Alpha 6 bet 4 integrin heterodimer is a componet of hemidesmosomes. *Proc Natl Acad Sci USA* 1990;87:88970–88974.

Suzuki M, Choi BH. The behavior of the extracellular matrix and the basal lamina during the repair of cryogenic injury in the adult rat cerebral cortex. *Acta Neuropathol (Berl)* 1990;80(4):355–361.

Van Winkle W, Jr. The fibroblast in wound healing. *Surg Gynecol Obstet* 1967;124:369.

Weiss P. The biological foundations of wound repair. *Harvey Lecture Series* 1985;55:13.

Whitby DJ, Ferguson MW. The extracellular matrix of lip wounds in fetal, neonatal, and adult mice. *Development* 1991;112:651–668.

52

Scar Revision

Dana Wolfe, Wesley Low, and Terence M. Davidson
*University of California, San Diego, School of
Medicine, San Diego, California*

PRINCIPLES OF WOUND HEALING AND SCAR FORMATION

A complete understanding of scar revision is possible only if one has a good grasp of the basic principles of wound healing and scar formation. Any wound that penetrates more deeply than the epidermis, whether inflicted by biologic, chemical, or physical injury, results in healing by scar formation. Initially an intense inflammatory reaction involves histamine, prostaglandins, complement, lymphokines, lipid peroxidases, the release of lysosomal enzymes, and numerous other cellular chemotactic substances. The cells that are attracted to the site of injury, particularly macrophages, produce substances that stimulate fibroblastic activity. The fibroblasts and epithelial cells then migrate along a scaffolding of fibrin strands constructed from coagulation and thrombus formation. Collagen is subsequently deposited in this matrix.

After extrusion from the fibroblasts and deposition in the matrix, collagen molecules aggregate into large fibrillar complexes by weak cohesive forces. Intra- and intermolecular covalent cross-links gradually form between reactive aldehyde groups, stabilizing the collagen complex and increasing the tensile strength of the matrix. The strength and integrity of the final repair are dependent upon this process.

After the initial period of wound healing, scar remodeling begins, a process that continues for years. As the collagen polymerizes, scar density increases. Wound contracture develops, usually weeks to months after the original injury, and may be disfiguring or disabling.

Several factors influence the remodeling process and affect the appearance of the final scar. Tension on a wound stimulates fibroblasts to secrete more collagenous proteins into the extracellular space, thereby increasing the scar size. If the noxious agent that originally produced the wound and induced the fibroproliferative inflammation is not absorbed or eliminated but remains as a source of chronic irritation, propagation of scar will result. Similarly, infection will prolong the inflammatory process, resulting in a less favorable scar. Hypoxia stimulates the synthesis and deposition of collagen, so poor oxygenation also impacts adversely on scar formation. Age and genetic factors also come into play.

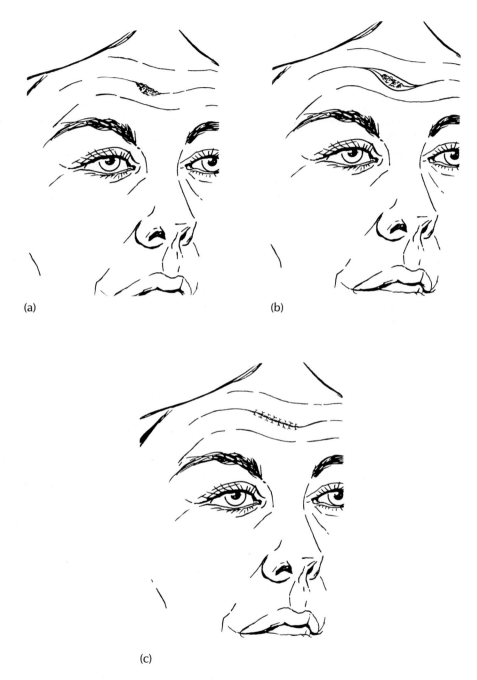

(a)

(b)

(c)

Figure 5 Simple fusiform excision demonstrating how the directional orientation of both ends of the excision can be modified so that the final scar will lie completely within a prominent skin crease.

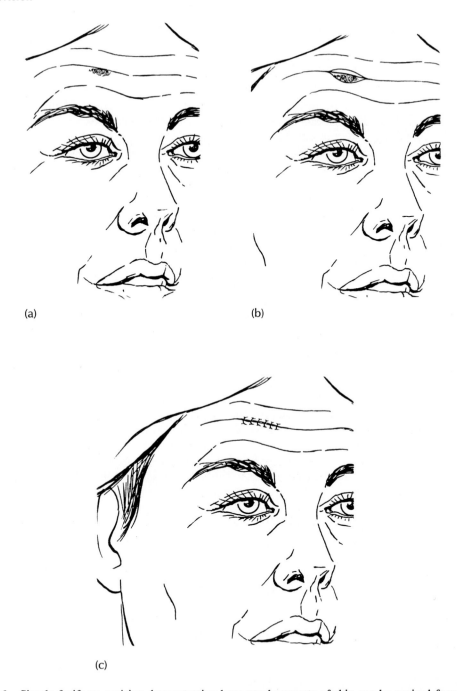

(a)

(b)

(c)

Figure 6 Simple fusiform excision demonstrating how equal amounts of skin can be excised from either side of a prominent skin crease producing a final scar that lies completely within that crease.

At this point the cuff of scar tissue along the advancing margin is finally excised and healthy skin approximated.

TISSUE EXPANDERS

Tissue expansion is a new surgical concept that involves the implantation of one or several inflatable silicone bags in the subcutaneous plane. A small dome connected by tubing is buried in the same plane and is injected with saline on a weekly basis, progressively stretching the overlying skin. Once sufficient excess skin has been obtained in this manner, the expander is removed and the lesion excised. The stretched skin (along with the underlying "capsule" that has formed around the expander) is advanced in a single stage to close the defect.

Expanders are therefore potentially useful for some of the same lesions as serial excision and may decrease the number of procedures required. However, careful preoperative planning is necessary, and the expander must be properly placed at the initial operation. There is also some risk of infection and extrusion. A separate incision is often required for placement of the expander, and the incision must be away from the area to be expanded. It is recommended that the placement incision be in nonscarred skin to minimize the risk of exposure and extrusion.

M-PLASTY

One problem that arises when excising broad scars is how to keep the resultant scar length to a minimum. In order to prevent protrusions or dog ears at either end, the lines of excision must be gradually tapered together so that they meet at an angle not exceeding 30°. In some cases this may result in an unacceptably long, straight scar and require excision by a large amount of normal skin.

By using an M-plasty, two small side-by-side 30° triangles of normal skin are excised, thereby reducing the total amount of skin to be removed and minimizing tissue protrusion. If the triangle of tissue in the middle of the M is then advanced centrally in a "Y-to-V" maneuver, the total central axis incisional length is further reduced. In addition, advancing these triangles centrally results in less overall tissue distortion with wound closure, since skin is being borrowed from both the longitudinal plane and the transverse plane (with respect to the central incision) (Fig. 7).

In addition to keeping incisions shorter while preventing tissue protrusions and distortions, M-plasties also camouflage. This concept is based on the ability of the eye to quickly perceive a straight line when even a portion of it is seen. If the line is broken into a series of short segments oriented in different directions, it is much more difficult for the eye to follow, even if the total length is now longer. This concept is the basis for more sophisticated scar-revision techniques.

Z-PLASTY

Z-plasty was one of the original techniques used for scar revision and is still the technique of choice for lengthening scars and altering their direction. It is ideal when used for linear scars that cross the junction of two aesthetic areas or are perpendicular to important FSTL, especially when the natural tissues are concave or convex, since this results in contracture formation and webbing or creasing.

A Z-plasty is basically two transposition flaps transposed over one another. In so doing, tissue is borrowed from an area of excess and transposed into an area of deficiency. The orientation of the scar is redirected by about 90°.

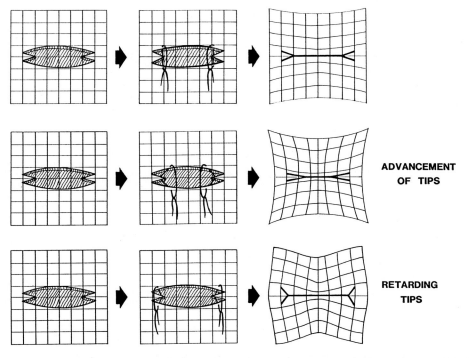

ADVANCEMENT OF TIPS

RETARDING TIPS

Figure 7 A fusiform wound closed with M-plasties at each end. Note that advancement of the M-plasty tips reduces tissue distortion in the vertical axis at the expense of additional distortion in the horizontal plane. When the tips are retarded the tissues become bunched at either end of the wound, and as more tissue must be borrowed from the vertical axis for closure, distortion is maximized in this direction.

First the scar is excised. This becomes the central limb of the Z. Two separate incisions are then made, beginning at each end of the central limb, which parallel each other at identical angles with the central limb. These incisions are called the lateral limbs, and the angles they make with the central limb define the Z-plasty (i.e., 60° Z-plasty, 30° Z-plasty, etc.).

The triangular flaps and the surrounding tissues are undermined and the flaps transposed. The additional length obtained is a function of the angle of the Z-plasty; the greater the angle, the greater the lengthening, but also the greater the amount of tissue distortion and protrusion. For this reason, surgeons rarely use Z-plasties of more than 60°.

Figure 8 illustrates the basic concept of Z-plasty. In planning and designing Z-plasties, one must pay careful attention to the lateral limb orientation, since the final scar orientation will be the same. As there are four different possible designs for the lateral limbs of any given Z-plasty, the one in which the lateral limbs most closely parallel the FSTL should be chosen. Figure 9 illustrates this point, showing both a correct and an incorrect choice of lateral limb placement.

COMPOUND Z-PLASTY

Sometimes more lengthening is necessary than can be obtained with a simple Z-plasty. The compound Z-plasty is done to avoid transposing very large flaps, resulting in long scars and substantial tissue distortion and protrusion. Several lateral limbs can be created, forming a number

SIMPLE 60° Z-PLASTY

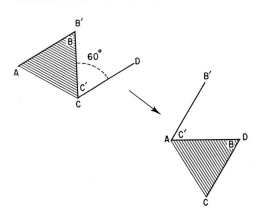

Figure 8 Simple 60° Z-plasty. Note that the orientation of the central incision is changed by 90° and that the orientation of the lateral limb incisions remains the same.

of triangular flaps, which can then be transposed. Four- and even six-flap Z-plasties can be interdigitated in this manner, resulting in a "zig-zag" type of scar (Fig. 10).

While not ideal for facial surgery, such compound Z-plasties can be useful in other areas of the body where significant lengthening is needed and appearance is less important. The tissue compressions and protrusions created by this method generally flatten with time.

SERIAL Z-PLASTY

An alternative to the compound Z-plasty for lengthening markedly contracted scars is the serial Z-plasty. First, two simple Z-plasty lateral limb incisions are made. Then several more incisions are made on either side of the central limb, parallel to the lateral limb incisions at the ends. Again, a zig-zag type of scar results after transposing the flaps (Fig. 11).

In addition to increasing the length along the long axis of an unfavorably oriented scar (while simultaneously changing the direction of that scar), this Z-plasty technique also camouflages long, straight scars by breaking them into several shorter segments. However, it does so at the expense of multiple incisions and possible tissue protrusion and distortion. For this reason, other techniques have been devised for revising scars by breaking them into smaller pieces without lengthening or distorting surrounding tissues.

RUNNING W-PLASTY

The rationale for running W-plasty scar revision is the concept of scar camouflaging by breaking the scar into short segments connected by acute angles. The scar is excised with a minimum of normal tissue, and a series of small side-by-side triangular flaps or serrations are cut into each wound edge. After undermining, the edges are advanced together with several deep, interrupted subcutaneous stitches placed at least 5 mm back from the edges. The triangular tips on one side are then interdigitated with the triangular notches on the opposing side. The skin closure is most

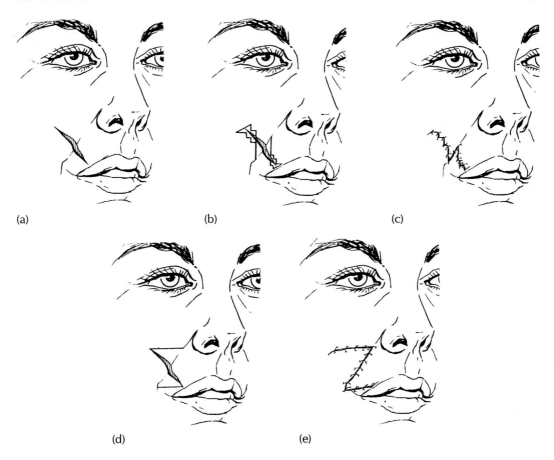

(a)   (b)   (c)

(d)   (e)

Figure 9 (a) Theoretical facial scar crossing an aesthetic border. (b,c) Appropriate way to deal with the scar using a running W-plasty. A Z-plasty is utilized at the site where the scar crosses the aesthetic border in order to change its directional orientation to conform to that of the border itself. (d,e) Incorrect way to deal with this scar. Although the central axis of the scar is changed to correspond to the direction of the aesthetic border, the lateral limb incisions are unacceptably long and do not parallel the favorable skin tension lines.

expeditiously performed using rapidly absorbable 6–0 chromic suture as a running, locked stitch. First, all flap tips on one side are sutured into position, then, crossing over, all the flap tips on the other side are similarly stitched into place. The result is an aesthetically favorable, zig-zag type scar. If desired, M-plasties can be used on the ends of these closures to minimize their length.

Properly done, no line should exceed 5 mm in length and no angle should exceed 90°. The eye tends to lose this type of scar at each corner as it goes off into healthy, nonscarred skin. As long as the angles are acute, the eye does not readily follow from one broken segment to the next. The camouflage thus produced results in a less visible scar despite an increase in the actual scar length.

COMPOUND Z-PLASTY   **SERIAL Z-PLASTY**

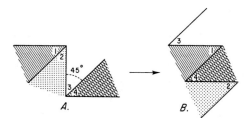

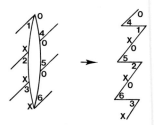

Figure 10 Compound Z-plasty. Two 45° lateral limb incisions are created at either end of the central axis, and when the triangular tissue flaps are transposed, a zig-zag scar results.

Figure 11 Serial Z-plasty. Note that multiple lateral limb incisions are created along the length of the central axis, and again a zig-zag scar is produced when the resultant tissue flaps are transposed as shown.

This technique may be used for excision of thin scars, wide scars, or curved scars. Two important technical points are:

1. Keep as many of the short segments as possible parallel to the FSTL.
2. When cutting the flaps on a curved scar, make the flaps on the outside of the curve broader based and less acutely angled in order to keep the number of flaps on each side equal.

The resultant disparity between flap size and their corresponding notches will become insignificant as the skin stretches and contracts during healing. If more flaps are accidently created on one side of the excision than on the other, one of the flaps on the deficient side is simply bisected, creating one additional flap and one additional notch, and the size disparity will dissipate with time (Figs. 12–14).

GEOMETRIC BROKEN LINE

This technique is a natural progression of the running W-plasty that, instead of a series of nearly identical triangular flaps, consists of a random pattern of constantly changing flaps, all variable in shape and size. It has the advantage of avoiding an easily recognized pattern. Once the eye has followed two or three zig-zags, the remainder of the scar can be easily detected and more readily perceived.

As with the running W-plasty, no segment should exceed 5 mm in length and all should parallel FSTL whenever possible. It is important that rectangular and square flaps be identical in size and shape to their respective recipient sites, so triangular flaps are superior along curved segments of scar.

The scar is excised and the flaps cut as a single step using a #11 blade. The edges are undermined, and wound closure is performed in the same manner as for running W-plasty.

The geometric broken-line technique can be used for straight, curved, short, or very long scars and is an effective camouflaging method. The surgery requires precise planning and accurate flap

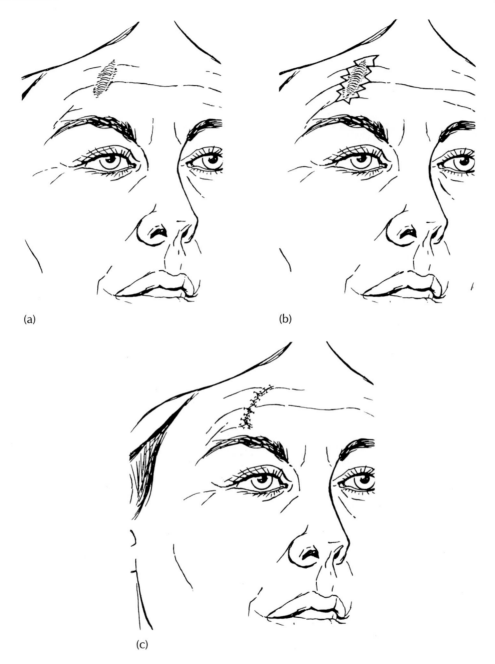

(a)

(b)

(c)

Figure 12 Running W-plasty. Note that a small M-plasty was utilized for closure at the inferior end of the wound.

design to ensure an even mesh of the two wound edges when the flaps are interdigitated. This planning is best done prior to anesthetic injections, which distort and blanch the tissues.

Figures 15 and 16 show two examples of geometric broken-line revisions. The actual techniques are superbly demonstrated on the videotapes *The San Diego Classics in Soft Tissue Surgery*.

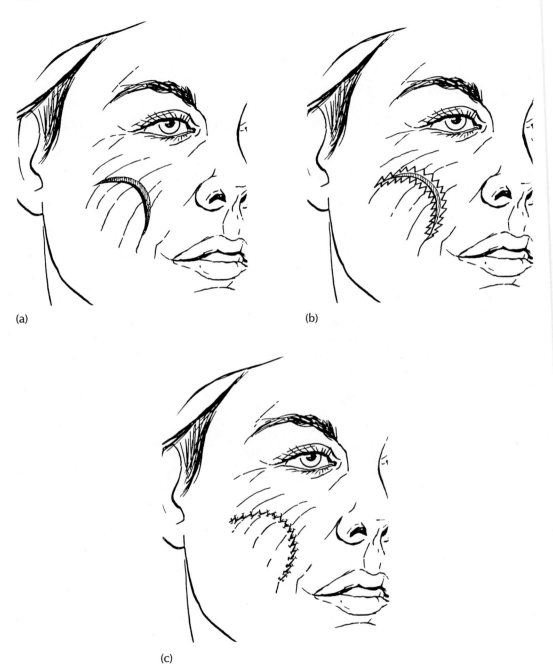

(a)   (b)

(c)

Figure 13 Running W-plasty. Note how the directional orientation and size of the triangles were altered in order to maintain an identical number of triangles on either side, and also to keep all incisions as parallel to the favorable skin tension lines as possible.

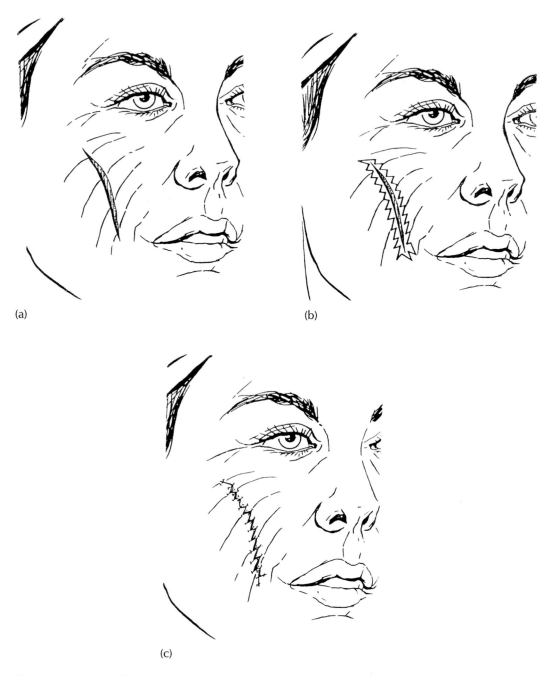

(a)

(b)

(c)

Figure 14 Running W-plasty. This again demonstrates how the orientation of the triangles is altered along the length of the scar to maintain a parallel orientation of the triangular incisions to the favorable skin tension lines. An M-plasty is used to facilitate closure at the inferior end of the wound.

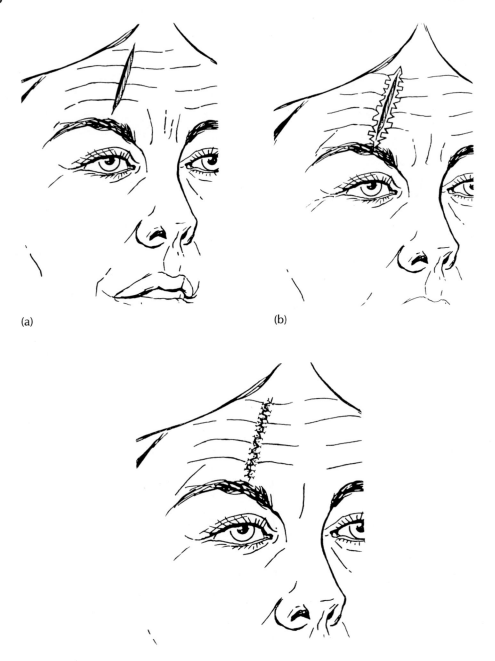

(a)   (b)

Figure 15 Geometric broken-line closure.

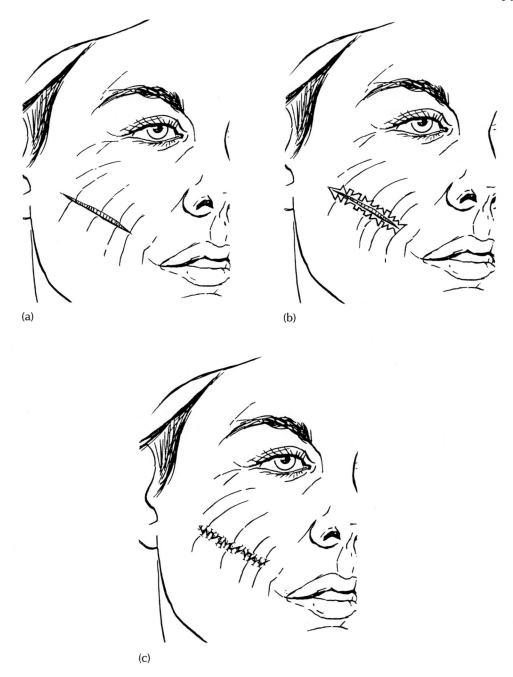

(a)

(b)

(c)

Figure 16 Geometric broken-line closure.

KELOIDS AND HYPERTROPHIC SCARS

These scars are caused by an imbalance between collagen deposition and degradation and probably represent different points along a continuum of excessive scar formation. Hypertrophic scars are thick and raised but generally remain within the boundaries of the original wound and often regress with time. Keloids extend beyond the boundaries of the original wound, invade surrounding tissues, and often recur after surgical removal.

Both are characterized histologically by an overabundant deposition of dermal collagen and biochemically by extremely high levels of proline hydroxylase activity and an increase in collagenase inhibitors. They are more likely to occur in younger patients and from wounds in thick skin, closed under tension. Keloids are more prevalent in the darker-skinned races, particularly in blacks.

Because of their tendency to recur, treatment of keloids is problematic. A wide range of treatment modalities have been advocated and several novel approaches are now being investigated, but at present it is unlikely that single modality treatment will render satisfactory results—combination therapy is generally more effective. In addition, a long period of frequent observation is mandatory, probably for at least 2 years following treatment, with additional intervention at the first sign of recurrence.

Surgical Excision

Many surgeons are reluctant to excise keloids because of a recurrence rate of about 55% following surgery alone. However, if certain general principles are adhered to and adjunctive modalities employed, results can be quite satisfactory. These general principles include sharp, minimally traumatic dissection technique, wound closure under minimal or no tension and good wound edge eversion, and use of nonabsorbable sutures which are removed as soon as possible after surgery. The use of tension-reducing measures, such as Z-plasty, or of camouflaging techniques is to be avoided, as they are likely to cause extension of the keloid. If necessary, it is acceptable to "core out" keloids and save part of the overlying skin if the wound cannot otherwise be closed without tension.

Corticosteroids

Intralesional corticosteroids can be used alone or in combination with surgery or other techniques, both to shrink and to prevent the recurrence of keloids. Corticosteroids are felt to work both by decreasing collagen synthesis and by increasing collagen degradation by decreasing the level of collagenase inhibitors.

Triamcinolone (Kenalog) is the most commonly used drug for this purpose, and it can be administered either with a needle and syringe or with a Dermajet. For many small keloids and most hypertrophic scars, a few Dermajet treatments repeated at 2-week intervals is all that is required. For some larger keloids, serial injections with a needle and syringe are necessary to deliver a sufficient steroid volume. In some cases up to 20 or 30 injections may be necessary to resolve the keloid. Often one is left with a large pouch of wrinkled, redundant skin, which can then be excised.

When used as an adjunct to surgery, presurgical intralesional injections should be performed about a month preoperatively with close follow-up after surgery. Injections should be continued at 2-week intervals at the first sign of recurrence. The maximum monthly dose of injected Kenalog is 120 mg for adults, 80 mg for children 6–10 years of age, and 40 mg for children 1–5 years of age. It is important that injections be made directly into the scar or keloid itself and not into the surrounding skin. Excessive use of steroids can result in thinning, atrophy, telangiectasias, and depigmentation and must be avoided. At the first signs of local steroid toxicity, further injections must be withheld.

Pressure

The use of pressure devices and garments is another method for preventing the development of hypertrophic scar and keloid. There are several theories on mechanisms responsible for the effect of pressure on maturing scars, but as yet it has not been fully elucidated.

Custom-tailored nylon compression garments have been used to prevent the development of excessive scarring and contracture in burn patients. Polyurethane sponges, foam splints, and polymethylmethacrylate molded splints have also been used to prevent keloid recurrence after treatment. These devices particularly lend themselves to use on the ear lobes following keloid excision but must remain in continuous use for at least 18 months to 2 years following surgery.

Radiation Therapy

Administration of external beam radiation therapy is the perioperative and postoperative period, up to a total dose of 1500–2000 rads, has been advocated to prevent postsurgical keloid recurrence. Its efficacy is probably due to the inhibitory effect on both fibroplasia and endothelial vascular budding.

Extreme caution must be exercised when giving radiation to keloids. There is a small but definite risk of developing cutaneous, thyroid, and other malignancies following its use. Some clinicians feel that it is never indicated for the treatment of benign conditions such as keloids. It probably never should be used in children or for abdominal or pelvic lesions in women of childbearing age.

Cryotherapy

Although cryotherapy is not an accepted first-line treatment for keloids, some provocative case reports have recorded impressive results with cryotherapy. However, others have reported poor results using this technique. In addition, cryotherapy is very prone to cause depigmentation due to the melanocytes' sensitivity to cold. At present it appears that cryotherapy may be a useful procedure in situations where other available modalities are contraindicated or ineffective, with great caution taken in non-Caucasian patients because of possible depigmentation.

Laser Surgery

Use of the CO_2 laser to excise keloids, alone or followed by intralesional corticosteroid injections, has produced good results in several preliminary studies and deserves further evaluation as a treatment for keloids. Theoretical advantages include sterilization, sealing of blood vessels up to 0.5 mm as it cuts, minimal necrosis of surrounding tissues, and sealing of nerve endings. The Nd:YAG laser may also prove to be useful in this regard.

Medical Therapy

Several medications, applied topically, orally, or injected locally, have been investigated and hold varying degrees of promise as either adjunctive or first-line models of therapy for keloids. These include oral tetrahydroquinone, oral asiatic acid (Medecassol), topical 0.05% retinoid acid solution, topical ZnO_2, oral β-amino propionitrile fumarate (BAPN) or penicillamine combined with colchicine, and antineoplastic agents such as nitrogen mustard, thio-TEPA, and methotrexate. Obviously, there is considerable potential for side effects and long-term toxicity with several of these agents, and these issues must be addressed and clarified before such agents can be used routinely in keloid therapy.

DERMABRASION

Even after a well-performed scar revision there are frequently minor irregularities which detract from an ideal result. Examples include fine scars which are not quite flush with the surrounding skin and the presence of subtle differences in texture and color from scar to healthy skin. In these situations, further improvement may be obtained by one, two, or occasionally more dermabrasions. Dermabrasion works to level out contour irregularities by bringing the level of healthy adjacent tissue down to the level of the scar. This also reduces color mismatch.

Before considering the use of dermabrasion, one must be certain that full maturation of the scar has occurred. This means a wait of at least 6 months, and often 1–2 years, following the last scar revision. However, some have gotten nice results with dermabrasion as early as 6 weeks postoperatively. Depressed scars, mild-to-moderate acne pitting, and fine wrinkles are all indications for dermabrasion. Raised, hypertrophic scars and otherwise normal but elevated scars are *not* appropriate for dermabrasion. Hypertrophic scars only proliferate more actively if abraded. Since dermabrasion is only good for lowering the height of normal tissue down to the level of a scar and not vice versa, treatment of elevated scars will only produce excessive thinning of the already very thin dermal and epidermal layers, with very little chance for satisfactory improvement.

Dermabrasion is the mechanical removal of the epidermis and some, but not all, of the dermis, leaving the skin appendages and the depths of the rete pegs intact. New epidermal cells then migrate across the exposed dermis within 3–7 days. A progressive thickening of the dermis and epidermis occurs over the next several months, but the original thickness is never attained—thus the effect of the dermabrasion is maintained. Areas of thick skin that are rich in skin appendages are therefore most amenable to dermabrading.

Before starting, the deepest portions of the scar are marked with ink or dye. After anesthesia (local or general) and freezing (with Freon, to provide a firm surface against which to work and to facilitate consistency in depth of abrasion), the skin is dermabraded down to the level of the inked marks, until the inked scar is just removed. At the edges, the level of planing is made progressively more superficial and careful feathering is performed peripherally to ensure a smooth transition to normal skin. Hemostasis is obtained with pressure (never cautery), a semiocclusive dressing is applied, and at 7–10 days the eschar will fall off and the skin can be washed.

BIBLIOGRAPHY

Amoils CP, Jackler RK, Lustig LR. Repair of chronic tympanic membrane perforations using epidermal growth factors. *Otolaryngol Head Neck Surg* 1992;107(5):669–683.

Bennett NT, Schultz GS. Growth factors and wound healing: Biochemical properties of growth factors and their receptors. *Am J Surg* 1993;165:728–737.

Bennett NT, Schultz GS. Growth factors and wound healing: Part II. Role in normal and chronic wound healing. *Am J Surg* 1993;166:74–81.

Boucek RJ. Factors affecting wound healing. *Otolaryngol Clin North Am* 1984;17:243–264.

Brown GL, Curtsinger LJ, Jurkiewicz M, et al. Stimulation of healing of chronic wounds by epidermal growth factor. *Plast Reconstr Surg* 1991;88(2):189–194.

Brown GL, Curtsinger LJ, White M, et al. Acceleration of tensile strength of incisions treated with EGF and TGF-α. *Ann Surg* 1988;208(6):788–794.

Brown GL, Nanney LB, Griffen J, et al. Enhancement of wound healing by topical treatment with epidermal growth factor. *N Engl J Med* 1989;321:76–79.

Brown LA, Pierce HE. Keloids: Scar revision. *J Dermatol Surg Oncol* 1986;12:51–56.

Carr-Collins JA. Pressure techniques for the Prevention of hypertrophic scar. *Clin Plast Surg* 1992;19(3):733–743.

Carrico TJ, Mehrhof AI Jr, Cohen IK. Biology of wound healing. *Surg Clin North Am* 1984;64:721–733.

Chvapil M, Koopmann CF. Scar formation: physiology and pathological states. *Otolaryngol Clin North Am* 1984;17:265–272.

Davidson TM. Lacerations and scar revisions. In Otolaryngology—Head and Neck Surgery. CW Cummings et al., eds. St. Louis, C.V. Mosby Co., 1986, pp. 289–311.

Davidson TM, Webster RC, Gordon BR. The principles and dynamics of local skin flaps. A self-instructional package from the Committee on Continuing Education in Otolaryngology (SIPAC). *Am Acad Otolaryngol* 1979;1–93.

Davidson TM, Webster RC. Scar revision. A self-instructional package from the Committee on Continuing Education in Otolaryngology (SIPAC). *Am Acad Ophthal Otolaryngol* 1977;1–97.

Davidson TM. Subcutaneous suture placement. *Laryngoscope* 1987;97:501–504.

Davies DM. Scars, hypertrophic scars, and keloids. *Br Med J* 1985;290:1056–1058.

Fina M, Baird A, Ryan A. Direct application of basic fibroblast growth factor improves tympanic membrane perforation healing. *Laryngoscopy* 1993;103(7):804–809.

Ketchum LD, Smith J, Robinson DW, et al. Treatment of hypertrophic scar keloid and scar contracture by triamcinolone acetonide. *Plast Reconstr Surg* 1966;38:209.

Kischer CW. The microvessels in hypertrophic scars, keloids and related lesions: A review. *J Submicrosc Cytol Pathol* 1992;24(2):281–296.

Mcgee G, Davidson J, Buckley A, et al. Recombinant basic fibroblast growth factor accelerates wound healing. *J Surg Res* 1998;45:145–153.

Nanney LB. Biochemical and physiologic aspects of wound healing. In *Cutaneous Surgery: Basic Surgical Concepts and Procedures*. RG Wheeland, ed. Philadelphia, W.B. Saunders, 1994, pp. 113–121.

Pastor JC, Calonge M. Epidermal growth factor and corneal wound healing. *Cornea* 1992;11(4):311–314.

Petroutsos G, Guinmaraes R, Pouliquen D, et al. Comparison of the effects of EGF, pFGF, and EDGF on corneal epithelium wound healing. *Curr Eye Res* 1984;3(4):593–598.

Pollack SV. Wound healing 1985: An update. *J Dermatol Surg Oncol* 1985;11:296–300.

Robson M, Phillips L, Thomason A, et al. Platelet-derived growth factor for the treatment of chronic pressure ulcers. *Lancet* 1992;339:23–25.

Schultz G, Cipolla L, Whithouse A, et al. Growth factors and corneal endothelial cells: Stimulation of adult human corneal endothelial cells mitosis in vitro by defined mitogenic agents. *Cornea* 1992;11(1):20–27.

Tritto M, Kanat IO. Management of keloids and hypertrophic scars. *J Am Podiatr Med Assoc* 1991;81(11):601–605.

Suggested Videotapes

The San Diego Classics in Soft Tissue Surgery. Webster RC, Davidson TM, Nahum AM. Scar Revision, Parts I, II and III. 1977.

53

Basic Laser Physics

Timothy J. Rosio
Marshfield Clinic, Marshfield, Wisconsin

Just a few years ago, dermatologic lasers were primarily employed by a handful of laser *cognoscenti*, who had made a serious academic and financial commitment to understanding their use. Rarely was one of the few existing laser types available to general, private dermatologists or residents. Today, increasing numbers and types of specialized lasers are accessible to a majority of practicing and training dermatologists, often without investment, through hospitals or other arrangements.

This laser windfall may be a mixed blessing. Many newer lasers employ wavelengths and high-intensity physical principles that appear easier to use but that place patients, staff, and physicians at higher risk of serious eye injury. Also, patients may be subjected to multiple, unsuccessful treatments when laser treatment, in general, or the particular wavelength or settings are inappropriate. Education is the key. A lack of background in laser physics impairs the reasoned application of lasers, purchase of the most cost-effective option by a practice or institution, and safe use by practitioners. This may intensify as health care reform shrinks resources and increases the "biznification" of medicine.

As a physician laser user (and decision maker or owner), you will be partially or largely responsible for practical, financial, and technical choices including selection, maintenance, growth, life cycle, and safety involving laser instruments; these and many other questions require a passing knowledge of "what's in the laser box." Since a single ideal laser does not yet exist, limited resources are a practical reality. This requires the laser user to decide whether to use available laser hardware on a tissue structure, pigment, vessel size, depth, or anatomic location to be treated.

On the other hand, the dilemma may be which laser first or next to purchase. The fact that the features of some lasers overlap to a degree, allowing, for example, a laser marketed for pigmented lesions to be promoted for vascular problems, makes this decision more complicated. Therefore, knowledge of laser physics and safety is cost-effective and practical in fiscal, therapeutic, and safety terms.

Optical Resonator Cavity

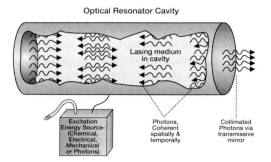

Figure 2 Schematic laser diagram. The lasing medium is confined within an optical cavity or resonator with reflective mirrors on opposing ends. A power supply excites resting state atoms to a high-energy state known as a "population inversion." The laser power supply "pumps" still more energy into the system, in the form of either direct current, radiofrequency, light, or other means. The result of energy pumping and continued stimulated emissions is "amplification," producing an extremely intense laser beam, a percentage of which exits through the partially transmissive mirror. (Reproduced with permission, © Timothy J. Rosio, M.D., Live Cutaneous Laser Surgery Workshop & Seminar.)

describes the photon's fixed rate of the speed of light and the inverse relationship between wavelength and frequency.

Visible light constitutes only a small segment of the wide range of EMR, sandwiched in between the most energetic ionizing gamma rays and x-rays at one end and the low-energy radio and microwaves (Fig. 3). The term "light" refers to the visible part of the EMR spectrum but will be used interchangeably with EMR for convenience.

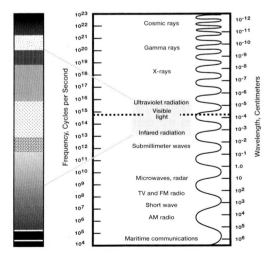

Figure 3 Electromagnetic radiation spectrum with visible wavelengths and frequencies. Visible light is only a small part of the EM spectrum, sandwiched in between the most energetic ionizing gamma rays at one end and the low-energy radio and microwaves at the other. Wavelength = 1/frequency × (c). (Reproduced with permission, © Timothy J. Rosio, M.D., Live Cutaneous Laser Surgery Workshop & Seminar.)

Laser Light Production

Laser production begins with a collection of specific atoms or molecules (lasing medium) confined within an optical cavity or resonator with reflective mirrors on opposing ends. A power supply furnishes energy to the predominantly resting state atoms, exciting the majority to a state known as a "population inversion," since excited-state atoms now predominate. Laser energy emission resonates back and forth, building up within the laser tube, continuing to stimulate more laser emissions. These stimulated emissions generate ever-increasing photons traveling in the same direction as the propagating beam and are therefore summated. Meanwhile, the laser power supply pumps still more energy into the system in the form of either direct current, radio-frequency, light, or other means. The result of energy pumping and continued stimulated emissions is amplification, producing an extremely intense laser beam. One mirror is partially transmissive, allowing egress of a percentage of the beam.

Lasers with similar average power and wavelength output may differ radically in power output vs. time (temporal emission or mode) (Fig. 4). The mode dramatically influences the laser's effects on chromophores. The laser mode depends on the type of power supply used for excitation and the lasing medium. Continuous wave (CW) lasers (e.g., argon) provide a constant power

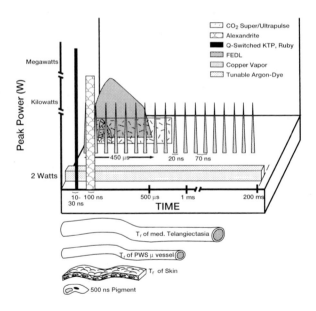

Figure 4 Thermal relaxation time related to power and exposure times of selected cutaneous lasers. Peak Power (W) and temporal delivery of lasers' energy result in characteristic energy profiles, which are superimposed here on a graphic plane, together with pictogram representation of relative thermal relaxation times (T_r) for small microvessels, moderate telangiectasias, skin, and pigment (melanosomes and small pigment granules). Exposures approximating T_r for the target selectively destroy it, and spatially confine damage to the target zone. Lower fluences with much longer exposures than T_r cause coagulation but also allow heat conduction to surrounding tissue, resulting in nonspecific epidermal and dermal damage (and possible visible scarring). Very brief (nanosecond) low-power pulses closely spaced (e.g., 2–5 kHz) are "quasi-continuous," e.g., copper vapor and non–Q-switched KTP lasers. The total energy contained in an individual pulse (area under the curve) is low despite a moderate peak power due to brief duration. (Reproduced with permission, © Timothy J. Rosio, M.D., Live Cutaneous Laser Surgery Workshop & Seminar.)

output over time. Quasi-continuous lasers deliver extremely short (nanosecond), weak pulses (low fluences) that must be summated over hundreds of thousands of milliseconds to have a clinical effect. Quasi-CW mode lasers have clinical effects comparable to CW lasers of similar average power. Pulsed lasers deliver moderately high fluences over milliseconds or microseconds (e.g., flashlamp dye lasers). Q-switched lasers produce extremely high fluences in milliseconds to nanoseconds, resulting in photomechanical effects, which can disrupt tattoo or melanocytic pigments.

Three Properties of Laser Energy

Ordinary light consists of photons with a variety of energies (frequencies or 1/wavelengths) traveling in multiple directions (Fig. 5).; photons of the same wavelength are not synchronized either in space or time (out of phase). Conversely, laser light photons are monochromatic (same wavelength and energies), travel in exactly the same direction with minimal divergence (highly collimated), and wave peaks and valleys are coherent (synchronized in time and space like a marching band, i.e., in phase). These three properties define laser light, conferring capabilities impossible for ordinary light.

Monochromaticity provides opportunity for strategic absorption selectivity (Fig. 6) via matching of laser wavelengths to desired chromophore targets and relative avoidance of other chromophores. Furthermore, ordinary polychromatic light wavelengths are refracted ('bent') to varying degrees as they pass through an interface to a medium of different optical density, e.g., air to water or glass. Thus, differential refraction results in a spread beam with diminished intensity (e.g., prisms and rainbows), while laser light maintains its directional focus and intensity all the way to the target.

Collimation emphasizes the high degree to which all photons are traveling in the same direction, allowing the intensity of the laser light to be maintained. This characteristic makes possible

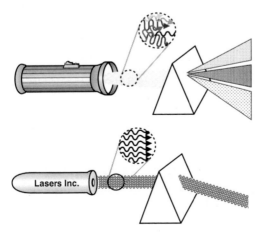

Figure 5 Laser versus incoherent light source characteristics. Ordinary light consists of photons with a variety of energies (frequencies or 1/wavelengths) traveling in multiple directions, out of phase. Conversely, laser light photons are monochromatic (same wavelength, therefore refracted in the prism to the same degree), travel in exactly the same direction with minimal divergence (highly collimated), and wave "peaks and valleys" are coherent, i.e., in phase. These three properties define laser light, conferring capabilities impossible for ordinary light. (Reproduced with permission, © Timothy J. Rosio, M.D., Live Cutaneous Laser Surgery Workshop & Seminar.)

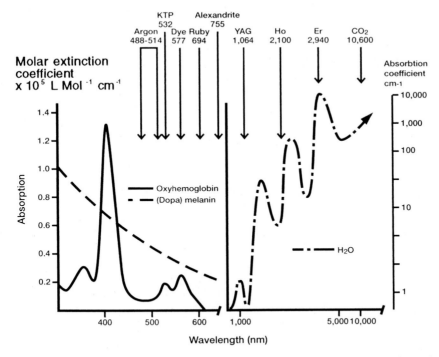

Figure 6 Laser and skin chromophore absorption. Laser photons encountering skin undergo absorption, transmission, reflection, and scattering. The relative probabilities of these continuous events depends on the tissue transmissibility and absorption efficiencies of the chosen wavelength and target tissues' competing chromophores. Depicted are the absorption profiles of the dominant skin chromophores and the main cutaneous laser wavelengths. (Reproduced with permission, © Timothy J. Rosio, M.D., Live Cutaneous Laser Surgery Workshop & Seminar.)

a beam that can travel immense distances, such as from the earth to the moon, and still be detectable. Directionality also makes spatial precision possible, such that tissues near the intended target may be avoided.

Coherence describes the synchronization of the electromagnetic waves that characterize laser light. Coherence underlies laser wave propagation and makes possible, for example, holography.

Laser Beam Spatial Configuration

Transverse Electromagnetic Mode (TEM)

Beam shape is critical to the dermatologic surgeon because it influences the power density that may be applied and the precision available. Is the curette a reasonable incisional tool? Conversely, would you choose a scalpel to ablate tissue? These questions highlight that for surgical lasers, similar to other surgical instruments, laser beam profile influences resurfacing, recontouring, and incisional surgery functions.

The spatial intensity distribution (profile) of a laser beam at the source depends on details of the optical resonator that produced it—mirror radius, spacing, or curvature—and lasing medium dimensions. Note that the beam profile at the target tissue may be similar to that at the source, or it may have undergone significant changes by the delivery system. The three most commonly

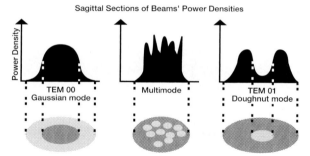

Sagittal Sections of Beams' Power Densities

Power Densities across beam profiles at the target

Figure 7 Transverse electromagnetic modes (TEM). Beam shape is critical to the dermatologic surgeon because it influences the power density that may be applied and the precision available. The three most commonly encountered spatial beam modes or configurations in dermatologic laser surgery are TEM_{00} (gaussian, fundamental), TEM_{01} (doughnut) and multimode. (Reproduced with permission, © Timothy J. Rosio, M.D., Live Cutaneous Laser Surgery Workshop & Seminar.)

encountered spatial beam modes or configurations in dermatologic laser surgery are TEM_{00} (gaussian, fundamental), TEM_{01} (doughnut), and multimode (Fig. 7).

The spot size of a radially symmetric (gaussian) beam is defined as that radius, r_{00}, which transmits 86% of the gaussian beam energy (Fig. 8):

$$r_{00} = \frac{0.9\lambda \times f_L}{D}$$

where f_L is the focal length of the lens and D is the diameter of the laser beam perpendicular to the axis of propagation (prior to lens transmission). Short-focal-length lenses, smaller-original-beam diameters, and shorter wavelengths all favor production of small spot sizes.

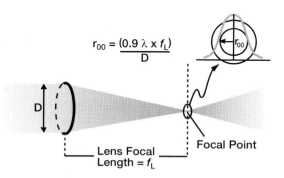

Figure 8 Laser spot size. The spot size of a radially symmetric (gaussian) beam is defined as that radius, r_{00}, which transmits 86% of the gaussian beam energy. $r_{00} = (0.91 \times f_L) \div D$, where f_L is the focal length of the lens and D is the diameter of the laser beam perpendicular to the axis of propagation (prior to lens transmission). Short-focal-length lenses, smaller original beam diameters, and shorter wavelengths favor production of small spot sizes. (Reproduced with permission, © Timothy J. Rosio, M.D., Live Cutaneous Laser Surgery Workshop & Seminar.)

The gaussian beam profile allows the smallest spot size, and therefore the highest peak power density, and is preferable for incisional work. In contrast, the TEM_{01} mode results in ~30% larger spot sizes, and thus a ratio of 0.56 of the power density available from the gaussian beam ($1:1.33^2 = 0.56$). For ablation at the same working distance, the cooler central spot of the doughnut beam and larger spot area may be partially compensated for by doubling the power output and scanning the beam with rapid, overlapping hand movements similar to the way in which one prevents grooving from the peripheral "tails" of the gaussian beam (Fig. 9).

Lasers may also produce more complex spatial beam patterns, such as multimode, characterized by many small rarefactions alternating with higher-power densities. Multimode, as in TEM_{01}, results in a slightly larger minimum spot size and may be seen in some solid-state lasers, e.g., YAG or ruby. However, the YAG laser is normally used with larger spot sizes and lower-power densities for coagulation or with an energy-intensifying contact fiber or sapphire tip for incisional work. Also, the Q-switched ruby and Q-switched YAG are used for delivery of large-spot-size pulses for photodisruption, as will be discussed later.

Delivery Methods

The spatial intensity distribution of the beam at tissue may be strongly influenced by the delivery system responsible for conduction of the beam from the laser source. These include items such as mirrors, lenses, optical fibers, and waveguides. Mirrors in articulated armatures, when correctly aligned, come closest to maintaining the original beam configuration. Optical fibers and waveguides result in a loss of collimation and produce a blunted spatial beam profile more similar to multimode, but which diverges much more rapidly. The laser surgeon should analyze data available on the beam profile at tissue, since alterations of the beam's spatial mode may result from delivery system attachments planned for use.

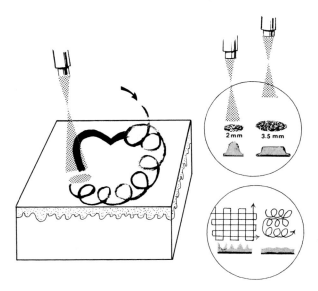

Figure 9 Depth control and tissue uniformity vary with resurfacing and recontouring technique. Different power profiles related to spot size are obtained from different hand piece-to-tissue distances. Tissue injury or removal uniformity is related to both beam profile and hand speed and direction of movement. Flat beam profiles, overlapping circles, and rapid scanning with alternating direction of highly regular, rapid hand movements are keys to excellent cosmetic laser surgery.

Basic Tissue Optics and Lasers

Four Fates for Laser Energy

Laser photons encountering skin are variably subjected to four fates: absorption, transmission, reflection, and scattering (Fig. 10). The relative probabilities of these continuous events depend on the transmissibility and absorption efficiencies of the chosen wavelength in the target tissues' competing chromophores (Fig. 6). In addition to absorption, variable scattering of wavelengths also influences outcome; highly energetic short wavelengths (290–400 nm) undergo strong scattering, while long wavelengths (600–1200 nm) are highly transmitted to depths of 2 mm or more.

A primary principle of photomedicine is that photon absorption must occur for a reaction to take place. But how deep will the photon travel? We know that the probability of sufficient photons being absorbed at the intended target declines exponentially with depth in a tissue because of attenuation. This is described qualitatively in Figure 11, which displays approximate relative penetration depths and combines calculated absorption values for IR and UV wavelengths with histologic research observations for more complicated visible wavelengths that consider selective clinical effects.

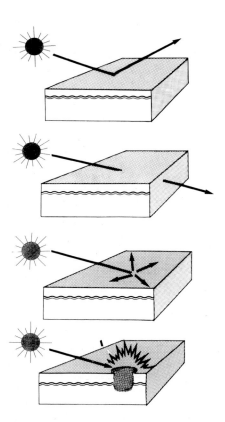

Figure 10   Four fates for laser energy. Photons and tissue interaction result in four potential outcomes: absorption, transmission, reflection, and scattering. The relative probabilities of these continuous events depend on the transmissibility and absorption efficiencies of the chosen wavelength in target tissues' competing chromophores. (Reproduced with permission, © Timothy J. Rosio, M.D., Live Cutaneous Laser Surgery Workshop & Seminar.)

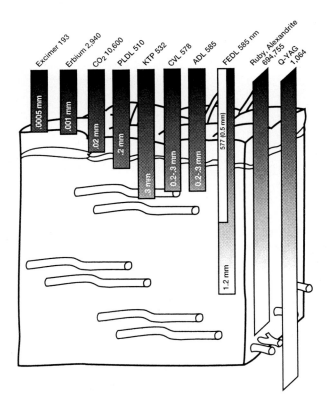

Figure 11 Relative laser wavelength penetration depths. The probability of sufficient photons being absorbed at the intended target declines exponentially with depth in a tissue because of attenuation. Approximate relative penetration depths for common wavelengths are displayed. Calculated absorption values for IR and UV wavelengths are used where absorption dominates, and histologic research observations are combined that consider selective clinical effects for more complicated visible wavelengths (scattering significant and many tissue variables). (Reproduced with permission, © Timothy J. Rosio, M.D., Live Cutaneous Laser Surgery Workshop & Seminar.)

Beer's Law

Photon absorption is described quantitatively by Beer's law, which shows that a fixed percentage of a beam of a given wavelength is absorbed per length as it travels through an ideally uniform (isotropic) tissue. Two common measures of a substance's absorption strength of a specific wavelength are (1) absorption length, or the distance wherein 63% of an incident beam is absorbed, and (2) extinction length, or the distance wherein 90% is absorbed. One extinction length is approximately 2.3 times the absorption length. The first 90% of a beam is absorbed in one extinction length; the remaining 10% undergoes 90% absorption in the second extinction length, etc. Experience has shown that minimum achievable tissue damage is between 1–2.3 times the absorption length for a specific wavelength. Beer's law is written as follows:

$$I_{(\chi)} = I_{(0)} \times 10^{\alpha\chi}$$

where $I_{(\chi)}$ is the transmitted intensity, α is the extinction length, and χ is the depth (cm) of penetration in the tissue. The absorption coefficient is commonly used to display relative absor-

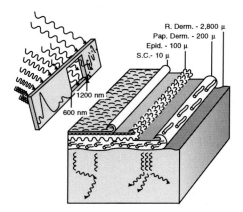

Figure 12 Four-compartment optical skin model. A four-compartment model of the skin, juxtaposed with the skin's major chromophores absorption spectra, is illustrated together with an optical window with minimal absorption from 600 to 1200 nm in all four compartments. Compartments and particular wavelengths fall into three categories:absorption dominant, transmissive/scattering dominant, and mixed. Most photomedicine takes place in the visible spectrum across multiple compartments where a mixture of absorption and scattering occurs. (Reproduced with permission, © Timothy J. Rosio, M.D., Live Cutaneous Laser Surgery Workshop & Seminar.)

bance by substances at varying wavelengths; it is derived from 1 divided by the absorption length (cm) and named μa, or given as absorbance (cm^{-1}).

An Optical Model of the Skin

A simple optical model has been used by Anderson and Parrish and others in efforts to explain and predict clinical laser–tissue interactions. This and other models are helpful gross approximations, since complex interrelationships between variables have so far defied attempts at precise models. I have illustrated my interpretation of such a mathematical model of the skin (Fig. 12) and juxtaposed the skin's nonmelanin major chromophore absorption spectra integrated with an optical window depicting minimal absorption from 600 to 1200 nm.

Optical skin compartments and particular wavelengths fall into three categories: (1) those with high absorption coefficients for a wavelength (absorption dominates), (2) compartments with low absorption coefficients for a wavelength (dominant scattering, transmission, and some reflection), and (3) particularly with visible wavelengths, compartments where much complicated photomedicine takes place with a balance of absorption and scattering present. Notably, the wavelength range 600–1200 nm may be considered as an "optical window" due to the paucity of absorption efficiency across these wavelengths by skin chromophores in all four compartments.

One may vary the skin model by assuming vitiliginous skin, or various melanized clinical conditions, with four layered compartments of varying thicknesses: stratum corneum (10 µm), epidermis (100 µm), papillary dermis (200 µm), and reticular dermis (2800 µm). The stratum corneum, by virtue of this thinness and lack of visible-range chromophores, transmits 95% of the entire visible spectra (only 5% remittance) for both white and black skin.

Epidermal Compartment

In the epidermal compartment, melanin is the only strong broad-band absorber of visible light from 400 to 600 nm (dramatically less and decreasing between 600 and 1200 nm). Melanin is responsible for 3 orders of magnitude variation in 400–600 nm light transmission between fair

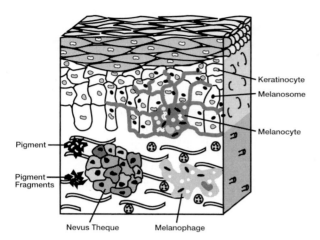

Figure 13 Pigmented optical model of the skin. Melanin may be distributed in the epidermal compartment in the basal layer as melanocytes and in the basal and suprabasal keratinocytes as transferred melanosomes. Superficial to deep dermal pigments include, for example, melanin in melanophages, compound and dermal nevi found alone or in theques, organic carbon, or other tattoo pigments. Any of these cells or pigment granules may be broken into smaller fragments by Q-switched photomechanical laser impulses. (Reproduced with permission, © Timothy J. Rosio, M.D., Live Cutaneous Laser Surgery Workshop & Seminar.)

and darkly pigmented skin types. Melanin may be found in the epidermal compartment in basal layer melanocytes and in the basal and suprabasal keratinocytes as transferred melanosomes (Fig. 13). Clinical examples of this superficial melanized compartment are found in ephelides (freckles), lentigos, junctional nevi, postinflammatory hyperpigmentation, superficial types of melasma (chloasma), and superficial café au lait macules. Junctional nevi overlap into the third (papillary dermal) compartment, in that they may have theques or nests of nevus cells below the basal layer as well as melanosomes in keratinocytes above. Postinflammatory hyperpigmentation may possess melanophages in the papillary dermis as well as hemosiderin.

Superficial Pigment and Vascular Lasers

Superficial pigment and vascular lasers include all the green and yellow light laser systems, including the argon, the KTP, the Q-switched KTP/YAG (532), copper vapor, the continuous-wave argon pumped dye laser, the flashlamp-excited green dye laser or pigmented lesion dye laser (PLDL), and the flashlamp-excited yellow dye laser (FEDL). These laser wavelengths transmit through water but penetrate the skin poorly, absorbed on average at a level of less than 0.1 mm by melanin or 0.02–0.5 mm by blood and to a lesser degree other tissue constituents. Deep pigment lasers include the ruby, alexandrite, and the Q-switched YAG (1064). They may also be used to treat superficial pigment, and will be discussed further.

Long temporal exposure to the wavelength from any of these lasers coagulates tissue widely. Short intense exposures on the order of nanoseconds to hundreds of microseconds allows thermal spatial confinement to superficial melanin and hemoglobin targets in the epidermis and papillary dermis. Exposures of greater than 10 msec may be well tolerated when a highly absorbing target intercepts the majority of photons and limits damage to the epidermis. The superficial pigment and vascular category of lasers is, therefore, ideal for treating these lesions in the epidermal compartment.

If one assumes that no melanin is in the epidermis, the vast majority of all visible light would be transmitted or forward-scattered to the next compartment—the papillary dermis. Nonvisible light spectra that are highly absorbed in tissue proteins or water will be mentioned below.

Papillary Dermis Compartment

The third compartment, representing the papillary dermis, has circulating soluble pigments in blood vessels that selectively absorb visible wavelength bands at 400–500 nm (bilirubin and carotenes) and at 400 and 520–600 nm (hemoglobins). These absorption bands are used to selectively thermolyze (heat-coagulate) the blood vessels, while sparing adjacent, poorly absorbing tissues, as mentioned above.

Papillary and Reticular Dermis Compartments

The papillary and reticular dermis comprising the third and fourth compartments is made of collagen fibers, which variably scatter visible wavelengths forward to a degree inversely proportional to wavelength (i.e., shorter wavelengths scatter more than longer wavelengths). Optical scatter explains why blue nevi—and the sky—appear blue. Because photons of wavelengths less than 600 nm are scattered or absorbed to such a degree, few will be transmitted past the superficial dermis. Conversely, wavelengths in the "optical window" are both absorbed less and scattered less. Therefore, approximately 1% of photons with wavelengths from 605 to 850 nm will be transmitted through chest wall dermis. This percentage may seem miniscule, but, recalling that tissue effects are time and energy dependent, if enough photons are delivered with high intensity in a short enough time period, they may be sufficient to have a dramatic effect on a selectively absorbing chromophore, even deep within the dermis. Examples of this are photo-disruption of melanocytic or tattoo pigment (decorative or traumatic).

Returning to a pigmented version of our optical skin model (Fig. 13), superficial to deep dermal pigments include, for example, melanin in melanophages, compound and dermal nevi, nevus of Ota, organic carbon, or other tattoo pigments. Reflectance spectra of melanin and black tattoo pigments suggest a rough correspondence in absorption profiles, with melanin showing less absorption over a range of wavelengths, particularly toward the longer end of the far-red and near-IR spectrum (Fig. 14). Professional tattoo pigments show a much greater variability in reflectance/absorption profiles associated with particular colors, most commonly reds, greens, and bright blues. The highest absorption (lowest reflectance) for reds is at 550–600 nm, while greens absorb best around 675–775 nm (Fig. 15). Hemosiderin is poorly absorbed by deep pigment wavelengths.

Deep Pigment Lasers

The deep pigment lasers are of extremely high intensity and short duration ("high fluence"). These are all Q-switched lasers, including the ruby, the Q-switched YAG, and alexandrite lasers. Q-switching (pulsing) results in such high-intensity photon delivery to tissue targets that photomechanical effects (fragmentation) are seen (Fig. 13). Surrounding tissues are protected from thermal injury. This occurs because delivery of the photons takes place over a period shorter than the thermal relaxation time of the target, i.e., before significant heat dissipation can occur.

Selective photothermolysis can occur in any chromophores that absorb these wavelengths efficiently enough, which includes most tattoo pigments over a broad range and, to some lesser degree, melanin pigment. The far-red and near-infrared wavelengths of these lasers are capable of penetrating several millimeters through the skin because of long-wavelength transmission and poor absorption by other chromophores. The Q-switched YAG infrared wavelength is less efficiently absorbed by melanin than shorter wavelengths (10% that of the ruby laser), however,

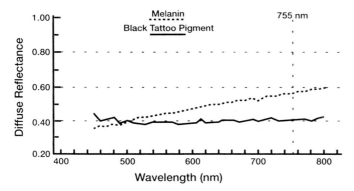

Figure 14 Reflectance spectra of melanin and organic carbon pigments. Reflectance spectra of melanin and black tattoo pigments reveal a rough correspondence in absorption profiles, but with melanin showing less absorption over a range of wavelengths, particularly toward the longer end of the far-red and near-IR spectrum. (Reproduced with permission of Candela Laser Corp.)

transmission efficiency is considerably greater so that a greater percentage of energy reaches the target.

Near-IR, YAG Wavelength

YAG (1060 nm) is minimally absorbed by any skin chromophore, including melanin; therefore, it is one of the most deeply penetrating wavelengths, being transmitted and scattered through all four compartments. Water absorbs minimal infrared energy up to wavelengths greater than 1200 nm of the skin model. The low absorptive affinity of the skin for YAG energy is demonstrated by the skin thickness (3 mm) required to absorb 90% of the beam energy, or the extinction length. Virtually all laser energy is absorbed within three extinction lengths within a tissue. The large extinction length for the YAG is borne out by observation that the beam expands three times after passing through just 2 mm of muscosa, resulting in a ninefold reduction in power density. The YAG energy is scattered throughout a tissue volume 300–900 times larger than CO_2 energy.

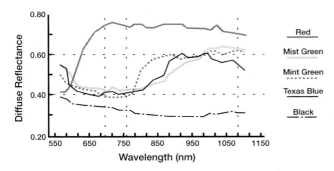

Figure 15 Reflectance spectra of colored professional tattoo pigments. Professional tattoo pigments show a much greater diversity in reflectance/absorption profiles for various colors, most notably reds, greens, and bright blues. Highest absorption (lowest reflectance) for reds is at 550–600 nm, while greens absorb best around 675–775 nm. (Reproduced with permission of Candela Laser Corp.)

Far-UV, Mid-IR

Further outside the visible spectrum lie the far-UV (e.g., 193 Excimer), mid-IR (2100–2940 Holmium and Erbium YAGs), and far-IR (10,600 nm CO_2) wavelengths. Far-UV is absorbed with extreme efficiency by tissue proteins (0.5–2 μm) and mid- to far-IR by tissue water in all compartments. The CO_2 wavelength is so efficiently absorbed that its extinction length is only 0.03 mm in tissue, 30–100 times less than the 3 mm for YAG in tissue water, which additionally undergoes marked scattering. The Holmium-YAG wavelength at 2100 nm falls at an absorption trough for water such that it penetrates 200 μm, the same as argon at 488 nm. This moderate water transmission, without absorption by hemoglobin, allows it to be used as an ablative tool capable of achieving hemostasis in a bloody fluid medium (e.g., joint surgery).

Spot Size

Spot size is another significant tissue optics variable. Optical scattering at small spot sizes diminishes dermal penetration depth when wavelength is held constant. A broad beam of photons undergoes random scatter such that the center portion of the beam may be slightly intensified relative to the average energy across the beam and may result in a slightly increased effective penetration depth. This phenomenon has been referred to as "tissue lensing." Meanwhile, photon density at the periphery of the beam is diminished or less intense. Small spot sizes with radii less than the wavelength's 50% penetration depth suffer markedly reduced penetration depth. For visible wavelength lasers, this effect is most notable at beam diameters of 1 mm or less. Penetration depth for visible spectra lasers is not significantly augmented at beam diameters greater than 3 mm.

Application of Basic Tissue Optics

In selective cutaneous laser surgery, we consider the simplified skin model just presented and find the degree to which specific targeting "fits" the pathology of our individual patients. It is then our objective to deliver light with chromatic, spatial, and temporal characteristics suggested by the model of sufficient magnitude to effect the desired change and minimize risk of unintended or undesirable side effects.

FORMULAS FOR QUANTIFYING LASER ENERGY

A number of terms and their mathematical expressions are crucial to quantify laser energy and its delivery in time and space. The physical importance of these definitions is that, for any given wavelength, the result of light–tissue interactions is both time and energy dependent. Use of a common, standard nomenclature helps us specify laser techniques and parameters that are reproducible, which facilitates research, communication, and practice.

Characterizing the physics of a laser delivery system and its tissue effects includes identifying wavelength, output power, power density, fluence, temporal and spatial beam profile, and finally optical-thermal interactions with tissue (reflection, transmission, absorption, scattering) with subsequent biological responses (damage and healing). See Figure 4 for the major types of laser energy output and temporal profiles.

Power

Power is the rate of photon output of the laser, described as watts equivalent to joules per 1 second, which may be likened to a liquid flow rate past a fixed point, e.g., liters per second. The formula for deriving power is:

Power = watts (W) = J/sec

i.e., power = energy/time.

Joules, or Total Beam Energy

The joule is the common unit used to quantify light energy. Joules relate to the number of photons in a beam, analagous to moles, which specify the number of particles in chemistry. Joules describe the total energy of a beam by the product of the photon flow rate (power in watts) and the amount of time in seconds. The formula for deriving joules is:

Joules = watts (W) × seconds = total beam energy

i.e., energy = power × time.

Power Density (Irradiance)

Power density or irradiance is the degree of photon concentration, intensity or density in a spot size in mm^2 at a given rate of delivery (Fig. 16). The more concentrated the photons, the more rapidly they will affect the tissue target. Returning to our liquid analogy, water may flow from

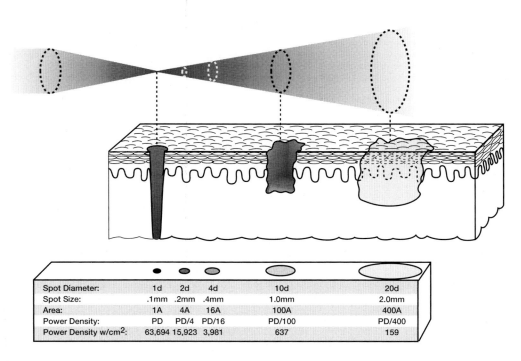

Spot Diameter:	1d	2d	4d	10d	20d
Spot Size:	.1mm	.2mm	.4mm	1.0mm	2.0mm
Area:	1A	4A	16A	100A	400A
Power Density:	PD	PD/4	PD/16	PD/100	PD/400
Power Density w/cm^2:	63,694	15,923	3,981	637	159

Figure 16 Spot size, power density, and tissue effect. The more concentrated the photons, the more rapidly they will affect the tissue target. The formula for power density, also known as irradiance, relates the flow rate of photons (W) per unit surface area of a circular spot of size (πr^2). Since area is a squared function, doubling the radius leads to a fourfold decrease in power density. Conversely, small decreases in spot size markedly increase power density, suitable for incisions or drilling (0.1-mm spot size). Defocusing to 1- to 3-mm spot size achieves ablation-sized spot tools and intermediate power densities. A very defocused beam 4–6 mm achieves lower power densities suitable for coagulation. (Reproduced with permission, © Timothy J. Rosio, M.D., Live Cutaneous Laser Surgery Workshop & Seminar.)

a large hose opening or be sprayed under pressure through a smaller opening at the same rate. The higher-pressure (more intense) spray will concentrate more water molecules upon its smallest target surface area (spot size). Similarly, a higher-power density beam is capable of doing more work on the smaller surface area. The formula for power density, also known as irradiance, relates the flow rate of photons per unit surface area of a circular spot of size (πr^2). Since area is a squared function, small increases in radius lead to marked decreases in power density, Conversely, small decreases in spot size markedly increase power density. The formula for deriving power density is:

$$\text{Power density} = \text{W/cm}^2 = \text{Power (W)} \times (100 \text{ mm}^2/\text{cm}^2) \div \pi r^2 \text{mm}^2$$

i.e., power density = power/circular beam area.

Fluence, Energy Density, or Energy "Dose"

Fluence may be thought of as the concentration of laser energy, i.e., total dose of beam energy related to the target surface area. Put another way, it is the product of power density and time. Since tissue effects are time and power-density dependent, one must know the independent terms, not just the final product; for example, a laser beam fluence = 100 J/cm^2 may be derived from either 100 W/cm^2 × 1 sec or 1 W/cm^2 × 100 sec. The former would vaporize tissue, while the latter would barely be perceived as warm. The formula for deriving energy density is:

$$\text{Fluence} = \text{J/cm}^2 = \text{W} \times \text{T/cm}^2 = \text{Power density (W/cm}^2) \times \text{Time}$$
$$= \text{Energy density or Energy dose}$$

i.e., fluence = power × time/area.

Average Power, Peak Power, and Duty Cycle

$$\text{Average power} = \text{Output power} \times \text{Duty cycle (\%)}$$

$$\text{Duty cycle} = \text{Laser "on-time"} \div \text{Total time}$$

i.e., laser on plus laser off time.

Some of laser surgery's greatest advances in recent years relate to achieving precise, reproducible, energy delivery in sufficiently short time periods to spatially confine damage to tissue targets while sparing adjacent tissue. Even expert surgeons' manual control of laser exposure time and energy has been shown to vary by orders of magnitude in vitro. Greater precision has been accomplished with a variety of laser hardware strategies to make laser exposure duration very predictable.

Laser types and designs vary dramatically in their basic power output, irradiance, and temporal delivery profiles. Power supplies and other electronic means may generate brief, extremely intense peak beam powers. Delivery systems may also interrupt the beam en route to the patient with electromechanical shutters to alter the quantity and temporal delivery of light. The most common terms used to describe these differences are shuttering and chopping, pulsing, superpulsing, and Q-switching (Fig. 4).

The basic terms used to describe temporally interrupted beams are total power, average power, exposure duration, interval, and duty cycle. A noninterrupted CW beam has a total power = average power. If the beam is interrupted by an interval time:

$$\text{Total on-time} = T_{\text{total}} = T_{\text{on}} + T_{\text{off}}$$

until the beginning of the next exposure. Duty cycle can be calculated as follows:

$$\text{Duty cycle} = \frac{(T_{total} - T_{off}) \times 100\%}{T_{total}}$$

The average power of a periodically interrupted beam is the product of peak power × duty cycle, e.g., 20 W × 25% duty cycle = 5 W average power. Note that the same average power may be obtained from markedly different combinations of peak powers and duty cycles. An average power of 5 W may be obtained from 200 W × 2.5% duty cycle, 100 W × 5% duty cycle, etc. Thus, the total or average power delivered by interrupted beams, whether they be shuttered or superpulsed, is a fraction derived from the percentage on-time multiplied by the peak power.

MANIPULATING POWER AND TIME PARAMETERS TO ACHIEVE SPECIFIC TISSUE EFFECTS

Shuttering or Chopping

Low- to moderate-power, moderate-duration exposures of 0.1–2.0 sec are most correctly referred to as shuttered, chopped, or gated exposures. Average power is reduced by the fraction of laser "on-time" or duty cycle that any time energy flow is cyclically interrupted. It is important to recognize the many clinically significant benefits achievable with conventional lasers operating in the shuttered mode. Reproducible, more precise laser effects are achievable, often with less patient discomfort and greater physician control. 20 W CO_2 lasers shuttered at 0.05 sec can achieve vaporization with spatial confinement of irreversible peripheral tissue damage to four to five times the CO_2 wavelength penetration depth of 20 μm. This approximates the benefits achieved with superpulsed lasers at a lower cost. Trade-offs may be less flexibility, slower working speed, and smaller spot size.

Pulsing

The term "pulsed" is reserved for extremely short laser emissions with very high peak energies orders of magnitude higher than its average power (e.g., flashlamp excited dye laser, or FEDL). However, even expert users will occasionally lapse into applying the term pulsed to describe low- to moderate-power, shuttered brief exposures on CW lasers. Laser manufacturers have frequently called timed exposures "pulses" on the controls of their CW argon, krypton, tunable-dye, and other lasers.

Three variables are used to characterize noncontinuous pulses of CO_2 laser energy as shuttered or chopped, superpulsed, or UltraPulse™, peak power, duration, and fluence (Fig. 17). For a fluence capable of vaporizing 1 cm^2 of skin, the chopped mode must have the longest-duration exposure because of its low peak power. The superpulse has a much higher peak power, therefore an equivalent fluence is reached with an extremely brief pulse duration repeated several times. The UltraPulse sustains the high peak power of the superpulse four to five times longer, obtaining the equivalent fluence in the fewest pulses.

Superpulsing

Superpulse is a term usually reserved for CO_2 lasers with brief, rapid microsecond pulses (hundreds to a thousand Hertz), capable of achieving ≥10 times higher peak powers than nonsuperpulsed lasers. CW-like results occur at rates approaching 1000 Hz, but at slower repetition rates in the hundreds of Hertz, minimal hemostasis and spatially confined thermal damage plus slower controlled working speeds are features of this type of system. Generally, small spot sizes (1 mm and less) ensure sufficient energy densities to achieve instant vaporization and spatial confine-

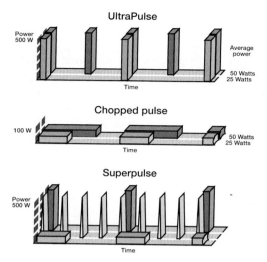

Figure 17 Chopped vs. superpulse vs. UltraPulse™. Three variables are used to characterize noncontinuous pulses of CO_2 laser energy as chopped, superpulsed, or UltraPulse: peak power, duration, and fluence. For a fluence capable of vaporizing 1 cm² of skin, the chopped mode must have the longest duration exposure because of its low peak power; the superpulse has a much higher peak power, therefore an equivalent fluence is reached with an extremely brief pulse duration repeated several times; the UltraPulse sustains the high peak power of the superpulse four to five times longer, obtaining the equivalent fluence in the fewest pulses. (Adapted with permission of Coherent Laser Corp.)

ment of thermal damage to 100 μm (0.1 mm) or less, allowing char-free tissue incision or ablation.

A new high-energy, radiofrequency-excited CO_2 laser dubbed the UltraPulse achieves spot sizes notably larger (3 mm) while delivering the 5 J/cm² critical energy density needed to achieve vaporization within the skin's thermal relaxation time (estimated at 600 μsec), or preferably within 1000 μsec (1 msec). are required to vaporize 1 g of water and, therefore, approximately the same for cutaneous tissue, which is 85% water. Note in Figure 4 the relative total energies (~1:5) ratio, areas under the curves) of the superimposed superpulse and UltraPulse waveforms. Both waveforms rise sharply; the Superpulse falls off slightly, then drops rapidly to zero. UltraPulse laser waveforms deliver more energy in one pulse, are more flattened indicating longer sustained peak power, until dropping to zero (Fig. 17).

Superpulsed lasers may be applied to wider area ablations, resurfacing similar to the UltraPulse, by employing several strategies, including mechanically scanning a small spot size at impact sites, just slightly offsetting the impulses, or using a larger spot size but superimposing several superpulses in less than the skin's longest thermal relaxation time of 1 msec.

Scanning

The principle of working at or above tissue vaporization threshold to minimize thermal injury is crucial to the application of laser resurfacing. At the time of this writing, the freehand use of miniscule spot sizes with individual pulses makes uniform controlled-depth, large-scale ablation difficult to achieve. However, small spot sizes in CW mode combined with rapid scanning is another practical approach to resurfacing and ablation to be discussed here.

So currently, two approaches offer an enhanced margin of safety and uniformity relative to traditional freehand continuous wave resurfacing. The two methods are high-energy-density pulses up to several mm in diameter, or scanning a high-power 0.2-mm CW beam very rapidly over the skin (i.e., SilkTouch™ Flashscan, Sharplan); the latter rapid scanning method allows brief tissue exposures and has reliably and practically obtained uniform ablation required for laser resurfacing. Both pulsing and scanning methods are capable in a single exposure of vaporizing 3 mm of tissue to a depth of 50–100 μm, with a limited zone of thermal necrosis of 50–150 μm. The SilkTouch scans the 0.2-mm beam through a 2- to 5-mm circular area in 0.2 sec (Fig. 18). Since software controls the scan area and shape, elliptical or other shapes and sizes are possible, facilitating hair transplant–recipient sites and other procedures.

Q-Switching

Q-switching produces extremely high photon intensities (mega to gigawatt peak powers) in extremely short durations (nanoseconds). This is accomplished by using a Pockels cell (polarizing gate) within the laser optical cavity to build up huge quantities of photons, which are suddenly released. Examples are the Q-switched ruby, alexandrite, and YAG lasers. The resultant massive power density results in photodisruption or photomechanical destruction of small objects with appropriate absorption coefficients and thermal relaxation times.

LASER–TISSUE INTERACTION CATEGORIES: FROM FUNCTIONAL TO ANATOMIC

Clinical effects of lasers occur by the interaction of laser fluence, time, and the relative absorption efficiencies of target chromophores operating under the principles discussed earlier. The physical changes that occur after photon absorption may be classified in three nonlinear functional categories: photochemical (low fluence), photothermal (moderate fluence), or photomechanical (very brief exposure, high fluence). The majority of past laser treatments have been of moderate fluence and poorly selective photothermal nature. Applications of very selective photo-

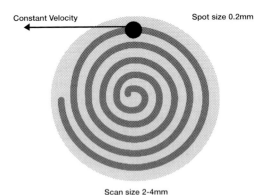

SilkTouch Flashscan

Constant Velocity

Spot size 0.2mm

Scan size 2-4mm

Figure 18 High-intensity scanning for resurfacing. A high-intensity CW beam is capable in a single exposure of vaporizing 3 mm of tissue to a depth of 50–100 μm, with a limited zone of thermal necrosis of <50 μm. The SilkTouch™ scans the 0.2-mm beam through a 2- to 5-mm circular area in 0.2 sec. (Reproduced with permission, Sharplan Lasers Corp.)

thermolysis, photomechanical (e.g., pigment and lithotripters), and photochemical (e.g., photo-dynamic therapy) mechanisms have increased recently.

Photochemical Principles

The chemical bonds of a tremendous number of common molecules are capable of absorbing a visible-range photon whose energy matches that needed to move the material's electrons to the next energy level (orbital). The total amount of energy therefore is exceedingly low. Photodynamic therapy (PDT) exploits this principle by using a chemical photosensitizer as an intermediary to maximize the reaction while selectively localizing the effect to specific target sites. The transitional energy is used to generate singlet oxygen, which is highly reactive and therefore exerts a destructive effect on cellular membranes. Lasers are used to generate not only monochromatic light, but large quantities of it that are consistent and may be easily quantified and delivered to varying delimited areas, if necessary via optical fibers.

Photothermal Principles

Photothermal effects range on a continuum from protein denaturation and coagulation ($>50°C$) to vaporization ($>100°C$), depending on the amount of energy, the delivery rate, and target size. However, very high-power (megawatt) and rapid ($\leq$ nanoseconds) pulsed energy delivery induces nonlinear photomechanical target disruption typified by Q-switched lasers. Cutaneous tissue may recover from brief exposures in excess of 50°C temperatures, thereby decreasing the likelihood or quantity of fibrosis. Absolute temperature and duration are both important in determining reversible laser thermal injuries.

Selective photothermolysis spatially confines irreversible thermal injury to the target tissue (e.g., vessels or pigment) while limiting heat diffusion injury to the surrounding stromal tissue (e.g., collagen, adnexal structures). Inadequate energy delivery or insufficient depth leads to treatment failure, whereas excessive energy delivery may result in scarring and pigmentary and textural changes. Selective photothermolysis surgery techniques operate either in the photothermal or photomechanical realm.

Photothermal effects on tissue depend upon the tissue temperature achieved (and total time): temperatures of $<50°C$ for brief periods may cause reversible thermal injury. Temperatures from 50 to 70°C cause irreversible thermal injury and coagulation; cells reaching 100°C vaporize when their tissue water boils. Prolonged or repeated subvaporization laser exposure over time heats and desiccates tissue and reduces it to carbon. The carbon residue cannot vaporize. It does absorb laser radiation and conducts heat, potentially damaging surrounding tissue and leading to a wider zone of thermal necrosis.

The time course of the elevated temperature is important too. Slow heat delivery achieves lower peak temperatures and conducts the heat injury to a broader area around the target before vaporization occurs. Conversely, high-intensity rapid delivery of energy reaches much higher temperatures for shorter periods of time and confines thermal injury closer to the target. Therefore, the surgeon attempting to work at lower energy densities beneath the threshold for vaporization will cause greater thermal necrosis; working at higher power densities restricts damage to the narrowest zone (Fig. 19).

Selective Photothermolysis and Thermal Relaxation Time

Among the first laser variables to be manipulated for a given laser wavelength was power density. In the 1980s, the emphasis turned to raising peak powers of selectively absorbed wavelengths and limiting exposure time; this strategy delivers photothermal energy to the target in less time than that required to lose 50% of the acquired heat, thus confining thermal damage.

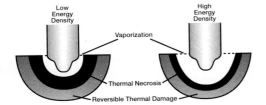

Figure 19 Thermal damage related to fluence and time. Slow heat delivery achieves lower peak temperatures and conducts the heat injury to a broader area around the target before vaporization occurs. Conversely, high-intensity rapid delivery of energy reaches much higher temperatures for shorter periods of time and confines thermal injury closer to the target. Therefore, the surgeon attempting to work at lower energy densities beneath the threshold for vaporization will cause greater thermal necrosis; working at higher power densities restricts damage to the narrowest zone. (Reproduced with permission, © Timothy J. Rosio, M.D., Live Cutaneous Laser Surgery Workshop & Seminar.)

In brief, absorption of sufficiently concentrated photons during periods equal to or less than a structure's thermal relaxation time minimizes thermal loss from conduction to its surroundings. Therefore, peak temperature is reached more quickly at a lower total energy, and less energy is wasted damaging nontarget tissues. Conduction dominates as the mechanism of heat transfer for tissue objects. Surface area is the prime determinant of conductive losses, confirming our experience that small objects exchange heat much faster than large objects (e.g., children gain or lose heat much faster than adults). These physical principles allow calculation of thermal relaxation time T_r, which varies most dramatically by the structure's diameter or thickness D (a squared function) (Table 1). Other terms include the ease of heat diffusion and constants. Note the marked difference in T_r for modest changes in structure size.

$$T_r = \frac{G(D^2C)}{K}$$

Thermal relaxation (cooling time) is proportional to the square of the vessel diameter. Essentially, T_r describes the period required for a structure to lose 50% of its elevated temperature, i.e., the absorbed photothermal laser energy. The FEDL was one of the first laser tools to specifically utilize this principle in tissue (Fig. 20). Subsequently, design of other lasers was based upon this principle for treating other problems with different chromophores, with radically different T_r values.

Photomechanical Disruption

Extremely high-intensity, very short pulses (e.g., nanoseconds) produce photomechanical effects resulting in disintegration of the target and minimal damage to surrounding tissues. An example

Table 1 Selected Cutaneous Target Thermal Relaxation Time (T_r) Values

Target	Diameter (μm)	T_r (nsec)
Melanosome	1	200
Erythrocyte	5	5,000
Microvessel	20	140,000
Microvessel (enlarged)	100	3,600,000

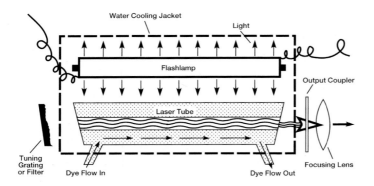

Figure 20 Flashlamp excited dye laser. FEDLs operate by storing high quantities of energy in a capacitor; sudden energy release powers a very brief intense flashlamp burst to excite laser production in rhodamine dye contained within the laser tube. Filters and resonators may be adjusted in series with the optical cavity to restrict wavelength and duration output to the currently desired 585 nm, 450 μsec. Neither setting is user-adjustable. (Reproduced with permission, © Timothy J. Rosio, M.D., Live Cutaneous Laser Surgery Workshop & Seminar.)

would be a ruby, alexandrite, or Q-switched KTP-YAG laser photodisrupting tattoo pigment particles or melanocytes by highly efficient absorption of massive quantities of photons (Fig. 21). This abrupt photothermal transfer generates nonlinear physical effects, including plasma formation (removal of atomic particle's electrons) and rapid expansion followed by contraction, that propagate mechanical forces (pressure wave) capable of fragmenting the absorbing particle. If the wavelength chosen is very selective for the absorbing chromophore, virtually complete spatial confinement of tissue injury to the target is possible.

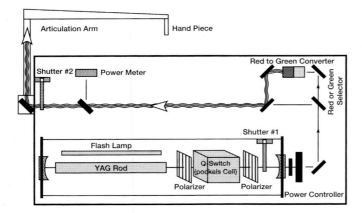

Figure 21 Q-switched KTP-YAG. Q-KTP-YAG adds a "Q-switch" mechanism and frequency-doubling crystal to a basic YAG laser. Similar to the well-known ruby laser, Q-KTP-YAG provides thousands of times greater peak energy in brief delivery time intervals (millions of watts equivalence, 10 nsec) providing selective photothermolysis capabilities, at 1064 or 532 nm, vs. the ruby's 694 nm. The Q-switch polarizing Pockels cell mechanism interrupts the optical path, allows a massive photon buildup and then sudden energy release, resulting in high peak power, short pulse width. (Reproduced with permission, © Timothy J. Rosio, M.D., Live Cutaneous Laser Surgery Workshop & Seminar.)

Laser–Tissue Interaction: Three Anatomic Categories

In contrast to the functional laser-tissue interaction categories just discussed, analyzing the physics of laser–tissue interaction allows applications to be viewed in three anatomic-level categories: whole organ, tissue-specific surgical lasers, and cell or subcellular specific.

1. *Organ Level*: The organ of skin is predominately water. Lasers such as the CO_2 and YAG (at moderate energy densities) are similar in affecting many different tissues indiscriminately by raising intracellular and extracellular water temperatures. Depending on the power density and beam size, the same laser may coagulate, cut, or vaporize large or small tissue volumes.
2. *Tissue Level*: Tissue-level laser treatments utilize selectively absorbed wavelengths in a specific tissue, such as vascular tissue, at moderate peak powers and short exposure durations. Other dissimilar tissues nearby are relatively unaffected by coagulation injury.
3. *Cell or Subcellular Level*: Extremely brief, high energy densities with specific wavelength matching to cell or subcellular organelles allow selective destruction on the cellular or subcellular level. Individual macrophage destruction in tattoos or melanosomes in pigmented cells exemplifies the most precise functional category of laser treatment.

MECHANISMS AND PHYSICS OF BASIC LASER TYPES

The comparative mechanisms by which current classical lasers and more recent arrivals function can be briefly illustrated by drawings and discussion of four lasers: the tunable argon dye laser (ADL), the flashlamp-excited dye laser, the metal vapor laser, and the Q-switched KTP-YAG laser. These four lasers illustrate a wide range of various modes of function, including temporal output (continuous wave, quasi-continuous, microsecond pulse, and extremely short Q-switched nanosecond pulse), lasing medium (gas ions, metal vapor ions, organic dye, and solid-state rare earth mineral–doped crystal), and means of excitation (direct current, secondary laser pumping, flashlamp). Two lasers exhibit very different methods of obtaining alternative wavelengths: the tunable dye laser, with multiple-wavelength secondary laser output, and the KTP-YAG, using frequency doubling to achieve a single alternate wavelength one-half that of the original.

Tunable Argon Dye Laser

The ADL begins with a basic gas tube laser mechanism—similar to the carbon dioxide laser, with argon ions constituting the lasing medium in an optical resonator containing inert gases—and is excited by direct current (Fig. 22). The resultant CW green beam contains both 488 nm blue and 514 nm green laser photons produced by argon. The argon laser is used as an optical energy–pumping source to excite a mixture or organic rhodamine dye molecules. The rhodamine dye mixture in turn emits secondary laser light in the yellow-to-red range. The yellow-range beam (577–585 nm) more closely matches the β-absorption peak of oxyhemoglobin. The specific mixture of rhodamine has been designed to emit a range of laser wavelengths (577–630 nm) when stimulated by the blue-green laser light. The precise wavelength is selected by adjusting the refraction angle of an optical crystal in the laser light path. The laser surgeon may "tune" or select any wavelength and time exposure within the range of the laser at any time, hence the designation tunable dye. This is in contrast to fixed-wavelength and fixed-pulse-duration dye lasers of the FEDL type, changeable only with major factory servicing modifications to the dye mixture, software, and possibly hardware.

The ADL produces laser light at modest power (1–3 W) as a continuous wave. Electromechanical timed shuttering (comparable to a camera) allows user-selectable exposure times rang-

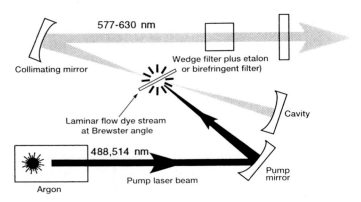

Figure 22 Tunable argon dye laser. The argon laser is used as an optical energy pumping source to excite organic rhodamine dye molecules. The rhodamine dye in turn emits a secondary laser light in the yellow to red range. (Reproduced with permission, © Timothy J. Rosio, M.D., Live Cutaneous Laser Surgery Workshop & Seminar.)

ing from 2.0 to 0.02 sec. In laser terminology low-power brief exposures are most correctly referred to as "shuttered" or "gated" exposures.

The blue-green or yellow-to-red laser light is delivered through an optical fiber or cable. Commonly this is coupled to a handpiece with interchangeable fixed-focal-length lenses to achieve different spot sizes; even more useful is a focusing handpiece that can produce spot sizes from 0.05 to 6 mm.

Optical cavity alignment is crucial to obtain normal power output. Significant movement of the laser may require a service call for mirror alignment or to replace very expensive light-conduction cables that may break when bumped or stretched. Dye replacement may only be necessary every 2–3 yr, depending on use, although every 6–12 months is advised by the vendor. This much less frequent dye-replacement rate (compared to FEDL systems) is due to less dye photodegradation at relatively low power argon laser pumping. The longevity, stability, relative simplicity, and large installed base of argon lasers make the cost of purchase, operation, and maintenance moderate compared to other lasers. Tunability allows use in photodynamic therapy but may require a different dye mixture for optimization of power and prolonged 630 nm output.

Flashlamp-Excited Dye Laser and Pigmented Lesion Dye Laser

FEDLs operate by storing high quantities of energy in a capacitor; sudden energy release powers a very brief intense flashlamp burst to excite laser production in rhodamine dye (Fig. 20). The rhodamine group allows selection of a dye with a specified wavelength output range. Filters and resonators may be adjusted in series with the optical cavity to restrict wavelength and duration output to the currently desired 585 nm, 450 μsec. Neither setting is user adjustable. An approximate 4–8 kW peak output is produced. Two main flashlamp designs (linear vs. coaxial) are available in clinical systems. Linear flashlamps excite the dye mainly from one direction, possibly aided by reflecting surfaces. A patented design claimed to be more efficient utilizes a coaxial flashlamp, which surrounds the dye medium with more uniform light.

A variation on the FEDL vascular layer used for treating superficial pigmented lesions is the pigmented lesion dye laser (PLDL), with parameters of 510 nm, 400 nsec pulse width, 0.5–1 Hz, and output of 3–5 J/cm^2. The latter parameters are suitable for some very superficial melanocytic lesions or red tattoo pigments.

The treatment beam is delivered by an optical fiber coupled to a fixed-focal-length handpiece with a 5-mm spot size at a rate of 0.5–1 Hz. A 2-mm handpiece and a finger-activated control (alternative to the standard foot pedal) are available. Newer models supply energy more rapidly, with a 7- to 10-mm spot size.

Software systems and electronic controls are used to assure safe and accurate energy densities. Software, hardware, or simultaneous problems can cause prolonged treatment interruptions and downtime ranging from 30 min to several days. Therefore, the more expensive service contracts with these lasers are indispensable. Long downtimes were common in early models (occasionally several per month). This is very disruptive to patient and physician scheduling. Current models are much more reliable, and scheduled preventative maintenance visits greatly reduce to a manageable level the frequency and severity of downtime.

The much higher peak energies used in FEDLs to excite the dye medium cause rapid photo-degradation, requiring fresh dye to maintain output levels. Replacement of dye containers should be considered, along with flashlamp replacement and maintenance visits. Competition in the marketplace has stimulated less frequent dye replacement, changes to the hardware, slightly lowering cost and increasing efficiency.

Quasi-Continuous Wave, Low-Average-Power, Metal Vapor Ion Laser

Copper vapor lasers (CVL) (Fig. 23) emit two harmonic wavelengths: 510.6 nm (green) and 578.2 nm (yellow) light. The yellow beam matches the β-absorption peak of oxyhemoglobin. The CVL uses vaporized copper ions as its lasing medium, generated from metal beads in a vaporization chamber. Electrical energy pumping leads to stimulated emission of extremely brief, very rapidly repeating, moderately high peak power, but low average power pulses. Power output is 2–3 W. Typical pulses have a duration of 15–20 nsec, frequency of 15 kHz (15,000/sec), interval of 70 nsec, peak energy of 90 μJ and a peak power of 5 kW. The minimal energy contained in any one brief pulse, together with the very rapid repetition rate, result in the classifi-

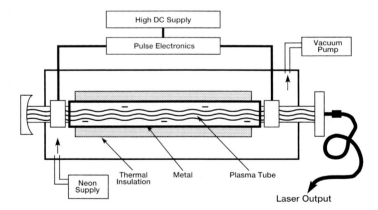

Figure 23 Metal vapor laser. The CVL uses vaporized copper ions as its lasing media. Electrical energy pumping leads to stimulated emission of extremely brief, very rapidly repeating, moderately high peak power, but low average power pulses. The minimal energy contained in any one 20-nsec pulse, together with the very rapid repetition rate, result in the classification of this as a "quasi-continuous" beam, with clinical effects comparable to CW lasers of similar wavelength. (Reproduced with permission, © Timothy J. Rosio, M.D., Live Cutaneous Laser Surgery Workshop & Seminar.)

cation of this beam as "quasi-continuous." Shuttered operation allows exposures from 0.05 to 2.0 sec. Variable-spot-size handpieces allow beam diameters from less than 0.5 mm to greater than 5 mm. Fiberoptic delivery is standard.

Metal vapor lasers must raise the temperature of the lasing medium. This has historically required long warm-up times, commonly 45 min. Interruption of the vaporization during treatment may require shorter but noticeable delays to resume treatment. Recently, Cu-Br systems have decreased these drawbacks. The system is not truly tunable but allows switching from yellow to green wavelength for treatment of epidermal melanocytic lesions. Another possibility is substitution of vaporization chamber components (at significant cost) to use a gold tube and produce 628 nm red light suitable for photodynamic therapy.

Solid-State Q-Switched KTP-YAG

KTP-YAG and Q-switched KTP-YAG lasers (Fig. 21) have at their core a crystalline rod composed of an yttrium-aluminum-garnet crystal, doped (incorporated) with a rare earth element known as neodymium (Nd). When the Nd is excited by a high-intensity optical pumping source such as a xenon flashlamp, 1060 nm laser light is generated. The YAG wavelength may be used as is or may be halved (by either a frequency doubling potassium titanyl phosphate (KTP) crystal or a photoacoustic method), resulting in 532 nm beam output. The green 532 nm beam comes close to the α-absorption peak of oxyhemoglobin. The KTP beam is quasi-continuous, similar to the CVL. Average power peak outputs may be from 5 to 20 W, and minor variations on the following beam specifications occur depending on the make and model. Typical beams have continuous appearing power peaks with duration of 150 nsec, frequency of 5 kHz (5000/sec), and interval of 200 nsec. While the intervals between pulses are three times longer than the CVL, thereby allowing some thermal relaxation, the total energy per pulse is insufficient to accomplish coagulation. Therefore, like the CVL, the energy from a train of pulses must be combined to achieve sufficient temperature for coagulation.

Shuttering and delivery aspects are similar to those for the CVL and ADL. Nd:YAG lasers are touted as solid-state lasers with few moving parts and minimal consumables. No dyes are used. Only the flashlamp-pumping source will need replacement based on use. Many systems are now primarily air-cooled, advantageous where plumbing difficulties exist or mobility is a factor. However, heat generation could be undesirable in smaller rooms or ones with less generous air-exchange and cooling rates. Stability and performance are felt to be strong due to infrequent alignment problems and service requirements. Robotized scanners may be attached for treating large areas with a point-by-point technique.

Q-switched KTP-YAG lasers (Q-YAG) begin with a frequency-doubled KTP-YAG laser; the addition of a Q-switch mechanism provides thousands of times greater peak energy delivery over much shorter time intervals (millions of watts equivalence, 10 nsec) providing selective photothermolysis capabilities at 1064 nm or 532 nm. The Q-switch Pockels cell mechanism interrupts the optical path by rotating the polarity of the laser light as long as power is supplied to the switch. A polarizing filter oriented 90° out of phase with the powered Pockels cell prevents release of optical laser beam. Deactivating the Pockels cell suddenly allows transmission of all of the now-parallel-phase laser energy through the polarizing filter in nanoseconds.

Delivery is through an articulated arm sytem, with a 2-mm spot size and repetition rate of 1–10 Hz. The Nd:YAG laser foundation makes this a solid-state laser with few moving parts without consumables. The flashlamp-pumping source will need replacement based on use, and due to the very high intensity of the beam, optics (chiefly lenses and their coatings) should be regularly inspected. This system is air-cooled. Stability and performance are felt to be strong due to infrequent alignment problems, a stable crystal, and claimed infrequent service requirements.

BIBLIOGRAPHY

Anderson RR, Margolis RJ, et al. Selective photothermolysis of cutaneous pigmentation by Q-switched Nd:YAG laser pulses at 1064, 532 and 355 nm. *J Invest Dermatol* 1989;93:28.

Anderson RR, Parrish JA. Microvasculature can be selectively damaged using dye lasers: a basic theory and experimental evidence in human skin. *Lasers Surg Med* 1981;1(3):263–276.

Arndt KA, Noe JM, et al. Laser therapy. Basic concepts and nomenclature. *J Am Acad Dermatol* 1981;5(6):649–654.

Ben-Barucg G, Fidler JP, et al. Comparison of wound healing between chopped mode-superpulse mode CO_2 laser and steel knife incision. *Lasers Surg Med* 1988;8:596.

Brunner F, Hafner R, et al. [Removal of tattoos with the Nd:YAG laser.] *Hautarzt* 1987;38(10):610–614

Chernoff G, Slatkine M, et al. SilkTouch: a new technology for skin resurfacing in aesthetic surgery. *J Clin Laser Med Surg* (in press).

Dover JS, Margolis RJ, et al. Pigmented guinea pig skin irradiated with Q-switched ruby laser pulses. Morphologic and histologic findings. *Arch Dermatol* 1989;125:43–49.

Fitzpatrick RE, Ruiz-Esparza J, et al. The depth of thermal necrosis using the CO_2 laser: a comparison of the superpulsed mode and conventional mode. *J Dermatol Surg Oncol* 1991;17:340.

Green HA, Burd E, et al. Skin graft take and healing after continuous wave CO_2, pulsed CO_2, 193 nm excimer, and holmium laser ablation of graft beds. *J Invest Dermatol* 1989;92:436.

Green HA, Burd EE, et al. Skin graft take and healing following 193-nm excimer, continuous-wave carbon dioxide (CO_2), pulsed CO_2, or pulsed holmium: YAG laser ablation of the graft bed. *Arch Dermatol* 1993;129(8):979–988.

Gravelink JM, Casparian JM, et al. Undesirable effects associated with treatment of tattoos and pigmented lesions with the Q-switched lasers at 1064 nm and 694 nm: the MGH experience. *Lasers Surg Med Suppl* 1993;5:270.

Hobbs ER, Bailin PL, et al. Superpulsed lasers: minimizing thermal damage with short duration, high irradiance pulses. *J Dermatol Surg Oncol* 1987;13:955.

Hulsbergen HJ, van Gemert M. Port wine stain coagulation experiments with a 540-nm continuous wave dye-laser. *Lasers Surg Med* 1983;2(3):205–210.

Keijzer M. Light distributions in artery tissue: Monte Carlo simulations for finite-diameter laser beams. *Lasers Surg Med* 1989;(9):148–154.

Lahaye CT, van GM. Optimal laser parameters for port wine stain therapy: a theoretical approach. *Phys Med Biol* 1985;30(6):573–587.

Lanzafame RJ, Naim JO, et al. Comparison of continuous-wave, chop-wave, and super pulse laser wounds. *Lasers Surg Med* 1988;8(2):119–124.

Laub DR, Yules RB, et al. Preliminary histopathological observation of Q-switched ruby laser radiation on dermal tattoo pigment in man. *J Surg Res* 1968;5:220.

McKenzie AL. How far does thermal damage extend beneath the surface of CO_2 laser incisions? *Phys Med Biol* 1983;28:905.

Polla LL, Jacques SL, et al. [Selective photothermolysis: contribution to the treatment of flat angiomas (port wine stains) by laser.] *Ann Dermatol Venereol* 1987;114(4):497–505.

Polla LL, Margolis RJ, et al. Melanosomes are a primary target of Q-switched ruby laser irradiation in guinea pig skin. *J Invest Dermatology* 1987;89:281.

Reid R. Physical and surgical principles governing carbon dioxide laser surgery on the skin. *Dermatol Clin* 1991;9(2):297–316.

Reid WH, McLeod PJ, et al. Q-switched ruby laser treatment of black tattoos. *Br J Plast Surg* 1983;36(4):455–459.

Rosio T. Cosmetic cutaneous laser surgery. In: *Cosmetic Dermatology*. London, Martin-Dunitz, 1994, pp. 509–540.

Sherwood KA, Murray S, et al. Effect of wavelength on cutaneous pigment using pulsed irradiation. *J Invest Dermatol* 1989;92:717.

Tan OT, Murray S, et al. Action spectrum of vascular specific injury using pulsed irradiation. *J Invest Dermatol* 1989;92:868.

Taylor CR, Anderson RR, et al. Light and electron microscopic analysis of tattoos treated by Q-switched ruby laser. *J Invest Dermatol* 1991;97:131.

Taylor CR, Flotte T, et al. Q-switched ruby laser (QSRL) irradiation of benign pigmented lesions: dermal vs. epidermal. *Lasers Surg Med Suppl* 1991;3:65.

Taylor CR, Gange RW, et al. Treatment of tattoos by Q-switched ruby laser. A dose-response study. *Arch Dermatol* 1990;126:893–899.

Tong AKF, Ton OT, et al. Ultrastructure: effects of melanin pigment on target specificity using a pulsed dye laser (577 nm). *J Invest Dermatol* 1987;88:747.

Van Gemert JMC, Jacques SL, et al. Skin optics. *IEEE Trans Biomed Eng* 1990;36:1146.

Van Gemert M, de Kleijn W, et al. Temperature behaviour of a model port-wine stain during argon laser coagulation. *Phys Med Biol* 1982;27(9):1089–1104.

Van Gemert MJC, Welch AJ. Time constants in thermal laser medicine. *Lasers Surg Med* 1989;9:405.

Venugopalan V. *Carbon Dioxide Laser Ablation of Biological Tissue: Effect of Pulse Repetition Rate on Mass Removal and Thermal Damage*. MIT Archives, 1990.

Venugopalan V, Nishioka NS, et al. The effect of CO_2 laser pulse repetition rate on tissue ablation rate and thermal damage. *IEEE Trans Biomed Eng* 1991;38(10):1049–1052.

Venugopalan V, Nishioka NS, et al. The effect of laser parameters on the zone of thermal injury produced by laser ablation of biological tissue." *J Biomech Eng* 1994;116(1):62–70.

Walsh JJ, Flotte TJ, et al. Pulsed CO_2 laser tissue ablation: effect of tissue type and pulse duration on thermal damage. *Lasers Surg Med* 1988;8(2):108–118.

Watanabe S, Anderson RR, et al. Comparative studies of femtosecond to microsecond laser pulses on selective pigmented cell injury in skin. *J Photochem Photobiol* 1991;53:757.

Welch AJ, Pearce JA, et al. Heat generation in laser irradiated tissue. *J Biomech Eng* 1989;111(1):62–68.

Yules RB, Laub DR, et al. The effect of Q-switched ruby laser radiation on dermal tattoo pigment in man. *Arch Surg* 1967;95:179–180.

Zweig AD, Meierhofer B, et al. Lateral thermal damage along pulsed laser incisions. *Laser Surg Med* 1990;10:262.

Zweig AD, Weber HP. Mechanical and thermal parameters in pulsed laser cutting of tissue. *IEEE J Quantum Electronics* 1987;10:1787.

54

Basic Laser Safety

Timothy J. Rosio
Marshfield Clinic, Marshfield, Wisconsin

SAFETY, THE GREAT INTANGIBLE

This chapter begins with the question: How does one achieve, or even describe, the intangible "safety" with lasers? Safety describes a nonevent, or the absence of an adverse occurrence. Accident rates or injury risk are described in statistics or probabilities, but as the saying goes, it's 100% if the complication happens to you! Is a 5% occurrence of minor laser injury (e.g., finger burns) less safe than a 0.1% occurrence of severe injuries (e.g., partial blindness)? Unfortunately, severe injuries like blindness often occur under circumstances very similar to those that have never caused a particular user injury before. These low-probability, high-impact events occur most often because expert users are lulled into disregarding safety standards or conversely because inexperienced personnel (e.g., students in research facilities) are unaware of proper protection.

Entire books have been written on laser safety. Laser safety may be discussed from a myriad of perspectives. To summarize, laser injury prevention and minimization relies on a multifactorial interaction between vendors, regulation standards, users, patients, staff, and facilities. But no hardware, regulation, or protocol provides complete safety. Laser safety is only achieved by a continuous state of safety-mindedness on top of safety mechanisms. This begins with knowledge of basic laser physics and tissue interaction, preferably obtained in a hands-on laser course, followed by a preceptorship with wavelengths and procedures to be used in practice.

We will first look at background information on laser safety standards, followed by laser hazards and organs at risk, dealing with the methods of laser injury and prevention. Then the procedural and technical steps to achieve and maintain a safe operating environment will be summarized.

LASER SAFETY STANDARDS AND GUIDELINES

Laser Device Hazard Classification

Lasers can be categorized in four main groups and a few subgroups, based on risk of injury potential from the beam. The criteria for classifying lasers into classes I, II, III, or IV are "the capability of the radiant energy of the laser system to injure health care personnel or the patient's body area other than the intended treatment sites, the environment in which the laser system is used, the personel who may use, or be exposed to, laser radiation, and the non-emission hazard associated with the laser."

It is important to note that safe limits have been defined partially through research on specific wavelengths under specific conditions and partially through calculation and extrapolation of an enormous number of combinations. Safe limits are associated with the term maximum permissible exposure (MPE), based on observations and calculations, plus a safety factor. It may be possible under certain extreme circumstances to cause injury with a certain laser despite meeting safety criteria from its laser hazard class.

Class I lasers are safe for viewing even for prolonged periods under normal circumstances. Normal circumstances preclude any additional beam intensification.

Class II lasers are of visible wavelength and low-output power that does not exceed the safe limits of radiation within 0.25 sec, the critical time period required for a nonsedated healthy person to blink or avert their gaze. Certain medical conditions or medications may impair the healthy aversion reflex, leading to the potential for visual damage. Such patients near these sources should be monitored and provided with well-secured passive eye protection, like opaque corneal shields, goggles, or tape-fixed dressings. Class II laser examples include the helium-neon (He-Ne) aiming beams on most CO_2 lasers and some radiotherapy devices.

Class III lasers must produce less than 0.5 W continuous energy, or for pulsed lasers less than 10 J/cm^2 in 0.25 sec. Class III lasers must not be capable of causing injuries from diffuse reflected beams. Subclass III-a could cause eye injury if further concentrated by additional optical attachments, e.g., parabolic mirrors or microscopes. Subclass III-b could cause eye injury by direct intrabeam viewing or nonconcentrating reflections.

Class IV lasers includes lasers with greater than 0.5 W power in 0.25 sec, or greater than 10 J/cm_2 or having a potential for eye damage from diffuse reflection. Unconcentrated beams are capable of causing severe eye injury from intrabeam viewing or combustion of materials in or near the operative field.

Regulation and Standards Agencies

A variety of organizations are involved in regulating laser safety standards or issuing safety guidelines. The American National Standards Institute (ANSI) has produced a periodically updated comprehensive guide to medical laser safety, referred to as Z136.3. Institutions are responsible for producing their own laser safety plan, which is customarily overseen by their representative laser safety committee, which in turn is charged with demonstrating effective compliance with the accepted standards of the Joint Commisssion for Accreditation of Health Care Organizations (JCAHO). Standards emphasize documentation of all aspects of the plan, including physician credentialing and education with specific lasers and procedures, safety protocols, and a quality assurance program reviewing outcomes and indicators. Demonstrations may be demanded onsite to prove effectiveness and familiarity with safety protocols.

The Food and Drug Administration (FDA) governs the approval of laser hardware and procedures and through the Center for Devices and Radiological Health (CDRH) regulates the manufacture of these devices. FDA maintains a list of approved laser wavelengths and applications. Similar to medications, companies are not allowed to promote a laser for an unapproved application (e.g., vascular treatment) despite other approved applications for the same laser (e.g., tattoo pigment).

The Occupational Safety and Health Administration (OSHA) deals with work safety hazards such as laser plume, chemical dyes used in certain lasers, etc. Review of this information is mandatory by law for the protection of employees and must be available to them in the form of Material Safety Data Sheets at any time. Additionally, local regulations are derived by individual states. One must check with the appropriate state government office for variable policies comprising registration, facility certification, site specifications and inspections, training and operating requirements, and reporting mandates to responsible agencies.

The American Society for Laser Medicine and Surgery (ASLMS) has produced guidelines on training and practice, which have influenced or been significantly incorporated into the published standards of the JCAHO and World Health Organization. ASLMS guidelines are available from the society, which is located in Wausau, Wisconsin.

Documentation and Quality Assurance

"If it isn't documented, it wasn't done" is the JCAHO maxim. Compliance with institutional and regulatory agency requirements is made feasible by series of checklists to ensure documentation and consistency with safety policies. Administrative and safety checklists may be grouped into categories and column headings, such as installation and inservice, credentials and privileges, and preoperative, operative, and postoperative. Much of this information should be cross-referenced for accessibility and accuracy between the patient's medical record, quality assurance reports, laser safety committee reports, and the essential laser logbook.

Information recorded should include:

> procedure time and date
> assistants and observers present
> pertinent health history and diagnosis
> laser wavelength and type
> average power
> temporal mode (CW, shuttered, pulsed, chopped, Q-switched, etc.)
> power density
> fluence, spot size
> spot profile at tissue (TEM mode)
> delivery system and accessories (fiber, arm, waveguide, etc.)
> pattern of beam application (e.g., superimposed on or overlapping spots, number of impulses, CW)
> time duration of treatment ('laser on-time')
> complications, etc.
> documentation of the informed consent, photographs, postop instructions and entry of information that laser log and checklists were completed, when, and by whom

Outcome information should be routinely recorded on the chart. Complications should be recorded and quality assurance informed with all pertinent information to facilitate quality improvement. Opportunities for procedural, technical, and hardware improvement can be realized from cumulating and analyzing quality assurance/improvement data.

LASER SAFETY HAZARDS

Basic laser safety hazards and concerns comprise:
 Protection of the eye and skin
 Avoidance of electrical shock
 Fire hazards, toxic gases, or infectious particles in the plume
 Avoidance of potential chemical injuries due to toxic or carcinogenic substances used in the
 operation of some lasers
 Laser safety hazards will be discussed individually below.

Eye and Skin Damage

Mechanisms of Eye and Skin Injury

The eye is more susceptible to harm in the course of using lasers than is any other organ or tissue. The relative risk to the eye exceeds all others due to its tremendous photon-concentrating ability upon the posterior segment. A 1 W laser beam forms an image 100,000 times brighter than the sun on the retina. The greatest focusing ability derives from the cornea and together with the 25% lens contribution multiplies light intensity 100,000 times! Even aphakic individuals are at risk, since 75% of light concentration occurs at the air–corneal interface. So small amounts of divergent or reflected laser energy, too weak to harm the skin, may nevertheless cause temporary or permanent damage to vision.

Retina

The visible and near-infrared spectrum (400–1400 nm) is mostly transmitted through the cornea, anterior chamber, lens, and vitreous, finally to be efficiently absorbed in the retinal pigment epithelium (Fig. 1). The rate of energy absorption and total quantity will determine whether injury will occur and severity. A substantial amount of 1060 nm radiation may be tolerated at a low-energy density by the lens due to its relative transparency to that wavelength, and therefore with minimal risk to it. However, it is the pigmented and vascular layers of the retina that are likely to absorb harmful energy densities, due to the combined focus of the cornea and lens, and the absorption efficiency of melanin and hemoglobin proximal to the delicate photoreceptors. Keep in mind that an injury in a 10° arc near the macula damages the fovea centralis, the central area responsible for visual acuity.

 Serious acute or subacute retinal injuries include retinal membrane formation, macular contraction, bleeding from rupture of retinal or choroidal vessels, nerve fiber damage, retinal hole with consequent scotoma (visual field defect), and retinal detachment, and any or all may lead to permanent blindness. Disruption of Bruch's membrane (Fig. 1) can cause acute retinal bleeding and detachment, or it may impair vision with neovascularization, similar to the uncontrolled blood vessel growth in severe diabetes.

 Chronic intense blue light exposure, too weak to cause acute injury, has been documented to destroy components of color vision. A photochemical breakdown of visual receptor pigments is the mechanism. Note that intense blue light is emitted from heating of char material by infrared lasers, which some believe should be filtered by tinted eye shields instead of completely clear lenses, yet another reason for good technique, including char removal during CO_2 surgery.

Cornea and Lens

The opposite ends of the spectrum, ultraviolet and far-infrared, are highly absorbed by protein and water, respectively, with potential for injuring the cornea and lens in the anterior half of the eye. The cornea is at acute risk from brief exposure to CO_2, holmium-YAG, erbium-YAG, and excimer lasers, with 10,600, 2000, 3000, and 193–351 nm, respectively. Corneal burns are very

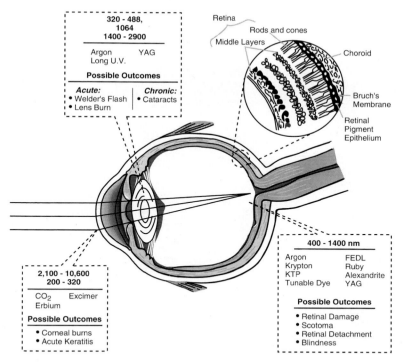

Figure 1 The specific sites of laser-induced ocular damage, listed by wavelength.

painful but usually heal rapidly. More severe burns may leave permanent scars, interfering with vision.

Less severe injuries for both the cornea and lens include acute keratitis ("welder's flash"), which is briefly painful and may cause enough pain, tearing, and swelling to disable a person for several days. Chronic effects of these wavelengths, and also argon, on the lens may induce cataracts.

Skin Injury and Possible Mutagenicity

Acute burns of the skin may occur from either direct or reflected energy. This may occur at any wavelength, while the depth and severity depends on the effects of wavelength, irradiance, and exposure time. Risk reduction is achieved by use of preset laser shuttered modes, correct power or energy settings, and operative safety protocols.

The mutagenicity of certain excimer wavelengths has been researched. KrF at 248 nm is excluded for human use due to this property. Several excimer wavelengths theoretically may have some risk but are believed to be less hazardous.

Eye Protection

Of the many factors considered for laser eye protection, wavelength absorption and optical density are paramount. Historically, the color of eyeglasses could be correlated with the wavelength they protected against. New materials have led to many lenses that are clear or of slight and variable tints. Lasers have increased in power or energy density. Therefore one must *read the* inscribed wavelength range of protection and optical density (Fig. 2). Optical density (O.D.) is

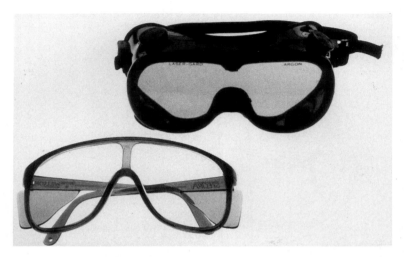

Figure 2 One should never assume the wavelength or O.D. of laser safety glasses. Color is not a reliable indicator of wavelength protection. Values should be inscribed on the glasses indelibly.

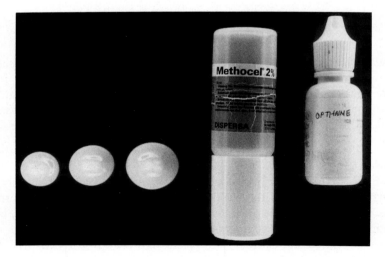

Figure 3 Corneal protectors used in laser surgery should cover the cornea, be opaque, and fit comfortably and snugly under the lids without migrating. They are placed after using topical anesthetic drops (e.g., Opthaine™) and lubrication with viscous methocellulose.

expressed in a logarithmic scale indexed to the decrease in transmitted light by a factor of 10 for each increase in the O.D. For example, a lens with an O.D. of 2 reduces ambient light for the specified wavelength 100-fold; one with an O.D. of 3 reduces it one thousand times. Maximum permissible exposure (MPE) data are available for common wavelengths and are ordinarily determined for the worst case scenario and an additional safety factor added. With increasing availability of multiwavelength lasers, many ask, why not produce glasses that protect against all common wavelengths? More is not always better. If the wavelength range is too broad, vision may be compromised, which is also dangerous.

Correct fit considers coverage from all angles. Gaps in the frame or between the frame and the face may allow damaging beam access to the eyes. Side shields may be added to many glasses to improve protection. Some adjustable lenses or larger goggles fit over prescription lenses to maintain corrected vision. All lenses should be routinely inspected for clarity and defects, including cracks and incipient breaks at temple joints and fixation of lens to frame. Many standard prescription lenses are adequate frontal protection for CO_2 lasers of low to average power. Note that even moderate-power CO_2 lasers can burn through plastic lenses in an instant when focused and that contact lenses are inadequate protection.

Patients may be allowed to wear glasses or goggles, particularly if the area of the body treated is away from the face and the wavelength is in the far infrared range. Since much laser surgery is accomplished near the patient's face, opaque goggles, wet gauze, or corneal shields after topical anesthetic is preferred (Fig. 3). Opacity is safer since the eye of the patient is likely to be nearer the focal point of the beam, beam deflection angles are more likely to be toward the patient, and the patient is less likely to be startled by any visual stimulus.

Eye Examinations and Treatment of Eye Injuries

Eye examinations for personnel working with lasers have been the subject of much controversy. Complications abound in attempting to differentiate laser-induced lesions from those of other causes; people may have congenital defects or suffer mild injuries without being aware of pain or visual field defects. Focal defects may go undetected by careful ophthalmologic testing even if the central 100 of vision corresponding to the macula is affected. Furthermore, except for serious injuries, which are immediately recognizable by the patient, no treatment is available. But what about mild cumulative exposures over a long period? Ophthalmologists were discovered to have decreased color sensitivity due to chronic unprotected slitlamp exposure to higher-energy blue wavelengths, which caused photobleaching of their cone photoreceptors. This can been prevented by switching to a softer green wavelength. No other group is exposed without eye protection in this manner.

Current recommendations vary by institution, with most following the World Health Organization guideline that no exam is needed unless there is an accidental exposure. An alternative approach recommended by Epstein Photomedicine Institute at Marshfield Clinic is to obtain a baseline eye exam of personnel who will work directly around lasers in operation and repeat the exam on termination or transfer as well as if an incident is reported. The eye exam consists of visual acuity, Amsler grid, anterior segment exam (cornea, iris, lens), and dilated fundus exam (retina). The Amsler grid utilizes very finely spaced lines, which help identify scotomas or defects in the central visual field, which could be caused by endogenous as well as exogenous injuries.

Figure 1 shows eye structures with potential injury sites affected by specific lasers and wavelengths in current use. Many of the newer lasers, for all their ease of use, are potentially more dangerous to the eye than their lower-energy-density predecessors. Clearly, knowledge of injury potential and precautions is required for all who work around lasers. Serious injuries have repeatedly occurred in laboratory settings where safety procedures are not known or followed by the primary personnel or part-time employees and visitors. Keep in mind that lower-power lasers can be as great a threat as high-power ones. Even a 1 W direct hit can damage the eye, in some cases through approved safety lenses!

Recent studies have quantified safety parameters and the likelihood of eye injury from CO_2 beams reflected off surgical instruments. Friedman et al. found that "with the use of eye protection or anodized instruments, there is extreme irreversible ocular hazard . . . within 12 cm of the eye" and a "potential for grade III irreversible corneal damage at reflected beam distances of 30 cm." Anodized instruments decreased the power of reflected laser beam 700 times. Friedman's assumptions of injury likelihood are based on ocular damage studies performed by Borland in 1971 on CO_2 wavelength injuries to rabbits. Mild injury causing temporary opalescence of the cornea (grade I) similar to welder's flash and snow blindness resolved in 24 hr. This may be treated with lubricants, antiinflammatory drugs, and cool compresses. Grade II injuries caused epithelial coagulation and loss, requiring 7 days to resolve without scarring. Such an injury may require topical steroids and lubricants with an antibiotic, along with compresses, and close follow-up. Grade III injuries were burns involving the substantia propria, which healed with full-thickness scar and visual loss. Treatment of this kind of injury would require corneal transplant after keratectomy.

Fire Prevention and Control

Preparedness is the key to fire prevention and control, since a large variety of items in or near the operative field may be ignited by contact with the beam. All items such should be either fireproof or fire resistant and prepared or dealt with in such a way as to minimize and contain flammability.

Flammable substances include patient and staff clothing, hair and operating room hair bonnets, drapes, gauze, cotton applicator sticks, prep solutions containing alcohols, acetone, or other combustible substances, plastics, ointments, oils (including certain make-ups), hair preparations (many even when dry, e.g., sprays, mousses), oxygen and many anesthetic gas mixtures, tubing used for endotracheal tubes, intravenous lines, and monitoring equipment. Methane bowel gas is of concern for intraabdominal or deeper rectal closed spaces, but generally is not a hazard for cutaneous surgeons operating in the perirectal area.

Preventive steps include restricting all but necessary clothing, drapes, and monitoring tubing, making sure that they are snug fitting and secured next to the body of staff and patients by tucking in, taping, securing with Velcro, snaps, or elastic bands. Flame-retardant materials should be employed in drapes and personnel clothing. Anesthesia and operating room personnel should know the surgeon's preference and operative field approach to locate materials and tubes unobtrusively. Thorough wetting of drapes and gauze adjacent to and underneath the target tissue field should be standard procedure. A basin of water or saline solution should be kept on the tray for rewetting of drapes, packing materials, etc., and for emergencies, along with a fire extinguisher rated for all types of potential fires (electrical, chemical, etc.).

Hair near the operative field should be either trimmed or restrained and preferably wet as often as needed with wet Telfa or saturated drapes. Even wet gauze can cause a flash fire in the presence of oxygen, therefore for eyes wet Telfa™ is preferable to wet gauze. I have found use of oil-free water-based gels (e.g., K-Y™) valuable in sticking down fly-away hair and maintaining protective moisture. Trimming or shaving hair avoids burning it and improves visualization and laser penetration to target. You may treat vascular lesions through gel applied to the eyebrow or frontal hairline margin without shaving. Certain hair products such as pomades and sprays containing petroleum-based vinyls and other coating substances are surprisingly flammable. I have seen a miniscule flash ignite a few hairs, which burned to the scalp like a fast-burning fuse!

Lightly wash hair and scalp on the operating table and wipe with towels to remove these residues.

Laser-resistant E.T. tubes and wrapping materials are available, and literature should be reviewed before using them. Clear masks, cannulae, and airway materials are not ignitable with visible light laser even in a 100% oxygen-enriched atmosphere, however, green and other colored airway devices can be ignited in the presence of oxygen. The most likely places for oxygen leaks are near the eye region, where a nose-sealing mask is used, near the nose when nasal cannulae are used, and near the mouth when using E.T. tubes.

Research has established the order of decreasing flammability as PVC tubing (149°F) > red rubber (intermediate) > Silastic tubing (700°F). Newer flame-retardant plastics are under investigation for their combination of greater stiffness and burning temperature than Silastic. Preferences and application demands prevent unanimity as to the ideal E. T. tube. Laser-resistant taping is advocated for nonmetallic tubes applied with one-half overlap; an inflatable cuff filled with methylene-blue or other visible nontoxic dye in sterile water provides a tight seal, decompression early warning, and ignition extinguishment.

An oxygen concentration of less than 30% after dilution by mixture with compressed air and nonflammable anesthetic gas is safest; also, flow rate should not be in excess of what is required. Nitrous oxide is an example of a gas as flammable as oxygen in effective concentrations, and halothane burns at high temperatures. The stream of escaping O_2 or other gases should be scavenged or at least diverted away from the operative field, if possible, to minimize support of ignition.

I frequently pack the rectum proximal to my removal of intra- or perirectal warts, more to gain control of mucosal walls, as backstop provision, and to prevent entrance of fecal material into the field than from concern about methane gas. Rectal packing material (combustible) should be thoroughly wet before use and lubricated only with oil-free substances (e.g., K-Y gel). The distal portion and retrieval string will need remoistening.

Ebonized or "brushed" diffuse reflectance instruments should be utilized in the operative field to minimize ricochet burns and potential ignition of combustible materials nearby. The laser should be placed in stand-by mode or turned off when not in immediate use.

Infectious and Toxic Airborne Hazards: Protection and Evacuation

Laser surgery hazards include toxic and infectious substances, which become airborne safety risks by vaporization and splatter, constituting the laser plume. Most of these irritating, toxic, potentially infectious, mutagenic, or carcinogenic foreign substances are produced by high temperatures or liberated by physical forces produced by lasers and electrocautery units. A few of the better-known chemical substances are also found in cigarette smoke and include benzene, carbon monoxide, creosols, formaldehyde, free radicals, ammonia, xylene, and hydrocyanide. Carbon particulate matter in smoke, often referred to as soot and causative in black lung, must also be considered. Tomita and Mihaski put laser smoke inhalation risk into perspective by noting that 1 g of CO_2 laser vaporized tissue inhaled is equivalent to smoking three cigarettes (six for electrocautery smoke).

Tissue particles from laser treatments may result from vaporization or ejection. Smoke evacuators (with adequate suction and filtration) held within 1 cm of the laser impact site may achieve greater than 98% efficiency in plume removal, but efficiency drops to 50% at 2 cm. Splattered or ejected particles traveling near sonic speeds are caused by rapid thermal expansion or pressure waves. Plume or ejected particles may contain intact DNA, and some studies have demonstrated transfer of viable microorganisms. However, the incidence of warts in CO_2 laser users is no greater than in the general population, indicating that the risks of viral transmission may be nil if precautions are taken.

Clearly, multistep and universal precautions must be taken to protect against airborne and fomite contactant exposures to potentially harmful substances associated with laser use. Safety points will be further elaborated later.

Smoke Evacuators

The smoke evacuator is the first-line protection against airborne substances. Doubling the distance from 1 to 2 cm from the laser site reduces evacuation efficiency by 50%. Proper integration and use of the following four components including maintenance is also required: vacuum unit, HEPA filter, ULPA filter, and charcoal filter (Fig. 4). The vacuum must be set high enough to capture all plume, yet not exceed the capacity of the filter series to capture airborne substances. HEPA (high efficiency particulate air) filters describe first-stage glass fiberglass or glass wool used to trap 0.3-μm particles and water vapor by physical blockage (interception and impaction) with greater than 99.97% efficiency. ULPA (ultralow particulate air) filters achieve trapping of particles of 0.1 μm size, but efficiency may vary depending on flow rate, and industry definitions appear up in the air. The activated charcoal filter is used for for toxic chemical and noxious odor absorption. Note that charcoal becomes useless once saturated or if air flow rate exceeds its capacity.

Smoke evacuator filters must be replaced prior to the weakest link becoming saturated, increasing resistance or reducing effectiveness. Units may be rated by time of use, which should be documented on the filter or by sensors that monitor components of the filter. Beware of excessively long tubing, folds or kinks in the tubing, and filter saturation from particularly high plume volume cases, which increases resistance and decreases flow rate. Either case may be indicated by the need to increase vacuum motor settings higher than 50–75% speed to maintain adequate plume evacuation. When in doubt, change the filter. You may request an exchange unit while yours is being serviced and evaluated.

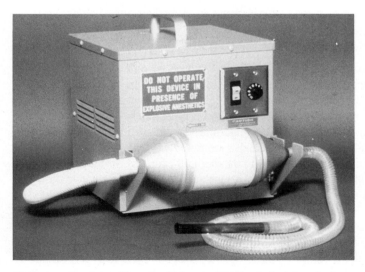

Figure 4 The laser filter should be specifically designed to fit the type of evacuator, rated for the airflow range of the evacuator, and hours of use safety scale marked on the filter. This classic smoke evacuator with HEPA and charcoal filter has been superceded by the addition of an ULPA filter, which increased filtering efficiency rating from 0.3 to 0.1 μm.

Masks

Filtering efficiency means that little if most air flows around (not through) a mask. A moldable nosepiece and flexible side panels that mold to the jaw and cheeks are required for a snug fit. Additional surface area provided by pleating and billowing the mask fabric greatly lowers breathing resistance through the mask. Comfortable fabric surfaces prevent irritation and encourage compliance, along with antifog and moisture-resistant features (Fig. 5).

Masks designed for laser use combine electrostatically charged synthetic fibers with traditional filtering mechanics of diffusion, interception, and inertial impaction to achieve 0.1 μm and smaller

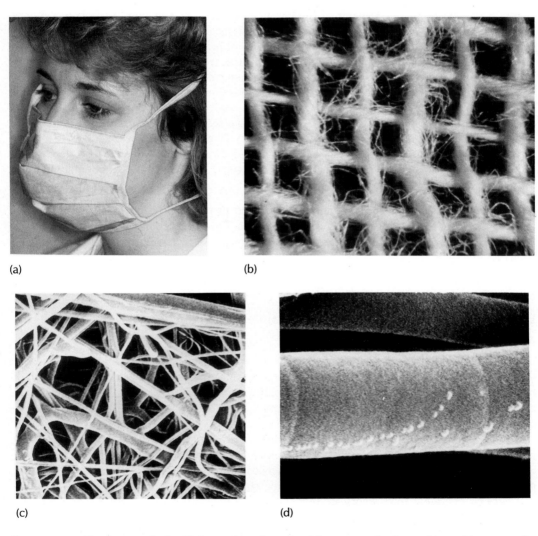

(a)   (b)

(c)   (d)

Figure 5   (a) The laser mask should fit snugly and comfortably at nose, cheeks, and jaw with no gaps for airflow around the mask. (b) Cloth mask II: ordinary cloth fiber masks have large spaces filtering only the largest debris and splatter. (c) Laser mask III: 500× enlargement of laser mask shows densely packed fibers capable of filtering 0.3-μm particles. (d) Laser mask IV: 10,000× enlargement of laser mask shows fiber capable of capturing 0.1-μm particles via electrostatic forces, which is dominant for charged particles of extremely low mass.

particle clearance. Combining these mechanisms increases efficiency and decreases breathing resistance. The laser surgeon and staff must understand that multiple factors govern mask-filtering function, and the safety benefits of a mask may not be realized without optimizing contour, surface area, comfort, and moisture saturation.

It is important that masks be changed between cases or if inadvertently splashed or wet, even during prolonged cases, when the mask may be moistened from respiration or sweating. Electrostatic charge filtering by mask fibers is eliminated when they are wet, thus lowering safety protection of the mask.

Tissue and Fluid Splatter

Lasers may splatter tissue fragments or fluid particles up to sonic velocities, especially the high-energy pulsed lasers increasingly used in removing pigment or resurfacing applications. Smoke evacuators, masks, goggles, and clothing are essential for protection. But manufacturers and users have offered or devised additional products to reduce risk from flying particles, including acrylic tubes, screens, and cones, which largely contain splatter or screen the user from direct flying fragments. Tubes and cones offer more complete protection than screens but should be pressed against the skin to seal.

Dressings may be applied prior to treatment. I have seen fragments penetrate through thin-membrane materials such as Tegaderm™ and Opsite™. Thicker gel membranes, e.g., Vigilon™, are more effective, particularly with the splatter-prone Q-switched YAG treatments. Despite some reduction in target visualization and energy density results, I recommend this for safety reasons.

Universal Precautions with Biohazard Contaminants

Cleaning, handling, and disposal of areas treated and items used during laser surgery is well outlined by OSHA and professional society guidelines. Specific attention should be paid to surfaces closest to the operative field, such as laser handpieces, protective clothing, lights, and light handles.

STEPS TO CONSISTENT RESULTS AND SAFETY

Environmental Design, Management, Maintenance, and Safety

Room and Door Location, Access, Keys

Selection of rooms in which to use lasers should allow implementation or modifications to achieve the many essential safety factors discussed throughout this chapter, including room access, warning signs, window protection, operating and traffic space, lighting sources, freedom from unexpected visitors and interruptions, fire prevention and burn treatment facilities, and smoke evacuation.

Laser rooms are preferably located in controlled-access locations or at least in low-traffic areas. Solitary doors to laser rooms are best to minimize possible entry points. Doors may open inward, outward, or recess or fold. However, laser-location planning should preclude the surgeon, patient, laser, or ancillary equipment from being struck by an abruptly opened door.

Locks on operating room doors are recognized as a potential hazard to the patient and staff. Therefore, interlocks that prevent laser operating room doors from opening while lasers are in use are seldom installed or employed. Rooms may be locked when not in use, and laser keys are best stored at a separate site rather than with the laser. Such steps control access to expensive and hazardous equipment, preventing unauthorized use and injury.

Space, Equipment, Foot Pedal Arrangement, and Clutter

Adequate space must be allocated for laser procedures. Handpiece, laser arm, or fiberoptic equipment must be able to move freely so as not to obstruct the surgeon during the procedure.

Foot pedals operating power tables, suction, cautery, dermabraders, etc., must not be confused with the laser, and vice versa. Rolling stools and chairs must not be capable of activating the laser foot pedal. A metal housing that restricts access to a carefully placed foot pedal is excellent insurance.

Operative Personnel and Observers

Just as nonessential equipment should be aggressively cleared from the perioperative area, so should observers. Each person present is subject to general risks of ocular, pulmonary, and cutaneous injury. Moreover, observers or operative personnel frequently lean on the surgical table or patient in their efforts to watch the procedure. Changing the relative position of equipment, operator, or laser target may lead to unintended tissue destruction, richochets, or other hazard to patient or medical staff members. If an emergency occurs, then the less crowded the perioperative area, the faster and more organized the response will be, whether rescue, evacuation, or both are needed.

Laser Warning Signs

Clear, uniform, laser warnings signs with adequate information are crucial to prevent personnel from entering an area with a potential vision hazard. Sign dimensions, letter size, color, etc. shall be in accordance with American National Standard Specification for Accident Prevention Signs (ANSI A35.1). Signs must display the word "Danger" prominently at the top and specify which wavelength is being used, and correct eyewear protection should be located near the sign. This practical consideration lessens the likelihood of personnel knocking on the door and then peeking around the door to ask for protective lenses.

Window Covers

Wavelengths transmissable through window glass must be prevented from leaving the operatory, placing passers-by at risk. Therefore, removable or fixed opaque shades or coverings need to be installed on internal or external windows for any rooms posing this type of risk. Removal of focusing lenses or other measures resulting in delivery of collimated beams dramatically increase the degree of risk, even at distance. Operatories several stories above the ground must still consider the presence of nearby rooms with facing unshielded windows as well as the possibility of a window washer.

Lighting

Lighting should be adequate for visualizing the operating field and all other areas of the room. Lights and armatures should not interfere with the laser armature or operator and assistants.

Electrical and Fiberoptic Hookups and Inspections

Lasers are electrically powered devices storing large amounts of energy capable of discharging even hours after all electrical sources are disconnected. This stored energy has been a source of electrocution of experienced operators inappropriately attempting to investigate or fix their laser, and even authorized repair personnel have been injured.

Proper connections require wiring up to electrical code wall receptacles, grounding, and laser device wiring and plugs. The enormous amount of current some lasers draw requires special wiring specified by the manufacturer, of which most laser users are unaware. Thus, moving some lasers may not be feasible without rewiring or at least determining wiring and receptacles to be compatible with device requirements.

Any defects in electrical wiring or worn spots should be reported and replaced. Areas of frequent bending or pressure from wheeled stools and the like begs for preventive maintenance. Small cracks may continue to function normally until meeting a metal surface or being dragged through a small puddle of water dripping from an instrument stand. Ground fault protection circuits and periodic electrical device leakage testing by trained personnel is insurance against unnoticed or invisible problems.

External fiberoptics from laser devices to handpieces are subjected to similar stresses as electrical wiring. Fibers more commonly cause a loss of delivered laser energy or a loss of precise pattern, which may lead to unintended target exposure when damaged. However, damaged connectors or fibers occasionally lead to potentially injurious laser exposure. If a disconnect leads to a collimated beam being loosed, the potential injury radius (nominal hazard zone) may be much greater than the usual treatment beam, which is strongly defocused after passing through the handpiece lens. Therefore, connectors with the handpiece and fiberoptic junctions with the laser device should be routinely inspected. We have found it helpful with some of our lasers to build an additional protection box to shield the fiber from physical trauma at its exit point.

Water Hoses and Connections

Many laser systems generate considerable heat during operation. This heat is either dissipated by external water cooling or through an internal heat exchanger to air. External water-cooled systems demand a critical volume and flow rate to function properly. Dangers include ruptures, leaks, disconnects, drain back-ups, sediment plugging internal or external to the laser, and interruptions in water delivery; any of these may lead to electrocution, short-circuit fire damage, water damage to electronics, overheating damage to key components resulting in fires, and physical injury from slipping. Quick-disconnect fittings tested for pressures and type of use at hand are indicated.

Minimum water flow pressure should be guaranteed; otherwise, laser protection circuits may shut down the system when someone on the same plumbing system uses water. Cleaning personnel should be warned against stressing electrical of plumbing connections or, for many laser systems, the laser system itself in any way. Preferably, water supplied for cooling is already sediment poor. However, filters and drains should be inspected periodically to prevent occlusion by debris or sediment.

Communications Devices

Hands-free communications should be incorporated into the laser operatory, allowing surgeons or other personnel to respond to questions without opening the door and to give clear instructions if and when entry is permitted and as well as to confirm safety precautions. Convenient communication into the operatory prevents garbled communications through or around the door.

The Laser Safety Officer

Who oversees and troubleshoots the broad variety of safety issues described here while the physician is concentrating on treating the individual patient? The laser safety officer (LSO) is an individual physician, nurse, or technician designated to monitor and manage the safe use of the laser in any particular case and who has the authority to discontinue laser use in a procedure if laser safety or standard of care requirements are not met. There may be several LSOs, who may be designated by the physician or operating room supervisor at the beginning of a case.

The LSO should be thoroughly familar with all basic principles concerning lasers and laser safety and additionally must accept responsibility for additional administrative duties. LSO administrative duties include reviewing all laser policies and procedures for adequacy and updating as required, documenting implementation and compliance with laser practice standard of care, instituting or updating a continuing staff laser education program, including in-services for new or modified equipment, and monitoring calibration, maintenance, and repair schedules.

Operative Procedures and Techniques

Prep Solutions

Prep solutions should be nonalcohol-based or allowed to dry completely. Iodophors may flash at high temperatures, especially if pooled near the operative site. I recommend removal of chlorhexidine scrub solutions with a water wash or blot due to a report of prolonged tracheobronchitis in laser surgery staff and physician who vaporized a surface area with this prep.

Nonreflective Instruments

Instruments used in the laser operative field (Fig. 6) should be brush finished, which adds many microsurfaces at varying angles; this prevents a concentrated beam from reflecting to nearby tissue with a high power density. Better than brushed finishes is ebonization, which combines a roughened black finish to avoid specular reflections of the beam. Note that a smooth black finish alone may still reflect far-infrared beams without significant absorption. Businesses provide new or refinish currently owned instruments with these specifications.

Spatulae or other flat, curved, and variable-shaped instruments may be used as backstops (Fig. 7) and tissue-controlling or protective tools. By placing a blocking instrument adjacent to or behind tissue to be excised or ablated, nearby tissue is protected.

Backstops and Heat Sinks

A wet dental roll or gauze may be placed in the naris or labial gingival sulcus overlapping the teeth to protect nearby structures such as nasal mucosa or tooth enamel during laser surgery. Wet large or small cotton-tipped applicators likewise provide a backstop function, which is easily manipulated, offer better tissue traction than metal or plastic instruments, and are more comfortable for the patient in unanesthetized areas. Packing material may be saturated with water, then coated with a water-based lubricant (no oil allowed!). Curettes are invaluable on the tray to remove charred tissue and to assess tissue character and depth, e.g., when treating warts.

Laser Calibration, Aiming Beam Coaxial Alignment Check, and Fiber Tips

Coaxial alignment checks of invisible beam lasers together with their aiming beams should be performed each day and whenever a laser has been moved from its previous location or sustained

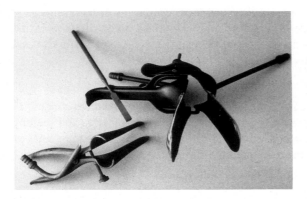

Figure 6 Instruments used in the laser operative field should be brush finish or, better yet, ebonized with with a rough black finish to avoid specular reflections of the beam. Businesses provide new or refinished previously owned instruments with these specifications.

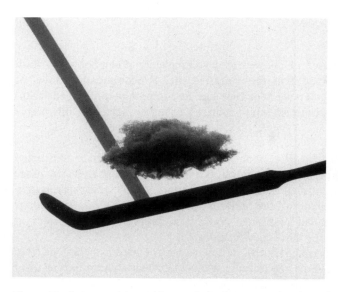

Figure 7   Laser excision with spatula backstop: nearby tissue is protected by a blocking instrument adjacent to or behind tissue to be excised or ablated.

a jar or impact to the laser. A tongue blade with a safe, light-colored backstop is regularly used with our carbon dioxide laser set at 20 W and 0.05 sec single pulse. If alignment is correct, the aiming beam travels through the tongue blade burn hole to reveal itself on the underlying backstop. If alignment is incorrect, the aiming beam remains on the anterior surface of the blade surface, somewhere adjacent to the entry hole. Fiber-tipped lasers should be checked at low aiming beam power on a light-colored surface and defocused. Significant beam asymmetry reveals the need to score and break, then clean the fiber. Q-switched lasers may use burn-paper to examine their impact profile.

Lens Focal Length

Short-focal-length lenses reduce power and energy densities in much shorter distances, thereby decreasing the zone of potential injury and severity of injury within a given distance in the operative field. Longer-focal-length lenses make it easier to maintain consistent beam size and power density while excising or ablating tissue.

Equipment and Operator Settings

Laser personnel are advised to use laser equipment whenever feasible in shuttered modes, to practice hand movements with the laser in stand-by prior to excising or ablating, and thereby to gain better control. Should the patient move or observers jar the surgeon, equipment, or patient, damage control will already have been initiated by the limited exposure.

Smoke Evacuator Use

The smoke evacuator should be maintained within 1 cm of the laser-treatment site. Tubes should be as short and straight as possible, the filter adequate for the procedure scheduled, and the vacuum setting in the medium range.

Physician and Staff Education

All laser-using physicians and staff members working around or with lasers should have a basic education in relevant laser biophysics and tissue effects, laser systems and their hazard classification, and laser safety protocols to prevent harm to themselves, other health care providers, and the patient.

Physician Education

Recommended ANSI and ASLMS standards of practice for physician use of lasers in medicine and surgery include both training and experience, which may be obtained in a combination of settings, including residency training, postgraduate training in courses and preceptorships, literature, and audio-visual learning aids. Comprehensive coverage of laser topics, the necessity of hand-eye coordination, and development of clinical judgment are considered so vital to good outcomes and safety that the total education should include (1) courses devoted to laser principles and safety, including physics, tissue interaction, clinical specialty topics, and hands-on experience with lasers (for a minimum total of 8–10 hr) and (2) a laser preceptorship with a minimum of 6–8 hr of observation with an expert and some hands-on involvement. Documentation of actual cases is very important.

Staff Education

Hospital and clinic nonphysician staff responsible for performing or assisting in laser procedures need a basic understanding of laser physics and tissue interaction; even more, they need in-services on laser hazards, accident prevention, adherence to principles of operatory environmental design, management, and safety as well as practice with safety protocols. In addition to organized didactic information, the following hands-on in-services/courses are vital: demonstrating laser systems to be used; connection, disconnection, cleaning, and maintenance of laser accessories (handpieces, lenses, scopes); gas tank or dye cannister handling and gauge interpretation; set-up and tear-down procedures; calibration; smoke evacuator use and filter changes; sterile and nonsterile draping of the laser for clean vs. truly sterile procedures.

The Laser Safety Officer

LSO's duties have been described above. Frequent laser and safety education updates are needed by the LSO to remain current with new technology, be aware of new regulatory guidelines, fulfill staff education duties, and work with quality assurance personnel to ensure compliance with institutional requirements.

The LSO should be thoroughly familar with all basic principles concerning lasers and laser safety and must accept responsibility for additional administrative duties as outlined above.

BIBLIOGRAPHY

AlHaddad S, Brenner J. Helium and lower oxygen concentration do not prolong tracheal tube ignition time during potassium titanyl phosphate laser use. *Anesthesiology* 1994;80(4):936–938.

Allinson RW, Thall EH, et al. Risk to the treating ophthalmologist when using the laser [letter]. *Arch Ophthalmol* 1991;109(8):1057–1058.

Baggish M. The effects of laser smoke on the lungs of rats. *Am J Obstet Gynecol* 1987;156.

Bollinger NJ, Schutz RH. *NIOSH Guide to Industrial Respiratory Protection*. U.S. Department of Health and Human Services, Centers for Disease Control, National Institute for Occupational Safety and Health, Division of Safety Research, 1987.

Borland RG, Brennan DH, et al. Threshold levels for damage of the cornea following irradiation by a continuous wave carbon dioxide (10.6 μm) laser. *Nature* 1971;234:151–152.

Brosseau LM, Evans JS, et al. Collection efficiency of respirator filters challenged with monodisperse latex aerosols. *Am Ind Hyg Assoc J* 1989;50(10):544–549.

Byrne PO, Sisson PR, et al. Carbon dioxide laser irradiation of bacterial targets in vitro. *J Hosp Infect* 1987;9(3):265–273.

Cadwell GH, Jr., Inc FF. *A Brief History of the Modern ULPA Filter.* Las Vegas, Institute of Environmental Sciences, 1985.

Chinn SD. Complications of laser surgery: safety, risks, and the plume. *Clin Podiatr Med Surg* 1992;9(3):763–779.

Davis RK, Simpson GT, II. Safety with the carbon dioxide CO_2 laser. *Otolaryngol Clin North Am* 1983;16(4):801–811.

Driver I, Taylor C. The effect of surface finish on the reflection of CO_2 laser beams from specula. *Phys Med Biol* 1987;32(2):227–235.

Epstein RH, Brummet RR, et al. Incendiary potential of the flashlamp pumped 585 nm tunable dye laser. *Anesth Analog* 1990;71:171–175.

Epstein RH, Halmi B. Oxygen leakage around the laryngeal mask airway during laser treatment of port-wine stains in children. *Anesth Analog* 1994;78:486–489.

Forster WK, Emmerich H, et al. [Induction of chromosome aberrations in human lymphocytes as a model for evaluating the mutagenic effect of excimer laser irradiation in ophthalmology.] *Fortschr Ophthalmol* 1991;88(4):377–379.

Frenz M, Mathezlioc F, et al. Transport of biologically active material in laser cutting. *Lasers Surg Med* 1988;8(6):562–566.

Friedman NR, Saleeby ER, et al. Safety parameters for avoiding acute ocular damage from the reflected CO_2 (10.6 microns) laser beam. *J Am Acad Dermatol* 1987;17(5 Pt 1):815–818.

Garden JM. Papillomavirus in the vapor of carbon dioxide laser-treated verrucae. *JAMA* 1988;259(8):1199–1220.

Gloster HM, Roenigk RK. Risk of acquiring human papillomavirus from the plume produced by the carbon dioxide laser in the treatment of warts. *J Am Acad Dermatol* 1995;32:436–441.

Goldman L. *Optical Radiation Hazards to the Skin. Safety with Lasers and Other Optical Sources: A Comprehensive Handbook.* New York, Plenum Press, 1983.

Goldman L. Some concerns about current laser surgery of condylomata acuminata [letter]. *J Am Acad Dermatol* 1988;18(4 Pt 1):744–745.

Laser safety eyewear. *Health Devices* 1993;22(4):159–204.

Laser use and safety. *Health Devices* 1992;21(9):306–310.

Liu BY, Rubow KL, et al. *Performance of HEPA and ULPA Filters.* Las Vegas, Institute of Environmental Sciences, 1955.

Lowe NJ, Burgess P, et al. Flashlamp dye laser fire during general anesthesia oxygenation: case report. *J Clin Laser Med Surg* 1990;

Mainster MA, Sliney DW, et al. Damage mechanisms, instrument design, and safety. *Ophthalmology* 1983;90:973.

Matchette LS, Vegella TJ, et al. Viable bacteriophage in CO_2 laser plume: aerodynamic size distribution. *Lasers Surg Med* 1993;13(1):18–22.

Mohr RM, McDonnell BC, et al. Safety considerations and safety protocol for laser surgery. *Surg Clin North Am* 1984;64(5):851–859.

Ott D. Smoke production and smoke reduction in endoscopic surgery: preliminary report. *Endosc Surg Allied Technol* 1993;1(4):230–232.

Patel KF, Hicks JN. Prevention of fire hazards associated with use of CO_2 lasers. *Anesth Anal* 1981;60:885–888.

Prendiville PL, McDonnell PJ. Complications of laser surgery. *Int Ophthalmol Clin* 1992;32(4):179–204.

Rodriguez JG, Sattin RW. Injuries as an adverse reaction to clinically used laser devices. *Lasers Surg Med* 1987;7(6):457–460.

Rupke G. Vigilance, education are keys to overcoming laser safety complacency. *Aorn J* 1992;56(3):523–525.

Seiler T, Bende T, et al. Side effects in excimer corneal surgery. DNA damage as a result of 193 nm excimer laser radiation. *Graefes Arch Clin Exp Ophthalmol* 1988;226(3):273–276.

Sosis MB, Dillon FX. A comparison of CO_2 laser ignition of the Xomed, plastic, and rubber endotracheal tubes. *Anesth Analg* 1993;76(2):391–393.

Sosis MB, Pritikin JB, et al. The effect of blood on laser-resistant endotracheal tube combustion. *Laryngoscope* 1994;104(7):829–831.

Toon S. Doctors using lasers risk problems without proper training. *J Occup Health Saf* 1988;57(7):30.

Vassiliadis A. *Ocular Damage from Laser Radiation. Laser Applications in Medicine and Biology.* New York, Plenum Press, 1971.

Wheeland RG, Bailin PL, et al. Use of scleral eye shields for periorbital laser surgery. *J Dermatol Surg Oncol* 1987;13(2):156–158.

55

CO_2 Laser

John Louis Ratz
Tulane University, Louisiana State University, and The Ochsner Clinic, New Orleans, Louisiana

Philip L. Bailin
The Cleveland Clinic Foundation, Cleveland, Ohio

The laser, introduced in the late 1950s, was first applied to medicine in the early 1960s. Cutaneous disease was one of the first areas in which lasers, primarily the argon laser, were applied. New lasers have been developed, and the argon, though far from obsolete, is no longer the predominant laser used in dermatology. This is due primarily to the evolution of the CO_2 laser and CO_2 techniques, which lend themselves particularly well to the skin. Two major reasons for increased use of the CO_2 laser in cutaneous and general medicine are its versatility and precision. It may be used for a variety of cutaneous entities because it vaporizes tissue precisely.

PRACTICAL CO_2 PHYSICS AND TISSUE INTERACTIONS

The CO_2 laser is structurally the same as lasers in general. The active medium is a mixture of CO_2, N_2, and He gases in a ratio of 1:1.5:4. In most instances, it is pumped by an electrical power source and is relatively efficient, eliminating the need for special electrical hookups and externally supplied cooling systems. Several manufacturers have developed CO_2 lasers that are pumped by radiofrequency waves. These *self-contained* lasers do not require an external supply of exhaustible gases and function for years before tube replacement is necessary. These lasers are smaller and eliminate the inconvenience of having to replace cumbersome gas canisters periodically. The low cost of tube replacement makes the self-contained systems particularly cost-effective.

Light produced by the CO_2 laser has a wavelength of 10,600 nm, which is in the far-infrared portion of the electromagnetic spectrum. As such, it is currently not available with fiberoptic delivery. The beam exiting the optical resonator must enter a mirrored delivery system. The most common type of mirrored system is the articulating arm now used on most CO_2 lasers (Figs. 1,2). Also available is a rigid wave-guide fiber, which is basically a hollow mirrored tunnel. Because of its rigidity, it may not offer any practical advantage over the articulated delivery systems. The mirrors in some of the articulated systems are adjustable, which allows for rela-

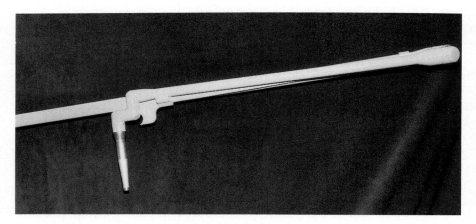

Figure 1 Articulating arm system for the CO_2 laser.

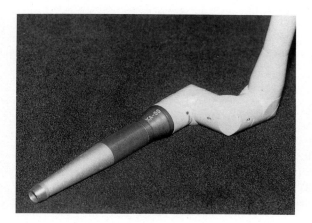

Figure 2 Terminal articulating knuckles and handpiece for typical CO_2 laser.

tively simple alignment of the laser beam. Fixed mirrored systems, on the other hand, have basically eliminated the need for such periodic alignments and because of this are far more mobile than the nonfixed systems.

Once formed, the CO_2 beam is transported down the mirrored system to the handpiece, which contains the lens apparatus. The lens is responsible for converging the parallel laser beam to its smallest spot at the focal length of the lens and divergence beyond focality (Fig. 3). The size of the spot at its focal point is a function of the lens and its optical properties. Various handpieces and lens systems offer a variety of focal lengths and spot sizes. Regardless of the system, the handpiece is usually on the end of an articulating knuckle.

The number and type of articulating knuckles, as well as the size and type of handpiece, all play a role in the mobility and maneuverability of the handpiece. Balanced, counterweighted arms make the procedure much less laborious for the surgeon, because the handpiece feels weightless and can be released while it is still in position over the surgical field. Innovations such as zoom or variable spot size handpieces offer little practical advantage, particularly to the experienced laser surgeon, but may be useful to the novice to reliably reproduce a specific spot size and power density. Aids are also available, such as stylus tips, which allow for tissue contact with the handpiece at the exact focal length, and angled mirrored tips to facilitate undercutting and undermining procedures.

Because the CO_2 beam is invisible, a coaxial red helium–neon (HeNe) laser beam is used as an aiming beam. In addition, some lasers may be equipped with controls to alter the intensity of this aiming beam.

The impact of the CO_2 laser beam on tissue results in almost total energy absorption. There is no transmission of CO_2 laser energy through tissue and virtually no scatter from the impact site. There is only 2–3% total energy reflection, both directly off the surface and indirectly off tissue contents such as adnexal structures. The nature of the laser–tissue impact is dependent on a number of variables, including (1) laser power level, (2) power density or irradiance (i.e., power concentration), (3) duration of interaction or impact, (4) relative water content of the target tissue, and (5) tissue temperature level resulting from the impact.

A tissue temperature of 100°C can be achieved instantaneously in appropriate tissue and with correct parameters. This level will transform all inter- and intracellular water into steam, resulting in tissue vaporization. This reaction is what the CO_2 laser has been predominantly used for. However, by adjusting the parameters, different tissue reactions can occur. If the tissue temperature is raised to approximately 70°C, protein denaturation will occur, which is likely to be ir-

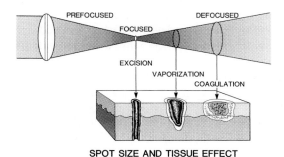

Figure 3   The lens within the handpiece converges the laser beam to its focal point, which then diverges into the defocused beam. At the focal point, a narrow, relatively deep impact is used for excision. In the defocused portion of the beam, there is decreasing depth of thermal destruction.

reversible. If the tissue temperature reaches 85°C, coagulation will result. This can be used to achieve hemostasis. If vaporization is achieved by elevating the tissue temperature to 100°C and the interaction is continued, the laser impacts on desiccated tissue. Further vaporization does not occur because the target is carbonized and functions as a heat sink. If laser treatment is continued on such a target, potentially high elevations in tissue temperature (>500°C) result. This conducts heat, causing thermal damage to surrounding tissue and usually unwanted and undesirable nonspecific thermal necrosis beyond the original laser impact. This interaction does not make optimal use of the CO_2 laser and its properties—that is, precise vaporization with minimal damage to surrounding tissue. Indiscriminate and inappropriate use results in undesirable scarring and thermal burns, about which some surgeons have complained. This type of wound can be avoided by *appropriate* use of the CO_2 laser.

Appropriate vaporization of tissue will result in little or no carbonization or char formation, although this may not be completely avoidable. The appropriate interaction is either broad (defocused, large impact spot) shallow vaporization or narrow (focused, small impact spot) penetrating vaporization (Fig. 3). The broad, shallow impact is useful for tissue ablation. The narrow penetrating impact allows for precise incisional surgery.

In addition to damage from the immediate impact, the CO_2 laser wound has other important characteristics. Blood vessels and lymphatics up to 0.5 mm in diameter are instantaneously sealed for relative hemostasis. This may provide some protection from lymphatic or hematogenous dissemination of tumor when excised with the CO_2 laser. Vaporized nerve endings are sealed. This may minimize neurotransmitter release, which may also minimize the sensation of pain. In addition, thermal damage of adjacent tissue can be minimized if the laser is used appropriately. In skin, peripheral thermal damage is limited to an area less than 50 μm (roughly the diameter of a basal cell) from impact. This not only improves the quality of wound healing and the resulting scar but can also maintain the histologic integrity of the tissue. This is particularly useful for histologic evaluation of tissue excised with the CO_2 laser.

CO_2 laser wounds develop little or no postoperative edema and little inflammatory response. This is beneficial for procedures in certain locations such as the meatal or perimeatal structures, since it reduces the chance for stenosis or stricture. It is very likely that fibroblast secretory activity and proliferation are greatly diminished, as has been shown in studies with other infrared systems. This may account for the quality of postoperative CO_2 laser wounds and the decreased incidence of hypertrophic scar formation when the laser is used properly. It may also account for the successful treatment of keloids and keloid-related conditions such as acne keloidalis nuchae with the CO_2 laser.

All CO_2 lasers can be set to deliver a predetermined power output (watts) to tissue. By convention, the wattage recorded on the control panel of the laser is that delivered to tissue. However, the wattage is of relatively little importance unless other parameters are taken into account at the same time. As an example, a power of 5 W delivered to tissue with an impact spot 10 mm in diameter will have very little effect on the tissue because of the dispersion of energy in such a broadly defocused beam. On the other hand, 5 W focused onto a 0.1-mm impact spot can easily be used to excise skin, because all of the power output is concentrated into a very small impact spot.

This dilution or concentration of power is the key to laser surgery. It reflects the amount of energy absorbed by the tissue. Power diluted over a broad surface area will result in little damage that penetrates tissue a minute amount. That same amount of power concentrated into a small spot will penetrate deeply. Power per unit of surface area is termed *power density* or *irradiance*. Divergence of a laser beam by the lens either concentrates or dilutes the power density when one is simply moving the beam into and out of focus (Fig. 3).

Power density, or irradiance, is the key to laser–tissue interaction and can easily be calculated when the power delivered to tissue and impact spot size are known. The formula for this calculation is:

$$\text{Power density} = \text{Irradiance} = \frac{W\,(\text{delivered to tissue})}{\pi r^2\,(\text{impact surface area})}$$

The area is calculated in cm^2, while most spot sizes are measured in mm. This conversion must be made before making the calculation. Power density or irradiance charts are generally available to make this determination without the need for calculation.

Another important factor that affects the laser–tissue interaction is time. If the laser beam is in contact with the skin for a longer time, it will result in greater tissue destruction. This time factor is included with the concept of energy fluence, which is a measure of the irradiance or power density delivered to tissue multiplied by the time of exposure in seconds:

Energy = Power $\times$ time

Fluence = Power density $\times$ time (sec)

Fluence = W-sec/cm^2

Fluence = J/cm^2

Fluence, like irradiance, can be adjusted by changing the treatment parameters. Both can be increased by increasing the power in a direct relationship. Conversely, the fluence is inversely proportional to the impact spot size: increased by decreasing the impact spot and decreased by increasing the impact spot. This inverse relationship varies by the square of the radius of the spot size and thus has the greatest influence on irradiance and fluence.

Fluence, unlike irradiance, is affected by time, and the relationship, like that for power, is a direct one. An increase in time will result in an increase in fluence, while decreasing the time of exposure decreases the fluence. Though power and time both have a direct and theoretically equivalent effect on fluence, in practice this is not the case. Theoretically, doubling either the time or the power would have the net effect of doubling the fluence. While this may be true, increasing the time causes more thermal damage, more charring, and less vaporization than does the equivalent increase in power. This needs to be taken into account when adjusting parameters.

CO$_2$ lasers are continuous emission lasers: they deliver their energy in a continuous beam, the duration of which is controlled with a foot switch. Alternatively, the impact can be delivered in pulses, the duration and rapidity of which are usually set at the control panel. Pulses are the result of a mechanical shutter and should not be confused with other types of pure pulsed lasers, which are systems not capable of continuous output. The mechanical pulsed delivery of the CO$_2$ laser can be useful for vaporization but is generally not applicable to excision. Superpulse is discussed below.

OPERATIVE PROCEDURE

The surgical site can be prepared as for any surgical procedure. However, the CO$_2$ laser is capable of igniting flammable materials. If alcohol-containing agents are used for preparation, time must be given for evaporation of the flammable substance. The blue flame of an alcohol fire might be difficult to detect on the surface of the skin but is quite capable of causing a severe burn on the patient or igniting the drapes or sponges.

It is helpful to outline the lesion or mark the planned excision. As for any surgical procedure, the tissue can be distorted by the injection of local anesthesia, thus obscuring the target. Epinephrine is not required for hemostasis but can be useful to prolong anesthesia. It is particularly beneficial when treating vascular lesions, such as port-wine stains, to prevent the rapid flush-out of anesthesia. Occasionally, epinephrine is helpful for excision in highly vascular areas. It adds an additional element of hemostasis, but these wounds must be watched for hemorrhage once the epinephrine's effect has ceased.

Since the CO_2 laser is only relatively hemostatic, back-up hemostatic measures such as hemostats, ties, and electrocautery should be available. Other ancillary equipment such as forceps, scissors, needle holders, etc., should also be on hand as should wet sponges, wet towels and drapes, cotton-tipped applicators, and hydrogen peroxide.

CO_2 Laser Vaporization

CO_2 laser vaporization is hemostatic ablation of tissue. During the procedure, the treated tissue is turned to steam, meaning the tissue temperature reaches 100°C. In order to achieve this, a power density of at least 150 W/cm^2 is necessary. Power and impact parameters can be adjusted to deliver such irradiance. For practical purposes, it is useful to work with a 2–3 mm impact spot size and an incident power of 5–10 W. These parameters are sufficient for the majority of cases.

Vaporization is possible with increased irradiance, but the additional power is not generally necessary. The increased irradiance may not necessarily speed up a procedure but can created unwanted deeper impacts, more char, and more surrounding thermal damage, particularly if the beam is advanced slowly over the target. Occasionally, however, vaporizing at increased irradiance can be beneficial. This is particularly true in desiccated or unhydrated tissue such as hyperkeratotic plantar skin or nail keratin.

Once appropriate parameters are selected and the site has been prepped and anesthetized, the lesion can be vaporized. This can be done in continuous fashion, which is preferred for larger lesions, or it can be done in single or repeated pulses. Pulsed delivery is recommended for the novice or for small lesions that require little total energy input, such as syringomas and xanthelasma. High-irradiance, ultra-short-exposure techniques are the optimal approach. However, conventional continuous-wave lasers do not provide pulse durations that are short enough.

Once a single pass has been made over the target lesion, char can easily be removed by swabbing the area with a hydrogen peroxide–soaked sponge or cotton-tipped applicator. The field should then be dried up with a dry sponge or applicator and the wound carefully examined for any remaining pathologic tissue. While this can be done macroscopically, magnifying loupes (2.5×) are useful and enhance inspection of the wound.

Normal vaporized dermis is a characteristic off-white color resembling the inside of an orange peel (Fig. 4). In most instances, residual lesional tissue can easily be distinguished from normal skin. Residual blood vessels from port-wine stains are still red, and tattoo pigment is brighter and quite obvious. Other types of residual pathologic tissue have a characteristic appearance, which, because of the hemostasis produced by vaporization, can quite readily be identified. Additionally, normal dermis shrinks or contracts when vaporized, while most epithelial lesions bubble. This further aids in identifying pathologic tissue. Residual pathology can then be revaporized. Following the second pass, the wound can be cleansed and examined again. This is repeated until all pathologic tissue has been removed.

The number of lesions amenable to CO_2 laser vaporization is quite extensive. Virtually any lesion that can be successfully ablated by cryosurgery or electrodesiccation can be vaporized with the CO_2 laser (Fig. 5). A partial list of lesions that have been successfully vaporized is given in Table 1.

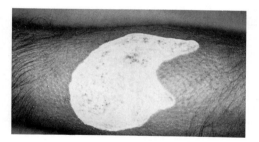

Figure 4 Normal tissue following CO_2 laser vaporization will have a characteristic off-white appearance, resembling the inside of an orange peel.

In a modification of the vaporization technique, the use of very low power output or even milliwatt output combined with short pulsing, superpulsing, or ultrapulsing has fostered the development of resurfacing techniques. Such techniques have been used in the treatment of fine line wrinkles when the laser is used alone or in combination with a trichloroacetic acid chemical peel.

CO_2 Laser Excision

CO_2 laser excision can be done with the precision of a scalpel and far greater hemostasis. The irradiance for excision is far greater than for vaporization. The appropriate irradiance will depend on the nature of the tissue; but, generally, irradiances of at least 50,000 W/cm^2 are required. Although excisions can be carried out at lower irradiances, unnecessary char and thermal damage usually result and wound closure is compromised. Exceptionally good excision can be done with a 0.1-mm impact spot size and power settings between 4 and 10 W, depending on the nature of the tissue. This results in an irradiance of 50,000–128,000 W/cm^2. The advent of the 0.1-mm spot has made CO_2 laser excision much more precise and easier to perform at lower power outputs than could be achieved with a 0.2-mm spot. The same irradiance can be obtained with 5 W and a 0.1-mm spot as with 20 W and a 0.2-mm spot.

Increasing the irradiance will increase the depth of the incision. Longer exposure will also increase the depth of the incision and will also increase char formation and unnecessary ther-

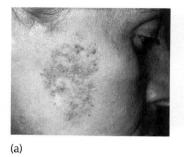

(a)

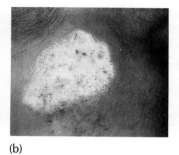

(b)

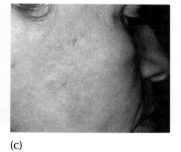

(c)

Figure 5 CO_2 laser vaporization of a port-wine stain that had failed to respond to argon laser photocoagulation. (a) Preoperatively. (b) Immediately postoperatively. (c) Four months later.

Table 1 Indications for CO_2 Laser Vaporization

Actinic cheilitis	Porokeratosis
Actinic keratoses	Port-wine stains
Adenoma sebaceum	Prurigo nodularis
Balanitis xerotica obliterans	Rhinophyma
Bowen's disease	Seborrheic keratoses
Dermatofibromas	Superficial basal cell carcinomas
Dystrophic nails	Syringomas
Kraurosis vulvae	Tattoos
Leiomyomas	Trichoepitheliomas
Lentigo maligna	Verrucous epidermal nevi
Lymphangiomas	Warts
Neurofibromas	Xanthelasma

mal damage. It is far better for the surgeon to incise at a constant speed and adjust the power to achieve the appropriate depth to minimize adjacent thermal damage.

The CO_2 laser excision is almost completely hemostatic, since small vessels 0.5 mm or less in diameter are sealed instantaneously. Larger vessels, up to approximately 1.5 mm, can be sealed by defocusing the laser beam to achieve coagulation. For larger vessels, ligation or electro-coagulation is required for hemostasis.

It is important to surround the surgical field by wet drapes or sponges to protect adjacent tissue from inadvertent or accidental laser damage. This is particularly important when the specimen is being undercut for removal. It is wise to place wet sponges behind the specimen in order to avoid inadvertent impact on adjacent tissue (Fig. 6).

Once the specimen has been removed, undermining can be done either directly with the CO_2 laser handpiece or with an angled-mirror endpiece (Fig. 7). Alternatively, undermining can be done in conventional fashion. The wound can be closed or allowed to heal by second intention.

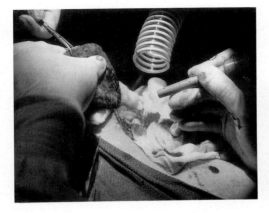

Figure 6 Surround the surgical field with wet sponges. Back up a laser excision with wet sponges to avoid a cut-through impact on adjacent tissue.

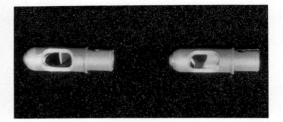

Figure 7 Angle tips are available for undercutting. These are capable of diverting the beam either 90 or 120 degrees from its original direction.

If necessary, a flap can be advanced or rotated into a laser wound or a graft can be used to cover the defect. The procedure for using a flap or graft in a laser-created wound is no different than that created by a scalpel. In addition, a laser-created wound that is closed primarily will have the same healing time as a scalpel-created wound. It has been shown that the tensile strength is slightly less in CO_2 laser wounds for the first 3 weeks but catches up in this time. The degree of tensile strength reduction can be significant when one is considering suture removal, especially when steroids are administered or other factors affect wound repair. In practical terms, CO_2 laser excision wound can be dealt with in the same way as a scalpel excision wound. Suture removal normally occurs as with a scalpel technique.

Although the laser can be used for any excision, it has distinct advantages in some situations. It is particularly useful in patients receiving anticoagulants or in highly vascular areas in which the hemostatic properties of the laser are advantageous.

CO_2 laser excision is indicated for the removal of keloids and keloid-related tissue such as acne keloidalis nuchae (Fig. 8). These cases have resulted in exceptional cure rates and low rates of recurrence compared with conventional treatment. This may be due, in part, to diminished postoperative inflammation and also to decreased fibroblast activity after infrared laser irradiation.

In addition, CO_2 laser wounds, because of their minimal peripheral thermal damage, retain their histologic integrity. Therefore, the CO_2 laser may be used in Mohs surgery, for which histologic integrity is mandatory.

The CO_2 laser has also been used advantageously for several cosmetic procedures. This includes CO_2 laser blepharoplasty, for which the laser replaces either scalpel or electrosection cutting in performing upper lid blepharoplasties, and transconjunctival lower lid blepharoplasties, resulting in far less postoperative edema and ecchymoses and allowing for more rapid recovery and return to normal activity. CO_2 laser excision can also be adapted for use in hair transplantation. While using the CO_2 laser to remove donor strips and for the creation of recipient slits for incisional slit grafting, intraoperative bleeding can be minimized without sacrificing graft integrity.

CO_2 laser excision has not gained universal acceptance. This is likely due to the initial awkwardness of the laser for novice laser surgeons. Poor technique results in broad excisions, margin desiccation, char formation, and unnecessary thermal damage.

ANCILLARY MEASURES

CO_2 laser surgery has unique ancillary requirements. Perhaps the most important is smoke evacuation. Because of evaporation, CO_2 laser surgery produces a large amount of malodorous steam. This steam requires evacuation by a suction system, which generally has replaceable filters that must be changed periodically. In addition, hoses, which must be large and flexible, and a handpiece are necessary to evacuate directly in the surgical field. This equipment must be on hand before a procedure can be carried out (Figs. 9,10). It is uncertain what organisms are viable in the laser plume, but human papillomavirus has been identified on filter materials. Inhalation of the plume is a theoretical mode of microbial transmission.

Eye protection is also mandatory for anyone in the room when the laser is in use. For the CO_2 laser, appropriate protection is provided by glass or plastic wraparound lenses. In most instances, normal eyeglasses are acceptable. Occasionally, where the procedure is close to the patient's eye, layered wet sponges or methacrylate or chromed metal protective scleral shields can be used for the patient's maximal protection (Fig. 11). Eye shields are used with topical anesthesia. The patient's eye must be protected for several hours to avoid inadvertent injury, since the protective blink reflex is temporarily lost.

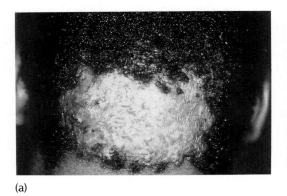

(a)

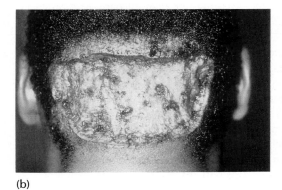

(b)

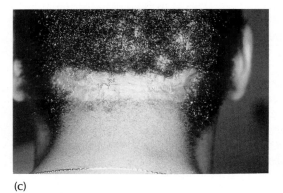

(c)

Figure 8 CO_2 laser excision of acne keloidalis nuchae. (a) Preoperatively. (b) Immediate postoperatively. (c) Three months later.

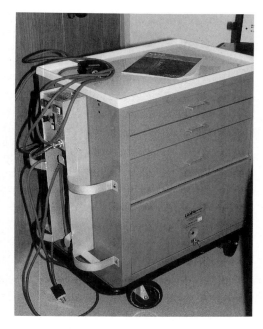

Figure 9,10   Several types of smoke evacuators are available and are necessary ancillary equipment.

Despite the possibility of reflecting the CO_2 laser beam off shiny surgical instruments and onto surrounding tissue, the use of blackened or anodized instruments for cutaneous laser surgery is unnecessary. Instruments should be out of the field during surgery. The laser beam is not conducted down a hemostat, as with electrocoagulation, to obtain hemostasis. Inadvertent impacts on surgical instruments are, therefore, rare. Whey they do occur, the power is dissipated rapidly and over a short distance so that damage to surrounding tissue is likely to be insignificant.

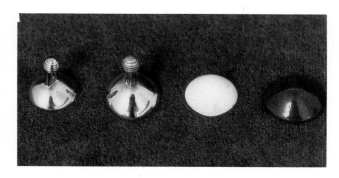

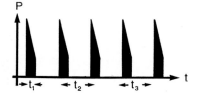

Terms

Pulse duration = t_1

Repetition rate = $\dfrac{1}{t_3}$ = frequency

Duty cycle = Pulse duration x repetition rate
= % "on"

Figure 11   Protective eye shields are available in a variety of sizes and types. The two shields on the left are chromed and designed specifically for laser use. The two methacrylate shields on the right are lightweight and relatively easy to insert.

Figure 12   Each superpulse impulse is of short duration but significant peak power. Each impulse is identical, and they follow one another in rapid succession. Several hundred impulses are delivered per second.

Although the CO_2 laser beam is a hemostatic instrument, it is only relatively hemostatic. Vessels larger than 1.5 mm, and occasionally even smaller vessels, require other forms of hemostasis. Ligation or electrocautery may be necessary for hemostasis and should be available at all times.

Many CO_2 lasers are equipped with a nitrogen or fresh air purge. This is a continuous flush of gas, either nitrogen from an external tank or ambient air, through the laser handpiece, distal to the lens, to keep debris and the plume away. This purge is devised to keep the lens clean. Periodic cleansing of the lens with acetone is effective and simple.

The CO_2 laser is equipped with a coaxial aiming beam from a helium–neon (HeNe) laser. This aiming beam can be turned off or its intensity reduced during the procedure so as not to interfere with the surgeon's field of vision. It is important to remember that the apparent impact spot size of the HeNe beam on tissue may not be the same as the impact spot size of the CO_2 laser beam. This is especially true when using a defocused beam. The HeNe beam should be used to indicate the center of the beam and does not represent the spot size.

SUPER-PULSED LASERS

Continuous-wave CO_2 lasers are available with different peak power outputs. For dermatologic use, a peak output of 25 W is considered satisfactory, particularly with a 0.2-mm spot handpiece. However, higher-output lasers are available, with powers as high as 100 W. These are useful for neurosurgery but are not particularly advantageous for cutaneous applications. Super-pulsed lasers have a peak power of several hundred watts. However, short pulses are delivered rapidly (i.e., in microseconds, nanoseconds, or picoseconds). A relatively long lag period follows the pulse before the next identical pulse (Fig. 12). Theoretically, this interval allows the tissue to recover from thermal damage before it is exposed to the next impact. This has been termed tissue relaxation time. These pulses occur several hundred times per second. The interpulse interval is usually longer than the pulse itself. Therefore, the duty cycle of these lasers—the percentage of time the laser is actually on—is commonly in the 10–20% range.

These lasers are promoted as being capable of cleaner cuts and vaporization, thus minimizing tissue thermal damage and speeding up operating time. However, the most beneficial power and pulse rate settings have not been determined, and no clear advantage has been shown in clinical testing. One might theorize that diminished tissue damage, though beneficial in some ways, may actually diminish several advantages of the continuous-wave CO_2 laser, such as hemostasis and sealing of cut nerve endings. Therefore, the super-pulsed laser remains unproven. It may prove advantageous for some procedures and less acceptable for others.

More recently developed superpulsed and ultrapulsed lasers present a different type of pulse profile, which comes much closer to the "perfect" profile. Such delivery appears to be a vast improvement over that of earlier superpulsed lasers. Hemostasis appears to be maintained, and charring and thermal damage seem to be minimized.

BIBLIOGRAPHY

Apfelberg DB. *Evaluation and Installation of Surgical Laser Systems*. New York, Springer-Verlag, 1987.

Bailin PL, Ratz JL. Use of the carbon dioxide laser in dermatologic surgery. In *Lasers in Cutaneous Medicine and Surgery*. JL Ratz, ed. Chicago, Year Book Medical Publishers, 1986, pp. 73–104.

Bailin PL. Lasers in dermatology. *J Dermatol Surg Oncol* 1985;11:328–334.

Bailin PL, Ratz JL, Lutz-Nagey L. CO_2 laser modification of Mohs surgery. *J Dermatol Surg Oncol* 1981;7:621–623.

Bailin PL, Wheeland RG. Carbon dioxide (CO_2) laser perforation of exposed cranial bone to stimulate granulation tissue. *Plast Reconstr Surg* 1985;75:898–902.

Bailin PL, Ratz JL, Levine HL. Removal of tattoos by CO_2 laser. *J Dermatol Surg Oncol* 1980;6:997–1001.

David LM. The laser approach to blepharoplasty. *J Dermatol Surg Oncol* 1986;14:741–746.

David LM, Grassborg E, Lask GP. Combined carbon dioxide laser resurfacing and TCA chemical peel. *Am J Cosmet Surg* 1992;9:153–158.

Fairhurst MV, Roenigk RK, Brodland DG. Carbon dioxide laser surgery for skin disease. *May Clin Proc* 1992;(1):49–58.

Finsterbush A, Rousso M, Ashur H. Healing and tensile strength of CO_2 laser incision and scalpel wounds in rabbits. *Plast Reconstr Surg* 1982;70:360–362.

Goldman L. Comparison of the biomedical effects of the exposure of human tissue to low and high energy lasers. *Ann NY Acad Sci* 1965;122:802–813.

Goldman L. Dermatologic manifestations of laser radiation. *Fed Proc* 1965;24 (suppl 14):92–93.

Huerter CJ, Wheeland RG, Bailin PL, Ratz JL. Treatment of digital myxoid cysts with carbon dioxide laser vaporization. *J Dermatol Surg Oncol* 1987;13:723–727.

Kantor GR, Wheeland RG, Bailin PL, et al. Treatment of earlobe keloids with carbon dioxide laser excision: A report of sixteen cases. *J Dermatol Surg Oncol* 1985;11:1063–1067.

Kantor GR, Ratz JL, Wheeland RG. Treatment of acne keloidalis nuchae with carbon dioxide laser. *J Am Acad Dermatol* 1986;14:263–267.

Olbricht SM. Use of the carbon dioxide laser in dermatologic surgery. A clinically relevant update for 1993. *J Dermatol Surg Oncol* 1993;(4):364–369.

Ratz JL. Laser therapy update. *Current Issues Dermatol* 1984;2:244–251.

Ratz JL. Carbon dioxide laser treatment of balanitis xerotica obliterans. *J Am Acad Dermatol* 1984;10:925–928.

Ratz JL. Laser applications in dermatology and plastic surgery. In *Surgical Applications of Lasers.* 2nd ed. JA Dixon, ed. Chicago, Year Book Medical Publishers, 1987, pp. 160–182.

Ratz JL, Bailin PL, Levine HL. CO_2 laser treatment of port-wine stains: A preliminary report. *J Dermatol Surg Oncol* 1982;8:1039–1044.

Ratz JL, Bailin PL, Wheeland RG. Carbon dioxide laser treatment of epidermal nevi. *J Dermatol Surg Oncol* 1986;12:567–570.

Ratz JL, McGillis ST. Treatment of facial acne scarring with the carbon dioxide laser. *Am J Cosmet Surg* 1992;9:181–184.

Roenigk RK, Ratz JL. CO_2 laser treatment of cutaneous neurofibromas. *J Dermatol Surg Oncol* 1987;13:187–190.

Roenigk RK. CO_2 laser vaporization for rhinophyma. *Mayo Clin Proc* 1987;62:676–680.

Wheeland RG, Bailin PL. Scalp reduction surgery with the carbon dioxide laser. *J Dermatol Surg Oncol* 1984;10:565–569.

Wheeland RG, Bailin PL, Ratz JL. Combined carbon dioxide laser excision and vaporization in the treatment of rhinophyma. *J Dermatol Surg Oncol* 1987;13:172–177.

Wheeland RG, Bailin PL, Reynolds OD, et al. Carbon dioxide (CO_2) laser vaporization of multiple facial syringoma. *J Dermatol Surg Oncol* 1986;12:225–228.

56

Dye Lasers in Dermatology

Jerome M. Garden and Abnoeal D. Bakus
Northwestern University Medical School, Chicago, Illinois

The proliferation of various medical lasers has made it difficult to remain well informed about their potential uses. The multiple claims made about these laser systems are confusing even for laser investigators. It is incumbent on all dermatologists to have a basic understanding of the principles of laser physics and tissue interaction in order to recognize which patients and cutaneous lesions may appropriately benefit from laser surgery.

Detailed articles are available in the literature describing basic laser physics. The interaction of laser energy with tissue, however, remains an area that continues to be defined. In this chapter, laser–tissue interaction will be discussed as it applies to the dye laser and its current and future role in dermatologic surgery.

Two types of dye lasers are currently used in dermatology. One type is flashlamp pumped and the other is argon laser pumped. Both lasers use organic dyes as the lasing material but are "energized" or pumped by either a flashlamp or argon laser energy source. Organic dyes permit these lasers to emit coherent light at varying wavelengths, depending on the organic dye used and the "tuning" or filtering of the laser emission to the desired wavelength. The flashlamp-pumped dye laser only delivers pulses of energy. The argon laser–pumped dye laser delivers a continuous wave that can be electromechanically shuttered to deliver the energy in pulses, or it can be attached to a robotized scanner mechanism, which emits the light in a predetermined pulsed pattern. The flashlamp-pumped dye laser is used for the treatment of benign cutaneous small blood vessel diseases and pigmented lesions, and the argon laser-pumped dye laser is used for both blood vessel and pigmented lesions and for photodynamic therapy. Photodynamic therapy is the use of exogenous photosensitizing agents and nonionizing light (usually laser light), mainly to treat malignant disease.

The dye laser in dermatology has been generally used to treat benign cutaneous blood vessel disease. This includes port-wine hemangiomas, telangiectasia, capillary hemangiomas, and small angiomatous processes. The laser can significantly lighten or eliminate these lesions while minimizing side effects. An analysis of several intrinsic laser parameters is fundamental to understanding why this laser is beneficial.

All lasers emit coherent light at specific wavelengths peculiar to the lasing material in the optical cavity (laser tube). To treat vascular lesions, the organic dyes used as the lasing material emit a light with a wavelength in the 570–600 nm range (yellow-orange light). The skin contains two major chromophores that are considered when choosing the optimal wavelength for interaction with the targeted blood vessels. The first is oxyhemoglobin, located in the red blood cell. Oxyhemoglobin is located intravascularly in high concentrations and has three absorption bands in the visible light range. The largest band, the Soret band, is at 418 nm, while the smaller bands are at 542 and 577 nm. The second chromophore of importance is epidermal melanin. Melanin absorbs maximally in the ultraviolet range. Throughout the visible and infrared range there is a dramatic decrease in absorption.

When selecting a specific wavelength, the choice should optimize absorption by the targeted structure while minimizing nonspecific or undesired absorption. For this reason, the dye laser is originally set at 577 nm when one is treating blood vessel processes. The 577 nm wavelength coincides with the oxyhemoglobin band, which has the longest wavelength in the visible range. Although the 418 nm band is the largest and, as such, would absorb well, it is also the band closest to the ultraviolet range. Melanin absorbs best in the shorter wavelengths and would better absorb photons emitted from the laser at the 418 nm emission wavelength compared to the longer 577 nm (Fig. 1). Thus, epidermal melanin absorption, as a potential barrier to the incoming laser light, is minimized with the longer wavelength. Also, for nonionizing wavelengths, the longer the wavelength, the greater the tissue penetration. This potentially allows for treatment of deeper cutaneous structures. Indeed, studies revealed that by changing the wavelength to the slightly longer 585 nm, blood vessel specificity could be maintained while increasing tissue penetration and clinical outcome.

The next important parameter for optimizing laser therapy of benign cutaneous blood vessel processes is the length of time the laser emits its light. As mentioned earlier, the argon laser--pumped dye laser can either emit the laser light continuously onto the tissue or as a solitary pulse of light for a predetermined length of time or in a set pulsed pattern by a robotized scanner. The flashlamp-pumped dye laser always emits in pulses as the flashlamp discharges and stimulates the organic dyes. A basic principle in laser emission is that the longer the tissue receives laser irradiation, the greater the potential absorption of laser energy.

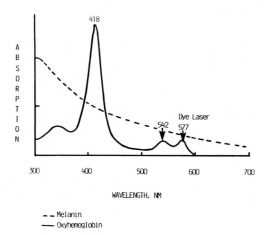

Figure 1 Absorption spectra of oxyhemoglobin and melanin.

For dye laser systems, the laser energy is mainly converted to thermal energy after chromophore absorption. Several other potential tissue changes may occur after laser impact, such as photodisruption, ablation, or plasma formation, but these reactions are nonexistent or noncontributory to the overall dye laser–tissue interaction. Specific changes are produced in tissue after laser-induced thermal–tissue reaction. If the tissue temperature increases mildly, reversible molecular changes will occur with no clinical outcome. As the temperature increases, irreversible tissue changes occur that are clinically apparent. These changes may be due to thermal necrosis or thermomechanical mechanisms such as water vaporization, which are accompanied by explosive phase change, volatilization of organic material, or acoustic and pressure wave formation.

These thermal events destroy and eliminate the targeted lesion. Selective thermal damage to the targeted vessels, with sparing of the surrounding tissue, can only be achieved through a process of thermal spatial confinement. As a structure is heated, the thermal energy initially remains contained in the heated structure. This process depends on the size, integrity, and heat-containment properties of the structure. Should the heating process remain for a long period of time, the structure may no longer be able to contain the heat, and it will diffuse into the surrounding environment. Thermal relaxation time reflects the ability of a structure to contain heat within itself. This factor can be calculated for cutaneous blood vessels and is helpful for predicting how much time the laser should irradiate the tissue to effect selective blood vessel thermal damage.

Thermal spatial confinement to the blood vessels can be achieved with a pulsed laser system (Fig. 2). The laser emits light for a predetermined time in a single pulse and, with preferential absorption of oxyhemoglobin, a conversion of light energy to thermal energy occurs. Only during the laser pulse is heat generated in the blood vessel. If the laser emits for a longer period of time than is necessary solely to achieve blood vessel damage, the perivascular area will begin to be heated. To maximize blood vessel thermal damage selectivity, the laser discharge should be less than the thermal relaxation time of the targeted blood vessel. Calculated times for blood vessels of the port-wine hemangioma are in the 1- to 10-msec range. If the laser pulse is shorter than this range, an optimal degree of thermal spatial confinement may be achieved.

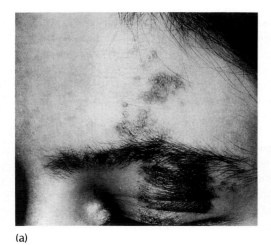 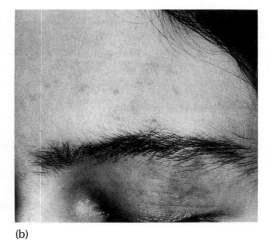

(a)   (b)

Figure 2   (a) Purple port-wine hemangioma in a 27-year-old woman. (b) After three pulsed dye laser treatments.

The argon-pumped dye laser pulsed mode exceeds this time frame. When used with a robotized scanner, the pulse durations have been reduced and are approaching the calculated msec range. The flashlamp-pumped dye laser is able to produce pulses within the desired times. Cutaneous blood vessel disease patients have been treated with the flashlamp-pumped system at the 400–500 µsec/pulse range. This is appropriately below the calculated 1–10 msec thermal relaxation time of the targeted vessels.

When pulses shorter than 500 µsec are used, although there is selective damage to the blood vessel, different mechanisms of damage occur. A rapid pulse of 1.5 µsec produces blood vessel–specific changes; however, the blood vessels have a shattered appearance with a relative lack of endothelial necrosis. This is attributed to rapid vaporization and phase expansion associated with quick incorporation of laser power. The slower 400- to 500-µsec pulses produce more diffuse endothelial necrosis, while thermal damage is still limited to the blood vessel. The less explosive nature of the longer pulse duration allows for more homogeneous endothelial thermal denaturation and necrosis. The clinical results reflect these manifestations of thermal-induced damage. The longer pulses are better able to lighten ectatic vessels than the more rapid pulses. Although the rapid pulses produce significant vascular fragmentation, the blood vessel is repaired and remains clinically unchanged.

After selecting an appropriate wavelength for the laser emission and pulse duration, the degree of blood vessel thermal damage selectivity has been dramatically increased. Another important parameter is the amount of laser energy emitted per pulse. The goal is to emit only the amount of energy necessary to cause the desired thermal events. Any additional energy may generate enough heat to damage the perivascular area. Clinical studies have revealed that only 5.00–8.50 J/cm^2 of energy are necessary to achieve the desired selectivity at a wavelength of 585 nm and pulse duration of 500 µsec.

A substantial increase in selective blood vessel damage occurs with this fundamental understanding of laser–tissue interaction. The flashlamp-pumped dye laser has produced very acceptable clinical results based on these principles. Histologic changes of both normal skin and port-wine hemangiomas reflect the increased therapeutic selectivity. Although there is intense purpura immediately after laser therapy at these settings, histologically there is no or rare extravasation of red blood cells. Instead, an intravascular coagulum of fused red blood cells and fibrin is apparent with diffuse endothelial cell necrosis. There is little evidence of perivascular damage. All collagen appears to be intact, with no thermal damage with electron microscopy. The epidermis is essentially unchanged with only focal areas of intercellular edema in the basal layer. After one month, biopsies of treated port-wine hemangioma reveal vessels of normal caliber.

The flashlamp-pumped dye laser has been used to treat thousands of patients with cutaneous blood vessel disease. The majority have had port-wine stains, and the remainder have had various telangiectatic or angiomatous processes. A pinprick sensation is associated with the impact of the laser light. This discomfort is generally tolerable in adults, so there is little need for anesthesia. Children, however, tolerate the procedure better after the use of topical anesthetics, sedation, or general anesthesia.

Port-wine stain patients are generally treated using the flashlamp-pumped dye laser at energies of 5.50–8.50 J/cm^2. The lower energies are usually reserved for pediatric cases. Test sites are placed with various energy levels over the lesion. Various anatomic sites differ in their response to the laser and need to be considered prior to therapy.

The intense purpura that occurs with laser impact resolves in 5–14 days in these patients. There may be some transient postinflammatory hyperpigmentation, which can be present for several more weeks. Hyperpigmentation over the lower extremities can be very prolonged, persisting for more than 12 months in some cases. Once the purpura resolves, the treated lesional area gradually fades over the next 6–10 weeks. It is for this reason that any retreatment of the lesion is postponed for 2–3 months. Patients less than 3 years of age may be treated at 2-month intervals, while those older may receive some benefit in waiting the additional month. Continued fading of the treated area has occurred even after 3 months in some of these lesions.

After the test sites have been evaluated, even large areas may be treated during one procedural session. It is not uncommon to be able to treated a lesion that covers one third to one half of the face. Almost always there is some residual lesion present after the first treatment. The same area may necessitate several treatment sessions in order to obtain the maximum therapeutic outcome. At least 75% of port-wine stains achieve 50% lesional lightening, with 50% of these lesions responding by at least 75%. These results can be achieved in three to five treatment sessions, with further procedures continuing to be beneficial. The pediatric patient responds more readily to therapy.

The most important clinical advance has been in the ability to accomplish the above lesional clearing while significantly reducing undesired side effects. There have been only occasional cases of permanent hypo- or hyperpigmentation, cutaneous atrophy, or depression. Even rarer have been the cases of cutaneous fibrosis or, especially, raised scarring. Even when adverse effects occur, they have been localized to small sections of the total treated areas.

Patients having very melanized skin, such as those with skin type V or VI or those with nodular lesions, respond less favorably to the flashlamp-pumped dye laser. Patients with hypertrophic lesions may be more responsive to other lasers used for the treatment of cutaneous vascular lesions, such as the argon-pumped dye in a continuous or pulsed mode or the copper vapor or krypton lasers. These lasers generally produce more nonspecific thermal damage, which can shrink involved tissues. However, with this added thermal dimension, there can be a loss of safety, especially in the pediatric population.

Although there have been only rare occurrences of scarring or induration with the flashlamp-pumped dye laser, this does not preclude their potential occurrence from increasing. As described earlier, even though the laser parameters have been significantly optimized to increase blood vessel damage selectivity, the events that produce the desired changes are thermomechanical. As such, it is always possible to sufficiently incorporate too much energy into the tissue, producing perivascular damage and clinical fibrosis. There appears to be a therapeutic energy window for these patients. If too much energy is incorporated into the tissue, there is a significant potential for an increase in scarring. If not enough energy is used, the clinical results are unapparent. When patients who have experienced minor skin changes, such as scattered focal hypopigmentation, are subsequently treated with lower energy doses, even these minor adverse effects do not recur.

Another cutaneous vascular lesion that has been successfully treated with the flashlamp-pumped dye laser is the capillary hemangioma. Flatter lesions have been totally eliminated, while rapidly growing lesions have stopped proliferating with therapy. Although almost all of these lesions eventually spontaneously regress during childhood, lesions that are present over anatomically important areas, such as periorificial, anogenital, or periorbital areas, or areas that are very apparent, may be candidates for laser therapy.

Response to the laser has been greatest with the superficial type of capillary hemangioma (Fig. 3). Deep or cavernous hemangiomas or mixed hemangiomas with a significant deep component do not respond well to the laser. Studies have revealed that superficial lesions 3 mm thick or less respond best. It appears that the limited laser penetration diminishes its effect on thicker lesions. It is not uncommon to have the superficial portion of mixed hemangioma respond effectively to the laser while the deep region continues to enlarge.

The dye laser appears to be able to beneficially treat almost all superficial small vessel cutaneous processes. These include telangiectasia, permanent erythema (Fig. 4) from such sources as trauma or rosacea, poikiloderma of Civatte, and papular and spider angiomas. Raised vascu-

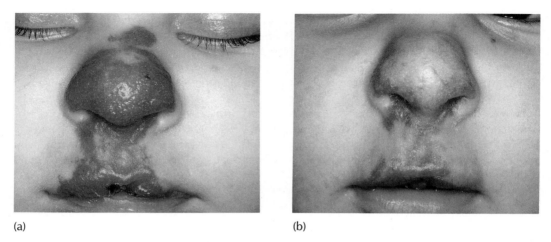

(a)   (b)

Figure 3 (a) Superficial hemangioma in a 2-month-old female. (b) After four treatments with the pulsed dye laser and a 3-month course of oral steroids. Child is 8 months old and 3 months off steroids.

lar processes such as cherry (senile) angiomas or pyogenic granulomas can be treated but are limited in their response by the thickness of the particular lesion. Although telangiectasia (Fig. 5) over the face respond very favorably to these lasers, spider veins over the lower extremities are therapeutically more problematic. Very small caliber veins have responded well, while the larger vessels are less responsive and have been associated with prolonged postoperative browning of the treated area.

Two other important cutaneous lesions have been treated with the flashlamp-pumped dye laser. The first is warts: regular, flat, periungual, and plantar verrucae (Fig. 6) have been successfully treated. The more keratotic lesions are less responsive but still have been eradicated with successive procedures. Plantar warts are the most resistive to this process. The mechanism of therapeutic action is not understood and may have to do with vascular destruction followed by necrosis of the infected epidermal cells. Higher energies are usually necessary to treat these lesions,

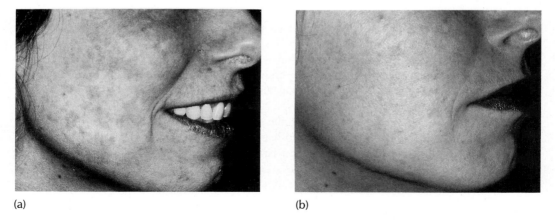

(a)   (b)

Figure 4 (a) Permanent erythema after accidental scalding with hot water as a child; patient is a 40-year-old woman. (b) After two pulsed dye laser treatments

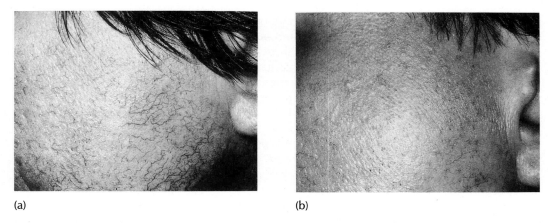

(a)   (b)

Figure 5   (a) Familial essential telangiectasia in a 41-year-old man. (b) After one pulsed dye laser treatment

producing scaling and crusting. The treated areas generally heal well, without the scarring often accompanying electrotherapy or carbon dioxide laser therapy.

Scar tissue not only exhibits decreased erythema, but also a reduction in lesional thickness when treated with the flashlamp-pumped dye laser. Originally recognized with the treatment of port-wine stains that had scarred from prior therapeutic modalities, this effect has been seen with scars induced from multiple sources. The reason behind the reduction in scar tissue thickness is unknown, with speculation as to effect on collagen production and/or the underlying scar vasculature.

When using the flashlamp-pumped dye laser at a 510 nm wavelength and a 300-nsec pulse duration, it is possible to selectively treat epidermal melanocytic-pigmented lesions. Such lesions as lentigines respond very well to the laser. The chosen wavelength is closer to the ultraviolet

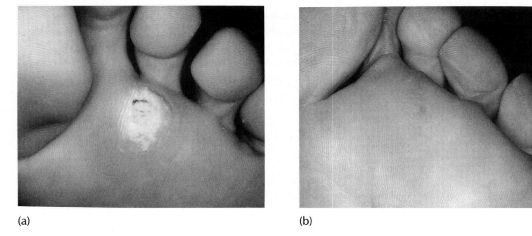

(a)   (b)

Figure 6   (a) Left plantar verruca in a 42-year-old female. Lesion present for 4 years and treated with topical acids, paring, and the CO_2 laser with persistence. (b) After three treatments with the pulsed dye laser and at 7-month follow-up.

range, where melanin has its most effective absorption and the pulse duration is rapid enough to maintain the thermal damage to the melanin containing cell structure. It is of interest that this laser at these parameters also has been used to treat red tattoo pigment. Although this process is dermal and dermal melanocytic processes do not appear to be affected by this laser, the red dermal tattoo pigment does respond. Perhaps after absorption, there is sufficient dermal inflammation in order to induce enough red tattoo pigment elimination to be clinically effective.

The dye laser has played a key role in the field of photodynamic therapy. Argon-pumped dye lasers emitting in a continuous mode from 630 nm (red light) to the mid-700 nm range have been used to irradiate cutaneous malignancies after the patient has received systemic photosensitizers. The systemic photosensitizer generally used for experimental evaluation in photodynamic therapy has been a hematoporphyrin derivative. A porphyrin dimer held together by an ether linkage, dihematoporphyrin ether, has been suggested as the active component of hematoporphyrin derivative and is now used for therapy.

Dihematoporphyrin ether is administered intravenously. A 48- to 72-hr waiting period is allowed for accentuated accumulation of the porphyrin into the tumor area relative to the skin. Porphyrins are selectively retained in tissue with rapid turnover, such as malignancies. The molecules can be activated by nearly all wavelengths of light in the visible and ultraviolet A (UVA) spectrum. However, the 630 nm wavelength range is used clinically, since there is greater penetration.

The phototoxic effect of porphyrin and laser light in the tumor is believed to occur at both the cellular and the tissue levels. Cellular membranes including the outer cell and nuclear membranes, as well as mitochondria, have been implicated. At the tumor level, the vasculature is believed to be the site of phototoxicity leading to tumor necrosis.

Several cutaneous malignancies have been treated, including basal cell carcinoma. The response has been varied, while the true efficacy still must be evaluated by controlled, well-designed studies. A significant adverse effect of therapy is a severe generalized photosensitization due to the systemic administration of porphyrin. The patient remains photosensitized to UVA and visible light for a minimum of 30 days. Although there is a preferential retention of the porphyrin in the tumor versus the skin, enough porphyrin still remains in the skin to cause persistent photosensitization.

Areas of research in the field of photodynamic therapy include other photosensitizers that may allow a greater relative tumor accumulation, topical or intralesional injection of dihemotoporphyrin ether to eliminate the generalized photosensitization, and the use of tumor-specific monoclonal antibodies that conjugate with photosensitizing agents. Treatment of other cutaneous hyperproliferative processes such as psoriasis and the development of new laser light–delivery systems that optimize laser parameters to enhance therapeutic selectivity are also being investigated.

BIBLIOGRAPHY

Alster TS, Kurban AK, Grove GL, Grove MJ, Tan OT. Alteration of argon laser-induced scars by the pulsed dye laser. *Lasers Surg Med* 1993;13:368–373.

Anderson RR, Parrish JA. Microvasculature can be selectively damaged using dye lasers: A basic theory and experimental evidence in human skin. *Lasers Surg Med* 1981;1:263–276.

Anderson RR, Parrish JA. Selective photothermolysis: Precise microsurgery by selective absorption of pulsed radiation. *Science* 1983;220:524–527.

Arndt KA, Noe JM, Northam DBC, Itzkan I. Laser therapy: Basic concepts and nomenclature. *J Am Acad Dermatol* 1981;5:649–654.

Ashinoff R, Geronemus RG. Capillary hemangiomas and treatment with the flashlamp pumped dye laser. *Arch Dermatol* 1991;127:202–205.

Ashinoff R, Geronemus RG. Flashlamp-pumped pulsed dye laser for portwine stains in infancy: Earlier versus later treatment. *J Am Acad Dermatol* 1991;24:467–72.

Berns MW, McCullough JL. Porphyrin sensitized phototherapy. *Arch Dermatol* 1986;122:871–874.

Dougherty TJ. Photoradiation therapy for cutaneous and subcutaneous malignancies. *J Invest Dermatol* 1981;77:122–124.

Dougherty TJ. Photosensitization of malignant tumors. *Semin Surg Oncol* 1986;2:24–37.

Dougherty TJ, Cooper MT, Mang TS. Cutaneous phototoxic occurrences in patients receiving Photofrin. *Lasers Surg Med* 1990;10:485–488.

Fitzpatrick RE, Goldman MP, Ruiz-Esparza J. Laser treatment of benign pigmented epidermal lesions using a 300 nsecond pulse and 510 nm wavelength. *J Dermatol Surg Oncol* 1993;19:341–347.

Garden JM, Bakus AD. Clinical efficacy of the pulsed dye laser in the treatment of vascular lesions. *J Dermatol Surg Oncol* 1993;19:321–326.

Garden JM, Bakus AD, Paller AS. Treatment of cutaneous hemangiomas by the flashlamp-pumped pulsed dye laser: Prospective analysis. *J Pediatr* 1992;120:555–560.

Garden JM, Burton CS, Geronemus R. Dye laser treatment of children with portwine stains. *N Engl J Med* 1989;321:901–902.

Garden JM, Geronemus RG. Dermatologic laser surgery. *J Dermatol Surg Oncol* 1990;16:156–168.

Garden JM, Tan OT, Kerschmann R, Boll J, Furumoto H, Anderson RR, Parrish JA. Effect of dye laser pulse duration on selective cutaneous vascular injury. *J Invest Dermatol* 1986;87:653–657.

Garden JM, Tan OT, Parrish JA. The pulsed dye laser: Its use at 577 nm wavelength. *J Dermatol Surg Oncol* 1987;13:134–138.

Geronemus RG. Pulsed dye laser treatment of vascular lesions in children. *J Dermatol Surg Oncol* 1993;19:303–310.

Goldman MP, Fitzpatrick RE, Ruiz-Esparza J. Treatment of portwine stains (capillary malformation) with the flashlamp-pumped dye laser. *J Pediatr* 1993;122:71–77.

Gonzalez E, Gange RW, Momtaz KT. Treatment of telangiectases and other benign vascular lesions with the 577 nm pulsed dye laser. *J Am Acad Dermatol* 1992;27:220–226.

Grekin RC, Shelton RM, Geisse JK, Frieden I. 510 nm pigmented lesion dye laser: Its characteristics and clinical uses. *J Dermatol Surg Oncol* 1993;19:380–387.

Lowe NJ, Behr KL, Fitzpatrick R, Goldman M, Ruiz-Esparza J. Flashlamp pumped dye laser for rosacea-associated telangiectasia and erythema. *J Dermatol Surg Oncol* 1991;17:522–525.

Lui H, Anderson RR. Photodynamic therapy in dermatology: Shedding a different light on skin disease. *Arch Dermatol* 1992;128,1631–1636.

Morelli JG, Tan OT, Garden J, Margolis R, Seki Y, Boll J, Carney JM, Anderson RR, Furumoto H, Parrish JA. Tunable dye laser (577 nm) treatment of portwine stains. *Lasers Surg Med* 1986;6:94–99.

Polla LL, Tan OT, Garden JM, Parrish JA. Tunable pulsed dye laser for the treatment of benign cutaneous vascular ectasia. *Dermatologica* 1987;174:11–17.

Rabinowitz L, Esterly N, ed. Anesthesia and/or sedation for pulsed dye laser therapy: Special symposium. *Pediatr Dermatol* 1992;9:132–153.

Renfro L, Geronemus R. Anatomical differences of portwine stains in response to treatment with the pulsed dye laser. *Arch Dermatol* 1993;128:182–188.

Swinehart JM. Hypertrophic scarring resulting from the flashlamp-pumped pulsed dye laser surgery. *J Am Acad Dermatol* 1991;25:845–846.

Tan OT, Carney JM, Margolis R, Seki Y, Boll J, Anderson RR, Parrish JA. Histologic responses to portwine stains treated by argon, carbon dioxide, and tunable dye lasers: A preliminary report. *Arch Dermatol* 1986;122:1016–1022.

Tan OT, Hurwitz RM, Stafford TJ. Pulsed dye laser treatment of recalcitrant verrucae: A preliminary report. *Lasers Surg Med* 1993;13;127–137.

Tan OT, Morelli JG. Kurban AK. Pulsed dye treatment of benign cutaneous pigmented lesions. *Lasers Surg Med* 1992;12,538–542.

Tan OT, Morrison P, Kurban AK. 585 nm for the treatment of portwine stains. *Plast Reconstr Surg* 1990;86:1112–1117.

Tan OT, Sherwood K, Gilchrest BA. Treatment of children with portwine stains using the flashlamp-pumped tunable dye laser. *N Engl J Med* 1989;320:416–421.

van Gemert MJC, Hulsbergen Henning JP. A model approach to laser coagulation of dermal vascular lesions. *Arch Dermatol Res* 1981;270:429–439.

Wilson BD, Mang TS, Cooper M, Stoll H. Use of photodynamic therapy for the treatment of extensive basal cell carcinomas. *Facial Plast Surg* 1990;6:185–189.

Wilson BD, Mang TS, Stoll H, Jones C, Cooper M, Dougherty TJ. Photodynamic therapy for the treatment of basal cell carcinoma. *Arch Dermatol* 1992;128:1597–1601.

57

Laser Treatment of Tattoos and Pigmented Lesions

Arielle N. B. Kauvar and Roy G. Geronemus
*New York University Medical Center and Laser and Skin
Surgery Center of New York, New York, New York*

Dramatic advances in the technological development of lasers over the course of the past decade have revolutionized the treatment of tattoos and a variety of benign pigmented lesions. The need for gross tissue excision or destruction has been substantially replaced by the selective removal of pigment particles and melanin within these lesions by pulsed lasers. Amateur and professional tattoos, as well as cosmetic, medicinal, and traumatic tattoos, can be cleared or lightened by these newer lasers with a minimal risk of scarring. Pigmented lesions treatable with these lasers include ephelides, solar lentigines, café-au-lait macules, nevi of Ota, and Becker's nevi. Melasma and postinflammatory hyperpigmentation respond variably to pulsed laser treatment.

The first lasers used to treat tattoos and pigmented lesions were continuous wave lasers that operate in the green (argon, 488–514 nm), red (ruby, 694 nm), and infrared (carbon dioxide, 10,600 nm) regions of the electromagnetic spectrum. These lasers produced nonselective thermal destruction of pigment-containing structures, often resulting in scar formation. The most dramatic advances in the technological development of lasers, as well as in our understanding of the mechanisms of laser–tissue interaction, came during the past decade. With the development of the concept of selective photothermolysis and high-peak-power, short-pulsed lasers, the damage caused by laser light could be effectively confined to specific targets, such as melanin and ink particles, without harming adjacent tissues, virtually eliminating the risk of scarring.

LASER–TISSUE INTERACTION

Laser light has several unique properties that make it ideal for targeting specific structures in the skin. Laser light is monochromatic (i.e., concentrated within 1 nm of a single wavelength) and can be focused into very small spot sizes. A biologic effect is produced when laser light is taken up by specific light-absorbing molecules in the skin called chromophores. Examples of such molecules include hemoglobin, melanin, tattoo ink, and water. Specific chromophore-containing skin structures, such as pigment particles or melanocytes, can be targeted with lasers by choosing a wavelength of light that is well absorbed by the particular chromophore but poorly absorbed by surrounding substances in the nearby tissues.

Before the advent of short-pulsed, high-energy lasers during the past decade, the continuous wave lasers used to destroy cutaneous vascular and pigmented lesions, including the argon, carbon dioxide, continuous wave, ruby, and neodymium:yttrium-aluminum-garnet (Nd:YAG) lasers, could not induce thermal destruction confined to specific skin structures. Heat produced within the targeted chromophores was conducted to adjacent tissues, making scarring a constant risk.

The concept of selective photothermolysis emerged in the 1970s, and with the application of this principle to laser development, newer-technology lasers were produced that could direct preferential injury to targeted tissue structures using very brief, selectively absorbed laser pulses. This technological advancement enabled lasers to remove vascular and pigmented lesions without damaging the surrounding skin.

Two principles must be satisfied in order to achieve selective photothermolysis of cutaneous structures. First, a wavelength of light must be chosen that provides acceptably selective absorption by the targeted chromophore. Second, the laser light must be produced with a pulse duration shorter than or equal to the thermal relaxation time of the targeted structure. The thermal relaxation time is the characteristic time for an object to lose heat energy to its surroundings. Therefore, with sufficiently brief pulses of laser light, the heat produced by the laser energy is contained wholly within the targeted structure, such as the melanosome or pigment particle, without diffusing to nearby tissues.

TATTOOS

Approximately 10 million Americans, or 5% of the population in the United States, are decorated by at least one tattoo. Traumatic tattoos resulting from vehicular accidents and firearms explosions and medicinal tattoos used to define radiation ports are also common. Tattooing with skin-colored pigments is used for the purpose of camouflaging vascular birthmarks, infraorbital hyperpigmentation, and unwanted decorative tattoos. The application of red, black, and brown pigments to eyebrows, lip lines, and cheeks simulating eyeliner, lipliner, and blush has become increasingly popular.

Many modalities have been used in the past to remove tattoos, including excisional surgery, acid applications, cryosurgery, dermabrasion, and salabrasion, but all result in undesirable scarring. Treatment of tattoos with a laser was first reported as having poor results by Goldman et al. in the 1960s using a continuous wave (500 msec pulse duration) ruby laser. Improved outcomes were then achieved by these same investigators using a very short-pulsed (20 nsec) Q-switched ruby laser, but these studies were then abandoned for some 20 years.

Continuous Wave Laser Treatment

Treatment of tattoos with two continuous wave lasers, the argon and carbon dioxide lasers, was explored in the 1980s. The carbon dioxide laser emits a continuous wave at 10,600 nm that is absorbed by its tissue chromophore, water. Tattoos are removed with the carbon dioxide laser by direct vaporization of pigment-containing tissue as well as thermal necrosis of adjacent tissue. Nonconfined thermal damage can be extensive and often leads to hypertrophic scarring (Fig.1) with the use of a continuous wave carbon dioxide laser. Scarring was only somewhat improved by the development of a superpulsed carbon dioxide laser that could be used in a pulsed mode, which ablates tissue more efficiently and therefore limits the nonspecific thermal damage to tissue.

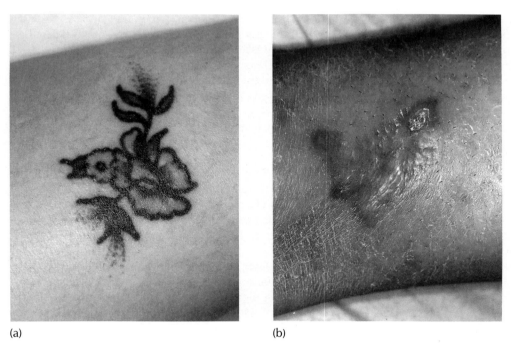

(a)   (b)

Figure 1   (a) Multicolored tattoo prior to treatment. (b) Hypertrophic scar after treatment with the carbon dioxide laser.

With either a continuous beam or repetitive pulse of 50–200 msec, power settings of 8–25 W are used to treat tattoos with the carbon dioxide laser. Repetitive treatments are necessary to effectively lighten or clear tattoos and appear to contribute to nonspecific tissue necrosis. In an effort to limit carbon dioxide laser exposure to one treatment session, a technique was devised whereby carbon dioxide laser vaporization of the tattoo to the level of the papillary dermis using powers of 10–15 W was combined with the application of 50% urea in hydrophilic ointment for 1–2 weeks. Cosmetic outcomes were still unpredictable with this technique.

The argon laser was initially used to treat tattoos because of the absorption by tattoo pigments of its 488 nm and 514 nm wavelengths. Nonspecific thermal damage resulting in scarring was seen with the argon laser because the 488 nm and 514 nm wavelengths are also absorbed by melanin and hemoglobin. The argon laser is used as a continuous beam or shuttered pulses of 50–200 msec with powers ranging from 1- to 3.5 W. As with the carbon dioxide laser, the long pulse duration of the argon laser allows extensive diffusion of heat from all absorbing tissue chromophores, and unacceptable scarring results.

Pulsed Laser Treatment

The recent development of high-peak-power, short-pulse-duration lasers based on the theory of selective photothermolysis allowed for excellent lightening or complete removal of tattoos with a minimal risk of scarring. Effective removal of tattoo pigments and excellent cosmetic outcomes with the Q-switched ruby laser were reported by Reid et al. in 1983 and subsequently confirmed by other investigators. Green, black, and blue pigments are well absorbed by the 694 nm red light of the ruby laser, and its pulsewidth is shorter than the thermal relaxation time of the ink particles found within tattoos. The latest models of the Q-switched ruby laser have a pulse duration of 20–40 nsec, spot sizes of 3–6.5 mm, and a pulse delivery rate of 1–2 sec (0.5–1 Hz).

Treatment of tattoos with the Q-switched ruby laser is usually performed at fluences of 6–10 J/cm^2. Immediately following the impact of the laser light on skin, the treated area turns greywhite (Fig. 2), followed by a wheal and flare reaction. Pinpoint bleeding and tissue splatter are common, especially when higher fluences are used. Hypopigmentation occurs in approximately 50% of treated patients and is usually transient (Fig. 3). Precautions used to protect the operator from contact with blood and tissue splatter include the use of a transparent film (e.g., Tegaderm or Vigilon) applied to the treatment site or plastic extender tubes placed over the laser's handpiece.

The 1064 nm Q-switched Nd:YAG laser operates in the near-infrared portion of the electromagnetic spectrum at 1064 nm and has a pulse duration of 10 nsec. At fluences of 6–12 J/cm^2, the 1064 nm Q-switched Nd:YAG laser effectively removes black and blue pigment. As with the Q-switched ruby laser, whitening of the treated area is the desired clinical response. The Q-switched Nd:YAG laser has available spot sizes of 1.5, 2, and 3 mm and a repetition rate of up to 10 pulses per sec (10 Hz).

In contrast to the 694 nm Q-switched ruby laser, it was thought that the longer 1064 nm wavelength of the Q-switched Nd:YAG laser would result in increased dermal penetration and decreased melanin absorption, thereby improving pigment removal and avoiding hyperpigmentation. Although less hyperpigmentation was noted with the Q-switched Nd:YAG laser than with the Q-switched ruby laser, the higher fluences and shorter pulsewidth of the Nd:YAG laser results in more tissue debris and bleeding. Safety precautions taken with the Nd:YAG laser include the use of transparent films and extender tubes as described for the Q-switched ruby laser. While the Q-switched ruby laser effectively removes black, blue, and green pigments, the Q-switched Nd:YAG laser can remove black and blue, but not green, ink. The number of treatments necessary to clear a dark-colored amateur or professional tattoo are generally the same with both lasers. A frequency-doubling crystal added to the 1064 nm Q-switched Nd:YAG halves its wavelength to 532 nm, producing laser light in the visible green spectrum. The 532 nm Q-switched Nd:YAG laser effectively treats red ink, but not black or blue pigments (Fig. 4).

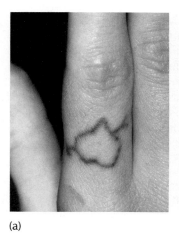 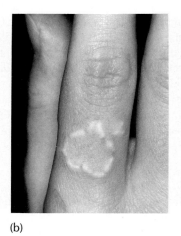 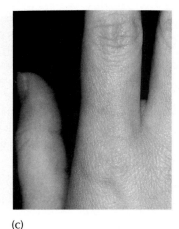

(a)   (b)   (c)

Figure 2 (a) Amateur tattoo prior to treatment with the Q-switched ruby laser. (b) Whitening of tattoo immediately following a treatment session. (c) Complete clearance after four treatment sessions with the Q-switched ruby laser.

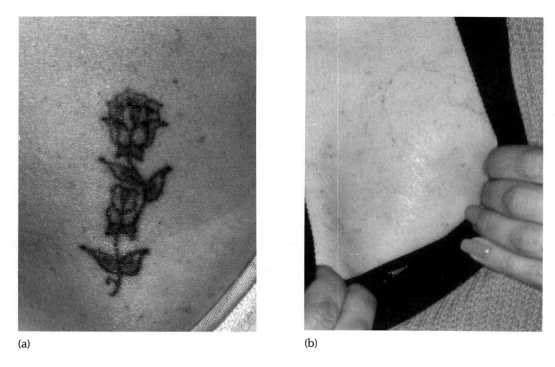

(a) (b)

Figure 3 (a) Professional tattoo on a woman's chest prior to treatment. Treatment took place with the 694 nm Q-switched ruby laser. (b) Complete clearance with transient hypopigmentation following seven treatment sessions.

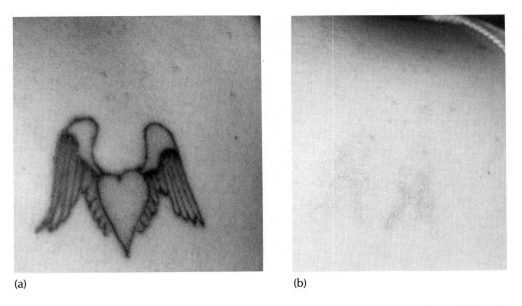

(a) (b)

Figure 4 (a) Multicolored professional tattoo prior to treatment. (b) Approximately 90% lightening after six treatment sessions with the Q-switched ruby laser for the black pigment and the Q-switched Nd:YAG laser for the red pigment.

The Q-switched alexandrite laser is the third Q-switched laser developed for the treatment of tattoos. This laser has a wavelength of 755 nm and a pulse duration of 100 nsec, as is delivered through a homogeneous 3 mm beam. The repetition rate of this laser is 1 Hz. Black, blue, and green pigments are effectively treated with the Q-switched alexandrite laser. Fluences of 6–10 J/cm^2 are used to treat tattoos. Clinically, epidermal lightening and slight tissue edema result immediately after laser impact, as is seen with the Q-switched ruby and Q-switched Nd:YAG lasers. Although hypopigmentation is a common side effect, occurring in approximately 50% of treated patients, it is usually transient and gradually resolves over a period of 1–12 months. When higher fluences are used, purpura, pinpoint bleeding, and tissue splatter occur. Red, purple, yellow, and orange pigments do not respond well to the Q-switched alexandrite laser.

The 510 nm flashlamp-pumped pulsed dye laser has a pulse duration of 300 nsec and was originally developed to treat superficial melanocytic lesions. This green light laser was found to effectively remove red tattoo pigments and variably lightens purple, yellow, and orange-colored tattoos.

At present, no one laser can remove all tattoo colors well (Table 1). Black, blue, and green inks are well absorbed by red and infrared light lasers (Fig. 5). The 694 nm Q-switched ruby, 1064 nm Q-switched Nd:YAG, and 755 nm Q-switched alexandrite lasers are all effective in eliminating black tattoo colors. In addition, green tattoo pigments are effectively treated with the Q-switched ruby and Q-switched alexandrite lasers, but not the 1064 nm Q-switched Nd:YAG laser. Red inks are not well absorbed by red or infrared light lasers, but are well absorbed by green light lasers. The frequency-doubled 532 nm Nd:YAG as well as the 510 nm pulsed dye laser, which are ineffective for dark tattoo pigments, are effectively absorbed by red tattoo inks. Purple, yellow, and orange pigments are often more difficult to eradicate and respond variably well to green, red, and infrared light lasers.

An in vitro agarose gel assay has recently been developed to examine the responsiveness of various color tattoo inks to Q-switched laser treatment. A spectrum of pigments used in amateur and professional, as well as cosmetic, tattoos were tested using this assay for their ability to absorb laser light from the 694 nm Q-switched ruby and the 1064 nm and frequency-doubled 532 nm Q-switched Nd:YAG lasers. We found that green tattoo pigments responded best to the Q-switched ruby laser, and red tattoo pigments responded best to the 532 nm Q-switched

Table 1 Response of Tattoo Colors to Pulsed Laser Therapy

Color	Q-switched ruby (694 nm)	Q-switched Nd:YAG (694 nm)	Q-switched Nd:YAG (532 nm)	Q-switched alexandrite (755 nm)	Pulsed green dye (510 nm)
Black—amateur	+ +	+ +	–	+ +	–
Black—professional	+ +	+ +	–	+ +	–
Blue	+ +	+	–	+ +	–
Green	+ +	–	–	+ +	–
Brown	+ +	+	–	+ +	–
Red	–	–	+ +	–	+ +
Yellow	+	+	+	+	+
Orange	+	+	+	+	+
Purple	+	+	+	+	+

+ +, Excellent response; +, moderate response; –, poor response.

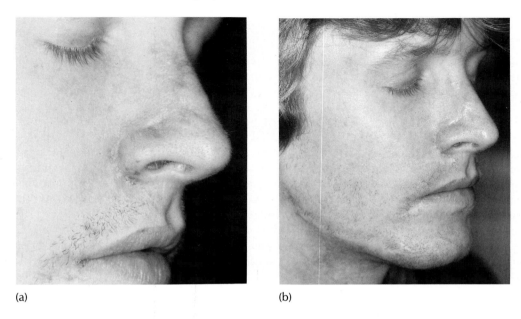

(a)   (b)

Figure 5 (a) Traumatic tattoo prior to treatment. (b) Approximately 90% lightening after four treatment sessions with the Q-switched ruby laser.

Nd:YAG laser, confirming our clinical experience. Some purple, yellow, and orange pigments responded well to the 532 nm Nd:YAG laser, while others were better absorbed by the Q-switched ruby or 1064 nm Q-switched Nd:YAG.

Several studies have compared the relative efficacy of different Q-switched lasers in treating the same tattoos. Although in many of these studies sample sizes were too small for accurate comparisons, certain trends have emerged from these investigations. The Q-switched ruby and 1064 nm Q-switched Nd:YAG are equally effective in removing black pigment. Black pigment removal is somewhat slower with the Q-switched alexandrite laser. The Q-switched ruby and Q-switched alexandrite lasers are more effective in the removal of green ink than the 1064 nm Q-switched Nd:YAG laser. More textural change and hyperpigmentation result from the 1064 nm Q-switched Nd:YAG laser, and more hypopigmentation results from the Q-switched ruby and Q-switched alexandrite lasers.

Several generalizations can be made concerning the treatment of tattoos with all of the Q-switched lasers. Although some patients can tolerate laser therapy of their tattoos without anesthesia, many patients desire local anesthesia, which is administered with injections of 1% lidocaine with epinephrine. To achieve 75–100% lightening of tattoos, amateur tattoos generally require 4–6 treatment sessions, while professional tattoos require 6–10 laser procedures. Laser treatments are usually performed at intervals of 4–8 weeks. The carbon-based and India ink pigments found in amateur tattoos appear to clear more easily than the organic dyes in professional tattoos. The greater density of ink placed in professional tattoos may also be a factor. Older tattoos usually require fewer treatments than newer tattoos, and distally placed tattoos are slower to respond than more proximal tattoos. These phenomena may relate to tattoo ink dispersion over time and the relative efficiency of lymphatic drainage in different anatomic locations.

Laser Therapy of Cosmetic Tattoos

Laser removal of cosmetic tattoos, especially those with skin-colored pink, tan, or white pigments, should be approached with caution. Immediate, irreversible darkening of cosmetic tattoos following Q-switched and pulsed laser treatment has recently been described (Fig. 6). Irreversible ink darkening has been documented to occur with the Q-switched ruby (694 nm), Q-switched Nd:YAG (1064 nm/532 nm), and pulsed green dye (510 nm) lasers, but it can occur with any high-energy, short-pulse-duration laser operating in the visible through near-infrared wavelengths. In only some cases was removal of the darkened ink possible with subsequent laser treatments. Patients who seek laser removal of cosmetic tattoos must be forewarned of this possible complication, and test sites should be performed before embarking on treatment of a large area.

Although the chemical mechanism of tattoo ink darkening is unknown, it is likely that conversion of ferric oxide (Fe_2O_3) to ferrous oxide (FeO) and/or other iron compounds is involved. Extreme temperatures, pressures, and free charge carriers induced by high-peak-power laser pulses presumably cause this conversion to ferrous oxide. In vitro tests have demonstrated the conversion of white, yellow, red, and brown pigments, composed of ferric oxide, to a gray-black color immediately following exposure to Q-switched ruby (694 nm) or Q-switched Nd:YAG (1064 nm/532 nm) lasers.

BENIGN PIGMENTED LESIONS

Continuous Wave Laser Treatment

Lasers have been successfully used to destroy pigmented lesions in the skin for over a decade. The first lasers used to treat pigmentation were the continuous wave lasers including the argon at 488 nm and 514 nm, the Nd:YAG at 1064 nm, the copper vapor laser at 510 nm, and the carbon dioxide laser at 10,600 nm. Of the continuous wave lasers, the argon laser has been used most successfully to treat pigmented lesions. Since melanin has a maximum absorption coefficiency in the 500–600 nm wavelengths, it readily absorbs the blue-green light of the argon laser. Small epidermal pigmented lesions, including lentigines (Fig. 7), seborrheic keratoses, and

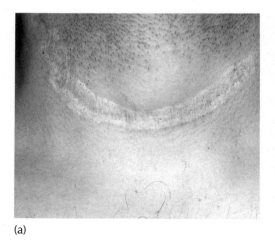
(a)

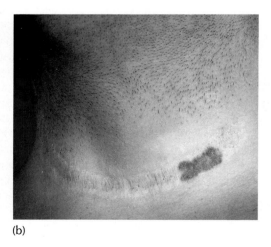
(b)

Figure 6 (a) A white cosmetic tattoo on the anterior neck applied to cover a thyroidectomy scar. (b) Immediate tattoo blackening was noted after Q-switched ruby laser exposure in a test area. Reprinted with permission from Anderson RR et al. Cosmetic tattoo ink darkening: a complication of Q-switched and pulsed-laser treatment. Arch Dermatol 1993;8:1010–1014.

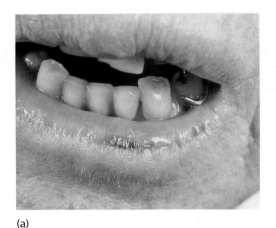
(a)

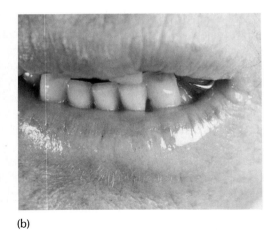
(b)

Figure 7 (a) Labial lentigo prior to treatment. (b) Complete clearance after treatment with the argon laser.

some junctional nevi, have responded well to the argon laser. The outcomes have been variable in treating larger lesions such as café-au-lait macules and Becker's nevi. More deeply pigmented processes, such as congenital nevi and nevi of Ota, have been partially lightened with the argon laser, but often with permanent pigmentary loss and textural change.

Continuous wave lasers should only be utilized for the removal of epidermal pigmentation. The long pulse duration of these lasers results in nonselective thermal destruction of tissue when dermal pigmented processes are targeted. Although epidermal pigmentation can be treated with somewhat improved therapeutic outcomes when the continuous wave lasers are used with the attachment of a robotized scanning device, pigmentary and textural alteration remain a risk.

Pulsed Laser Treatment

The concept of selective photothermolysis has also been applied to the development of lasers for the removal of pigmented lesions. Selective destruction of melanosomes is possible by using high-peak power laser pulses that are shorter than the 1-μsec thermal relaxation time of these 1-μm structures. Many different wavelengths may be used in treating pigmented lesions since melanin absorbs well from the ultraviolet to the near-infrared portions of the electromagnetic spectrum. The deep red portions of the visible spectrum provide the highest degree of selectivity for melanin absorption because hemoglobin absorbs poorly at these wavelengths. The 694 nm wavelengths of the Q-switched ruby (40-nsec pulsewidth) laser is nearly ideal in this respect. The Q-switched ruby laser was the first laser to demonstrate effective removal of dermal pigmentation without scarring. The 1064 nm Q-switched Nd:YAG (10 nsec pulsewidth) as well as the 755 nm Q-switched alexandrite (100 nsec pulsewidth) lasers also function in the red and near-infrared portion of the spectrum. These lasers are capable of inducing selective photothermolysis of deeper pigmented processes that extend into the dermis, as well as superficial lesions, because longer wavelengths of light are required to penetrate deeper into the skin.

Relatively higher melanin absorption and moderate hemoglobin absorption occur in the less selective blue-green portion of the visible spectrum. Lasers employing these shorter wavelengths are used to treat superficial pigmented lesions. Selective destruction of melanosomes has been demonstrated with the 351 nm excimer laser (20 nsec pulsewidth), 510 nm pulsed dye (300 msec pulsewidth) laser and 532 nm frequency-doubled Q-switched Nd:YAG (10 nsec pulsewidth) laser.

Immediately following the impact of pulsed and Q-switched lasers on a pigmented lesion, the skin develops a grey-white discoloration, which usually lasts for 20 min. In addition, localized purpura formation may occur with the 510 nm pulsed dye laser. It appears that the skin whitening is related to gas formation that accompanies the fragmentation of melanosomes secondary to rapid thermal expansion, shock waves, and localized cavitation.

Fluences used for the treatment of epidermal pigmented lesions are generally 4–6 J/cm^2 for the Q-switched ruby, 2–4 J/cm^2 for the 532 nm Q-switched Nd:YAG, and 2–4 J/cm^2 for the 510 nm pulsed dye laser. When deeper pigmented processes extending into the dermis are treated, the Q-switched ruby and 1064 nm Q-switched Nd:YAG lasers are typically used at maximal fluence. When treating more darkly pigmented individuals, fluences need to be reduced for all lasers so as to avoid prolonged or permanent hypopigmentation, and test spots should be performed to assess the clinical response. Maximal lightening of treated lesions occurs at 3–6 weeks, and successive treatments should be performed following this time interval. When required, anesthesia can be administered with injections of 1% lidocaine with epinephrine.

Excellent clearing of simple lentigines (Fig. 8), solar lentigines, labial lentigines, and ephelides, or freckles, has been obtained with the Q-switched ruby, 510 nm pulsed dye, and 532 nm frequency-doubled Q-switched Nd:YAG lasers in one to two treatment sessions. Histologically, the hypermelanosis is present in the basal layer of the epidermis and is therefore amenable to treat-

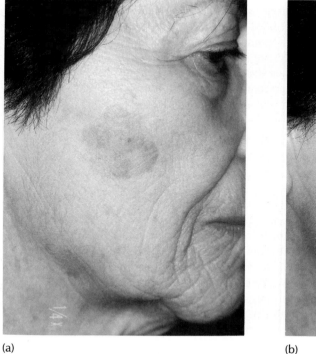
(a)

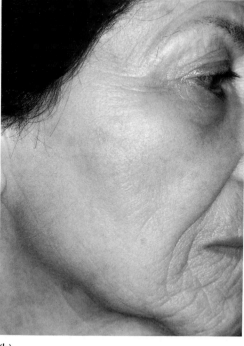
(b)

Figure 8 (a) Solar lentigo on the cheek of a woman. (b) Complete clearance after treatment with the Q-switched ruby laser.

ment with the shorter-wavelength green light lasers, as well as the red and infrared lasers. Lentigious processes that should also respond well to these pulsed and Q-switched lasers include the Peutz-Jeghers, Moynahan, and leopard syndromes.

Café-au-lait macules are tan-to-brown macules or patches that occur with an incidence of up to 14% in the population. These lesions are typically an isolated finding, but may be associated with a variety of cutaneous syndromes, including von Recklinghausen's disease, Albright's syndrome, and Marfan syndrome. Since the hypermelanosis is present in the basal layer in these lesions, café-au-lait macules may be treated with both green and red or infrared light lasers. Café-au-lait macules have been effectively cleared (Fig. 9) with the 510 nm pulsed dye, Q-switched ruby, and 532 nm Q-switched Nd:YAG lasers. A subset of café-au-lait macules hyperpigment before clearing, some café-au-lait macules recur after a 1- to 2-yr period, and when café-au-lait macules respond well to laser therapy, multiple treatment sessions are necessary.

Becker's nevi are tan-to-brown patches ranging from 2 to 40 cm in diameter that appear during childhood or early adulthood. Histologically, basal layer hyperpigmentation and an increased number of melanocytes are found. These hamartomatous lesions are also characterized by sebaceous gland hyperplasia and enlarged pilar apparati, and, clinically, hypertrichosis is often present. Similar to the café-au-lait macules, Becker's nevi have responded variably to treatment with the 510 nm pulsed dye, Q-switched ruby, and Q-switched Nd:YAG lasers.

Nevus spilus is a pigmented lesion comprised of junctional or compound nevi within a background field of macular café-au-lait pigmentation. The response of this lesion to pulsed and Q-switched lasers is not predictable, and multiple treatment sessions are necessary when it does respond to laser therapy.

Melasma is an acquired hypermelanosis of the face usually associated with pregnancy or oral contraceptive therapy. Two types of melasma are found on histologic examination and can be

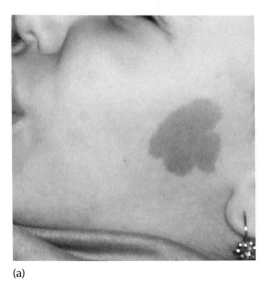 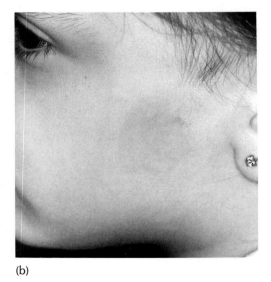

(a)   (b)

Figure 9 (a) Café au lait macule on the cheek of a child prior to treatment. (b) Approximately 90% lightening after five treatments with the Q-switched ruby laser.

clinically differentiated by Wood's light examination. The epidermal type is characterized by highly melanized melanosomes in the basilar and suprabasilar layers. In the dermal type, melanophages are scattered throughout the dermis in addition to the epidermal hyperpigmentation. Although a variety of different laser systems including the pulsed green dye, Q-switched ruby, Q-switched Nd:YAG, and Q-switched alexandrite lasers have successfully cleared melasma, repigmentation is common. Postinflammatory hyperpigmentation and postinflammatory hemosiderin deposition following sclerotherapy also respond variably to pulsed laser treatment.

Nevus of Ota is a benign congenital oculocutaneous melanosis of the dermis that consists of a grayish-blue discoloration of the face in the distribution of the first and second branches of the trigeminal nerve. These lesions occur most commonly in Asians, with an estimated incidence of 1–2% in the Japanese population, and other races are variably affected. Nevi of Ota fall within the spectrum of blue nevi and are characterized histologically by elongated, bipolar melanocytes scattered throughout the upper half of the dermis. Because of the intradermal location of melanocytes, the shorter-wavelength green light lasers, including the 510 nm pulsed dye laser and the 532 nm Q-switched Nd:YAG, are ineffective in lightening these lesions. Excellent results with complete or partial clearing without scarring (Fig. 10) have been obtained using the Q-switched ruby laser and the 1064 nm Q-switched Nd:YAG laser to treat nevi of Ota. These lesions also respond well to the Q-switched alexandrite laser. Nevus of Ito is a lesion that clinically and histologically resembles the nevus of Ota, but is found on the shoulder or upper arm in the distribution of the supraclavicular and lateral brachial cutaneous nerves. Nevi of Ito and blue nevi

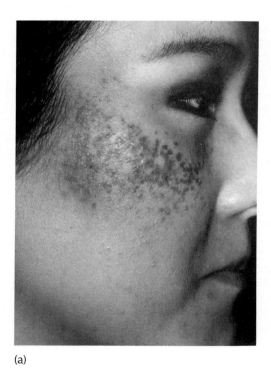 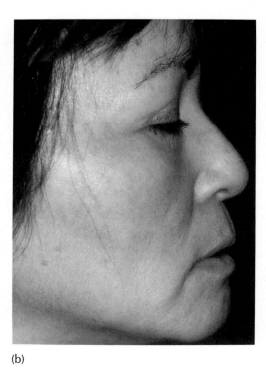

(a)   (b)

Figure 10 (a) Nevus of Ota prior to treatment. (b) Approximately 90% lightening after five treatments with the Q-switched ruby laser.

should also respond well to treatment with the Q-switched ruby, 1064 nm Q-switched Nd:YAG, and the Q-switched alexandrite lasers.

Removal of benign melanocytic nevi is often sought for cosmesis. Laser eradication of melanocytic nevi without scarring offers considerable advantages over conventional surgical techniques, particularly for lesions located in cosmetically important sites. Common acquired nevi usually appear after the first 6 months of life, and most develop in adolescence and early adulthood, during which time crops of new lesions may arise.

Histologically, melanocytic nevi are composed of collections of melanocytes present in the epidermis (junctional nevi), dermis, (intradermal nevi), or both (compound nevi). The shorter-wavelength green light lasers are ineffective modalities for treating lesions with dermal melanocytes. The 694 nm Q-switched ruby laser was reported to be effective in removing 12% (9 out of 74) of benign melanocytic nevi in a Japanese population. Histologic evaluation of nevi treated in this study revealed that lesions with junctional nests responded well, while nevi with middermal nests failed to respond to treatment with the Q-switched ruby laser. A preliminary histological study of the response of common acquired melanocytic nevi in eight patients to the Q-switched ruby laser revealed no evidence of residual nevus cells in two nevi, a decreased number of nevus cells in five nevi, and no change in the number of nevus cells in one nevus. Although more detailed investigations are necessary, the Q-switched ruby laser appears to be effective in clearing some of these lesions both clinically and histologically. The 755 nm Q-switched alexandrite laser and the 1064 nm Q-switched Nd:YAG laser, which also operate in the red to near-infrared portions of the spectrum, should be similarly effective.

Much controversy exists concerning laser treatment of melanocytic nevi, and treatment of these lesions should be undertaken with caution. Studies have shown that Q-switched ruby laser treatment can eradicate histological evidence of melanocytes junctional nevi, but nevus cells often remain in compound and intradermal nevi. Since residual melanocytes can remain following laser therapy, this treatment cannot reduce the risk of developing melanoma in these lesions. Nonetheless, partial removal of common acquired melanocytic nevi is routinely performed using conventional surgical techniques. Acquired dysplastic melanocytic nevi should not be treated because these lesions are potential histogenic precursors of melanoma and markers of increased melanoma risk.

Another area of debate concerns laser treatment of small and large congenital nevi. Small congenital nevi have a diameter of 1–3 cm and occur in approximately 1 of 100 births. These lesions are present with a greater-than-normal frequency in patients with malignant melanoma. Large congenital nevi are usually 5–20 cm in diameter, but they may involve larger surface areas of the body. When most of the trunk is involved, the lesion is called a giant hairy bathing-trunk nevus. Although the incidence of malignant melanoma arising in large congenital nevi is unknown, the lifetime risk has been reported to vary from 4 to 20%. Since congenital nevi extend into the deep reticular dermis, it is unlikely that treatment with the 694 nm Q-switched ruby, 1064 nm Q-switched Nd:YAG, or 755 nm Q-switched alexandrite laser could destroy all of the nevus cells. Laser treatment, therefore, is unlikely to prevent the development of melanoma in these lesions. For congenital nevi that are not amenable to surgical excision, some physicians find that dermabrasion of the superficial portion of the nevus for improved cosmesis is an acceptable procedure. Laser treatment of a congenital nevus poses similar risks in this respect by removing only the superficial component of nevus cells, but the cosmetic outcome is likely to be superior, with less chance of permanent scarring or textural change. Although controversial, laser treatment of small congenital nevi or portions of large congenital nevi located in cosmetically important areas may be an appropriate modality in cases when surgical excision is an impractical consideration.

BIBLIOGRAPHY

Anderson RR, Geronemus R, Kilmer, SL, et al. Cosmetic tattoo ink darkening: a complication of Q-switched and pulsed-laser treatment. *Arch Dermatol* 1993;8:1010–1014.

Anderson RR, Margolis RJ, Wanatabe S, et al. Selective photothermolysis of cutaneous pigmentation by Q-switched Nd:YAG laser pulses at 1064, 532, and 355 nm. *J Invest Dermatol* 1989;93:28–32.

Anderson RR, Parrish JA. Microvasculature can be selectively damaged using dye lasers: a basic theory and experimental evidence in human skin. *Lasers Surg Med* 1981;1:263–276.

Anderson RR, Parrish JA. Optical properties of human skin. In *The Science of Photomedicine*, JD Regan, JA Parrish, eds New York, Plenum Press, 1982, pp. 147–194.

Anderson RR, Parrish JA. The optics of human skin. *J Invest Dermatol* 1981;77:13–19

Anderson RR, Parrish JA. Selective photothermolysis: precise microsurgery by selective absorption of pulsed radiation. *Science* 1983;220:524–527.

Apfelberg DB, Laub DR, Maser MR, et al. Pathophysiology and treatment of decorative tattoos with reference to argon laser treatment. *Clin Plast Surg* 1967;28:745–748.

Apfelberg DB, Laub DR, Maser MR, et al. Update on laser usage in treatment of decorative tattoos. *Lasers Surg Med* 1982;2:169–171.

Apfelberg DB, Manchester GH. Decorative and traumatic tattoo biophysics and removal. *Clin Plast Surg* 14:243–251.

Apfelberg DB, Maser Mr, Lash H. Argon laser treatment of decorative tattoos. *Br J Plast Surg* 1979;32:141–144.

Apfelberg DB, Maser MR, Lash H, et al. The argon laser for cutaneous lesions. *JAMA* 1981;245:2073–2075.

Apfelberg DB, Maser MR, Lash R, et al. Comparison of argon and carbon dioxide laser treatment of decorative tattoos: a preliminary report. *Ann Plast Surg* 1985;14:6–8.

Apfelberg DB, Maser MR, Lash H, et al. Expanded role of the argon laser in plastic surgery. *J Dermatol Surg Oncol* 1983;9:145–151.

Apfelberg DB, Maser MR, Lash H. Extended use of the argon laser for cutaneous lesions. *Arch Dermatol* 1979;115:719–721.

Apfelberg DB, Rivers J, Maser MR, et al. Update on laser usage in treatment of decorative tattoos. *Lasers Surg Med* 1982;2:169–177.

Ashinoff R, Geronemus R. The Q-switched ruby laser in the treatment of pigmented lesions of the mucous membranes. *J Am Acad Dermatol* 1992;27(5):809–812.

Ashinoff R, Geronemus RG. Rapid response of traumatic and medical tattoos to treatment with the Q-switched ruby laser (abstr). *Lasers Surg Med* 1992;4(suppl):71.

Ashinoff R, Levine V, Tse Y, et al. Removal of pigmented lesions: Comparison of the Q-switched ruby and neodynium:YAG lasers (abstr). *Lasers Surg Med* 1994; 14(suppl 6):50.

Bailin PL, Ratz JL, Levine HL. Removal of tattoos by CO_2 laser *J Dermatol Surg Oncol* 1980;6:997–1001.

Bailin PL, Ritzpatrick, RE, Geisse JK. Successful treatment of blue, green, brown and reddish-brown tattoos with the Q-switched alexandrite laser (abstr). *Lasers Surg Med* 1994;14(suppl 6):52.

Beacon JP, Ellis H. Surgical removal of tattoos by carbon dioxide laser. *J R Soc Med* 1980;73:298–301.

Brady SC, Blokmanis A, Jewett L. Tattoo removal with the carbon dioxide laser. *Ann Plast Surg* 1978;2:482–484.

Buncke HR Jr, Conway H. Surgery of decorative and traumatic tattoos. *Plast Reconstr Surg* 1957;20:67–69.

Chai KB. The decorative tattoo: its removal by dermabrasion. *Plast Reconstr Surg* 1963;32:559–563.

Chapel TA, Tavafoghi V, Mehregan All. Becker's melanosis: an organoid hamartoma. *Cutis* 1981;27:405.

Clabaugh W. Removal of tattoos by superficial dermabrasion. *Arch Dermatol* 1968;98:515–521.

Crowe FW, Scnull WJ. Diagnostic importance of cafe-au-lait spot in neurofibromatosis. *Intern Med* 1953;91:758.

Curcio JA, Petty CC. The near infrared absorption spectrum of liquid water. *Lasers Surg Med* 1988;8:108–118.

Dixon J. Laser treatment of decorative tattoos. In *Cutaneous Laser Therapy: Principles and Methods*. KA Arndt, JM Noe, S Rosen, eds. New York, John Wiley and Sons, 1983, pp. 201–211.

Dover JS, Smoller Br, Stein RS. Low-fluence carbon dioxide laser irradiation of lentigines. *Arch Dermatol* 1988;124:1219–1224.

Finley JL, Arndt KA, Noe J, et al. Argon laser-port-wine-stain interaction immediate effects. *Arch Dermatol* 1984;120:613–619.

Finley JL., Barsky SH, Geer DE, Kamat BR, et al. Healing of port-wine stains after argon laser therapy. *Arch Dermatol* 1981;117:486–489.

Fitzpatrick R. Comparison of the Q-switched ruby, Nd:YAG and alexandrite lasers in tattoo removal (abstr). *Laser Surg Med* 1994;14(suppl 6):52.

Fitzpatrick RE, Goldman MP. Tattoo removal using the alexandrite laser (755 nm, 100 ns). *Arch Dermatol* (in press).

Fitzpatrick RE, Goldman MP, Ruiz-Esparza J. Laser treatment of benign pigmented epidermal lesions using a 300 nsecond pulse and 510 nm wavelength. *J Dermatol Surg Oncol* 1993;18:341–347.

Fitzpatrick RE, Goldman MP, Ruiz-Esparza J. The use of the alexandrite laser (755 nm, 100 psec) for tattoo pigment removal in an animal model. *J Am Acad Dermatol* 1993;28:745–750.

Garden JM, Tan OT, Kerschmann R, et al. Effect of dye laser pulse duration on selective cutaneous vascular injury. *J Invest Dermatol* 1986;87:653–657.

Geronemus RG. Q-switched ruby laser therapy of nevus of Ota. *Arch Dermatol* 1992;128:1618–1622.

Goldberg D. Benign pigmented lesions of the skin, treatment with the Q-switched ruby laser. *J Dermatol Surg Oncol* 1993;19:376–379.

Goldberg D. Treatment of pigmented and vascular lesions of the skin with the Q-switched Nd:YAG laser. *Lasers Surg Med* 1993;13(suppl 5):55.

Goldman MP, Fitzpatrick RE. Treatment of benign pigmented cutaneous lesions. In *Cutaneous Laser Surgery: The Art and Science of Selective Photothermolysis.* St. Louis, Mosby, 1994, pp. 106–141.

Goldman L, Hornby P, Meyer R. Radiation from a Q-switched laser with a total output of 10 megawatts on a tattoo of a man. *J Invest Dermatol* 1965;44:69–71.

Goldman L, Nath G, Schindler G, et al. High-power neodymium-YAG laser surgery. *Acta Derm Venereol (Stockh)* 1987;53:45–49.

Goldman L, Rockwell RJ, Meyer R, et al. Laser treatment of tattoos: a preliminary survey of three year's clinical experience. *JAMA* 1967;201:163–66.

Goldstein N, Penoff J, Price N, et al. Techniques of removal of tattoos. *J Dermatol Surg Oncol* 1979;5:901–910.

Goyal S, Dover JS, Arnt KA. Comparison of 1064 nm (neodymium:YAG), 694 nm (ruby) and 532 nm (frequency-doubled neodymium:YAG) Q-switched laser treatment of tattoos (abstr). *Laser Surg Med* 1994;14(suppl 6):52.

Greenwald J, Rosen S, Anderson RR, et al. Comparative histological studies of the tunable dye (at 577 nm) laser and argon laser: the specific vascular effects of the dye laser. *J Invest Dermatol* 1981;77:305–310.

Grekin RC, Shelton RM, Geisse JK, et al. 510 nm pigmented lesion dye laser. *J Dermatol Surg Oncol* 1993;19:380–387.

Grevelink JM, Flotte TJ, Anderson KK. Comparison of alexandrite, Nd:YAG and ruby lasers in treating tattoos (abstr). *Lasers Surg Med* 1994;14(suppl 6): 52.

Grossman MC, Anderson RR, Flotte J, et al. Laser treatment of cafe-au-lait macules (CALM): a clinicopathological correlation (abstr). *Laser Surg Med* 1994;14(suppl 6):49.

Haneke E. The dermal component in melanosis naeviformis Becker. *J Cutan Pathol* 1979;6:53.

Hruza GJ, Dover JS, Flotte TJ, et al. Q-switched ruby laser irradiation of normal human skin: histologic and ultrastructural findings. *Arch Dermatol* 1991;127:1799–1805.

Kasai K, Notodihardjo HW. Analysis of 200 nevus of Ota patients who underwent Q-switched Nd:YAG laser treatment (abstr). *Lasers Surg Med* 1994; 14(suppl 6):50.

Kauvar AB, Schiff T, Geronemus RG. Prediction of tattoo pigment response to Q-switched laser therapy using an in vitro assay (abstr). *Lasers Surg Med* 1994;14(suppl 6):63.

Kilmer SL, Anderson RR. Clinical use of the Q-switched ruby and the Q-switched Nd:YAG (1064nm and 532 nm) lasers for treatment of tattoos. *J Dermatol Surg Oncol* 1993;19:330–338.

Kilmer SL, Lee MS, Grevelink JM, et al. The Q-switched Nd:YAG laser (1064 nm) effectively treats tattoos: a controlled dose-response study. *Arch Dermatol* 1993;129(8):971–978.

Kopf AW, Levine IJ, Rigel DS, et al. Prevalence of congenital-nevus-like nevi, nevi spili, and cafe-au-lait spots. *Arch Dermatol* 1985;121:766

Kopf AW, Weidman AI. Nevus of Ota. *Arch Dermatol* 1959;85:145.

Landthalder M, Haina D, Waidelich W, et al. A three-year experience with the argon laser in dermatotherapy. *J Dermatol Surg Oncol* 1984;10:456–461.

Levine V, Geronemus R. Tattoo removal with the Q-switched ruby laser and the Nd:YAG laser: a comparative study (abstr). *Lasers Surg Med* 1993;5(suppl):53.

Margolis RJ, Dover JS, Polla LL, et al. Visible action spectrum for melanin-specific selective photothermolysis. *Lasers Surg Med* 1989;9:389–391.

McBurney EL. Carbon dioxide laser treatment of dermatologic lesions. *South Med J* 1978;71:795–798.

McBurney EI, Leonard GL. Argon laser treatment of port-wine hemangiomas clinical and histologic correlation. *South Med J* 1981;74:925–930.

McDaniel D. Clinical usefulness of the Hexascan. *J Dermatol Surg Oncol* 1993;19:312–319.

McGillis ST, Bailin PL, Fitzpatrick RE, et al. Successful treatment of yellow, orange, red, violet/purple, tan and flesh tattoos with the 510 nm pulsed dye laser (abstr). *Lasers Surg Med* 1994;14(suppl 6):52.

Murphy GF, Shepard RS, Paul BS, et al. Organelle-specific injury to melanin-containing cells in human skin by pulsed laser irradiation. *Lab Invest* 1983;49:680–683.

Ohtsuka H, et al. Ruby laser treatment of pigmented skin lesions. *Jpn J Plast Reconstr Surg* 1991;44:615.

Oshiro T, Maruyama Y. The ruby and argon lasers in the treatment of naevi. *Ann Acad Med Singapore* 1983;12:388–395.

Piggot Ta, Norris RW. The treatment of tattoos with trichloracetic acid: experience with 670 patients. *Br J Plast Surg* 1988;41:112–117.

Polla LL, Margolis RJ, Dover JS, et al. Melanosomes are a primary target of Q-switched ruby laser irradiation in guinea pig skin.

Reid WH, McLeod PJ, Ritchie A, et al. Q-switched ruby laser treatment of black tattoos. *Br J Plast Surg* 1983;36:455–459.

Reid WH, Miller ID, Murphy MJ, et al. Q-switched ruby laser treatment of tattoos: a 9-year experience. *Br J Plast Surg* 1990;43:663–669.

Reid R, Muller S. Tattoo removal by CO_2 laser dermabrasion. *Plast Reconstr Surg* 1980;65:717–719.

Resnick S. Melasma induced by oral contraceptive drugs. *JAMA* 1967;199:95–98.

Rhodes AR. Neoplasms: benign neoplasma, hyperplasias, and dysplasias of melanocytes. In *Dermatology in General Medicine*. 4th ed. TB Fitzpatrick, AZ Eisen, E Wolff, et al., eds. New York, McGraw Hill, 1993.

Ruiz-Esparza J, Goldman MP, Fitzpatrick RE. Tattoo removal with minimal scarring: the chemo-laser technique. *J Dermatol Surg Oncol* 1989;14:1372–1376.

Sanchez NP, Pathak MA, Sato S, et al. Melasma: a clinical, light microscopic, ultrastructural and immunoflorescent study. *J Am Acad Dermatol* 1981;4:698–702.

Scheibner A, Kenny G, White W, et al. A superior method of tattoo removal using the Q-switched ruby laser. *J Dermatol Surg Oncol* 1990;16:1091–1098.

Seneviratne J, Sheehan-Dare RA, Cotterill JA. Can the Q-switched ruby laser eradicate benign melanocytic naevi? Results of a preliminary histological study (abstr). *Lasers Surg Med* 1994;14(suppl 6):50.

Sherwood KA, Murray S, Kurban AK, et al. Effect of wavelength on cutaneous pigment using pulsed irradiation. *J Invest Dermatol* 1989;92:717–720.

Stenn KS, Arons M, Hurwitz S. Patterns of congenital nevocellular nevi: a histologic study of 38 cases. *J Am Acad Dermatol* 1983;9:388.

Tan OT, Morelli JG, Kuihan AK. Pulsed dye laser treatment of benign cutaneous pigmented lesions. *Lasers Surg Med* 1992;12:538–542.

Tan OT, Murray S, Kurban AK. Action spectrum of vascular specific injury using pulsed irradiation. *J Invest Dermatol* 1989;92:868–871.

Taylor CR, Anderson RR, Gange RW, et al. Light and electron microscopic analysis of tattoos treated by Q-switched ruby laser. *J Invest Dermatol* 1991;97:131–136.

Taylor CR, Gange RW, Dover JS, et al. Treatment of tattoos by Q-switched ruby laser. *Arch Dermatol* 1990;126:893–899.

Tong AKF, Tan OT, Boll J, et al. Ultrastructural effects of melanin pigment on target specificity using pulsed dye laser (577 nm). *J Invest Dermatol* 1987;88:747–752.

Waner M, Dinehart S. Lasers in facial plastic and reconstructive surgery. In *Lasers in Otolaryngology—Head and Neck Surgery*. RK Davis, ed. Philadelphia, WB Saunders, 1990, pp. 156–191.

Wheeler ES, Miller TA. Tattoo removal of split thickness tangential excision. *West J Med* 1988;124:272–274.

58

Laser Treatment of Telangiectasia

Mitchel P. Goldman and Richard E. Fitzpatrick
University of California School of Medicine and Dermatology Associates of San Diego County, Inc., San Diego, California

INTRODUCTION

The term *telangiectasia* refers to superficial cutaneous vessels visible to the human eye. These vessels measure 0.1–1.0 mm in diameter and represent a dilated venule, capillary, or arteriole. Telangiectasia that are arteriolar in origin are small in diameter, bright red in color, and do not protrude above the skin surface. Those that arise from venules are wider, blue in color, and often protrude above the skin surface. Telangiectasia arising at the capillary loop are often initially fine, red lesions but become larger and purple or blue with time because of venous backflow from increasing hydrostatic pressure.

Telangiectasia have been subdivided into four categories based on clinical appearance: (1) simple or linear, (2) arborizing, (3) spider, and (4) papular (Fig. 1). Red linear and arborizing telangiectasia are very common on the face, especially the nose, midcheek, and chin. These lesions are also seen relatively frequently on the legs. Blue linear and arborizing telangiectasia are most commonly seen on the legs but may also be found on the face. Spider telangiectasia arise from a central arteriole and can occur on any cutaneous surface. Papular telangiectasia are frequently part of genetic syndromes, such as Osler-Weber-Rendu syndrome, and also are seen in collagen vascular diseases.

All forms of telangiectasia are thought to occur through the release or activation of vasoactive substances under the influence of a variety of factors, such as anoxia, hormones, chemicals, infection, and physical factors, with resultant capillary or venular neogenesis. Telangiectasia of the face are most commonly seen in patients with fair complexion (Type I and Type II skin).

Portions of this chapter are abstracted with permission from M.P. Goldman and R.E. Fitzpatrick, eds. *Cutaneous Laser Surgery: The Art and Science of Selective Photothermolysis*. St. Louis: Mosby, 1994.

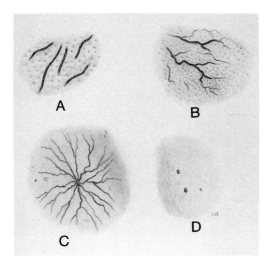

Figure 1 Four types of telangiectasia: (A) simple, (B) arborized, (C) spider, (D) papular. (From Goldman MP, Bennett RG. Treatment of telangiectasia: a review. *J Am Acad Dermatol* 1987;17:167.)

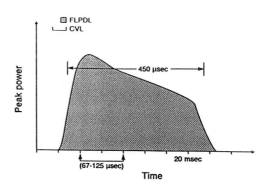

Figure 2 Graphic comparison of peak power output from flashlamp-pumped pulsed dye laser and copper vapor laser (From Goldman MP, Fitzpatrick RE. *Cutaneous Laser Surgery: The Art and Science of Selective Photothermolysis*. Mosby, St. Louis, 1994, p. 24.)

These lesions are especially common on the nasal alae, the nose, and midcheeks and are probably due to persistent arteriolar vasodilation resulting from vessel wall weakness. They are worsened by damage to the surrounding connective and elastic tissue from chronic sun exposure or the use of topical steroids. There is a definite familial or genetic component to these lesions. Rosacea may be an accompanying condition.

THE VASCULAR LASERS

Argon Laser

The argon laser was the first laser developed for vascular lesions, but it has been largely replaced by more specific lasers, which are both more effective and less likely to produce adverse effects. Difficulties associated with the argon laser result from three factors: short wavelength, small spot size, and prolonged exposure time. The shorter wavelengths of this laser (488 or 514 nm) are absorbed more heavily in the epidermis and superficial dermis, causing nonvascular damage. Increasing the wavelength from 514 to 585 nm will cause deeper vascular damage at fluences 64–186 times lower. The small spot size is another factor limiting penetration. A large spot size effectively increases penetration due to the effects of light scattering in the epidermis and superficial dermis. As a comparison, the 5-mm spot size of the flashlamp-pumped pulsed dye (FLPD) laser penetrates substantially deeper than the 0.1- to 1-mm spot size of the argon laser at identical power densities. Third, the continuous operation of the laser forces the physician to manually control the fluence to a specific area of the skin by moving the handpiece. This limits reproducibility from treatment to treatment and from physician to physician. Since argon laser irradiation, even when using the safest parameters, is several orders of magnitude removed from the ideal, the risk of hypertrophic/atrophic scarring and pigmentary change must be explained to the patient.

Nevertheless, if the argon laser is to be used for the treatment of telangiectasia, our recommendation is to use minimal power and pulsed delivery as described by Cosman and Fitzpatrick and Feinberg. In short, a 1-mm-diameter spot size is pulsed at 0.05 sec and moved across the telangiectasia as the power is increased from 0.4 W until minimal blanching occurs (usually between 0.6 and 1.2 W). This becomes the median parameter for the test patch, which should include laser powers up to 0.4 W above and below this median. However, even this technique results in a nonspecific dermal-epidermal burn, since visible blanching as an endpoint denotes epidermal protein denaturization. Our favorable clinical experience with short exposure times of 0.05 sec has been confirmed by others who note less hypopigmentation and atrophy.

In order to limit heat diffusion with the argon laser, robotized scanning laser handpieces have ben utilized. The use of this device has been reported to be successful in the treatment of facial and leg telangiectasia when the telangiectasia are densely present in interlacing mats. This technique is effective and greatly reduces the risk of adverse response, but it is not well suited for individual or widespread isolated telangiectasia.

Because of the adverse sequelae from argon laser treatment of vascular lesions, lasers having more specific absorption characteristics for intravascular oxyhemoglobin (HbO_2), the treatment target, have been developed. In vitro studies demonstrate HbO_2 in red blood cells to be the absorbed target at 577 nm. Endothelial cells are also damaged at this wavelength independent of red blood cell absorption, but in the presence of HbO_2, this effect is minimal. This led to the development and use of argon-pumped dye, copper vapor, and krypton lasers.

Argon-Pumped Dye Laser

This is a continuous wave laser, though mechanically shuttered pulses as short as 20 msec are achievable. Beam size may be varied from 50 μm to 6.0 mm. Yellow light (577-595 nm) is usually chosen for treatment of vascular lesions. The tracing technique using a 100-μm beam with this laser has been used extensively and advocated by Scheiber and Wheeland as a technique that produces good to excellent results with minimal risk in a variety of cutaneous vascular lesions, including facial telangiectasia. The proper endpoint of treatment is disappearance of the vessel, not blanching, blistering, or charring. Because the tracing hand motion cannot be accurately quantified, treatment parameters are difficult to teach except by direct monitoring. The very small spot size limits penetration depth, as previously discussed. In addition, this technique is more tedious and time consuming than the FLPD laser, even when one becomes a skilled operator. Multiple treatments are usually required, with hypopigmentation rarely occurring. The laser may be used as well with a robotized scanning device if large areas of matted telangiectasia are to be treated. However, multiple treatments are still required with a scanner in order to eliminate the hexagonal appearance of treated and cleared vessels that results from a single treatment session.

Copper Vapor Laser

The copper vapor laser (CVL) has also been promoted for treatment of telangiectasia and portwine stains in adults. This laser is not considered safe or effective in children. The copper vapor laser has a wavelength of 510 and/or 578 nm, which is pulsed at 20 nsec with a repetition rate of 15,000 Hz. This is an appropriate wavelength to selectively treat vascular lesions (578 nm), but each 20 nsec pulse is too short and does not deliver enough energy to treat vascular lesions (2.4 mJ/pulse compared to 0.5-2 J/pulse with the FLPD laser). It therefore must be used in a train of pulses to coagulate vascular lesions (Fig. 2). The train of pulses at 15,000 Hz results in additive thermal damage and reacts in tissue as if it were a continuous beam. The net tissue effect of this laser is very similar to that of the argon-pumped dye laser. To provide a larger safety margin, a mechanically shuttered pulse, a mechanical scanner, or a very small spot size (100 μm) is necessary to prevent unwanted thermal diffusion. It must be remembered that non-specific epidermal and dermal damage does occur with the use of this laser.

Krypton Laser

The latest addition to the yellow light lasers is the krypton laser. This laser produces wavelengths of 521, 530, and 568 nm. When used in treating vascular lesions, the two green bands are filtered out, yielding a beam of pure yellow light (568 nm). This energy can then be delivered in a manner identical to the argon dye and copper vapor lasers using a tracing technique or a robotic scanner. The beam size is less than 1 mm in diameter and is delivered as a continuous beam that may be pulsed at high rates. One problem with this laser is the low energy output. Since this system has only recently been developed, long-term studies on its efficacy are not yet available.

Flashlamp-Pumped Pulsed Dye Laser

In addition to target-specific wavelengths, Anderson and Parrish's theory of selective photothermolysis also relies on the pulse duration to limit thermal diffusion by keeping the laser pulse shorter than the time necessary to allow heat to spread from the treated target to surrounding tissue (thermal relaxation time). This theory led to the development of the flashlamp pulsed dye (FLPD) laser, which has been very successful in treating the small ectatic vessels of port-wine stains in addition to telangiectasia and other vascular lesions.

The theory of selective photothermolysis is the basis for the FLPD laser, having a wavelength of 585 nm and a pulse duration of 450 μsec. Initial studies on normal skin confirmed the validity of this theory and stressed the importance of pulse duration. Subsequent clinical studies confirmed the efficacy of this laser for treatment of lesions in both children and adults. Though Candela's original FLPD wavelength was set at 577 nm, it was later changed to 585 nm in order to increase penetration into the dermis without loss of vascular specificity. Although blood absorbs 585 nm light about half as efficiently as it absorbs 577 nm light, 585 nm light will coagulate larger vessels than will 577 nm at a given depth with a 5% blood volume because of deeper penetration of laser energy. In addition, deeper vessels absorb laser energy at longer wavelengths.

Another laser parameter, spot size, also contributes to the ultimate outcome of laser interaction with tissue. Although a decrease in spot size results in a larger increase in laser fluence and vice versa for a large spot size, mechanisms responsible for clinical effects are more complex. Tan et al. found that a 1-mm-diameter spot size affected blood vessels only in the most superficial vascular plexus (0.2 mm from the dermal-epidermal junction), even though extremely high fluences (27 J/cm^2) were needed to produce purpura. Here, purpura resolved quickly since only superficial damage occurred. They hypothesize that a 1-mm spot size alters dermal components, changing the refraction of tissue, which alters distribution and scattering of laser fluence. Although a 1-mm diameter spot could affect deeper dermal vessels, extensive nonspecific damage occurred as compared to 3- and 5-mm-diameter spot sizes. Clearly, nonlinear changes in the optical behavior of tissue occur through manipulation of laser scatter.

Although the superiority of the FLPD laser over other vascular lasers is clearly established with respect to both safety and efficacy, adverse effects can occur. Hypopigmentation can occur in treated areas in darkly pigmented patients. Persistent hypopigmentation is more common on the neck, legs, and chest. Persistent hyperpigmentation may also occur from sun exposure to healing skin as well as from hemosiderin deposited in the dermis from resolving purpura. These effects are particularly prominent from treating vascular lesions on the legs. Finally, although very rare, hypertrophic scarring has been reported with high laser fluences. Two of 92 adults with facial telangiectasia developed dermal atrophy with normal skin texture on the nose, nasolabial folds, and malar regions, which lasted at least 6 months. These areas were treated with a 1-mm spot diameter at a fluence of 7 J/cm^2. We have also seen two patients with localized hypertrophic scars treated with a 5-mm-diameter spot size at 7.5–8.0 J/cm^2 on the anterior chest and shoulder. In our patients, trauma to the treated area within 24 hr of treatment was reported by the patient with the shoulder lesion. Laser fluence, lesion location, and posttreatment care are all important factors that may contribute to the risk of scarring when using the FLPD laser.

TELANGIECTASIA

Facial Telangiectasia

Patients with telangiectasia of various types present for treatment primarily because of cosmetic concerns. Therefore, it is important that the procedure be relatively risk-free without unsightly scarring. In addition, facial telangiectasia often carry an unjustified social stigma, implying alcoholism. It is thus understandable why patients are distressed by this otherwise benign condition. Treatment of large vessels on the nasal ala or nasal alar groove is difficult and often leads to noticeable scarring when conventional methods are used. We have found the FLPD laser to be a powerful and effective tool in the treatment of these lesions virtually without the risk of scarring or other permanent skin changes.

One study reports a 77% response rate to FLPD laser treatment of adult facial linear telangiectasia. Although vessel diameter was not measured, larger, blue vessels were less responsive than smaller red vessels. Although thermal relaxation time in larger-diameter telangiectasia are longer and deoxygenated hemoglobulin has a wavelength of 545 nm, the 77% response rate may also be due to the lower fluences used (6–6.5 J/cm^2) and a 1-mm-diameter spot size, which produces less targeted energy as described previously. Our published series shows 97.5% of 182 patients achieving good to excellent results, indicating resolution of more than 50% of the treated lesions in one or two treatments (Fig. 3). Fourteen percent of patients showed a good and 83.5% an excellent response. In 152 of these 182 patients, over 75% of their telangiectasia were removed. Scarring did not occur in any patient. In all patients, the skin texture remained unchanged. As expected, all patients experienced a transient bluish-purple discoloration at the treatment site, which resolved spontaneously in 10–14 days. This discoloration was well tolerated by our patient population, who were all informed in advance of its occurrence. They could therefore modify

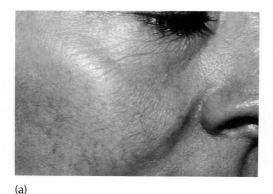 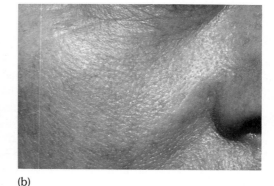

(a)   (b)

Figure 3   (a) A 56-year-old woman with extensive telangiectasia on the cheeks. (b) Six months after one treatment with the FLPD laser at 7.25 J/cm^2. A total of 45 5-mm-diameter pulses were given to the entire right cheek.

their social and business schedules accordingly. Typically, make-up foundation was used to camouflage the purpura approximately 3–5 days after treatment. Even though no anesthesia was used, patients experienced only mild to moderate discomfort in 93% of the cases.

Most patients (62%) require only one treatment, although further improvement and a better response will occur with more than one treatment. Skin pigment type does not have a measurable influence on response to treatment. The largest percentage of patients with an excellent response were treated with fluences above 7 J/cm^2 (93% vs. 78% for 6 J/cm^2). There was a noticeable trend towards increasing effectiveness with increasing fluence, but this is balanced by the fact that a higher fluence may result in a greater risk of nonspecific thermal injury.

A 2-mm spot size is now available from Candela Laser Corporation for their FLPD laser. Geronemus and Greken (reported in Candela Laser Corporation brochure, 1992) reported clearing in 70% of 35 patients with linear telangiectasia using this small spot size to minimize posttreatment purpura. There were no cases of scarring, skin texture change, or hypopigmentation. Reduced purpura was the major advantage. However, high fluences of 8.5–9.5 J/cm^2 were needed to produce vessel clearing.

It is our impression that vessels larger than 0.2 mm in diameter require multiple treatments. Vessels larger than 0.4 mm in diameter are poorly responsive to FLPD laser treatment and may be best treated with sclerotherapy alone or with the photoderm VL™ (Energy Systems Corporation, Newton, MA) or in combination with one of the continuous output lasers as previously described. Though treatment is tolerated well by patients without the use of anesthesia, it may be prudent to offer the use of topical anesthetic creams such as EMLA^R (Astra, Sweden) or 30% Xylocaine in acid mantle base, or possibly intermittent nitrous oxide with careful attention to the fire hazards of an oxygen-enriched treatment environment when large areas are to be treated.

The CO_2 laser has been used for treatment of facial telangiectasia. Because tissue destruction is nonselective with this laser, occurring by vaporization of water within cells, the skin surface and dermis overlying the telangiectasia as well as the vessel are destroyed. Because of this nonselective action, the CO_2 laser has no advantage over electrosurgery in the treatment of telangiectasia.

The argon laser has been commonly used for treatment of facial telangiectasia. Treatment parameters have varied: laser powers of 0.8–2.9 W, exposure times of 50 msec, 0.2 sec, 0.3 sec, and continuous and spot sizes of 0.1 and 1 mm have been used. Although the success rate of treatment of facial telangiectasia has been reported to be good to excellent in 65–99% of patients treated, pitted and depressed scars, hypopigmentation, hyperpigmentation, and recurrence of veins have been noted. One area of particular concern has been the nasal ala and nasolabial crease, where a depressed scar has been relatively common, though with time, resolution gradually occurs.

The copper vapor laser is also effective for treating facial telangiectasia (Fig. 4). Excellent results are achieved in 45–50% of patients, with fair to poor results achieved in 26–31% of patients. The CVL usually produces epidermal blistering in the first 48 hr with edema during the first 3 days and epidermal crusting for 7–14 days. A comparison of the CVL with the FLPD laser in 10 adults with facial telangiectasia resistant to electrosurgical therapy demonstrated no difference in efficacy or adverse sequelae. However, Dinehart reports a 10% incidence of transient hyperpigmentation with the CVL. Whether this represents melanin or hemosiderin is unknown. A second study comparing these two lasers in 12 adults with facial telangiectasia demonstrated no significant difference in efficacy between the two lasers. All subjects required two treatments to obtain desirable results with either laser. Treatments required similar time for both lasers. However, healing time was longer for the FLPD laser and patients preferred the thin linear crusting of the CVL to the purpura of the FLPD laser.

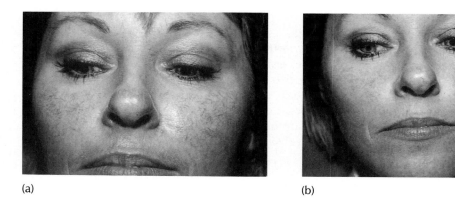

(a)   (b)

Figure 4 (a) Woman with extensive facial telangiectasia before treatment. (b) After two treatments with the CVL, each of 30-min duration 8 weeks apart. (Courtesy of Sue McCoy, M.D.)

When used with the modulating influence of a secondary shuttered pulse or scanning device, the risk of adverse response is further minimized without significant change in clinical effectiveness. In a comparison of 144 patients treated with the point-by-point technique with 105 patients treated by the Hexascan, French investigators determined that the incidence of hypertrophic scarring to be less than 1% with the Hexascan group versus 7% in the point-by-point group. Treatment time was also reduced to 20% of the point-by-point time. Patient treated by Hexascan also experienced less pain, with local anesthesia rarely required. The balance between these two results (vessel obliteration and adverse healing) must be weighed and the treatment technique altered to be consistent with the goals of treatment.

Both the CVL and the 577 nm argon-pumped dye laser offer reasonable alternatives to the FLPD laser, with the potential advantage of causing less visible crusting over treated vessels instead of purpura. However, it must be recognized that there is some perivascular thermal damage with both lasers that can cause scarring and hypopigmentation. They are also generally more time-consuming to operate. These three lasers are all superior to the argon laser, which, although successful with expert technique, must be used with discretion. The carbon dioxide laser has no advantage over electrosurgery and in our opinion should not be used for treating facial telangiectasia.

Spider Telangiectasia

Spider telangiectasia typically appear in preschool and school-aged children. The peak incidence appears to be between ages 7 and 10 and as many as 40% of girls and 32% of boys less than 15 years old have at least one lesion. The incidence in healthy adults is around 15%. The difference between these stated incidences implies that 50–75% of childhood lesions regress. However, this is not easily observable, as most lesions seem to persist without change and become a source of cosmetic concern when present on the face.

Treatment in the past included electrocautery and the argon laser. Both modalities have the disadvantage of being painful and prone to causing punctate scarring. In addition, recurrence is common if treatment is done lightly in order to avoid scarring. The FLPD laser has proven to be a very effective treatment for these benign lesions and is our recommended treatment modality.

Geronemus reported 100% success without any adverse sequelae in 12 children treated with the FLPD laser for facial spider telangiectasia.

We retrospectively evaluated the response to treatment with the FLPD laser in 23 children with 55 spider telangiectasias. In our practice, lesions were treated at energy fluences between 6.5 and 7.5 J/cm^2 (mean 6.9 J/cm^2). One or two pulses were given to the central punctum of the "spider," with additional pulses with a 10% overlap given to the radiating "arms" of the lesion if the lesion was over 5 mm in diameter. Local anesthesia was not utilized. Seventy percent of lesions resolved completely with one treatment. Twelve lesions required a second treatment for complete resolution. The remaining five lesions not treated a second time had an average clearance of 78% (Fig. 5).

Our results confirm the safety and effectiveness of the FLPD laser in treatment of childhood facial telangiectasia. Spider telangiectasia respond equally well in adults, with 93% of patients having total resolution with one treatment between 6.5 and 7 J/cm^2.

Generalized essential telangiectasia generally occurs on the legs, but it may also involve other cutaneous surfaces. Various treatments have been proposed that have a variable efficacy. Tan and Kurban have recently reported successful treatment with the FLPD laser at fluences of 6 J/cm^2. We have also treated four patients with the FLPD laser at fluences ranging from 6 to 7.5 J/cm^2. Two patients responded with total resolution, while two patients had almost no improvement in their appearance (Fig. 6). We believe that intrinsic factors in these patients may preclude predictable results and recommend performing a patch test on these patients.

Rosacea-associated telangiectasia and erythema respond well to treatment with the FLPD laser. We have reported good to excellent results in 24 of 27 patients (89%). In addition to the cosmetic improvement resulting from elimination of the vascular component of this disorder, treatment with the FLPD laser also appears to alter the pathophysiology of this condition as a decrease in papule and pustule activity occurs in up to 59% of patients. After FLPD laser treatment, patients who responded to treatment with elimination of the vascular component required less or no topical or systemic antibiotic therapy to maintain disease resolution. Anecdotal reports from Tan confirm our more formal evaluations.

In assessing the overall success and potential risk of each laser that has been used in the treatment of facial telangiectasia, we believe that the FLPD laser provides the most effective and risk-

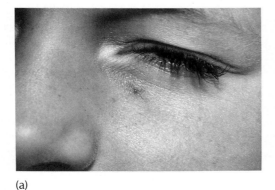
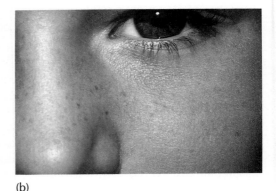

(a)   (b)

Figure 5   (a) Eight-year-old boy with spider telangiectasia on the cheek for over one year. (b) After FLPD laser treatment at 7.0 J/cm^2. A total of five 5-mm-diameter pulses were given to the central punctum and radiating vessels.

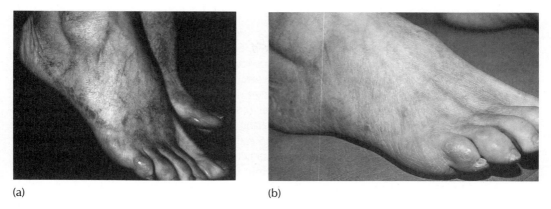

(a)   (b)

Figure 6 (a) Extensive pedal telangiectasia. (b) Three months after two treatments with the FLPD laser at 7.25 J/cm^2. A total of 84 5-mm-diameter pulses were given in the first treatment with an additional 115 5-mm-diameter pulses given 3 months later. (From Goldman MP. *Sclerotherapy Treatment of Varicose and Telangiectatic Leg Veins*, 2nd ed. Mosby, St. Louis, 1995, p. 341.)

free results. However, purpura resulting after treatment is an inconvenience that must be recognized in advance and allowed for in scheduling treatment.

Leg Telangiectasia

Unsightly or symptomatic venulectases and/or telangiectasias on the legs occur in 29–41% of women and 6–15% of men in the United States. These smaller vessels are most often directly or indirectly connected to larger reticular or varicose "feeding" veins. A family history of varicose or telangiectatic leg veins ranges from 43–90%. Approximately one third of patients first note the development of these veins during pregnancy. Between 20 and 30% of patients developed these veins prior to pregnancy, with 18% of women noting the onset while ingesting progestational agents. Therefore, the development of "spider leg veins" is probably a partially sex-linked, autosomal dominant condition with incomplete penetrance and variable expressivity.

Even though up to 53% of patients have associated symptoms with these veins, the most common reason patients seek treatment is cosmetic. Therefore, any treatment that is effective should be relatively free of adverse sequelae. Unfortunately, all forms of treatment to date have some side effects. The most common method for treating leg telangiectasia is sclerotherapy. Up to 30% of patients treated with sclerotherapy will develop postsclerosis pigmentation and/or telangiectatic matting. Postsclerosis hyperpigmentation is caused by the extravasation of erythrocytes through sclerotherapy-damaged or destroyed vessels. This is more likely to occur if sclerosing agents of excessive strength are utilized but may occur with optimum treatment. Telangiectatic matting is also thought to be related to the use of excessively strong sclerosing agents with the development of "excessive" perivascular inflammation or "excessive" thrombus formation. This adverse reaction usually resolves within 6 months but, if persistent, is usually recalcitrant to further sclerotherapy treatment.

Various lasers have been utilized in an effort to enhance clinical efficacy and minimize the adverse sequelae of sclerotherapy. Unfortunately, most have also been associated with adverse responses far in excess of those associated with sclerotherapy. This is related both to the non-specificity of the laser used and the lack of treatment of the "feeding" venous system.

Varicose veins most likely lead to the development of telangiectasia either through associated venous hypertension with resulting angiogenesis or vascular dilatation and/or through an associated increased distensibility of the telangiectatic vein wall. Although telangiectasia associated with varicose veins may appear at first as erythematous streaks, with time they turn blue. Often they are directly associated with underlying varicose veins so that the distinction between telangiectasias and varicose veins becomes blurred. Fifty percent of patients with blue reticular veins demonstrate reflux from incompetent calf perforating veins. In this scenario, treatment of the feeding varicosity results in treatment of the distal telangiectasia. A direct connection from telangiectasia to the deep venous system in 2 of 15 radiographed patients has also been demonstrated. Finally, when no apparent connection exists between deep collecting or reticular vessels, the telangiectasia may arise from a terminal arteriole or arteriovenous anastomosis.

Leg telangiectasia may be associated with underlying venous disease even when there are no obvious reticular or varicose veins. Twenty-three percent of patients without clinically apparent varicose veins examined with duplex imaging and venous Doppler demonstrated incompetence of the superficial venous system. This study demonstrates the need for a clinical and/or noninvasive diagnostic work-up in patients who present with telangiectatic leg veins and also reinforces the view that "spider" leg veins arise from underlying varicose veins via venous hypertension.

The venules in the upper and middermis usually run in a horizontal orientation. The diameter of the postcapillary venule ranges from 12 to 35 μm. Collecting venules range from 40 to 60 μm in the upper and middermis and enlarge to 100–400 μm diameter in the deeper tissues. One-way valves are found at the subcutis (dermis)–adipose junction on the venous side of the circulation. The free edges of the valves are always directed from the smaller to larger vessel, so blood flows towards the deeper venous system. Thus, with venous hypertension, blood flow is reversed from valvular incompetence.

Histologic examination of simple telangiectasia demonstrates dilated blood channels in a normal dermal stroma with a single endothelial cell lining, limited muscularis, and adventitia. Most leg telangiectasia measure between 26 and 225 μm in diameter. Electron microscopic examination of "sunburst" varicosities of the leg has demonstrated that these vessels are widened cutaneous veins. They are found 175–382 μm below the stratum granulosum. The thickened vessel walls are composed of endothelial cells covered with collagen and muscle fibers. Elastic fibers are also present.

Unlike leg telangiectasia, the ectatic vessels of a port-wine stain are arranged in a loose fashion throughout the superficial and deep dermis. They are more superficial (0.46 mm) and much smaller than leg telangiectasia, usually measuring 10–40 μm in diameter. This may explain the lack of efficacy reported by many physicians who treat leg telangiectasia with the same laser parameters as port-wine stains.

Since, in the vast majority of cases, spider veins are in direct connection to underlying varicose veins either directly or through tributaries, treatment should first be directed to "plugging" the leaking high-pressure outflow at its point of origin. An appropriate analogy is to think of spider veins as the fingers and the feeding varicose vein as the arm. Treatment should first be directed to the feeding "arm" and only if necessary directed to the spider "fingers." There are a number of advantages to this systematic approach. When performed in this manner, spider veins often disappear without direct treatment. The larger feeding vein is both easier to cannulate and less likely to rupture with injection of the sclerosant, thus minimizing the extent of extravasated red blood cells and sclerosant. Theoretically, this method should minimize treatment complications. A complete discussion of sclerotherapy treatment is presented in another chapter. Treatment should proceed from largest to smallest vessel. By adhering to these principles, patients will receive cost-effective, efficient, and logical care.

Laser Treatment of Leg Telangiectasia

Carbon Dioxide

The CO_2 laser has been used for the obliteration of venules and telangiectatic vessels. The rational for using the CO_2 laser in the treatment of telangiectasia is to produce precise vaporization without significant damage to tissue structures adjacent to the penetrating laser beam. However, the skin surface, as well as the dermis overlying the blood vessel, is destroyed. CO_2 laser penetration of vessels has also been reported to cause occasional brisk bleeding from the vessel, which required pressure bandages for 48 hr. Pain during treatment is moderate to severe but of short duration. All reported studies demonstrate unsatisfactory cosmetic results. Treated areas show multiple hypopigmented punctate scars with either minimal resolution of the treated vessel or neovascularization adjacent to the treatment site. Because of this nonselective action, the CO_2 laser is of no advantage over the electrodesiccation needle and has not been successfully utilized in treating leg telangiectasia.

Neodymium:YAG

The Nd:YAG laser at 1060 nm has also been used to treat leg telangiectasia. The average depth of penetration in human skin is 0.75 mm, and reduction to 10% of the incident power occurs at a depth of 3.7 mm. Thus, this laser should be well suited to treat blood vessels within the middermis. However, the wavelength is absorbed by water and to a certain degree by melanin and hemoglobin and has a continuous beam. Therefore, like the CO_2 laser, tissue damage is relatively nonspecific. Apfelberg treated leg telangiectasias with the Nd:YAG laser equipped with a 1.5-mm sapphire contact probe. Treatment complications included linear hypopigmentation and depressions overlying the skin of the treated vessel.

Argon

Argon laser treatment of telangiectasia or superficial varicosities of the lower extremities often results in purple or depressed scars. In a report of 38 patients treated by Apfelberg et al., 49% had either poor or no results from treatment; only 16% had excellent or good results. In addition, almost half of the patients had hemosiderin pigmentation. In another series, Dixon et al. noted significant improvement in only 49% of patients. They speculated that after initial improvement, incomplete thrombosis, recanalization or new vein formation produced reappearance of the vessels after 6–12 months.

In an effort to enhance therapeutic success with leg vein sclerotherapy, the argon laser has been used to interrupt the telangiectasia every 2–3 cm prior to injection of a sclerosing agent. Eleven of 16 patients completed treatment. Two patients developed punctate depigmented scars, and three patients developed hyperpigmentation. However, 93.7% of patients were reported to have "satisfactory" results. Cooling the skin simultaneously with argon or argon dye (577 nm and 585 nm respectively), laser treatment has been demonstrated to produce improvement in 67% of leg telangiectasia 1 mm in diameter. This may be secondary to temperature-related vasomotor changes in blood flow. Overall, argon laser therapy appears to be not only relatively ineffective in treating leg telangiectasias, but is also associated with an unacceptably high risk of adverse sequelae.

Flashlamp Pulsed Dye Laser

As previously described, the FLPD laser is highly efficacious in treating cutaneous vascular lesions. The potential depth of vascular damage is estimated to be 1.5 mm at 585 nm. Therefore, it can penetrate to reach the typical depth of leg telangiectasia. However, telangiectasia over the lower extremities have not responded as well, with less lightening and more posttherapy hyperpigmentation. This may be due to the larger diameter of leg telangiectasia as compared to dermal vessels in port-wine stains or to the failure to recognize the importance of high-pressure vascular flow from feeding reticular and varicose veins, as well as anatomic differences in the vessels.

Polla et al. treated 35 superficial leg telangiectasias with the FLPD laser. The exact laser parameters were not given, except that vessels were treated an average of 2.1 times with a maximum of four separate treatments. These vessels were described as being either red-purple and raised or blue and flat. No mention was made regarding the association of reticular or varicose veins or vessel diameter. Fifteen percent of treated vessels had greater than 75% clearing with 73% of treated areas showing little response to treatment. The only lesions that responded at all were red-pink "tiny" telangiectasia. Almost 50% of the treated patients developed persistent hypo- or hyperpigmentation.

It is difficult to compare the clinical and experimental results of laser treatment of leg telangiectasia with those of port-wine stains. The former typically do not report the diameter, location, or type of vessel treated. In addition, no mention is made of "feeding" varicosities or of postlaser compression. Therefore, we systematically examined the clinical effects of various powers of the FLPD laser in specific leg telangiectasia. We chose red telangiectasia less than 0.2 mm in diameter and vessels arising as a function of telangiectatic matting for examination since these vessels are the most difficult to treat with standard sclerotherapy techniques.

The FLPD laser produces vascular injury in a histologic pattern that is different than that produced by sclerotherapy. In the rabbit ear vein, approximately 50% of vessels treated with an effective concentration of sclerosant demonstrated extravasated red blood cells. With FLPD laser treatment, extravasated red blood cells were apparent in only 30% of vessels treated. Thus, the FLPD laser may produce less posttherapy pigmentation because of a decreased incidence of extravasated red blood cells.

The etiology of telangiectatic matting is unknown but has been thought to be related either to angiogenesis or a dilatation of existing subclinical blood vessels by promoting collateral flow through arteriovenous anastomoses. One or both of these mechanisms may occur. Obstruction of outflow from a vessel (the end result of successful sclerotherapy) is one of the most important factors contributing to angiogenesis. In addition, endothelial damage leads to the release of histamine and other mast cell factors, which promotes both the dilatation of existing blood vessels and angiogenesis. Thus, sclerotherapy by its very mechanism of action provides the means for new blood vessel formation to occur. Indeed, it is remarkable that one does not see a higher incidence of postsclerosis telangiectatic matting with sclerotherapy treatment.

Telangiectatic matting has not been reported to be a side effect of argon, FLPD, and/or dye laser treatment of any vascular disorders. This may be due to the production of intravascular fibrin that occurs during laser treatment. This is believed to occur through thermal alteration of fibrin complexes. Fibrin deposition has been demonstrated to promote angiogenesis. Interestingly, sclerotherapy-induced vascular injury has not been associated with the appearance of fibrin strands. Therefore, either factors other than those associated with the absence of fibrin deposition or the intravascular consumption of fibrin-promoting factors must limit angiogenesis in laser treatment of cutaneous vascular disease.

Another possible mechanism for the absence in telangiectatic matting in laser-treated blood vessels may be a decrease in perivascular inflammation. Rabbit ear vein treatment with the FLPD laser results in a relative decrease in perivascular inflammation as compared to vessels treated with sclerotherapy alone. Multiple factors associated with inflammation have been demonstrated to promote both a dilatation of existing blood vessels and angiogenesis.

The above-mentioned theoretical advantages and methods for treating leg telangiectasia with the FLPD laser were examined in 30 female patients. Telangiectasia measured less than 0.2 mm in diameter and were red in color. Thirteen of 101 telangiectatic patients were noted to have an associated reticular "feeding" vein 2–3 mm in diameter, which was not treated. Seven patients with 25 patches of telangiectatic matting after previous sclerotherapy were also treated.

FLPD laser 5-mm-diameter spots were overlapped slightly with every effort made to treat the entire vessel. After treatment, a chemical ice pack (Kwik Kold, American Pharmaseal Co., Valencia, CA 91355) was applied to the treated area until the laser-induced sensation of heat resolved (5–15 min). Thirty-nine telangiectatic patches, chosen randomly, were treated with laser energies between 7.0 and 8.0 J/cm^2 and compressed with a rubber "E" compression pad (Vascular Products Ltd., Bristol, England BSI 4DZ) fixed in place with Microfoam 100-mm tape (3M Medical-Surgical Division, St. Paul, MN 55144). A 30–40 mmHg graduated compression stocking was then continuously worn over this dressing for approximately 72 hr.

As hypothesized, telangiectatic matting and persistent pigmentation did not occur with FLPD laser treatment of leg telangiectasia. Post-FLPD–induced hyperpigmentation completely resolved within 4 months in these patients. There were no episodes of cutaneous ulceration, thrombophlebitis, or other complications. However, hypopigmentation was noted in one women with very tan skin treated for telangiectatic matting. The laser impact sites usually remained hypopigmented for 6 months. Brown hyperpigmentation usually occurred and lasted 1–6 months.

With FLPD laser treatment, the most effective fluence appears to be between 7.0 and 8.0 J/cm^2. At these laser parameters, approximately 67% of telangiectatic patches completely faded within 4 months (Fig. 6).

There appears to be no difference in the response to FLPD laser treatment between linear leg telangiectasia and telangiectatic matting vessels. In these seven patients with 25 sites treated, 72% of the treated sites completely faded at laser fluences between 6.5 and 7.5 J/cm^2. Telangiectatic matting vessels did not respond to treatment in only one patient with four areas of matting. Less than 100% resolution occurred in 16% of treated areas.

The reason for the greater efficacy of treatment in our report as compared to others may be due to the rigid criteria by which patients were selected for treatment. Our patients who responded well to treatment had red telangiectasia <0.2 mm in diameter without associated "feeding" reticular veins.

The FLPD laser is an effective modality for treating red leg telangiectasia ≤0.2 mm in diameter. FLPD laser treatment is efficacious for both essential telangiectasia and vessels of telangiectatic matting. This form of treatment alone has a remarkably low incidence of adverse sequelae. The optimal clinically useful laser energy is between 7.0 and 8.0 J/cm^2. Treatment is most efficacious if all vessels larger than 0.2 mm in diameter, especially varicose and reticular feeding veins, are treated first with sclerotherapy.

Photoderm VL™

In an effort to maximize efficacy in treating leg veins greater than 0.2 mm in diameter, a novel pulsed light source is now available. Leg venules are substantially larger and have thicker walls than the ectatic vessels in port-wine stains and hemangiomas. Therefore, thermal heat diffusion from absorbed red blood cells require longer times to effectively damage the vein wall (approximately 1–10 msec). In addition, since leg veins are located deeper in the dermis than telangiectasia, a longer wavelength and/or protection of the epidermis and superficial dermis from thermal damage is necessary for ideal treatment.

Optical properties of blood are mainly determined by the absorption and scattering coefficients of its various oxyhemoglobin components. Figure 7 shows the oxyhemoglobin absorption and scattering coefficient depth of penetration into blood. The main feature to note in the curve is the strong absorption at wavelengths below 600 nm with less absorption at longer wavelengths. However, a vessel that is 1 mm in diameter absorbs more than 67% of light even at wavelengths longer than 600 nm. This absorption is even more significant for blood vessels 2 mm in diam-

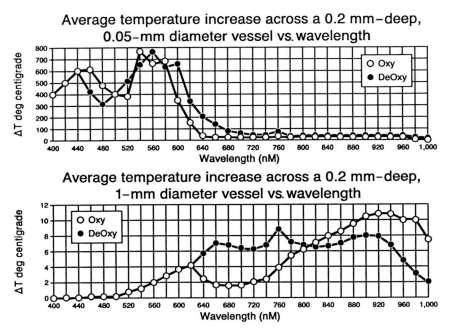

Figure 7 Average temperature increase across a cutaneous vessel as a function of wavelength for two extreme cases: a shallow capillary vessel and a deeper (2 mm depth), larger-diameter (1 mm) vessel. Note the dramatic shift in the optical wavelength as a function of vessel depth and diameter. (From Goldman MP, Fitzpatrick RE. *Cutaneous Laser Surgery: The Art and Science of Selective Photothermolysis.* Mosby, St. Louis, 1994, p. 23.)

eter. Therefore, utilizing a light source above 600 nm would result in deeper penetration of thermal energy without negating absorption by oxyhemoglobin. This is because the absorption coefficient in blood is higher than that of surrounding tissue for wavelengths between 600 and 1200 nm.

Pain or nonspecific epidermal damage are largely a function of the temperature that the skin reaches at the end of the exposure pulse. Higher temperatures yield greater damage and greater pain. As longer-wavelength light penetrates deeper into the skin, exposure to the same energy density of longer wavelengths will cause a similar increase in temperature with less epidermal damage and pain. This is true with a wavelength up to 1.2 μm. At longer wavelengths, there is a gradual increase in the absorption coefficient due to water absorption with practically zero transmission at 10.6 μm (similar to the absorption of CO_2). At that point, all energy is absorbed in a very thin layer of skin (on the order of 10 μm), with the resulting temperature for a given energy density added to maximum.

Theoretically, a phototherapy device that produces an incoherent light as a continuous spectrum longer than 575 nm should have multiple advantages over a single wavelength laser system. First, both oxygenated and deoxygenated hemoglobin will absorb at these wavelengths. Second, blood vessels located deeper in the dermis will be affected. Third, thermal absorption by the exposed blood vessels should occur with less overlying epidermal absorption.

Utilizing these theoretical considerations, a pulsed light source radiating in the 515–1200 nm range (Energy Systems Corporation, Inc., Newton, Massachusetts) was used at varying energy fluences (5–20 J/cm²) and various pulse durations (3–15 msec) to treat the dorsal marginal rabbit ear vein ranging in size from 0.4 to 0.8 mm in diameter. The rabbit ear vein was then ana-lyzed. Variable degrees of intravascular coagulation occurred with all tested parameters. A pulse duration of 5 msec at 15 J/cm^2 produced the most specific vascular damage, with evidence of partial vessel fibrosis at 28 days. All higher pulse diameters produced nonspecific dermal co-agulation. Therefore, this experimental treatment modality has the potential for treating human venectasias 0.4–2.0 mm in diameter. Clinical trials using various parameters with the Energy Systems Corporation photo light source photoderm™ VL including multiple pulses of variable du-ration, have recently been completed and confirm the clinical efficacy of this device.

BIBLIOGRAPHY

Achauer BM, VanderKam VM. Argon laser treatment of the face and neck: 5 years' experience. *Lasers Surg Med* 1987;7:495.

Alderson MP. Spidre naevi—their incidence in healthy school children. *Arch Dis Child* 1963;38:286.

Anderson AR, et al. The optics of human skin. *J Invest Dermatol* 1981;77:13.

Anderson RR, Parrish JA. Microvasculature can be selectively damaged using dye lasers: a basic theory and experimental evidence in human skin. *Lasers Surg Med* 1981;1:263.

Anderson RR, Parrish JA. Selective photothermolysis: precise microsurgery by selective absorption of pulsed radiation. *Science* 1983;220:524.

Apfelberg DB, ed. *Atlas of Cutaneous Laser Surgery*. New York, Raven Press, 1992.

Apfelberg DB, et al. Study of three laser systems for treatment of superficial varicosities of the lower ex-tremity. *Lasers Surg Med* 1987;7:219.

Apfelberg DB, Maser MR, Lash H. Argon laser management of cutaneous vascular deformities: a prelimi-nary report. *West J Med* 1976;124:99.

Apfelberg DB, Maser MR, Lash H, et al. Use of the argon and carbon dioxide lasers for treatment of su-perficial venous varicosities of the lower extremity. *Lasers Surg Med* 1984;4:221.

Ashton N. Corneal vascularization. In *The Transparency of the Cornea*. S. Duke-Elder, ES Perkins, eds. Oxford, Blackwell, 1960,

Bean WB. *Vascular Spiders and Related Lesions of the Skin*, Springfield, IL, Charles C Thomas Co., 1958.

Bodian EL. Sclerotherapy. *Sem Dermatol* 1987;6:238.

Bohler-Sommeregger K, Karmel F, Schuller-Petrovic S, et al. Do telangiectases communicate with the deep venous system? *J Dermatol Surg Oncol* 1992;18:403.

Braverman IM. Ultrastructure and organization of the cutaneous microvasculature in normal and pathologic states. *J Invest Dermatol* 1989;93:2S.

Braverman IM, Keh-Yen A. Ultrastructure of the human dermal microcirculation. IV. Valve-containing col-lecting veins at the dermal-subcutaneous junction. *J Invest Dermatol* 1983;81:438.

Carruth JAS, van Gemert MJC, Shakespeare PG. The argon laser in the treatment of port-wine stain birth-mark. In *Management and Treatment of Benign Cutaneous Vascular Lesions*, OT Tan, ed. Philadelphia, Lea and Febiger, 1992,

Chess C, Chess Q. Cool laser optics treatment of large telangiectasia of the lower extremities. *J Dermatol Surg Oncol* 1993;19:74.

Corcos L, Longo L. Classification and treatment of telangiectases of the lower limbs. *Laser* 1988;1:22.

Cosman B. Role of retreatment in minimal-power argon laser therapy for port-wine stains, *Lasers Surg Med* 1982;2:43.

Dinehart S. The copper vapor laser for treatment of cutaneous vascular and pigmented lesions. *J Dermatol Surg Oncol* (in press).

Dinehart SM, Waner M. Comparison of the copper vapor and flashlamp-pulsed dye laser in the treatment of facial telangiectasia. *J Am Acad Dermatol* 1991;24:116.

Dixon JA, Rotering RH, Huethner SE. Patient's evaluation of argon laser therapy of port-wine stain, deco-rative tattoos, and essential telangiectasia. *Lasers Surg Med* 1984;4:181.

Dolsky RL. Argon laser skin surgery. *Surg Clin North Am* 1984;64:861.

Duffy DM. Small vessel sclerotherapy: an overview. In *Advances in Dermatology*. Chicago, Yearbook Medical Publishers, 1988, p. 221.

Dvorak HF. Tumors: wounds that do not heal: similarities between tumor stroma generation and wound healing. *N Engl J Med* 1986;315:1650.

Engel A, Johnson ML, Haynes SG. Health effects of sunlight exposure in the United States: results from the first national health and nutrition examination survey, 1971–1974. *Arch Dermatol* 1988;124:72.

Fajardo LF, et al. Hyperthermia inhibits angiogenesis. *Radiat Res* 1988;114:297.

Faria JL de, Moraes IN. Histopathology of the telangiectasias associated with varicose veins. *Dermatologia* 1963;127:321.

Fitzpatrick RE, et al. Treatment of facial telangiectasia with the flash pump dye laser. *Lasers Surg Med* (suppl) 1991;3:70.

Fitzpatrick RE, Feinberg JA. Low dose argon therapy of port-wine stains. *ICALEO '83 Proc* 1984;6:47.

Folkman J, Klagsbrun M. Angiogenic factors. *Science* 1987;235:442.

Frazzetta M, Palumbo FP, Bellisi M, et al. Considerations regarding the use of the CO_2 laser: personal case study. *Laser* 1989;2:4.

Garden JM, Tan OT, Kerschmann R, et al. Effect of dye laser pulse duration on selective cutaneous vascular injury. *J Invest Dermatol* 1986;87:653.

Geronemus RG. Treatment of spider telangiectases in children using the flashlamp pumped pulsed dye laser. *Pediatr Dermatol* 1991;8:61.

Glassberg E, et al. The flashlamp-pumped 577 nm pulsed tunable dye laser: clinical efficacy and in vitro studies. *J Dermatol Surg Oncol* 1988;14:1200.

Goldman MP. Complications and adverse sequelae of sclerotherapy. In *Sclerotherapy Treatment of Varicose and Telangiectatic Leg Veins*. MP Goldman, ed. St. Louis, Mosby-Yearbook, 1991,

Goldman MP, et al. Pulsed dye laser treatment of telangiectasia with and without sub-therapeutic sclerotherapy: clinical and histologic examination in the rabbit ear vein model. *J Am Acad Dermatol* 1990;23:23.

Goldman MP, Bennett RG. Treatment of telangiectasia: a review. *J Am Acad Dermatol* 1987;17:167.

Goldman MP, Fitzpatrick RE. Pulsed-dye laser treatment of leg telangiectasia: with and without simultaneous sclerotherapy. *J Dermatol Surg Oncol* 1990;16:338.

Goldman MP, Fitzpatrick RE, Ruiz-Esparza J. Treatment of spider telangiectasia in children. *Contemp Pediatr* (in press).

Goldman MP, Kaplan RP, Duffy DM. Postsclerotherapy hyperpigmentation: a histologic evaluation. *J Dermatol Surg Oncol* 1987;13:547.

Gonzalez E, Gange RW, Momtaz K. Treatment of telangiectases and other benign vascular lesions with the 577 nm pulsed dye laser. *J Am Acad Dermatol* 1992;27:220.

Greenwald J, et al. Comparative histological studies of the tunable dye (at 577 nm) laser and argon laser: the specific vascular effects of the dye laser. *J Invest Dermatol* 1981;77:305.

Kaplan I, Peled I. The carbon dioxide laser in the treatment of superficial telangiectases, *Br J Plast Surg* 1975;28:214.

Landthaler M, et al. Laser therapy of venous lakes (Bean-Walsh) and telangiectasias. *Plastic Reconstr Surg* 1984;73:78.

Lowe NJ, et al. Flashlamp pumped dye laser for rosacea-associated telangiectasia and erythema. *J Dermatol Surg Oncol* 1991;17:522.

Lowe NJ, Burgess P, Borden H. Flash pump dye laser fire during general anesthesia oxygenation: case report. *J Clin Laser Med Surg* 1990;8(2):39.

Lyons GD, Owens RE, Moriney DF. Argon laser destruction of cutaneous telangiectatic lesions. *Laryngoscope* 1981;91:1322.

Majewski S, et al. Angiogenic capability of peripheral blood mononuclear cells in psoriasis. *Arch Dermatol* 1985;121:1018.

McDaniel DH, Mordon S. Hexascan: a new robotized scanning laser handpiece. *Cutis* 1990;45:300.

Merlen JF. Red telangiectasias, blue telangiectasias. *Soc Franc Phlebol* 1970;22:167.

Miami A, Rubertsi U. Collecting venules. *Minerva Cardioangiol* 1958;41:541.

Mordon SR, et al. Comparison study of the "point-by-point technique" and the "scanning technique" for laser treatment of port-wine stains. *Lasers Surg Med* 1989;9:398.

Mortemedi M, Welch AJ, Tan OT, et al. Non-linear changes in optical behavior of tissue during laser irradiation. *Lasers Surg Med* 1987;7:72.

Murdock L, Waner M, Griffin E. The treatment of vascular and pigmented malformations with a copper vapor laser. Presented at the International Conference Photodynamic Therapy and Medical Laser Applications, London, 1988.

Nakagawa H, Tan OT, Parrish JA. Ultrastructural changes in human skin after exposure to a pulsed laser. *J Invest Dermatol* 1985;84:396.

Neumann RA, Leonhartsberger H, Bohler-Sommeregger K, et al. Results and tissue healing after copper-vapour laser (at 578 nm) treatment of port wine stains and facial telangiectasias. *Br J Dermatol* 1993;128:306.

Orenstein A, Nelson JS. Treatment of facial vascular lesions with a 100 μ spot 577 nm pulsed continuous wave dye laser. *Ann Plast Surg* 1989;23:310.

Oster J, Nielsen A. Nuchal naevi and intracapsular telangiectases. *Acta Paediat Scand* 1970;59:416.

Ouvry PA, Davy A. The sclerotherapy of telangiectasia. *Phlebologie* 1982;35:349.

Pickering JW, Walker EP, Butler PH, et al. Copper vapor laser treatment of port-wine stains and other vascular malformations. *Br J Plast Surg* 1990;43:273.

Pickering TW, van Gemert MJC. 585 nm for the laser treatment of port-wine stains: a possible mechanism (letter). *Lasers Surg Med* 1991;11:616.

Polla LL, et al. Tunable pulsed dye laser for the treatment of benign cutaneous vascular ectasia. *Dermatologica* 1987;174:11.

Redisch W, Pelzer RH. Localized vascular dilatations of the human skin: capillary microscopy and related studies. *Am Heart J* 1949;37:106.

Rotteleur G, et al. Robotized scanning laser handpiece for the treatment of port-wine stains and other angiodysplasias. *Lasers Surg Med* 1988;8:283.

Ryan TJ. Factors influencing the growth of vascular endothelium in the skin. *Br J Dermatol* 1970;85(suppl 5):99.

Sadick NS. Treatment of varicose and telangiectatic leg veins with hypertonic saline: a comparative study of heparin and saline. *J Dermatol Surg Oncol* 1990;16:24.

Scheibner A, Applebaum J, Wheeland RG. Treatment of port-wine hemangiomas in children. *Lasers Surg Med* 1989;1(suppl):42.

Scheibner A, Wheeland TG. Argon-pumped tunable dye laser therapy for facial port-wine stain hemangiomas in adults—a new technique using small spot size and minimal power. *J Dermatol Surg Oncol* 1989;15:277.

Scheibner A, Wheeland RG. Use of the argon-pumped tunable dye laser for port-wine stains in children. *J Dermatol Surg Oncol* 1991;17:735.

Tan TT, Carney JM, Margolis R, et al. Histologic responses of port-wine stains treated by argon, carbon dioxide, and tunable dye lasers: a preliminary report. *Arch Dermatol* 1986;122:1016.

Tan OT, Kerschmann R, Parrish JA. Effect of skin temperature on selective vascular injury caused by pulsed laser irradiation. *J Invest Dermatol* 1985;85:441.

Tan OT, Kurban AK. Noncongenital benign cutaneous vascular lesions: pulse dye laser treatment. In *Management and Treatment of Benign Cutaneous Vascular Lesions*. OT Tan, ed. Philadelphia, Lea and Febiger, 1992,

Tan OT, Mortemedi M, Welch A, et al. Spot size effects on guinea pig skin following pulsed irradiation. *J Invest Dermatol* 1988;90:877.

Tan OT, Murray S, Kurban A. Action spectrum of vascular specific injury using pulsed irradiation. *J Invest Dermatol* 1989;92:868.

Tan OT, Sherwood K, Gilchrest BA. Treatment of children with port-wine stains using the flashlamp-pulsed tunable dye laser. *N Engl J Med* 1989;320:416.

Tan OT, Stafford TJ, Murray S, et al. Histologic comparison of the pulsed dye laser and copper vapor laser effects on pig skin. *Lasers Surg Med* 1990;10:551.

Thibault PK. Copper vapor laser and microsclerotherapy of facial telangiectases. *J Dermatol Surg Oncol* 1994;20:48.

Thibault P, Bray A. Cosmetic leg veins: evaluation using duplex venous imaging. *J Dermatol Surg Oncol* 1990;16:612.

Tretbar LL. The origin of reflux in incompetent blue reticular/telangiectasia veins. In *Phlebologie '89*. R Davy, R Stemmer eds. London, John Libby Eurotext, Ltd, 1989, p. 95.

van Gemert MCJ, et al. Can physical modeling lead to an optimal laser treatment strategy for portwine stains? In *Laser Applications in Medicine and Biology*. Vol. 5. ML Wolbarsht, ed. New York, Plenum Publishers, 1991, pp. 109–275.

van Gemert MJC, Hulsbergen-Henning JP. A model approach to laser coagulation of dermal vascular lesions. *Arch Dermatol Res* 1981;270:429.

Waner M, Dinehart S. Lasers in facial plastic and reconstructive surgery. In *Lasers in Otolaryngology Head and Neck Surgery*, RK Davis, S Shapstray, eds. Philadelphia, WB Saunders, 1989,

Waner M, Dinehart SM, Wilson MB, et al. A comparison of copper vapor and flashlamp pumped dye lasers in the treatment of facial telangiectasia. *J Dermatol Surg Oncol* 1993;19:992.

Weiss RA, Weiss MA. Resolution of pain associated with varicose and telangiectatic leg veins after compression sclerotherapy. *J Dermatol Surg Oncol* 1990;16:333.

Wenzl JE, Burgert EO. The spider nevus in infancy and childhood. *Pediatrics* 1964;33:227.

Wokalek H, et al. Morphology and localization of sunburst varicosities: an electron microscopic and morphometric study. *J Dermatol Surg Oncol* 1989;15:149.

59

Treatment of the Aging Face

Henry H. Roenigk, Jr.
Northwestern University Medical School, Chicago, Illinois

Why is aging skin and especially the aging face so important to patients and dermatologists? What causes aging skin? Who is making this an important issue? The media certainly puts great emphasis on youth, good looks, and smooth young healthy skin to sell everything from cosmetics to beer to automobiles. Who is pushing this need to get treatment for your small wrinkles? Is it driven by the pharmaceutical companies or cosmetic companies that make large profits on products to rid us of wrinkles? Is it a real issue with a health-conscious public that is looking for the fountain of youth? How should the dermatologist be prepared to deal with patients who want treatment for their aging faces?

ETIOLOGY OF AGING SKIN

There have been several good reviews on aging skin, such as Hurleys "Skin in Senescence," which is an excellent mix of science and therapy as we know it today. Kligman, who has influenced the literature on aging skin, stated that "growing old" represents a most intriguing set of biological events in all species but in humans creates both physical and psychologic problems. Despite its obvious importance, aging has only recently stimulated more intense scientific interest.

Skin aging has two distinct components. One is intrinsic aging: those clinical, histologic, and physiologic changes that occur in the skin throughout the body of all individuals with the passage of time, perhaps beginning at birth, perhaps beginning at age 20, perhaps being accelerated in the latter decades of life. Intrinsic aging is genetic in origin. Some of the changes in the skin and muscles are influenced by genetic factors (e.g., skin of redheads of Irish descent, or black skin of African Americans). Some facial muscle changes may also be influenced by intrinsic factors.

The second component of aging skin is actinic radiation, which accounts for the pathologic term "photoaging skin" (Fig. 1). Exposure to ultraviolet radiation (UVR), especially UVB (290–320 nm), is the principal environmental insult responsible for photoaging. Longer wave-

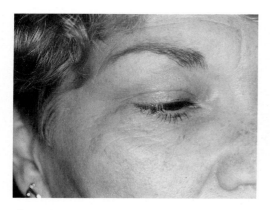

Figure 1   Photoaging skin with fine wrinkles around the eye.

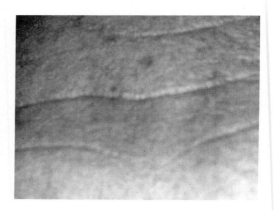

Figure 2   Deep brow lines.

lengths of UVR or UVA (320–400 nm) also participate in photoaging, especially its effect on the dermis, and may act synergistically with UVB in photoaging and photocarcinogenesis. Shorter wavelengths of UVR, such as UVC (200–290 nm), are not contributors, since they do not penetrate the earth's atmosphere.

PHOTOAGING

Clinically

Clinically, photoaged skin appears wrinkled and has a nodular, leathery surface which is frequently blotchy (Fig. 2,3). In extreme cases, deep furrows appear in a rhomboid geometric pattern on the posterior neck; this has been described as *cutis rhomboidalis elastosis.* The skin has a yellow to reddish hue and has been referred to as "red neck." Conversely, chronologically aged skin is unremarkable in its clinical appearance, with a smooth, unblemished surface with some loss of elasticity. The clinical manifestations are usually referred to as wrinkles, sagging skin, and furrow (Figs. 4–6).

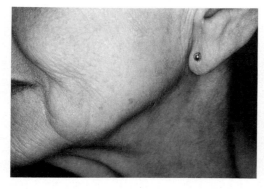

Figure 3   Deeper wrinkles and sagging of skin on lateral cheek.

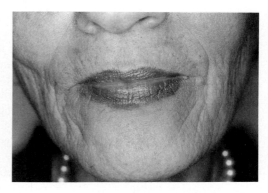

Figure 4   Deeper wrinkles and fat atrophy of both cheeks. Perioral wrinkles.

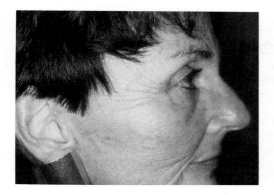

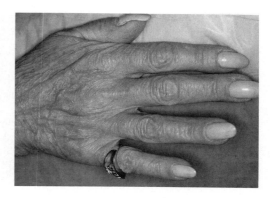

Figure 5 Deep furrows and sagging of lateral facial skin in a patient who has already had one face lift procedure.

Figure 6 Atrophy and wrinkling of skin of hand of older person.

Less common manifestations of chronic sun damage include dryness, rosacea, seborrheic keratoses, spider nevi, superficial varicose veins, pterygia, ectropion, arcus senilis, and certain changes in the mouth. Eventually, precancerous (actinic keratosis) and cancerous tumors (basal cell carcinoma and squamous cell carcinoma) develop.

Cellular and Molecular

The cellular and molecular mechanisms of cutaneous aging have only been clarified in part. Genetic factors are believed to have a major influence on aging. Ultraviolet radiation damages primarily keratinocytes, melanocytes, and fibroblasts in the skin through production of free radicals, i.e., atoms, ions, or molecules with an unpaired electron. Superoxide free radicals so formed can result in DNA breaks, damage cell membrane lipids, and interfere with cell enzymes. Free radical–clearing enzymes such as catalase, glutathione peroxidase, and superoxide disumutase help to deter or correct such damage and thus may modify the rate and degree of aging, although such palliative influence may still be more theoretical than actual.

Histology

Aging skin has distinct characteristics microscopically and physiologically. Changes are apparent in all skin layers and cells, in melanocytes, Langerhans cells, hair follicles, in sebaceous, eccrine, and apocrine glands, in the lymphatic and blood vessels, and in cutaneous innervation. Methods available for assessment of the physical and functional state of skin, including noninvasive techniques, have recently been discussed.

A thinning of the viable epidermis, basal keratinocyte heterogeneity, and a flattening of the dermal-epidermal junction are the most characteristic histologic changes associated with chronologically aged skin. Epidermal thinning is believed to reflect, in part, the well-accepted idea that epidermal proliferation decreases with age.

The most profound differences between chronological and photoaging are found in the dermis. Chronologically aged dermis generally has diminished amounts of eosinophilic material, and fibroblasts appear shrunken and smaller. This is in contrast to the photoaged dermis, which has a wide band of eosinophilic material (grenz zone) just beneath the epidermis. Beneath the grenz zone, there is a marked accumulation of abnormally stained elastic fibers organized into amorphous masses, telangiectatic vessels, and the presence of perivenular, histiocytic-lymphocytic infiltrate, along with numerous mast cells. Table 1 lists the histological features of aging skin, whereas the major physiological changes in aging skin are listed in Table 2.

Table 1 Histologic Features of Aging Human Skin

Epidermis	Dermis	Appendages
Flattened dermal/epidermal junction	Atrophy (loss of dermal volume)	Depigmented hair
Variable thickness	Fewer fibroblasts	Loss of hair
Variable cell size and shape	Fewer mast cells	Conversion of terminal to vellus hair
Occasional nuclear atypia	Fewer blood vessels	Abnormal nail plates
Fewer melanocytes	Shortened capillary loops	Fewer glands
Fewer Langerhans cells	Abnormal nerve endings	

Source: Gilchrest BA. *Skin and Aging Processes*. Boca Raton, FL, CRC Press, Inc., 1984.

Dermatoheliosis, or the effects of chronic sun damage on skin, is primarily extrinsic aging, which is preventable. The clinical and histologic features of dermatoheliosis have been summarized by Gilchrest in Table 3.

Classification

Glogau has prepared a very useful classification to help the dermatologist direct treatment to the aging face. The four categories are primarily based on age and severity of chronic photoaging changes in the skin (Table 4).

TREATMENT OF THE AGING FACE

The practice of dermatology has changed, with an increased emphasis on cosmetics and the prolongation and restoration of a youthful appearance. Television news programs present stories on the "latest cure for wrinkles." Many women's magazines promote the supposedly safe, easy, and free of side effects "quick cure" for wrinkled or older looking skin. Having been

Table 2 Functions of Skin That Decline with Age

Cell replacement
Injury response
Barrier function
Chemical clearance
Sensory perception
Immune responsiveness
Vascular responsiveness
Thermoregulation
Sweat production
Sebum production
Vitamin D production

Source: Gilchrest BA. *Skin and Aging Processes*. Boca Raton, FL, CRC Press Inc., 1984.

Table 3 Features of Actinically Damaged Skin

Clinical abnormalities	Histologic abnormality	Presumed pathophysiology
Dryness (roughness)	Minimal stratum corneum irregularity	Altered keratinocyte maturation
Actinic keratoses	Nuclear atypia; loss of orderly, progressive keratinocyte maturation; irregular epidermal hyperplasia and/or hypoplasia; hypoplasia; occasional dermal inflammation	Premalignant disorder
Irregular pigmentation		
Freckling	Reduced number of hypertrophied, strongly dopa-positive melanocytes	Reactive hyperplasia and later loss of functional melanocytes
Lentigenes	Elongation of epidermal ridges; increase in number and melanization of melanocytes	
Guttate hypomelanosis	Absence of melanocytes	
Dermis		
Wrinkling, fine surface lines	None detected	Alterations in dermal and matrix and fibrous proteins
Deep furrows, stellate pseudo-scars	Absence of epidermal pigmentation, altered dermal collagen	Loss of functional melanocytes, reactive collagen deposition by fibroblasts
Elastosis (fine nodularity and or coarseness)	Nodular aggregations of fibrous to amorphorous material in the papillary dermis	Overproduction of abnormal elastin fibers
Inelasticity	Elastotic dermis	Altered elastin fibers
Telangiectasia	Ectatic vessels often with atrophic walls	Loss of connective tissue support
Venous lakes	Ectatic vessels often atrophic walls	Loss of connective tissue support
Purpura (easy bruising)	Extravasated erythrocytes	Loss of connective tissue support
Appendages		
Comedones (maladie de Favre et Racouchot)	Ectatic superficial portion of the pilosebaceous follicle	Loss of connective tissue support
Sebaceous hyperplasia	Concentric hyperplasia of sebaceous glands	Increased mitotive and functional responsiveness of glandular tissue

Source: Gilchrest BA. *Skin and Aging Processes.* Boca Raton, FL, CRC Press, Inc., 1984.

Table 4 Glogau's Classification of Photoaging of the Face

Type I: "No Wrinkles"
Early photoaging
   mild pigmentary changes
   no keratoses
   minimal wrinkles
Patient age: twenties or thirties
Minimal or no makeup

Type II: "Wrinkles in Motion"
Early to moderate photoaging
   early senile lentigines visible
   keratoses palpable but not visible
   parallel smile lines beginning to appear
Patient age: late thirties or forties
Usually wears some foundation

Type III: "Wrinkles at Rest"
Advanced photoaging
   obvious dyschromia, telangiectasia
   visible keratoses
   wrinkles even when not moving
Patient age: fifties or older
Always wears heavy foundation

Type IV: "Only Wrinkles"
Severe photoaging
   yellow-gray color of skin
   prior skin malignancies
   wrinkled skin throughout, no normal skin
Patient age: sixth or seventh decade
Can't wear makeup—"cakes and cracks"

---

brainwashed by such misrepresentations, the patient presents to the dermatologist with great and often unrealistic expectations for a cure that will save their marriage or help make a sale at work the next day. The dermatologist's responsibility is to help the patient sort out these fables and real treatment options, then recommend what the patient really needs and is safe. Carefully done scientific studies for many of these treatments are lacking. Frequently, there are conflicts of interest and significant monetary gain in selling certain plans/procedures to create a new youthful image. Physicians often sell products in their offices in which they have a financial investment. Dermatologists should know the limits of the treatments and procedures they perform. They should be willing to refer patients to other surgeons with skills in the more advanced surgical treatments of the aging skin.

SUNSCREENS

Sunscreens may prevent sun-related skin damage and solar aging if the product used has a high sun-protection factor (SPF) and blocks UVA, but only if the product is used early in life and on a regular basis. SPF is defined as the ratio of the least amount of UVB energy required to produce a minimal erythema reaction (MED) through a sunscreen product to the amount of energy required to produce the same erythema without any sunscreen application. Sunscreen with an SPF of 15 or more not only prevents UV damage, but solar-damaged skin of experimental animals will repair itself if these same sunscreen products are used when UV exposure is given. Education of the public by dermatologists and their national organizations (American Academy of Dermatology, American Society for Dermatologic Surgery) is very important.

MOISTURIZERS

Dry skin has been confused with aged skin. Dry skin can occur at any age, but it worsens with age. The constant use of moisturizers will help keep the skin hydrated and smooth. Dry skin is more prone to itch, becoming inflamed, produce eczema, and get secondary bacterial infection.

The majority of moisturizers, cosmetic or pharmaceutical, are mixtures of oils, water, and an emulsifying agent that is used to keep the oil and water in suspension. Perfumes, preservatives, and other ingredients that enhance the cosmetic elegance or chemical stability of a product may be added. The emollient may be either an oil-in-water or a water-in-oil emulsion. When the continuous phase is water, oil is in the disperse phase, and vice versa. When moisturizers are applied to the skin surface, some of the water is absorbed by the stratum corneum, but most of it evaporates while the nonvolatile oil remains on the surface, acting as a lubricant. One example of a moisturizer often used by dermatologist is 12% ammonium lactate.

ALPHA HYDROXY ACIDS AND TOPICAL TRETINOIN

Alpha hydroxy acids (AHAs) have been the hottest addition to the cosmetic industry in the last several years. Most cosmetics with AHAs sold in department stores and beauty salons contain 3–6% AHA. Some cosmetologists are using up to 30% concentrations to do mini face peels without medical supervision. Some physicians—again those with financial interest in the companies producing AHAs—are encouraging nonmedical professionals to do these mini peels. Some physicians have cosmetologists in their offices doing 50–70% AHA peels.

Moisturizers such as 12% ammonium lactate change the dry skin stratum corneum from a disorganized group of cells with cracks and fissures to a more compact organized arrangement of cells. AHA treatment of dry skin results in the thinning of the stratum corneum and maintenance of a compact, well-organized stratum corneum for a short period of time after treatment is discontinued. AHAs remove a portion of the dry skin type of stratum corneum, and they might improve the stratum corneum's ability to protect against environmental insults.

The histological profile noted after AHA treatment has similarities to that achieved with topical tretinoin treatment. Topical tretinoin results in a marked thickening of the viable epidermis, compaction of the stratum corneum, and an increase in glycosaminoglycans. One of the differences between AHAs and tretinoin is that after treatment with ammonium lactate, the stratum corneum of AHA-treated skin retains its "basketweave" appearance, whereas the tretinoin-treated skin modifies the stratum corneum, yielding a thinner and more compact horny layer.

AHAs modestly thicken the viable epidermis and increase the deposition of glycosaminoglycans in the dermis. These changes are not accompanied by clinical or histologic signs of irritation and/or inflammation. Clinical studies have shown a benefit from AHAs, but double-blind controlled studies are lacking. Glycolic acid 70% peels (Table 5) can produce improvement in mild photoaging, acne, and melasma (Figs. 7–14). With respect to treating aging skin, a combination of topical tretinoin and AHAs might represent the treatment of choice.

Originally used in the treatment of acne, topical tretinoin or all-*trans* retinoic acid was first proposed for management of the effects of photoaging in 1986 by Kligman et al. Structural and functional improvement was observed after several months of applying a 0.05% and later a 0.1%

Table 5 Glycolic Acid Peel

Glycolic acid 50–70%
Skin Prep
  alcohol
  acetone
Neutralize 3–10 min
Repeat weekly 6×

tretinoin cream as compared to a control preparation. An increase in epidermal thickness, decreased keratinocyte atypia, altered and more uniform distribution of melanin granules, and increased collagen and fibroblast activity in the dermis were seen histologically. Four different effects have been emphasized, namely, increased epidermal thickness, increased thickness of the granular layer, decreased melanin content, and compaction of the stratum corneum. Clinically, a smoother texture with loss of or diminution of fine wrinkling was the most striking change described (Figs. 15,16). A faint erythema, lightening of lentigines, and perhaps improvement in deeper, more coarse wrinkling has also been described. The improvement appeared to be maximal after 6–10 months, although some patients felt that still further clearing occurred with longer use. Tretinoin can be used on nonfacial areas, such as the neck, upper anterior chest and back, forearms, and hands, but it tends to be more irritating and may accordingly be less effective on these sites. The required maintenance use of tretinoin suggests that the improvement seen is only temporary and results from simple irritation and edema. Goldfarb et al. and Marks have shown in double-blind placebo-controlled studies that tretinoin cream improved extrinsic aging with improvement in fine and coarse wrinkles, brown spots, and roughness. Weinstein et al. in a large multicenter trial showed similar effects with tretinoin 0.05% and 0.01% in a new emollient cream. Histologic changes also confirmed previous studies. The possible complications of long-term use of topical tretinoins are not known, although none have been seen in acne patients.

SOFT TISSUE AUGMENTATION

Soft tissue augmentation is a technique in which a substance is injected under the skin. It is used to correct wrinkles, depressions, and acne scarring. This treatment has continued acceptance and

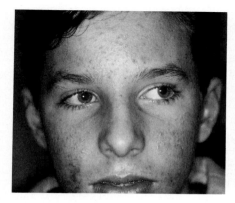

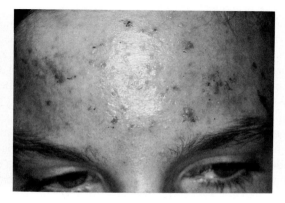

Figure 7 Patient with severe comedo type acne.

Figure 8 After several treatments with glycolic acid 70% peel to face.

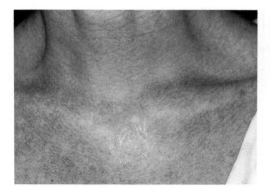

Figure 9 Photoaging skin of anterior chest before glycolic acid peel.

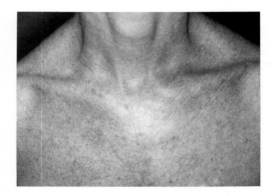

Figure 10 One week after 70% glycolic acid peel.

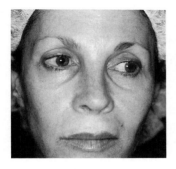

Figure 11 Photoaging skin of face before glycolic acid peel.

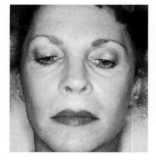

Figure 12 After 70% glycolic acid peel, the skin is smoother and has improved texture.

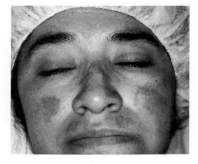

Figure 13 Melasma of both cheeks.

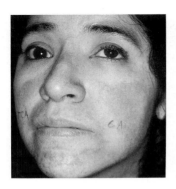

Figure 14 After treatment of melasma with 70% glycolic acid peel.

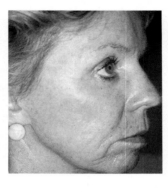

Figure 15 Photoaging skin and fine wrinkles, sagging skin.

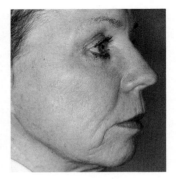

Figure 16 After topical tretinoin for 4 months, there is improvement in texture and fine wrinkles but no change in sagging skin.

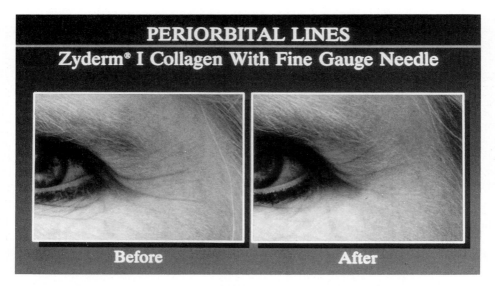

Figure 17 Before and after Zyderm I treatment of periorbital fine wrinkles.

widespread use. There are several choices of injectable substances. Among the collagen treatments, Zyderm (bovine) collagen may be injected to soften wrinkles (Fig. 17,18). Zyderm collagen is used for the correction of superficial (Figs. 19,20) to medium-depth wrinkling. Zyplast collagen (glutaraldehyde cross-linked bovine collagen) is used to treat deeper scars, furrows, creases, and wrinkles (Figs. 21,22). The effects generally last 3–12 months. Two skin tests are necessary before injecting collagen into the skin in large amounts.

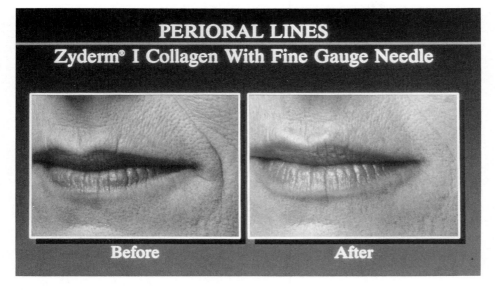

Figure 18 Before and after Zyderm I treatment of perioral wrinkles.

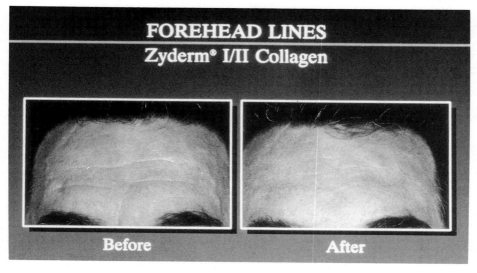

Figure 19 Before and after treatment of deeper brow lines with Zyderm I/II.

Fibrel, a gelatin matrix implant activated by the patient's own blood products, is also used to correct scars, in addition to the treatment of wrinkles. A series of treatments is normally necessary, as are skin tests.

Microlipoinjection (fat injection or autologous fat) involves fat extracted from one part of a patient's body (thigh, abdomen) and injected into the area of depression in another part. Evidence is being gathered to determine the longevity of these benefits. In studies at Northwestern

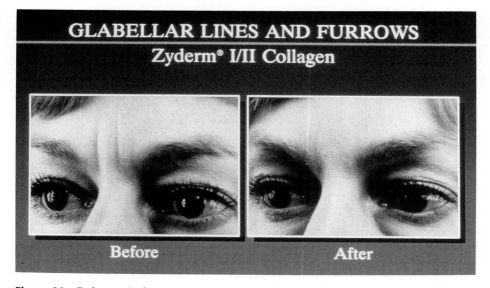

Figure 20 Before and after treatment of glabellar lines and furrows with Zyderm I/II.

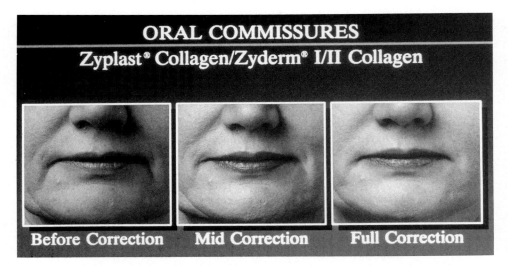

Figure 21 Before and after treatment of oral commissures with Zyplast (Zyderm I/II).

University, we found that in some areas, fat transplantation will last for over 6 years. This is especially true in the forehead, where there is bone below the skin. The advantage of fat transplant is that there are no allergic reactions, because the patient's own fat is used.

CHEMICAL PEEL

Chemical peeling has become a very popular way to remove wrinkles of the face, hands, and chest, along with other changes of photoaging. Chemical peeling, also known as chemexfoliation

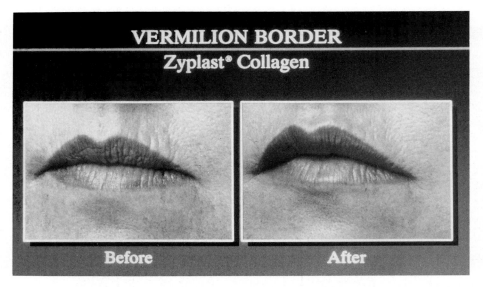

Figure 22 Before and after treatment of vermilion border wrinkles with Zyplast giving a smoother fuller lip.

Table 6 Chemical Peeling Agents

Trichloracetic acid 25, 35, or 50%
Jessner's solution
Alpha hydroxy acids
Glycolic acid 70%
Pyruvic acid
Phenol Baker/Gordon
Combinations

or dermapeeling, is used to improve the skin's appearance as well as to remove precancerous lesions. A chemical solution (Table 6) is applied to the skin that causes it to blister and peel. The new, regenerated skin is usually smoother and less wrinkled than the photodamaged skin.

Although used primarily for cosmetic purposes, this procedure is also used therapeutically. Cosmetic indications for chemical peel include wrinkles caused by aging, sun damage, or hereditary factors; superficial acne scarring; and irregular pigmentation of skin, including freckles and lentigines. Melasma that occurs in women during pregnancy or while taking birth control pills can also be improved. Precancerous conditions such as actinic keratosis also respond well to treatment. Chemical peel is sometimes done in conjunction with other surgical procedures, such as rhytidectomy (face lift). Examples of patients with severe photodamage and multiple actinic keratoses show the benefit of chemical peel in reversing these changes (Figs. 23–35).

Chemical peeling with Baker's phenol (Table 7) solution is an effective method for removal of severe wrinkles. Limitations are hypopigmentation and toxicity resulting from systemic absorption of phenol.

Results from chemical peels are consistent if the procedure is done properly. The best results are seen in younger patients with early changes due to photoaging, but improvement can also be seen in older patients with more extensive wrinkling.

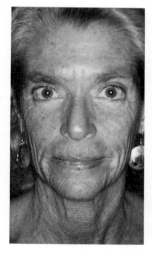 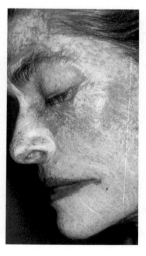 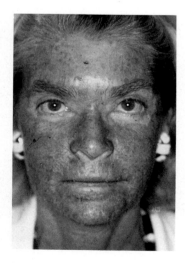

Figure 23 Severe photo-aged skin and deep wrinkles and sagging of skin.

Figure 24 TCA 50% full-face peel applied.

Figure 25 Four days after 50% TCA peel with fine crusting.

Table 7 Deep Peel—Baker's Phenol

Phenol 88% USP	3 ml
Croton oil	3 gtt
Septisol soap	8 gtt
Distilled water	2 ml

CRYOPEEL

Spot freezing of actinic keratosis on the face is a very common procedure and works well with minimal scarring or hypopigmentation. Full-face cryopeeling can eliminate precancerous lesions and also improve the texture, wrinkles, and pigmentary problems associated with photoaging.

Chiarello described this technique, which results in moderate to marked swelling similar to chemical peel but results in smoother-textured skin and fewer wrinkles. Examples of two of Chiarello's patients are shown in Figures 26–39.

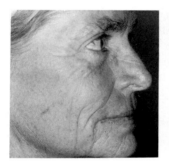

Figure 26 Before TCA peel.

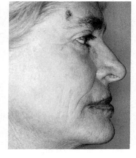

Figure 27 After TCA peel.

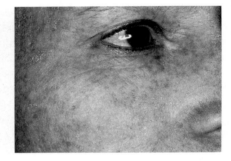

Figure 28 Severe photoaging and multiple actinic keratoses in young woman.

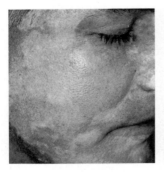

Figure 29 Immediately following 50% TCA peel.

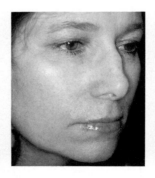

Figure 30 Two months after TCA peel.

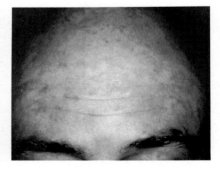

Figure 31 Severe photoaging and multiple actinic keratoses of forehead and scalp.

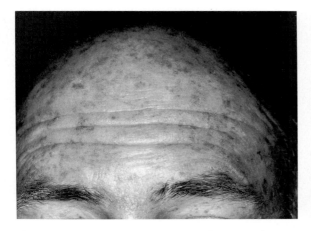

Figure 32 Crusting during healing of TCA 50% peel.

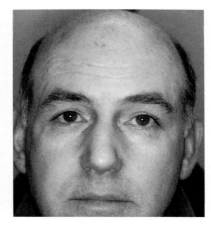

Figure 33 Two months after TCA peel.

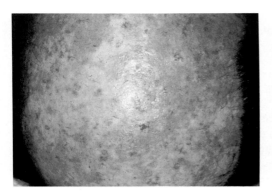

Figure 34 Scalp during TCA peel.

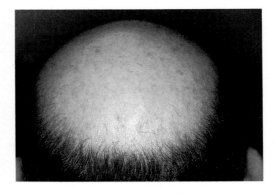

Figure 35 Scalp 2 months after TCA peel.

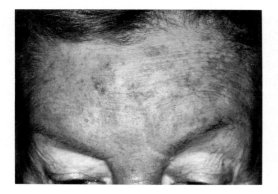

Figure 36 Forehead with severe actinic damage.

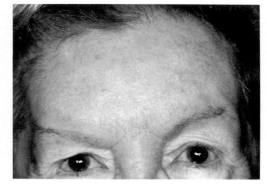

Figure 37 Three months after cryopeel of forehead.

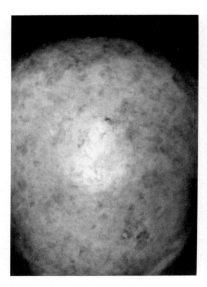 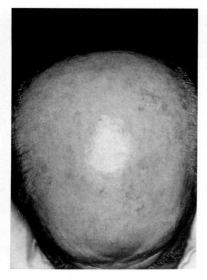

Figure 38 Scalp with sever photo-aging and multiple actinic keratoses.

Figure 39 Two months after cryopeel of scalp.

DERMABRASION

Dermabrasion, or surgical skin planing, is a procedure in which the dermatologic surgeon freezes the patient's skin and then abrades the skin with a rotary instrument. This abrasive or planing action is used to improve the skin's contour as new collagen and epidermis replace the abraded skin. The new skin generally has a smoother appearance.

Dermabrasion was originally a method of treating acne scars. It has been used to treat a variety of conditions, including hypertrophic scars, traumatic scars, actinically damaged and wrinkled skin, and pigmentary abnormalities. Among the cosmetic indications for dermabrasion are acne scars, fine wrinkling, scar revision, melasma, and perioral wrinkles.

The details of the technique, equipment, postoperative care, etc., are covered in review articles. In dermabrasion, as opposed to chemical peel, there are several important points to remember. Dermabrasion is often performed on young, healthy 18-year-olds with acne scars. These individuals usually heal quickly after dermabrasion and do not often have medical problems. They are normally happy with the results. The same is not true when dealing with older patients. When doing a dermabrasion on older patients, preoperative sedation must be a concern. Patients should not be sedated as heavily because of the potential risk of cardiac and respiratory problems. Cardiac evaluation should be done. Physicians must be cautious of medications and other medical problems. Additionally, older patients have thin skin, and the healing process is slower.

There is a difference between chemical peel and dermabrasion for photoaging skin: dermabrasion can go deeper. Physician technique controls the depth, though it is more of an advantage when treating scars than when treating aging skin. Sometimes, however, especially with brow lines, there are deeper wrinkles than a chemical peel can erase, but dermabrasion can achieve a clearing of brow lines. The operator controls the depth, which is the obvious advantage. Postoperatively, however, healing is somewhat slower with dermabrasion—the erythema persists longer. Dressings are necessary for a dermabrasion but not with a chemical peel and chemical peeling is usually less expensive than dermabrasion.

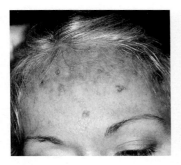 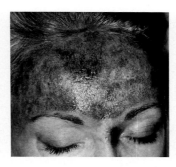 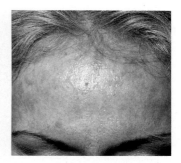

Figure 40 Severe photodamage and multiple actinic keratoses of forehead.

Figure 41 During dermabrasion of forehead.

Figure 42 Six months after dermabrasion of forehead.

Dermabrasion for aging skin is nothing new. Burks, who is the father of dermabrasion, wrote about this in the 1950s and did some studies in New Orleans at that time. He dermabraded only one side of some patients and followed them up, noting a marked difference in the two sides of the patient.

Chemical peeling will not always eradicate extensive actinic keratoses. One patient had had several liquid nitrogen treatments that did nothing to eradicate multiple actinic keratoses of the forehead due to sun damage (Fig. 40). Just her forehead was dermabrased, with excellent results (Fig. 41); she has been followed for the past 10 years (Fig. 42). Prior to dermabrasion, she was getting one or two actinic keratoses every month and since that time gets one or two per year.

A physician who was given all of the options, including dermabrasion and chemical peel, opted to have a full-face dermabrasion for multiple actinic keratoses and areas of actinic damage (Fig. 43). Soon after the dermabrasion, the brow lines seem to be eliminated, but once the edema is gone, the brow lines and nasal lateral folds return. However, the skin has an improved surface, and one year postoperative he has not had any recurrence of actinic keratoses or fine wrinkles (Fig. 44).

One of the potential problems of doing a dermabrasion is that in going deeper to obtain a better texture, the color of the skin is often lightened. With a full-face dermabrasion, there can be quite a color difference between the skin of the face and neck. These lines can usually be covered with some makeup, and sometimes a chemical peel of the neck will blend the color better. In general, patients don't mind the color difference.

One of the areas of the face that we have been particularly interested in has been the upper lip, which has been a difficult area to treat with chemical peeling unless full-strength phenol is used to eradicate the deep lines. There is a risk to treating that area because hypertrophic scars or keloids and hypopigmentation can occur. Topical tretinoin has very little effect in this area. Phenol peeling of the whole face does well and gives a fairly good result. Baker's peel does a very nice job for the whole face when used with tape, but many dermatologists don't like to do phenol peels. Full-strength phenol, open to lips only, can give good results. A large series of 54 patients from Sweden with perioral wrinkles had good results from dermabrasion. One patient had a good result from a chemical peel with 50% TCA (Fig. 45) in all areas except the perioral area (Fig. 46). We then did a dermabrasion of just the perioral area (Fig. 47), and one year later it was greatly improved (Fig. 48). Another patient received collagen injections to the lips every 6 months for years (Figs. 49,50). Selective dermabrasion of lip (Figs. 51–53) resulted in good and permanent results.

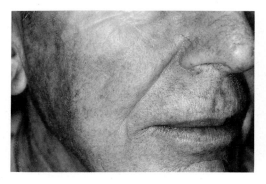

Figure 43 Severe actinic keratoses of face before dermabrasion.

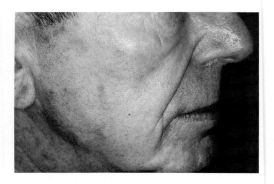

Figure 44 Six months after full-face dermabrasion.

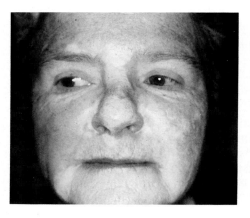

Figure 45 During TCA full-face peel for wrinkles.

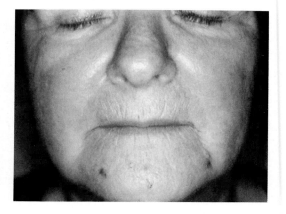

Figure 46 All areas of face improved after TCA peel except perioral area.

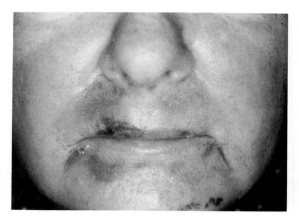

Figure 47 One week after dermabrasion of perioral area.

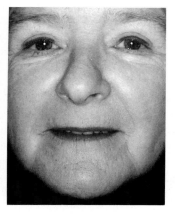

Figure 48 One year after combined TCA peel and dermabrasion of perioral area.

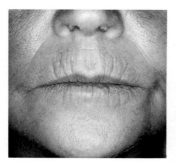
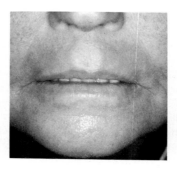
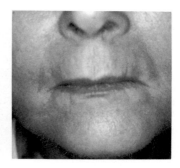

Figure 49 Perioral wrinkles treated with Zyderm in past.

Figure 50 Three months after dermabrasion of perioral area only.

Figure 51 Wrinkles of perioral area.

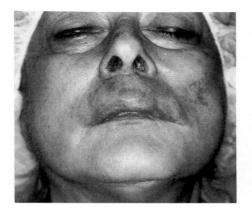
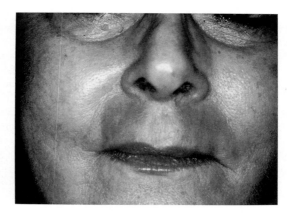

Figure 52 During dermabrasion.

Figure 53 Two months after dermabrasion of lips only.

In summary, there is more concern today about aging and increased interest in how technology can prevent or correct the effects of aging. The dermatologist has many different methods of approaching the problem. Topical application of moisturizers, sunscreens, tretinoin, and alpha hydroxy acids is something all dermatologists can advise to patients at risk. Procedures such as soft tissue augmentation and cryopeel are commonly done by most dermatologists. Chemical peeling and dermabrasion are often performed in the dermatologist's offices with excellent results, and both procedures have become more popular in recent years. Depending on their skills and training, physicians may choose to perform advanced procedures such as blepharoplasty and face lifts.

BIBLIOGRAPHY

Bhawan J, Gonzalez-Serva A, Nehal K, et al. Effects of tretinoin on photodamaged skin. *Arch Dermatol* 1991;127:666–672.

Cerimele D, Celeno L, Serri F. Physiological changes in aging skin. *Br J Dermatol* 1990;122(suppl 35):13–20.

Chiarello SE. Full face cryo (liquid nitrogen) peels. *J Dermatol Surg Oncol* 1992;18:329–332.

Engel A, Johnson ML, Haynes SJ. Health effects of sunlight exposure in the United States. *Arch Dermatol* 1988;124:72–79.

Gilchrest B. Cellular and molecular changes in aging skin. *J Geriatr Dermatol* 1994;2(1):3–6.

Gilchrest BA. *Skin and Aging Processes*. Boca Raton, CRC Press, 1984, pp. 1–120.

Glogau RM. Chemical peeling and aging skin. *J Geriatr Dermatol* 1994;2(1):30–35.

Goldfarb MT, Ellis CAN, Voorhees JJ. Topical tretinoin: its use in daily Practice to reverse photoaging. *Br J Dermatol* 1990;122(suppl 35):87–91.

Hurley HJ. Skin in senescence: a summation. *J Geriatr Dermatol* 1993;1(2):55–61.

Kligman A. Psychological aspects of skin disorders in the elderly. In *Aging Skin. Properties and Functional Changes*. JL Leveque, PG Agache, eds. New York, Marcel Dekker, 1993, pp. 275–284.

Kligman AM, Grove GL, Hirose R, Leyden JJ. Topical tretinoin for photodamaged skin. *J Am Acad Dermatol* 1986;15:836–859.

Lauker RM. Structural aspects of intrinsic vs photoaging. *Proc 18th World Congress* 1992;825–828.

Lauker RM. Topical Therapy of Aging Skin. *J Geriatr Dermatol* 1994;2(1):20–23.

Leveque JL, Agache PG, ed. *Aging Skin: Properties and Functional Changes*. New York, Marcel Dekker Inc., 1993.

Marks R, Lever L. Studies on the effects of topical retinoic acid on photoaging. *Br J Dermatol* 1990;122 (suppl 35): 93–95.

Pinski K, Roenigk HH Jr. Autologous fat transplantation-long term follow-up. *J Dermatol Surg Oncol* 1992;18:179–184.

Pinski K, Roenigk HH Jr. Long term follow-up of fat transplantation. In *Surgical Dermatology. Advances in Current Practice*. Roenigk R, Roenigk HH, eds. London, Martin Dunitz, 1993.

Ridge JM, Siegle RJ, Zuckerman J. Use of α-hydroxy acids in the thrapy for photoaged skin. *J Am Acad Dermatol* 1990;23:932.

Roenigk HH Jr. Dermabrasion: state of the art. *J Dermatol Surg Oncol* 1985;11(3):306–314.

Taylor CR, Stern RS, Leyden JJ, Gilchrest BA. Photoaging/photodamage and photoprotection. *J Am Acad Dermatol* 1990;22:1–15.

Van Scott E. Alpha-hydroxy acids: procedures for use in clinical practice. *Cutis* 1989;43:222–228.

Weinstein GD, Nigrac TP, Pouchi PE, Savin RC et al. Topical tretinoin for treatment of photodamaged skin. A multicenter study. *Arch Dermatol* 1991;127(5):659–665.

Yaar M, Gilchrest BA. Cellular and molecular mechanisms of cutaneous aging. *Dermatol Surg Oncol* 1990;16:915–922.

Yarborough JM Jr. Dermabrasion surgery: state of the art. *Clin Dermatol* 1987;5(4):75–80.

60

Soft Tissue Augmentation

Jeffrey L. Melton
Loyola University of Chicago, Maywood, Illinois

C. William Hanke
Indiana University School of Medicine, Indianapolis, Indiana

Interest in the augmentation of soft tissues has increased markedly in recent years. Increased emphasis on youthful appearance, as well as a much broader range of therapeutic options available, has fueled enthusiasm for soft tissue augmentation. The ideal material for soft tissue augmentation would provide consistent long-lasting correction, have a low incidence of adverse effects, and be easily procurable, inexpensive, and easily placed at the desired depth with minimal trauma to tissues. No currently available material meets all of these criteria. Each filler material has its own indications, as well as relative advantages and disadvantages. The most favorable outcome results from proper selection of indication, material, and technique and thus depends upon familiarity with each of the currently available options for treatment.

COLLAGEN-BASED FILLER MATERIALS

Zyderm® and Zyplast®

Zyderm I, Zyderm II, and Zyplast (Collagen Corporation, Palo Alto, CA) are bovine-derived collagen implants. In 1981 Zyderm I became the first injectable filler substance to be approved by the FDA for use in soft tissue augumentation. Zyderm II and Zyplast were approved for use in 1983 and 1985, respectively. All three products have enjoyed extensive use compared to other materials currently available (Fig. 1). Both Zyderm and Zyplast contain 95% type I collagen and 5% type III collagen. Zyderm I, Zyderm II, and Zyplast have collagen concentrations of 35 mg/cc, 65 mg/cc, and 35 mg/cc, respectively. Although Zyplast is of a lower concentration, it is cross-linked with glutaraldehyde, resulting in less shrinkage of the implant after placement. Zyderm I, Zyderm II, and Zyplast are each available in 0.5 or 1.0 cc tuberculin syringes. Zyplast is now also available in a 2.0 cc syringe. The implant material is in suspension in normal saline and 0.3% lidocaine. The implant is injected using a 30 or 32 gauge needle, causing only minimal patient discomfort.

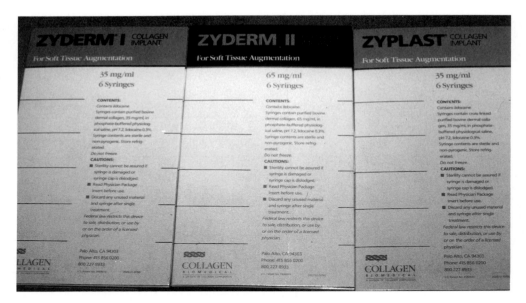

Figure 1   Bovine collagen implants are packaged as Zyderm I, Zyderm II, and Zyplast.

Contraindications, Hypersensitivity, and Skin Testing

Recommendations regarding skin testing are changing. Although the antigenicity of the bovine collagen molecule is lessened by pepsin digestion of the telopeptide regions, hypersensitivity reactions do occur. Three percent of the population are hypersensitive to a single Zyderm skin test (Fig. 2). In addition, a small group of patients who initially have a negative skin test will have a positive skin test on the second challenge. Therefore, several investigators have advocated routine use of a second test ("double skin testing") in order to identify these additional patients hypersensitive to the preparation prior to initiating treatment. In fact, double skin testing is rapidly becoming the standard of care. The skin tests are generally performed 4 weeks apart. Each is evaluated at 48–72 hr to check for transient positive reactions. Skin testing for Zyderm I, Zyderm II, and Zyplast are all performed with the same material, a specially packaged implant syringe, which contains 0.1 cc of bovine collagen implant. The material is injected intradermally on the volar forearm. The patient is evaluated at 48–72 hr and at 4 weeks after placement. When double skin testing, the second implant is commonly placed on the opposite arm. Evaluation is repeated as above. If no reaction occurs, treatment can be initiated. A positive skin test is manifest as local erythema and/or induration at the treatment site persisting more than 6 hr. It may be advisable to repeat a single skin test if a 2-yr period has elapsed since any skin testing or treatment if further implantation is contemplated.

Indications and Technique

In addition to a positive skin test, personal history of autoimmune disease such as rheumatoid arthritis, lupus erythematosus, or dermatomyositis are contraindications to treatment. Patients allergic to other bovine products or to lidocaine should not be treated. Patients with many allergies or atopy should be treated with caution.

Zyderm I and Zyderm II are best suited for more superficial defects and are placed in the upper dermis (see Table 1). Common indications for Zyderm I and Zyderm II include melolabial

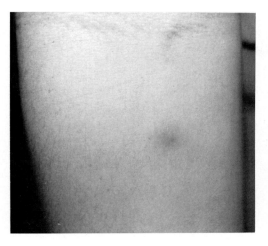

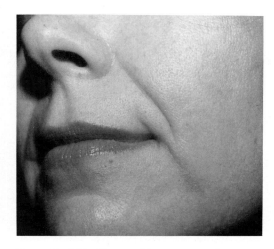

Figure 2 Approximately 3% of prospective patients will exhibit a positive pretreatment skin test. This is a contraindication to treatment.

Figure 3 This 40-year-old woman sought correction of deep nasolabial furrows.

lines, upper lip wrinkles, oral commissural lines, glabellar frown lines, superficial transverse forehead lines, and secondary cheek wrinkles. Zyderm I can be used in very small amounts to treat crow's-feet. Proper papillary dermal placement of Zyderm I is characterized by immediate white blanching of the skin. Overcorrection of most defects (except crow's-feet) with Zyderm is desired because the implant loses 66% of its volume in vivo, whereas Zyderm II loses 33%. Because Zyplast only loses 20% of its volume in the short term, defects can be fully corrected to the surface level without observable blanching. If skin blanches immediately after Zyplast injection, the injection has been misplaced in the papillary dermis or too much implant material may have been injected. Zyplast should be implanted in the mid to lower reticular dermis. It is effective for deeper creases and distensible scars. Common indications for Zyplast® are deeper marionette lines, perioral lines, nasolabial furrows, and broadly based undulating scars (Figs. 3–6). Sharply demarcated "ice pick"-type acne scars are difficult to improve with bovine collagen implants or with any other dermal filler material. Some patients have full-thickness, combination defects characterized by superficial wrinkles overlying deep furrows. In such patients a "layering technique" is often utilized: Zyderm I or Zyderm II is placed superficially over a more deeply placed Zyplast implant.

Table 1 Comparison of Filler Materials

Product	Site of placement	Duration of correction (site dependent)
Zyderm I, Zyderm II	Dermis	4–12 months
Zyplast	Reticular dermis	4–12 months
Autologous collagen	Mid-dermis, reticular dermis	Similar to above
Fibrel	Mid-dermis, reticular dermis	Months to years
Hylan Gel	Superficial to deep dermis	Uncertain
Gore-tex	Mid- to deep dermis	Uncertain, presumably long
Autologous fat	Subcutaneous fat	Months to years

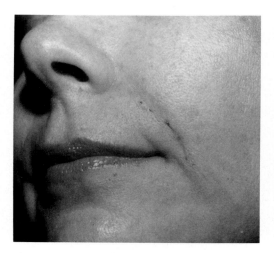

Figure 4 The patient has had 0.5 cc Zyplast placed in the reticular dermis in the nasolabial areas on each side of the face.

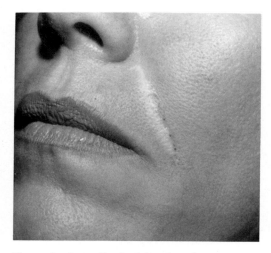

Figure 5 Immediately following Zyplast placement, 0.5 cc Zyderm I has been placed in the papillary dermis on each side. The white blanche from Zyderm I will resolve within 30 min.

Patients should be advised to discontinue nonsteroidal anti-inflammatory agents, including aspirin, as well as other anticoagulants for 10 days prior to treatment. Makeup and surface debris is removed from the skin with soap and water or isopropanol. It is often helpful to treat in the sitting position in order to accurately identify soft tissue defects when gravitational effects are present. Tangential lighting, usually from above, is used to accentuate subtle soft tissue defects.

Results

The duration of cosmetic improvement depends upon both the degree of facial movement at the site of implant and the material used. Nasolabial folds may require retreatment every 6 months,

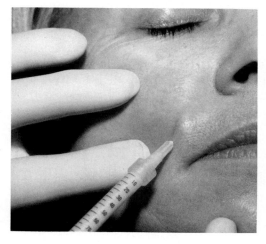

Figure 6 Zyplast should be injected at the level of the reticular dermis. This results in an observable swelling, but not a white blanche.

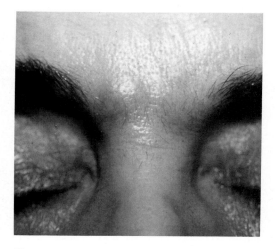

Figure 7 An allergic treatment site reaction from Zyderm I may take 6 months to resolve.

while scars in a less animated area may sustain significant cosmetic improvement for up to 2 years. Loss of correction has been determined by Stegman and others to be due to implant migration to the subcutis after 6–9 months.

Adverse Reactions

Adverse reactions of both an allergic and nonallergic nature occur. Nonallergic adverse reactions include surface deformities, bruising, infection, intermittent swelling, and local necrosis. Bruising occurs most readily in patients who have a history of easy bruising or who are taking medications with anticoagulant effects. Surface deformities or "beading" occur when placement is too superficial for the product or the site treated. This most commonly occurs in very thin areas of the dermis where the margin for error is small. For example, the thin-skinned crow's-foot area of the external canthus cannot tolerate overcorrection with Zyderm; Zyplast should not be used for the crow's-foot defect. Surface deformities do resolve, albeit slowly over several months. Infection is rare following Zyderm or Zyplast treatment. Local necrosis of the skin results from laceration or compression of the vasculature and occurs most frequently in the glabellar area.

Allergic-treatment-site reactions can occur after one or even two negative skin tests. Red, indurated, pruritic papules or streaks develop at the treatment site (Fig. 7). The reaction often resolves spontaneously by 6 months but can occasionally last longer. These patients have anti-Zyderm antibodies and should have no further treatment with the product. Very rarely a cystic-abscess reaction may occur. This is more commonly seen with Zyplast implant. The abscesses at the Zyplast implant sites will drain sterile purulent material for several months before healing, sometimes with permanent scarring. A very small group of patients who have been treated with Zyderm or Zyplast have developed polymyositis or dermatomyositis. A Food and Drug Administration (FDA) panel reviewed data on these patients on October 25, 1991, and the experts concluded that there is no significant statistical or biological evidence of risk for connective tissue disease in patients treated with bovine collagen implants.

Fibrel®

Fibrel (Mentor H/S Inc., Santa Barbara, CA) is an alternative collagen implant approved by FDA for soft tissue augmentation. Specifically, it was approved for treatment of scars in 1988 and age-related wrinkles in 1990. The collagen in Fibrel is porcine derived. The Fibrel treatment kit contains sterile absorbable gelatin powder, epsilon aminocaproic acid, and 0.5 cc normal saline (Fig. 8). The materials are mixed with the patient's serum (0.5 cc) or with lidocaine or normal saline. The fate of Fibrel after placement in the dermis has been compared to that of normal thrombus formation and dissolution. The gelatin provides a matrix, which traps fibrinogen and other clotting factors and also serves as a template for the synthesis of new collagen. Rapid dissolution of the thrombus is prevented by the antifibrinolytic effects of epsilon aminocaproic acid. Normal wound healing proceeds, completely replacing the gelatin matrix implant with new collagen over a 90-day period.

Contraindications, Hypersensitivity, and Skin Testing

Patients who have a history of autoimmune disease, keloids, anaphylactoid reactions or allergy to Fibrel components are not candidates for this treatment. A skin test (the powder mixed with normal saline only, no serum) is placed on the flexor aspect of the forearm and is evaluated at 4 weeks. A positive skin test, manifest by erythema and induration, is a contraindication to treatment with Fibrel. In clinical trials only 1.9% of patients had a positive skin test.

Indications and Technique

Many distensible postacne scars and deep to moderate age-related wrinkles can be treated successfully with Fibrel. Due to the relatively higher viscosity of Fibrel, a larger-gauge needle is

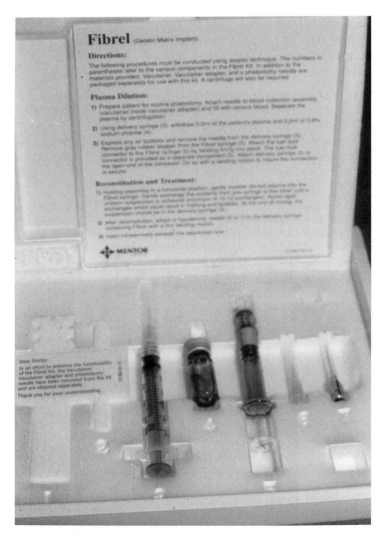

Figure 8 The Fibrel treatment kit consists of absorbable gelatin powder, 0.9% sodium chloride, delivery and mixing syringes, and two needles for injection.

required (27 gauge). Fibrel does not flow easily through smaller needles. Superficial wrinkles require papillary dermal placement of the implant, which is difficult with a 27 gauge needle. The best results for wrinkles are usually achieved in the melolabial folds and oral commissures. Broadly based, poorly circumscribed, slightly depressed acne scars also respond well to Fibrel treatment. Prior to treatment the area is cleansed with soap and water and then an alcohol wipe. Significant discomfort accompanies the infiltration of Fibrel. Therefore, areas to be augmented are first infiltrated with local anesthetic. It is advisable to delineate sites of placement with a marker pen before the administration of local anesthetic. If this is not done, tissue distortion caused by local anesthetic will make Fibrel placement difficult. It is also helpful to wait 15 min before injecting Fibrel, so that equalization of anesthetic within the tissue minimizes distortion. The multiple puncture technique is most commonly used. The needle is advanced through the defect, then Fibrel is injected as the needle is pulled back toward the entry site. To prevent excessive leakage of the product, placement should not be too close to the site of needle insertion. The implant is placed in the reticular dermis. Overcorrection of scars and wrinkles by 50–100% is desirable. Placement of the proper amount of material is accompanied by a subtle blanching of the skin surface. A specialized 20 gauge custom cutting needle is provided for the treatment of bound down scars. The sharp cutting needle allows release of thick dermal bands and creates small pockets for the placement of Fibrel.

Results

Milliken et al. reported that 55% of scars treated with Fibrel maintained significant correction for 5 years. In this series only 35% of the original correction was lost by 5 years. Duration of correction of wrinkles is related to the dynamic nature of the site. Interestingly, Monheit recently reported that Fibrel is equally effective whether mixed with lidocaine or with a patient's serum. Allergic reactions are distinctly rare with Fibrel. Most adverse reactions are transitory and nonallergic in nature. Mild local swelling of the treated area is common. Swelling begins immediately after placement and spontaneously resolves over 1–3 days (Fig. 9). Occasionally some swelling persists for up to 3 weeks. Superficial irregularities are seen when Fibrel is inadvertently placed superficially and/or in excess amount. Bruising is more common than with Zyderm because of the larger needle required for Fibrel placement. Local necrosis in the glabellar area has also been seen with Fibrel.

Autologous Collagen

Hypersensitivity to foreign (xenograft) materials has prompted an investigation into the use of autologous material for soft tissue augmentation. Both collagen and fat have been employed for

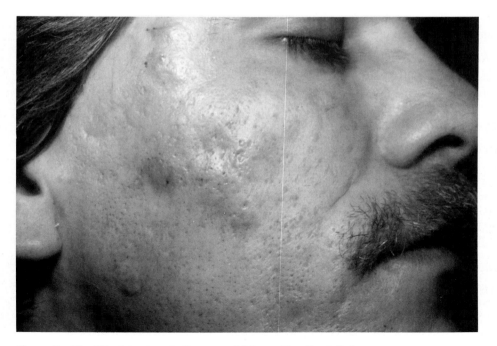

Figure 9   The Fibrel treatment site may exhibit swelling for 1–3 days.

this purpose. The advantage is a lack of hypersensitivity. The disadvantage is increased effort to harvest and prepare the material. Several advances have been made in this area.

Lipocytic Dermal Augmentation

Fournier has developed a technique for the harvest, preparation, and placement of collagen derived from liposuction. Collagen-rich material from fibrous subcutaneous fat septae is isolated from the liposuction aspirate by adding distilled water, freezing, and then thawing the emulsion. The adipocytes are ruptured in the process, and two fractions result: an oily triglyceride fraction and a collagen-rich connective tissue fraction. After decanting the lipid fraction, the collagen-rich material can be used for dermal augmentation. Coleman used the term "lipocytic dermal augmentation" to describe the method.

Contraindications, Hypersensitivity, and Skin Testing

No hypersensitivity reactions have been reported with the use of autologous collagen, and pre-treatment skin testing is unnecessary. Autologous collagen may be successfully used in patients who are allergic to bovine collagen and are not candidates for Fibrel. No contraindications, other than to the liposuction procedure itself (usually only a minimal procedure is required), are known.

Indications and Technique

The indications for augmentation with autologous collagen are similar to bovine collagen or Fibrel. The material is injected into the deep dermis or at the junction of the dermis and fat. Autologous collagen is viscous and requires injection through a 22 gauge or larger needle. This necessitates local anesthesia. A larger needle also makes it difficult to place the material at a particular dermal depth with precision. Autologous collagen is ideal for filling deeper depressions in the melolabial fold on the chin. Autologous collagen has also been used for lip augmentation. Zoochi reported that the duration of correction of autologous collagen is similar to bovine collagen. Coleman has described the histopathologic course of events following dermal placement of autologous collagen. An initial inflammatory response is later replaced by cellular fibrosis and expansion of the dermis.

Adverse Reactions

The 22 gauge needle causes more bruising than occurs with smaller needles. The larger percutaneous puncture sites may be visible for days or weeks following treatment.

Autologen®

Autologen (Autologen Technologies Inc., Boston, MA) is human dermal collagen processed for soft tissue augmentation. The source of the material is excess skin removed from the patient during a prior surgical procedure such as abdominoplasty, breast reduction, hair transplantation, face lift, or excision. Tissue specimens are frozen at $-160°C$ and are mailed to the company for processing, which consists of pulverizing and centrifuging the material. The collagen is suspended in a syringe containing buffered normal saline and then mailed back to the physician for injection. The concentration of collagen in the suspension is approximately 50–120 mg/cc.

Contraindications, Hypersensitivity, and Skin Testing

Skin testing is not routinely performed, and hypersensitivity reactions have to our knowledge not been reported. No contraindications are known. No allergic reactions occurred in 400 patients treated by 50 physicians. Autologen may be used in patients who are allergic to bovine collagen or to Fibrel.

Indications and Technique

These are similar to bovine or porcine collagen.

Results

Correction may last up to 18 months. During processing, the in vivo structure of collagen is apparently preserved. It is hypothesized that this preservation results in a greater resistance of Autologen to degradation when compared to bovine collagen.

Adverse Reactions

Adverse reactions are similar to nonallergic adverse reactions to bovine collagen including local swelling and bruising. A 27 gauge or larger needle is required to inject Autologen.

NON–COLLAGEN-BASED FILLER MATERIALS

Hylan Gel

Hyaluronic acid is a normal polysaccharide component of the connective tissue intracellular matrix. Hylan Gel (Biomatrix, Inc., Ridgefield, NJ) is an insoluble cross-linked hyaluronic acid derivative that is currently in clinical trials for dermal augmentation. Hylan Gel has also been used as a vitreous replacement, for cataract replacement, for treatment of urinary incontinence, in drug delivery, and for joint lubrication in rheumatoid arthritis and arthroscopic surgery.

Contraindications, Hypersensitivity, and Skin Testing

Hyaluronic acid is a polysaccharide that has an identical chemical structure in all species. In clinical trials, hypersensitivity to Hylan Gel has not been observed. Hylan Gel has not been shown to be immunologically reactive in other clinical uses. Pretreatment skin testing is not required.

Indications and Technique

Hylan Gel has been used to treat selected wrinkles and distensible scars. Severe wrinkling is not an indication. The material may be injected into the superficial and/or deep dermis. It flows easily and can be molded manually. Clinical trials began in 1991.

Results

In preclinical guinea pig studies, Hylan Gel was identifiable in test sites at 12 months. In human clinical studies, correction was maintained in 50% of treatment sites at 18 weeks after placement.

Adverse Reactions

Complications have been minor and include mild erythema, discomfort, local swelling, punctate injection marks, and bruising. All seem to resolve rapidly.

Gore-tex®

Recently, Gore-tex (W.L. Gore and Associates, Flagstaff, AZ), or polytetrafluoroethylene, has been investigated for use as a dermal filler material. Gore-tex has been used for some time in other implant applications, principally as a vascular graft. Another more recent use of Gore-tex is as an implant material placed next to bone to promote growth of bony tissue for filling of bony dental or facial defects. Gore-tex has been used as a surgically placed soft tissue filler in a patch, strut, or sheet form and more recently in a suturelike form. As a linear dermal filler material, it is used primarily for linear defects, such as the nasolabial groove. The suturelike material is threaded through a specialized needle. Local anesthesia is required. The introducing needle is advanced through the defect at the middermal level. The material is then trimmed to appropriate length, and fine sutures are placed at entry sites so that ends of the material do not extrude. Few clinical data are available at this time regarding the safety and efficacy profile of Gore-tex as a dermal filler substance. Advantages would include ready availability and, presumably, lengthy duration of correction.

Autologous Fat Transplantation

Atrophy of subcutaneous fatty tissue occurs in certain sites as parts of the aging process. Areas commonly affected are the temples, upper lip, and central cheeks. Similarly, aging results in deepening of the furrows in the nasolabial fold, glabella, and subcommissural areas. Extraction and reinjection of autologous fat developed as an adjunct to liposuction. Fournier described his method of "microlipoextraction and injection" in 1986. Subcutaneous fat is harvested in a minimally traumatic fashion with a 13 gauge needle attached to a syringe. The procedure is done under local anesthesia. In contrast to the other materials discussed in this chapter, fat is transplanted into the subcutaneous tissue, rather than in the dermis.

Contraindications, Hypersensitivity, and Skin Testing

Hypersensitivity to autologous fat has not been reported, and pretreatment skin testing is unnecessary. No known contraindications exist.

Indications and Technique

The major determinant of fat graft survival, and thus duration of correction, is vascularity of the recipient site. The survival of autologous fat under poorly vascularized skin grafts or in areas of posttraumatic fibrosis is limited. Well-vascularized facial soft tissue defects fare better and are the main indication for the technique. Autologous fat can be used to replace adipose tissue loss in the temples, upper lip, cheeks, nasolabial fold, glabella, and subcommissure areas. Autologous fat injection has also been used to rejuvenate atrophic dorsal hands and for breast augmentation.

Large volumes of autologous fat for injection are harvested as a byproduct of body liposuction. However, the small volumes normally required for transplantation can be harvested in a minimal procedure under local anesthesia. The best donor sites are the abdomen in men and the outer hip in women. The canula entry site is anesthetized with 1% lidocaine with 1:100,000 epinephrine using a 30 gauge needle. Oral sedation is optional and rarely required if only donor material is being sought. The donor site is prepped and draped. The subcutaneous tissue is infiltrated locally to tumescence (firmness) with a solution of 0.1% lidocaine and 1:1,000,000 epinephrine. The fat is harvested with a 13 gauge needle or blunt-tipped microcanula. Only syringe suction is needed. The plunger of the syringe is pulled back and yellow fat is aspirated using an advance/withdrawal motion in a roughly horizontal subcutaneous plane. Ten cc of yellow, nonbloody fat can be harvested in 60 sec. After the appropriate amount of material has been harvested, the syringes are placed tip down in a holding rack. The aqueous portion spontaneously separates from the fat in 5 min. The lower, nonlipid portion is expelled and discarded. Fat may be washed with normal saline or with Ringer's solution prior to injection.

The recipient site is prepped, draped, and infiltrated with 1% lidocaine. The autologous fat is injected into the subcutaneous tissue. A 16 gauge needle is commonly used. The needle is advanced into the defect and the fat is injected as the needle is withdrawn toward the site of entry. An overcorrection of approximately 100% is sought, and the implant is molded into place. Ice cold compresses are applied intermittently for several hours after treatment.

Results

Roughly 40–60% of autologous fat remains 1 year after injection. Several repeat injections at 3- to 6-month intervals result in maximum correction. Definitive improvement seems to occur after repeated injections. Often the most marked improvement occurs only after the second or third injection.

Adverse Reactions

Recipient site tenderness occurs and may remain for several months. Bruising and swelling of the treatment site occur and remain present for 1–2 weeks. Infections have been reported. Pre- and/or postoperative antibiotics are often prescribed. Permanent unilateral vision loss following autologous fat transplant to the glabella has been reported.

BIBLIOGRAPHY

Coleman WP. Collagen filler substances. In *Cosmetic Surgery of the Skin*. WP Coleman, CW Hanke, TH Alt, et al., Philadelphia, BC Decker, 1991, pp. 99–102.

Coleman WP, Lawrence N, Sherman RN, Reed RJ, Pinski KS, et al. Autologous collagen—lipocytic dermal augmentation: a histopathologic study. *J Dermatol Surg Oncol* 1993;19(11):1032–1040, 1993.

Elson M. Soft tissue augmentation of periorbital fine lines and the orbital groove with Zyderm-I and fine-gauge needles. *J Dermatol Surg Oncol* 1992;18(9):779–782.

Elson MC. The role of skin testing in the use of collagen injectable materials. *J Dermatol Surg Oncol* 1989;15:301–303.

Grosh SK, Hanke CW, Devore DP, et al. Variables effecting the results of xenogenic collagen implantation in an animal model. *J Am Acad Dermatol* 1985;15:792–798.

Hanke CW, Coleman WP. Collagen filler substances. In *Cosmetic Surgery of the Skin*. WP Coleman et al., eds. Philadelphia, BC Decker, 1991, pp. 89–93.

Hanke CW, Higley HR, Jolivette DM, et al. Abscess formation and local necrosis after treatment with zyderm or zyplast collagen implant. *J Am Acad Dermatol* 1991;25:319–326.

Kassimir J. Autologen. Washington, DC, 52nd Annual Meeting of the American Academy of Dermatology, 1993.

Klein AW. In favor of double skin testing. *J Dermatol Surg Oncol* 1989;15:263.

Maas CS, Gnepp Dr, Bumpous J, et al. Expanded polytetrafluorethylene (Gore-Tex soft-tissue patch) in facial augmentation. *Arch Otolaryngol Head Neck Surg* 1993;119(9):1008–1014.

Melton JL, Hanke CW. Soft-tissue augmentation. New Techniques and recent controversies. In *Surgical Dermatology*. RK Roenigk, HH Roenigk, eds. London, Martin Dunitz, 1993, pp. 448–449.

Millikan LE, Banks K, Parkail B, et al. A 5-year safety and efficacy evaluation with Fibrel in the correction of cutaneous scars following one or two treatments. *J Dermatol Surg Oncol* 1991;17:223–229.

Monheit GD. Fibrel. Washington, DC, 52nd Annual Meeting of the American Academy of Dermatology, 1993.

Peer LA. The neglected "free fat graft," its behavior and clinical use. *Am J Surg* 1956;40:92.

Petroff MA, Goode Rl, Levet Y, et al. Gore-Tex implants: applications in facial paralysis rehabilitation and soft-tissue augmentation. *Laryngoscope* 1992;102(10):1185–1189.

Piacquadio DJ. Hylan gel. Washington, DC, 52nd Annual Meeting of the American Academy of Dermatology, 1993.

Richter AW, Ryde EM, Zetterman EO. Non-immunogenicity of a purified sodium hyaluronate preparation in man. *Int Arch Allergy* 1988;59:45–48.

Spira M, Liu BC, Xu ZL, et al. Human amnion collagen for soft tissue augmentation—biochemical characterizations and animal observations. *J Biomed Mater Res* 1994;28(1):91–96.

Stegman SJ. Collagen implants. In *Dermatologic Surgery*. RK Roenigk, HH Roenigk, eds. New York, Marcel Dekker, 1989, pp. 1313–1336.

Teimourian B. Blindness following fat injections (letter). *Plastic Reconstr Surg* 1988;89(2):361.

Wetmore SJ. Injection of fat for soft-tissue augmentation. *Laryngoscope* 1980;90:50.

61

Dermabrasion

Henry H. Roenigk, Jr.
Northwestern University Medical School, Chicago, Illinois

HISTORY

Kromayer described his cylindrical knives for punching scars, tattoos, pigmentation, abscesses, hair, nevi, and other defects in 1905. Later he described rasps or burrs with either clockwise or counterclockwise rotation for scar removal to which he attached motor-driven instruments from the dental clinic. He adapted his punches and rasps to perform "scarless operations," which were described in his book *Cosmetic Treatment of Skin Complaints*. Kromayer showed that healing of wounds occurs beneath a scab without obvious cicatrization if the injury does not penetrate the reticular dermis. Freezing the skin with carbon dioxide snow and ether spray provided rigidity as well as anesthesia suitable for dermabrading.

Iverson reported successful removal of traumatic tattoos with sandpaper in 1947. This technique had several disadvantages, primarily bleeding, which obscured the operative field, and, subsequently, foreign body silica granuloma. Kurten, who was a dermatologist, reawakened interest in wire brush motor-driven dermabraders using refrigeration for anesthesia in 1953. He reported improvement in acne scars, seborrheic and actinic keratoses, tattoos, wrinkles, keloids, traumatic scars, adenoma sebaceum, nevi, and lichenoid plaques. Orentreich, who worked with Kurten, popularized dermabrasion and refined much of today's equipment. Burke's textbook, *Wire Brush Surgery in the Treatment of Certain Cosmetic Defects and Diseases of the Skin*, published in 1956, gave credibility to dermabrasion as an accepted procedure. There have been minor modifications in techniques since then. The author and others have used dermabrasion to treat non–acne-related lesions such as trichoepithelioma, epithelioma adenoides cysticum, and others.

Dermabrasion reached its peak in popularity in the 1950s. There was criticism of the procedure in the 1960s and early 1970s, but with the renewed interest in dermatologic surgery in the past 25 years, dermabrasion has become more popular. Dermabrasion and related procedures, such as chemical peel, soft tissue augmentation, and scar revision, are now routine dermatologic surgical procedures.

INDICATIONS

Dermabrasion was developed as a method of treating acne scars. It has been used to treat a variety of problems including hypertrophic scars, traumatic scars, actinically damaged and wrinkled skin, and correction of pigmentary abnormalities. Among the cosmetic indications for dermabrasion are acne scars, fine wrinkling, scar revision, melasma, perioral pseudorhagades, and tattoo removal.

There are many other therapeutic reasons for selecting dermabrasion: epidermal nevus, epithelioma adenoides cysticum, rhinophyma, nevus angiomatosus, syringoma, adenoma sebaceum, keloids, discoid lupus erythematosus, actinic keratosis and solar elastosis, seborrheic keratosis, basal cell carcinoma, and Darier's disease. Hanke provided a list of 50 conditions that have been treated with dermabrasion (Table 1).

The correction of old and new scars by dermabrasion is very effective. Superficial sharply demarcated scars can often be completely removed, while soft saucerlike depressions can be improved but not eliminated (Fig. 1). Emphasize to the patient that improvement is expected, but do not promise to eliminate all scars. Dermabrasion will soften sharp edges and improve the craterlike appearance of these scars caused by shadows in the depression. Deep ice-pick–type scars will require scar revision by punch excision and suturing, punch elevation, or punch grafting prior to dermabrasion. Dermabrasion can also be used for cysts or to marsupialize epithelialized sinuses when chronically infected. In another chapter, Yarborough shows that scars from excisional surgery or trauma can be dermabraded 6–8 weeks after sutures are removed to camouflage these wounds by forming a more natural epidermal surface. Older wounds do not respond

Table 1   Various Entities Treated with Dermabrasion

Postacne scars	Adenoma sebaceum
Traumatic scars	Neurotic excoriations
Smallpox or chickenpox scars	Multiple trichoepitheliomas
Rhinophyma	Darier's disease
Professionally applied tattoos	Fox-Fordyce disease
Amateur-type tattoos (India Ink)	Lichenified dermatoses
Blast tattoos (gunpowder)	Porokeratosis of Mibelli
Multiple seborrheic keratoses	Favre-Racouchot syndrome
Multiple pigmented nevi	Lichen amyloidosis
Actinically damaged skin	Verrucous nevus
Age- and sun-related wrinkle lines	Molluscum contagiosum
Active acne	Keratoacanthoma
Freckles	Xanthalasma
Pseudofolliculitis barbae	Hemangioma
Telangiectasia	Leg ulcer
Acne rosacea	Scleromyxedema
Chloasma	Striae distensae
Vitiligo	Early operative scars
Congenital pigmented nevi	Hair transplantation
Syringocystadenoma papilliferum	(elevated recipient sites)
Nevus flammeus	Linear epidermal nevus
Keloids	Syringoma
Dermatitis papilaris capilliti	Angiofibromas of tuberous sclerosis
Lupus erythematosus	Chronic radiation dermatitis
Basal cell carcinoma	Xeroderma pigmentosum
(superficial type)	Lentigines

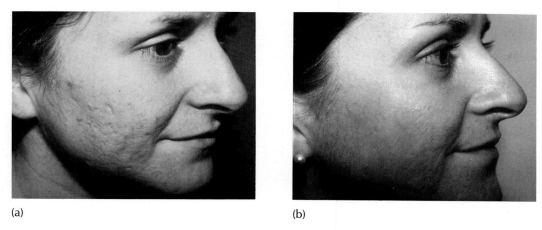

(a)   (b)

Figure 1   (a) Acne scars on cheek. (b) After dermabrasion (1 month).

as well unless they are reexcised, followed by dermabrasion. Dermabrasion has become a tool for treatment of photoaging skin (see Chap. 59).

EQUIPMENT

Proper outpatient operating room facilities must be available to perform dermabrasion. The room should be well ventilated and air conditioned. Most dermatologists perform dermabrasion in an office surgical unit separated from general offices or an ambulatory surgical center. Hospitalization with general anesthesia is not necessary and only adds to the expense of the procedure. There should be a versatile operating table capable of placing the patient in several different positions. Adequate lighting and proper emergency equipment should be available. The patient's past medical history and current medications should be noted. The operator and assistant wear surgical gowns and gloves. A plastic face shield and mask is worn for protection from blood and tissue particles that spray.

Several different dermabraders are available (Table 2). The older type have a flexible coil that protects rotating cables driven by an electric motor. The operative portion may be mounted on a stand or placed on a table. Rotating speed is controlled with a foot switch that goes from 800 to 12,000 rpm. Air-driven units use compressed gas. These units reach speeds of 40,000–60,000 rpm, are much easier to use, and achieve greater depth of planing.

Hand engines, developed in the past 15 years, are popular because they are small, hand-held engines that are quiet and easy to maneuver. The Bell Hand Engine and Osada models can reach rotational speeds of 18,000–35,000 rpm in both directions, depending on the model. A rheostat adjusts the speed, which can also be controlled with a foot pedal. The combination of rotational speed of the machine, abrading attachment, and pressure applied by the operator allows rapid planing.

Nitrogen-driven machines, such as the Stryker unit, are well built, provide excellent torque, and reach 50,000 rpm easily. The handpiece is larger than the hand engine. It is necessary, however, to store and replace large tanks of nitrogen. The engine with the greatest rotational speed is the high-speed Schreuss (Derma III) machine. This unit rotates at 15,000–60,000 rpm and retains a strong torque. The handpiece is larger than other units and more difficult to maneuver.

Table 2   Instruments Used in Dermabrasion

Dermabraders
  Motor-driven
    Bell International Hand Engine
    Mill-Bilt Equipment Company
    Robbins Instrument Company
    Dremel Power Tool #370 (hand-held unit)
  Air-driven
    Stryker Company
Dermatomes
  Laminar dermal reticulotomy
    Davis, Davol, or Brown dermatomes
  Schreuss (Derma III) machine
    Schumann Precision Manufacturer
Brushes
  Diamond fraises
  Wire brush
  Small contoured fraises
    Robbins Instrument Company

The abrading end pieces for dermabrasion are either the diamond fraise, wire brush, or serrated wheel. Diamond fraises are stainless steel wheels on which diamond chips of different grades of coarseness (regular, coarse, or extra coarse) are bonded. Most experienced surgeons use the coarse or extra-coarse fraises. The cylinder type comes in various widths and diameters, while other shapes, such as the pear, are helpful in specific locations (Fig. 2).

The wire brush is a stainless steel wheel with wires arranged at an angle. The wires of the brush cut deeply and rapidly in frozen skin. Most experienced surgeons prefer the wire brush, but for the novice these are much harder to control and can gouge easily. The wire brush should

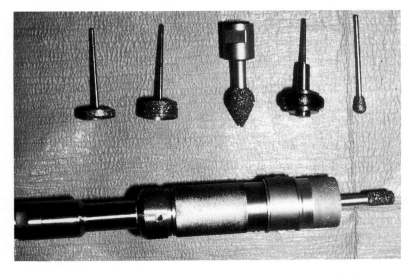

Figure 2   Stryker handpiece and various diamond fraises and wire brushes.

be used for the deep scars and the diamond fraise to feather the edges or plane more smoothly than an area treated with the wire brush.

PATIENT SELECTION AND PREOPERATIVE WORK-UP

The preoperative consultation is extremely important. You must tell the patient clearly what to expect from the procedure, as well as get a feel for what he or she really understands. List alternative procedures such as chemical peel, cryosurgery, or collagen implants. The use of photographs to demonstrate the procedure, as well as before and after pictures including that of complications, may be helpful in the consultation. This discussion should be documented in the chart.

Patients who seek cosmetic surgery to improve their appearance for a variety of personal reasons have unique personalities. The surgeon must have a basic understanding of psychology and specifically the psychopathology of the cosmetic surgery patient. Therapeutic dermabrasion may relieve some of the pressure to achieve perfect results (Fig. 3). Avoid promoting dermabrasion and list the other options available and the complications that can occur. There are adjunctive procedures that are often combined with dermabrasion, and these should be carefully covered in the consultation. The physician must decide who is a good candidate and if a reasonable improvement can be expected. Avoid the patient who has a minimal scar and cannot tolerate what seems like a slight blemish. Also, avoid patients critical of care given by previous physicians. The patient's criticism may be valid, but you too may be unable to live up to the patient's expectations.

Preoperative work-up includes a medical history, specifically other medication (especially aspirin) and diseases such as hepatitis, HIV infection, venereal disease, and recurrent herpes

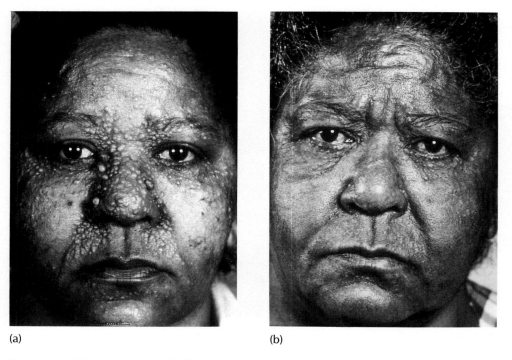

(a)   (b)

Figure 3   (a) Multiple trichoepithelioma. (b) After dermabrasion, note natural repigmentation.

simplex. Evaluate atypical scars from previous surgery that may be predictive of poor results. Laboratory evaluation includes complete blood cell count, serum chemistry values, and bleeding time. Other tests include evaluation of hepatitis B antigen and antibody and HIV III antibody titers. These are done to protect the surgeon and staff.

ANESTHESIA

Preoperative medication should relax the patient and reduce pain since most dermabrasions are done with local anesthesia. Intramuscular Demerol (50–100 mg) and intravenous Valium (10–20 mg) provide sedation, although other agents may be used. These can also be given during the procedure by keeping an intravenous line open. The blood pressure, pulse, and heart rate should be monitored continuously. A pulse oximeter is necessary for all patients under heavy sedation. Ibuprofen or corticosteroids may help reduce edema and bleeding. Preoperative topical retinoic acid may reduce the incidence of milia postoperatively and enhance wound healing.

For small areas, it is preferable to use a local anesthetic field block. Nerve blocks with lidocaine may be used on the central face, based on the distribution of facial sensory nerves. Approximately 3 ml of lidocaine is injected bilaterally at the supraorbital notch, supratrochlear region, infraorbital foramen, and mental foramen.

Tumanescent anesthesia may be useful in dermabrasion and can eliminate nerve blocks and cryanesthesia. This takes more time to deliver to the entire face.

Prechilling of the skin with ice packs enhances the anesthetic effect of hydrocarbon sprays used for topical cryoanesthesia. The skin is sprayed by the assistant in a circular motion for 10–20 sec until it becomes frigid and develops a white frost (Fig. 4). Freezing too aggressively will

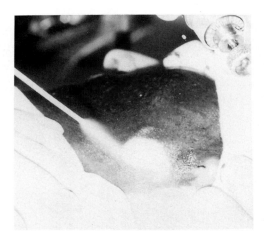

Figure 4 Spray cryoanesthesia to a small area prior to dermabrasion.

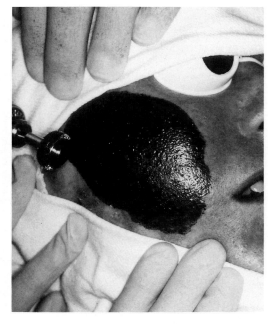

Figure 5 Area of dermabrasion painted with gentian violet; goggles on eyes and face draped with towels.

result in deep cryonecrosis in the dermis, especially over the mandibular bone. The area to be sprayed is usually not greater than 2–3 cm. Towels may be used to protect the adjacent skin.

The choice of spray anesthesia is important. Ethyl chloride is the oldest agent and is not used much because it is explosive and inflammable, has general anesthetic properties, and requires a blower for rapid evaporation. Frigiderm and Fluro-Ethyl are freon 114 and freon 114 plus ethyl chloride, respectively. They generally freeze the skin surface to –42°C in 25 sec, according to work done by Hanke. Other topical cryoanesthetic agents that contain pure freon 111 and 112 can freeze to –67°C and result in much more tissue necrosis. The risk of unpredictable hypertrophic scarring is greater with these sprays. The risk is greatest in areas overlying a bone, such as the mandibular ramus, zygomatic arch, malar eminence, and bossing of the chin and forehead. Frigiderm and Fluro-Ethyl are the preferred agents for cryoanesthesia.

General anesthesia is used more frequently by nondermatologic surgeons. Except for special circumstances, this only adds to the risk, cost, and time to do this procedure. The vast majority of dermabrasions are done in office surgical suites.

TECHNIQUE

There are many variations on the technique. Dermabrasion requires at least one assistant to help with freezing and to hold the skin taut. Both operator and assistant should wear gowns, rubber gloves, and plastic face shields. The assistant should wear cotton gloves over rubber gloves to protect the fingers. Cotton towels are preferred over gauze, which easily gets caught in the wire brush. The area to be abraded is painted with gentian violet (Fig. 5). This not only serves as a guide, but gentian violet deep in the scars also indicates whether the abrasion has gone the sufficient depth to obliterate them. Vaseline and goggles are used to protect the patient's eyes, ears, and nose. The patient lies supine on the table. Adequate ventilation and a cool ambient temperature of 62°F will help when freezing the skin.

Dermabrasion of the face is usually done in sections: four on each cheek, two on the chin, two on the nose, two on the upper lip, and three on the forehead. Spraying and abrading one area at a time, the surgeon starts at the outermost and dependent areas and moves toward the central and upper areas of the face. The operator moves the brush or fraise over the frozen skin with firm, steady, back-and-forth strokes and even pressure. In areas with deeper scars, more pressure may be applied. Dermabrasion is done in anatomic units, so it is usually done to the natural folds of the face (nasolabial fold, hairline, or submandibular) (Fig. 6). This is done to avoid obvious lines of demarcation that can occur with spot dermabrasion. A chemical exfoliant, such as 30–50% trichloroacetic acid, may be applied to adjacent unabraded areas (lower eyelids and upper lip) to help blend these lines. Pigment changes may result from procedures, and combining the two can result in both hypo- and hyperpigmentation in different areas. Localized dermabrasion of a small area of scarring is also risky because texture and pigment changes may be readily apparent. Although the trunk is usually not dermabraded, lesions on arms and legs may respond well.

POSTOPERATIVE CARE AND DRESSING

The author has tried many types of dressings in more than 30 years of performing dermabrasion. For the past 10 years the dressing of choice has been Vigilon.

Vigilon (Bard/Hermel) appears to fulfill more criteria for the ideal wound dressing than any of the other wound dressings. It is composed of 4% polyethylene oxide and 96% water in a colloidal suspension on a polyethylene mesh support. Prior to application, a polyethylene film is removed from the side of the dressing that will cover the wound. Vigilon, unlike other oc-

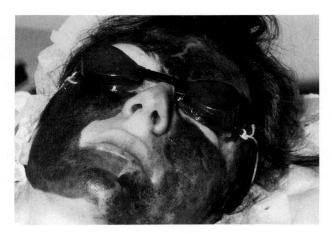

Figure 6   Immediately after dermabrasion of one half of face and laser abrasion of the other half.

clusive dressings, permits a moist environment while allowing for absorption of wound exudate. It is also nonadherent. The Vigilon is changed daily.

Pinski evaluated these new dressings in a bilateral comparison study of patients undergoing full-face dermabrasion. Occlusive dressings act by preventing dehydration to allow rapid epithelial migration. Healing time or reepithelialization is reduced by as much as 50%. Vigilon may be the best dressing to use following dermabrasion. It should be changed daily. Reepithelialization will occur in 5–7 days without crusting compared to 10–12 days when crusts are allowed to form.

Op-site was the first in a series of newly developed, thin, transparent, semipermeable, synthetic polyurethane membranes to be used as a wound dressing. Several others have been introduced, including Bioclusive (Johnson & Johnson), Tegaderm (3M), and Ensure (Deserat). Each is a thin, elastic film, transparent and permeable to air and water vapor without being porous. They do not adhere to the wound, but stick to intact skin and conform to the curves of the face. The membrane protects nerve endings like a second skin, giving immediate pain relief. They keep the wound moist and prevent eschar formation, thus providing optimal conditions for reepithelialization.

The patient is given written instruction for postoperative care. Pain medication such as acetaminophen with codeine is helpful. Systemic antibiotics (dicloxacillin 250 mg four times a day) and a short course of prednisone starting at 40 mg/day and tapering in one week are useful in reducing infection and postoperative edema.

The patient is seen in 24 hr for a dressing change. The Vigilon dressing is then changed on a daily basis at home. The patient should be evaluated regularly at 7, 14, and 30 days—more often if necessary (Figs. 7–9).

Avoidance of sun is important after dermabrasion. Sun exposure may easily burn the new skin and will predispose to postinflammatory hyperpigmentation (Fig. 10).

COMPLICATIONS AND CONTRAINDICATIONS

Among the most common complications are hyperpigmentation, hypopigmentation, keloids, gouging of skin, herpes simplex, milia, persistent erythema, and telangiectasia.

Erythema is expected in the postoperative period, but it may persist for weeks or months along with some telangiectasia. Milia formation is very common and can easily be corrected with

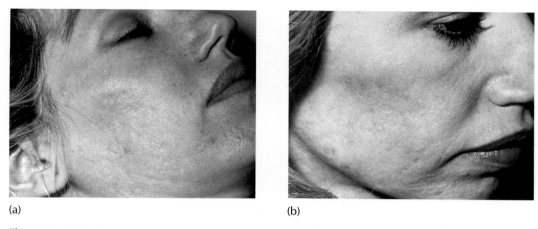

(a)   (b)

Figure 7   (a) Acne scars on cheek. (b) After dermabrasion (3 months).

abrasive soaps or simple extraction. Pinpoint electrodesiccation can also be used. The use of topical retinoic acid prior to and after dermabrasion may reduce the incidence of milia. Milia may be more common with the new occlusive wound dressings.

Hypertrophic scars or keloids may occur in a small number of patients. A personal or family history of keloid formation is a relative contraindication. Black patients tend to form keloids more frequently. The use of refrigerants, especially on the mandible, may be partially responsible (Fig. 11). Atypical keloids develop in atypical locations such as the buccal skin after dermabrasion of patients still on or having recently taken isotretinoin (Accutane). Patients now wait 6 months to 1 year after stopping Accutane before the procedure. Treatment of these scars with intralesional triamcinolone is helpful. Topical steroids may be used early for suspicious areas of hypertrophic scars.

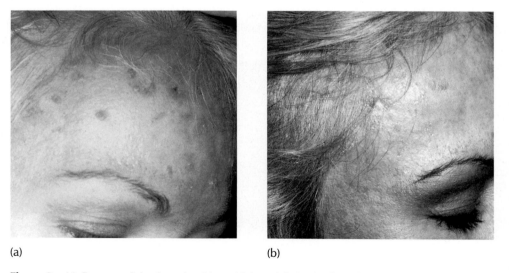

(a)   (b)

Figure 8   (a) Severe actinic elastosis with multiple actinic keratosis, prior to dermabrasion. (b) Five months postabrasion.

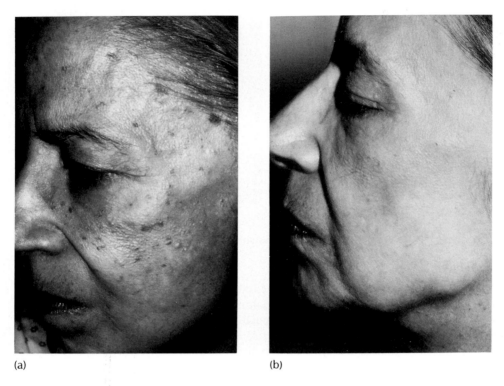

(a)   (b)

Figure 9   (a) Multiple seborrheic keratosis and aging skin. (b) Three years after dermabrasion.

Patients with a history of recurrent cold sores, possibly herpes simplex, should be approached with caution. The surgeon should avoid dermabrasion in the trigger areas of previous herpes simplex. Oral acyclovir (Zovirax), 200 mg five times a day for 3 days before and until the skin has reepithelialized, should be given prophylactically. If disseminated herpes simplex develops, hospitalization and intravenous acyclovir are indicated (Fig. 12).

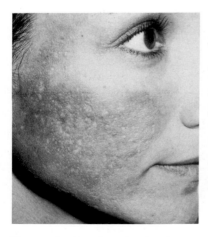

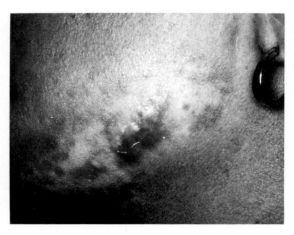

Figure 10   Postdermabrasion hyperpigmentation.

Figure 11   Hypertrophic scarring of mandibular area
following dermabrasion.

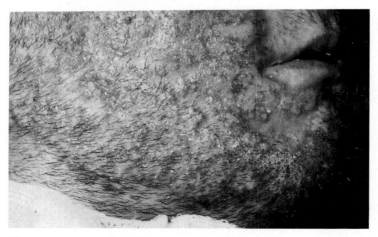

Figure 12 Acute disseminated herpes simplex into area of dermabrasion.

Hypopigmentation and hyperpigmentation are common but usually temporary. Pigmentary problems are more common in dark-skinned patients (skin types IV–VI). It is most noticeable at the edges of the dermabrasion or in spot dermabrasion. Postinflammatory hyperpigmentation usually fades in several months, and no treatment is necessary. Topical hydroquinone 4% may be helpful.

Acne will occasionally recur after dermabrasion, although most patients with minimally active disease will actually improve. Infection with *Staphylococcus* and *Pseudomonas* occurs occasionally and needs prompt topical and systemic therapy.

Dermabrasion is usually contraindicated in patients with chronic radiodermatitis, pyoderma, herpes simplex, psychosis, severe psychoneurosis, alcoholism, xeroderma pigmentosum, verrucae planae, or burn scars.

COMBINED PROCEDURES

Larger, deeper scars that do not respond well to dermabrasion alone may be treated in other ways. Punch excision with a circular punch can be sutured closed. Occasionally, the depressed scar can be elevated flush to the surface of the surrounding skin and held in place with tape. In addition, punch excision of the scar with a full-thickness punch graft replacement taken from the post-auricular area will fill these defects. Dermabrasion is usually then done 6 weeks after these procedures have corrected the deeper scars to smooth the skin surfaces.

Bovine collagen (Zyderm I or II or Zyplast) or medical-grade fluid polydimethylsiloxane (silicone) may be used to augment soft depressions remaining after dermabrasion. Dermabrasion should probably be done just to eliminate as many scars as possible. Zyderm or Fibril or even autologous fat implants can then be used to fill out the remaining scars. Zyderm will last only 6–18 months. Fibril and Zyplast last somewhat longer; fat implants may be more permanent. Fat transplants have been used in recent years to correct the soft shallow larger scars not corrected by dermabrasion. The correction of acne scars is not as permanent as can be achieved with dermabrasion. Dermabrasion can safely be done on patients who have previously received collagen or silicone injections.

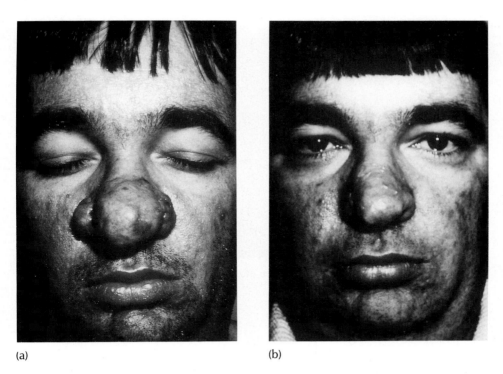

(a)   (b)

Figure 13   (a) Rhinophyma. (b) After treatment with combined electrosurgical excision and dermabrasion.

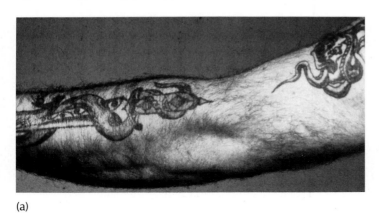

(a)

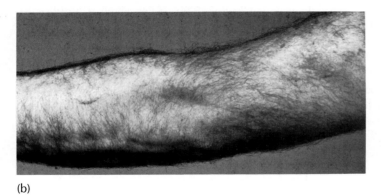

(b)

Figure 14   (a) Tattoo of left arm. (b) After dermabrasion with very little scarring.

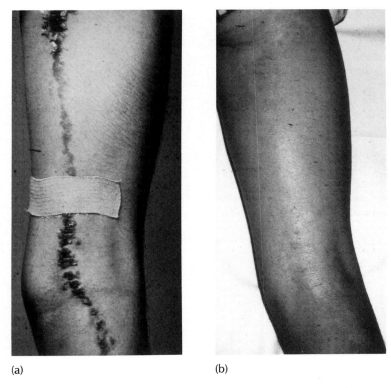

(a)   (b)

Figure 15   (a) Epidermal nevus of the leg. (b) After dermabrasion.

LASERBRASIONS

The CO_2 laser has been used to perform dermabrasion. The newer, rapidly pulsed, well-controlled CO_2 lasers have provided a new dimension to skin resurfacing in the past 1–2 years. This laser vaporizes tissue without bleeding and possibly with less pain than the standard dermabrasion instruments. The CO_2 laser has been suggested as ideal for treatment of multiple trichoepitheliomas, rhinophyma, epidermal nevi, syringomas, neurofibromas, and tattoos. These problems have all been treated satisfactorily with standard dermabrasion as well (Figs. 13–15). Since the CO_2 laser may be successfully used to treat keloids, the incidence of keloid formation may be less with the CO_2 laser. Controlling the depth of vaporization by the laser requires experience but could be done by computer. The lines of demarcation appear more sharp with the CO_2 laser, and blending, which can be done so well by dermabrasion, may be more difficult with the CO_2 laser. The new superpulse CO_2 lasers (Sharplan's Silktouch and Coherent Ultra Pulse) have recently gained popularity in the resurfacing of the skin for wrinkles and acne scars. Comparison studies need to be done before the value of laserbrasion can be shown to be comparable to dermabrasion.

BIBLIOGRAPHY

Burks JW. *Wire Brush Surgery*. Springfield, IL, Charles C Thomas, 1956.
Burks J. *Dermabrasion and Chemical Peeling, in the Treatment of Certain Cosmetic Defects and Diseases of the Skin*. Springfield, IL, Charles C Thomas, 1979.
Hanke CW, O'Brian JJ, Solow EB. Laboratory evaluation of skin refrigerants used in dermabrasion. *J Dermatol Surg Oncol* 1985;11:45–49.

Kromayer E. Die Heilung der Akne durch in Neves Norbenlases Operationsverfahren. Das Stanzen. *Illustr Monatsschr Aerztl Polytech* 1905;27:101.

Kurtin A. Corrective surgical planing of skin. *Arch Dermatol Syphilol* 1953;68:389–397.

Pinski JB. Dressings for dermabrasion: Occlusive dressings and wound healing. *Cutis* 1986;37:471–476.

Roenigk HH Jr. Advanced cosmetic procedures. *Cutis* 1994;53:211–216.

Roenigk HH Jr. Dermabrasion and aging skin. *J Geriatr Dermatol* 1994;2(1):24–29.

Roenigk HH Jr. Dermabrasion for miscellaneous cutaneous lesions (exclusive of scarring from acne). *J Dermatol Surg Oncol* 1977;3:322–328.

Roenigk HH Jr. Dermabrasion for rejuvenation and scar removal. In *Cosmetic Dermatology*. R Baron, H Maibach, eds. London, Martin Dunitz, 1994.

Roenigk HH Jr. Dermabrasion: rejuvenation and scar revision. In *Surgical Dermatology*. R Roenigk, H Roenigk, eds. London, Martin Dunitz, 1992, pp. 509–516.

Roenigk HH Jr. Dermabrasion: state of the art. *J Dermatol Surg Oncol* 1985;11:3:306–314.

Roenigk HH Jr. Scar camouflage using dermabrasion. *Facial Plast Surg* 1984;1:3:249–257.

Schultz BC, Roenigk HH Jr. Debrisan as a postoperative dressing after dermabrasion. *J Dermatol Surg Oncol* 1979;5:971–974.

Stegman SJ, Tromovitch TK. Dermabrasion equipment. In *Cosmetic Dermatologic Surgery*. Chicago, Year Book, 1984.

62

Glycolic Acid Chemical Peel

Lawrence S. Moy
University of California, Los Angeles, California

Romulo Mene
Private Practice, Rio de Janeiro, Brazil

Chemical peels are used for a variety of reasons. Certain peels are designed to penetrate deeper and cause longer healing times but also cause deeper levels of improvement. Phenol and trichloroacetic acid have been used and studied extensively. More recently, glycolic acid has become an established superficial peeling agent.

GLYCOLIC ACID

Glycolic acid causes a superficial chemical peel that can have beneficial effects on photodamage (wrinkles, actinic keratoses, solar lentigines, rough texture), acne, keratoses, and ichthyoses. Table 1 lists skin conditions that may be cleared or improved with glycolic acid. Glycolic acid is used repetitively to achieve positive results. In addition to the additive effect, repeated peels also have fewer side effects than a single deeper chemical peel.

Alpha hydroxy acids are a class of compounds derived from various fruits and foods and are therefore sometimes called fruit acids. Glycolic acid is naturally found in sugar cane. The principal structure of glycolic acid ($CH_2OHCOOH$) is composed of an alpha hydroxy group, the carboxyl carbon, and both carboxyl oxygens all lying in the same plane. Other alpha hydroxy acids include malic acid from apples, tartaric acid from grapes, citric acid from citrus fruits, and lactic acid from sour milk.

Glycolic acid's effect on corneocytes can be demonstrated by improvement of a variety of epidermal lesions, including ichthyosis, seborrheic keratoses, verrucae vulgaris, acne, and actinic keratoses. In addition, wrinkles, solar lentigines, pigmentation, and solar elastosis may be improved.

The mechanism by which glycolic acid affects wrinkles and hyperpigmentation may relate to its similarity to ascorbic acid. Ascorbic acid, a derivative of alpha hydroxy acid, has been shown to stimulate collagen production and possibly decrease melanin production. As with ascorbic acid, glycolic acid may also have clinical relevance as an antixodant, and it protects against the ef-

Table 1   Skin Conditions Treated with
Glycolic Acid

General photodamage
Actinic keratosis
Solar lentigines
Acne
Acne scars
Postinflammatory hyperpigmentation
Melasma
Xerosis
Icthyosis
Keratosis pilaris

fects of ultraviolet radiation. Glycolic acid may also affect wrinkles by its effects on glycosaminoglycans and other ground substances, and it may stimulate the production of collagen in fibroblasts. This is in contrast to other peeling agents, such as trichloroacetic acid (TCA) and phenol, that damage the skin and cause a thickened zone of papillary dermal collagen proportional to the damage. For glycolic acid, crusting and tissue necrosis can be minimized while still improving many skin conditions. In a mini pig study, 12% lactic acid was shown to deposit as much new papillary collagen as 25% TCA or 25% phenol after 21 days. Histologic studies of topical retinoic acid have suggested similiar effects.

Glycolic acid can penetrate as well as other chemical peels. When a 50–70% solution is left on the skin for 15 min, a depth of necrosis occurs that is comparable to 35% and 50% TCA. With shorter exposures, 50% and 70% glycolic acid will cause less depth of damage than 35% TCA.

HISTOLOGIC CHANGES AFTER CHEMICAL PEEL

Histologic studies have been done to analyze the effects of chemical peels on the different layers of the skin. Wounding and healing after chemical peel have been noted to be identical to those caused by dermabrasion including cellular and connective tissue destruction in the papillary dermis. A thin crust composed of keratin, necrotic keratinocytes, and a proteinaceous precipitate forms later. Epidermal regeneration typically occurs after 2–7 days. After 2 weeks, the epidermis is completely healed with partially reformed rete ridges. In addition, dermal thickening with fibroblast proliferation and new collagen deposition has been observed in the papillary dermis. This new dermal collagen deposition probably accounts for most of the cosmetic improvement and rejuvenation of the skin.

Biopsies show horizontally arranged new collagen with a predominance of fibroblasts 2–3 weeks after chemical peels. The sun-induced elastotic changes with basophilic degeneration and homogenization of collagen disappear, and the zone of new collagen remains for up to 1 year. Finely wrinkled, actinically damaged skin is benefited most by treatment with superficial peels. Subsequent biopsies performed after chemical peeling demonstrate both a reduction in the melanosis of the epidermis and fewer melanocytes at the dermal-epidermal junction. A long-term histologic study on phenol peels showed that the same new, horizontally arranged collagen deposits seen in the papillary dermis are maintained for at least 12 years and may be permanent.

PROCEDURE

Skin preparation is crucial to consistent and successful peeling in the office. The skin-preparation steps will determine the depth and the control of the chemical peel. Improper preparation can give minimal, insufficient, or uneven results. Overzealous preparation can deepen the chemical peel below the penetration level needed for the specific patient. Even though glycolic acid chemical peels are known to be superficial, glycolic acid can cause deeper necrosis of dermal layers and unanticipated deeper peeling.

Cleansing the skin is typically performed with a gauze or cotton pad. Alcohol is probably the easiest and most consistent skin-preparation cleanser, and cleansing should be done twice to properly prepare the skin.

It is recommended that 50% and 70% solutions of glycolic acid be applied. These are the concentrations in a gel formulation initially described as therapeutically beneficial. Our experience has been that these concentrations are best and can be used for a large variety of skin conditions and disorders. Lower-concentration glycolic acid chemical peels are available but have not yet shown sufficient therapeutic benefits or undergone sufficient research or combined clinical experience. The methods described here are for using gel formulations of 50% and 70% glycolic acid, which have given consistent therapeutic benefits with minimal side effects.

Unlike other chemical peels, glycolic acid is time dependent. Therefore, the preparation should not have any runoff and should adhere to the skin surface during the peel time period. The peel should be carefully timed from the first contact of glycolic acid with the skin until it is washed off. The peel may take longer if the skin condition requires deeper penetration and if the patient's skin tolerates the peel well.

To apply the peel after skin preparation, a stiff, horsehair brush or large cotton applicator should be used. A very liberal amount of glycolic acid peel should be put on the applicator, after which the glycolic acid should be lightly brushed on the skin. The recommended method is to start on one cheek and completely cover that anatomical unit, then apply around the forehead to the other cheek and down to the chin. The central face should be treated last. Glycolic acid peels do not cause frosting; thus, using this pattern ensures that the whole face is uniformly covered. Application over the face should take 15–20 sec.

Certain areas can be reapplied or rubbed more firmly with the glycolic acid gel. It is not recommended to rub the glycolic acid in further than the initial application unless treating a specific lesion or area. Keratotic lesions or deeper furrows are typical lesions that will be rubbed in further during the peeling time.

Using a stiff, horsehair brush with tight hairs, the thick glycolic acid chemical peel can be applied on the upper eyelid within 2 mm of the lid margin. This causes mild stinging but improves periocular results. Keep water-saturated gauze nearby to rinse out any glycolic acid that may enter the eye. Because glycolic acid is not dangerous to the eye, this wicking procedure is sufficient. The wet gauze is placed at the lid margin, and residual glycolic acid mixed with tears is absorbed by the gauze and removed from the eye.

Timing of the glycolic acid gel peel is very important. Glycolic acid effects are dependent on the time of contact of the peel solution. Proportionally, the longer that the glycolic acid stays on the skin, the deeper the penetration and peeling of the skin. For deeper skin conditions, including actinic elastosis, actinic keratoses, and acne scars, 70% glycolic acid gel is left on for 4–8 min. For more superficial problems, such as acne and melasma, 2–5 min of 50% glycolic acid gel is recommended. Sensitivity can vary significantly, so the length of time for a glycolic acid chemical peel must be individual.

Complete neutralization is very important for glycolic acid. Unlike TCA, glycolic acid activity is not dissipated during the peeling action. Complete removal is required after the timed application. It is highly recommended to remove the peel in three steps, to stop the reaction, and to ease comfort of the skin. First, with a water-soaked gauze, excess glycolic acid should be removed from the skin. This will not absolutely stop the reaction, but will lift off a majority of the gel. Then, a buffered cleansing lotion should be applied. This acts as a neutralizer and is buffered to stop the reaction and inactivate glycolic acid on the skin. Additionally, the neutralizer cools the skin to give comfort from the mild stinging and heat caused by the glycolic acid chemical peel. The neutralizer ensures that the peel is stopped. Finally, the patient is asked to rinse off the excess glycolic acid and neutralizer from the skin. It is not sufficient to have the patient rinse off without the neutralizer, because it should not be the patient's responsibility to completely remove and inactivate the peel. The neutralizer can also be used in TCA peels because of the comfort it gives to the skin.

POSTPEEL CARE

Postpeel care includes preventing infection and minimizing inflammation. Various products are used including antibiotic ointments, Prep H®, petroleum, and other agents. A complex of iodine-bromine (Iobrom Gel®) has been very successful. It is a potent antimicrobial agent and a mild drying agent that is ideal for epidermal wounds. Glycolic acid chemical peels are superficial peels that remove full-thickness epidermis, but typically will not peel into the papillary dermis. Iobrom gel is an agent that may increase healing, decrease inflammation, and prevent superficial infections. The patient is instructed to wash with cool water and a mild, soapless cleanser. Sunscreens are applied over the postpeel healing agent when the patient leaves the office and then reapplied regularly for 2 weeks. The patient is instructed not to apply their daily home glycolic acid products or topical retinoic acid for 2–4 days, depending on the depth and reaction of the glycolic acid chemical peel. The application of glycolic acid–containing products immediately on the peel can cause deeper, unwanted peeling reactions and problems.

DAILY LOTIONS

Glycolic acid formulations are a useful adjunct to chemical peels. The use of lotions at 8–15% concentrations can help accelerate the effects of glycolic acid chemical peels. In addition, daily application of lotions can maintain the beneficial effects of the chemical peel.

Efforts should be made to use an effective set of glycolic acid products. It is best to use a formulation line that is compatible with the therapeutic needs of the patient. The important qualities for such products include strength, specific intent (e.g., pigment, acne), and compatibility with glycolic acid chemical peels. There have been reported problems with chemical peels and daily lotions not produced by experienced manufacturers. Experience in the production of glycolic acid is required to ensure that irritation is minimized and the product will be effective. Many of the effectiveness claims of such products have not been substantiated.

To obtain the proper effect of the glycolic acid peeling agents, it is recommended to begin the daily home lotions 2 weeks before the first peel. This regimen is helpful for several reasons:

1. The patients' commitment is assessed for postpeel care. If the patient is not dedicated enough to use the daily products, then he or she may not be a proper peel candidate.
2. The 2 weeks of using the glycolic acid lotion conditions the skin to give a more even peel and increases the skin's tolerance for the glycolic acid procedure. This is analogous to the application of retinoic acid 2 weeks before dermabrasion and TCA.
3. Any reaction or sensitivity to the daily lotions will predict reactions that may result from the glycolic acid chemical peel.

Glycolic acid formulations for home use have helped accelerate and maintain the positive benefits of the glycolic acid chemical peel. By combining products or increasing the potency of the glycolic acid, these lotions can be tailored to the patient. For photodamage, increasing the concentration of the daily cream or lotion may increase the dermal effect by increasing collagen and glycosaminoglycan deposition, especially at the proper pH. For pigmentation, a mixture of several bleachers and glycolic acid appears to synergistically slow melanocytic activity and increase effectiveness. A study of acne has demonstrated beneficial effects from combinations of glycolic acid with other topical acne agents.

REACTIVITY TO GLYCOLIC ACID

Sensitivity to home products can manifest itself in several different ways. Stinging upon immediate application is common. This reaction will usually last a few days and then subside with continual use. For therapeutic products, the stinging should be expected and patients should be forewarned. In addition, the daily products can cause erythema, dryness, and peeling. For the majority of patients, the peeling effect is not desired for the daily lotions. Occasionally, patients with extreme sensitivity can develop acneiform papules soon after starting the products. In the case of any of these reactions, it is suggested that the patient stop the product temporarily and use a milder glycolic acid lotion.

Complications of the glycolic acid chemical peels are uncommon and usually can be avoided. First, determine which patients may be more sensitive to the peels. Then, be present with the patient throughout the peel procedure to manage problems.

Possible side effects are hyperpigmentation, postpeel erythema, and, rarely, irregular surface texture. The side effects that occur will resolve after a short time or can be treated with specific topical agents. Table 2 lists possible side effects from chemical peels. Hyperpigmentation can occur in patients with a tendency to pigment, including darker skin types and patients with melasma. Erythema long after a peel is uncommon. A mild cortisone cream applied to the area very early will commonly clear the erythema. Irregular surface texture is a "step-off" lesion that occurs when the peel is significantly uneven in a given area. The most common areas for this irregular healing are the upper cheek, upper nose, and perioral areas. Promoting rapid healing with Iobrom and other agents is advantageous, and with time the lesions will heal well. Further superficial peels will also smooth these areas.

CLINICAL INDICATIONS

Glycolic acid chemical peels can be used for a variety of skin conditions. Used properly, glycolic acid can be comparable in effectiveness to other commonly used chemical peels. In addition, glycolic acid can be selectively used on a wider variety of skin types than other chemical

Table 2 Possible Side Effects of Glycolic Acid

Hyperpigmentation
Hypopigmentation
Persistant erythema
Herpes simplex flare
Impetigo
"Step-off," irregular scarring

peels. It is necessary to repeat the glycolic acid peel to achieve the desired clinical results. However, glycolic acid chemical peels typically require less time to heal. Therefore, for the patient who prefers not taking an extended time to heal and tolerates repeat visits, glycolic acid chemical peels can be ideal. Glycolic acid is especially desirable if the patient does not want it known that a specific treatment was performed, because glycolic acid will cause gradual improvement and little postoperative disfigurement that has to be explained socially.

Glycolic acid has not been generally accepted as effective for the removal of deep photodamage. Maximizing the concentration of the glycolic acid combined with a consistent pattern of repeated peels and a strong concentration of the daily glycolic acid creams can give positive results in deep wrinkles. These results are proportional to maximally applying high concentrations of glycolic acid. Deep wrinkles can be improved without causing necrosis besides epidermolysis. However, compared to other conditions, glycolic acid chemical peels must be applied longer and allowed to react deeper when used for deep wrinkles. It is important to use the thick 70% glycolic acid gel. A thin or water-based glycolic acid chemical peel will often penetrate unevenly and cause "hot" spots where the peel penetrates too deeply.

Figure 1 shows a 73-year-old female with significant, deep creases on her lower cheeks who had a series of 20 70% glycolic acid chemical peels in a little over a year. Dramatic improvement can be seen in the deep creases. The depth of the wrinkles is raised, the skin is smoother, and the tone is improved.

Glycolic acid chemical peels can be beneficial for superficial cutaneous sun damage with lentigines and fine cross-hatched wrinkles. These patients can be peeled with 70% glycolic acid, but caution must be taken not to peel too deeply. Some patients with superficial and minimal photodamage can react more than anticipated to the glycolic acid, and timing is very important.

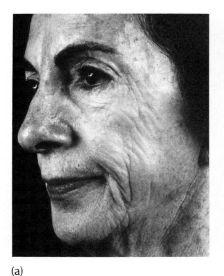
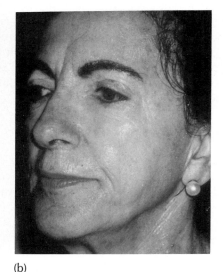

(a)   (b)

Figure 1 (a) This patient had deep creases on the cheeks and around the mouth from excessive sun exposure for many years. Glycolic acid peels were used because the patient requested short healing times. A series of more than 15 70% glycolic acid chemical peels were performed over 1 year. The peels were left on for 8–10 min. (b) This picture was taken 1 year after the series of glycolic acid chemical peels. Deep creases and wrinkles around the eyes, on the cheeks, and most prominently around the mouth are greatly improved and stay improved.

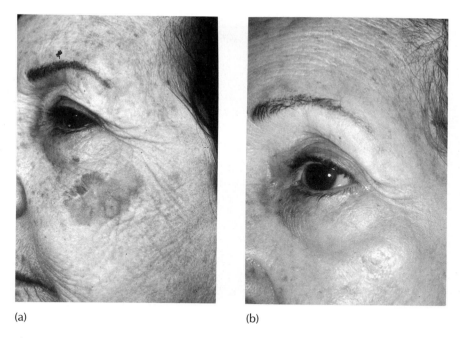

(a)   (b)

Figure 2 (a) This elderly patient had features of general photodamage composed of solar lentigines, wrinkles, rough texture, and sallow skin. The patient was treated with 70% glycolic acid chemical peels for 6 months and daily lotions. The peels were left on for 6–8 min. (b) After the treatments, the photodamage problems are greatly improved and cleared. The skin surface is markedly even and smooth.

As photodamage becomes more significant, with deeper creases and prominent lentigines, the skin's tolerance to the 70% glycolic acid peel increases dramatically (Fig. 2). The application time of the peel can be increased so the penetration can be enhanced.

Acne can be well controlled with glycolic acid chemical peels because they are extremely active comedolytics. Glycolic acid chemical peels penetrate deeply into the comedo, causing exfoliation of retention hyperkeratoses. Clinically, the exfoliative process can be seen by the dull whitening that will center only around acne lesions and comedomes immediately after glycolic acid peels. Within 1 or 2 days, the lesions with the whiteness will open and drain.

On the face, 50% glycolic acid gel works best (Figs. 3,4). The gel consistently penetrates the pores and acne lesions. Short contact time of 1–3 min is required. Leaving the peel on too long can be a problem because it penetrates too much and causes uneven and unwanted epidermolysis. Usually, acne patients are young, with thin, nonphotodamaged skin that can be sensitive to chemical peels. To affect deeper lesions, it is necessary for patients to use daily home products.

On the back, 70% glycolic acid chemical peels are one of the few treatments that can effectively lift deep cysts and plugs to the surface. Epidermolysis and whitening around the pores and acne lesions is more helpful on the back than on the face. The peel is left on for 4–8 min.

Acne scarring can also be improved by repeated glycolic acid chemical peels. The shallow, uneven scars will become smooth with several chemical peels. Some pore-type scars will also be tighter and improved. Ice-pick scars and deeper, concave scars will not be appreciably improved. Dermabrasion and deeper chemical peels may be needed. Glycolic acid chemical peels appear to be more effective in improving the acne scars when active inflammatory acne lesions are being treated.

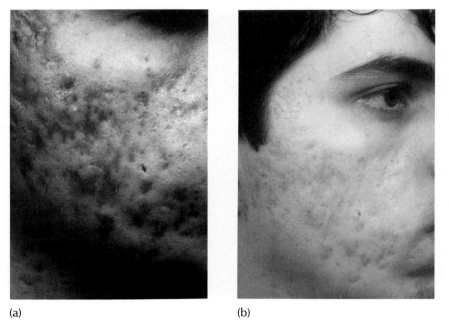

(a)   (b)

Figure 3 (a) This male had severe acne composed of acne papules, large comedomes, and large cysts. Intense areas of erythema are located on the cheeks. A series of four 50% glycolic acid chemical peels were performed over a 3-month period. The peels were left on for 3–5 min. (b) After the glycolic acid peels, the comedomes and cysts have opened and cleared dramatically. In addition, the scars that were apparent before the treatment have also smoothed and cleared.

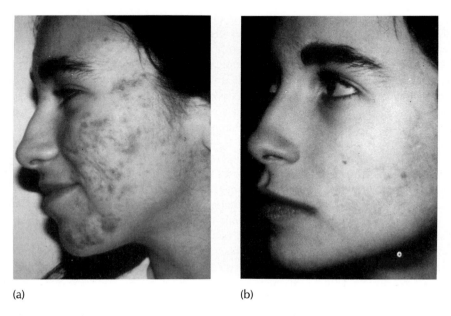

(a)   (b)

Figure 4 (a) This young female had extremely inflammatory acne with very large cysts across the cheeks. She had no to little improvement with other treatment regimens, including oral antibiotics. She had three 50% glycolic acid chemical peels over 2 months. Each peel was left on 2–4 min. (b) The acne cleared very well with repeated glycolic acid chemical peels. All the cysts have cleared without residual problems.

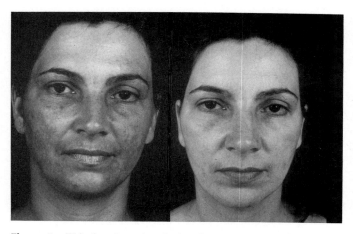

Figure 5 This female patient had melasma lesions noted by the symmetrical facial distribution of the pigmentation. The lesions were recalcitrant to other bleaching agents. A series of five 50% glycolic acid chemical peels were used along with a glycolic acid bleacher. The lesions cleared after 3 months of treatment. Sunscreen application was also used during the treatment time.

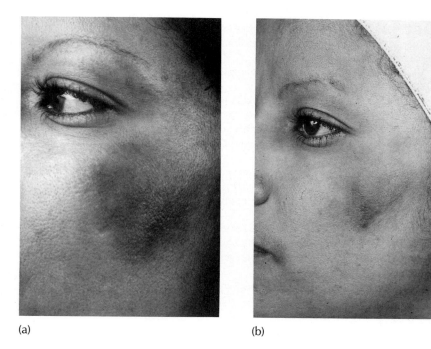

(a)   (b)

Figure 6 (a) This patient had a distinct area of melasmic pigmentation for several years. Use of retinoic acid had worsened the area with deeper hyperpigmentation after increased sun exposure. Two 50% glycolic acid chemical peels with a daily glycolic acid bleacher over 6 weeks was used. (b) The glycolic acid treatments significantly cleared the lesion within 6 weeks. The well-defined lesion on the cheek became indistinct and lightened.

Glycolic acid chemical peels can be very effective in the treatment of pigmentation. Using 50% glycolic acid chemical peels and maximal home therapy, pigmentation can be significantly lightened with minimal risk of hyperpigmentation from the chemical peel or photosensitivity from the treatments.

Melasma is caused by a combination of melanocytic sensitivity to estrogen and sun exposure. As can be seen in Figure 5, glycolic acid chemical peels will lighten the pigmented lesions. A possible mechanism of action for glycolic acid to decrease pigmentation is through the tyrosinase model if the glycolic acid can penetrate to the layers of pigmentation in the skin. Figure 6 shows a patient who had used topical retinoic acid that caused darker pigmentation after sun exposure. After 1 month of home products and one 70% glycolic acid chemical peel, the pigment improved.

As can be seen from the examples of clinical improvements with glycolic acid chemical peels, an assortment of skin types have been successfully treated. Although other chemical peels such as TCA can be used on darker skin types, glycolic acid can be used more consistently with less risk of hyperpigmentation.

BIBLIOGRAPHY

Ayres S III. Superficial chemicosurgery: its current status and its relation to dermabrasion. *Arch Dermatol* 1991;89:395–403.

Baker TJ, Gordon JL. Chemical face peeling and dermabrasion. *Surg Clin North Am* 1971;51:387–401.

Baker T, Gordon H, Mosienko P, Seckinger DL. Long-term histological study of skin after chemical peel and dermabrasion. *Plast Reconstr Surg* 1974;53:522–525.

Behin F, Feverstein SS, Marovitz WF. Comparative histological study of mini-pig skin after chemical peel and dermabrasion. *Arch Otolaryngol* 1977;103:271–277.

Brodland DG, Cullimore KC, Roenigk RK, Gibson LE. Depths of chemexfoliation induced by various concentrations and application techniques of trichloroacetic acid in a porcine model. *J Dermatol Surg Oncol* 1989;15:967–971.

Brody HJ, Hailey CW. Variations and comparisons in medium-depth chemical peeling. *J Dermatol Surg Oncol* 1989;15:953–963.

Coleman WP, Futrell JM. The glycolic acid trichloroacetic acid peel. *J Dermatol Surg Oncol* 1994;1:76.

Collins PS. The chemical peel. *Clin Dermatol* 1987;5:57–74.

Ditre CM, Griffin TD, Murphy GF, Van Scott EJ. Improvement of photodamaged skin with alpha hydroxy acid (AHA): a clinical, histological, and ultra-structural study. *Dermatology 2000 Congress*. Vienna, May 18-21, 1993, p. 175.

Haas JE. The effect of ascorbic acid and potassium ferricyanide as melanogenesis inhibitors on the development of pigmentation in Mexican axolotols. *Am Osteopath* 1974;73:674.

Kligman AM, Baker TJ, Gordon HL. Long-term histologic followup of phenol face peels. *Plast Reconstr Surg* 1985;75:652–659.

Kligman AM, Grove GL, et al. Topical retinoin for photoaged skin. *J Am Acad Dermatol* 1986;15:836–859.

Mackee GM, Karp FL. The treatment of post-acne scars with phenol. *Br J Dermatol* 1959;64:456–459.

Mandy SH. Tretinoin in the preoperative and postoperative management of dermabrasion. *J Am Acad Dermatol* 1986;15:878–879.

Moy LS. Glycolic acid superficial peels. In *Atlas of Cutaneous Surgery*. J. Robinson, ed. Philadelphia, W.B. Saunders, 1995.

Moy LS, et al. Glycolic acid peels for the treatment of wrinkles and photoaging. *J Dermatol Surg Oncol* 1989;19:243–246.

Moy LS, et al. Use of AHAs add new dimensions to chemical peeling. *Cosmet Dermatol* 1990;3:32–34.

Murad H, et al. Study shows that acne improves with glycolic acid regimen. *Cosmet Dermatol* 1992:32–35.

Newton MD, Jeffrey GA. Stereo chemistry of the alpha-hydroxycarboxylic acids and related systems. *J Am Chem Soc* 1977;99:2413–2421.

Perricone NV. An alpha hydroxy acid acts as an antioxidant. *J Geriatr Dermatol* 1994;1:101–104.

Pinnell SR, et al. Induction of collagen synthesis by ascorbic acid: a possible mechanism. *Arch Dermatol* 1987;123:1684–1686.

Rees RD. Chemabrasion with special reference to rehabilitation of the aging face. *Geriatrics* 1965;20:1039–1047.

Ridge JM, Siegle, Zuckerman J. Use of alpha hydroxy acids in the therapy for photoaged skin. *J Am Acad Dermatol* 1990;23:932.

Spira M, Dahl C, Freeman R, et al. Chemosurgery—a histological study. *Plast Reconstr Surg* 1970;45:247–253.

Stegman SJ. A comparative histologic study of the effects of three peeling agents and dermabrasion on normal and sun damaged skin. *Aesthetic Plast Surg* 1982;6:123–135.

Stegman SJ. A study of dermabrasion and chemical peels in an animal model. *J Dermatol Surg Oncol* 1980;6:490–497.

Stegman SJ, Tromovitch TA. chemical peels in cosmetic-dermatologic surgery. In *Cosmetic Dermatologic Surgery*. SS Stegman, TA Tromovitch, RG Glogau, eds. Chicago, Year Book, 1984, pp. 27–46.

Uitto, Fazio MJ, Olsen DR. Cutaneous aging, molecular alterations in elastic fibers. *J Cutan Aging Cosmet Dermatol* 1988;1:13–26.

Van Scott EJ, Yu RJ. Alpha hydroxy acids: therapeutic potentials. *Can J Dermatol* 1989;1(5):108–112.

63

Chemical Peel with Resorcin

Serge M. Letessier
Hôpital Saint Louis, Paris, France

In 1882 Unna, a German dermatologist, pointed out the properties of substances such as salicylic acid, phenic acid, trichloroacetic acid, and metaoxyphenol or resorcin. They were called *lepismatiques*, from the Greek "lepiso," which means to peel. Resorcin has been widely used for a century in France as described by Unna. Its effects are constant and the results predictable depending on the concentration and time of application to the skin. Because it is so reproducible, resorcin is a reliable chemexfoliant for chemical peeling.

EFFECTS OF RESORCIN ON THE SKIN

Resorcin separates stratum corneum and the most superficial layers of the epidermis from the deeper ones. The split seems to occur in the stratum granulosum. If this effect were the only one, the results would be temporary and unacceptable. A deeper inflammatory reaction, demonstrated by histologic sections, is associated with vasodilation visible 6 hr following the application of resorcin.

A week later, the exfoliation ends. One notices:

1. Increased mitosis in the stratum germinativum
2. Prolonged vasodilation of dermal vessels
3. Proliferation of fibroblasts
4. A thickened papillary dermal band

These are due to increased density of glycosamines in the intracellular space. A higher concentration of elastic fibers occurs in the deep dermis. The dermal changes are still visible 4 months later, with the exception of vasodilation. The epidermis is thicker, especially if actinically damaged skin with a thinner epidermis has been peeled.

INDICATIONS

Acne

Chemical peeling with resorcin is especially effective with medical therapy for acne, when some folliculitis and inflammation still remain (Fig. 1). It will reduce small depressed scars and will debride the skin deeply enough to remove closed comedones. Resorcin peeling may be done on the back, while other approaches such as dermabrasion are contraindicated because of poor healing (Fig. 2).

Actinically Damaged Skin

Actinic damage is a major indication for resorcin peeling. Pigmented macules, keratoses, and poikiloderma are solar changes that respond well. Atrophic epidermis thickens while the dermis regains some of its elasticity. This results in a more homogeneous, youthful appearance of the skin (Fig. 3). Unsatisfactory results may be peeled again 3 months later. Pits, depressed or wide scars, and deep wrinkles are unresponsive to resorcin peeling.

MATERIAL

In the past, Unna's paste contained 10, 20, or 30% resorcin and was applied in gradually increasing concentrations. Resorcin, 50%, is now used:

Resorcin	40 g
Zinc oxide	10 g
Ceyssatite	2 g
Benzoin axungia	28 g

Excessive erythema is avoided by the axungia. The zinc oxide and ceyssatite (a clay-bearing soil) are effective drying agents. They make the preparation homogeneous to allow an even peel.

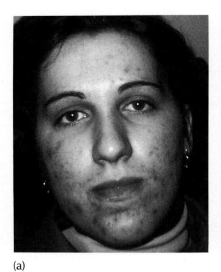
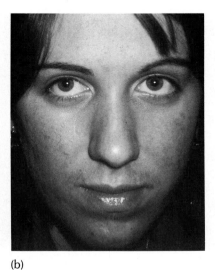

(a)   (b)

Figure 1 Acne on the face. (a) Prepeel. (b) Postpeel.

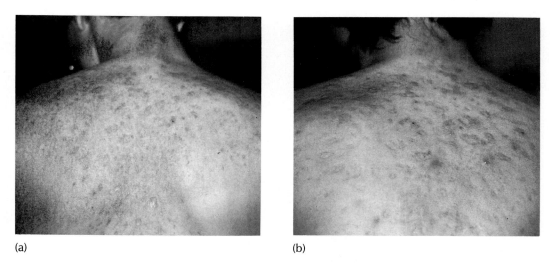

(a) (b)

Figure 2 Acne on the back. (a) Prepeel. (b) Postpeel.

PROCEDURE

Treatment may be tested behind the ear to assess reactions or allergies to resorcin. Allergies are unusual but do occur. The paste is applied behind the ear over an area 4 cm² and is left on for 15 min. The test site is checked 4 days later. The skin may be erythematous but not pruritic or vesicular. If the test site is satisfactory, the peeling of the face can proceed.

Unna's paste is applied with gloved fingers, first on the forehead and then on the whole face, 1–2 cm beyond the horizontal margin of the mandible and avoiding the eyebrows, ears, and mucosal surface of the lips (Fig. 4). The paste is spread by gentle massage, so peeling will be more homogeneous.

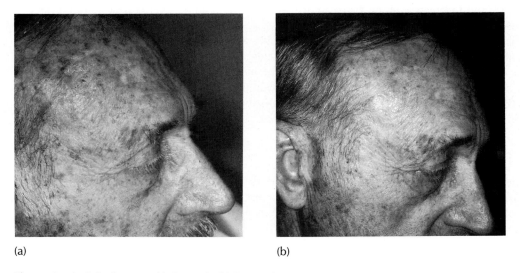

(a) (b)

Figure 3 Actinic damage. (a) Prepeel. (b) Postpeel.

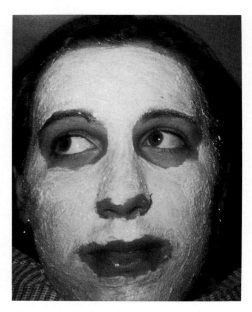

Figure 4 Application of paste.

The treatment schedule should be as follows. On the face: first day—25 min; second day—30 min; third day—35 min. On the back: first day—50 min; second day—60 min; third day—70 min.

The paste may be applied for variable lengths of time. For example, 5–10 min or less is required for some patients who are very sensitive. The paste becomes softer and is removed with a spatula or tongue depressor. The skin is wiped with a dry compress, leaving a gray film that will form the "resorcin membrane." It is better first to remove the paste on areas where the skin is thinner and to finish with the forehead or chin. If the area to be treated is large (the back), it is preferable to do it in two parts.

The patient should lie down for 30 min, especially when the paste is applied for the first time. Patients should be watched for syncope when getting up because of hyperemia produced by the paste. For some patients, a mild analgesic may be indicated for burning that occurs later.

A successful peel is obtained partially by dehydration of the epidermis, which will split the granular layer and produce a homogeneous exfoliation. Therefore, rehydration of skin by water, milk, or cream is absolutely avoided until desquamation is completed.

POSTOPERATIVE CARE

Patients should minimize physical activity for 8–10 days. After the fourth day following the first application, epidermis begins to desquamate in the peribuccal region because it is the most mobile area of the face. A good peel results in a resorcin membrane. The membrane is thick and dense, causing stiffness. It will make opening the mouth and cheek movement difficult.

When all the epidermis is gone, the skin is pink. Appendageal pores are sometimes dilated, so the patient should be aware of this. The result should not be assessed for at least 1 month. Since the skin is fragile at this point, hydrating creams may be used for protection and comfort. Sunscreens (SPF > 15) should be applied three times a day after exfoliation is completed until the end of the second or third month, depending on the patient's skin pigmentation.

SIDE EFFECTS

Resorcin peeling is very reliable. Complications are rare when allergy testing is done properly and postoperative instructions followed. Secondary hyperpigmentation is more frequent in dark-complexioned patients and women taking oral contraceptives. This may be treated by Kligman's bleaching solution (triamcinolone, hydroquinone, retinoic acid) for 3 weeks. If resorcin peeling is done appropriately, scars, atrophy, achromia, and general toxicity do not occur.

BIBLIOGRAPHY

Aron Brunetiere R. *Précis de Dermatologie Corrective* (édition SIVI).

Ayres S III. Superficial chemosurgery in treating aging skin. *Arch Dermatol* 1962;85:385–393.

Ayres S III. Dermal changes following application of chemical cauterants to aging skin: Superficial chemosurgery. *Arch Dermatol* 1960;82:578.

Stegman SJ. A comparative histologic study of the effects of three peeling agents and dermabrasion on normal and sun-damaged skin. *Aesth Plast Surg* 1982;6:123–135.

Unna PG. Thérapeutique générale des maladies de la peau.

64

Chemical Peel with Trichloroacetic Acid

Randall K. Roenigk
Mayo Clinic/Foundation and Mayo Medical School,
Rochester, Minnesota

Sorrel S. Resnik
University of Miami School of Medicine, Miami, Florida

James F. Dolezal
Creighton University, Omaha, Nebraska

Trichloroacetic acid (TCA) has been used as a chemexfoliant for the treatment of warts, keratoses, and photoaging, and as a cauterant for many years. Ayres first delineated the use of TCA as therapy for aging skin, however, its use in dermatology has been documented in the British literature from 1926. There are now many cosmetic and therapeutic indications for TCA chemexfoliation that correspond to the heightened interest in facial chemical peeling. Various application techniques and combinations with other procedures are now used (Table 1).

Depending on the concentration of TCA, it will chemically destroy the epidermis and upper dermis, causing a sluff of dead skin within 5–7 days. Cytologically atypical keratinocytes in patients with extensive photodamage and actinic keratoses are replaced by normal cells derived from the adnexae. Dermal collagen begins regeneration within 2–3 weeks. The remodeling of collagen fibers, including homogenization of the superficial dermal collagen and increased elastic staining, continues for up to 6 months. This is based principally on the concentration of TCA. These histologic changes are essentially permanent.

INDICATIONS

Treatment of actinic keratoses and photodamage are the principal indications for facial chemical peel (Table 2). Treatment of actinic keratoses may decrease the incidence of basal and squamous cell carcinoma as well as make facial skin feel more smooth and less dry or irritated. Other common methods of epidermal destruction such as cryotherapy are effective, but in some cases the number of actinic keratoses is so extensive that more complete treatment is warranted. TCA chemical peel also compares favorably with 5-fluorouracil cream for extensive actinic damage because of the need for prolonged application and the severe dermatitic reaction that results with application of the cream. It is not uncommon that patients using 5-fluorouracil cream will not complete a therapeutic trial. TCA chemical peel is applied by the physician and is normally performed once.

Table 1 Types of Chemical Peel with TCA

Superficial peel with 20% TCA w/v (single or repeated)
Intermediate peel with 30–40% TCA w/v
Deep peel with 45% TCA w/v (or higher in special cases)
Tape occlusion (more superficial peel)
TCA plus tretinoin cream (pre- and postoperatively)
TCA plus 5-FU
TCA plus Jessner's solution
TCA plus solid CO_2
TCA plus dermabrasion (chemabrasion)
TCA plus phenol
Focal treatment with 50–80% TCA w/v
Other agents sometimes added: emulsifiers (soap), lactate,
  glycolic acid, pyruvate, resorcinal (Unna's paste),
  salicylic acid

The cosmetic benefit obtained after chemical peel for photoaging is due to the decrease in mild to moderate wrinkling of facial skin by new collagen formed in actinically damaged, solar elastotic dermis. TCA improves fine cross-hatched facial rhytids and moderately deep, perioral wrinkles as well. However, the deepest rhytids caused by muscles of facial expression or excessively lax skin will not respond well to chemical peel with TCA at standard concentrations.

Indications for TCA chemical peel also include solar-induced pigmentary disorders, especially lentigo simplex. Other pigmentary problems such as postinflammatory hyperpigmentation or melasma may respond, but the results are highly variable and the condition may be worsened. A test patch is suggested in these cases, and patients should be cautioned about variable results. Many patients ask about chemical peel for acne scarring, but our experience is that most of these patients are better served by dermabrasion. Another common request is for treatment of dilated pilosebaceous pores for which TCA peels are also not very effective.

Table 2 Indications for Facial Chemical
Peel with TCA

TCA commonly used and effective
  Actinic keratoses
  Lentigo simplex
  Photoaging—solar elastosis
  Rhytids (superficial to medium depth)
TCA occasionally used and variably effective
  Acne scars (superficial or distensible)
  Alopecia areata
  Dilated pilosebaceous pores
  Melasma
  Neurotic excoriations
  Post inflammatory hyperpigmentation
  Rosacea
  Seborrheic dermatitis
  Telangiectasia
  Vitiligo

Table 3 TCA Formulation at Mayo Clinic

Concentration	Formulation
Mayo 60% (45% w/v)	TCA (crystals) 60 g per 100 ml distilled H_2O
Mayo 50% (40% w/v)	TCA (crystals) 50 g per 100 ml distilled H_2O
Mayo 35% (30% w/v)	TCA (crystals) 35 g per 100 ml distilled H_2O
Mayo 20% (18% w/v)	TCA (crystals) 20 g per 100 ml distilled H_2O

TCA crystals should meet the standards of United States Pharmacopeia (USP) XXI.

FORMULATION OF TCA

Chemical peeling with TCA is a versatile, elegant procedure. The concentration is chosen by the operator and reliably correlates with the depth of dermal damage. However, more than one method has been used to formulate TCA solutions, causing confusion in the literature (Tables 3,4). Standard concentrations of TCA at Mayo (Table 3) are 20, 35, and 50%, with occasional need for 60% TCA, which corresponds with 18, 30, 40, and 45% w/v. Higher concentrations of TCA cause unacceptable scarring on facial skin and animal models. Gynecologists routinely use 70% TCA w/v to treat vaginal and cervical condyloma. However, the moist mucosal surface effectively reduces the concentration, so submucosal damage is less and scar does not result. Scar likely would occur if 70% TCA w/v were applied to the face.

There has been concern about the appropriate method of formulating TCA. The standard pharmaceutical method of calculating and labeling the strength of any solution in which a solid is dissolved in a liquid is the weight in volume method. The number of grams contained in 100 ml of solution equals the concentration (% w/v).

Some authors of recent publications and studies have utilized an alternate formula in preparing TCA (addition of 100 ml distilled water to the stated number of grams) and have erred by equating the concentration so obtained to be the same as the number of grams added (it is not). The only way that the actual concentration (%) of such a solution can be determined is by analysis, or by measuring the final volume and calculating the actual concentration by standard pharmaceutical methods. For example, if 50 g of TCA crystals were added to 100 ml of distilled water, the final volume is approximately 126 ml, which is a 40% w/v solution (calculation: 50/126), not a 50% solution.

Although it is unclear where this error may have originated, the reader should be aware that some papers have incorrectly identified the strengths they used. The difference between such formulations can cause a significantly different depth of chemexfoliation. All concentrations in this chapter refer to the actual w/v strength used, regardless of the manner in which they may have originally been reported (unless otherwise stated, Mayo formulation.)

Table 4 Comparing Formulations of TCA Solutions

Weight TCA (g)	Volume water to make 100 ml (%) w/v	Volume water to make 100 g results in volume of (ml)	Add 100 ml water actual resulting volume of (ml)
25	25	90 (27.8%)	112 (22.3%)
30	30	88 (34%)	116 (25.9%)
35	35	86 (40.7%)	119 (29.4%)
40	40	82 (48.8%)	123 (32.5%)
50	50	79 (63.3%)	126 (39.7%)

Many physicians feel that TCA at concentrations above 35% w/v is more liable to cause scarring. We commonly use 40% TCA w/v but have not had a substantial scar and refer to this as a 50% TCA peel (Mayo formulation—Table 3).

TCA is not light sensitive and may be stored refrigerated or nonrefrigerated in clear or amber glass or TCA-resistant plastic containers for at least 23 weeks, providing the solution is not contaminated. At least one manufacturer has analyzed maintenance of potency of solutions 20–100% w/v through 2 years.

The histologic descriptions that follow are based on the formulations listed in Table 3. Communication between the physician and pharmacist is important to avoid complications, and communication between practitioners should be standardized. To avoid ambiguities, all TCA solutions should be fully labeled according to the method used. If a recipe is used, the recipe should be on the label. If the standard pharmaceutical method is used, it should be labeled % w/v.

PROCEDURE

In many ways, the preoperative consultation is more important than the procedure itself. Application of a solution of TCA requires little technical skill, while accurate medical and psychological evaluation requires years of experience. It is most important to choose the appropriate patients. The preoperative consultation is a learned art, as the clinician must not only determine a patient's candidacy for chemical peel on the basis of physical findings, but must also judge his or her motivation and ability to handle emotionally the postoperative disfigurement. Medically appropriate candidates for chemical peel may have little interest in this procedure because it is cosmetic. Conversely, some patients who have normal skin, because of their concern about cosmetic appearance, are willing to try anything, including chemical peel, for the perceived benefit. Chemical peeling results in a superficial burn that takes months to heal completely. The residual erythema that typically lasts 2–3 months after a moderate or deep TCA chemical peel can be anxiety provoking or depressing for an ill-prepared patient who expects rapid results quickly. In some cases, a superficial TCA peel or a less aggressive alpha hydroxy acid–type peel might be more appropriate.

The physician should also emphasize to the patient the importance of avoiding the sun for 6 months postoperatively. In temperate climates, patients may prefer to have a chemical peel in the fall or winter, when they are less likely to be outside. If the potential outcome is questionable, a small test patch can be performed on facial skin in a relatively hidden site (although this is routinely unnecessary).

Patients may be prepared with tretinoin (0.05 or 0.10% Retin-A® cream) applied two times a day for 2 weeks. This is used for mild debridement of the stratum corneum, including hypertrophic actinic keratoses. It may also mildly degrease the skin, as it decreases the activity of facial sebaceous glands. The patient should not apply make-up, moisturizer, hair conditioners, mousse, or hairspray for 24 hr preoperatively. Oils on the skin prevent transepidermal penetration of TCA.

A tray is prepared with the following material: bottles containing appropriate concentrations of TCA, cotton-tipped applicators, square cotton gauze, and a small glass cup to hold quantities of the TCA. A readily accessible container of sterile water should be available as a rinse in the event of an accidental eye splash.

The face is scrubbed with acetone for 10 min until the sebaceous oils have been thoroughly removed. When this step is complete, the skin feels like fine sandpaper. The small scales on the face turn white because the oil has been removed. The eyes are protected with an antibiotic ointment, gauze pads, and hypoallergenic tape or goggles. Oral or intramuscularly administered sedatives may be used. Local anesthetic is not required.

A cotton-tipped applicator is moistened with TCA and rolled against the wall of the glass cup to remove excess fluid. The TCA is applied to an area of skin approximately 2 × 3 cm by firmly rubbing the moistened applicator in a circular or linear fashion. Once the skin has been treated, it slowly changes color, becoming whitish-gray as a result of chemical coagulation of the epidermis (Fig. 1). This color change is called a "frost." The frost appears more rapidly with high concentrations of TCA and may not appear with low concentrations, especially if the skin has not been adequately degreased. The cotton-tipped applicator is used once and discarded. After the acid is applied, a gauze pad is used to blot (not wipe) excess TCA. After the acid is applied, SSR uses alcohol swab to neutralize any excess reaction. A new cotton-tipped applicator and swab are used at each site. A new cotton-tipped applicator and gauze are used at each site.

The acid stings moderately when applied and correlates with the concentration of TCA. The pain crescendos, normally peaking approximately halfway through the procedure. Dry, cool compresses are helpful to soothe the discomfort, as is a patient hand-held fan. Some practitioners like to perform chemical peel in a specific pattern by peeling anatomic units of the face in the same order for all patients. Typically some anatomic facial subunits require different concentrations of TCA (i.e., forehead, cheeks, chin—40% w/v; eyelids—18% w/v). As a matter of habit, for example, one might start with the highest concentration to be used on the forehead followed by the cheeks, chin, nose, ears, lips, and eyelids (lowest concentration). The moistened cotton-tipped applicator is kept away from the eyes at all times. When the eyelids are being treated, particular care is used to avoid seepage of excess TCA onto the sclera. Ophthalmic antibiotic ointment placed on the eye before peeling the eyelids helps protect against accidental chemical scleral burn.

Immediate postoperative care includes a thin coat of antibiotic ointment covered with a hydrogel dressing e.g., Vigilon® applied directly to the skin, sometimes omitting antibiotic ointment). This causes immediate relief from the burning sensation. Occasionally the hydrogel dressing is applied during the procedure if the pain in previously treated areas becomes intolerable. This

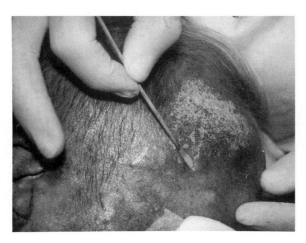

Figure 1 40% TCA w/v applied with cotton-tipped applicator. Note "frost," fine scale on untreated area due to acetone scrub, and eye protection.

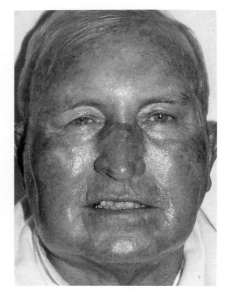

Figure 2 One day after 40% TCA w/v peel. Note edema. Skin has yet to exfoliate.

probably rapidly decreases ("neutralizes") the effective concentration of TCA and thereby hinders the chemical destruction. A face mask is fashioned from multilayered gauze placed over the hydrogel dressing and left intact for one day. In some cases, a short-acting corticosteroid is given intramuscularly [betamethasone (Celestone®), 1 cc] to minimize edema. The patient is instructed to sleep with the head elevated and to avoid excessive activity. Most patients go home and sleep or relax until the follow-up appointment the next day. One day postoperatively patients may be quite swollen (Fig. 2).

The dressing is changed twice daily. This includes soaks with water or dilute peroxide and reapplication of the antibiotic ointment (or plain petroleum jelly on the first post-op day after each washing). Patients often can manage this on their own or can come to the office for dressing changes. Reepithelialization is normally complete within 1 week, at which point wound care can stop, with the exception of lubrication and sunscreens. TCA peels of lower concentrations may reepithelialize quicker (those in the 10–20% w/v range may not completely sluff the epidermis). Diffuse erythema lasts up to several months for deeper TCA peels, but cosmetics may be used after 1 week. Some examples of patients treated for photoaging, actinic keratoses, and lentigo simplex are shown in Figures 3–6.

HISTOLOGIC EFFECTS OF TCA ON THE SKIN

The depth of wounds created by various concentrations and application techniques of TCA have been evaluated by several researchers using human and animal models (Table 5). The therapeutic effects of TCA are destruction of the epidermis and dermis with subsequent reepithelialization from epidermal appendages and new collagen formation (Figs. 7,8). The depth of the wounds caused by various dilutions of TCA are of paramount importance to its therapeutic efficacy.

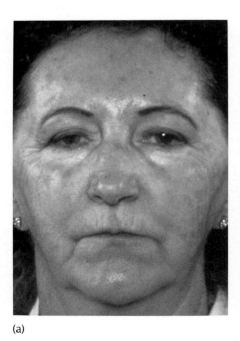 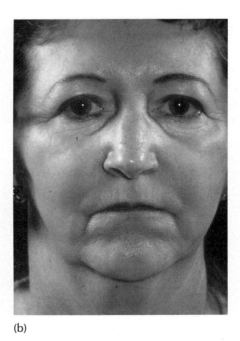

(a)   (b)

Figure 3 (a) Prior to peel using 40%, 30%, and 18% TCA w/v in different anatomic subunits. (b) Seven months postoperative.

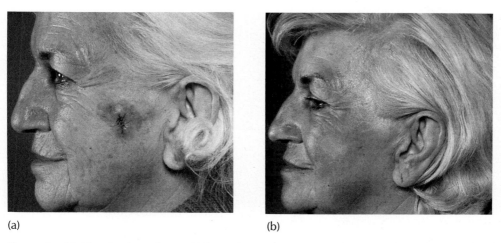

(a) (b)

Figure 4 (a) Note lentigo prior to 40% TCA w/v peel. (b) Five months postoperative.

IMMEDIATE EFFECTS

The depth of tissue necrosis increases with the concentration of TCA (Table 5). The concentration of a TCA solution used for actinic keratoses should be at least 30–40% w/v, which is required for complete removal of the epidermis and superficial dermis, allowing reepithelialization by appendageal keratinocytes. The appropriate concentration of TCA used for facial rejuvenation depends on the desired effect. A solution of 18% TCA w/v results in epidermal exfoliation. This is well tolerated, but the degree of rejuvenation is less, relatively short term, and superficial. Serial applications (weekly or biweekly) of 18% TCA w/v may directly or indirectly in-

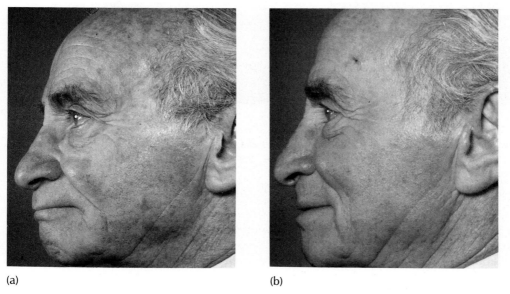

(a) (b)

Figure 5 (a) Solar elastosis, actinic keratoses, and lentigines prior to 40% TCA w/v peel. (b) Six weeks postoperative.

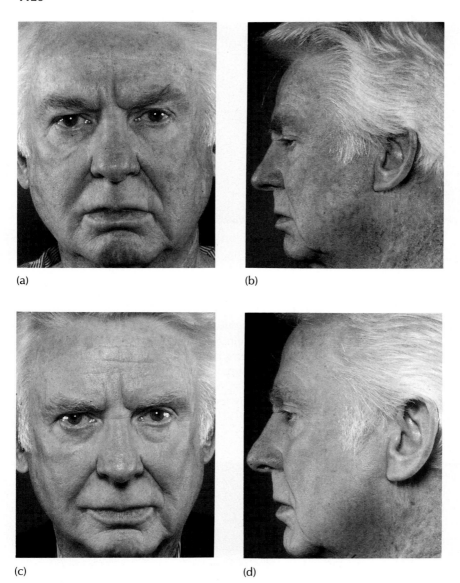

(a)   (b)

(c)   (d)

Figure 6 (a) Prior to 40% TCA w/v to forehead, cheeks, chin, nose, ears; 30% TCA w/v to upper and lower lips; 18% TCA w/v to upper and lower eyelids. Front view. (b) Side view. (c) Six months postoperative. Front view. (d) Side view.

duce remodeling of the papillary dermis because of the repeated caustic damage to temporarily thinned epidermis.

Solutions of 30 and 40% TCA w/v cause not only replacement of the epidermis but also longer-lasting dermal changes. Histologically, 0.3–0.5 mm of dermal necrosis results (Fig. 9). There is an associated reduction in fine and medium-depth facial wrinkles. There are no reports of the clinical use of 80% TCA (Mayo formulation) for facial rejuvenation procedures. Because

Table 5 Depth of Dermal Necrosis Produced by Treatment with 60% TCA, 100% Phenol, or Baker's Formula With and Without Tape Occlusion[a]

Treatment	Wound thickness (mm)		Depth of scar at 60 days (mm)	
	Not occluded	Occluded	Not occluded	Occluded
Non–sun-damaged skin				
60% TCA	0.27	0.36	0.35	0.25
100% Phenol	0.41	0.41	0.38	0.41
Baker's mix	0.6	0.65	0.41	0.40
Sun-damaged skin				
60% TCA	0.5	0.4	0.5	0.45
100% Phenol	0.55	0.4	0.5	0.53
Baker's mix	0.63	0.85	0.57	0.9

[a]Formulation method not specified.
Source: Modified from Stegman, 1982.

of dermal necrosis noted in experimental studies (0.8–0.9 mm depth), scarring would likely result (as was noted clinically in animal studies) and would be cosmetically unacceptable.

Tape occlusion for chemical peeling has in the past been thought to increase the depth of penetration of TCA. Increased penetration and a deeper peel after skin occlusion with tape may occur with phenol (Baker's formula). In several studies, it has been confirmed that occlusion of TCA

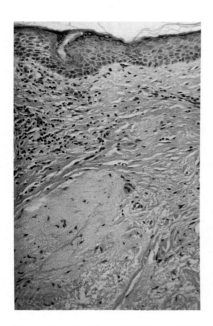

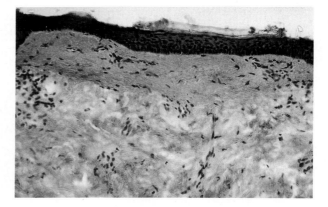

Figure 7 Histology (H&E × 40) 3 months after 40% TCA w/v in a human. Note fibroblasts forming new collagen in papillary dermis. Also note persistent nodule of solar elastosis in reticular dermis, deeper than peel penetrated.

Figure 8 Histology (H&E × 40) one year after 40% TCA w/v in a human. Note band of mature new collagen that overlies blue stain scar damage.

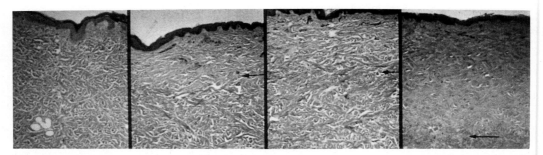

Figure 9   Histology (H&E × 40) of porcine skin 24 hr after application of TCA. Arrows indicate depth of necrosis. Open technique. Left to right: 20%, 25%, 50%, 80% TCA (Mayo formulation).

with tape reliably decreases the depth of dermal necrosis (Fig. 10). In a porcine model at all TCA concentrations tested, the occluded technique produced significantly less necrosis than the unoccluded technique (Table 6). Hypothetically, less dermal necrosis in the occluded specimen could be the result of interstitial humidificaton (Fig. 11). Occlusion accomplishes this by the prevention of transepidermal water loss, which leads to increased interstitial water content in the epidermis and dermis. Therefore, the effective concentration of TCA is decreased or more rapidly "neutralized." However, even in the open technique (no tape used), wounds are covered with antibiotic ointment followed by a hydrogel dressing. Therefore, some occlusion may result. Occlusion 20–30 min after application of TCA may not be as important as what happens immediately after application of the TCA solution.

In addition, there is histologic benefit to pretreating the skin with tretinoin cream for 2 weeks and acetone immediately preoperatively. Although both drugs degrease the skin, they also thin and dedifferentiate the epidermis, including the stratum corneum, which may contain hypertrophic actinic keratoses. The depth of damage in the skin correlates directly with the concentration of TCA and is constant. Thinning the epidermis causes relatively deeper dermal necrosis at a given concentration (Fig. 12). The effect on the epidermis is relatively short lived. The longer-lasting dermal effect is usually preferable. Higher concentrations of TCA might be used in place of preparing the skin with tretinoin and acetone but would likely cause some variable results, risking a scar.

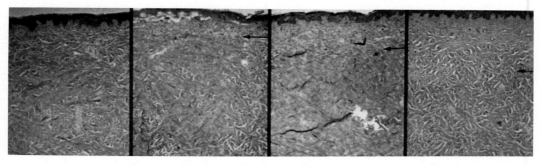

Figure 10   Histology (H&E × 40) of porcine skin 24 hr after application of TCA by closed technique (tape occlusion). Arrows indicate depth of necrosis. Left to right: 20% (no necrosis noticeable), 35%, 50%, 80% TCA (Mayo formulation). Depth of necrosis less at all concentrations compared with Figure 9.

Table 6 Depth of Necrosis in a Porcine Model at Various Concentrations of TCA

| TCA concentration (%) | Depth of necrosis (mm) | | |
(Mayo method)	Unoccluded technique	Occluded technique	Difference
20 (18% w/v)	0.044	0	—
35 (30% w/v)	0.2555	0.075	0.180
50 (40% w/v)	0.500	0.178	0.322
80	0.983	0.633	0.350

Source: Modified from Brodland et al., 1989.

Long-Term Effects

In long-term histologic studies of TCA on porcine skin, test sites have been treated with 20, 35, 50, and 80% TCA (Mayo formulation) and either tape-occluded or unoccluded techniques, in addition to serially applied 20% TCA (Mayo formulation) on six occasions over 9 weeks. Biopsy specimens have been obtained over a 28-week period. Specimens stained with hematoxylin and eosin and sel Giemsa microscopically showed epidermal changes, which include thinning and orthokeratosis of the stratum corneum at 4 weeks after treatment with TCA. This change is transient. At 8 and 28 weeks, the stratum corneum is similar to its baseline status. The change in the epidermal thickness is variable, depending on the concentration of TCA, the time of the biopsy, and the application technique.

At 24 hr and 4 weeks, collagen is distinctly basophilic, representing the zone of necrosis. Collagen is altered at 8 and 28 weeks, as the staining tends to be much more pale in the superficial dermis, and the level of dermal necrosis much less distinct. The bundles are haphazardly organized, smaller, and fragmented and have less well-defined borders.

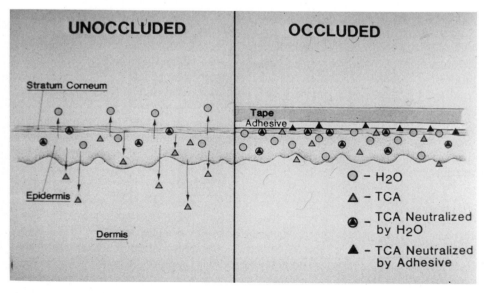

Figure 11 Theoretically, occlusion increases interstitial water causing a relative decrease in TCA concentration causing less necrosis.

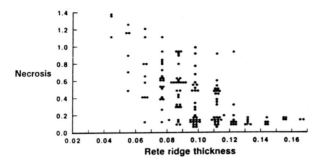

Figure 12   Thicker epidermis causes less dermal necrosis at a given concentration. Supports pretreatment with tretinoin and acetone to thin or equalize the epidermis (specifically the stratum corneum).

The number of fibroblasts is increased in the superficial dermis at 4, 8, and 28 weeks in skin treated with 30% TCA w/v or higher concentrations. These fibroblasts appear histologically to be metabolically active and are characterized by abundant basophilic cytoplasm. Solutions with high concentrations of TCA induce a greater number of fibroblasts than low concentrations. At 28 weeks, the number of fibroblasts remains greater than that at baseline.

Elastic fibers are histologically unchanged in skin treated with 18% TCA w/v and the serial application technique. However, skin treated with higher concentrations have a decrease in the quantity of elastin (stained with sel Giemsa) at 4 and 8 weeks. At 28 weeks, the amount of elastin is increased. The depth of these alterations in elastin correspond roughly to the depth of basophilic necrosis. The morphology of new elastic fibers at 28 weeks shows no characteristic pattern and range from short, thin fragments to long, branching, thick fibers.

The long-term (28 weeks) histologic effects vary depending on the concentration used and the application technique. Serial applications of 18% TCA w/v have very little long-term effect. However, further clinical investigation of the serial application of 18% TCA w/v is warranted because there are some short-term histologic changes. Specimens treated with 35, 50, and 80% TCA have definite alterations, which persist. Generally, the degree of histologic alteration increases in proportion with the increase in TCA concentration. The histologic effects were most intense with 80% TCA. Scar and pigmentary alteration (decreased pigment) are clinically evident in porcine skin treated with solutions of 80% TCA but not in skin treated with 35 and 50% TCA (Mayo formulations). When the long-term histologic effects of tape-occluded and unoccluded techniques were compared, the tape-occluded specimens have significantly less long-term histologic alteration than the unoccluded specimens. This finding is consistent with that seen at 24 hr after treatment.

COMPLICATIONS

The complications of TCA chemical peel, when performed by a skilled operator, are rare and tend to be minor or easily corrected (Table 7). Superficial bacterial pustulation and eczematization may rarely occur as early complications and are managed with appropriate antibacterial therapy. Routine postoperative care includes topical antibiotic ointment or petroleum jelly applied after cleansing with dilute peroxide (a standard wet dressing technique). Latent herpes simplex virus may reactivate, so patients with this history should be treated prophylactically with oral antiviral agents (2–5 days prior and 5 days after).

Table 7   Potential Complications of TCA Peels

Accentuation of telangiectasia, nevi, and pores
Bacterial infection
Hyperpigmentation (usually superficial peels, dark skin)
Hypopigmentation (usually deep peels)
Milia
Persistent erythema
Reactivation of herpes simplex
Scar (neck, hands, lips)
Sensitivity to sun, wind, temperature change

Milia frequently form early in the postexfoliation period but are easily treated with incision and drainage or mild abrasive scrubs and otherwise resolve spontaneously. Hyperpigmentation and hypopigmentation are the most common long-term problems (Figs. 13,14). Generally, hyperpigmentation is more likely to occur after superficial peels, whereas hypopigmentation may occur after deep peels. These problems occur more commonly in patients with darker complexion.

Scars may occur on skin less richly endowed with cutaneous adnexa such as the dorsal aspects of the hand. Scar formation may also occur in certain sites due in part to greater skin movement during normal activity, such as the lip and neck, associated with interdigitation of muscle fibers with the skin. We normally do not perform chemical peel of the face unless lower concentrations of TCA are used or when using other formulations (such as alpha hydroxy acids) that typically cause only epidermolysis. Hypertrophic scars may form on the face, but keloids are rare.

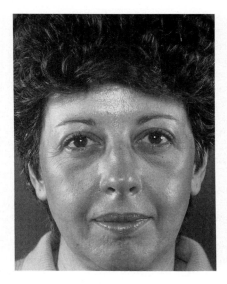   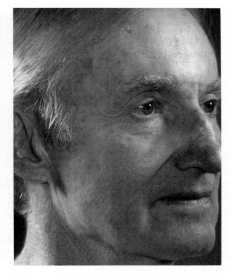

Figure 13   Postinflammatory hyperpigmentation at 3 months after 35% TCA w/v peel.

Figure 14   Postinflammatory hypopigmentation at one year after 50% TCA w/v peel.

Table 8 Advantages of TCA Peels

Few medical contraindications
Elegant (adjust depth of necrosis by concentration of TCA)
No allergic reactions
No systemic toxicity
Scarring rare at standard concentrations
Wound-healing time shorter than with 5-fluorouracil cream (better compliance)
More practical than repeated cryotherapy for patients with extensive actinic keratoses

Full-thickness skin loss, as reported in some cases of phenol chemical peel, have not been reported with TCA chemical peel. Other complications include accentuation of telangiectasias, apparent enlargement of pores, darkening of pigmented nevi, persistent erythema, and increased sensitivity to wind, sunlight, and temperature variation.

ADVANTAGES OF TCA AS A SOLO AGENT FOR CHEMICAL PEEL

The goal of facial chemical peeling is to achieve not just a deeper peel, but the appropriate peel for the patient. Various solutions used for facial chemical peel have been employed as each clinician tries to achieve "better" results, but these formulations need to be studied scientifically to establish their safety and efficacy. It is also important to know how a TCA solution is formulated. TCA as a solo agent for facial chemical peel has been tested and used for decades as a safe, effective, elegant, regularly reproducible method for treating common problems associated with photoaged skin (Table 8). Higher concentrations of TCA and phenol may cause full-thickness chemical burns, leaving long-lasting scars. However, when standardized techniques are used, it is possible to quantify the therapeutic effects and reliably predict the outcome.

BIBLIOGRAPHY

Ayres S III. Superficial chemosurgery in treating aging skin. *Arch Dermatol* 1962;85:385–393.

Baker TJ. The ablation of rhitides by chemical means. A preliminary report. *J Fl Med Assoc* 1961;48:451.

Brodland DG, Cullimore KC, Roenigk RK, et al. Depths of chemexfoliation induced by various concentrations and application techniques of trichloroacetic acid in a porcine model. *J Dermatol Surg Oncol* 1989;15:967–971.

Brodland DG, Roenigk RK. Trichloroacetic acid chemexfoliation (chemical peel) for extensive premalignant actinic damage of the face and scalp. *Mayo Clin Proc* 1988;63:887–896.

Brody HJ. *Chemical Peeling*. St. Louis, MO, Mosby-Yearbook, Inc., 1992.

Brody HJ, Hailey CW. Medium-depth chemical peeling of the skin: a variation of superficial chemosurgery. *J Dermatol Surg Oncol* 1986;12:1268–1275.

Coleman III, WP, Futrell JM. The glycolic acid trichloroacetic acid peel. *J Dermatol Surg Oncol* 1994;20:76–80.

Heria O, Nemeth AJ, Taylor JR. Tretinoin accelerates healing after trichloroacetic acid chemical peel. *Arch Dermatol* 1991;127:678–682.

Lober CW. Chemexfoliation—indications and cautions. *J Am Acad Dermatol* 1987;17:109–112.

Matarasso SL, Salman SM, Glougau RC, et al. The role of chemical peeling in the treatment of photo damaged skin. *J Dermatol Surg Oncol* 1990;16:945–954.

Monash S. The uses of diluted trichloroacetic acid in dermatology. *Urol Cutan Rev* 1945;49:119.

Monheit GD. The Jessner's + TCA peel: a medium depth chemical peel. *J Dermatol Surg Oncol* 1989;15:945–950.

Morrow DM. Chemical peeling of the eyelids and periorbital area. *J Dermatol Surg Oncol* 1992;18:102–110.

Resnik SS, Lewis LA. The cosmetic uses of trichloroacetic acid peeling in dermatology. *South Med J* 1973;

Resnik SS, Lewis LA, Cohen BH. Trichloroacetic acid peeling. *Cutis* 1976;17:127–129.

Roberts HL. The chloroacetic acids: a biochemical study. *Br J Dermatol* 1926;38:323, 375.

Spinowitz AL, Rumsfield J. Stability-time profile of trichloroacetic acid at various concentrations and storage conditions. *J Dermatol Surg Oncol* 1989;15:874–875.

Spira M, Gerow FJ, Hardy SB. Complications of chemical face peeling. *Plast Reconstr Surg* 1974;54:397.

Stegman SJ. A study of dermabrasion and chemical peels in an animal model. *J Dermatol Surg Oncol* 1980;6:490.

Stegman SJ. A comparative histologic study of the effects of three peeling agents and dermabrasion on normal and sun damaged skin. *Esthet Plast Surg* 1982;6:123.

Van Scott EJ, Yu RJ. Hyperkeratinization, corneocyte cohesion and alpha hydroxy acids. *J Am Acad Dermatol* 1984;11:867.

Wang B, Carey WD. Chemical peeling as adjuvant therapy for facial neurotic excoriations. *J Am Acad Dermatol* 1994;30(4):669–670.

Zelickson AS, Mottaz JH, Weiss JS, et al. Topical tretinoin in photo aging: an ultrastructural study. *J Cut Aging Cosmet Dermatol* 1988;1:41.

65

Combination Chemical Peels

William P. Coleman, III
Tulane University School of Medicine, New Orleans, Louisiana

Harold J. Brody
Emory University School of Medicine, Atlanta, Georgia

Medium-depth chemical peels are those that penetrate to the upper or middermis. This depth of injury can be achieved by using a single agent such as 50% trichloracetic acid (TCA) or undiluted phenol. Alternatively, dermal wounding can be accomplished by using a combination of two milder chemical agents. The first chemical is applied to cause destruction of the epidermis. If the treatment were stopped at this point, this would result in a superficial (epidermal) peel. However, when the second agent is applied, it wounds into the dermis by penetrating rapidly through the injured epidermis.

Normally 35% TCA, when used as a solo agent, will not cause significant dermal injury. However, after pretreatment with solid carbon dioxide ice, Jessner's solution, or glycolic acid, the 35% TCA penetrates more easily through the damaged epidermis. The combination of two superficial peeling agents to achieve medium-depth wounding is called combination chemical peeling. Combination chemical peels have been shown to be quite reliable and predictable in achieving medium-depth chemical peeling. Reports of complications have been rare when compared to the use of solo agents for dermal peels.

SOLID CARBON DIOXIDE ICE PLUS TCA CHEMICAL PEEL

Carbon dioxide ice has been used in block form to produce superficial peeling for over 50 years. When this cryosurgical pretreatment is followed by application of 35% TCA, a medium-depth peel can be achieved.

After cleansing the skin with a bacteriostatic agent (e.g., povidone-iodine) followed by alcohol, the skin is scrubbed with acetone for 3 min. Superficial and deeper scars, wrinkles, and keratoses are mapped on a diagram. Then, a hand-size block of solid CO_2 ice is dipped in a solution composed of three parts acetone and one part alcohol so that the dry ice will move easily over the skin (Fig. 1).

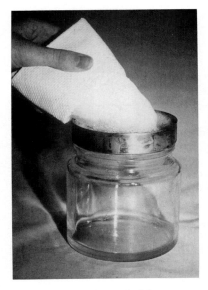

Figure 1 Dipping of CO_2 cut to hand size into a 3:1 solution of acetone:alcohol.

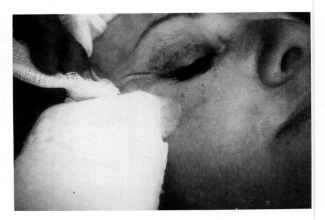

Figure 2 Hard application of CO_2 to periorbital area for treatment of fine rhytides.

The length of contact with the skin determines the depth of injury. This can be conveniently divided into mild pressure (3–5 sec), moderate pressure (5–8 sec), and hard pressure (8–15 sec). The edges of scars can be frozen even more deeply to obtain maximal smoothing through increased penetration of TCA. Periorbital rhytides or seborrheic keratoses can be frozen moderately hard for additional penetration of the TCA.

Certain portions of the face such as the upper forehead and the glabella may be more sensitive to pain from the icing (Figs. 2,3). Electrical or hand-held fans reduce discomfort as well as help to disperse acetone vapors.

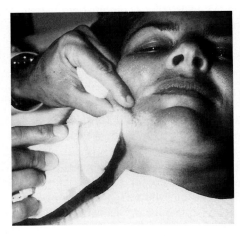

Figure 3 Hard application of CO_2 to a scar.

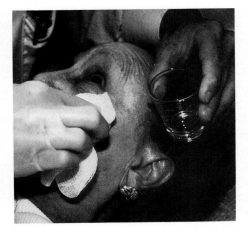

Figure 4 Application of TCA with single 4 × 4 gauze pad.

After pretreatment with the CO_2 ice, the skin is wiped with a dry gauze pad and 35% TCA is applied using cotton-tipped applicators or gauze 4 × 4 pads (Figs. 4,5). Fifty percent TCA can be used to soften the edges of scars or solitary lesions such as keratoses or deeper wrinkles. Large areas treated with 50% TCA after CO_2 ice risk hypertrophic scarring, especially in the perioral area.

Burning usually subsides within a few minutes, especially after application of ice packs or cold gel packs. After the patient is comfortable, individual areas may be retreated with 35% TCA if deeper penetration is desired. However, increased application of TCA increases the risk of scarring.

It is crucial when using the solid CO_2 ice plus TCA chemical peel that the physician plan ahead and diagram exactly which areas require deeper treatment. This allows the process to proceed smoothly, avoiding physician indecision. This will also help to minimize patient discomfort. This peel is very successful in removing actinic keratoses and improving fine wrinkles. It is the only peel that can flatten the edges of depressed scars by virtue of the physical CO_2 adjuvant. It is also useful for reducing hyperpigmentation. It is not used on Fitzpatrick skin types V and VI (Figs. 6,7).

Histologic studies of medium-depth combination peels with the combination of solid carbon dioxide ice followed by TCA indicates a depth of injury greater than TCA alone. Stegman observed a Grenz zone of normal-appearing expanding papillary dermis after chemical or abrasive wounds. He found that the thickness of this Grenz zone varied with the strength of the wounding agent used and the depth of the wound. Below this Grenz zone a band of thick elastotic-like fibers and glycosaminoglycans was identified. The thickness and intensity of staining of this band also increased with the depth of the wounding. Ninety days after the CO_2 ice plus 35% TCA peel, there was a significant papillary dermal Grenz zone and a wide dermal elastotic band (Fig. 8).

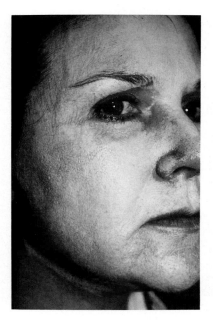

Figure 5 Uniform frost of the skin after TCA application. Overcoating to force a solid white color on every square centimeter is not required.

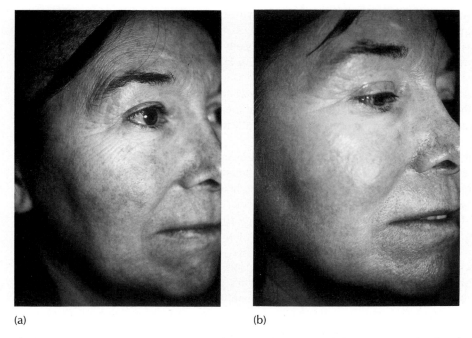

(a)   (b)

Figure 6 (a) Fitzpatrick type II, photoaging III patient with actinic keratoses, splotchy pigmentation, and fine periorbital rhytides. (b) 90 days post-CO_2 hard followed by TCA 35% showing improvement of skin quality and easing of periorbital rhytides.

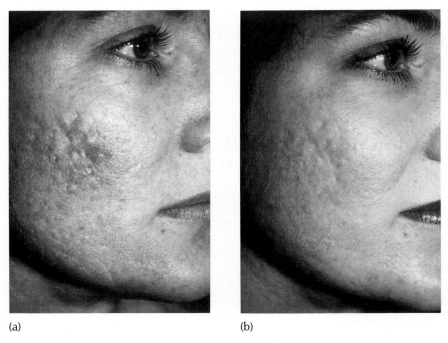

(a)   (b)

Figure 7 Improvement of depressed scarring with CO_2 hard followed by TCA 35% to edge of scars and TCA 35% to entire remaining area.

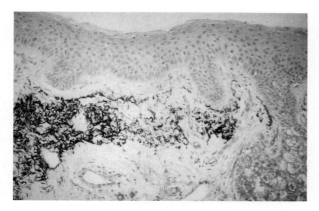

Figure 8 Elastic staining 90 days after a CO_2 plus TCA 35% peel shows a papillary dermal Grenz zone and a mild dermal elastic band.

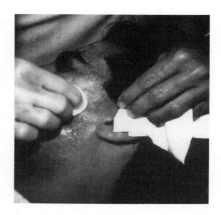

Figure 9 Application of a single coat of Jessner's solution with a single cotton ball.

JESSNER'S SOLUTION PLUS TCA CHEMICAL PEEL

Dr. Max Jessner combined 14 g each of resorcinol, salicylic acid, and lactic acid with enough ethanol to make 100 cc of solution. This formula was designed to lower the concentration of each of these wounding agents and decrease toxicity. (Resorcinol in repetitive usage can cause thyroid depression and syncope, while salicylic acid in prolonged contact can lead to tinnitus). The solution is unstable unless stored in a dark bottle. (Use of this combination has also been termed "Combes' peel" after Dr. F. C. Combes.)

The effect of Jessner's solution on the skin is modulated by the application of successive coats. Increasing the number of coats increases the injury and depth of penetration. It is usually applied with a sable brush or liberal applicator. No neutralization or dilution is required. This approach produces a superficial peel within the epidermis.

Jessner's solution can be combined with TCA to produce a combination chemical peel. After degreasing the skin with an alcohol or acetone scrub, Jessner's solution is applied with a cotton ball, two cotton-tipped applicators, or sable brush to the entire face using only one coat (Fig. 9). A very light frost usually results. Next, 35% TCA is applied evenly using cotton applicators or a single gauze pad as described previously (see Fig. 4). This solution should be applied evenly. Individual areas may be retreated to achieve deeper penetration for an actinic keratosis or deeper wrinkle.

After a consistent frost has developed, cold saline compresses or an ice pack can be applied to make the patient comfortable. Once the frost has appeared, cool solutions help to ease the burning but have no effect on depth of penetration of the peel.

The Jessner's plus 35% TCA combination chemical peel is useful for treatment of actinic damage, pigmentary dischromias, and fine wrinkling. Histologically it produces a slightly thinner Grenz zone and elastotic band than the solid CO_2 ice plus 35% TCA peel (Fig. 10).

GLYCOLIC ACID PLUS TCA CHEMICAL PEELS

Glycolic acid (nonbuffered, 70%) has been shown to be an effective agent for achieving superficial chemical peeling. When this agent is applied to the skin and then diluted with water after 2 min, it will usually cause erythema and subsequent desquamation. Histologically, application

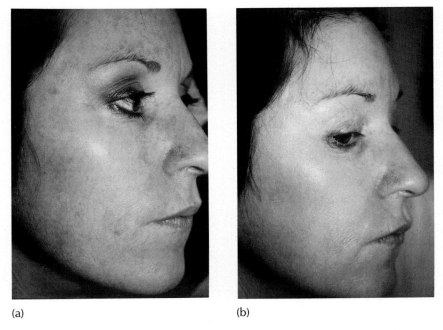

(a)   (b)

Figure 10   (a) Fitzpatrick type I, photoaging II patient with freckling, early lentigines, and melasma. (b) Good resolution of pigmentary dyschromias after peel with JS applied with cotton ball followed by TCA 35% with single 4 × 4 gauze applicator.

of this chemical produces epidermolysis. Glycolic acid has become quite popular in recent years as a solo agent for achieving superficial chemical peeling.

When glycolic acid is applied in the method previously described and then followed by application of 35% trichloracetic acid, the injured epidermis allows deeper penetration of the TCA. This is the basis of the glycolic acid plus trichloracetic acid combination peel.

This approach is used without acetone or alcohol defatting of the skin. After bacteriostatic soap cleansing, the 70% glycolic acid is applied uniformly over the entire area to be peeled with a large cotton-tipped applicator. After 2 min the acid is diluted by flushing with copious amounts of water. The reversal of the glycolic acid should be done in the same order as its application proceeding segmentally from cosmetic unit to cosmetic unit. This allows a uniform time of contact with the glycolic acid for each area of the face. After the acid is diluted, the patient is asked if any burning areas still remain. These portions of the face may not have been sufficiently reversed and require additional applications of water.

The skin is then dried with a 4 × 4 gauze, and 35% TCA is painted on the same cutaneous areas with a 2 × 2 gauze square with moderate pressure and friction. In areas where deeper penetration is desired, the acid is applied with greater friction. This is useful for achieving deeper peeling over lentigines, seborrheic keratoses, and other epidermal lesions. After 4 or 5 min a consistent frost develops over the treated areas. The skin can then be soothed by application of water. Water does not reverse or modify the effect of TCA once frosted but cools the skin and usually reverses any burning. However, application of water prior to complete frosting may dilute the TCA and hamper uniform peeling.

Patients usually experience burning and stinging during the application of both acids. This is worse with TCA, but can be relieved some by using hand-held fans or cold gel packs. Patients are discharged with prescriptions for mild analgesics.

Histologic studies have shown that the glycolic acid plus trichloroacetic acid combination peel is similar to the Jessner's plus TCA chemical peel. A narrow Grenz zone is produced in the upper dermis. This deposition of new collagen fibers correlates with clinical improvement of minor wrinkles. Deep wrinkles and scars are usually not improved by this approach. Such defects would require reticular dermal injury such as that achieved with dermabrasion.

The glycolic acid plus trichloracetic acid combination peel is usually quite effective in eliminating epidermal and upper dermal pigmentation (Fig. 11). It can be used successfully in darker-skinned individuals (Fitzpatrick types V and VI) by utilizing pre- and posttreatment with hydro-Jinones and tretinoin to minimize postinflammatory hyperpigmentation.

NONFACIAL PEELING

CO_2 ice, Jessner's solution, or glycolic acid is usually combined with 35% TCA when combination peels are used on the face. However, nonfacial areas such as the back, upper chest, arms, and legs are better peeled using 20% TCA after the superficial wounding agent. The skin in these areas heals more unpredictably, and the more superficial approach is safer. Some patients can tolerate 35% TCA after glycolic acid on the arms, but this should only be done after previously employing lower concentrations of TCA and observing each patient's individual clinical response.

The neck is the most difficult area of the skin to peel. Necks can develop persistent erythema, which may lead to hypertrophic scars even after application of 20% TCA alone without any skin preparation or prior use of a superficial agent. For this reason it is wise to perform superficial peels on a patient's neck initially and only then to proceed with deeper subsequent peels as their clinical response warrants.

POSTOPERATIVE CARE

The three combination chemical peels described above produce injury in the upper to middermis. This must be remembered when planning a postoperative regimen that will maximize wound

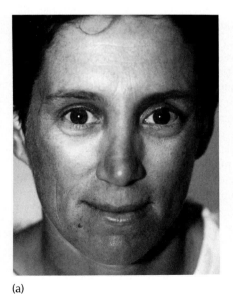
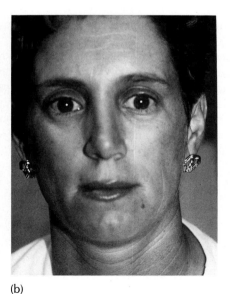

(a)   (b)

Figure 11 (a) Fitzpatrick type II, photoaging II patient with freckling and melasma. (b) Good improvement 30 days after 70% glycolic acid reversed after 2 min followed by 35% TCA applied with a 2 × 2 gauze.

healing (Fig. 12). Emollients should be used for the first several days postoperatively. A bland emollient ointment such as petrolatum, Aquaphor, or Preparation H is applied four times daily after the patient rinses the skin with lukewarm tap water or antiseptic (e.g., povidone-iodine) compresses. Biologic dressings offer no advantage and are not recommended.

After 3 or 4 days a mild soap (e.g., Dove) can be added to this regimen to cleanse off the emollients more thoroughly. Patients should be instructed not to scrub or pick at the skin but to wash it gently. Once reepithelialization is complete, within 6–7 days, the heavy emollient is discarded and a soothing moisturizer is substituted. Eucerin® cream with sunscreen is an excellent choice. If the patient experiences some burning when using a moisturizer, it should be discontinued for a day or two and the emollient ointment used again until healing has progressed. Women can resume make-up foundation after 7 or 8 days. This allows patients to return to an active social life. However, erythema may not entirely disappear for up to 1 month postoperatively, and it may be patchy in nature. If focal areas remain extremely erythematous, then they should be treated with topical steroids or steroid-impregnated tape to prevent such persistent erythema from developing into a hypertrophic scar. If scars do develop, then treatment with intralesional steroids or silastic sheeting may be required.

Some patients have a tendency to develop postinflammatory hyperpigmentation after a combination chemical peel. Patients should be observed for this possibility within 3–4 weeks postoperatively. If the skin begins to turn somewhat brown, topical hydroquinones can be used to reverse this tendency. Hydroquinone creams are generally more soothing to newly peeled skin but may be less effective than hydroquinone gels or alcohol solutions, which can be employed later as the skin tolerates. Sunscreens must also be used as soon as tolerated. Many sunscreen formulations burn newly peeled skin. Generally creamy lotions are more soothing and should be used early and then replaced by water-resistant gels and alcohol-based solutions later.

Many patients will benefit from a program to maintain the effects of their combination chemical peel. This may include the application of tretinoin and alpha hydroxy acids such as glycolic acid and lactic acid. These agents may be introduced one at a time 4–6 weeks after the combination chemical peel. If burning is encountered, they should be discontinued and tried again several days later. Tretinoin use should be individually titrated, and stronger formulations may be gradually introduced as tolerated. Alpha hydroxy acid creams can be used soon after healing and later used as gels when tolerated.

Because combination chemical peels injure the dermis, clinical and histologic recovery may not be complete for up to 90 days. For this reason the peel should not be repeated for at least 3 months postoperatively. In some cases clinical signs such as erythema will indicate that healing is not complete and repeeling would be unwise even at 3 months. Most patients do not require repeeling during the first few years after a combination chemical peel.

Some patients, however, may benefit from a touch-up of certain areas that did not adequately respond to the peel. This can sometimes be done using dermabrasion or a localized repeat peel. Other patients will enjoy repetitive superficial peels to maintain the effects of the deeper peel. These superficial peels may be repeated as soon as 3 months after the initial peel and continued as the patient requires. The benefits of these are improved texture and a "fresher" look to the skin.

CONCLUSION

Three different proven approaches are available for combination chemical peeling that provide reliable and consistent medium depth chemical peel injury. Physician and patient preference will determine which of these approaches are chosen. All typically provide improvement of skin color, actinic damage, and wrinkles with minimal potential for complications.

BIBLIOGRAPHY

Bloom RF. Combined peels tackle actinic keratoses. *Dermatol Times* 1991;19:25.

Brody HJ. *Chemical Peeling.* St. Louis, Mosby, 1992.

Brody HJ. Variation and comparisons in medium depth chemical peeling. *J Dermatol Surg* 1989;15:953–963.

Brody HJ, Hailey CW. Medium depth chemical peeling of the skin: a variation of superficial chemosurgery. *J Dermatol Surg Oncol* 1986;12:1268–1275.

Coleman WP III, Futrell JM. The glycolic acid-trichloroacetic acid chemical peel. *J Dermatol Surg Oncol* 1994;20:76–80.

Monheit GD. The Jessner's & TCA peel: a medium depth chemical peel. *J Dermatol Surg Oncol* 1989;15:945–950.

Moseley JC, Katz SI. Acne vulgaris: treatment with carbon dioxide slush. *Cutis* 1972;10:429–431.

Moy LS, Murad H. Use of AHAs adds new dimensions to chemical peeling. *Cosmet Dermatol* 1990;3:32–34.

Slagel GA, McMartin SL. Chemical face peels. *J Assoc Milt Dermatol* 1984;10:38–43.

Stegman SJ. A comparative histologic study of the effects of three peeling agents and dermabrasion on normal and sun-damaged skin. *Aesth Plast Surg* 1982;6:123–135.

Van Scott EJ. Alpha hydroxy acids: procedures for use in clinical practice. *Cutis* 1989;43:222–228.

66

Chemical Peel with Phenol

E. Gaylon McCollough and Brian P. Maloney
*University of Alabama Medical School and the
McCollough Plastic Surgery Clinic, P.A., Birmingham, Alabama*

Phillip R. Langsdon
University of Tennessee College of Medicine, Memphis, Tennessee

Phenol-based peeling formulas have been used to treat aged and actinically damaged skin since the late 1800s. They are regarded as the deeper peeling agents because their tissue penetration is greater than most other peeling agents and clinically the results are generally more dramatic.

The authors' preferred formula combined with a moist dressing technique has yielded favorable results for over 25 years. The formula is as follows:

Phenol U.S.P. 88%	3 ml
Croton oil	3 drops
Septisol soap	8 drops
Distilled water	2 ml

With this technique, there is no tape placement, mask removal, or powder-induced crust formation. We believe that this method reduces the risk of postoperative scarring and is more convenient and comfortable for the patient. The results of this technique have been gratifying.

The depth of tissue injury is thought to depend upon the concentration of the phenol. Phenol concentrations of less than 80% act as keratolytic agents, penetrating deeply into the dermis. At concentrations greater than 80%, phenol acts as a keratocoagulant, thus decreasing the penetration of the agent. In the above formula, phenol acts as a keratocoagulant despite its concentration of less than 80%.

Croton oil acts as a vesicant, helping to disrupt the keratin layer. Septisol soap is included as a surfactant—reducing surface tension and allowing deeper penetration of the other agents. Water is added to create the desired concentration of the emulsion.

In our experience, results with this method are comparable to that attained using a tape mask. If a deeper peel is indicated in a particular region, more peel solution may be applied. The exfoliative and irritative agents in the formula are effective almost immediately. We contend that the application of additional solution produces further maceration and a greater depth of peel [achieved by taping in the "classic" (mask) method of face peels].

We generally prepare the formula prior to each application, but the solution can be stored in an amber glass bottle for short periods of time. Constantly agitating the formula during application of the peel ensures that the proper concentration is applied to the region being treated. The formula is an emulsion and will otherwise separate.

Phenol, the principal ingredient in the formula, is toxic to some tissues and organs, and therefore cautions are advised. High blood levels result in hepatotoxicity, nephroticity, and cardiotoxicity. For these reasons, good hydration and adequate time spacing (15–20 min) between peeling of each aesthetic region are keys to maintaining blood levels at subtoxic levels. As always, patient tolerance varies and the risk of drug sensitivity and allergic reactions exists.

Resuscitative equipment and emergency medications should be available. When peeling more than one third of the face, intravenous fluids should be started prior to the peel procedure and continued throughout the operative period. Dangerous cardiac arrhythmias can occur. We have seen a variety of toxic arrhythmias, although we have never encountered a situation in which emergency measures were required. When peeling more than one third of the face, the patient's cardiac status should be monitored so the surgeon can be aware of arrhythmias that may develop.

INDICATIONS

The surgical approach to the aging face often includes chemical face peeling as an adjunct to improve the surface facial appearance (Table 1). For example, several months after blepharoplasty (3 months or more), the fine wrinkles around the eyes can be improved by chemexfoliation. Also, rhytidectomy is frequently combined with a perioral peel, which is performed at the completion of the procedure.

Superficial acne scarring can be improved somewhat with peeling. Deep ice pick–type scars from acne, however, are best treated by dermabrasion, staged punch grafts, or scar revision combined with dermabrasion.

Superficial pigmented lesions such as lentigines or freckles may be improved by chemical peel. We have had satisfying results treating freckles. However, these lesions may disappear for a short period of time only to reappear to varying degrees later (see Fig. 1). The response of freckles or lentigines to chemexfoliation is related to the depth of the melanocytes. For this reason we try to inform patients that the removal of pigmented lesions is somewhat unpredictable.

Wrinkled, leathery, actinically damaged skin usually responds well to this exfoliative procedure. However, a person with fair complexion, thin skin, and fine rhytids may be the best candidate. The fair complexion reduces color contrast at the margin of the treated areas. Dark-skinned individuals, on the other hand, are more likely to demonstrate pigment irregularities since the peel usually causes some degree of hypopigmentation (see Fig. 2).

When the entire face is affected by the signs of aging and sun damage (i.e., seborrheic and actinic keratoses), a full face chemical peel combined with superficial curettage is an ideal treat-

Table 1   Indications for Chemical Peel with Phenol

Acne scarring, superficial
Actinic keratosis
Aging face (combined with other rejuvenation procedures)
Freckles
Lentigines
Rhytids
Seborrheic keratosis
Solar elastosis

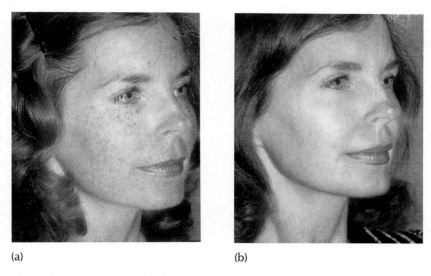

(a)   (b)

Figure 1 (a) Patient with freckling. (b) After phenol peel.

ment. Isolated keratoses can be treated by simple curettage combined with localized chemical exfoliation or electrodesiccation. When the entire face is involved with keratoses, the ideal treatment may be the peel, thus eliminating multiple, isolated surgical treatments, or repeated applications of 5-fluorouracil. Preliminary observations indicate no advantage of laser exfoliation over the traditional chemexfoliation techniques herein discussed.

CONTRAINDICATIONS

The dark-skinned patient is generally not an ideal candidate for deep chemical face peel. Postoperative pigment abnormalities may be more likely to occur. Since the skin is usually some-

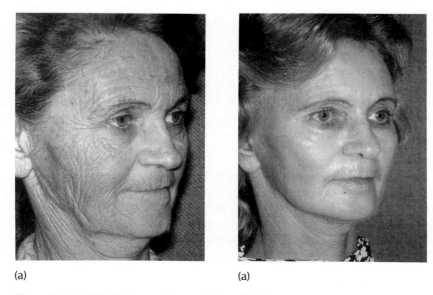

(a)   (a)

Figure 2 (a) Wrinkled, sun-damaged skin. (b) After phenol face peel.

Table 2   Relative Contraindications to Chemical Peel

Associated use of epinephrine-containing local anesthetic
Cardiac disease
Dark-skinned patient
Hepatic disease
Herpetic lesions (fever blisters), active
Medications (estrogen, progesterone)
Psychological (unrealistic, unreliable patients)
Renal disease
Skin of the neck

what lighter after a peel, there would be greater discrepancy in skin color between the peeled and nonpeeled areas. Spotty, pigmentary aberrations might also be more apparent on the dark-skinned patient (Table 2). It would appear that these conditions may be technique-specific and due to nonuniform oil removal and/or application of the peel solution.

Caution should be used when peeling the neck and chest. Superficial and medium-depth agents are generally more appropriate. Although we feather over the angle of the mandible when performing a full face peel, we generally do not peel down onto the neck skin with a phenol-based solution. Caution is advised in patients who have had multiple facial surgical procedures.

Caution is advised when peeling patients with renal, hepatic, or cardiac disease due to the phenol component of the peel. If a patient has significant problems with any of these organ systems, we obtain a medical consultation. Our preoperative work-up includes studies that may reveal an abnormality in the liver or kidney in patients who have a negative history. Since epinephrine can exacerbate cardiac arrhythmias, it is probably wise to limit or avoid using an epinephrine-containing local anesthetic.

If the patient gives a history of fever blisters or herpes simplex, there is a high likelihood that these will recur in the postoperative period. We may proceed with a chemical face peel after having explained this possibility to the patient and treat prophylactically with acyclovir. The patient with an *active* herpetic lesion may experience a spread of these lesions over the entire area peeled. For this reason we treat the condition until it is under control before performing the peel.

Estrogen and progesterone may exacerbate postoperative pigmentary changes. The patient should make an attempt to abstain from any hormonal replacement therapy or use of birth control pills for at least 6 months postoperatively. If the patient needs hormone therapy to control symptoms such as hot flashes or irritability, they should be made aware of possible hyperpigmentation.

PREOPERATIVE CONSIDERATIONS

Patients should have a clear understanding of the procedure prior to undergoing treatment. Printed information about the procedure and the perioperative period is helpful for patients prior to the consultation. The patient is asked to study the material and write down questions. During the consultation, the procedure, limitations, risks, alternative methods of treatment, complications, and postoperative care are reviewed. In addition, the patient is encouraged to ask any questions he or she may have concerning the procedure. The patient should be aware that there will be some alteration of the texture and color of the skin.

Both the patient and the family should be aware of the skin's expected appearance for the first few days after chemexfoliation. Despite written and verbal explanations by the physician and staff about the expected appearance, the patient or family members may be unpleasantly surprised at the immediate postoperative appearance (Fig. 3).

Preoperative photographs are important. These include full face, lateral, and oblique views. In special areas such as the perioral and periorbital regions, close-up photographs should be taken. It is helpful to have photographs in the operative suite during the procedure.

We generally perform the chemical face peel in an outpatient surgical suite. When the patient arrives, the surgical consent is reviewed. The face is then washed three times with a mild, nonoily soap such as Neutrogena®. This is thoroughly rinsed prior to the procedure.

Preoperative oral medications, if more than one third of the face is to be peeled, include cephalexin 500 mg, diazepam 20 mg, Dramamine 200 mg, and prednisone 40 mg. Acyclovir 200 mg is included if the patient has a history of herpes simplex. For regional peels involving less than one third of the face, only buffered aspirin and acetaminophen-hydrocodone (Oxycodone) tablets are given orally. An intravenous line is started. Diazepam is given intravenously in 2-mg increments also to aid with sedation during the administration of the local anesthesia. Generally the amount of intravenous diazepam is 10–20 mg. If further sedation is required, hydromorphone (0.5 mg) can be used intravenously. The local anesthesia reduces pain both during and after the peel.

Local infiltration of anesthesia, when the peel is restricted to a single aesthetic unit, usually consists of a mixture of 0.25% Marcaine and 1% Xylocaine. If a full face peel is to be performed, we use the same combination to anesthetize the forehead, the initial region peeled, and then switch to plain 0.25% Marcaine for the remainder of the face.

Sponges (2" × 2") tightly folded on a hemostat are used to cleanse the patient's face gently with the acetone. The face is now ready for application of the peel. Cleaning with acetone improves the likelihood of a smooth peel because the facial oils prevent adequate chemical penetration. When cleansing has been inadequate, skip areas will appear during the postoperative

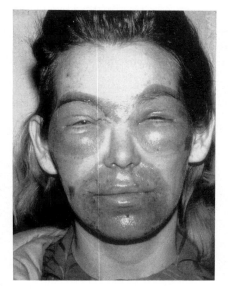

Figure 3 Significant postoperative swelling. This patient is shown 19 hr postperiorbital and perioral peel.

period where the peel has not penetrated satisfactorily. Cleansing is very important to obtaining good results.

PROCEDURE

When applying the peel solution, one should immediately note the development of a white frost, provided the treated areas have been properly cleansed and the surface oils removed with acetone. If the white frost does not develop, facial oils probably have not been adequately removed. The area should be recleansed with acetone (Fig. 4).

The peel is applied with a wooden cotton-tipped applicator. The applicator is dipped into an amber glass bottle containing the peel. The applicator is gently rolled against the inside of the neck of the bottle to remove the excess peel solution. Extensive amounts of solution may be blotted onto a 4 × 4 sponge. The surgeon and assistant stand on opposite sides of the table. The assistant holds the amber glass bottle that contains the formula, constantly agitating it to keep the emulsion uniformly mixed, to ensure that the proper concentration is applied to each region. The surgeon and the assistant should stand above a line that passes horizontally through the patient's eyes when peeling superior to that line. Likewise, they should stand inferior to the horizontal line when peeling the lower eyelids or lower face. This is done to prevent the peel solution from crossing the patient's eyes.

Diluting the peel formula may result in deeper tissue penetration than intended. If the peel formula inadvertently contacts an area that has already been peeled or is not intended to be peeled, one could intensify the peel by diluting the solution with saline or water. Quickly touching the areas with an absorbent gauze sponge may remove some of the peel solution. Conversely, if the peel solution is spilled or dripped into the eye, rapid irrigation with copious amounts of mineral oil should be performed. Caution is advised when peeling around the eyes. Any tears that may occur in the medial and lateral canthal areas should be removed with dry cotton-tipped applicators. This reduces the possibility of diluting the peel in the periorbital region and prevents the reflux diffusion of phenol into the eye.

If a full face peel is being performed, the procedure progresses by treating one aesthetic unit at a time. There should be a 15- to 20-min delay between treating aesthetic units. For instance, the forehead is peeled first, the right cheek second, left cheek third, perioral region fourth, periorbital region fifth, and any nasal peeling occurs last. When one is peeling forehead skin,

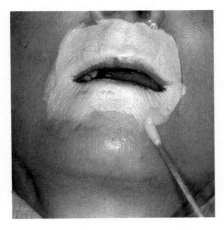

Figure 4 Development of the white frost.

the formula is feathered into the hair of this region, including the frontal hairline, sideburns, and the eyebrows. Failure to do this may result in a demarcation line between the peeled and unpeeled areas. We have not encountered any hair loss as a result of feathering into hair-bearing regions (Fig. 5). When peeling the cheeks, we feather the formula into the sideburn, onto the lobule of the ear, as well as gently over the angle of the mandible (Fig. 6). We are cautious not to peel too far down onto the neck. The risk of scarring may be greater in this area with a deep-peeling agent.

When peeling the perioral region, the formula is applied 2–3 mm onto the vermilion of the lips. This prevents a demarcation line from developing around the mouth. Should this occur, reapplication of the peel at a later date may help. If the lips contain deep creases, we break an unused applicator stick and use the frayed wooden end to apply extra peel directly into the deeper rhytids (Figs. 7,8).

The surgeon and the assistant stand caudal to the patient's eyes when peeling the lower eyelids. The cotton-tipped applicator should be a little drier when peeling the periorbital region because the skin is thinner. The patient is asked to look superiorly, thus stretching the lid skin, and the peel is applied to within 2–3 mm of the lower lid margin. When peeling the upper eyelids, the surgeon and the assistant stand cephalic to the eyes. The patient's eyes are closed and the surgeon elevates the brow. This tightens the upper lid skin. The peel formula is applied within 2–3 mm of the upper lid margin (Figs. 9,10). While the surgeon is applying the peel to the periorbital region, an assistant stands ready with a bottle of mineral oil in case the solution should come in contact with the eye. It is not unusual for the burning sensation around the eyes to cause tearing. Both the surgeon and the assistant should pay particular attention when peeling this region. An assistant should be ready with a dry cotton-tipped applicator to remove any tearing in the medial or lateral canthal areas. Tears are blotted immediately to prevent the diffusion of any peel solution into the patient's eyes. This also prevents dilution of the peel on the thin lid skin, avoiding a deeper peel than intended.

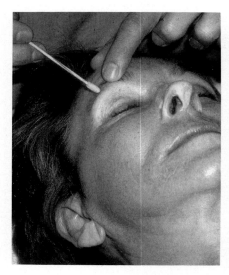

Figure 5 Feathering into the eyebrow. When one is peeling the forehead and cheeks, the hairline and sideburns should be feathered.

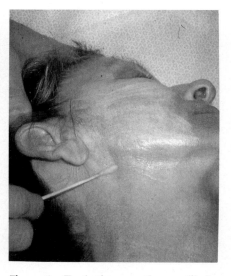

Figure 6 Feathering over the mandibular angle. Be careful not to peel down onto the neck.

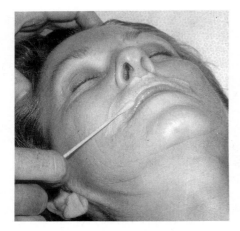

Figure 7 The peel is carried 2–3 mm into the pink vermilion of the lips.

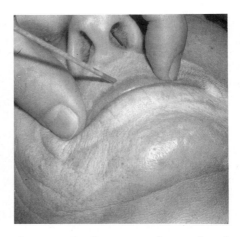

Figure 8 Small amounts of extra phenol may be applied to the deep rhytids.

POSTOPERATIVE CONSIDERATIONS

Application of phenol peel is usually accompanied by a stinging or burning sensation for 15–20 sec. This subsides for 15–20 min and then returns for 6–8 hr. Acetaminophen-oxycodone (Hydrocodone) or oxycodone tablets may be taken every 3–4 hr as needed for pain. Diazepam (5 mg) may also be used for the patient's comfort. Cephalexin (500 mg orally, two times daily) is given as a prophylactic measure. Upon completion of the procedure, the intravenous line is maintained and fluids are administered for 2 hr at a rate of 500 ml/hr. Then the rate is decreased to 100 ml/hr for another 2 hr.

We do not tape the skin or apply bulky dressings over peeled areas. We may allow the patient to use cool saline compresses on the cheeks to help relieve pain. The morning after the pro-

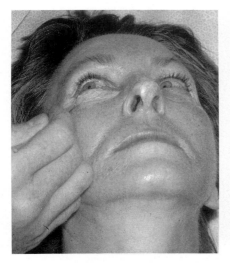

Figure 9 When one is peeling the lower lid, the patient looks superiorly to help tighten the lid skin.

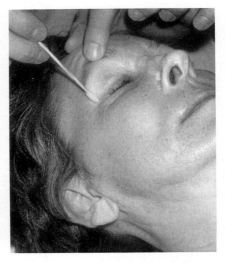

Figure 10 The eyes are closed and the brow is lifted to tighten any redundant skin when peeling the upper eyelid.

cedure the patient may experience little or no pain. However, there may be some discomfort associated with edema and desquamation while following the cleaning protocol. The patient's skin is usually an ashen gray color. The first signs of desquamation may be apparent in 24 hr. If a periorbital peel has been performed, the eyes may be swollen shut. After a perioral peel, there may be significant protrusion of the lips. Swelling may worsen on the second postoperative day, but after the third or fourth day, this begins to subside. The patient usually needs reassurance during the immediate postoperative period (Fig. 3).

Wound care begins the first preoperative day. The patient is instructed to shower four times daily. After each shower a thick layer of Bacitracin ointment is now used. Most patients report that this feels soothing. This is continued for at least the first week. Desquamation usually continues for 7–10 days, but wound care should be continued until epithelialization is complete. After 10–14 days, the patient is usually well healed. In the early postoperative period, some patients complain of dry skin and may need to continue using a moisturizing agent. The new skin is very delicate, especially in the early stages. The patient is instructed not to pick any desquamating skin from the cheeks. Crusts are removed by repeated tap water cleansing and the application of cream to lubricate the skin. This allows crust to shed atraumatically. If desquamating skin is pulled off, one can convert a second-degree defect into a third-degree defect, resulting in scar formation. We have found the topical application of mycolog cream useful for erythema and persistent redness.

The intense pink color present in the postoperative period gradually fades in 8–12 weeks. After 6 weeks patients should be encouraged to use sunscreens (SPF 15) daily, and direct sunlight should be avoided during the healing period. This minimizes postinflammatory pigment changes. Sunlight, heat, cold, or wind could be damaging to the newly formed skin. The patient generally may return to work in 2 weeks as long as this does not involve any outdoor activities. We prefer that patients wait until they have been examined before applying cosmetics. Generally, by the second postoperative week, a water-based makeup can be used.

COMPLICATIONS

The cardiotoxic effects (arrhythmias) of phenol are the most common complications seen. Hepatotoxicity and nephrotoxicity can also occur. The procedure therefore requires cardiac monitoring and adequate hydration with intravenous fluids. Arrhythmias can occur within minutes after the application of phenol, especially in particularly sensitive patients or when more than one third of the face is peeled within 10–15 min. If arrhythmias occur, peeling should be discontinued until normal sinus rhythm has returned for a full 15 min. We usually recommend consultation with an internist for patients with abnormal liver or kidney function studies. Phenol-induced cardiotoxicity may be more pronounced in those patients who have liver or kidney disease, requiring prolonged detoxification. Arrhythmias are also more likely to occur in patients with preoperative cardiac arrhythmias or when epinephrine-containing local anesthetics are used.

Herpetic ulcerations may occur in patients who are herpes simplex carriers. Patients who have had fever blisters in the past are given acyclovir 200 mg orally every 4 hr. This is done preoperatively and continued for 6–7 days as a prophylactic measure. Patients who have active herpes ulcerations are advised to delay peeling until the lesions have healed. Peeling can be performed in the presence of an active lesion if it is sealed and distant from the area to be treated. Herpetic eruptions may occur in any location on the face, but do so most commonly around the mouth. Should this develop in the postoperative period, topical acyclovir ointment is added to the treatment program. Prophylactic antiviral ointments may be applied to the eyes as well. However, in our experience, we have not found this to be necessary and have observed no ocular complications. We have not seen any permanent skin defects develop as a result of herpetic ulcerations (Fig. 11).

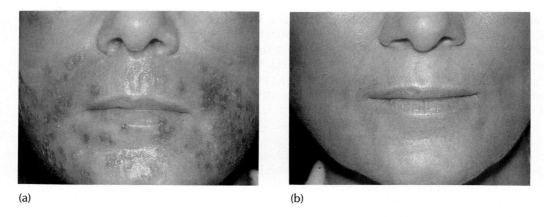

(a)   (b)

Figure 11   (a) Herpes simplex eruption 9 days after peel. (b) Resolution without residual defect. Photo 5 months postpeel.

If pigment alterations occur, they usually do so within 3–6 months. In fair-skinned individuals, the demarcation line between the peeled and nonpeeled areas is minimal. The feathering technique is used at the junctions of the treated and nontreated areas, such as the angle of the jaw, the hair-bearing regions, and the vermilion area of the lips. This is done in order to decrease the contrasting color and texture. When doing regional peels, it is especially important to feather into surrounding areas. The patient should be prepared to accept the pigment irregularities in exchange for smoother skin.

The tendency to develop hyperpigmentation may be exacerbated if the patient is exposed to sunlight, takes estrogen, or becomes pregnant within the first 6 months after the peel. This may be treated with a cream made of Eldoquin Forte® (15 g) plus Retin A® 0.1% (15 g) applied at bedtime and increased as tolerated. Spotty hyperpigmentation may result from an uneven application of the peel, inadequate preparation with acetone, or if the patient experiences postpeel erythema syndrome. Should this occur, the area can be repeeled or dermabraded in about 3 months. Hypopigmentation, on the other hand, is more common and expected following a deep peel or prolonged healing. The conditions should be viewed as side effects of the procedure rather than a complication.

Prolonged erythema can occur in some individuals. There appear to be both intrinsic and extrinsic causes of postpeel erythema. Peeling may unmask a subclinical skin disorder such as eczema or lupus. Contactants such as hairspray, fragrance, makeup, printer's ink, bleach, and cotton balls are the cause in some people. Treatment includes systemic and topical steroid preparations. Erythema may last for several months postoperatively but it is not a permanent problem. Hydrocortisone cream (2½%) can be used twice a day for 2 weeks and then once a day if erythema is a prolonged problem. Scarring has been a very rare occurrence. Temporary hypertrophy in the perioral area, forehead, and periorbital areas is treated successfully with topical steroids in the early stages. Once thickening occurs, intralesional Kenalog (10–20 mg/ml) injections can be used. If hypertrophic scarring does not resolve, traditional scar revision procedures and emotional support can help. A good doctor-patient relationship is important. Patients should know that surgical scar revision techniques can generally improve most scars, but we have not seen this problem with our patients (Figs. 12,13).

Wound infections are extremely rare when the maskless technique of chemexfoliation as long as the patient faithfully follows postoperative wound care instructions. One elderly patient de-

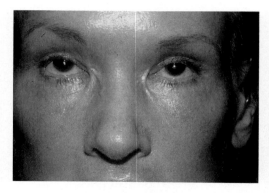

Figure 12 Patient peeled elsewhere by "exodermatology" and taping. Medial canthal scarring is apparent.

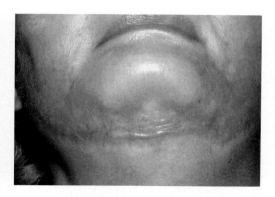

Figure 13 Patient referred for treatment of neck scarring after peel.

veloped a full facial pyoderma from which *Pseudomonas* was cultured as a result of not washing her face for several days postoperatively as instructed. The patient was vigorously debrided and the situation resolved without any residual defect (Fig. 14).

Milia may develop within the first 4–6 weeks after chemexfoliation. They usually subside with proper cleaning. If they persist, an 18-gauge needle can be used to uncap the pore. Recurrence is rare.

Inadequate removal of facial rhytids should not be considered a complication. It can be a result of an inadequate application of the peel solution, inadequate removal of facial oils, or simply deep rhytids that require additional peeling. However, some rhytids simply cannot be removed. Perfection is very rarely obtained with any cosmetic procedure. Repeeling, dermabrading, la-

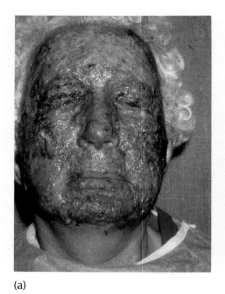

(a)

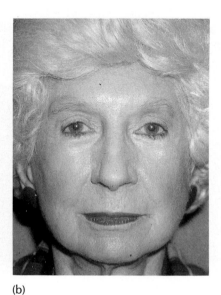

(b)

Figure 14 (a) Patient who failed to follow postoperative cleaning protocol developed full facial infection. (b) Resolution and good result with adequate cleaning.

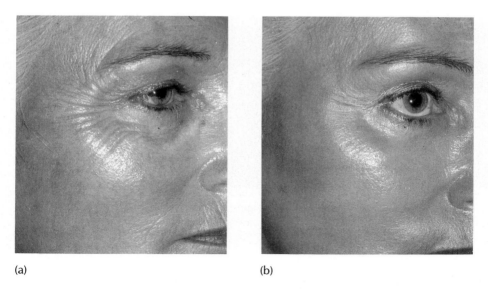

(a)   (b)

Figure 15   (a) Preoperative peel. (b) After periorbital peel. Some residual rhytids are still present.

ser resurfacing may provide additional improvement. The deep creases and folds in the forehead and nasolabial folds cannot be removed by chemexfoliation, and the patient should be informed of this preoperatively. We have had some improvement in the deep forehead grooves by combining dermabrasion and peeling at the time of initial treatment. Peeling should be done first.

REGIONAL PEELS IN COMBINATION WITH FACIAL SURGERY

We perform a number of regional peels in conjunction with facial surgery. Patients undergoing blepharoplasty should understand that the procedure will not remove fine wrinkling around the eyes. It is often necessary to perform a periorbital peel 3–6 months postoperatively. Patients who

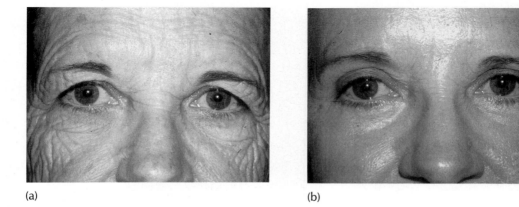

(a)   (b)

Figure 16   (a) Before blepharoplasty, facelift, and peel. (b) After blepharoplasty, facelift, and peel.

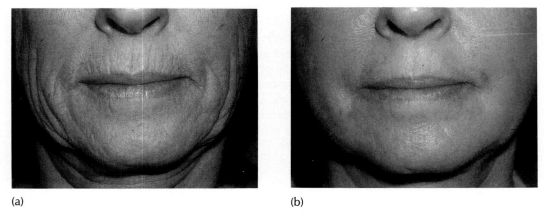

(a)   (b)

Figure 17   (a) Before perioral peel. (b) After perioral peel.

undergo rhytidectomy often require a peel in the perioral region at the completion of the procedure in order to obtain improvement around the month. Simultaneous peeling over areas that have been undermined is risky, and we generally advise against the combination. If the undermined area needs to be peeled, this can be done after healing is complete. A periorbital peel may be performed with a facelift if blepharoplasty is not being performed. A full face peel can be done 3–6 months postrhytidectomy. Peeling over an undermined area could result in the development of full-thickness skin loss and hypertrophic scarring (Figs. 15–18).

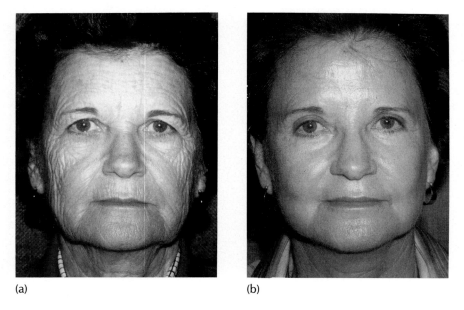

(a)   (b)

Figure 18   (a) Before facelift, blepharoplasty, full face peel. (b) Postoperative appearance.

CONCLUSION

Chemexfoliation is a time-tested method of skin rejuvenation. When properly carried out, in the appropriate patient it can lead to gratifying and lasting improvement.

Skin resurfacing with chemical agents can be performed as isolated procedures or in conjunction with a variety of other techniques and procedures. As is the case with all surgery, results seem to be directly related to both the skill and experience of the operator and the individual subject's propensity to heal in the expected manner.

Unfavorable outcomes can often be either avoided or minimized by attention to detail and compliance with accepted courses of procedure. Preoperative counseling and close postoperative monitoring are essential to maintaining a good doctor–patient relationship

BIBLIOGRAPHY

Baker TJ, Gordon HL. The ablation of rhitides by chemical means—preliminary report. *J Florida Med Assoc* 1961;48:451.

Beeson WH, McCollough EG. Chemical face peeling without taping. *J Dermatol Surg Oncol* 1985;11:985–990.

Maibach HI, Rovee DT. *Epidermal Wound Healing*. Chicago, Year Book Medical Publishers, 1972.

McCollough EG, Hillman RAI. Chemical face peel. *Otolaryngol Clin North Am* 1980;13:353–365.

67

Postsurgical Cosmetics

Zoe Diana Draelos
Bowman Gray School of Medicine, Winston-Salem, North Carolina

The postsurgical patient emerges with a new self-image whether the surgery was therapeutic or cosmetic. The patient may view the therapeutic surgery as deforming and experience a period of depression during which he or she withdraws from social situations with family and friends. Even when an elective cosmetic procedure is performed, there is a brief time during which uncertainty about the positive outcome of the surgery may cause emotional problems for the patient. The physician should anticipate these postsurgical difficulties and provide counseling.

Appropriate counseling should include expected time to healing and wound care instructions. The patient should thoroughly understand what changes are expected in the surgical site and are part of the normal healing process. Warning signs indicating problems and requiring medical evaluation should also be discussed.

Another often overlooked area of postsurgical counseling is helping patients maximize their appearance during and after the healing process. This counseling should include recommendations for appropriate skin care routines and the use of cosmetics. The patient should understand how to select appropriate cleansers, moisturizers, and sunscreens. Camouflage techniques should also be discussed, whether they are employed on a temporary or a permanent basis. Postsurgical cosmetics and skin care products are important for both the physical and the emotional well-being of the patient following surgery.

SKIN CHANGES IN THE POSTSURGICAL PATIENT

In the postsurgical patient skin no longer functions as a barrier to the external environment. Therefore, all applied substances have much greater access to the dermal vasculature. This increases the probability of experiencing adverse reactions to topical products, including irritation (stinging, burning, itching, tingling), sensitization, and urticaria. Products must be carefully selected to meet the strictest standards to hypoallergenicity in the postsurgical patient. Unusual erythema, vesiculation, or urticaria in and around the postsurgical site suggest adverse reactions to topically applied material.

POSTOPERATIVE WOUND CARE AND COSMETICS

Cosmetics should not be applied to wounds that are healing by either first or second intention immediately following surgery. This generally is not a problem since cosmetics will not adhere to skin until the serous drainage from the wound has stopped. Premature application of cosmetics can create a foreign body reaction.

Facial foundations are pigmented lotions or creams that are applied to the face to hide blemishes and create an even skin tone. They are especially useful in the postsurgical patient to mask erythema and bruising. They are composed of titanium dioxide, a covering agent, and iron oxide pigments. Both of these substances represent powders that could act as foreign bodies and impede wound healing by initiating an inflammatory response or milia formation. Therefore, facial foundations and all other cosmetics should be avoided until reepithelialization has occurred or the sutures have been removed.

TOPICAL THERAPEUTICS

Topical therapeutic agents may be used during the postsurgical period to enhance wound healing. Commonly employed topical products include antibiotic preparations and corticosteroids. The absence of an intact stratum corneum requires careful selection of postsurgical topical agents.

Topical antibiotics with the least sensitizing potential should be selected. Therefore, neomycin, a cause of allergic contact dermatitis, and polymixin B, a mast cell degranulater, should be avoided. Less sensitizing antibiotics such as polysporin, bacitracin, erythromycin, and mupirocin should be recommended for topical use. Patients who experience delayed wound healing should be patch-tested for topical antibiotic sensitivity.

Topical corticosteroids may also be used to decrease inflammation during the postsurgical period. Ointment preparations are preferred over gels, creams, and emollients as they have a petrolatum base and are less likely to contain cutaneous irritants, such as propylene glycol. Anhydrous, or water-free, preparations do not require high preservative concentrations, thus eliminating another potential source of irritancy or sensitization. Statistically, corticosteroids preserved with parabens have the least sensitizing potential, while products preserved with Kathons sensitize patients most often.

SKIN CARE PRODUCT SELECTION

Physicians should provide patients with a grooming routine during the postoperative period designed to optimize wound healing. Cleanser, moisturizer, and sunscreen products should be selected for each patient's individual requirements.

Cleansers

Cleansers used during the postoperative period should be nonirritating to minimize damage to newly formed epithelium. Immediately postoperative, lukewarm water may be the only cleanser required. As serum crusting begins, a synthetic detergent soap (e.g., Dove, Cetaphil, Oil of Olay, Basis, etc.) gently cleanses without overdrying the skin. Synthetic detergent soaps are generally labeled as "beauty bars."

Lipid-free cleansing lotions (e.g., Cetaphil, Aquanil), used with or without water, can also gently cleanse a wound. They do not possess substantial antibacterial properties, however. In surgical sites where bacterial contamination may be a problem, deodorant soaps containing triclosan (e.g., Dial) may be appropriate. Some beauty bar soaps are available that are antibacterial (e.g., Lever 2000) and may be helpful in some patients.

Moisturizers

Moisturizer use is important for the postsurgical patient since the barrier to transepidermal water loss is absent. This allows free water evaporation from the skin creating a tight sensation accompanied by pruritus. Furthermore, desiccation impedes wound healing, which proceeds most rapidly in a moist environment.

Immediately after surgery, pure white petroleum jelly may be the best moisturizer. It is an excellent occlusive, thus trapping moisture within the skin. It is used as a negative control for dermatologic patch testing because its irritation and sensitization potentials are low. Furthermore, it is extremely economical. Drawbacks to petroleum jelly are its greasy appearance, odor, and ability to stain natural fiber fabrics.

Once reepithelialization has begun, oil-in-water formulations may be substituted and are more cosmetically elegant. Creams should be selected over lotions since they are better moisturizers and are less likely to contain irritants. Products should be chosen for their paucity of ingredients. Therefore, creams with fragrances, herbal or biological additives, and specialty ingredients should be avoided until complete healing has occurred.

Sunscreens

Sun exposure to the surgical site should be avoided after surgery as the skin has lost its ability to adequately protect against photodamage. Postinflammatory hyperpigmentation may also result. Many patients will continue their daily activities, which may include casual sun exposure. All chemical sunscreening agents (PABA esters, cinnamate derivatives, benzophenones, etc.) are potential causes of both irritant and allergic contact dermatitis.

The physician may suggest a "chemical-free" sunscreen, but these contain titanium dioxide, which may result in a foreign body reaction. These products should not be used until reepithelialization is complete or sutures have been removed.

COSMETIC SELECTION

Cosmetics available for camouflage purposes in the postsurgical patient include foundations, cover creams, and color correctors.

Foundations

Facial foundations are designed to add color, cover blemishes, and blend uneven facial color. Postsurgical patients commonly have residual erythema for 2 weeks to 6 months following the procedure depending on the type of surgery, speed of healing, and skin color of the patient. Facial foundations are an excellent method of camouflaging postsurgical erythema.

Facial foundations used for blending erythema do not require the coverage necessary for surgical camouflaging. These products generally contain a high concentration of titanium dioxide and oils and can be purchased at any retail store. Table 1 lists a variety of appropriate products.

Table 1 Facial Foundations for Postsurgical Patients

Foundation	Formulation	Color selection	Purchase site
Waterproof Creme Makeup (Max Factor)	Cream	Medium	Mass merchandiser
Workout Makeup (Clinique)	Cream	Fair to medium	Cosmetic counter
Soft Finish Compact Makeup (Estee Lauder)	Cream/Powder	Fair to medium	Cosmetic counter
Flawless Finish (Elizabeth Arden)	Cream/Powder	Medium to dark	Cosmetic counter
Advanced Formula Liquid Compact (Ultima II)	Cream/Powder	Fair to medium	Cosmetic counter
Matte Deluxe Cream/Powder Foundation (Germaine Monteil)	Cream/Powder	Fair to medium	Cosmetic counter
Dual Finish Creme/Powder Makeup (Lancome)	Cream/Powder	Fair to dark	Cosmetic counter
Perfect Finish Cream Makeup (Fashion Fair Cosmetics)	Cream	Dark	Cosmetic counter

Cover Creams

Cover creams are also facial foundations, but they are designed to provide opaque cover, thus completely obscuring the underlying skin. They are formulated as creams, sticks, and compressed powders. Cream and stick formulations may be waterproof, while the compressed powders are not water resistant. Table 2 lists examples of currently available cover creams.

Color Correctors

Color correctors are liquid or cream facial foundations in specialty colors designed to aid in blending of unwanted skin tones. They contain additional pigments to produce colors of green, purple, orange, peach, pink, etc. Their use will be more fully discussed later.

Table 2 Postsurgical Cover Creams

Trade name	Company address
Corrective Concepts	Pattee Products European Crossroads 2829 West Northwest Highway Dallas, Texas 75220
Coverette	Ben Nye Company, Inc. 5935 Bowcroft Street Los Angeles, California 90016
Covermark	Lyda O'Leary 1 Anderson Avenue Moonachie, New Jersey 07074
Cover Tone	Fashion Fair Cosmetics 820 South Michigan Avenue Chicago, Illinois 60605
Cream Makiage	Il-Makiage PO Box 1064 Long Island City, New York 11101
Dermablend	Dermablend Corrective Cosmetics PO Box 3008 Lakewood, New Jersey 08701
Dermaceal	Joe Blasco Cosmetics 1708 Hillhurst Avenue Hollywood, California 90027
Dermacolor	Kryolan Corporation 132 Ninth Street San Francisco, California 94103
Natural Cover	LS Cosmetics PO Box 32203 Baltimore, Maryland 21208
Veil	Atelier Esthetique 386 Park Avenue South Suite 209 New York, New York 10016

BASIC CAMOUFLAGE TECHNIQUES

Postsurgical cutaneous defects can be divided into pigmentation abnormalities and contour abnormalities. Surgery may also destroy appendageal structures resulting in the absence of cutaneous texture and landmarks.

Pigmentation Abnormalities

Pigmentation abnormalities can be corrected by the use of facial foundations, cover creams, and color correctors. Facial foundations of the type listed in Table 1 can be used if the pigmentation problem is minor erythema, hypopigmentation, or hyperpigmentation. If bruising, depigmentation, or dark hyperpigmentation is present, then a cover cream of the type listed in Table 2 should be selected.

Cover creams, also known as surgical camouflaging cosmetics, require special application and removal techniques. They are completely opaque and can cover any underlying pigmentation problem if a quality product is selected. In order to obtain high coverage, long wearability, and waterproof qualities, proper application is essential.

Prior to application of the cosmetic, a proper color match should be determined. The stock cosmetic color closest to the patient's natural skin color should be selected and a small amount scooped from the jar onto the back of the patient's hand. The back of the hand is an excellent surface for warming the stiff cosmetic and blending the appropriate color. Additional makeup colors can be blended with a cosmetic spatula until the desired color is obtained. All hues present in the patient's skin should be represented, but it is better not to blend more than three colors.

Once the final color has been obtained, it is dabbed (not rubbed) over the face. Application should begin over the central face with blending into the hairline, over each tragus, and down beneath the jawline. No lines of demarcation should be present where cosmetic application has stopped. It is important to dab the cosmetic, since rubbing may remove foundation applied earlier. Foundation does not adhere to facial scars as well, since appendageal structures are decreased or absent.

The cover cream must now be set with a translucent powder. The powder is pressed into the foundation to impart a matte finish and waterproof characteristics. The foundation may require some touch-up, but surgical facial foundations are designed to wear 8 hr, and most colored cosmetics applied on top of the surgical foundation wear better than when applied directly to the skin.

An alternative to an opaque surgical cover cream is the use of color correctors. Color correctors are applied under a facial foundation to avoid the use of surgical cosmetics. They are based on the principle of complementary colors. For example, red pigmentation defects can be camouflaged by applying a green color corrector foundation. The blending of red skin with green foundation yields a brown tone, which can be readily covered by a more conventional facial foundation. Yellow skin tones can be blended with a complementary colored purple foundation to also yield brown tones. Bluish bruising can be camouflaged with a peach or orange colored corrector.

Contour Abnormalities

Contour abnormalities represent areas of hypertrophy or atrophy within the surgical scar. Contour defects cannot be masked with foundations, cover creams, or color correctors and may accentuate contour abnormalities with a shiny finish.

High and low skin areas are camouflaged by shading. Contour camouflaging is based on the principle that dark areas recede while light areas project. Thus, a depressed scar will appear darker than the surrounding skin simply due to the shadows created. Conversely, a hypertrophied scar will appear lighter than the surrounding skin due to the lack of shadows. A lighter cosmetic, either a facial foundation or a blush, can be applied to depressed scars while a darker cosmetic, either a facial foundation or blush, can be applied to hypertrophied scars. Achieving a good cosmetic result requires some artistic skill and practice. Fortunately, poor results can be easily removed. Patients left with chronic contour abnormalities may wish to seek the services of a paramedical camouflage artist who can assist them in cosmetic selection, color blending, and cosmetic application.

Recreating Cutaneous Texture and Landmarks

Many procedures, such as Mohs micrographic surgery, flaps, or grafts, destroy appendageal structures, thus creating skin of different texture once healing has occurred. Furthermore, surgery requiring removal of significant amounts of normal tissue may remove folds and contours on the face that create important landmarks, such as the nasal groove, nasolabial fold, chin crease, etc. Camouflage techniques are also available to restore these cutaneous textures and landmarks.

Scarred skin may be devoid of hair. If the male beard is missing in a key area on the face, cover creams alone will not be able to adequately reproduce the color or texture of beard stipple. Beard stipple can be added by dipping a coarse sponge into black theatrical powder and then pressing the sponge into the surgical foundation.

If there are areas where it is critical to more accurately reproduce hair, such as the eyebrow area, a prosthesis can be constructed. Crepe wool, yak hair, and human hair are three materials from which missing eyebrows can be created. Crepe wool is a wool-like material that is inexpensive and available in a wide variety of colors. Yak hair and human hair give more realistic results but are more expensive and require greater application skill. The fibers can be glued with spirit gum on a daily basis to the affected area, or a permanent prosthesis can be constructed, if necessary.

Skin folds, wrinkles, bags, jowls, or pouches are actually painted on the face. Powdered or cream colors in various shades of gray, red, and brown are used to artistically create these landmarks and minimize the appearance of the facial deformity. More detailed discussion of the techniques used can be obtained from texts on stage makeup.

SPECIFIC CAMOUFLAGE TECHNIQUES

Specific camouflage techniques are used following dermabrasion and face peels, cryosurgery and electrosurgery, laser surgery, incisional surgery, liposuction, and fat transfer.

Dermabrasion and Face Peels

Dermabrasion and face peel patients have temporary erythema, which can be easily camouflaged with a superior facial foundation of the type listed in Table 1. These are oily foundations and will help smooth skin scale. The foundation should not be applied, however, until reepithelialization has occurred. Once the reddish skin hues have faded to pink, the patient may resume his or her normal foundation. For individuals with longstanding vibrant red skin tones, especially following a vigorous dermabrasion, a green color corrector may be used under the foundation to aid in camouflage.

Cryosurgery and Electrosurgery

Cryosurgery and electrosurgery usually induce localized wounding that is allowed to heal by second intention. Once a serum crust has formed, a dab of cover cream can be applied to the area and blended with the patient's usual facial foundation. If erythema is persistent following reepithelialization, a green color corrector may be used under the foundation.

Laser Surgery

Flashlamp yellow dye sites are noted for bruising. Purplish-red bruising is best camouflaged with a green color corrector under foundation, while bluish bruising is best camouflaged with an orange color corrector under foundation. As the bruise resolves and the yellowish-brown hemosiderin pigments become apparent, a purple color corrector may be used.

Incisional Surgery

Incisional surgery creates scars that are generally permanent. If extensive Mohs micrographic surgery is performed or if a graft or flap is required, contour and pigmentation abnormalities may occur. These patients generally do best with a surgical facial foundation listed in Table 2. If the scarring is severe, the patient should receive professional instruction in application of the product. Lightening of depressions and darkening of hypertrophic areas may be needed to minimize contour abnormalities. Cutaneous textures and landmarks can be recreated, as previously discussed.

Liposuction and Fat Transfer

Liposuction and fat transfer are also known for postsurgical bruising. The same techniques as discussed for laser surgery apply here.

SUMMARY

It is important for the dermatologist to make the postsurgical patient comfortable with his or her new image following surgery. This entails counseling the patient on postoperative wound care, the appropriate use of skin care products, cosmetic selection, and camouflage techniques, if appropriate. The dermatologist who has knowledge in these areas can improve both patient satisfaction and ultimately the final result.

BIBLIOGRAPHY

Allsworth J. *Skin Camouflage*. Cheltenham, England, Stanley Throes Ltd, 1985.
Buchman H. *Stage Makeup*. New York, Watson-Guptill.
Cash TF, Cash DW. Women's use of cosmetics. *Int J Cosmet Sci* 1982;4:1.
Draelos ZK. Cosmetic camouflaging techniques. *Cutis* 1993;52(6):362–364.
Draelos ZK. *Cosmetics in Dermatology*. Edinburgh, Churchill Livingstone, 1990.
Rayner V. *Clinical Cosmetology*. Albany, Milady Publishing, 1993.

68

Sclerotherapy

Mitchel P. Goldman
*University of California School of Medicine and Dermatology
Associates of San Diego County, Inc., San Diego, California*

Sclerotherapy as a treatment for varicose and telangiectatic leg veins is becoming increasingly popular in the United States. This treatment originates from the mid-1800s when various solutions were injected into varicose veins. Unfortunately, because of aseptic techniques and solutions, these early treatments often resulted in major complications and the procedure was abandoned. At the turn of the century, intravenous treatment for syphilis was noted to produce sclerosis in injected veins and physicians once again thought of injecting varicose veins.

Early reports on this treatment were enthusiastic and the basic principles of treatment were established. Linser in 1916 first recommended postsclerotherapy compression to limit thrombosis and excessive phlebitic reactions. McAusland in 1939 promoted injection into "empty veins." He described the necessity for beginning treatment by closing the saphenofemoral junction before treating distal varicosities. He also developed the concept of "minimal sclerosing concentration," using sodium morrhuate froth to treat venulectases and telangiectasia and more concentrated sodium morrhuate to treat larger veins. However, general surgeons who had previously been practicing sclerotherapy became disenchanted with this technique because of allergic reactions to sclerosing solutions, difficulty in accurately diagnosing reflux points, and difficulty in applying compression dressings for long periods. In addition, with the onset of World War II the surgeon's expertise was directed towards more serious problems and less to cosmetic concerns. Arterial surgery was rapidly evolving, and sclerotherapy of varicose veins, indeed the treatment of venous disease in general, became less glamorous and, perhaps more importantly, less financially rewarding.

However, primarily in Europe and to some extent in the United States, both surgeons and medical physicians, including dermatologists, continued refining sclerotherapy techniques. Less toxic synthetic sclerosing solutions (sodium tetradecyl sulfate, described by Reiner in the United

Reprinted with permission from Martin/Dunitz, London, from *Surgical Dermatology Advances and Current Practices*, Martin Dunitz, 1993.

States) were being used with greater efficacy and less morbidity. The concept of prolonged compression was advanced by Sigg, Orbach, and Fegan. Also, more accurate methods for diagnosing points of high-pressure reflux (Doppler ultrasound) were developed. The foundation for proper technique was established.

Why then is sclerotherapy treatment becoming popular now? Present-day interest has arisen through the publication of many articles in the dermatologic literature and, more importantly, from publication in the lay press. Only within the past few years have patients begun to take an active role in their medical care. Patients are unwilling to submit to the morbidity and scarring process of ligation and stripping operations of the past. They are demanding cosmetic treatment. They are also unwilling to accept a physician's advice that they should not worry about "minor" leg pains. Sclerotherapy offers the vast majority of those who suffer from both the symptoms and cosmetic embarrassment of varicose veins an affordable and practical treatment. This chapter will describe three "advances" in sclerotherapy treatment. These are advances not because they are new, but because they are newly popular—proper diagnosis prior to treatment, optimal choice of sclerosing solutions and concentrations, and ideal compression techniques to limit sclerophlebitis, recanalization, and complications.

PRESCLEROTHERAPY EVALUATION

To appreciate the fundamentals of noninvasive diagnostic techniques, an understanding of the anatomy and pathophysiology of varicose and telangiectatic veins is required. Since this is beyond the scope of this chapter the reader is referred to a recent textbook. In short, the venous system is just that—a "system" of veins. Flow through the venous system is directed towards the heart by one-way valves, which are present in all veins below the dermal–epidermal junction. Under external compression through various muscle pumps, especially the calf and foot pumps, blood is propelled through the veins. Respiratory actions which decrease intraabdominal pressure suck blood into the abdominal veins. Vis-a-tergo and osmotic gradients propel blood through venulectases. This orchestrated flow can only occur if the valvular system is competent. With valvular destruction or venous dilatation, one-way flow is replaced by retrograde flow, resulting in venous hypertension. Because veins are intricately connected, venous hypertension is distributed throughout the venous system, resulting in a cascading breakdown of one-way flow.

Dermal and superficial venulectases have anastomotic connections with larger subcutaneous veins (Fig. 1). An elegant radiographic study of cadaver veins illustrates the intricate connections between superficial and deep veins through multiple perforator veins (Fig. 2): "perforator" because connections between the superficial and deep system occur through veins that perforate the fascial covering of the deep venous system. Therefore, to alleviate venous hypertension, one must first cut off the most proximal point of abnormal reflux. Various physical and noninvasive diagnostic techniques have been developed to find this point. It is here that treatment should begin.

Physical Examination

Visual observation and palpation are the obvious first steps in presclerotherapy evaluation. Patients' legs should be exposed in their entirety. At times, a bulging dilatation of an incompetent junction between the deep and superficial system can be missed (Fig. 3). A diagram of the visual varicosities and telangiectasias is made on a standard form with notation of bulges and fascial defects (Fig. 4).

Although fascial defects usually overlie incompetent perforator veins, these defects may only be associated with perforator veins 50–70% of the time. To detect fascial defects it is best to have the patient lie on his or her back and elevate the leg. After a few minutes the medial leg

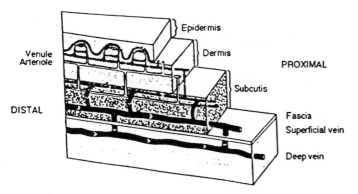

Figure 1 Schematic diagram of the cutaneous and subcutaneous vascular plexus. (Reproduced with permission from Goldman MP. *Sclerotherapy Treatment of Varicose and Telangiectatic Leg Veins*. St. Louis, Mosby-Yearbook Inc., 1991.)

is massaged distal to proximal. With practice the examiner's finger will fall into depressions within the subcutaneous tissue. These depressions are marked. If only a few depressions are felt, one then allows the patient to stand while holding pressure on these points. If the varicose vein fails to reappear, the examiner then releases each finger one at a time, distal to proximal, and notes the point at which the vein recurs. This point represents the site of the most distal incompetent perforating vein (Fig. 5). In the patient with an incompetent saphenofemoral junction, the test is just as simple.

Trendelenburg first described a physical examination technique for diagnosing incompetence at the saphenofemoral junction (SFJ). In short, the superficial veins of the leg are emptied by raising the leg 60° above the horizontal. A tourniquet is placed at the proximal thigh to occlude superficial veins and the patient stands. If the superficial varicosity fails to refill within 20 sec, the test is positive and the etiology of venous reflux is at the SFJ. If the vein refills within 20

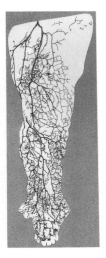

Figure 2 Radiographic demonstration of the superficial venous system. (Reproduced with permission from Taylor et al., 1990.)

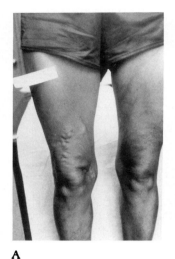 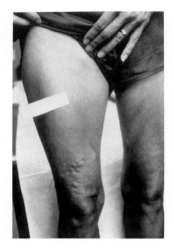

A   B

Figure 3 (A) This patient sought treatment because of an obviously enlarged varicose vein in her thigh. (B) Further inspection revealed a varix at the saphenofemoral junction (arrow) indicative of insufficiency. (Courtesy Anton Butie.) (Reproduced with permission from Goldman MP. *Sclerotherapy Treatment of Varicose and Telangiectatic Leg Veins*. St. Louis, Mosby-Yearbook Inc., 1991.)

sec, one should look for incompetent perforating veins in the distal calf, knee, and thigh (Fig. 6).

Another physical examination technique is a modified Perthe's test. To determine if superficial varicosities are necessary for venous return, the patient is fitted with a 30–40 mm Hg gradu-

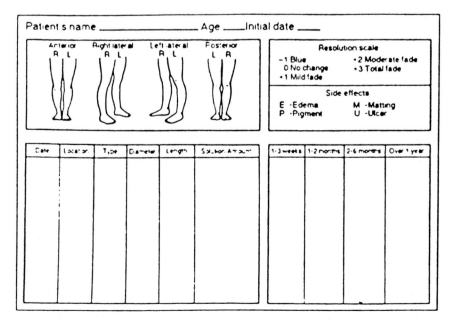

Figure 4 Diagrammatic chart notes and follow-up notes. (Reproduced with permission from Goldman MP. *Sclerotherapy Treatment of Varicose and Telangiectatic Leg Veins*. St. Louis, Mosby-Yearbook Inc., 1991.)

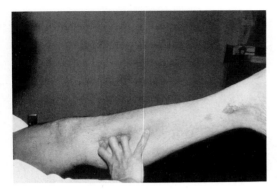

A

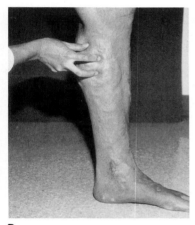

B

Figure 5 (A) Compression of fascial defects indicating "points of control" of incompetent perforating veins with the leg elevated. (B) When the patient stands, the varicose vein remains collapsed while pressure is maintained over control points and distends when the control points are released. (Courtesy Helane Fronek.) (Reproduced with permission from Goldman MP. *Sclerotherapy Treatment of Varicose and Telangiectatic Leg Veins.* St. Louis, Mosby-Yearbook Inc., 1991.)

ated compression stocking and/or a tourniquet is applied at the proximal thigh. This degree of compression will occlude the superficial veins. If the leg feels better or does not become painful after walking for 15–30 min, adequate flow is present in the deep venous system.

Noninvasive Diagnostic Techniques

The venous Doppler is as indispensable for the phlebologist as the stethoscope is for the cardiologist. The Doppler ultrasound transmits sound waves to a recorder or audio system, which are reflected off blood cells traveling through a specific vein. This provides information on both the direction of blood flow and its velocity. By performing various physical maneuvers, one can then determine the presence of deep venous thrombosis, deep venous valvular insufficiency, and superficial venous valvular insufficiency. A complete description of this examination technique is found elsewhere.

Patients who should be evaluated with Doppler ultrasound are those with varicose veins large enough to be hemodynamically significant. Since spider telangiectasia commonly occurs over an

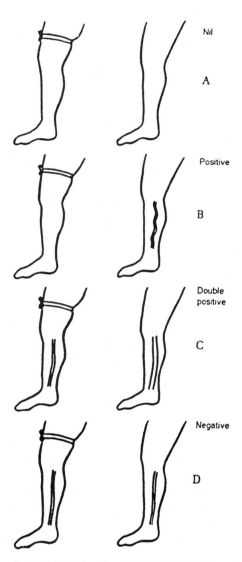

Figure 6 Interpreting the Brodie–Trendelenburg test. (A) Nil—no distension of the veins for 30 sec both while the tourniquet remains on and also after it is removed implies a lack of reflux. (B) Positive—distension of the veins only after the tourniquet is released implies reflux only through the saphenofemoral junction (SFJ). (C) Double positive—distention of the veins while the tourniquet remains on and further distention when it is removed implies reflux through perforating veins as well as the SFJ. (D) Negative—distension of the veins while the tourniquet remains on and no additional distension once it is removed implies reflux only through perforating veins. (Courtesy Helane Fronek.) (Reproduced with permission from Goldman MP. *Sclerotherapy Treatment of Varicose and Telangiectatic Leg Veins*. St. Louis, Mosby-Year-book Inc., 1991.)

incompetent perforating vein, a radiating flare of telangiectasia from a central point may also indicate an incompetent perforator vein. Although there is no substitute for sound clinical judgment, recommendations for performing a venous Doppler examination include:

1. Patients with varicosities greater than 4 mm in diameter.
2. Any varicosity over 2 mm in diameter extending throughout the calf or thigh.
3. Any varicosity extending into the groin or popliteal fossae.
4. When a "starburst" cluster of telangiectasia is present, especially if it is over the usual points of perforating veins (mid-posterior calf, medial knee, medial mid-thigh, medial distal calf).
5. Patients with a history of deep vein thrombosis and/or thrombophlebitis.
6. Patients who have undergone previous venous surgery or sclerotherapy with poor results or recurrence of varicosities.

The deep venous system is evaluated at three sites for the presence of acute or chronic damage to the valvular system by thrombosis or phlebitis. One listens for normal one-way flow at the junction of the femoral and iliac veins in the groin, in the popliteal vein in its fossae, and in the posterior tibial vein in the medial malleolar region. Patients are best examined in a warm room lying down. A spontaneous continuous venous signal near the arterial signal should be heard over all of the above-mentioned veins unless venoconstriction is present from low temperature or emotional excitation. Augmentation of the venous signal is performed by applying pressure distal to the Doppler probe. Lack of augmentation should be heard if pressure is applied proximal to the probe.

The first point in examining the superficial system is the saphenofemoral junction (SFJ). The Doppler probe is placed on the anterior medial thigh a few centimeters below the groin crease. The long saphenous vein (LSV) is located by moving the probe along the thigh while performing a short series of compressions on the medial distal thigh to augment flow. When it is located, competence of the LSV is established by eliciting one-way flow through augmentations. The patient then performs a Valsalva maneuver. If significant flow occurs down the LSV lasting longer than a few seconds, the SFJ in incompetent. This can be confirmed through duplex examination (described below). A wide range of accuracy for venous Doppler examination of SFJ incompetence has been reported, which probably reflects the experience of the examiner. At times, competent iliac vein valves or occlusion with Valsalva from the inguinal ligament may give a false-negative examination. Overall, the accuracy ranges between 80 and 100%.

A similar sequence of augmentation and release is then performed over any other visible varicose veins to determine if they are competent and if the incompetence arises from the SFJ. In addition, Doppler examination permits a fairly accurate tracing of the varicose vein origin, which aids in determining if reflux comes from the LSV or short saphenous vein. Atypical reflux may also occur through incompetent pelvic varicosities or anatomic anomalies described elsewhere. Finally, fascial defects are examined for evidence of perforator vein incompetence. Augmentation maneuvers will produce the loudest amplitude changes over the pathological perforator veins. These points should be treated first with sclerotherapy.

Light reflection rheography [(LRR), photoplethysmography] offers a simple technique for "physiologically" evaluating the efficiency of the calf muscle pump. With this instrument, a light source illuminates a small area of skin, which by convention is located 8–10 mm above the medial malleolus. An adjacent photoelectric sensor measures light reflectance, which correlates with cutaneous blood volume. The patient sits with the knee bent at a 80–70° angle and raises the toe 10 times in synchrony with the machine to empty the superficial venous plexus through the calf pump. The photoelectric cell measures the time until cutaneous blood volume returns to

baseline [refilling time (RF)]. By convention, a RF of <25 sec indicates venous valvular insufficiency. If a shortened RF occurs, the test is repeated after applying a tourniquet above or below the knee at 40–60 mmHg. This effectively prevents reflux from the superficial venous system. If the RF normalizes, a presumptive diagnosis of hemodynamically significant incompetent superficial veins can be made. If the RF remains abnormal, the deep venous system may be damaged and sclerotherapy should not be performed without further evaluation.

The LRR can also be used to assess the efficacy of sclerotherapy treatment. Successful treatment will normalize the LRR RF. An abnormal RF after sclerotherapy treatment should alert the physician to more closely evaluate the superficial venous system for additional incompetent perforator veins, or recanalized sclerosed veins. Figure 7 is a useful guide to LRR evaluation and treatment.

Duplex sonography is the most advanced (and expensive) modality for evaluating the patient prior to sclerotherapy. This modality combines the utility of venous Doppler with pictorial information from sonography. As a screening tool, duplex sonography evaluates the deep venous system for evidence of thrombosis. Most perforating veins can be accurately localized, and the degree of junctional reflux can be quantified. During treatment, duplex sonography can aid the physician in placing the sclerosing solution accurately within the desired vein. In addition, augmentation maneuvers can be used to determine if effective sclerosis occurs with injection. Posttreatment, duplex sonography can be used to evaluate the degree of endofibrosis and recanalizations in sclerosed veins. Although duplex sonography is not indicated for the majority of varicose vein patients, its availability enhances the quality of a sclerotherapy practice.

SCLEROSING SOLUTIONS

The goal of sclerotherapy treatment is to destroy the endothelium producing endosclerosis with resorption of the resulting fibrotic process. The key event is endothelial destruction. Too little destruction leads to thrombosis without fibrosis and early recanalization. Too much destruction leads to vascular dehiscence with resulting extravasation of red blood cells and sclerosing solution into perivascular tissues. This produces hyperpigmentation through hemosiderin-laden macrophages and may also produce cutaneous necrosis through direct toxic effects on dermal tissue. In addition, excessive inflammation may stimulate angiogenic and vasodilatory effects, which may lead to telangiectatic matting. Therefore, one must choose the appropriate sclerosing solution and, most importantly, the appropriate concentration of solution. Sadick has coined the term minimal sclerosant concentration (MSC) through an evaluation of the effectiveness of different concentrations of hypertonic saline (HS). Studies utilizing the rabbit ear vein have also determined MSCs for a variety of sclerosing solutions. Table 1 summarizes recommended MSCs for various vessel diameters.

Every sclerosing solution has its own inherent advantages and disadvantages (Table 2). Although the author personally utilizes four different sclerosing solutions at various concentrations in his practice to tailor treatment to the particular patient, excellent results can be achieved with any sclerosing solution. Space does not permit a complete discussion of each type of sclerosing solution; this appears elsewhere. It is also inappropriate to discuss the rationale for using FDA-approved versus non–FDA-approved solutions. This section will present a summary of the three types of sclerosing solutions—detergent solutions, osmotic agents and chemical irritants.

Detergent Solutions

Sodium morrhuate (SM) (Scleromate, Palisades Pharmaceuticals Inc., Tenafly, NJ) is a mixture of sodium salts of the saturated and unsaturated fatty acids present in cod liver oil. As with all

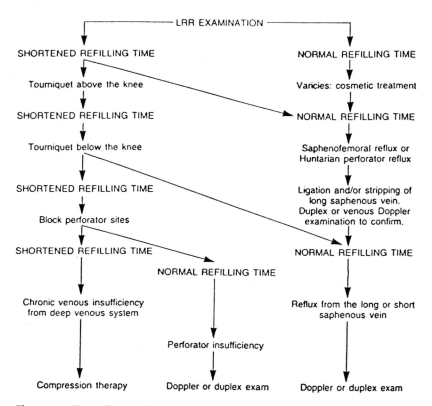

Figure 7 Flow diagram for light reflection rheography as an aid to planning treatment. (Modified from Neumann HAM, Boersma I. Light reflection rheography: a noninvasive diagnostic tool for screening venous disease. *J Dermatol Surg Oncol* 1992;18:125–130.)

detergent solutions, SM acts to damage endothelial membranes through alterations of cell surface lipids. The disadvantages of SM consist primarily of extensive cutaneous necrosis when it is inadvertently injected perivascularly and allergic reactions. Anaphylactic reactions have occurred within a few minutes of injection or more commonly when injections are repeated after a few weeks. Anaphylactic reactions have rarely been fatal. Of note is that there have been no reports of allergic reactions involving SM in the recent medical literature. Gallagher describes treating 20,000 patients over 25 years with one anaphylactic reaction 15 years ago and 20 anaphylactoid reactions, all with favorable outcomes. Sodium morrhuate is approved by FDA for sclerosis of varicose veins. However, because of its extremely caustic nature, it is not recommended for treating telangiectasias.

Ethanolamine oleate (EO) (Etholamin, Block Drug Company, Piscataway, NJ) is a synthetic mixture of ethanolamine and oleic acid with an empirical formula of $C_{20}H_{41}NO_3$. The oleic acid component is responsible for the inflammatory action. Oleic acid may also activate coagulation in vitro by release of tissue factors and Hageman factor XII. Although EO is mainly used in the United States for sclerosis of esophageal varices, it is commonly used in Australia for sclerotherapy of varicose veins.

Ethanolamine oleate is thought to have a decreased risk of allergic reactions compared to SM or sodium tetradecyl sulfate. Anaphylactic shock has been reported following injection in a

Table 1 Relative Potency of Sclerosing Solutions (minimal sclerosant concentrations)

Vein diameter (mm)	Sclerosing solution
<0.4	Scleremo 1:1
	Polidocanol 0.25%
	Sodium tetradecyl sulfate 0.1%
	Scleremo 100%
	Polidocanol 0.5%
	Variglobin 0.1%
	Hypertonic saline 11.7%
	Sclerodex
	Ethanolamine oleate 2%
	Sodium morrhuate 1%
0.6–2	Sodium tetradecyl sulfate 0.25%
	Polidocanol 0.75%
	Variglobin 1.0%
	Hypertonic saline 23.4%
	Ethanolamine oleate 5%
	Sodium morrhuate 2.5%
3–5	Polidocanol 1–2%
	Sodium tetradecyl sulfate 0.5–1.0%
	Variglobin 2%
	Sodium morrhuate 5%
>5	Polidocanol 3–5%
Perforating vessels	Sodium tetradecyl sulfate 2–3%
Saphenopopliteal and saphenofemoral junction	Variglobin 3–12%

Source: Goldman. By permission of Mosby-Yearbook, Inc.

Table 2 Sclerosing Agents

	Active ingredient	Allergic reaction	Necrosis	Pain
Osmotic agents				
Hypertonic saline	18–30% saline	None	Occasional[b]	Moderate
Sclerodex[a]	10% saline + 5% dextrose	None	Occasional	Mild
Chemical irritants				
Scleremo	Chromated glycerin	Rare	Very rare	Moderate
Variglobin	Polyiodinated iodine	Rare	Frequent	Moderate
Detergents				
Sodium morrhuate[a]	Fatty acids in cod liver oil	Occasional	Frequent[b]	Moderate
Sotradecol[a]	Sodium tetradecyl sulfate	Occasional	Occasional[b]	Mild
Aethoxysklerol[c]	Polidocanol	Very rare	Very rare[b]	None
Etholamin	Ethanolamine oleate	Occasional	Occasional	Mild

[a]Approved for use by the Food and Drug Administration.
[b]Concentration dependent.
[c]Not approved for use in the United States.
Source: Goldman. By permission of Mosby-Yearbook, Inc.

number of patients. Generalized urticaria occurred in about 1 out of 400 patients, clearing with antihistamines.

Some degree of nonspecific red blood cell hemolysis may also occur with its use. A hemolytic reaction occurred in 5 out of 900 patients with injection of over 12 ml 0.5% EO per patient per treatment session. Acute renal failure with spontaneous recovery followed injection of 15–20 ml EO in two women.

Sodium tetradecyl sulfate (STS) [Sotradecol, Elkins Sinn, Cherry Hill, NJ), sodium 1-isobutyl-4-ethyloctyl sulfate plus benzoyl alcohol 2% (as an anesthetic agent)] is a synthetic long-chain fatty acid salt of an alkali metal with detergent properties. It is commonly used worldwide as a sclerosant for varicose and telangiectatic veins. Sodium tetradecyl sulfate, presently approved for use by FDA for vein sclerosis, has a number of disadvantages. Epidermal necrosis frequently occurs if concentrations over 0.5% are even slightly extravasated. Occasional anaphylactic shock and, more commonly, generalized urticaria and edema or diffuse maculopapular eruptions have been noted.

Polidocanol (POL) [hydroxypolyethoxydodecane, Aethoxysklerol, Chemische Fabrik Kreussler & Co GmbH, Wiesbaden-Biebrich, Germany) is a urethane anesthetic (compounds with an $-NHCO_2-$ linkage). Unlike the two main groups of local anesthetics, the esters (procaine, benzocaine, and tetracaine), and the amides (lidocaine, prilocaine, mepivacaine, procainamide, and dibucaine), POL lacks an aromatic ring. The actual active substance is an aliphatic molecule composed of a hydrophilic chain of polyethylene glycolic ether and a liposoluble radical of dodecylic alcohol. Polidocanol is a weaker detergent type of sclerosant than STS. Experimental studies indicate that its sclerosant power is about 50% that of STS. Polidocanol is unique among sclerosing agents in that it is painless to inject (when the solution, which contains 5% alcohol, is diluted) and will not produce cutaneous ulcerations even with intradermal injection of a 1% solution. Allergic reactions have only been reported in four patients with an estimated incidence of 0.01%. In addition, patients who are allergic to STS do not develop an allergic reaction with POL.

Osmotic Solutions

Hypertonic saline (HS) (sodium chloride 23.4%, Lymphomed Inc., Rosemont, IL), unlike detergent sclerosing solutions, acts nonspecifically to destroy all cells (intra- and extravascular) within its osmotic gradient. Therefore, osmotic agents are very damaging to all cellular tissues, readily producing ulceration if injected (or with seepage) extravascularly. In addition, osmotic agents are rapidly diluted in a blood-filled vein, losing potency within a short distance of injection. Thus, these agents are not recommended for treating veins larger than 1–2 mm in diameter. Unadulterated HS is not an allergen. An annoying adverse effect of its use is unpleasant stinging on injection and 5 min or so of muscle cramping immediately following injection. Pain and cramping can be minimized by using MSC.

Heparsol (20% hypertonic saline, 100 units/ml heparin, and 1% procaine) was patented by Foley in 1975 for microinjection of "venous blemishes." He believed that adding heparin helped prevent thrombi in larger vessels, with procaine decreasing the immediate pain and cramping from injection. Recently, Sadick, in a randomized, blinded, 800-patient study, found no benefit for adding heparin to HS.

Sclerodex (SX) (Dextroject, Ondee Laboratory Ltd, Montreal, Quebec, Canada) is a mixture of dextrose 250 mg/ml, sodium chloride 100 mg/ml, and phenethyl alcohol 8 mg/ml (as a local anesthetic/preservative) and is mainly used in Canada for sclerosis of telangiectasias. It is essentially a midpotency hypertonic solution with a mechanism of action similar to that of HS. It is best reserved for vessels less than 1 mm in diameter. Mantse notes one allergic reaction in

500 patients treated with SX, an incidence of 0.2%. Like HS, it is slightly painful on injection and occasionally produces superficial necrosis.

Chemical Irritants

Polyiodide iodide (PII) (Varigloban, Chemische Fabrik Kreussler & Co., Wiesbaden-Biebrich, Germany; Variglobin, Globopharm, Switzerland; Sclerodine, Omega, Montreal, Canada) is a stabilized water solution of iodide ions, sodium iodine, and benzyl alcohol. The active sclerosing ingredient is iodine, with sodium and potassium increasing its water solubility. Benzyl alcohol is added as a preservative/stabilizer. The sclerosing effect is from direct destruction of endothelium. The entire vessel wall is destroyed through defusion at the point of injection. It is neutralized within a few seconds by binding to different blood components, especially proteins, and thus its sclerosing effect is lost within a centimeter or two. Polyiodide iodide is primarily used for large varicosities including the saphenofemoral junction. Paravenous injections produce extensive tissue necrosis. Fortunately, PII is painful when injected outside a vein so that improper injection technique is immediately apparent. To prevent nonspecific damage, the concentration, not the volume, of solution is increased to enhance sclerosing power.

Chromated glycerin, 72% (SCL) (Scleremo, Laboratories E Bouteille, Limoges, France), is a polyalcohol with a mechanism of action similar to that of PII. It provokes endothelial lesions without desquamation of endothelial cells in plaques. Its clinical efficacy has been shown to be dose dependent with a very low incidence of adverse sequelae. In the dorsal rabbit ear vein, undiluted SCL appears to be equivalent in potency to 0.25% polidocanol. The relatively weak sclerosing power of SCL corresponds to its promotion as a mild sclerosant. Pigmentation and cutaneous necrosis are exceedingly rare. The disadvantages of SCL include high viscosity and local pain with injection. These drawbacks can be partially overcome by dilution with 1% lidocaine without epinephrine. Hypersensitivity is very rare. Hematuria accompanied by ureteral colic can occur transiently following injection of over 10 ml undiluted SCL. Ocular complications, including blurred vision and partial vision field loss, have been reported by a single author with resolution in less than 2 hr.

POSTSCLEROSIS COMPRESSION

Postsclerosis compression is perhaps the most important advance in sclerotherapy treatment of varicose veins since the introduction of relatively safe synthetic sclerosing agents in the 1940s. Primarily, compression eliminates a thrombophlebitic reaction and substitutes a 'sclerophlebitis' with the production of a firm fibrous cord. For compression to be effective it must be given in a graduated manner to prevent a tourniquet effect. Higher proximal external pressures will cause retrograde blood flow with further dilatation of distal superficial veins. However, localized increase in pressure can be given with foam pads or cotton balls which will increase pressure under the pad by 15–50% (Fig. 8). A complete discussion of graduated compression appears elsewhere.

Compression serves at least five purposes. First, compression, if adequate, may result in direct apposition of the treated vein walls to produce more effective fibrosis. Therefore, sclerosing solutions of lesser strength may be successfully utilized. Second, compressing the treated vessel will decrease the extent of thrombus formation, which inevitably occurs with the use of all sclerosing agents, thereby decreasing the risk for recanalization of the treated vessel. Third, a decrease in the extent of thrombus formation may also decrease the incidence of postsclerosis pigmentation. Fourth, the limitation of thrombosis and phlebitic reactions may prevent the appearance of telangiectatic matting. Finally, the function of the calf muscle pump is improved by the physiological effect of a graduated compression stocking. This improved efficiency promotes

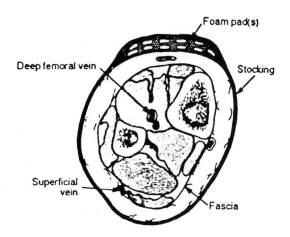

Figure 8 Schematic cross-section of a superficial varicose vein compressed with a foam rubber pad under a compression stocking. Note that superficial varicosities lateral to the foam rubber pad are only slightly compressed, and veins deep to the fascia are not compressed. (Reproduced with permission from Goldman MP. *Sclerotherapy Treatment of Varicose and Telangiectatic Leg Veins*. St. Louis, Mosby-Yearbook Inc., 1991.)

emptying of the superficial veins into the deep system, thereby decreasing their diameter. In addition, by externally supporting untreated large veins, compression stockings will narrow vein diameters, restoring valve function and decreasing retrograde blood flow. External pressure will also retard the reflux of blood from incompetent perforating veins into the superficial veins. In short, compression sclerotherapy is now the standard practice for the treatment of varicose veins.

Compression is also advocated for treating leg telangiectasia. Although one study has found that superficial telangiectasias require up to 80 mmHg for complete closure, graduated compression has a number of potential benefits. First, since telangiectasias are fed by veins of larger diameter, compression (via Laplace's law) will produce a greater decrease in luminal diameter of larger feeding veins, decreasing inflow into distal telangiectasias. In addition, if a direct connection exists between telangiectasias and the deep venous system, which has been demonstrated in 13% of patients radiographically, compression will ensure rapid dilution of sclerosant from deep veins, thereby preventing endothelial or valvular damage with subsequent thromboembolic complications. Finally, graduated compression, while not totally closing telangiectasia luminal diameter, will decrease the lumen. A decreased luminal diameter will limit thrombus formation and its resulting complications as demonstrated in a multicenter study.

SUMMARY

The treatment of varicose and telangiectatic leg veins can be approached in a logical, systematic fashion (Table 3). Instead of merely the injection of as many veins as possible in a given period of time, "venous regions" or entire abnormal superficial venous networks on the leg can and should be injected in a single session. Although patients will require differing amounts of time with this systematic approach, with experience, accurate estimations can be made ensuring optimal productivity. It is illogical for physicians to only treat large veins or small veins. A phlebologist (sclerotherapist) should strive to appreciate the venous system as a complete "system." With this understanding, we will be best able to render optimal care. Hopefully, this will

Table 3 Sclerotherapy of Varicose Veins—Sequence of Events

1. Physical examination
2. Venous Doppler/light reflection rheography
3. If abnormal, consider duplex scanning or varicography
4. Eliminate high-pressure inflow points
   (a) Saphenofemoral—popleteal junction
   (b) Incompetent perforators
5. Sclerotherapy of large-diameter varicose veins
6. Sclerotherapy of communicating or reticular veins which feed "spider" telangiectasias
7. Sclerotherapy of "spider" telangiectasias
8. Yellow light laser treatment of remaining fine telangiectasias and arteriolar telangiectasias

Source: Modified from Goldman. By permission of Mosby-Yearbook, Inc.

prevent present-day entnusiasm for sclerotherapy to disappear as it did in the 1940s so that the wheel will not have to be "reinvented" in the future.

BIBLIOGRAPHY

Allan JC. The micro-circulation of the skin of the normal leg, in varicose veins and in the post-thrombotic syndrome. *S African J Surg* 1972;10:29.

Beesley WH, Fegan WG. An investigation into the localization of incompetent perforating veins. *Br J Surg* 1970;57:30.

Bohler-Sommeregger K, Karnel F, Schuller-Petrovic S, et al. Do telangiectases communicate with the deep venous system? *J Dermatol Surg Oncol* 1992;18:403–406.

Braverman IM. Ultrastructure and organization of cutaneous microvasculature in normal and pathologic states. *J Invest Dermatol* 1989;93:28.

Dick ET. The treatment of varicose veins. *NZ Med J* 1966;65:310–313.

Fegan WG. The complications of compression sclerotherapy. *The Practitioner* 1971;207:797–799.

Fegan WG. Compression sclerotherapy. *Ann R Coll Surg Engl* 1967;41:364.

Fegan WG. Continuing uninterrupted compression technique of injecting varicose veins. *Proc R Soc Med* 1960;53:837–840.

Fegan WG. Continuous compression technique of injecting varicose veins. *Lancet* 1963;2:109–12.

Fentem PH, Goddard M, Godden BA, et al. Control of distension of varicose veins achieved by leg bandages as used after injection sclerotherapy. *Br Med J* 1976;2:725.

Foley WT. The eradication of venous blemishes. *Cutis* 1975;15:665–668.

Foote RR. Severe reaction to monoethanolamine oleate. *Lancet* 1944;2:390–391.

Fronek H. Noninvasive examination of the patient before sclerotherapy. In *Sclerotherapy treatment of varicose and telangiectatic leg veins*. MP Goldman, ed. St. Louis, Mosby-Yearbook, 1991, pp. 108–157.

Fronek H, Fronek A, Saltzbarg G. Allergic reactions to sotradecol. *J Dermatol Surg Oncol* 1989;15:684.

Gallagher PG. Varicose veins—primary treatment with sclerotherapy: a personal appraisal. *J Dermatol Surg Oncol* 1992;18:39–42.

Glaxo, Inc., Ethanolamin injection 5%, product information. 1988.

Glaxo Pharmaceuticals. Product insert. Research Triangle Park, NC, 1989.

Goldman MP. A comparison of sclerosing agents: clinical and histologic effects of intravascular sodium morrhuate, ethanolamine oleate, hypertonic saline (11.7 percent), and sclerodex in the dorsal rabbit ear vein. *J Dermatol Surg Oncol* 1991;17:354–362.

Goldman MP. Compression hosiery and elastic bandages. In *Sclerotherapy Treatment of Varicose and Telangiectatic Veins*. MP Goldman, ed. St. Louis, Mosby-Yearbook, 1991, pp. 158–182.

Goldman MP. *Sclerotherapy Treatment of Varicose and Telangiectatic Leg Veins*. St. Louis, Mosby-Yearbook, 1991.

Goldman MP, Beaudoing D, Marley W, et al. Compression in the treatment of leg telangiectasia. *J Dermatol Surg Oncol* 1990;16:322–325.

Goldman MP, Bennett RG. Treatment of telangiectasia: a review. *J Am Acad Dermatol* 1987;17:167–182.

Goldman MP, Kaplan RP, Duffy DM. Postsclerotherapy hyperpigmentation: a histologic evaluation. *J Dermatol Surg Oncol* 1987;13:547–550.

Goldman MP, Kaplan RP, Oki LN, et al. Sclerosing agents in the treatment of telangiectasia: comparison of the clinical and histologic effects of intravascular polidocanol, sodium tetradecyl sulfate, and hypertonic saline in the dorsal rabbit ear vein model. *Arch Dermatol* 1987;123:1196–1201.

Harridge H. The treatment of primary varicose veins. *Surg Clin North Am* 1960;40:191–202.

Heberova V. Treatment of telangiectasias of the lower extremities by sclerotization. Results and evaluation. *Cs Dermatol* 1976;51:232–235.

Hoare MC, Royle JP. Doppler ultrasound detection of saphenofemoral and saphenopopleteal incompetence and operative venography to ensure precise saphenopopleteal ligation. *Aust NZ J Surg* 1984;54:49–52.

Hughes RW Jr, Larson DE, Viggiane TR, et al. Endoscopic variceal sclerosis: a one-year experience. *Gastrointest Endosc* 1982;28:62.

Hutinel B. Esthetique dans les scleroses de varices et traitement des varicosites. *La Vie Medicale* 1978;20:1739–1743.

Imhoff E, Stemmer R. Classification and mechanism of action of sclerosing agents. *Soc Franc Phlebol* 1969;22:143–148.

Jaquier JJ, Loretan RM. Clinical trials of a new sclerosing agent, aethoxysklerol. *Soc Franc Phlebol* 1969;22:383–385.

Lewis KM. Anaphylaxis due to sodium morrhuate. *JAMA* 1936;107:1298.

Linser P. Ueber die konservative Behandlung der Varicen. *Med Klin* 1916;12:897.

Lufkin H, McPheeters HQ. Pathological studies on injected varicose veins. *Surg Gynecol Obstet* 1932;54:511–517.

McAusland S. The modern treatment of varicose veins. *Med Press* 1939;201:404–410.

McIrvine AJ, Corbett CRR, Aston NO, et al. The demonstration of saphenofemoral incompetence; Doppler ultrasound compared with standard clinical tests. *J Surg* 1984;71:509–510.

Mantse L. A mild sclerosing agent for telangiectasias. *J Dermatol Surg Oncol* 1985;11:9.

Martin DE, Goldman MP. A comparison of sclerosing agents: clinical and histologic effects of intravascular sodium tetradecyl sulfate and chromated glycerin in the dorsal rabbit ear vein. *J Dermatol Surg Oncol* 1990;16:18–22.

Miyake H, Kauffman P, de Arruda Behmer O, et al. Mechanisms of cutaneous necrosis provoked by sclerosing injections in the treatment of microvarices and telangiectasias: experimental study. *Rev Ass Brasil* 1976;22:115–120.

Nebot F. Quelques points tecniques sur le traitement des varicosites et des telangiectasies. *Phlebologie* 1968;21:133–135.

Neumann HAM, Boersma I. Light reflection rheography: a non-invasive diagnostic tool for screening venous disease. *J Dermatol Surg Oncol* 1992;18:425–430.

O'Donnell TF Jr, Burhand KG, Clemenson G, et al. Doppler examination vs clinical and phlebologic detection of the location of incompetent perforating veins. *Arch Surg* 1977;112:31.

Orbach EJ. A new approach to the sclerotherapy of varicose veins. *Angiology* 1950;1:302.

Ouvry PA. Telangiectasia and sclerotherapy. *J Dermatol Surg Oncol* 1989;15:177–181.

Ouvry P, Arlaud R. Le traitement sclerosant des telangiectasies des membres inferieurs. *Phlebologie* 1979;32:365–370.

Ouvry P, Davy A. Le traitement sclerosant des telangiectasies des membres inferieurs. *Phlebologie* 1982;35:349–359.

Passas H. One case of tetradecyl-sodium sulfate allergy with general symptoms. *Soc Franc Phlebol* 1972;25:19–26.

Perthes G. Über die operation der Unterschelkenvaricen nach Trendelenburg. *Dtsh Med Wehrschr* 1895;21:253.

Pravas C-G. *CR Acad Sci* 1853;236:88.

Raj TB, Goddard M, Makin GS. How long do compression bandages maintain their pressure during ambulatory treatment of varicose veins? *Br J Surg* 1980;67:122.

Reid RG, Rothnie NG. Treatment of varicose veins by compression sclerotherapy. *Br J Surg* 1968;55:889–895.

Reiner L. The activity of anionic surface active compounds in producing vascular obliteration. *Proc Soc Exp Biol Med* 1946;62:49.

Sadick NS. Sclerotherapy of varicose and telangiectatic leg veins: minimal sclerosant concentration of hypertonic saline and its relationship to vessel diameter. *J Dermatol Surg Oncol* 1991;17:65–70.

Sadick NS. The treatment of varicose and telangiectatic leg veins with hypertonic saline: a comparative study of heparin and saline. *J Dermatol Surg Oncol* 1990;16:24–28.

Schultz-Ehrenburg U, Hubner H-J. *Reflux Diagnosis with Doppler Ultrasound.* New York, FK Schattauer Verlag, 1989.

Scleremo Product Information. Laboratoires E. Bouteille, 7 rue des Belges, 8100 Limoges, France, 1987.

Sigg K. The treatment of varicosities and accompanying complications. *Angiology* 1952;3:355.

Somerville JJ, Brown GO, Byrne PJ, et al. The effect of elastic stockings on superficial venous pressures in patients with venous insufficiency. *Br J Surg* 1974;61:979–981.

Stemmer R. *Sclerotherapy of Varicose Veins.* St. Gallen, Switzerland, Anzonie & Cie, 1990, pp. 6–8.

Stother IG, Bryson A, Alexander S. The treatment of varicose veins by compression sclerotherapy. *Br J Surg* 1974;61:387–390.

Struckman J, Christensen SJ, Lendorf A, et al. Venous muscle pump improvement by low compression elastic stockings. *Phlebology* 1986;1:97–103.

Taylor GI, Caddy CM, Watterson PA, et al. The venous territories (venosomes) of the human body: experimental study and clinical implications. *J Plast Reconstr Surg* 1990;86:185–213.

Townsend J, Jones H, Williams JE. Detection of incompetent perforating veins by venography at operation. *Br Med J* 1967;3:583.

Trendelenburg F. Über die Unterbindung der Yena Saphena Magna bei Unterschelkenvaricen. *Beitr Z Klin Chir* 1891;7:195.

Wallois P. Incidents et accidents de la sclerose. In *La Sclerose des Varices.* 4th ed. R Tournay, ed. Paris, Expansion Scientifique Francaise, 1985, pp. 297–319.

Wenner L. Anwendung einer mit Athylalkohol modifizerten Polijodidjonenlösung bei Skleroseresistenten Varizen. *VASA* 1983;12:190–192.

Wenner L. Sind Endovarikose hamatische Ansammlungen eine Normalerscheinung bei Sklerotherapie? *VASA* 1981;10:174–176.

69

Hair Transplantation

James Bernard Pinski
Northwestern University Medical School, Chicago, Illinois

Hair replacement by multiple punch autografts was described by Orentreich in 1959. Since then, the technique has undergone considerable refinement, which has improved the cosmetic and therapeutic benefits. Hair transplantation is the most common operation performed on men. It is estimated that more than one million bald patients have elected to have this procedure.

Androchronogenetic alopecia (a term used by Orentreich) or male pattern baldness depends upon the interaction of androgens, age or time, and genetics. Dihydrotestosterone, acting on genetically predisposed hair follicles, produces miniaturization of hair with resultant baldness. There are approximately 100,000 hairs on the average scalp, but up to 50% can be lost before thinning is noted.

The success of hair transplantation is based on transplanted hair follicles that will behave as they did in their original habitat and continue to grow. They are unresponsive to dihydrotestosterone. Grafts taken from areas susceptible to dihydrotestosterone (e.g., as too high or low on the occiput) will be lost (Fig. 1).

The following information will largely reflect the author's approach unless otherwise noted. There are many variations, but in the end the result speaks for itself. A good hair transplant is not noticed but a poor result is always apparent.

PREOPERATIVE EVALUATION

Prior to scheduling a patient for hair transplantation, consultation is essential. The patient must be carefully evaluated and the procedure explained in great detail so that the patient will totally understand what is involved. The best candidates for hair transplantation have sufficient donor hair of adequate density. Age is not a determining factor, as long as the patient is in good health. Those with light-colored or gray hair appear to have denser hair since there is less contrast between hair and scalp (Figs. 2,3). This is also true of those with thick, curly hair since it tends to cover up more area (Figs. 4,5).

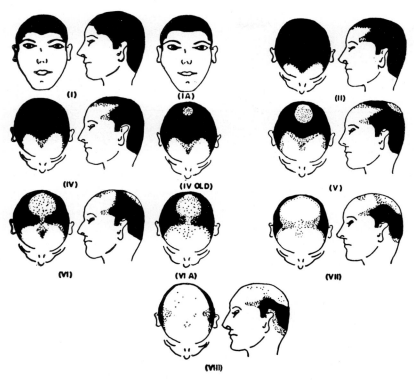

Figure 1 Patterns of male androgenic alopecia.

The question of when to start hair transplantation is difficult to answer. Many start when there is sufficient alopecia that can be corrected and before it is apparent that the patient has lost a great deal of hair. Thus, the healing wounds can be covered by the existing hair. It is also important to start hair transplantation while the patient is relatively young. Hair is important to a young person with an active social life and who is trying to forge ahead in the business world. At the other end of the spectrum, there are those in their sixties and seventies who desire hair transplantation and in whom very good results have been achieved.

Prior to surgery, laboratory studies are performed. These include a complete blood count, serum chemistry profile, syphilis screen, coagulation studies, hepatitis screens, and a test for acquired immunodeficiency syndrome. Patients who have abnormal results of laboratory studies must be evaluated medically prior to surgery.

Preoperatively patients are placed on phytonadione (vitamin K) 5 mg twice daily beginning 1 week prior to surgery and continuing through the day of surgery. The author finds that this has reduced the incidence of bleeding and helped with coagulation. Prior to surgery, erythromycin 500 mg twice daily is instituted and continued for 1 week postoperatively. In addition, the patient receives 1 ml (6 mg) betamethasone intramuscularly at the time of surgery. This is most important in reducing edema and postoperative inflammation.

INSTRUMENTATION

The original trephines or punches used for hair transplantation surgery were hand-held, and the surgeon twisted and pushed or just pushed downward to cut the graft (Fig. 6). One of the most

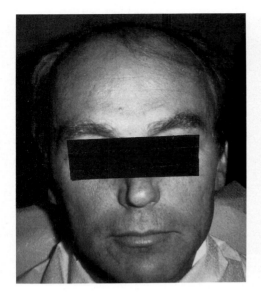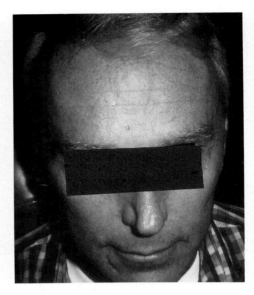

Figure 2,3 Light-colored or gray hair gives the appearance of being denser since there is less contrast between hair and scalp. Scalp is shown pre- and posttransplantation.

significant advances in hair transplant surgery was the development of the power punch. Superior-quality grafts and thus more hair growth are obtained while at the same time enhancing patient comfort during the procedure. There are several power units available (Figs. 7,8). Operate the unit at approximately 5000–6000 rpm or one third of the maximum speed. A rapid revolution rate causes heat or physical injury to the peripheral follicles.

The power punch must operate without vibration or wobble, which could occur as a result of motor movement of the power tool within the housing but most commonly occurs as a result

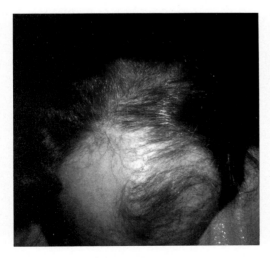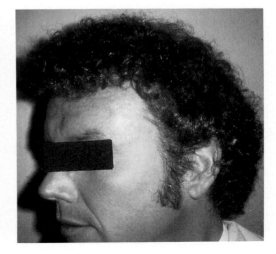

Figure 4,5 Coarse, curly hair looks thicker since it covers more area. Scalp is shown pre- and posttransplantation.

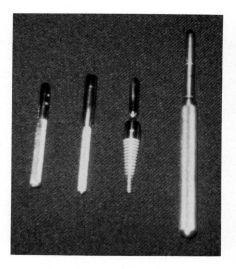

Figure 6 Various hand punches. Left to right: 1 and 2—Orentreich; 3—Stough; 4— long handle.

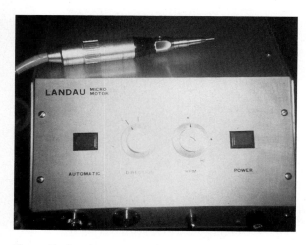

Figure 7 Landau power unit.

of defects in the punch itself. A slight bend in the shaft of the punch due to resharpening, the shaft being placed eccentrically on the hub of the punch, or the shaft not being perpendicular to the hub of the punch may cause wobbling, which will result in coning or peripheral damage to the plug. To check for wobbling, run the power unit at its lowest speed.

Patients prefer the power punch over the hand punch. With the hand punch, the patient will feel pressure as the punch is pushed into the scalp and a crunching sensation, which can be likened to chewing a carrot. This can be eliminated with the power punch. Grafts produced by the power punch are both subjectively and objectively superior to those of the hand punch. They tend

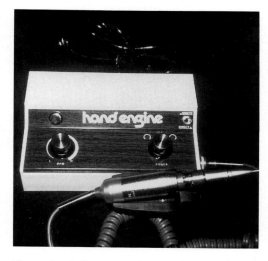

Figure 8 Bell power unit.

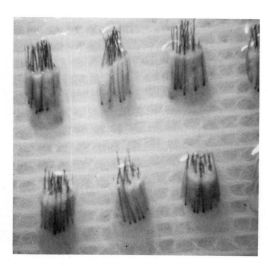

Figure 9 Superior-quality grafts are produced by the power punch.

to be more uniform and wider at both top and bottom, contain more viable hairs, and have less peripheral beveling and coning (Fig. 9).

It is important that the punch be exquisitely sharp or else the graft will be distorted, beveled, and torn at the periphery. The best quality punches or trephines are the Australian punches. They are made of carbon steel and have both internal and external bevels on the cutting edge and are polished internally as well as externally. Grafts cut with a dull punch are small, rough, and conical with the wide end on the skin surface (Fig. 10). Distortion of the graft is caused by the blunt punch indenting the skin and spreading the underlying tissues. A sharp punch cuts without pressure, and the grafts are broader at the base than at the skin surface. It is also important to use a sharp punch at the recipient sites; otherwise, the hole produced may be conical. This will cause compression of the graft and may result in less than perfect growth or perhaps curly hair because of pressure.

ANESTHESIA

It is not necessary to administer preoperative sedatives, but if requested, diazepam 5 or 10 mg orally or intravenously can be given. If the patient is subject to vasovagal syncope, an intramuscular injection of atropine, 1/150 grain, is useful. The predominant anesthetic used is 1 or 2% lidocaine with epinephrine 1:100,000. The epinephrine is essential to reduce bleeding. No more than 25 ml of 2% lidocaine should be administered to avoid toxicity. Bupivacaine 0.5% with epinephrine 1:200,000 may be added in small amounts at the anterior edge of the recipient site

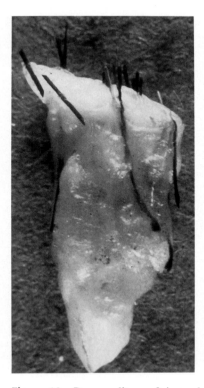

Figure 10 Poor-quality graft is produced by a dull punch, a hand punch, or not using saline to firm the donor area. (Courtesy of Tom Alt, M.D.)

and the inferior border of the donor area to prolong the duration of anesthesia. Lidocaine and bupivacaine are both supplied in 1.8 ml carpules that are inserted into a dental-type syringe to which a 30-gauge needle is attached.

PREOPERATIVE CONSIDERATIONS

It is important to plan each surgical session in advance. Efficient technique and able assistance are essential; otherwise, the procedure takes an inordinate amount of time. Prior to beginning surgery, a hairline is outlined. The proposed hairline must be suitable for the remainder of the patient's life. Therefore, it must not be too low and take into account temporal recession that may occur in the future. It is best to err on the conservative side, since it is always easier to lower the hairline than to attempt to remove transplants once they have been inappropriately placed.

Prior to surgery, each recipient site is premarked with a cotton-tipped applicator with gentian violet (Figs. 11,12). Others use a marking pencil or a dull punch and an ink pad. An area

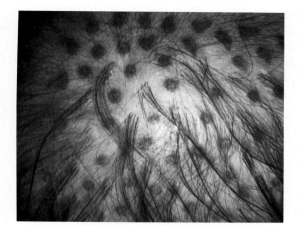

Figure 11

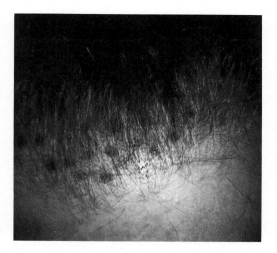

Figure 11,12   Recipient sites premarked for both spacing and direction.

of hair-bearing scalp, usually from the occipital area, is clipped so that the hairs are cut short to the scalp, but not shaved. It is important to leave a sufficient length of hair available to determine the angle at which the hair emerges from the scalp, so that the punch may be directed parallel to this (Figs. 13,14). Some operators will use a rectangular donor area and remove four or five rows of 15 or 20 grafts per row (Fig. 15). Others use one or two long rows and suture the donor site postoperatively (Fig. 16).

PROCEDURE

The average frontal hairline is five to six rows deep and requires at least four sessions of 4-mm grafts placed into a 3.5-mm recipient holes (Figs. 17,18). This differential between graft and recipient site results in a close approximation as the graft tends to shrink when removed from the scalp, and the recipient site tends to expand. There are variations when a 0.25-mm differ-

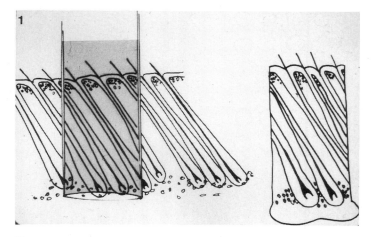

Figure 13

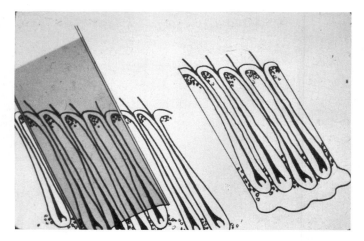

Figure 13,14   The angle of the punch after it penetrates the dermis should correspond to the angle of the hair as it emerges from the skin in order to obtain maximum growth from the graft. (Courtesy of Peter Goldman, M.D.)

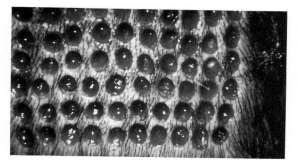

Figure 15 Rectangular donor site.

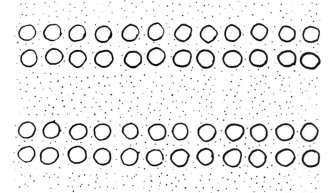

layered DONOR site technique

Figure 16 Layered donor site technique.

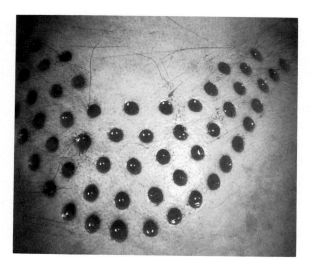

Figure 17 First session of 60 3.5-mm holes in recipient site.

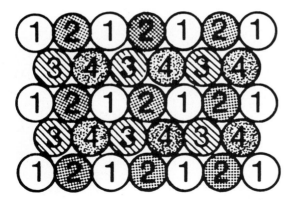

Figure 18 Pattern illustrating four (1,2,3,4) sessions for frontal hairline producing confluence of grafts.

ential or a 0.75-mm differential is required. To maintain adequate vascular supply, intact skin approximately 3.5 mm in diameter is left between each graft. A pattern should be followed so there is adequate space between each graft during each session. Spaces should be left between each graft and an empty row between each row after the first session. In the second session, grafts fill the spaces between the first grafts; the third and fourth sessions will fill between the rows. It takes at least four sessions to approximate the grafts in any given area (Figs. 19–21).

Grafts are placed at an acute angle of 20–30 degrees, producing a shingled effect as the hair grows. Keeping the hair low to the scalp and growing forward results in a natural appearance and greater coverage (Fig. 22).

The power punch has led to the production of superior-quality grafts that contain more viable hairs, have less peripheral beveling and coning, are wider at both top and bottom, and result

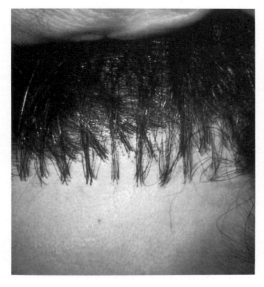

Figure 19 First session: spaces between each graft and an empty row between each row.

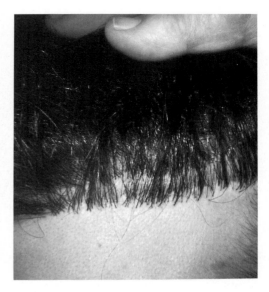

Figure 20 Second session: filling between each graft.

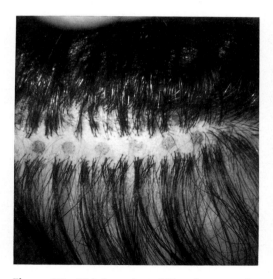

Figure 21 Third session: filling between the rows.

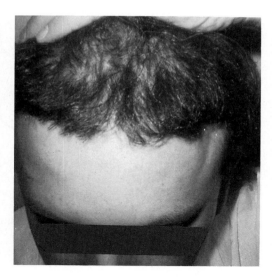

Figure 22 Shingling effect produced by placing the hair low to the scalp and growing forward to give a natural appearance and greater coverage.

in much better growth (Figs. 23,24). One might mistakenly think that because of the rapid spinning of the power punch, it need not be as sharp as the hand punch. The punch must be exquisitely sharp or else the plug will be distorted, beveled, and torn at the periphery.

In addition to an exquisitely sharp, power-driven punch, sufficient tissue turgor is essential to obtain good grafts. This is accomplished by dermal and subcutaneous injection of normal saline solution into the donor site. The amount of saline required for sufficient tissue turgor varies with each patient and surgical area, but it is injected until the donor area is distended as much as possible. Since the site is anesthetized, the saline injection is painless. The saline is absorbed

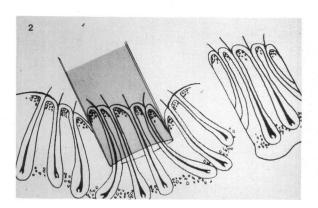

Figure 23 Distortion of donor site occurs with a dull punch, a hand punch, or without saline infiltration, resulting in a poor graft. (Courtesy of Peter Goldman, M.D.)

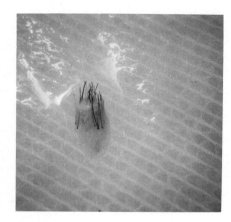

Figure 24 An ideal graft.

rapidly (approximately 1½–3 min). Therefore, only a small portion of the donor site is infiltrated at a time and grafts taken. Depending upon the speed of the surgeon, as many as 15 grafts can be harvested in that period of time. The total amount of saline used may vary from 60 to 150 ml per patient.

Saline infiltration firms the skin surface, which then resists the application of pressure while the graft is cut. The hair follicles are not bent while the grafts are cut, and there is less chance of damaging follicles at the periphery of the plug. If the donor site is not firm, the graft will be distorted by the cutting pressure. The pressure required to cut is inversely proportional to the degree of sharpness of the punch. Try to obtain a perfectly cylindrical graft with little or no lip.

One must make the graft parallel to the hair shafts so as not to transect hair follicles. The hand punch allows you to begin perpendicular to the scalp and then angle in with the follicles. The power punch should start at the proper angle to the hair shafts, because cutting occurs too rapidly to allow a change of direction after one begins. This may result in grafts that are slightly oval rather than round at the surface. The recipient holes are also cut at an acute angle to the surface of the scalp; thus the grafts fit well. The angle of the hair in adjacent areas of the scalp often varies, and it is necessary to check constantly that the grafts are made parallel to the hair shafts.

To remove a graft from the donor site, gently grasp it at the epidermis and trim any fibrous attachment with an iris scissors. Do not avulse a graft, since trauma will cause scarring and follicles may be lost. When handling the graft with forceps, be certain always to grasp it gently at the epidermis or upper dermis. Do not squeeze the graft. Never grasp a plug at the lower dermis or subcutaneous fat: hair bulbs could be traumatized. When trimming the subcutaneous fat, it is best to be conservative. Do not trim too much fat, thereby exposing the matrices. It is better to leave too much rather than too little subcutaneous fat.

Once they have been removed, keep the grafts moist in saline in a Petri dish at all times. Do not allow them to dry out in the process of trimming the grafts and awaiting insertion into the receptor sites. In an effort to increase the viability of the grafts and perhaps to reduce telogen effluvium, a plastic cup filled with a nontoxic gel and placed in a freezer until frozen is a convenient receptacle for the saline-filled Petri dish.

The characteristics of an ideal graft are (1) parallel to hair shafts, (2) follicles not transected, (3) perfect cylindrical shape, (4) glistening, smooth sides, and (5) minimal or no lip. To obtain perfect grafts, one must use a power-driven, sharp punch at moderate speed with firm saline infiltration. In this manner, the pressure exerted in performing the punch is minimized and distortion of the skin is reduced.

Following removal of the donor grafts and the discarded skin from the recipient site, hemostasis is obtained, and the scalp is cleansed with hydrogen peroxide. The grafts are then inserted into the recipient sites. Hairs are placed in an anterior direction, and the best grafts are put into the most strategic locations, usually anterior and on the part side.

The majority of transplant surgeons do not routinely suture the donor site. However, recent publications by several authors have rekindled interest in primary closure of the donor site defect. This may allow a greater number of grafts to be harvested, decreased scarring, and less chance of postoperative bleeding. However, this may produce an effect similar to scalp reduction in reverse since it pulls together the donor site, thus stretching the bald area of the crown.

POSTOPERATIVE CARE

Telfa and antibiotic ointment are placed over the grafts and donor site. This is covered with 4" × 4" or 4" × 8" gauze and a Kling or Conform pressure dressing (Fig. 25). Spray adhesive is used on recipient sites by some surgeons in place of the pressure dressing. The dressing

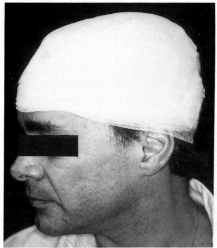
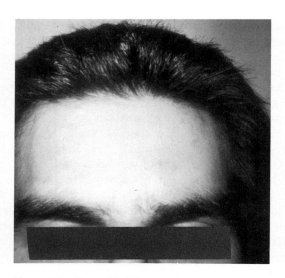

Figure 25   Pressure dressing.   **Figure 26**   Natural hairline.

is left on overnight, and the patient returns the next morning to have the dressing removed. The scalp is cleansed and the grafts checked to determine if any have become dislodged or turned in a wrong direction. A crust will form over each graft and remain for approximately 3 weeks. Hair in the grafts is shed by the fourth week and regrows in 10–16 weeks.

MINIGRAFTS AND MICROGRAFTS

One problem with hair transplantation is the tendency to produce a hairline that is too abrupt and too thick. A natural hairline is not really a line but a transitional zone between the bald skin of the forehead and the thick, uniform density of the frontal forelock (Fig. 26). Micro- and minigrafts are used to soften the frontal hairline. This makes it less abrupt and reduces the tufted effect. Nordstrom described in 1981 a technique in which 4 mm grafts were cut longitudinally to obtain grafts containing two to four follicles each. For years, smaller grafts obtained with 2-, 2.5-, and 3-mm trephines were used to soften the frontal hairline.

Micro- and minigrafting to soften the frontal hairline has become increasingly popular. Some hair transplant surgeons are now advocating that the entire replacement be done with micrografts and minigrafts or even all micrografts. The transplanting of 1000 micrografts in one session is now being accomplished. However, it may be that the excitement over micro- and minigrafting has swung the pendulum too far in that direction, and if one is seeking good density, 3.5- or 4.0-mm grafts are essential and micro- and minigrafts are better utilized in the anterior hairline to produce the desired aesthetic result. Micro- and minigrafts are also desirable in the correction of female pattern hair loss where the patient is thin but not bald. These smaller grafts can be placed between the existing hair to increase the density.

Minigrafts, consisting of three or more hairs, may be obtained by sectioning 4.5-mm grafts into halves and the halves into quarters with a Gillette blue blade in a holder (Figs. 27,28) and the graft resting on a firm surface, such as a wooden tongue blade. Magnification is necessary so the cutting is accurate. The minigraft is placed in the scalp after a slash wound is created with

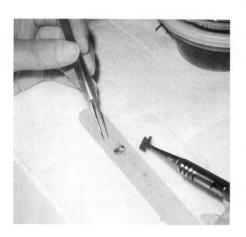

Figure 27 Cutting minigrafts.

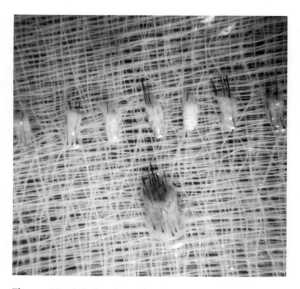

Figure 28 Minigrafts and a 4-mm graft.

a #15 scalpel blade at a point slightly anterior to or between the spaces in the hairline. The quartered graft can be inserted into this slash wound, held open by a cross-action jeweler's forceps, and directed in an anterior fashion. The wound heals without scarring and the hairs appear very natural (Fig. 29). A micrograft consists of one or two hairs and may be obtained by teasing intact hairs from the periphery of a standard graft (Figs. 30,31).

A far superior method for obtaining micro- and minigrafts from the donor area is by use of the double, triple, or quadruple bladed knife (Fig. 32). With this instrument one is able to cut

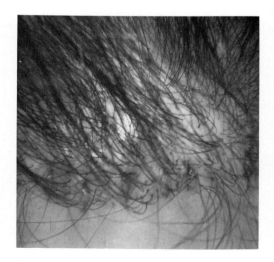

Figure 29 Mini- and 4-mm grafts growing and new minigrafts in place.

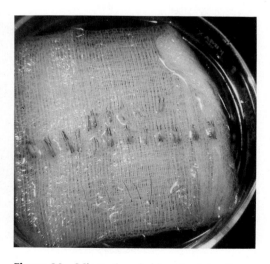

Figure 30 Micro- (one hair) and minigrafts.

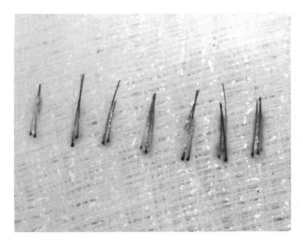

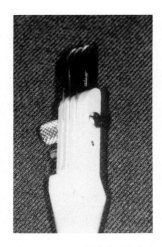

Figure 31   Micrografts (two hairs). (Courtesy of Emanuel Marritt, M.D.)

Figure   32   Triple-bladed
scalpel.

a single, double, or triple strip of hair-bearing tissue (Figs. 33,34). The strip is then sliced, similar to a loaf of bread (Fig. 35). The width of the slice determines the size of the minigraft or the production of micrografts (Fig. 36). Superior quality minigrafts can be produced in this fashion than can be bisected or quadrisected from larger grafts. One cannot punch small grafts as accurately as the margin of error greatly increases as the diameter of the graft decreases.

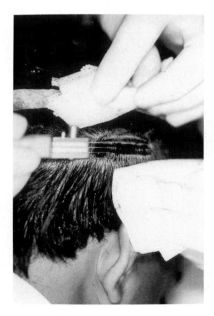

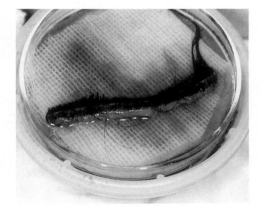

Figure 33   Double strip.

Figure 34   Double strip in saline.

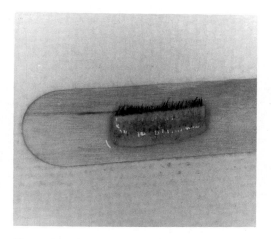

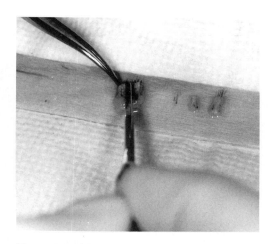

Figure 35   Strip on firm surface (tongue blade).   **Figure 36**   Slicing the strip.

Harvesting by the strip method also is most useful in obtaining additional mini- and micrografts from a previous punch graft donor site that was not sutured. After removing the strips, the hair follicles are harvested by slicing and the scarred areas discarded. This procedure will also diminish a scarred donor site as the resulting defect is sutured.

As mentioned previously, minigrafts can be placed into slash wounds created by a #15 scalpel blade, holes made by 1.0, 1.25, 1.50, etc. trephines, or by a small Sharptome microsurgical knife (Fig. 37). 16- or 18-gauge Nokor Becton Dickinson vented needles can be used to create the receptor hole for micrografts (Fig. 38).

Marritt described the use of stainless steel dilators for micro- and minigraft recipient sites (Fig. 39), which provide hemostasis, dilatation, and make placement of these grafts easier. Most importantly, the dilators offer a more efficient method of micro- and minigrafting and improve the organization of the procedure. Not all operators use dilators, but I personally find them indispensable. 16-gauge needlelike dilators are used for micrografting and various-sized spatulalike dilators are used for minigrafting. As the dilator is removed, the hole remains open long enough for the graft to be easily inserted without trauma (Figs. 40–42).

COMPLICATIONS

Complications following hair transplantation are rare. Postoperative bleeding from a donor site is not a frequent problem. Usually pressure applied to the wound after removal of the donor graft is sufficient. If bleeding persists, a cotton-tipped applicator dipped into epinephrine 1:1000 can be inserted into the bleeding socket. If this fails to produce hemostasis, the wound can be sutured. A hemostatic, collagen sponge (Helistat) is also useful. The sponge is 6 mm × 6 mm, white, pliable, and nonfriable. The collagen sponge promotes hemostasis by rapidly absorbing blood through a three-dimensional porous matrix that acts as a supporting framework for aggregation of platelets, which disintegrate and release coagulation factors that, together with plasma factors, enable the formation of fibrin. The spongy structure provides additional strengthening of the clot.

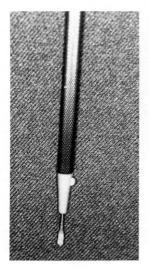

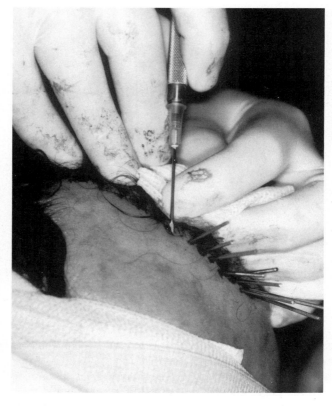

Figure 37 Sharptome surgical knife.

Figure 38 Nokor needle.

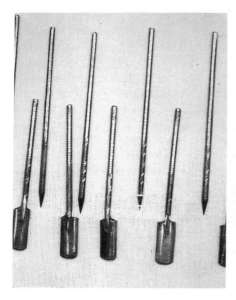

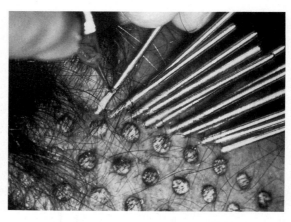

Figure 39 Needlelike microdilators and spatulalike minidilators. (Courtesy of Emanuel Marritt, M.D.)

Figure 40 Micrograft dilators in place. (Courtesy of Emanuel Marritt, M.D.)

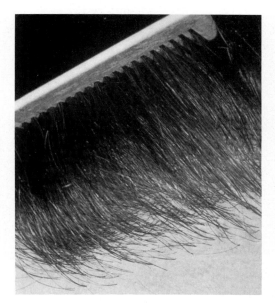

Figure 41 Micrografts growing. (Courtesy of Emanuel Marritt, M.D.)

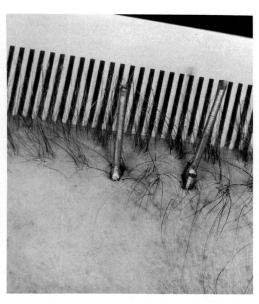

Figure 42 Minigraft dilators in place.(Courtesy of Emanuel Marritt, M.D.)

If bleeding persists from a donor site wound, one or two Helistat sponges are inserted with an Adson forceps and held in place with gentle pressure from a cotton-tipped applicator. Bleeding is controlled within 2–5 min. The sponge is absorbable and can be left in place. The author has not observed delayed healing, granuloma formation, or infection with the use of Helistat. In several weeks, when the entire donor site has healed by second intention, it is not possible to determine any gross difference between a Helistat and a non-Helistat wound.

Bleeding is rarely a problem in the recipient area since the grafts act as a tamponade. Because the scalp is so vascular, infection is extremely uncommon, especially when prophylactic antibiotics are used (Fig. 43). Arteriovenous malformations may occur during wound healing in either the recipient or donor sites. Postoperative edema may occur when one is transplanting the frontal area of the scalp, especially following the first session. This can be diminished with the use of systemic corticosteroids. Pain in the postoperative period is minimal and responds to mild analgesics. Hypesthesia can occur as a result of cutting peripheral nerve endings. Sensation usually returns in 2–3 months.

Sparse growth and scarring are usually due to poor technique (Fig. 44), as is cobblestoning or elevation of the grafts. Elevated grafts can be corrected by electrodesiccation, shaving with a scalpel, or dermabrasion.

Telogen effluvium, with regrowth in approximately 3 months, will occur (Fig. 45). This is not a complication; rather, it is expected as part of wound healing. Some believe this can be minimized by the application of minoxidil during the postoperative course.

Be conservative and do not attempt to place too many grafts in an area at one time. If the blood supply is compromised, poor growth, scarring, and even sloughing can occur (Fig. 46). Most importantly, the surgeon must have a sense of aesthetics to complement his or her technical skill (Fig. 47).

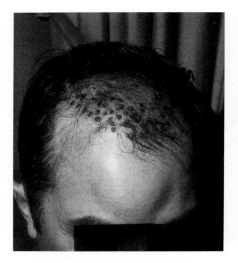

Figure 43 Beta-hemolytic streptococcal infection prior to use of prophylactic antibiotics. Patient is a pediatrician, and the source of infection was one of his patients.

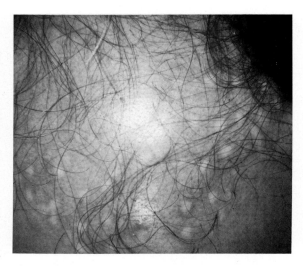

Figure 44 Sparse growth and scarring.

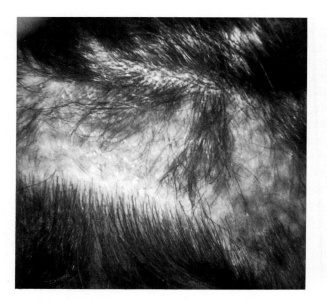

Figure 45 Telogen effluvium in donor site.

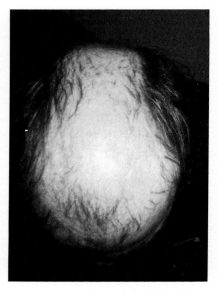

Figure 46 Creation of 220 grafts in one session resulted in slough. Treated with skin graft.

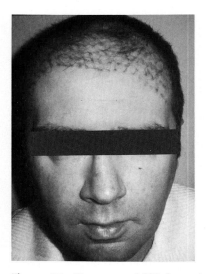

Figure 47 Placement of 100 (horror) grafts illustrating absence of aesthetics.

The art and science of hair transplantation has come a long way since its introduction. Both technique and instrumentation, as well as aesthetic considerations, have greatly improved, thus offering the patient a vastly superior cosmetic result that will last a lifetime.

BIBLIOGRAPHY

Alt T, Sr. Evaluation of donor harvesting techniques in hair transplantation. *J Dermatol Surg Oncol* 1984;10:799.

Bendl B. Troubles with power punches in hair transplantation. *J Dermatol Surg Oncol* 1977;3:594.

Hill T. Closure of the donor site in hair transplantation by a cluster technique. *J Dermatol Surg Oncol* 1980;6:190.

Lepaw M. Aids in cutaneous and hair transplant surgery. *J Dermatol Surg Oncol* 1983;9:273.

Marritt E. Single hair transplantation for hairline refinement: a practical solution. *J Dermatol Surg Oncol* 1984;10:962.

Morrison I. An improved method of suturing the donor site in hair transplantation surgery. *Plast Reconstr Surg* 1981;67:378.

Nordstrom R. "Micrografts" for improvement of the frontal hairline after hair transplantation. *Aesth Plast Surg* 1981;5:97.

Orentreich N. Autografts in alopecias and other selected dermatologic conditions. *Ann NY Acad Sci* 1959;83:463.

Pierce H. Improved method of closure of donor sites in hair transplantation. *J Dermatol Surg Oncol* 1979;5:475.

Pinski J. How to obtain the "perfect" plug. *J Dermatol Surg Oncol* 1984;10:953.

Sturm H. The benefit of donor site closure in hair transplantation. *J Dermatol Surg Oncol* 1984;10:987.

Unger W. A new method of donor site harvesting. *J Dermatol Surg Oncol* 1984;10:524.

70

Single Hair Grafting

Dow B. Stough, IV
*University of Arkansas Medical Sciences, Little Rock,
and The Stough Clinic, Hot Springs, Arkansas*

Francisco J. Jimenez
The Stough Clinic, Hot Springs, Arkansas

Hair transplantation using single hair grafting (SHG) is by no means a new technique. In 1943 Hajime Tamura wrote an article in the Japanese scientific literature about the technique of single hair grafting. Tamura excised a strip of donor hair from the occipital scalp by an elliptical incision and created single hair recipient sites using a thick injection needle, a concept identical to current practice. Tamura stated in this article that "it is better if the grafts are as small as possible; the reason is that if the grafts are big, the hair will grow in bundles in a very unnatural appearance. Therefore, the best way is to conduct single hair grafting entirely, because grafted hairs cannot be distinguished from their natural grown hairs" (translation courtesy of Dr. Shiro Yamada).

Tamura's article passed unnoticed for decades by European and American hair surgeons. If it had had more impact in the literature, the evolution of hair restoration surgery might have been significantly different.

For more than 20 years, since the initial works by Orentreich, hair transplant surgeons have employed trephines or punches to harvest large round grafts (4 mm in diameter) in hair restoration procedures. In the 1980s a number of authors began to describe their experiences with minigrafts. Since then, the popularity of smaller grafts has increased significantly. Two main reasons account for this shift: better long-term cosmetic results, including undetectability and a natural look achieved by single hair grafts, and the refinement of instruments that allow for easier harvesting, cutting, and graft placement.

The yield of hair growth after SHG has been addressed by Limmer, who demonstrated a survival rate for one or two hair grafts of 95% if they are transplanted 2 hr after removal and kept in chilled isotonic saline at 4°C. The survival decreases with the length of time between removal at donor site and implantation in the recipient sites, but even after 24 hr the survival rate is still relatively high (79%).

Single hair grafting, like any other combination of minigrafting, is a surgical technique that, once mastered, allows the physician to obtain reproducible results. The surgical technique itself is relatively straightforward; however, in order to achieve optimum results, it is important to select the proper candidates and to aesthetically distribute the grafts.

SELECTION OF THE CANDIDATE AND PLANNING THE SESSION

Two factors must be taken into consideration when evaluating a patient as a possible candidate for SHG: (1) patient expectations and (2) the degree of alopecia and hair quality.

Patient Expectations

It must be clear to the patient that the main goal of SHG is to frame the face. Framing the face returns the center of the attention to the face and not to the upper one third of the face. It is important to remind the patient about the goals of SHG before and after each session. Patient satisfaction can be a moving target; once it is achieved, a new and higher standard develops. There will never be enough hair for the patient if he or she is not properly educated in this matter. If the patient is looking for a significant increase in density, SHG is not the procedure of choice.

On the other hand, the patient should be informed that SHG is the most natural and undetectable hair restoration procedure. One of the main concerns of patients is that the transplant will look odd, artificial, or clumpy. A natural appearance can be achieved by using SHG, which mimics the natural distribution pattern. Since single hair grafts are placed into 18-gauge needle slits, little or no scarring is created in the recipient bed. Occasionally, small delling or indentations can be seen with single hair graft transplanted sites.

Degree of Alopecia and Hair Quality

The best candidates for the use of SHG have advanced or total alopecia of the frontal and/or crown region (Norwood type VI and VII). In these patients, the results of this approach constitute a diffuse, thinned look (Figs. 1,2). Patients with an ample quantity of retained native, nontransplanted hair may fail to notice any increase in volume, and thus are less suitable candidates. Realistic counseling prior to transplantation is essential.

A number of hair characteristics are important in the selection process and planning of a hair restoration procedure: the color of the hair, the hair/skin color match, the texture or caliber of the hair, and the curliness. While these factors are especially important when using bigger grafts (more than 2 mm in diameter), their influence in the selection of candidates is significantly minimized with SHG. For example, a hair transplant in a patient with black straight hair and white skin may look pluggy with 2-mm grafts but natural with SHG. All types of hair are suitable for SHG; therefore, it is the degree of alopecia that ultimately defines the better candidate.

NUMBER OF SINGLE HAIR GRAFTS PER SESSION

For a number of years, we have been using SHG to recreate a frontal hairline that looks natural and undetectable. Once we started to dissect large numbers of single hair grafts in a relatively short period of time, we realized that the whole transplantation procedure could be done using only SHG. This approach involves the utilization of a large number of grafts (1500–4000) over four to six sessions (400–1000 single hair grafts per session).

Graft numbers are limited by the degree of alopecia and by the quantity and quality of technical personnel available to dissect and plant the grafts. The harvesting and placement of single hair grafts require substantially more technical skills and hours of labor than the traditional big grafts. One experienced technician can produce 200–300 single hair grafts per hour.

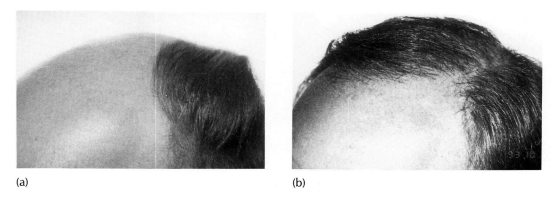

(a)　　　　　　　　　　　　　　　　　(b)

Figure 1 (a) Preoperative photograph of a patient with alopecia Norwood type IV. (b) Same patient after five sessions of SHG averaging 600 single hair grafts per session. This approach provided a thin, mature coverage.

In the last few years there has been a trend to move to megasessions, i.e., transplanting a large number of grafts per session (1000–2000). Megasessions with up to 2500–3000 grafts per session can be performed, but problems encountered when those numbers are reached include fatigue of the patient and personnel, need for additional technicians, increased procedure time, and problems in maintaining anesthesia. In addition, very dense packing of grafts may affect the vascular supply to the point of decreasing the rate of graft survival, but scientific data to prove or deny this hypothesis are still lacking.

SURGICAL TECHNIQUE

Excision of the Donor Site

Depending on the density of the donor area and the number of single hair grafts desired to be transplanted, a length of donor area is trimmed and marked to be excised (Table 1). In persons

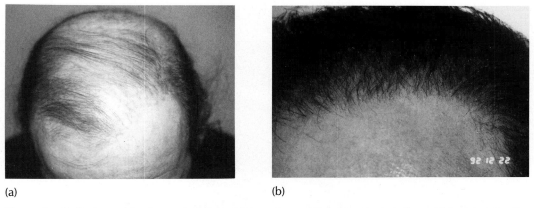

(a)　　　　　　　　　　　　　　　　　(b)

Figure 2 (a) Patient with advanced alopecia Norwood type VI before single hair grafting. (b) After five sessions. Notice the natural look and undetectability of this hair transplant using only single hair grafts.

Table 1 Harvest Length Requirements for Single Hair Grafts Based on Graft Quantity Desired

Desired number of single hair grafts	Required length (cm)[a]
50	1
100	2
150	3
200	4
300	6
400	8
500	10
600	12
700	14
800	16
900	18
1000	20

[a]Figures are based on triple-bladed knife, 2-mm spacers, and patient with average hair density.

with a normal donor density we are able to obtain 50 single hairs from a strip 1 cm long and 4 mm wide. Therefore, we obtain a strip 10 cm long to transplant 500 single hair grafts per session and a 15 cm strip to transplant 750 single hair grafts.

Ten minutes prior to surgery, 15 cc of 0.5% lidocaine with 1:200,000 epinephrine is administered to the donor area. Immediately before excision 20 cc of saline solution is injected for dermal turgor.

The best method to harvest the donor area for single hair grafting is to excise a long strip of occipital hair-bearing scalp. This can be done by using a conventional scalpel or a multiple blade knife (Fig. 3). The authors prefer the use of a triple blade knive with 2-mm spacers, thereby obtaining two long strips, each of them 2 mm wide (Fig. 4). The thinness and relative ease in handling the narrow strips facilitates the dissection of the single hair grafts (Fig. 5). The authors acknowledge comparable results with the freehand single-bladed approach.

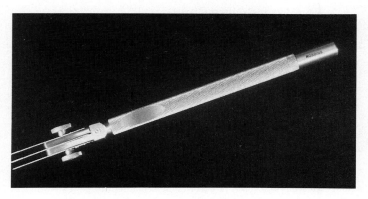

Figure 3 Triple bladeholder with 2.0-mm spacers. (Courtesy Robbins Instruments Co., Chatham, New Jersey.)

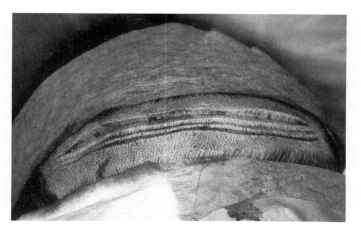

Figure 4 The donor site immediately after incision with the triple bladed knive.

The use of the triple bladed knife requires some expertise in order to avoid as much transection of the hair shafts as possible. The knife is held parallel to the patient's hair follicles but not perpendicular to the skin, because this would result in a degree of hair shaft transection. The depth of insertion of the knife blade should be approximately 5 mm into the scalp, enough to reach a depth of 1–2 mm below the terminus of the hair follicles. A deeper incision results in greater frequency of transection of arteries and therefore is not desirable. After the incision is made the ends are contoured with a single surgical scalpel to produce an elliptical pattern. The strips are cut from their base using sharp scissors, hemostasis is obtained, and the wound is closed with staples. Polysporin ointment is applied to the wound bed and the area is covered with a nonadherent dressing (e.g., Telfa®) and Reston® foam packing.

Graft Preparation

The transplantation of hundreds of single hair grafts is a time-consuming procedure that requires a team effort, with the hair transplant surgeon acting as the coordinator of this team. The role that the technicians play in the graft preparation is crucial.

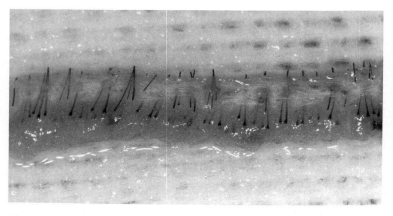

Figure 5 A thin strip of hair showing parallel alignment of hairs. Notice minimal hair shaft transection.

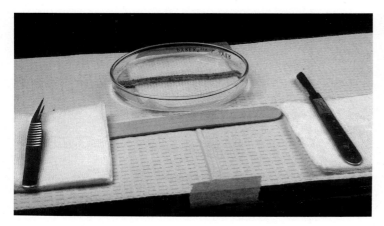

Figure 6 Instruments used to dissect the single hairs: scalpel with a #10 Personna blade, jeweler's forceps (Van Sickle Co., Bedford, TX), and a tongue blade.

The strips are separated from each other and emersed in Petri dishes containing chilled isotonic saline at 2–4°C. Surgical technicians then prepare the single hair grafts by sectioning follicles from the strips, working toward the center of the strip. All grafts are sectioned using a #10 surgical blade and jeweler's forceps (Fig. 6). The yield of grafts depends on the density of hair present in donor tissue. Excess tissue may be trimmed from single follicles if density is low (Fig. 7).

Recipient Site Preparation and Graft Insertion

While the dissection of the single hairs proceeds, the recipient scalp can be anesthetized. We routinely perform a bilateral supraorbital nerve block, which will anesthetize the frontal and anterior half of the scalp. The local infiltration of the scalp is then started using 10 cc of 0.5% lidocaine with 1:200,000 epinephrine. Fifteen to thirty minutes before making the incisions, the

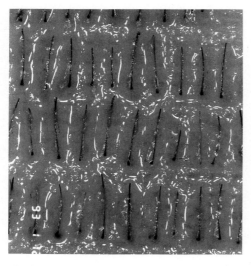

Figure 7 Rows of single hair grafts placed on a Petri dish after dissection.

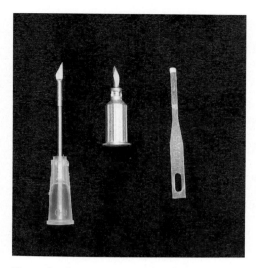

Figure 8 Instruments to make slits for single hair graft placement. Left to right: NoKor needle, Yeh needle, and #61 Beaver blade. All three instruments produce similar slit incisions for the placement of single hair grafts.

recipient site is infiltrated subcutaneously with a mixture of 12 cc of saline and 0.1 cc of epinephrine 1:1000 to reduce the bleeding.

A variety of instruments have been used to make the slits for single hair recipient sites, including #15 and #11 blades, 18 gauge needles, No-Kor needles, #61 Beaver blade, and Yeh needle. We prefer either the 18 gauge No-Kor needle, the #61 Beaver blade, or the Yeh needle (Fig. 8). The No-Kor needle has a sharp lance tip and can be used to quickly and easily create large numbers of single-stab incision sites. The Yeh needle is a solid needle with a sharp, pointed, beveled tip, which facilitates the penetration of the skin. This needle is only 6 mm long and cannot penetrate deeper, thus providing precise depth control (13).

The single hair grafts are inserted using a finer version of jeweler's forceps, originally designed for microvascular surgery. The placement of these tiny grafts into the small, tight slits is technique-sensitive and requires considerable experience. Care is also required to avoid follicular damage. While the results are often undetectable, this technique does not completely negate all long-term consequences. Further balding may require multiple sessions and a lifelong commitment to hair transplantation.

BIBLIOGRAPHY

Brandy DA. A new instrument for the expedient productions of the minigrafts. *J Dermatol Surg Oncol* 1992;18:487.

Brandy DA, Meshkin M. Utilization of No-Kor needles for slit-micrografting. *J Dermatol Surg Oncol* 1994;20:336–339.

Jiminez F, Stough DB IV. The Yeh needle: a depth controlled solid needle for single hair recipient sites. Abstract presented at the Meeting of the International Society of Hair Restoration Surgery, Toronto, Canada, September 1994.

Limmer BL. Survival of minigrafts as a function of time from removal at the donor site to implantation in the recipient scalp site. Abstract presented at the Meeting of the International Society of Hair Restoration Surgery, Toronto, Canada, September 1994.

Marritt E. Patient selection, candidacy and treatment plan for hair replacement surgery. *Facial Plast Surg Clin North Am* 1994;2:39–46.

Marrit E. Single hair transplantation for hairline refinement: a practical solution. *J Dermatol Surg Oncol* 1984;10:962–966.

Norwood OT. Patient selection, hair transplant design, and hairstyle. *J Dermatol Surg Oncol* 1992;18:386–394.

Orentreich N. Autografts in alopecias and other selected dermatologic conditions. *Ann NY Acad Sci* 1959;83:463.

Rassman WR. The science of hair density/consequences of dense packing of grafts in megatransplant session. Abstract presented at the Meeting of the International Society of Hair Restoration Surgery, Toronto, Canada, September 1994.

Stough DB IV. Hair transplantation by the feathering zone technique: new tools for the nineties. *Am J Cosmet Surg* 1992;9:243.

Stough DB. Single hair grafting for advanced male pattern alopecia. *Cosmet Dermatol* 1993;6:11–15.

Tamura H. Hair grafting procedure. *Jpn J Dermatol* 1943;53.

Uebel CO. Micrografts and minigrafts: a new approach for baldness surgery. *Ann Plast Surg* 1991;27:476–487.

71

Scalp Reduction

Henry H. Roenigk, Jr.
Northwestern University Medical School, Chicago, Illinois

HISTORY

Advancement and rotation flaps, as well as serial excision, have been used in the reconstruction of scalp defects or cicatricial alopecia for half a century. Blanchard and Blanchard presented the first scientific paper on the correction of male pattern baldness using serial excisions of bald scalp in 1977. Unger and Unger described the first large series in 1978. Schultz and Roenigk reported on the use of scalp reduction for treatment of scarring alopecia. Alt described the paramedian incision, a variation on the technique. Other variations have been described over the years including mini-reductions, scalp reduction following tissue expansion, or use of tissue expanders at the time of surgery and scalp lifting as described by Brandy. The combination of scalp reduction and hair transplantation is the most common surgical approach to extensive male pattern alopecia. Scalp reduction is also helpful for a variety of scalp conditions, such as aplasia cutis congenita, burn scars, cutis verticis gyrata, discoid lupus erythematous, pseudopelade, lichen planopilaris, traction alopecia, nevus sebaceous of Jadassohn, and localized morphea scleroderma (en coup de sabre).

PREOPERATIVE CONSULTATION

Time spent during the consultation may be more important to the outcome of the operation than the surgery itself. Once one has determined that the alopecia is amenable to surgery, the patient's motivation, expectations, and medical history are carefully assessed. It is important to screen out inappropriate patients. A thorough medical history is taken and laboratory studies should include a complete blood count, serum chemistry screen, coagulation studies, and screens for hematogenously transmitted infection including hepatitis and human immunodeficiency virus (HIV). If the patient is a suitable candidate for surgery, the procedure is outlined and related questions are answered. The use of pamphlets, videotapes, and photographs are helpful for patient education.

First decide if the patient has adequate hair for transplantation. Take into consideration what the patient wishes, unless it will result in an abnormal appearance. Consider personal grooming habits. Work with a hair stylist who may suggest a new style that will complement the procedure. The patient may be better served by the combination of scalp reduction and hair transplantation. Scalp flaps and tissue expanders and other options should be discussed. Medical treatment (minoxidil, or Rogaine) and other options (toupees) should be discussed for completeness. It is not uncommon for patients seeking hair replacement surgery to be well informed from the lay press and consultations with other surgeons.

There is controversy over whether scalp reduction should be done prior to or after hair transplantation. The donor area is less dense after scalp reduction, since it reduces the number of hairs per graft. If hair transplantation is done first, distortion of the frontal hair line can be expected by subsequent scalp reduction.

Testing laxity of the scalp gives more indication of how much scalp can be removed (Fig. 1). Sometimes during surgery more can be removed than planned if it is adequately undermined. Scalp reduction is usually performed as either a midline sagittal excision or a paramedian excision. The midline excision results in equal tension from both parietal sides of the scalp. If several reductions are performed, the previous scar will be excised, so only one long scar in the midline will result. The midline excision is, thus, nothing more than a large excision. After scalp reduction, hair transplants can be done to create the hairline. This will now require fewer grafts. Hair transplant grafts can also be used to cover the scar from scalp reduction.

Besides using photographs, it is helpful to draw a picture of the scalp and then sketch changes, showing exactly what the patient can expect after each procedure. The time between each procedure is important. At least 6 weeks and preferably 3 months are needed between scalp reduc-

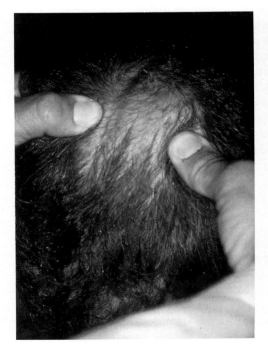

Figure 1   Testing for laxity of scalp.

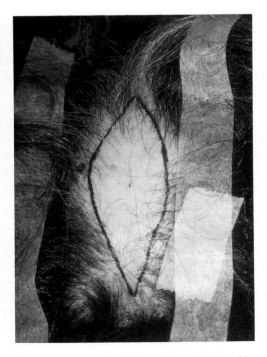

Figure 2   Planned excision of the scalp by midline technique.

tion. As little as 2 weeks is needed between hair transplants. Micrographs and minigraphs can be done once regrowth is well established.

PREOPERATIVE MANAGEMENT

Scalp reduction may be done in an office surgical suite with sterile technique. It is impossible to sterilize the unshaven scalp, but patients should be prepped and draped and the surgeon fully gloved and gowned during surgery. Cardiac monitoring and establishment of intravenous access for sedation may be desired. Preoperative sedation with diazepam 10–20 mg intravenously can be given slowly over the length of the procedure. Demerol 50–100 mg intramuscularly can also be added. The scalp is cleansed with Hibiclens or Betadine scrub followed by alcohol.

Tumanescent lidocaine 0.05% with epinephrine 1:1,000,000 and no sodium bicarbonate is the standard anesthetic. Some patients require 1% lidocaine with epinephrine 1:100,000 for complete anesthesia. For anesthesia of longer duration, dilute the lidocaine with bupivacaine HCl (Marcaine). A cephalic ring block should be performed. The ring should encompass the excision and anticipated area of undermining. The injection should be in the dermis and the superficial subcutaneous fat, not the subgaleal space. The rings of anesthesia generally extend to 1.0 cm above the ear and posteriorly to the occiput. The ring is then completed along the opposite side and anteriorly along the frontal hairline. Keep the ring low at the ears and high at the occiput. Lidocaine 1% should also be injected along the incision lines for vasoconstriction as well as anesthesia. With tumanescent anesthesia about 250 ml of solution is needed for a scalp reduction.

TECHNIQUE

The patient can be in a sitting position with a neck support or in the prone position with the head supported. The excision is planned and outlined with gentian violet (Fig. 2). An area the length of the alopecic scalp (10–14 cm) and between 2.0 and 4.0 cm wide is standard. The excision should not extend anteriorly beyond the proposed frontal hairline. Only one side of the ellipse is incised down to the galea. Hemostasis is obtained with electrocautery, and suction may be necessary. The edges of the incision are everted so that large vessels can be quickly and easily cauterized. The larger vessels are at the level of the galea and deep dermal plexus.

Undermining may be done with large Metzenbaum scissors or a similar instrument, like the Iconoclast developed by Ralph Luikart. Blunt dissection is also done with the index and second finger to free adhesions over the periosteum. Undermining should be done to the anterior hairline, the ears or below, and the lambdoid ridge. This is done in the subgaleal plane, because there is little bleeding, and the galea is used for deep suturing. Occasionally, there are some perforating vessels, but generally there is a thin, avascular fibrous stroma between the galea and the calvarium.

Pull the parietal scalp toward the midline so the incision overlaps. This maneuver can be accomplished manually or with towel clips and is done to estimate the amount of skin that can be excised. If this is inadequate, further undermining can be undertaken at this point, an adjustment can be made in the amount of skin excised, and the second incision line moved accordingly if necessary.

The second side of the excision is then cut and skin removed (Fig. 3). Hemostasis is obtained as previously described, and the wound is ready for closing. Towel clips are placed along the suture line to hold the wound together (Fig. 4). The galea closure can then easily be done without tension. The clips are removed once the galea has been closed. There should be no tension on the skin closure, since this may result in necrosis and wound dehiscence.

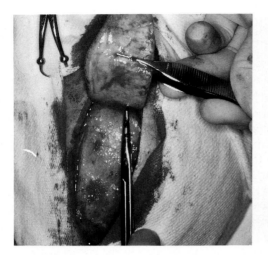

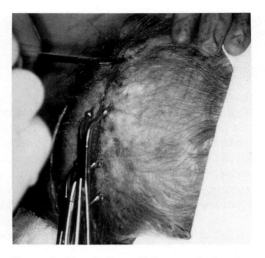

Figure 3 Completing the excision.   **Figure 4** Towel clips pull the wound edges together.

The galea may be closed with 2–0 Vicryl or 2–0 catgut on an OS-4 cutting needle. Interrupted sutures are used, but the knot may be placed above the galea for tighter closure. Staples are preferred for the skin since they are nonreactive and are left in for 3 weeks (Fig. 5). A wound dressing is optional. Many patients do not require a dressing, but a head wrap may be applied for 12–24 hr.

If there is too much tension on the wound prior to closure of the galea, galeotomies can be performed. These are parallel incisions through the galea. One or two incisions on either side of the excision are performed through the galea to the subcutaneous fat with a #15 Bard-Parker blade or a 75-S Beaver blade. When procedures are properly planned, with adequate undermining, galeotomies are seldom used today. If there is difficulty in getting the excision to close, relax-

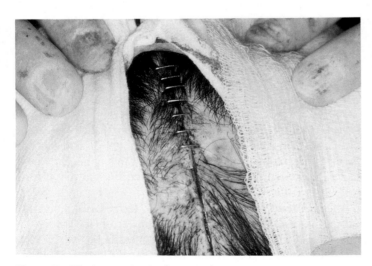

Figure 5 Placing staples in the wound.

ing incisions may be done 1–2 cm from the wound or in the hair above both ears. The relaxing incision is made through the galea. The central excision is closed and then the relaxing incisions are closed.

DESIGN OF THE SCALP REDUCTION

Midline Sagittal

The midline sagittal excision is the most common design used for scalp reduction (Figs. 6–13). The scalp has more mobility and elasticity laterally; therefore, this excision is easiest to perform. Major vessels close to the ear are avoided. The previous scalp reduction scar is removed so the patient has only one scar in the midline. There is an unnatural part in the midline that will extend into the occiput and may be objectionable. This can be avoided by everting the skin edges of the excision and positioning hair to grow through the scar (Fig. 14). Hair transplanted into and around the scar can also be used for camouflage (Figs. 15–17). There can also be a dog ear effect in the frontal or posterior part of the midline scar. This can be corrected later with a lateral extension of the scar.

Distortion of the frontal hairline should be expected. If hair transplants are done first, pulling back the lateral portions of the hairline must be carefully planned ahead of time. If a hairline already exists, scalp reduction will pull both temporal areas posteriorly and create a recession that may not please the patient.

Paramedian

The paramedian scalp reduction advocated by Alt is crescent- or S-shaped (Figs. 18–20). The inferior incision is several millimeters superior to the existing hairline. The scar is less noticeable than the midline excision. It is easier to undermine, but it limits undermining on both sides,

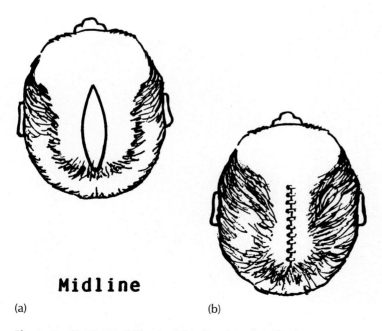

Midline

(a)   (b)

Figure 6   Standard midline excision for alopecia reduction.

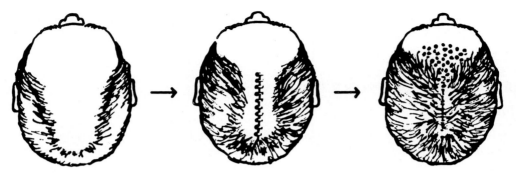

Figure 7 Midline approach combined with hair transplant grafts.

as in the midline excision. There is a greater risk of bleeding from transection of the larger vessels near the ear. The paramedian excision can be done on both sides of the scalp with subsequent reductions, but a narrow strip of central scalp will receive blood supply from only the supraorbital and supratrochlear arteries. The risk of avascular necrosis and skin slough is increased. The paramedian incision should be done after the donor plugs are harvested from the supraauricular and temporoparietal areas. This provides grafts with maximum hair density. There is less distortion of the frontal hairline with the paramedian excision than the midline excision. It is also more difficult to estimate the amount of scalp that may be removed with the paramedian excision.

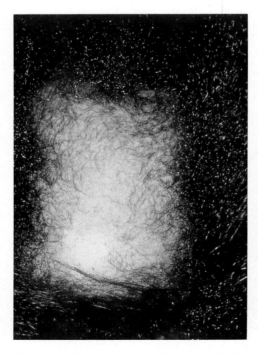

Figure 8 Vertex alopecia with a natural hairline.

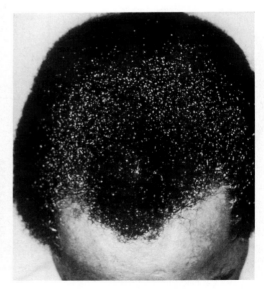

Figure 9 Appearance after three scalp reductions. Note the retraction of the hairline in a bitemporal recession pattern.

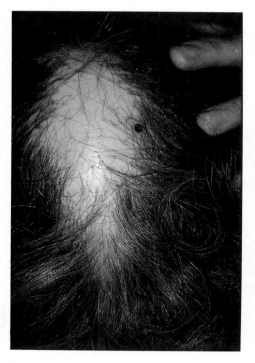

Figure 10 Scalp reduction planned in a woman with scarring alopecia.

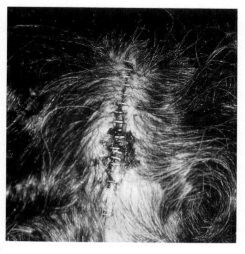

Figure 11 Completed scalp reduction of scarring alopecia in Figure 10.

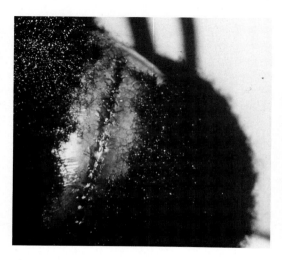

Figure 12 Scalp reduction of burn scar.

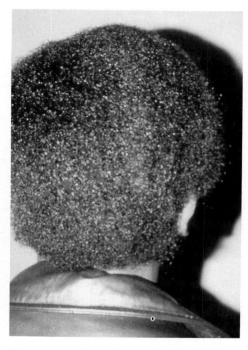

Figure 13 Completed scalp reduction of burn scar in Figure 12.

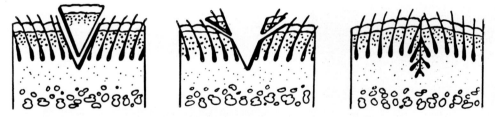

Figure 14 Wound edges are cut so that the hair grows through and hides the scar of scalp reduction in the posterior scalp.

Y or Mercedes Patterns

This pattern is useful for vertex baldness (Fig. 21). If this is the only area of alopecia, a Y or Mercedes excision is the best approach. Each section of the excision may be done separately and closed before one proceeds to the next. There is risk of tip necrosis when there is tension on the wound, since this becomes a three-cornered, three-directional advancement flap. Relaxing incisions cannot be done if there is difficulty closing, so it is better to let a small gap heal by second intention, which can be revised later.

Brandy "Scalp Lifting"

Maryola in 1983 first described an extensive type unilateral scalp reduction with extensive undermining of the entire hair-bearing portion of the scalp on one side. Bradshaw in 1985 then

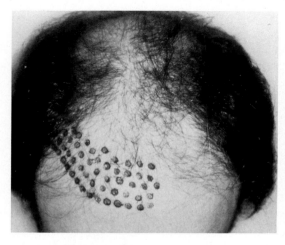

Figure 15 Establishment of a hairline with hair transplants.

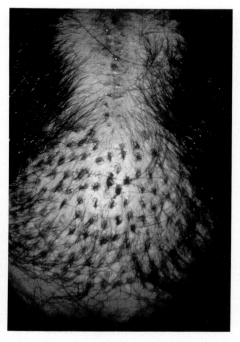

Figure 16 Completed scalp reduction and hair transplantation.

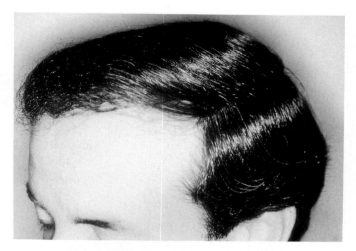

Figure 17 Six months after hair transplants in Figure 16.

described the bilateral lateral scalp reduction. Brandy has popularized the procedure, which he refers to as "scalp lifting."

Recently concern has been expressed at hair-replacement meetings about the incidence of serious postoperative complications, including necrosis of large areas of the scalp. Bradshaw and Maryola have both reported a high incidence of postoperative necrosis, while Brandy reports a complication rate of only 6.5% in 168 cases when occipital arteries are not ligated prior to surgery. Most surgeons who do scalp-reduction surgery feel that the bilateral lateral reduction is too extensive a surgical procedure with unacceptable risks compared to other, more standard scalp reductions.

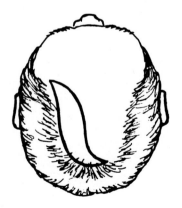

Paramedian

Figure 18 Paramedian, crescent, or S-shaped incision.

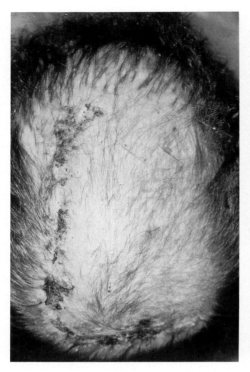

Figure 19 Hair transplants completed. Para-median scalp reduction.

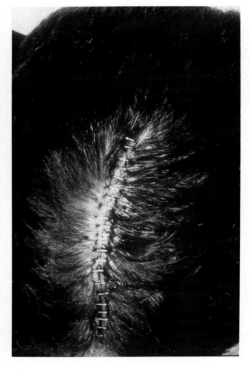

Figure 20 Completion of several scalp reductions results in complete coverage of scalp with hair.

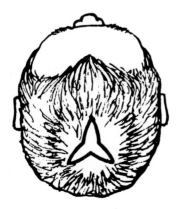

Mercedes

Figure 21 Y-shaped or Mercedes incision.

Scalp Reduction with Tissue Expansion

The concept of tissue expansion prior to excision was developed by Radovan. The technique has been applied to many areas of the skin to create flaps of tissue to cover defects. The technique has been applied to male pattern alopecia and cicatricial alopecia.

Miniscalp Reduction

Unger uses dozens of 4- to 6-mm punch biopsies to remove a bald area and then sutures them closed. This reduces the alopecia and is a simple technique that any dermatologist could perform. It is especially helpful when the alopecia is not complete and one wishes to spare patches of hair-bearing scalp.

POSTOPERATIVE CARE

Antibiotics (erythromycin or penicillin) may be given 24 hr before surgery and continued for 7–10 days. Immediately after the surgery, the area is cleaned, dried, and combed. Postoperative photos are taken, and the patient is allowed to see the results. A dressing is not necessary unless there is minor bleeding. A turban pressure dressing may be used for 24 hr. Staples are left in place for 3 weeks.

Postoperative pain is common after a scalp reduction and is much more severe than with hair transplantation. The pain is due to tightness of the scalp. This is more severe after the first scalp reduction than after subsequent reductions. It lasts about 24 hr and may require narcotic analgesics for relief. Short-acting systemic steroids may be used to reduce swelling and pain.

COMPLICATIONS

Bleeding

There is usually very little bleeding with scalp reduction, most of which is due to small vessels in the dermal plexus. The CO_2 laser, Shaw scalpel, or skin clips may be used to minimize bleeding. Most bleeding is controlled with manual pressure and stops in 10 min. Often very little cautery is required.

Profuse bleeding may occur when one is undermining and one of the larger vessels is transected. This can be avoided by blunt dissection with a finger or an Iconoclast. If a vessel is cut, pack the area with gauze soaked in epinephrine 1:1000 and apply pressure for 5–10 min. Repeat this procedure if bleeding persists. Arterial bleeding may require another incision near the source to allow you to visualize and clamp the vessel. Complete hemostasis is important to prevent formation of a hematoma.

Hematoma

If there is persistent bleeding after closure, a hematoma may form. Excess activity by the patient may also be responsible. It is best to drain a hematoma within 24 hr. This speeds healing and prevents secondary infection. Look carefully for signs of persistent bleeding and close the wound again. If a hematoma is not evacuated, it may result in pain, hair loss, or infection and take several months to resolve. Sodium bicarbonate in tumanescent anesthesia may contribute to hematoma, and thus we eliminate it from our local anesthetic in scalp surgery.

Infection

Infection is not common when one is using prophylactic antibiotics. If the closure is tight, with resulting ischemia in the suture line (Fig. 22), it may become secondarily infected. This is treated topically with antiseptic soaks and debridement. A second procedure will eliminate areas of tissue necrosis and scar.

Temporary Hair Loss and Stretch Back

Temporary hair loss due to the trauma from the surgery (telogen effluvium) commonly occurs 1–2 weeks after scalp reduction (Fig. 23). The patient should be made aware of this, and documentation with photographs is helpful. It is necessary to schedule subsequent scalp reductions after regrowth has occurred (about 3 months) so that normal hair follicles are not removed.

Nordstrom coined the term "stretch back" to refer to a stretching of the scalp and an increase in the area of alopecia after scalp reduction. He found that up to half of the benefit of scalp reduction could be lost due to stretch back. Unger and others have studied this phenomenon and feel that it is much less common. (Unger found that 91.1% of all patients had less than 7% stretch back.) It is possible that several other factors may be mistaken for stretch back, including progressive male pattern baldness, tension or wound tightness, temporary telogen effluvium, and widening of the scar if there is too much tension on the scalp.

Nonclosure

The initial scalp reduction should be conservative (2–3.5 cm wide rather than 4–5 cm). It is better to do an extra procedure than to close a wound too tightly or perform lateral relaxing incisions

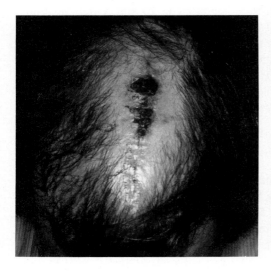

Figure 22 Necrosis of incision from tension.

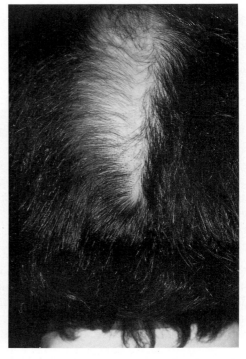

Figure 23 Telogen effluvium following scalp reduction.

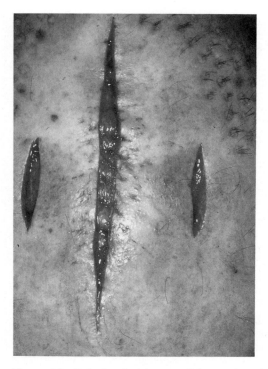

Figure 24 Relaxing incision parallel to scalp reduction.

(Fig. 24). Keep the skin that has already been excised available in saline. If all else fails, a free graft may be used to close a gap in the incision. The key to scalp reduction is proper planning, adequate anesthesia, and extensive undermining.

Wound Dehiscence

Wound dehiscence is rare but occurs if there is too much tension after closure, resulting in necrosis. Because staples are nonreactive, they can be left in place for 3 weeks. By this time, the wound is well healed and there is little chance for separation.

Suture Reactions

Using a large gauze suture in the galea or placing suture too close to the skin results in sero-sanguineous cysts, suture granuloma, and small pockets of infection along the incision line. Confining the suture to the galea and tying the knots so that they are buried below the galea will minimize this problem. Spitting suture should be removed and fluid accumulations drained. The wound will heal promptly.

BIBLIOGRAPHY

Alt TH. History of scalp reductions and paramedian methods. In *Hair Transplant Surgery*. 2nd ed. Norwood OT, Shiell RC, eds. Springfield, IL, Charles C Thomas, 1984, pp. 221–244.

Alt T. Scalp reduction. *Cosmet Surg* 1981;1:1–19.

Alt T. Scalp reduction as an adjunct to hair transplantation. *J Dermatol Surg Oncol* 1980;6:1011.

Blanchard G, Blanchard B. Obliteration of alopecia by hairlifting: A new concept and technique. *J Natl Med Assoc* 1977;69:639–641.

Blanchard G, Blanchard B. La réduction de la tonsure (détonsuration): Concept nouveau dans le traitement chirurgical de la calvitie. *Union Med Care* 1976;105:618–624.

Bell ML. Role of scalp reduction in the treatment of male pattern alopecia. *Plast Reconstr Surg* 1982;69:272–277.

Bosley LL, Hope CR, Montroy RE. Male pattern reduction (MPR) for surgical reduction of male pattern baldness. *Curr Ther Res* 1979;25:281–287.

Bosley LL, Hope CR, Montroy RE, et al. Reduction of male pattern baldness in multiple stages. *J Dermatol Surg Oncol* 1980;6:498–503.

Brandy DA. A new surgical approach for the treatment of extensive baldness. *Am J Cosmet Surg* 1986;3:19–25.

Brandy DA. The effectiveness of occipital artery ligations as a priming procedure for extensive scalp lifting. *J Dermatol Surg Oncol* 1991;17:946–949.

Hirtzing GS, Sadid NS. A new technique for curvilinear scalp reduction. *J Dermatol Surg Oncol* 1989;15:1108–1112.

McCray MK, Roenigk HH. Scalp reduction for correction of cutis aplasia congenita. *J Dermatol Surg Oncol* 1981;7:655.

McCray MK, Roenigk HH Jr. Cosmetic correction of alopecia. *Am Fam Pract* 1983;28:207.

Nordstrom REA. Hair replacement—special issue. *Facial Plast Surg* 1985;2:167–290.

Norwood OT, Shiell RC. Scalp reductions. In *Hair Transplant Surgery*. 2nd ed. Norwood OT, Shiell RC, eds. Springfield, IL, Charles C Thomas, 1984, pp. 163–200.

Norwood OT, Shiell RC, Morrison ID. Complications and problems of scalp reduction. In *Hair Transplant Surgery*. 2nd ed. Norwood OT, Shiell RC, eds. Springfield, IL, Charles C Thomas, 1984, pp. 201–220.

Roenigk HH Jr. Combined surgical treatment of male pattern alopecia. *Cutis* 1985;570–577.

Schultz BC, Roenigk HH Jr. Scalp reduction for alopecia. *J Dermatol Surg Oncol* 1979;5:808.

Stegman S, Tromovitch T. Scalp reduction for alopecia. In *Cosmetic Dermatologic Surgery*. Chicago, Year Book Publishers, 1983, pp. 109–130.

Unger MG, Unger WP. Management of alopecia of the scalp by a combination of excision and transplantations. *J Dermatol Surg Oncol* 1978;4:670.

Unger MG. Postoperative necrosis following bilateral lateral scalp reduction. *J Dermatol Surg Oncol* 1988;14:541–543.

Unger MG. Scalp reduction. *Clin Dermatol* 1992;10:345–355.

72

Scalp Flaps

Richard W. Fleming and Toby G. Mayer
University of Southern California School of Medicine,
Los Angeles, California

There has been a tremendous evolution in hair replacement surgery over the past 30 years. Each patient should have the opportunity to make an educated decision about surgery depending upon his or her needs and expectations. In our practice we use all techniques but place emphasis on the transposition flaps, which we believe are best for most patients.

HISTORY

Scalp flaps were initially used for reconstructive surgery during the nineteenth century. Passot first described the use of small lateral temporoparietal flaps for the treatment of male pattern baldness. In 1957, Lamont described a similar procedure for hair replacement of the anterior hairline. These reports were essentially unnoticed. Juri refined and extended flap surgery to establish it as a relatively safe and very effective procedure for extensive aesthetic hair replacement. Since 1969, he has used temporoparietal-occipital flaps to treat alopecia. His results were reported in 1972 at the First International Congress on Aesthetic Plastic Surgery and later published in 1975. Other surgeons, including Fleming and Mayer, Kabaker, and Fournier, began to use this flap. Fleming and Mayer described in 1981 a modification of the Juri flap that resulted in a more natural hairline configuration without blunting of the frontal temporal recession. Juri described another flap for correction of occipital baldness based on the postauricular or occipital artery.

Elliott described in 1977 a flap similar to that used by Lamont, which differs from the Juri flap by being shorter, narrower, and random patterned rather than axial. Unfortunately, with this method each flap (one from each side) gives only 1 inch of hair in the frontal region of the scalp. Heimberger presented his short nondelayed flap for the treatment of frontal baldness. The authors modified the design, especially of the hairline of the short flap, and presented their 5-yr results in 1981.

Harii et al. were the first in 1974 to describe free scalp flaps to replace cicatricial alopecia in the temporal region. Juri in 1979 and Ohmori in 1980 described a free flap done with microvascular anastomosis, but this has little practical application for an elective cosmetic procedure at the present time.

Nataf and others described superior-based preauricular and postauricular flaps. These superiorly based flaps rarely reach the midline in most individuals. Marzola described his technique using extensive scalp reductions followed by the superiorly based flap to achieve the increased length necessary to reach the midline and beyond. Further use of Marzola's flap was reported by Brandy in 1986.

Fleming and Mayer improved the Juri flap using the irregular trichopoytic hairline. In 1982 they described a method of delaying the recipient area before rotation of the second flap and in 1984 suggested the use of a temporary graft in the donor site or tissue expansion to prevent elevation of the postauricular hairline. These modifications of Juri's original design have resulted in the Fleming/Mayer (F/M) flap. We published our experience with replacement surgery emphasizing scalp flaps in 1992.

FLEMING/MAYER FLAP (MODIFIED AFTER JURI)

The original Juri flap is a twice-delayed flap, 4 cm in width, based on the posterior branch of the superficial temporal artery (Fig. 1). It has been suggested that no delay or one delay is possible. However, there is increased risk of flap necrosis. Juri's initial report in 1975 was based on extensive experience in more than 400 cases. The basic technique has remained unchanged. The original Juri flap has been modified to create the F/M flap.

Our flap retains the following elements of Juri's original design:

1. The flap is based on the superficial temporal artery.
2. Two delays are always performed.
3. When possible, the flap is designed to span the entire bald area.
4. Flap design also allows a full-length second flap to be taken from the opposite side of the scalp.

Our flap differs from Juri's original description in the following ways:

1. The flap varies in width from 3.75 to 4.50 cm.
2. The superior portion of the flap is irregular, corresponding to the new hairline design.
3. The frontotemporal recession is not blunted. Therefore, the hairline does not have a rounded or apelike appearance.
4. Scalp reductions are almost always performed before flap rotation except in patients with only frontal baldness or those with an extremely tight scalp.
5. Tissue expansion with the Fleming/Mayer expander is often used in conjunction with flap surgery.
6. A skin graft is frequently placed to help close the donor defect so the postauricular hairline is not elevated.
7. An additional delay is always done at the anterior margin of the recipient sight in conjunction with delays for the second flap.
8. Forehead lifting is performed in combination with the Fleming/Mayer procedure in many patients.

Design

First the posterior branch of the superficial temporal artery is located by palpation or with a Doppler flowmeter. The inferior edge of the flap starts at a point approximately 3.0 cm above

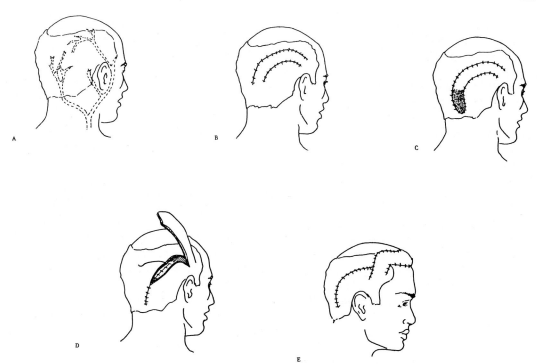

Figure 1 (A) Arterial blood supply to the central and posterior scalp. (B) First delay. Parallel incisions made as shown and wound closed. (C) Second delay, 1 week later. The tail of the flap is incised, undermined, and closed. (D) Transposition of the flap 1 week later. The flap is lifted from the donor site and the donor wound closed without excess tension. (E) Bald frontal scalp excised and flap sutured in place.

the root of the helix (Fig. 1). The superior edge begins 4.0 cm anterior and superior to this point at an angle of 30–45 degrees to horizontal, so the flap is centered over the superficial temporal artery. The lines of incision extend posteriorly and superiorly through the temporoparietal region and curve inferiorly into the occipital scalp, approximately 4 cm apart, for the entire length of the flap. Future alopecia should be anticipated when planning the flap so that the superior edge of the flap, which will establish the new frontal hairline, is not taken from an area where further hair loss may occur. The length of the flap is determined by measuring the distance from the point of rotation across the hairline to the contralateral fringe and adding 3.0–4.0 cm. The excess is lost within the dog ear at the point of rotation.

The distal two thirds of the flap become the new hairline. Therefore, the design of this portion of the flap must correspond to the proposed hairline. The configuration of the hairline is a matter of aesthetic judgment, but a slight curve with some temporal recession, creating a temporal gulf, is preferable. Blunting or rounding the temporal gulf will create an unnatural hairline that is difficult to conceal. The superior point of the hairline is the junction of the frontal and temporal hairlines. The midpoint of the hairline is never placed higher than the temporal gulf.

Technique

The flap is outlined with a skin marker, and the hair is moistened and secured with rubber bands. The hair is not cut along the proposed incisions, since this detracts from the immediate benefits of an established hairline.

The first two delay procedures are done in the office with local anesthesia. The area is locally infiltrated with lidocaine 1% with epinephrine 1:100,000. Neither the flap nor its base should be injected at any time. Intravenous sedation for the occasional apprehensive patient is helpful. In the first delay procedure (Fig. 1), incisions are angled, parallel to the hair follicles, three fourths of the length of the flap and closed with staples. The dressing is removed the next morning, the scalp is shampooed, and the patient can resume normal activities.

One week later, the second delay procedure is done. The tail of the flap is elevated from underlying tissue and perforating vessels that penetrate the scalp posterior and inferior to the galea severed. The incisions are again closed with staples. A drain is placed at the inferior aspect of the incisions. The patient has a bandage in place the evening after surgery, which is removed the next morning.

Two weeks after the first delay procedure, the flap is rotated into place. The office operating suite is used and general endotracheal anesthesia administered. The surgical field is anesthetized with lidocaine 0.5% with epinephrine 1:200,000. The flap is elevated in the subgaleal plane and kept moist at all times with saline solution. The inferior margin of the donor defect is raised in the subgaleal plane until the lower limit of hair-bearing skin is reached. Then the dissection is continued subcutaneously. The postauricular skin is elevated to the helical rim, and the dissection is carried into the neck as necessary to close the donor defect without tension. The frontal hairline incision is done while beveling the blade inferiorly. This corresponds with the angle of the cut on the superior border of the flap done parallel to the hair to avoid transection of follicles. The frontotemporal skin posterior to this incision is elevated deep to the galea so that it can be rotated posteriorly and inferiorly to help close the donor wound.

A Jackson-Pratt drain is placed through a postauricular stab wound. The margins of the donor defect are approximated with 0-polydioxanone interrupted inverted galeal suture and staples in the epidermis. It is important that the flap not be closed under extreme tension to avoid necrosis of hair-bearing scalp (Fig. 2). A full-thickness skin graft may be placed so that the postauricular hairline is not elevated. The graft is later removed after scalp laxity returns (Fig. 3).

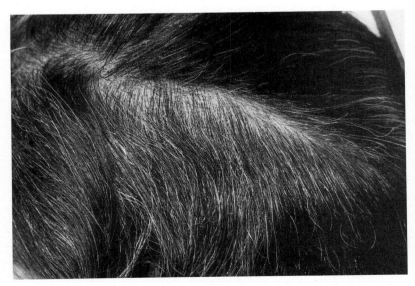

Figure 2   Hair is pulled back to expose 1- to 2-mm scar in parieto-occipital scalp after F/M donor defect closure.

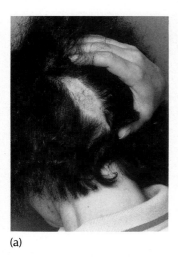
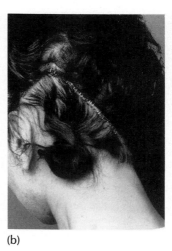

(a)   (b)

Figure 3   (a) Patient after removal of flap that was rotated to establish a new hairline. A small skin graft was placed in the back of the donor closure to avoid tension on the scalp. The surrounding hair hides the donor graft. (b) The small graft has been removed after the scalp has regained its normal elasticity.

Two millimeters of the anterior border of the flap is deepithelialized and the flap sutured to the forehead with a 5-0 polypropylene suture (Fig. 4). Hair will grow from follicles buried beneath the skin closure, establishing a new hairline and camouflaging the scar. An appropriate amount of frontal scalp is removed. Penrose drains are placed along the posterior margin of the flap. The remaining incisions are closed without tension with staples.

A nonadhesive dressing and gauze fluffs are left in place for 4 days. The drains are removed the day after surgery. Hairline sutures are removed 6 days postoperatively and staples 1 week later.

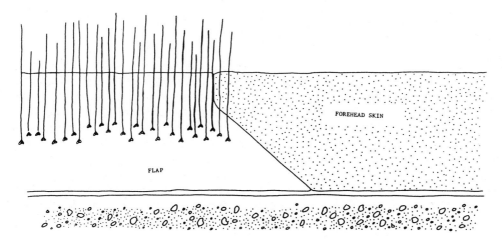

Figure 4   Hairline closure: cross section through junction of flap and forehead skin. Anterior border of flap is deepitheliazed. The growth of hair from follicles buried beneath the wound closure established a new hairline and camouflages the scar.

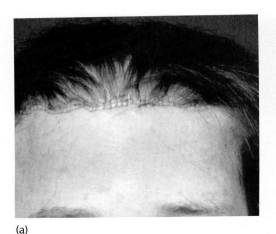   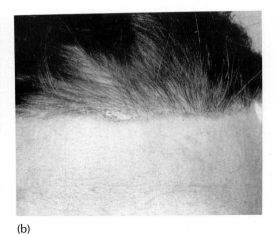

(a)   (b)

Figure 5 (a) Patient 6 days after surgery with hair combed back immediately before removal of hairline sutures. Small bump or "dog ear" present at end of hairline. (b) Same patient 3 weeks after surgery with redness along hairline and decrease in size of dog ear. Dog ear is easily concealed with surrounding hair until it is revised 6 weeks after flap rotation.

Morbidity

Eyelid and forehead edema occurs commonly after procedures performed in the frontal region of the scalp including punch grafts. This problem has been eliminated by use of short-acting oral steroids. Patients are given methylprednisolone, 24 mg, the day of surgery. The dosage is gradually tapered off over the next 5 days. There may be tenderness of the ear on the donor side that persists for a few days due to sensitivity of the cartilage after surgical manipulation. Swelling and ecchymosis of the lateral aspect of the neck in the area of undermining will occur as well. Patients should avoid strenuous activities for approximately 3 weeks postoperative.

A dog ear occurs along the anterior margin of the flap at its base because the flap is rotated back upon itself to establish the hairline. The size of the dog ear, which is almost always present after F/M flaps, will decrease markedly after several weeks. Hair within the flap is used to cover the dog ear until it is revised at 6 weeks (Fig. 5).

Additional Procedures

Six weeks after rotation of the flap, the dog ear is divided at the junction of frontal and temporal hairlines. The divided ends are rotated posteriorly and superiorly (Fig. 6). If necessary, a second flap may be rotated from the opposite side 3 months after the initial flap rotation. A 3- to 4-cm patch of bald skin is left between the two flaps and is later removed with scalp reduction and stretching of the anterior flap (Fig. 7). Total or near-total excision of bald skin on the crown can be accomplished with scalp reduction and further stretching of the posterior flap (Fig. 8). Two 4.0-cm flaps usually cover 12 cm of alopecia and occasionally more in those with a loose scalp. Combined with occipital scalp reduction, most patients have total excision of bald skin and replacement with uniformly dense hair-bearing scalp. A third (retroauricular or occipital) flap, as described by Juri, has not been necessary in the authors' experience.

Complications

Complications of the F/M flap are classified into two groups: those occurring in patients with normal scalp circulation and those in patients with compromised or impaired scalp circulation.

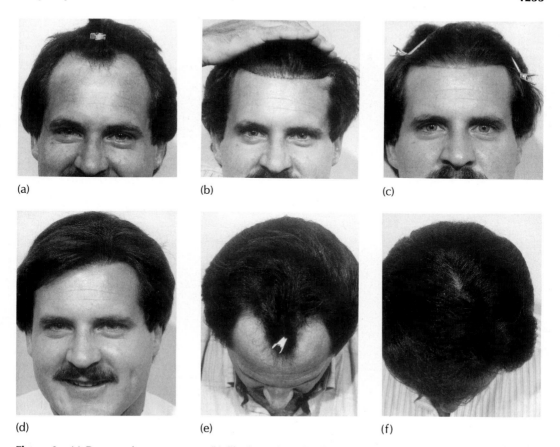

(a) (b) (c)

(d) (e) (f)

Figure 6 (a) Preoperative appearance. (b) Six days after F/M flap rotation with dog ear present, left temple. (c) Patient after removal of dog ear 6 weeks after flap rotation, with hair retracted. (d) Patient 7 weeks postoperative with hair styled. (e) Preoperative appearance. (f) Postoperative appearance.

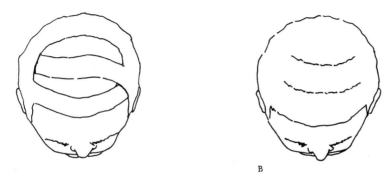

A B

Figure 7 (A) A second flap can be transferred from the opposite side 3 months later or when baldness progresses in the future. (B) Bald skin left between the flaps and in the crown can be excised and the flaps stretched to eliminate bald skin and replace it with hair-bearing scalp.

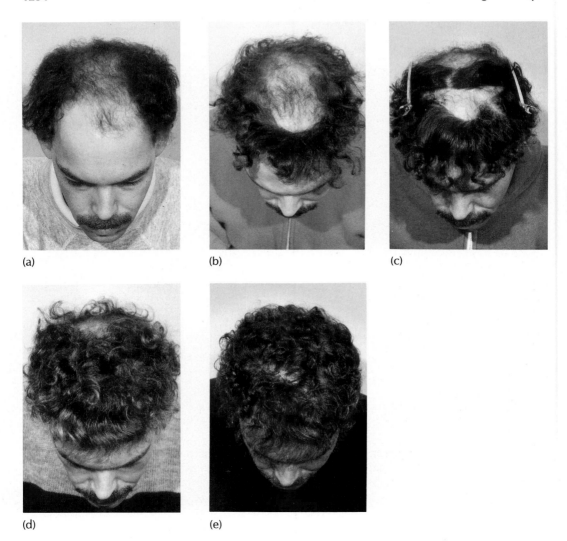

(a)   (b)   (c)

(d)   (e)

Figure 8 Patient with excessive baldness extending into the crown. (a) Preoperative appearance. (b) After one F/M flap. (c) After second F/M flap. (d) After reduction between flaps. (e) After reduction posterior to second flap with total elimination of alopecia.

Patients with Normal Circulation

The possibility of serious complications compromising the final result does exist. This has occurred twice in the authors' experience of more than 3000 Juri flaps in patients with normal scalp circulation. Necrosis or permanent hair loss along any portion of the flap or donor wound closure is rare. The F/M flap technique is not done on patients who smoke cigarettes because of possible vascular compromise. One of the patients who developed flap necrosis had denied his two-pack-a-day smoking habit. Flap loss may be corrected by rotation of small flaps from the contralateral side.

Very small areas of permanent hair loss in the flap or the donor area are rare in the authors' experience. If this occurs, the bald spot can be excised after wound maturation. Temporary telogen at the distal end of the flap is occasionally seen. Hair growth resumes in 2–3 months. Telogen effluvium occurs to a minor extent in the donor area in approximately 5% of patients. On rare occasions, hair loss can be significant, but the hair always regrows if the scalp circulation is normal.

The most common complications in patients referred to our office are poor hairline design, prominent hairline scarring, and donor area hair loss, usually with necrosis. These complications can be avoided with careful planning and meticulous surgical technique.

Patients with Compromised Circulation

Many patients need reconstructive surgery and may have compromised vascular supply. These patients may have had punch graft transplantation, scalp reductions, nylon fiber implantation with infection, face lifts with ligation of the superficial temporal artery, or trauma. These patients carry greater risk because of their impaired circulation.

In the authors' series of patients with compromised circulation, five patients had necrosis of the distal portion of the flap. Three of these patients had previously undergone hair transplantation. The punch graft donor scars had decreased circulation in the distal 2–3 cm of the flap. The resultant alopecia was excised and replaced with a small flap from the opposite side. The other two patients were women who had had superficial temporal artery ligation as a part of face lift surgery. These patients had no superficial temporal artery traceable with a Doppler, and only 20% of the normal amount of bleeding was present at the first and second delay procedures. In both patients, the flaps were absolutely normal prior to transposition. One patient developed 3.0 cm of necrosis that was corrected with a small flap from the opposite side, with an excellent cosmetic result.

In the other patient, the complication was treated with advancement of the flaps as well as partial augmentation with punch grafts. This demonstrates the importance of having a viable branch of the superficial temporal artery within the flap. Even though the flap may not appear compromised prior to transfer, necrosis may occur. Patients without a superficial temporal artery should have small flaps or punch grafts because of the possibility of necrosis using the F/M flap.

The incidence of temporary telogen in the donor area in this group is much higher. Two patients had almost total temporary hair loss in the parietal occipital region. There is regrowth of hair in approximately 2 months.

In summary, nonsmoking patients with normal circulation can expect good results from scalp flaps done by experienced surgeons. The incidence of necrosis and permanent hair loss is extremely small.

Advantages

There are several aspects of the F/M flap that make it more desirable to patients. Frontal alopecia is eliminated within 2 weeks (Fig. 9). This takes up to 1 or 2 years with punch grafting. Density of the hair is greater and more uniform than with punch grafts. The "row-of-corn" appearance is avoided (Fig. 10). The density makes hair styling easier, since patients do not have to create the appearance of density. Hair may be parted through the flap, or the hairline may be exposed (Fig. 11,12). Good results are obtained in black patients with curly hair as well. With few exceptions, there are no restrictions to hair styling after this procedure. Temporary hair loss that accompanies punch grafting is rare with flaps. When it does occur, the area of telogen is easily covered by surrounding hair.

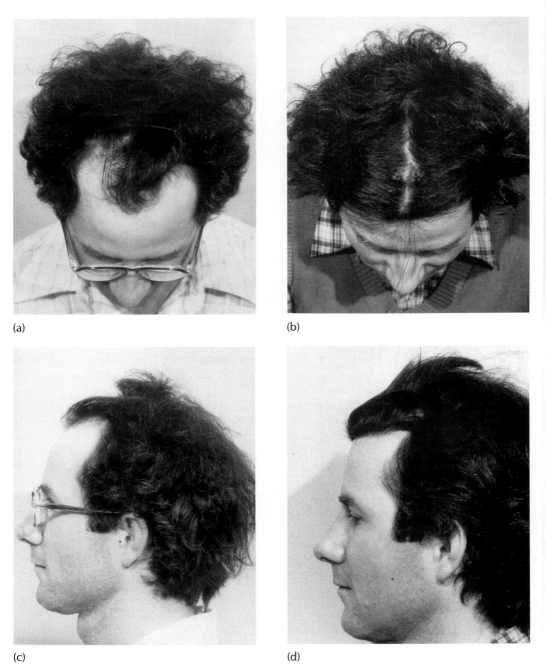

(a)

(b)

(c)

(d)

Figure 9   Thirty-year-old patient with frontal baldness and thinning of frontal tuft. (a) Preoperative appearance, head down. (b) Postoperative appearance: F/M flap with head down shows excellent density and continuity with remaining hair. A second flap is available for future use, if necessary, from the opposite side. (c) Preoperative profile. (d) Postoperative appearance 8 weeks after F/M flap rotation.

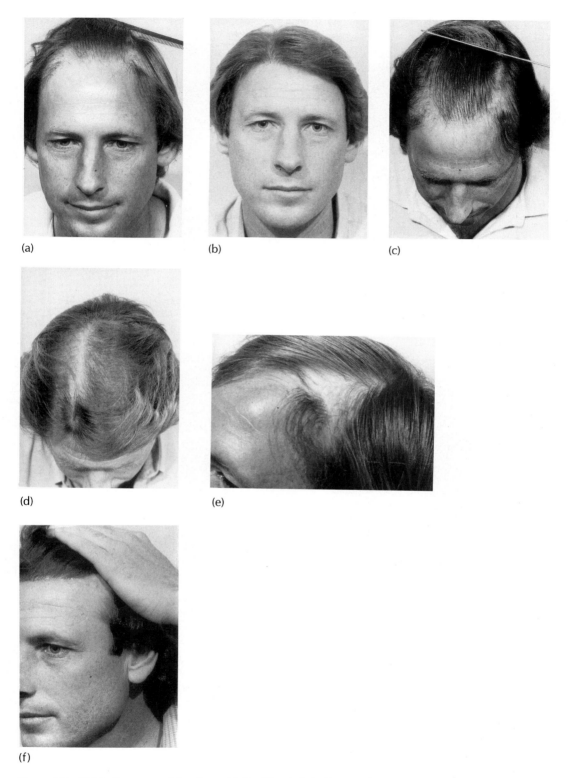

Figure 10 Thirty-three-year old patient with fine blonde hair who previously had undergone bilateral punch grafts and strip grafts in both temples. (a) Preoperative appearance. (b) After F/M flap. (c) Preoperative appearance. (d) Postoperative. (e) Preoperative close-up, left forehead and temple. (f) Postoperative appearance with hair held back 7 weeks after excision of strips and grafts and reconstruction with F/M flap.

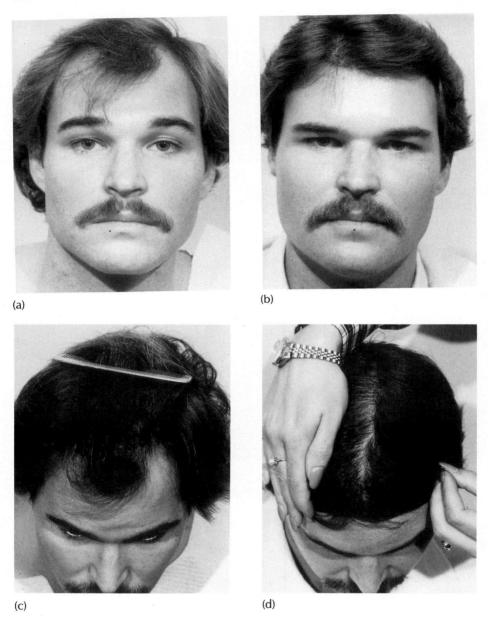

(a)

(b)

(c)   (d)

Figure 11 Twenty-three-year-old patient with frontal baldness. (a) Preoperative appearance. (b) Postoperative appearance: normal uniform density of hair allows patient to part through flap. (c) Preoperative appearance. (d) After one F/M flap. Second flap is available if baldness extends over top of head at a later date.

The hairline scar will be hidden by hair growing through and in front of the hairline incision (Fig. 13). Without this refinement in the hairline, the scar anterior to the hairline would be noticeable. The patients in Figure 13 have the old straight hairline, which is softened using an irregular design (Figs. 14,15). Some patients will also have micrografts placed at the hairline

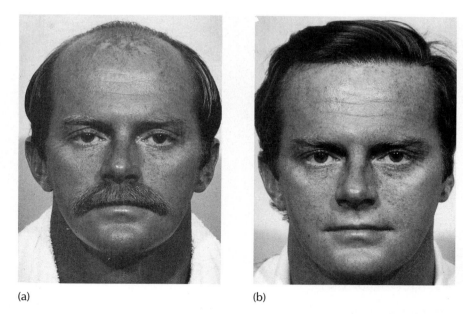

(a)   (b)

Figure 12 (a) Preoperative appearance. (b) Appearance 8 weeks after F/M flap with hair combed back to expose hairline.

(Fig. 16). Two F/M flaps combined with scalp reductions result in the greatest possible excision of bald skin and replacement with the largest amount of hair-bearing skin of uniform density.

Disadvantages

Approximately 6 days' rest at home is required postoperatively, so the disability accompanying this procedure is greater than that with punch grafts. The surgery is more extensive, but fewer procedures are necessary. The risk of serious complications is more likely than with punch grafts and must be clearly explained to the patient. There is a change in hair direction: it is directed posteriorly instead of growing anteriorly. However, there are fewer styling restrictions than with punch grafts because of increased hair density, a nontufted hairline, and the ability to comb the hair back or part the hair in the flap.

OTHER SCALP FLAPS

The F/M flap is most commonly performed for hair replacement surgery and scalp reconstruction because of its versatility. A large amount of bald skin can be removed in a single procedure. Other scalp flaps have limited application but are designed for specific areas of alopecia.

Inferiorly Based Temporoparietal Flaps (Modified by Fleming and Mayer)

Design

Temporoparietal flaps are narrower, shorter, inferiorly based flaps that are nondelayed and narrower than F/M flaps. They do not extend across the entire forehead. A second flap may be rotated from the contralateral side to complete the hairline (Fig. 17).

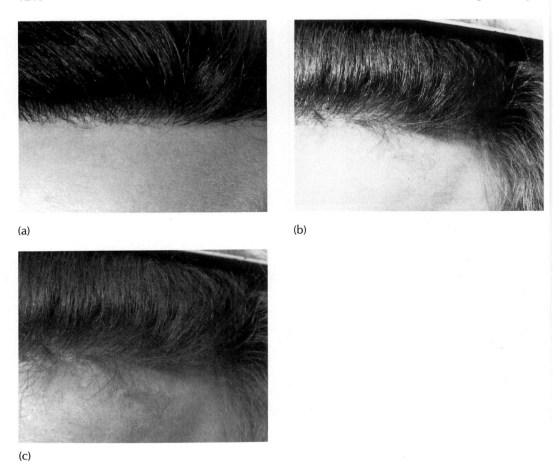

(a)   (b)

(c)

Figure 13   Three hairlines in patients with different hair color and texture all shown more than 1 year after surgery. Postoperative appearance shows hair growth through the undetectable scar and normal uniform density of the flap hairline.

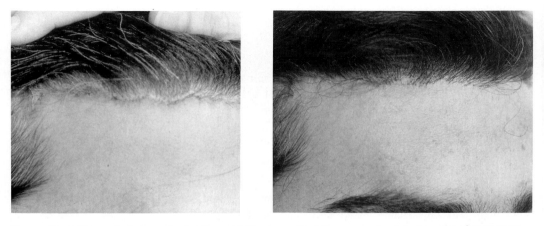

Figure 14   (a) Irregularly irregular hairline. (b) Close-up of hairline approximately 8 weeks after surgery.

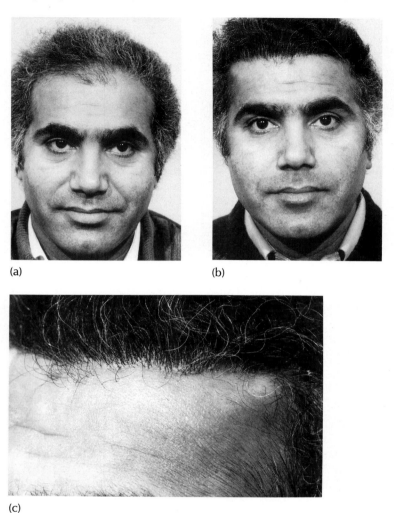

(a)

(b)

(c)

Figure 15   (a) Patient with thick, dark hair. (b) After one F/M flap with hairline created in an irregularly irregular fashion. (c) Close-up view of irregular hairline.

Some authors have designed the flap without regard to the artery, and therefore its vascular supply is at risk. All scalp flaps should be axial whenever possible. This maneuver ensures maximum survival of the sensitive hair follicles and does not generally compromise flap design or make the procedure more difficult.

The incision is gently curved posteriorly and superiorly over the ear and then inferiorly into the parietal or anterior occipital region. The first flap is cut long enough to extend beyond the midpoint of the new hairline, so there is less risk of hair loss in the tail of the shorter second flap. Furthermore, it is better to err on the side of making the flaps longer than to be caught

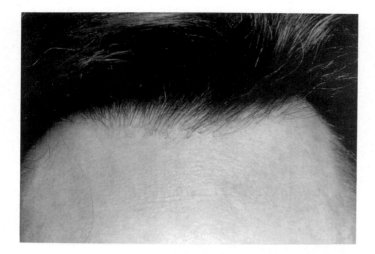

Figure 16 The irregular design of the flap has softened the abruptness of the newly established hairline. Micrografts are present to further soften or feather the hairline.

with flaps that are too short and, therefore, fail to join. The distal end of the first flap is designed to dovetail with the flap from the opposite side at an angle of 45–60 degrees. This angle will prevent the scar from being seen at the junction of the two flaps. The base of the flap should be well within the temporal incision, especially in young patients. The width of the flap is 2.5–3 cm throughout its length.

The authors' design of the inferiorly based temporoparietal flap differs from previous designs. As stated earlier, the base of the flap is axial. Narrowing the base of the flap and performing a delay procedure has been described, but this is rarely done by the authors. Narrowing the base of the flap decreases dog-ear formation but may cause flap ischemia, necessitating the delay step. The pedicle, however, is the source of blood supply, and decreasing the width is risky. There are safer techniques to minimize the dog ear. The proximal incision of the flap is gently curved. A more horizontal flap design results in a larger dog ear. The distal 3.0 cm is straight to meet the corresponding straight line at the tail of the second flap to avoid a notch in the hairline when two distinctive curves meet at the junction of the flaps.

The flaps are transposed 2 weeks apart. If distal necrosis of the first flap occurs, the second flap may be delayed and extended to complete the hairline. Necrosis of the second flap is much more difficult to reconstruct.

Surgical Technique

The procedure is performed in an office operating suite under light general anesthesia and local anesthesia with lidocaine 0.5% and epinephrine 1:200,000. Basic principles are the same as described for the F/M flap. Even though this is a smaller flap, the inferior border of the donor

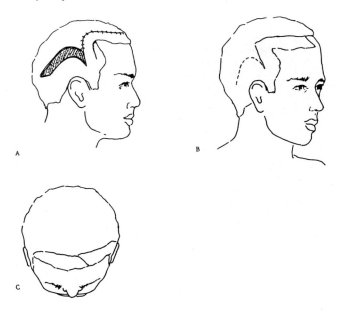

Figure 17 Inferiorly based temporoparietal flaps. (A) Well-defined frontotemporal recession without blunting. Only one flap is done at a time. (B) Flap has been transposed and the donor area closed along the dotted line. (C) Two weeks later, a second flap on the opposite side is used to complete the hairline. Scalp reduction and stretching of the short flaps will eliminate small areas of remaining frontal baldness.

defect should be undermined to the posterior surface of the auricle and down into the neck in order to achieve a tension-free closure. Score the hairline on the contralateral side with a scalpel when the first flap is rotated to ensure symmetry when the second flap is transposed 2 weeks later. The dog ear is smaller and not as stiff. It may completely resolve in 2–3 months but can be revised 6 weeks postoperatively if necessary by splitting the flap at the junction of the frontal and temporal hairline and rotating the two cut ends superiorly and posteriorly. Two or three months after the flaps have been rotated, they can be stretched with scalp reductions to increase coverage by about 25% (Fig. 18).

Morbidity

Tenderness and tightness over the lateral scalp and upper neck last about 1 week. Strenuous activity is restricted for 3 weeks, but normally the patient returns to work 1 week after the procedure. Short-term oral steroids have eliminated forehead and eyelid edema that occurs when surgery is done in the frontal region of the scalp. Hair on the flap covers the dog ear until it resolves or is revised.

Complications

Infection, hematoma, and temporary or permanent hair loss are possible but rarely occur. Necrosis and permanent hair loss, whether in the flap or donor area, would be the most serious complication. In the authors' experience with short-flap procedures, there was only one instance of distal hair loss (1.5 cm in a second short flap that had been traumatized postoperatively). When necrosis occurs in the distal portion of the second flap, it is more difficult to correct than with the F/M flap because hair loss is in the center of the hairline. Correction of the problem could be done by excising the area of alopecia, then rotating and advancing the flaps medially to ob-

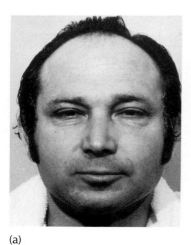 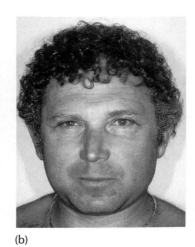

(a)   (b)

Figure 18   (a) Preoperative 42-year-old patient with limited frontal baldness. (b) Appearance 3 months after rotation of two temporoparietal flaps. Stretching of the flaps with one scalp reduction totally eliminated the baldness.

tain complete closure. Alternatively, punch grafting could be done, with a less desirable cosmetic result. Careful handling of the flap means no pressure or twisting the base combined with tension-free closure to ensure that the incidence of necrosis is low.

Disadvantages

The important disadvantage of temporoparietal flaps is that they provide only one fourth of the coverage of two F/M flaps. Therefore, if alopecia is present 3 cm posterior to the anterior frontal scalp, one must rely on scalp reduction and punch grafts. One cannot achieve total or near-total hair replacement with two temporoparietal flaps as with two F/M flaps followed by scalp reductions when alopecia is or will be more advanced.

Superiorly Based Temporal and Parietal Flaps

Superiorly based preauricular and postauricular flaps were described by Nataf in 1976. These flaps (Fig. 19) provide anteriorly directed hair growth. A long postauricular flap can reach the midline if the temporoparietal fringe is high enough.

The preauricular flap is useful only for partial hairline completion, since the flap rarely reaches the midline. Marzola's technique utilizes extensive scalp reduction to stretch the occipital scalp superiorly and anteriorly. The donor area can be lengthened and, at the same time, the intertemporal (hairline) distance is shortened. This preauricular flap may reach the midline and beyond if scalp laxity permits adequate reduction before flap rotation. The flaps are 2.5–3.0 cm in width at the base and narrowed to 2.0–2.5 cm inferiorly. The average length is approximately 12–15 cm.

These flaps have only one advantage over the others—the hair grows in an anterior direction. This would be desirable if it were not for the following important disadvantages:

1. The F/M flap and most other inferiorly based flaps are axial flaps. The superiorly based temporoparietal flaps are random flaps and, therefore, more susceptible to necrosis. For this reason, the delay procedure is done to prevent necrosis.

(a)

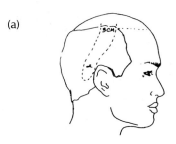 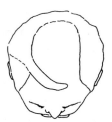

POSTAURICULAR FLAP

(b)

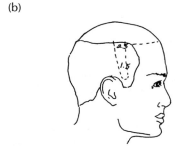 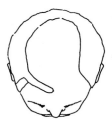

PREAURTICULAR FLAP

Figure 19 (a) Postauricular flap. This superiorly based flap must be narrow in order to close the donor area. (b) Preauricular flap superiorly based. It is usually shorter than a postauricular flap and is difficult to reach the midline.

2. The hair at the distal end of these flaps is taken from the preauricular hair just above the sideburn and is often of poor quality and low density.
3. If distal necrosis occurs, it results in alopecia in the center of the hairline that is more difficult to correct.
4. The temporal hairline is pulled posteriorly to close the donor defect and will appear more receded.
5. Incisions made along the temporal hairline result in scars that may be more noticeable, especially with further temporal recession.
6. The donor defect can be difficult to close because it is vertically oriented. The F/M flap and the inferiorly based temporoparietal flaps are horizontal.
7. Superiorly based flaps rarely reach the midline unless combined with scalp reduction. Punch grafts can be done to complete the hairline. The dissection is quite formidable and should be carried out only by those with extensive experience in scalp surgery.

8. The most important drawback to superiorly based flaps is the same as that with the short, inferiorly based temporoparietal flap. Only 2.0–2.5 cm of hair in the frontal scalp is eliminated. The remaining alopecia posteriorly must be treated with scalp reduction or punch grafting. The authors feel that the final results do not compare with two F/M flaps.
9. Even with scalp reduction, there is still a major problem with divergence of hair growth around the reduction scar in the midscalp.

These flaps are applicable in the following situations:

1. Patients with only mild frontal baldness
2. High, superior, and anteriorly placed temporal hairline
3. Good hair quality in the temporal scalp including the preauricular area
4. Our modification of the superiorly based flaps includes the use of a rectangular tissue expander placed in the temporoparietal scalp prior to flap elevation and rotation.

The only advantage of this technique is the ability to provide anteriorly directed hair within the flaps. The many disadvantages limit its application.

Free Scalp Flaps

Harii, Juri, Ohmori, and others have described microvascular anastomosis for transposition of scalp flaps. The main advantage of free scalp flaps is proper orientation of hair growth. The microsurgical dissection and vascular anastomosis involve a longer, technically more difficult procedure. The risk of total flap loss is much greater than with axial transposition flaps.

Random Scalp Flaps

Random flaps have limited application, especially for the treatment of significant male pattern baldness. These flaps are smaller, but there is no formula by which we can design a random flap with total assurance that it will survive. Preoperatively, it is important to evaluate the patient to rule out vascular disease or the presence of traumatic or surgically induced compromise of scalp circulation. Fluorescein or Doppler ultrasound may be used to evaluate the amount of blood flowing through a flap. However, the interpretation of these tests is frequently difficult in delineating possible skin loss, let alone trying to determine the viability of sensitive hair follicles.

Random flaps should be used only when absolutely necessary. The infinite variations of alopecia occasionally make these flaps worthwhile (Fig. 20). In young men, the possibility of future male pattern baldness that could result in the exposure of surgical scars should be considered. Tissue expansion in many cases is a safer alternative than random transposition flaps, although patient acceptance is sometimes difficult.

PATIENT SELECTION

To present our philosophy in an organized fashion, the following discussion of scalp flaps is based on the extent of male pattern baldness. The treatment of alopecia secondary to other causes is too variable and extensive to discuss in this chapter.

When possible the authors prefer the use of scalp flaps in surgical treatment of male pattern alopecia. There are few absolute medical contraindications to hair replacement surgery; however, the medical condition of the patient is more critical when doing transposition flaps. A history of cardiovascular disease, hematologic disorders, or prior surgical complications should be thoroughly investigated. Diabetic patients and cigarette smokers may be poor risks because of impaired peripheral circulation affecting the flap. If the circulation is compromised secondary to

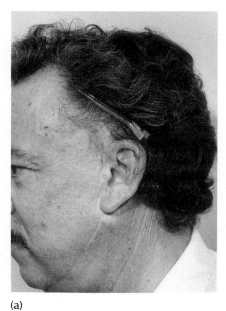 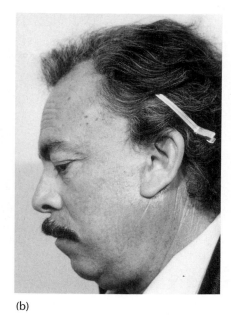

(a)   (b)

Figure 20 (a) Fifty-six-year-old man with loss of inferior tuft of temporal hair after facelift surgery. (b) Superiorly based random flap is rotated anteriorly to replace lost hair.

trauma or previous surgery, this cicatricial alopecia is best treated with hair-bearing scalp flaps, since blood supply is provided by the flap pedicle. Punch grafts can be done on scar tissue, but the growth is often diminished due to impaired circulation.

Hair density is important for punch grafting. For patients with low-density hair, flap procedures are advantageous since hair is not lost and hair redistribution is uniform. Furthermore, there may be difficulty concealing the tufted appearance or change in hair texture associated with punch grafting. We consider this procedure a second choice. The success of any technique, however, depends on the surgical experience of the surgeon. The use of scalp flaps, punch grafts, and tissue expansion must be applied individually to patients with unusual patterns of alopecia.

The first useful classification of male pattern baldness was published by Hamilton in 1951 and is repeated in this text in the chapter on hair transplantation. In 1973, Norwood simplified his classification, organizing baldness into seven categories plus a variant type. Norwood stated that classification is essential to an organized, systematic study of male pattern alopecia. The authors have chosen to simplify the classification further (Fig. 21):

> Class I: Frontal baldness only, with or without an anterior tuft
> Class II: Frontal and midscalp baldness with no thinning of the crown
> Class III: Frontal to occipital baldness
> Class IV: Crown baldness only

Class I

The most important consideration prior to surgical hair replacement is the evaluation of the amount of existing baldness, the potential for progressive alopecia, and the quality of the donor area. In general, patients with fully established frontal baldness that will not progress can be treated with the F/M flap, the nondelayed temporoparietal flaps, or superiorly based tempo-

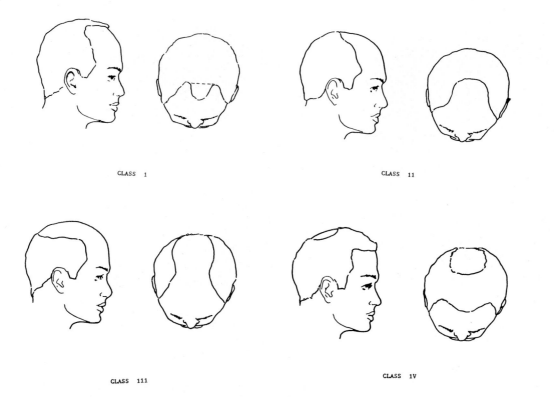

CLASS 1   CLASS 11

CLASS 111   CLASS 1V

Figure 21   Simplified classification of male pattern baldness.

ral or temporoparietal flaps. One F/M flap can be done with immediate, total hair replacement for alopecia limited to the frontal scalp (Fig. 22). The hair within the flap has normal uniform density without a change in texture. Class I alopecia may also be treated with two short flaps, superiorly or inferiorly based (Fig. 23). However, creation of two short flaps involves more work for both the patient and surgeon than one F/M flap. The advantages and disadvantages of these flaps have been discussed previously.

Class II

This is the least common balding pattern. Scalp reduction is of benefit in these patients to decrease midscalp baldness. Two F/M flaps may also be done with or without scalp reduction. Short flaps combined with scalp reduction and punch grafting give suboptimal results.

Class III

The overwhelming majority of male patients have or eventually will have class III pattern baldness. Often patients with this degree of hair loss are not satisfied with punch grafts. The supply of donor grafts is usually not adequate to achieve an ideal result. Therefore, grafts are concentrated at the hairline and on the part side of the scalp. This is done in conjunction with scalp reduction, so that hair can be combed over portions of the scalp where fewer grafts are placed. Another alternative is to leave the crown bald, utilizing all of the grafts at the hairline and the

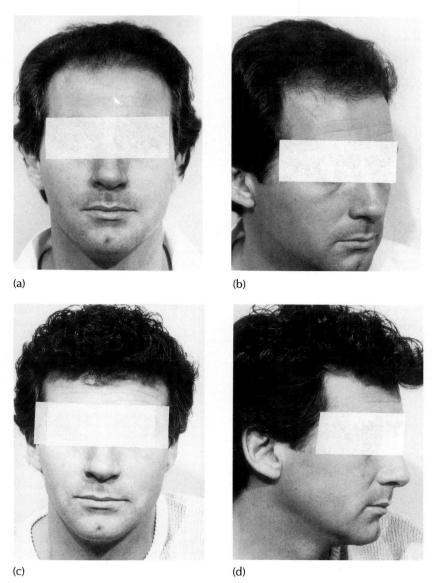

(a)

(b)

(c)

(d)

Figure 22 (a,b) Preoperative appearance of man with limited frontal baldness. (c,d) After one F/M flap: note freedom of styling after flap surgery.

anterior portion of the scalp. Although alopecia is not totally eliminated, the bald area is decreased, with maximum concentration of grafts anteriorly and a natural pattern of residual alopecia at the crown. Scalp reduction should be considered for these patients. A significant amount of bald scalp can be excised in patients with average scalp laxity.

Two F/M flaps combined with scalp reduction to stretch the flaps will eliminate the baldness in most class III patients (Fig. 24). This can be accomplished even in those with low-density fine hair (Fig. 25). Total or near-total elimination of the baldness can be achieved with two larger Juri flaps followed by scalp reduction (Fig. 26).

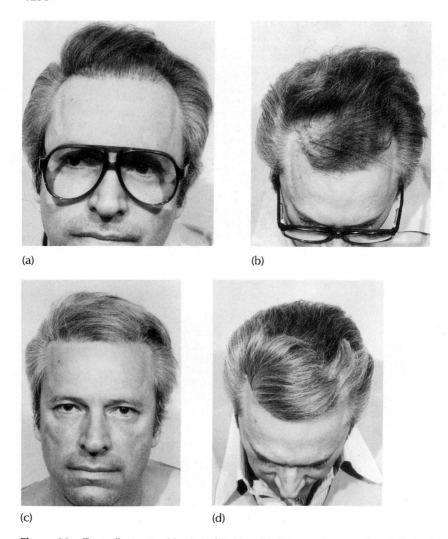

(a)

(b)

(c)

(d)

Figure 23 Forty-five-year-old man with frontal baldness who was dissatisfied with the results of punch grafting. (a,b) Lack of density with punch grafts preoperatively. (c,d) Appearance after two inferiorly based temporoparietal flaps. When short flaps were used, scars within the posterior donor scalp secondary to punch graft harvesting were avoided.

Short flaps may be used for class III alopecia, but this technique provides only 1–1.5 inches of hair in the frontal scalp and leaves a large bald area that must be treated with scalp reduction and punch grafting (Fig. 27). Few men have adequate scalp laxity to eliminate most of the baldness behind the flaps. It does not make sense to do flaps anteriorly followed by reductions and transplantations. Patients who lack sufficient donor area for a F/M flap may have an acceptable but less desirable result with short flaps followed by reductions and transplants. Short flaps may be a prudent choice for patients who have punch graft donor scars in the occipital scalp that will compromise blood supply in the distal end of the F/M flap. In carefully selected patients who have a limited donor area with excellent density or a very tight scalp, tissue expansion prior to F/M flap rotation is a good alternative.

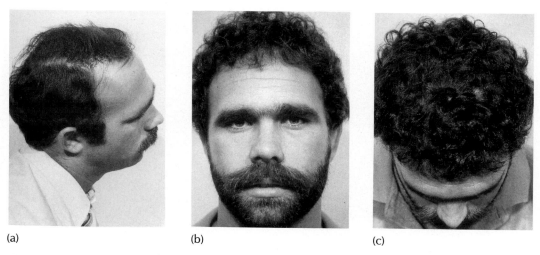

(a) (b) (c)

Figure 24 Twenty-eight-year-old patient after nylon implantation of the scalp from the hairline to the occiput. Patient has chronic infection and scarring. (a) Preoperative appearance. (b,c) Postoperative result after two F/M flaps and scalp reduction. Scarred and infected scalp is eliminated and replaced with normal hair.

Class IV

The F/M flap (Fig. 28) or an axial transposition flap based on the postauricular or occipital artery may be used for baldness limited to the crown. The F/M flap is the procedure of choice because the donor defect, oriented horizontally, is easier to close. In addition, after flap rotation, hair growth is in the normal posterior, inferior direction.

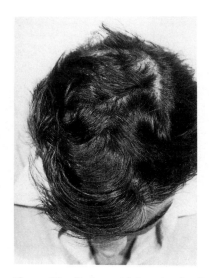

Figure 25 Patient with low-density fine hair after F/M flap procedure. No loss of hair thickness occurred with flap technique.

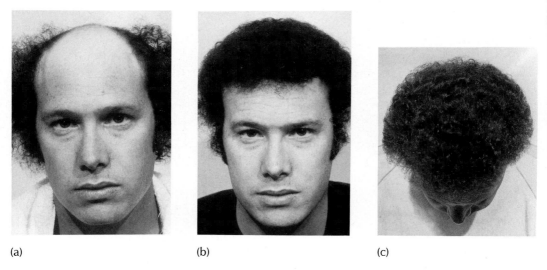

(a) (b) (c)

Figure 26 Thirty-three-year-old patient treated with two F/M flaps and scalp reduction. (a) Preoperative appearance. (b,c) Postoperative result.

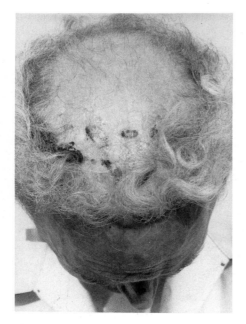

Figure 27 Patient after two short flaps with necrosis. The only option is scalp reduction and punch grafting, with a less desirable result.

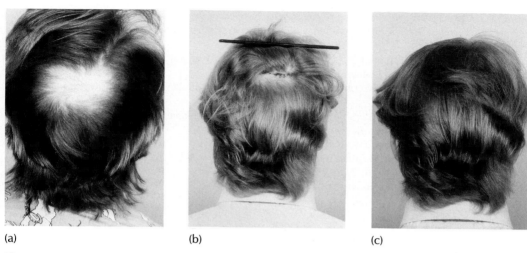

(a)   (b)   (c)

Figure 28 (a) Baldness limited to crown. (b) One F/M flap. Hair is pulled back to expose residual alopecia that can be eliminated with scalp reduction. (c) Hair is styled 10 days after surgery.

BIBLIOGRAPHY

Brandy DA. The bilateral occipito-parietal flap. *J Dermatol Surg Oncol* 1896; (Sept.).

Dunham T. A method for obtaining a skin flap from the scalp and a permanent buried vascular pedicle for covering defects of the face. *Ann Surg* 1893;17:677.

Elliott RA. Lateral scalp flaps for instant results in male pattern baldness. *Plast Reconstr Surg* 1977;60:699.

Fleming RW, Mayer TG. Scalp flaps in the treatment of male pattern baldness. In *Hair Transplant Surgery*. 2nd ed. OT Norwood, RC Shiell, eds. Springfield, IL, Charles C Thomas, 1984, pp. 278–314.

Fleming RW, Mayer TG. Scalp flaps-reconstruction of the unfavorable result in hair replacement surgery. *Head Neck Surg* 1985;7:315.

Fleming RW, Mayer TG. Short versus long flaps in the treatment of male pattern baldness. *Arch Otolaryngol* 1981;107:403–408.

Hamilton JB. Patterned loss of hair in man: Types and incidence. *Ann NY Acad Sci* 1951;53:708.

Harii K. Hair transplantation with fee scalp flaps. *Plast Reconstr Surg* 1974;53:410–413.

Heimburger RA. Single-stage rotation of arterialized scalp flaps for male pattern baldness. *Plast Reconstr Surg* 1977;60:789.

Hunt HL. *Plastic Surgery of the Head, Face, and Neck*. Philadelphia, Lea & Febiger, 1926.

Juri J. Use of parieto-occipital flaps in the surgical treatment of baldness. *Plast Reconstr Surg* 1975;55:456.

Juri J, Juri C, Arufe HN. Use of rotation scalp flaps for treatment of occipital baldness. *Plast Reconstr Surg* 1978;61:23.

Juri J, Juri C, Ohmori K, et al. Colgajo libre temporo-parieto-occipital para el tratamiento de la calvicie. *Cir Plat Argent* 1979;3:2.

Kabaker SS. Experience with parieto-occipital flaps in hair transplantation. *Laryngoscope* 1978;88:73.

Kabaker SS. Flap procedures in hair replacement surgery. In *Skin Surgery*. Epstein E and Epstein E Jr, eds. Philadelphia, WB Saunders, 1987, pp. 299–319.

Lamont ES. A plastic surgical transformation: Report of a case. *West J Surg Obstet Gynecol* 1957;65:164.

Lauzon G. Transfer of a large, single, temporo-occipital flap for treatment of baldness. *Plast Reconstr Surg* 1979;63:369.

Marzola M. An alternative hair replacement method. In *Hair Transplant Surgery*. 2nd ed. OT Norwood, RC Shiell, eds. Springfield, IL, Charles C Thomas, 1984, pp. 315–324.

Mayer TG, Fleming RW. *Aesthetic and Reconstructive Surgery of the Scalp*. St. Louis, MO, Mosby, 1992.

Mayer TG, Fleming RW. Hairline aesthetics and styling in hair replacement surgery. *Head Neck Surg* 1985;7:286.

Mayer TG, Fleming RW. Hair transplants and hair bearing flaps in scar camouflage. In *Facial Scars*. R Thomas, R. Holt, eds. St. Louis, MO, CV Mosby, 1988.

Nataf J, Elbaz JS, Pollet J. Etude critique des transplantations de cuir chevelu et proposition d'une optique. *Ann Chir Plast* 1976;21:199.

Norwood OT. *Hair Transplant Surgery*. Springfield, IL, Charles C Thomas, 1973.

Ohmori K. Free scalp flap. *Plast Reconstr Surg* 1980;65:42.

Passot R. *Chirurgic Esthetique Pure*. Paris, G. Doin and Cie, 1931.

Rizzetto-Stubel A, Ellenbogen R. Male Baldness: Immediate single-stage rotation of very long arterialized temporo-parieto-occipital flaps. *Plast Reconstr Surg* 1986;77:215.

Stough DB, Cates JA. Transposition flaps for the correction of baldness: A practical office procedure. *J Dermatol Surg Oncol* 1980;6:286.

73

Scalp Expansion for Male Pattern Baldness

Ernest K. Manders
*The Milton S. Hershey Medical Center, Pennsylvania State Hospital,
Hershey, Pennsylvania*

Marc Friedman
Private Practice, Kenner, Louisiana

Though recession of the anterior hairline is a male secondary sex characteristic, few men find this change flattering or desirable. For some individuals, especially those who develop a significant degree of baldness at an early age, the change in appearance may affect their self-image. Restoration of normal hair distribution has been attempted by treatment with medicines, devices, and operations such as hair transplants, scalp reduction, and flaps. Now with the advent of soft tissue expansion, there is a new modality for reducing or entirely eliminating male pattern baldness.

Soft tissue expansion has precedent in nature. Expansions of the scalp by untreated hydrocephalus is a familiar observation, but its implications were never realized. Lewis et al. reported a case of a patient with a gigantic epidermal inclusion cyst of the scalp that foretold the degree of expansion that would later be possible using implanted soft tissue expanders.

Though Dr. Charles G. Neumann carried out the first controlled soft tissue expansion using an implantable device in 1956, his idea was lost. Doctor Neumann only attempted the expansion once, and none of his colleagues had the insight to pursue this idea.

Independently Dr. Chadomir Radovan developed a device that was totally implantable. It was used to remove a tattoo in 1976. Doctor Radovan's device was constructed with a self-sealing injection port attached to a silicone silastic elastomer envelope by a length of Silastic (Dow Corning) tubing. The envelope was backed by a stiffer material so that the base of the soft tissue expander was defined. The entire device was implantable and filled by injection of sterile saline, and thus suitable for intravenous use, through a small-gauge needle into the self-sealing injection port. Large soft tissue expansions were accomplished over weeks to months with gradual distention.

Expansion of the scalp was pioneered at the Hershey Medical Center in 1982. Soft tissue expanders could be placed in the subgaleal plane over the calvaria of children and adults and inflated to allow reconstruction of massive scalp defects. Little blood loss was encountered in the areolar plane of dissection and few complications recurred. Its original use was to replace skin grafts following resection of neoplasms and trauma or for areas of alopecia following burns. Soft tissue expansion proved very successful.

It was inevitable, in view of these successes, that the technique would be applied to the treatment of male pattern baldness. Now a number of workers have shared their experiences, and even in this short space of time, an evolution of technique is already evident. Several articles have been written on the use of soft tissue expansion in the scalp. Several articles described the use of soft tissue expansion to eliminate male pattern baldness, including expanders of conventional design and newer designs such as the differential expander. Expansion has been used for creation of larger Juri temporoparieto-occipital flaps and scalp advancement flaps for treating male pattern baldness.

PROCESS OF SOFT TISSUE EXPANSION

Soft tissue expansion is accomplished by inserting a Silastic envelope into a subgaleal plane beneath the scalp. The subgaleal plane is a natural plane of loose areolar tissue and can be entered and opened with little blood loss. Dissection is aided by the use of blunt instruments such as a Hegar dilator, a Van Buren male urethral sound, and a malleable retractor. With care and a little experience, the subgaleal plane can be entered rapidly and opened safely in a matter of minutes.

The subgaleal plane preserves the inherent blood supply and innervation of the scalp. If the incision used to place the soft tissue expanders is carefully chosen, there will be no significant interruption of the vascularity or innervation of the scalp.

The expanders used have either remote ports attached to the soft tissue expander by a length of tubing or integrated injection ports that are part of the envelope of the expander. The self-sealing injection ports work well in either location. Surgeons beginning their soft tissue experience may feel more comfortable using expanders with injection ports remote from the envelope. With time, however, the surgeon will find that, particularly in scalp reconstructions, it is advantageous to use an expander with an integrated injection port because both its placement and especially its removal are much easier. The tubing and remote injection port of the remote port design are invested by fibrous tissue. This may be difficult to dissect open for removal of the port and tubing.

Jackson and coworkers from the Mayo Clinic have reported that remote injection ports of soft tissue expanders may be left dangling on their tubing outside the scalp. This has been identified as a great aid in the soft tissue expansion of the scalp in children. Neumann first described this 30 years ago, but this is the first confirmation of the safety of this approach. This has not been used in patients seeking reconstruction for aesthetic reasons because the ports would be an unwanted anomaly. Patients do well with soft tissue expanders with conventional remote or integrated ports. Several patients have even been able to inject their own integrated ports without incident.

The process of soft tissue expansion begins approximately 2 weeks following expander insertion. Patients are much more comfortable if no saline is placed in the soft tissue expanders at the time of insertion. The wound is sufficiently healed by 2 weeks that the expansion can typically begin, even if the incision overlies the implant. Sterile isotonic saline is injected through the injection port. A small-gauge needle, typically a 23-gauge scalp vein needle, is inserted through the skin into the injection port. After the needle penetrates the skin, there is an initial resistance as the Silastic roof of the injection port is penetrated, and then it stops advancing when it reaches the base. If the needle is moved from side to side there will be grating, which is palpable to the operator and often audible, particularly for the patient. This is due to the needle rubbing against the stainless steel backing of the injection port.

The injection port of isotonic saline progresses until the patient reports a sense of tightness. The expansion proceeds cautiously with instillation of saline to not exceed 40 mmHg. By monitoring the intraluminal pressures of many patients undergoing soft tissue expansion, patients typically sense tightness at 40–50 mmHg of pressure. The soft tissues surrounding the expander relax, and typically within minutes the intraluminal pressure of the expander drops to 40 mmHg or below. Measurement of intraluminal pressure is of value, but with experience it is not mandatory. The surgeon familiar with the technique can inject appropriate amounts of saline if he or she listens to the patient and carefully palpates the soft tissue over the expander.

Patients are usually injected at weekly intervals. Some patients have aggressively injected themselves at 4-day intervals. This will lead to more rapid expansion. It will also, however, risk tissue necrosis and exposure of the expander. All patients should be counseled that soft tissue expansion is labor-intensive and takes weeks to months to accomplish for major tissue replacement. It is vital that patients know that the process cannot be rushed.

To secure cooperation, measure the width of the defect to be replaced. Then give the patient a measuring tape to take home. For most patients, a prediction can be made of the amount of expansion required for the treatment of male pattern baldness through scalp expansion. The patient can then measure the increasing distance from ear to ear at home and can thereby be an integral part of the team working to eliminate his problem.

Patients should be told that the process may take 3–4 months or longer and depends on the frequency with which they can be injected and their own particular tissue characteristics. We do not tell our patients that it depends on their ability to tolerate pain. There is no doubt that some patients have accelerated their expansions by living with hours of discomfort on the day of injection. This is an unwise practice, and we emphasize that there should be no pain at any time during the process of scalp reconstruction through expansion except in the immediate postoperative period following placement of these soft tissue expanders.

As the expansion progresses, patients will become increasingly aware of the change in their appearance. Every effort is made to support them psychologically. Urge patients to share an honest explanation of what is going on with curious onlookers who may inquire about their appearance. Patients are often supported by the comments of others who respect their attempt at improving their appearance and self-image. Patients need to know that others who look on are, in general, sympathetic. They need to know that some people will joke childishly. When counseling them for surgery, ask them to consider how they will cope with this aspect of the expansion process.

The appropriate time to advance tissue is determined by measurements indicating that a sufficient arc of tissue has been generated. The soft tissue expansion advancement is less painful than placement of the implant, and it can often be done under local anesthesia if the patient is so inclined. Therefore, operating room and anesthesia charges can be significantly reduced. Sutures are left in for approximately 2 weeks following scalp advancement, except at the anterior hairline, where they may be removed as early as a week after surgery.

It is surprising to many who have operated on the scalp that the galea will accommodate soft tissue expansion so readily. In fact, the galea can be expanded to remarkable size, and there is no need to perform galeotomies in an attempt to assist or accelerate this change. Incising the galea into the subcutaneous tissue where the vessels and nerves lie is an unnecessary risk.

The hair follicles will spread apart during the course of expansion, and, therefore, the hair density is somewhat reduced. Over the scalp this is not a practical problem. The scalp can be expanded by a factor of 2 before any diminution in hair density becomes apparent. Even with larger expansions, the resulting hair density is quite acceptable in the typical patient.

During the course of expansion the hair density will appear less than the ultimate result. There are three reasons for this. First, the hair shafts exit the scalp in an altered direction so one looks down the length of the shaft rather than from the side. This makes the hair look thinner. Second, as the expansion becomes large and the scalp over the expander bears the weight of the patient's head on a pillow, some hair can be rubbed out at night. To prevent this, patients wear stocking caps after about 6 weeks of expansion. Third, a group of patients may experience some telogen effluvium. This is probably due to the excessive local pressure on the follicle. This has been a bigger problem in patients who have undergone home expansion and have been too aggressive with their injection schedule. Hair loss during expansion has regrown for all scalp expansions and has had an adequate density following advancement and reconstruction.

Austad and Pasyk have studied the mitotic index of expanded soft tissues and noted a very high labeling index in the areas of hair follicles. An increase in guinea pig hair growth has been documented during expansion and has also been reported by Austad and Pasyk. An increase in the cell proliferation rate of the hair matrix in expanded pig skin has also been noted by Cherry. During the typical soft tissue expansion of the scalp, hair grows vigorously. Patients let their hair grow longer during expansion since this helps conceal the change in contour.

It is important to emphasize that soft tissue expansion will not reverse androgenetic hair loss. If the scalp that has been expanded is destined to develop alopecia, it will do so as time passes. The surgeon must use an advancement flap design that will remedy this. The midline closure has been a good choice for this reason.

The histologic changes of soft tissue expansion have been observed in both animals and humans. They have not been adequately related to intraluminal injection pressures. Experience has shown that there is virtually no change in the thickness of scalp subjected to a gradual soft tissue expansion. In laboratory animals, hyperplasia of the epidermis, thinning of the dermis, and thinning of the underlying fat has been demonstrated. Certainly thinning of the underlying fat is a common observation, but this discrepancy in thickness is made up by a fibrous capsule that surrounds the soft tissue expander. It is not necessary to excise this capsule; in fact, there is no step-off or depression at the line of closure. Furthermore, neovascularization around the capsule increases the blood supply to the expanded flap. It should be preserved and not incised or excised in the typical case.

In the author's series of adults who have had soft tissue expansion for reconstruction of alopecia due to traumatic defects or for aesthetic reasons, a depression or deformity of the skull attributable to pressure from the overlying expander has not been seen. Two children have had bony ridges that appeared at the edge of the soft tissue expanders, but these have rapidly disappeared following removal of the implant and scalp advancement. Alteration of calvarial shape caused by soft tissue expansion has not occurred.

DESIGN OF SOFT TISSUE EXPANSION

The design of soft tissue expansion for the elimination of male pattern baldness has evolved. Kabaker placed soft tissue expanders of conventional design under the temporoparietal scalp. The expanded scalp was advanced over the vertex. The advancing flaps meet at the midline, but, using conventional expanders that generated hemispheric flaps, a midline V-shaped deformity resulted. This was filled by hair transplantation anteriorly. An alternative is to use longer soft tissue expanders and an occipital midline incision, as advocated by Manders et al.

A geometric approach should be sought for the elimination of male pattern baldness. Ideally, incisions should be inapparent. Because of the uncertain progression of male pattern alopecia, the solution should allow for revision or correction of future hair loss. Do not cause irreversible damage by transecting the blood supply and innervation of normal scalp skin.

Many patients seeking the elimination of baldness have hippocratic (type VI) baldness or incipient hippocratic baldness and require more than advancement of the anterior hairline. The solution has been to expand the remaining temporoparieto-occipital scalp on both sides and advance toward the midline and anteriorly at the same time. If there is a forelock behind which we can camouflage the anterior incision, we preserve it. Hair transplantation or minitransplants can be done at the patient's request to camouflage the anterior incision. It should be noted, however, that this technique is not meant to require hair transplantation in the typical patient.

The soft tissue expansion is accomplished by insertion of two soft tissue expanders of special design. They are differential expanders (Dow Corning, Wright, Arlington, TN), so the portion of the expander that lies under the temporoparietal scalp will expand more than the part of the expander under the occipital scalp (Figs, 1,2). This is important because the gap to be bridged is larger anteriorly. The expanders come as a pair, which meet in the midline posteriorly or overlap slightly. This allows circumferential expansion, which is critically important. Even the occipital scalp will advance forward 6–7 cm. This gives additional length, allowing more anterior advancement of the temporal scalp. The soft tissue expanders are made in an open sigmoid shape so that they follow the natural curve of the hair-bearing scalp: more caudal posteriorly, and more cephalad above the ear and anteriorly.

As the expansion proceeds, differential expansion becomes evident as the expander volume approaches 400 ml. Expansion proceeds to reach a total arc from ear to ear (or the side of the head anterior to the ear) of 60 cm. Typically the arc should approximate 52 cm, depending on the width of alopecia. As expander volumes approach 700 ml, the differential expansion becomes quite obvious. Despite the advancement operation, the scalp will fall forward very nicely, reconstituting the anterior hairline and eliminating the area of alopecia on top of the head.

PREOPERATIVE MANAGEMENT

Prior to surgery, all patients are counseled carefully. It is determined whether this treatment is a realistic approach for them (Fig. 3). Alternatives are discussed, including psychotherapy, wearing a hairpiece, minoxidil treatments, hair transplantation and temporoparieto-occipital flaps, and doing nothing. With surgery, emphasis is placed on the period of transient deformity that lasts perhaps 2 months. The resultant scars are described in detail, and patients are encouraged to talk with previous patients so that they may learn what to expect. They are told that there will

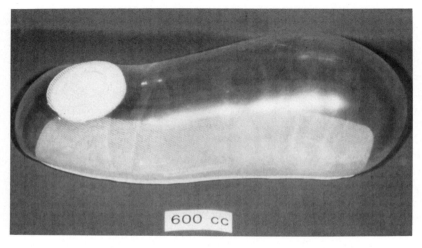

Figure 1   The differential expander that will enlarge more at its anterior end.

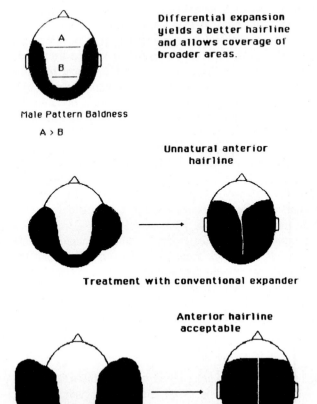

Differential expansion
yields a better hairline
and allows coverage of
broader areas.

Male Pattern Baldness

A > B

Unnatural anterior
hairline

Treatment with conventional expander

Anterior hairline
acceptable

Treatment with a differential
expander

Figure 2 Rationale for differential expansion. Conventional hemispheric flaps fall short of the desired anterior hairline. Differential expansion allows more anterior expansion and the entire hair-bearing scalp moves forward.

also be a widening of the sagittal scar on top of the head, and this may approach 1.0–1.5 cm in width. It may appear wider because the hair exits the scalp directed away from the incision. Generally the anterior incision does very well, but they are told that a minor revision of lateral dog ears may be necessary.

Some patients have unrealistic expectations. They may believe that baldness has crippled them and denied them normal opportunities in life. These patients need psychiatric evaluation and may not be good candidates for surgery.

INSERTION OF SOFT TISSUE EXPANDERS

Soft tissue expanders may be placed in a subgaleal pocket utilizing only local anesthesia. Fifty milliliters of 0.5% lidocaine with epinephrine 1:200,000 is mixed with an equal volume of 0.5% bupivacaine with epinephrine 1:200,000. To this 100 ml anesthetic mixture an additional 100 ml

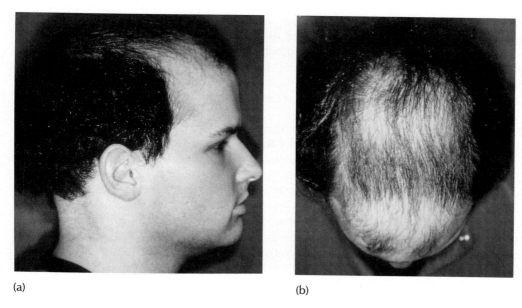

(a)

(b)

Figure 3 Preoperative photographs.

of isotonic saline is added, and the resultant mixture (0.125% lidocaine, 0.125% bupivacaine, and epinephrine 1:400,000) is injected. Some patients will request intravenous sedation. Two techniques have been used by the authors. Initially a ring block of the scalp beginning with a block of supratrochlear and supraorbital nerves was done. The subcutaneous injection of local anesthesia was extended around to the auricular temporal nerve anterior to the ear. The injection was continued above the ear and posterior to the occiput to accomplish a complete ring block of the scalp. This proves very effective. A mixture of lidocaine and marcaine was used. The intended line of incision in the scalp, the posterior midline over the occiput, is also infiltrated for hemostasis.

The newer technique causes less discomfort to the patient. Simply instill local anesthetic solution into the subgaleal space where the pocket will be dissected under hair-bearing scalp. Begin in the occipital region, injecting the skin intended for the midline incision over the occiput. Through this then enter the subgaleal plane and infiltrate with several injections from the occiput to the anterior hairline. This results in excellent anesthesia, and the epinephrine in the anesthetic solution helps to maintain hemostasis.

The patient is then moved to the operating room where suitable monitoring procedures are available. Intravenous access is established, and the patient is prepped and draped. All patients are instructed to shampoo with a soap of their choosing the night before and the morning before surgery. In the operating room the scalp is painted with povidone-iodine solution. The skin is tested with a pin to determine its sensitivity. When adequate anesthesia is established, a 5-cm midline incision is made over the occiput. The incision begins near the top of the hairline.

Hooks are used to retract the skin margins, and the incision is carried down to the pericranium. The pericranium itself is not incised. When the loose areolar plane is identified, the knife is turned so that the blade is uppermost. The back of the knife is swept across the pericranium, which opens the subgaleal space. It is especially important to use a sharp approach over the occiput where the scalp is adherent.

After the occipital scalp is elevated, a blunt dissector such as the Van Buren male urethral sound is introduced and the dissection carried forward. It is completed with a large malleable retractor at least 6 cm wide, approximately the width of the base of the expander. The cavity is dissected all the way to the anterior temporal hairline but not beyond.

A suction drain is inserted through the occipital scalp on each side and placed in each cavity. Saline is used for irrigation to remove fragments of hair, and then the soft tissue expanders are inserted.

There is a right and a left expander to fit the hair distribution on the right and left sides of the head. The expander is introduced completely free of loose hair and without saline. It is gently pushed forward and should slide into position with relative ease. A trial expansion is carried out after the operator's finger has been swept over the injection port to ensure that there is nothing folded over it (Fig. 4). If a remote injection port is used, the trial expansion may proceed while the injection port lies outside the wound. Approximately 50–100 ml sterile isotonic saline is injected and placement of the expander assessed. When it is evident that the expander is appropriately placed under the hair-bearing scalp, the saline is completely evacuated, and the expander for the other side inserted and tested with a trial inflation in a similar fashion. The wound is closed with interrupted 3-0 nylon galeal sutures followed by a running 4-0 nylon skin suture. Sutures are removed in 2–3 weeks.

Postoperatively, the patient has some pain. These patients are hospitalized for observation overnight, although outpatient status is possible for some. The drains are typically removed in 2–3 days. Expansion is begun in 2 weeks.

Postoperatively there will be some swelling around the forehead, and the majority of patients will have a small amount of ecchymosis of the lower lids. Patients should be reassured that this is expected and will resolve in 2 weeks.

EXPANSION

Approximately 2 weeks after insertion of the expanders, inflation is begun. A scalp vein needle is very helpful because it allows mobility without dislodging the needle or lacerating the expander

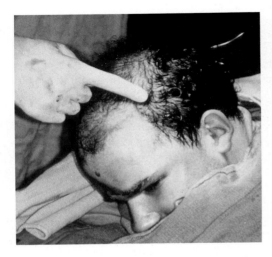

Figure 4 Trial inflation at the time of insertion to ensure proper placement.

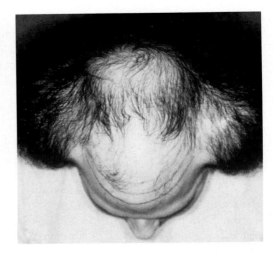

Figure 5 Expansion is completed. Horizontal lines are drawn to aid in symmetry. Note the differential expansion.

envelope. The scalp vein needle assembly is especially useful in those patients performing expansions on themselves at home.

Because one expander will impinge on the other, raising its pressure, it is important to inject one expander first one week and then the contralateral expander first in the next week. Typically, 40 ml can be injected into each expander each week. Some patients will appreciate a sense of tightness before 40 ml is injected; and in such cases, the injection should be stopped early. The patient is instructed to say when he begins to feel a sense of tightness. Initially 15–20 ml may be all that is injected on each side.

All patients return to the clinic for the first three postoperative injections. They are given the chance to perform the expansion, and if they do it well and feel confident under direct supervision, they may begin self-expansion at home. Patients who contemplate home expansion are taught to palpate the injection ports with their index fingertips. They wash their hands prior to needle insertion and prep the skin and their fingertips with an alcohol sponge. They use their fingertips to guide the needle to the dome. This has been quite successful. The appropriate patient can perform self-expansion with relative ease. However, only those patients who are eager to adopt this regimen are allowed to perform home expansion.

All patients are monitored by phone and office visits every 3–4 weeks so that pressures can be measured and the experience can be reviewed. It is important to emphasize the necessity of slow expansion so that risks are minimized.

Expansion continues until there is an arc of expansion adequate to cover the area of alopecia (Fig. 5). Typically the arc across the top of the head from ear to ear is 34 cm. If, for example, the area of alopecia is 14 cm across, to cover the midline one would need 34 cm plus 14 cm, or 48 cm, of expanded hair-bearing skin.

In addition, however, the scalp must advance forward. Because of the circumferential expansion there will be a 6- to 7-cm advancement of the occipital scalp. The temporal scalp is tethered by the hairline. It has been the authors' approach not to incise much laterally at the temporal hairline so that the scar is minimized. This limits the amount of advancement of the temporal scalp. The incision in the forehead is limited to 6–7 cm from the midline on each side. Because of this, it is usually desirable to have several centimeters extra for advancement of the anterior hairline. Therefore, 52 cm would be a typical ear-to-ear distance for a patient with a defect of 14 cm. This will establish an acceptable anterior hairline while allowing removal of all the bare scalp on the top of the head.

ADVANCEMENT

When the arc of expansion is appropriate, the patient is brought to the operating room for advancement. This operation is typically done under local anesthesia. It is less painful than the insertion of the soft tissue expanders, and patients will typically experience only minimal discomfort postoperatively.

There are two alternatives for administration of local anesthesia. Lidocaine and bupivacaine with epinephrine is mixed and administered as either a ring block or as local infiltration atop the scalp. Begin with bilateral supraorbital and supratrochlear nerve blocks and infiltrate along the edge of the expanders on the head. Next a wheal is created across the top of the head along the midline to the occipital incision. If the occipital incision has not spread, it is left untouched. If it has widened, it will be injected and excised. The patient is positioned on his stomach with his chin on his hands and the scalp is prepped with povidone-iodine solution, as during the first operation.

The first incision goes from the occipital scar, over the vertex in the midline, and down to the subgaleal plane. The capsule is encountered and opened with electrocautery using a blunt blade, and the expander is removed. The scalp is then moved forward and great care taken to release the capsule anteriorly at the temporal hairline. A giant pleat can now be taken up to approximate the edge of the scalp on the right to that on the left. Marking is completed, and the resection of bare scalp is begun posteriorly (Fig. 6). Every 3–4 cm the scalp is approximated and fixed with staples. The incision is carried forward so that there are two long rabbit ears of scalp hanging free (Fig. 7). Next the anterior hairline is sketched, and the temporal scalp moved forward over the operator's thumb to determine exactly how far forward it will easily move. The scalp and the redundant forehead are marked as a lateral triangle for removal. Next the forehead is incised and the anterior border of the forehead created by excision of bare scalp and the lateral triangle of forehead in the temporal recession.

The specimen is removed and the incision closed anteriorly with interrupted stitches of 4–0 nylon in the galea and running 6–0 nylon suture in the skin (Fig. 8). Closure over drainage is generally advisable. The drains can be removed in 1 or 2 days.

Postoperatively the patient's hair is shampooed and a foam dressing applied. Pressure helps to minimize forehead swelling, although there still may be some. Ecchymosis commonly occurs on the third or fourth day after surgery.

POSTOPERATIVE CARE

One week after surgery the sutures in the anterior hairline are removed. Two weeks postoperatively the midline staples are removed.

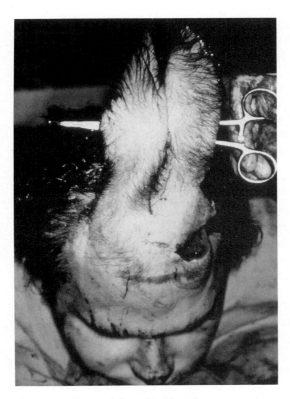

Figure 6   The excision of bald scalp.

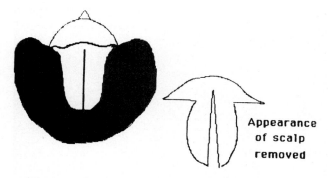

Figure 7 Diagram shows the incisions developed and the appearance of the excised scalp.

Ecchymosis will resolve, and the scars will become less obvious anteriorly. If there is a dog ear laterally, it is best to watch this for 4–6 weeks. It can be revised later. The patient should be instructed that the midline scar, which may be inapparent initially, will widen. All sagittal scars seem to widen, although they widen more in some patients that in others. The patient should be informed that this can be narrowed with a simple excision, if desired, at a future date. Patients may shower and shampoo the day after surgery and every day thereafter until sutures are removed.

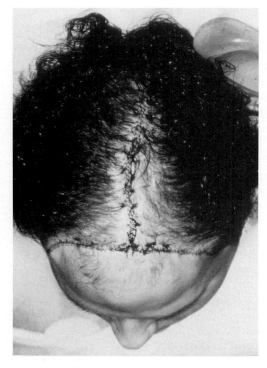

Figure 8 Closure.

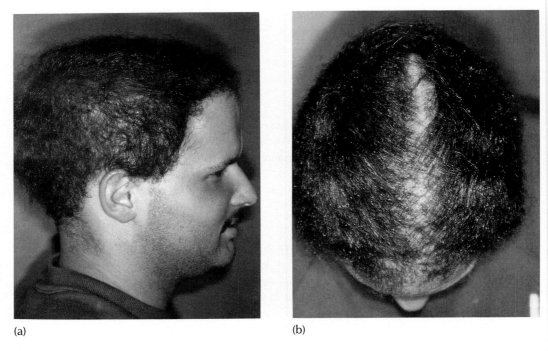

(a)   (b)

Figure 9   Appearance several weeks postoperatively.

ADVANTAGES

The advantages of soft tissue expansion for the elimination of male pattern baldness are obvious. The chief advantage is that adjacent soft tissue is used for reconstruction, with minimal change of the normal anatomy. The hair distribution is not obviously altered, so the "toothbrush" appearance of hair transplantation is avoided. There is no donor site, as required for hair transplantation, nor is there a potential for devascularizaton and denervation, as with the temporoparieto-occipital flaps. The operation can easily be modified, should alopecia progress, with a midline excision if needed in the future.

Patients tolerate this procedure well, and they cope with the period of transient deformity successfully. This procedure is not meant for every patient with male pattern baldness. For those who are well motivated, it is a solution that results in great patient satisfaction (Fig. 9). A successful reconstruction is accomplished in approximately 4 months.

The method is safe and effective when done by someone well versed in this procedure. Complications include point necrosis, bleeding, and infection but are generally easily managed. From the patient's standpoint, the procedure is relatively cost-effective. It is anticipated that this will be an increasingly common means of treatment for male pattern baldness in the future.

BIBLIOGRAPHY

Anderson RD. Expansion-assisted treatment of male pattern baldness. *Clin Plast Surg* 1987;14:477.

Austad ED. Tissue-expansion techniques. *Arch Dermatol* 1987;123:588.

Austad ED, Pasyk K, McClatchey KD, et al. Histomorphologic evaluation of guinea pig skin and soft tissue after controlled tissue expansion. *Plast Reconstr Surg* 1982;70:704.

Austad ED, Thomas SB, Pasyk K. Tissue expansion: Dividend or loan? *Plast Reconstr Surg* 1986;78:63.

Kabaker SS, Kridel RWH, Krugman ME, et al. Tissue expansion in the treatment of alopecia. *Arch Otolaryngol Head Neck Surg* 1986;112:720.

Lewis SR, Blocker TG, Eade GG. Problems of scalp reconstruction. *Plast Reconstr Surg* 1957;20:133.

Manders EK, Au VK, Wong RKM. Scalp expansion for male pattern baldness. *Clin Plast Surg* 1987;14:469.

Manders EK, Graham WP, Schenden MJ, et al. Skin expansion to eliminate large scalp defects. *Ann Plast Surg* 1984;12:305.

Manders EK, Schenden MJ, Furrey JA, et al. Soft-tissue expansion: Concepts and complications. *Plast Reconstr Surg* 1984;74:493.

Neumann CG. The expansion of an area of skin by progressive distension of subcutaneous balloon. *Plast Reconstr Surg* 1957;19:124.

Radovan C. Tissue expansion in soft-tissue reconstruction. *Plast Reconstr Surg* 1984;74:482.

Roenigk RK, Wheeland RG. Tissue expansion in cicatricial alopecia. *Arch Dermatol* 1987;123:641–646.

74

Liposuction Surgery

Rhoda S. Narins
New York University Medical Center, New York, New York

Its origins dating back to the early and mid 1970s, liposuction (suction-assisted lipectomy, lipolysis, lipoplasty) has come of age. Within 15 years an explosion in concepts, applications, instrumentation, and anesthesia has occurred. The author was introduced to liposuction by Doctors Yves-Gerard Illouz, Pierre Fournier of Paris, and Giorgio Fischer of Rome in the clinic and office of Dr. Illouz in Paris in 1982. Dr. Illouz, by modifying the sharp, hollow aspiration tube of Fischer and designing a blunt cannula and using a "wet technique" and injecting hypotonic saline solution into the tissue preoperatively, made the extraction of fat safe. Blunt surgical aspiration of the adipose bulk allowed preservation of septae in which vessels, lymph channels, and nerves survived. The local injection of fluid diminished bleeding considerably. Dr. Illouz also popularized liposuction at various medical meetings. The next important advance in liposuction was in 1986 with the development of the tumescent technique of local anesthesia. Changes have occurred in cannula size and design, in progressing from indirect to direct to criss-cross approaches to removal of fat, to smaller incision areas, to advances in the administration of anesthetic solutions and to using various combinations of taping and updated garments, etc. The idea of using larger cannulas in deep areas and the development of tiny cannulas that enable one to work more superficially without causing rippling has added the technique of "liposculpture" to that of liposuction.

Focal reduction, circumferential reduction, and volume reduction, as well as the treatment of obesity, continue to evolve. In order to comply with OSHA standards, disposable tubing and canisters, as well as viral filters have been developed (Fig. 1).

Deformities of fat exist in different anatomic locations for a variety of reasons. Some are considered evolutionary caloric storehouses, others facial and genetic configurations, and still others to be hormonally controlled. Concepts of beauty change, but today large accumulations of adipose tissue are considered unsightly among many of the world's peoples. The development of a surgical method of changing genetically and hormonally controlled fat contours that does

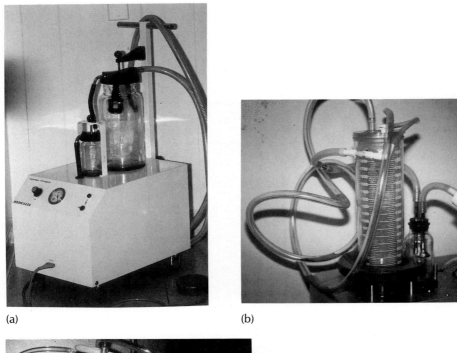

(a)   (b)

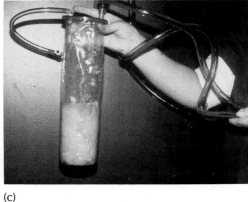

(c)

Figure 1   (a) Old 1982 machine. (b) New machine with disposable tubing and viral filter. (c) Fat with no blood.

not produce the long, undesirable, and significantly unaesthetic scars of block lipectomy with skin resection (dermolipectomy) is thus of great import.

PATIENT SELECTION AND RISK MANAGEMENT

The applicability of this technique has steadily expanded to include young and old, male and female patients, and both aesthetic and reconstructive challenges. Studies are underway in diabetics, hypertensive patients, and in serial procedures for the obese. Liposuction is appropriate for any individual with an indication for the procedure who can tolerate the pre-, intra-, and postoperative stresses and risks and who accepts realistic limitations.

Preoperative photographs are mandatory, and patients refusing these should be categorically denied any intervention. The necessity for possible "touch-up" procedures should be mentioned, the charge for such being each surgeon's decision.

Candidates undergoing tumescent liposuction procedures require no general anesthesia. Usually they receive some type of IM and/or PO sedation, along with local tumescent anesthesia. When patients are first seen in consultation, the procedure is gone over with them in detail, and they are examined to see if they are good candidates for this surgery. The medical history, including a history of bleeding, medication, allergies, etc., is taken.

Once it has been determined that the patient is a good candidate for this surgery by evaluation of his or her objectives and the realistic goals that can be achieved from the examination of fat and skin turgor, then possible complications and other risks and benefits and options are discussed with the patient. If the patient decides to go ahead with the procedure, a Polaroid picture is taken; blood pressure, urine, and blood tests, including a CBC, SMAC, PT, PTT, HEP C surface antibody, HEPB surface antigen, and HIV tests, are done. All medical problems must be evaluated individually. Any patient taking systemic medication of import is evaluated by his or her family physician prior to the procedure. Preoperative directions are discussed, including avoidance of all salicylates and nonsteroidal anti-inflammatories 2 weeks prior to surgery. Forms are given to the patient with extensive preoperative and postoperative instructions, and pre- and postoperative pictures of other patients are reviewed to give a good idea of what can be expected.

Patients must be told that this is not a procedure to correct striae, spider veins, skin turgor, or cellulite. This is a contouring procedure. Deformities and unusual prominence of anatomic bony structures must be evaluated and discussed with the patient.

Most patients are extremely realistic about the results that they can achieve. If they are already nearly perfect, you can give them a perfect contour, but most patients, especially those who are older and who have had children and whose skin is somewhat loose, will find that liposuction surgery gives extremely gratifying results with very little scarring or morbidity. Most patients are happy to look better in clothing and have a nicer contour. The consultation is perhaps the most important part of the procedure because picking the right patient is extremely important. A good consent form and operative flow sheet are necessities when dealing with risk management.

EQUIPMENT

The sine qua non of liposuction is the introduction of cannulas of varying lengths and designs through small apertures in the skin. These allow removal of adipose tissue while sparing some neurovascular septae and arcades of connective tissue between overlying and deeper elements. A series of tunnels fan out along arcs from each incision point, varying in size and depth by individual requirements. Each fat-containing area has varied entrance points, and each surgeon his or her own favorites.

Cannulas

Many new cannulas are available at the present time, and it is important to use a blunt, less aggressive cannula with the opening further away from the distal tip of the cannula when you are beginning liposuction surgery (Fig. 2). As you gain more experience, more aggressive tips can be used, and some of my favorite cannulas are the Klein sizes 10, 12, and 14 (akin to needle sizes) in various lengths and 2-, 3-, and 4-mm cannulas of either the Lamprey, Cobra, Pinto, or Cook designs. There are many others available and it is good to train at a hands-on meeting where you can use several of these and pick your favorites. The original Illouz cannulas I used were blunt and went up to size 10, which now looks enormous. With these larger cannulas it

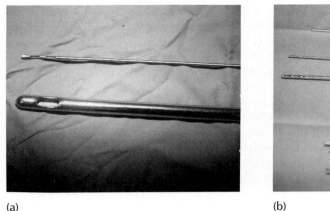
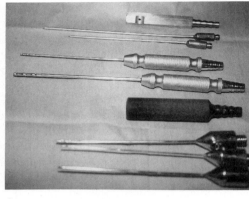

(a)   (b)

Figure 2   (a) Old Illouz "10" cannula compared to new Klein "12" cannula. (b) Multiple other cannulas.

was important to stay deep in the fatty tissue so as not to get rippling. Much finer adjustments (liposculpture) can be achieved with the smaller cannulas. Larger cannulas up to size 6 can still be used occasionally where there is a great amount of adipose tissue to remove the deeper bulk. Multiple cannulas are used on every patient. Cannulas vary by (1) length, curvature, and diameter, (2) the number, size, and placement of apertures, (3) the bluntness, rounding, or flattening of tips, and (4) the placement of one or more apertures ventrally, on the sides, close to, or more distant from, the end. The size and type of grasping handle—round or angled, large or small, smooth or textured—is a matter of individual preference and comfort. Some means of identifying the orientation of the cannula is necessary so that the surgeon does not unknowingly turn the orifice upward and damage the dermis with resultant cicatrization. The relationship of diameter of cannula handles to the transparent tubing diameters varies, so there may be some problem in adapting a particular tubing to a particular cannula handle and/or the machine. Progressively graded attachments are available to allow adaptation of varying manufacturers' diameters. Single handles with interchangeable tips are also available, some of which are adaptable for fat transplantation.

Pulse Oximeter

A pulse oximeter is a useful adjunct to measure the oxygen saturation as toxicity to lidocaine is related to decreased oxygen. Because patients are awake, the surgeon can just tell them to take a deep breath if the level decreases (Fig. 3).

Aspiration Pump and Tubing

A variety of manufacturers in several countries now produce aspiration pumps that develop negative air pressures approaching 30 inches (1 atm) negative pressure. This reference point is sought by the instrument makers, but adequate suction for some areas may be obtained with readings as low as 15–18 inches.

Today's canisters are either disposable as a unit or come with removable/disposable bags. The tubing is also disposable, and a viral filter is used and changed according to direction. Dr. Pierre Fournier has developed a syringe technique and can aspirate thousands of cubic centimeters by hand without using a pump at all.

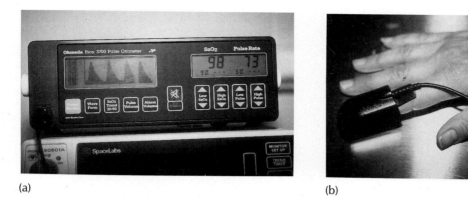

(a)   (b)

Figure 3   (a) Pulse oximeter. (b) Oximeter applied to finger.

ANESTHESIA ADMINISTRATION

Most dermatologic surgeons use the tumescent technique. Several methods of administering tumescent anesthesia are available. For large areas, many of us have progressed from 60 cc syringes attached to a three-way stopcock to the Klein infiltrator to using a pressure cuff around the bag of anesthesia to an electric infiltration pump. The author has used all of these methods, and although each gives the desired results, the easiest to use is the electric pump. These machines were first developed in the 1990s and make the administration of anesthesia much more simple. Tumescent anesthesia is made up in 1000 cc bags of normal saline, which are then attached by IV tubing to either a spinal needle or infiltrators with showerlike heads (Fig. 4).

ANESTHESIA

Preoperative sedation runs the gamut from using nothing for smaller areas in nonanxious patients such as the neck, knees, lipomas, etc., to using PO diazepam to IM meperidine, promethazine, and/or midazolam. These methods are used by most dermatologic liposuction surgeons, but some surgeons use other methods of anesthesia such as general anesthesia, epidural or IV sedation, especially when the procedure is done in the hospital or with a nurse anesthetist or anesthesiologist present. The author uses IM meperidine, promethazine, and midazolam and PO diazepam preoperatively.

Since 1982 when liposuction was first introduced into the United States and when I first started doing the procedure, the greatest advance has been that of tumescent liposuction introduced by Dr. Jeffrey Klein, a dermatologic surgeon. Drs. Patrick Lillis and William Coleman and the author have further advanced the use of this technique. The benefits of the tumescent technique are the lack of bleeding with no need for transfusion, the practically painless as well as long-lasting anesthetic effect, the increased safety to the patient because the risks of general anesthesia are avoided, and the fact that anesthetic solution itself provides fluid replacement. This has made liposuction surgery a safe and wonderful procedure for the patient. The author used general and epidural anesthesia and/or IV sedation with an anesthesiologist from 1982 until 1987 when Dr. Klein sent the equipment to administer the tumescent anesthetic with a note to "try it once." The author did try it and because of its superiority has not used any other since.

The anesthetic is made up in 1000 cc bags of normal saline, the formulas for which can be found in Tables 1 and 2. There are various adaptations of this formula. The reported margin of

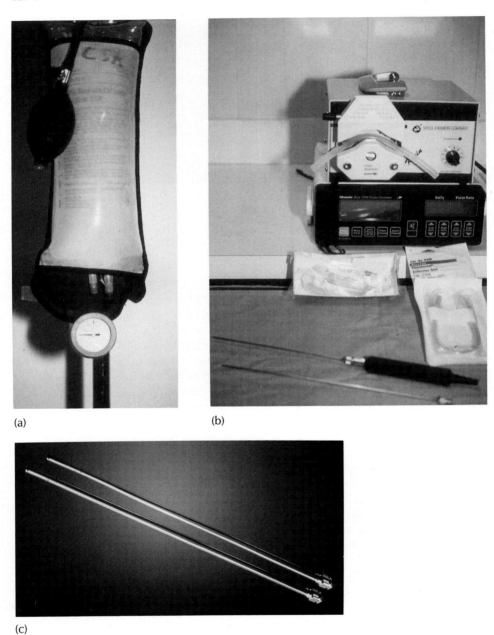

(a)   (b)

(c)

Figure 4 (a) Bag contains anesthesia surrounded by pressure cuff. (b) Electric pump for anesthesia. (c) Infiltrator to deliver anesthetic solution.

safety is 35 mg of lidocaine/kg of body weight. However, by the time this book is published the safety levels may have been moved higher. When 50 cc of 2% lidocaine is used per 1000 cc bag, lidocaine is present in 0.1% with 1/1,000,000 epinephrine. The total amount of lidocaine administered is 1000 mg. When 50 cc of a 1% solution of lidocaine is added to the saline with 1 cc of epinephrine, you have a 0.05% solution of lidocaine with a total of 500 mg per bag,

Table 1 Formula for Anesthetic with 0.1% Lidocaine

Ingredient	Amount (cc)
Normal saline 0.9%	1000
Lidocaine 2%	50
Epinephrine 1/1000	1
Bicarbonate 8.4%	12.5
Triamcinolone acetonide 10 mg/cc	1

and epinephrine is kept at 1/1,000,000. In very sensitive areas like the abdomen, buttock, inner thighs, and knees, one should try to use the 0.1% solution. If many areas are being treated and one needs to conserve anesthesia, then use the 0.5% lidocaine in the less sensitive areas such as the lateral thigh, arms, neck, etc.

The anesthetic can be given using a three-step procedure with the incision marks injected first with a syringe and a 30-gauge needle. The second step is the injection through the incision areas of small amounts of the solution under low pressure using a spinal needle in a radial fashion. The third step is to inject a lot of anesthetic to get the tumescent effect using a spinal needle or an infiltrator. The tissue is filled with anesthetic so that it is fairly firm. This three-step procedure provides a practically painless way to administer the tumescent anesthetic solution.

PREOP PROCEDURE

Having bathed with an antiseptic antimicrobial skin cleanser for 7 days preoperatively, the patient reports to the office wearing loose-fitting clothing that can be easily removed and replaced. The patient has washed his or her hair that morning and is given postoperative support garments by the nurse.

It is important to weigh the patient. If an occasional patient should gain a large amount of weight after surgery, the weight gain will be distributed over the body and not accumulate in the surgical area, though extra fat may appear to make the surgical results not as aesthetically attractive. It is most important as previously stressed to take photographs of the patient so that they can be checked at 3- and 6-month intervals, and Polaroids may be placed on the operatory wall so they can be referred to during surgery.

Once the patient is weighed and photographed, the areas including all incision areas are marked using an indelible marking pen, with the patient in a standing and sitting position (Fig. 5). Several systems of marking gradations of excess fat have evolved, and each doctor will adopt the most comfortable one. Once the areas have been marked and mapped, the surgeon must not deviate from that after the patient is supine or prone. These markings are gone over with the patient.

Table 2 Formula for Anesthetic with 0.05% Lidocaine

Ingredient	Amount (cc)
Normal saline 0.9%	1000
Lidocaine 1%	50
Epinephrine 1/1000	1
Bicarbonate 8.4%	12.5
Triamcinolone acetonide 10 mg/cc	1

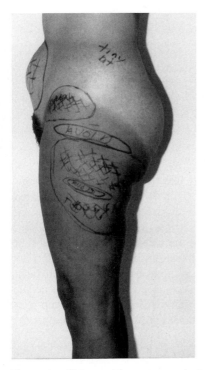

Figure 5 Skin marking preoperatively.

All of the patient's questions are answered, and the consent sheet is then signed. At this time the patient receives any preoperative medications. The patient should go to the bathroom, otherwise he or she will have to go during the procedure because of the large amounts of fluid injected.

TECHNIQUE

A bactericidal prep is used, and the patient is then guided to a power table draped with a sterile sheet. Sterile drapes with apertures are used, which help to insulate and reduce heat loss. Some surgeons prewarm the solution to body temperature in a microwave so that the patient doesn't feel so cold. The tumescent anesthetic is then administered through incisions made in the premarked areas with a stab from an 11 blade. The apertures are generally only 2–4 mm in length. Some surgeons use few incisions, while others use a gridwork with multiple, tiny incisions both to deliver the anesthetic and to remove fat.

The author waits 15–30 min after the anesthetic is delivered before performing liposuction surgery. Deeper areas are done first in a radial criss-cross fashion with the larger cannulas. With the noncannula grasping hand (Fournier's "thinking, educated hand"), the surgeon guides the cannula to those areas from which adipose tissue is to be systematically removed within a prearranged pattern using a series of pistonlike movements at varying depths to accomplish the liposculpturing process. Limits are determined by the preoperative markings, the surgeon's estimate of how much fat should be removed from a particular area, and visual observation of the quality of aspirant and assessment of the amount of blood loss occurring. With the tumescent technique the amount of blood loss is minimal. Liposuction should be performed in criss-cross channels, using larger cannulas more deeply to begin with and smaller cannulas more superficially for liposculpturing. It is believed that not only is the procedure a debulking procedure, but the fibrous tissue that forms afterwards also retracts the skin. A windshield wiper–like sweeping movement is never allowed in any part of the body except the submental area (and even its use there is the subject of controversy). Preservation of some neurovascular septae is imperative to preclude cavity formation with the attendant risks of hematoma, seroma, infection, and significant postoperative deformity.

In defatted areas residual palpable masses of fat may be noted. Smaller cannula with either more aggressive or flatter aspirating tips may be directed into these residual islands. Peripheral mesh undermining may then be performed using solid rods or smaller cannula with or without suction.

Fischer observed that postoperative surface irregularities seem more frequent along the horizontal than the vertical axis of the body. The major aspiration should therefore be along vertical lines where possible, utilizing the criss-cross technique.

Prior to the use of tumescent anesthesia, the safe amount of fat to remove was generally considered to be less than 2000 cc. However, with the use of large amounts of anesthetic fluid volume used, many surgeons routinely remove between 2000 and 4000 cc, with 2500 cc being the average removed at any one time.

Many surgeons no longer suture all incision sites. During the procedure a lot of fluid drains, so if you do decide to suture with either a subcutaneous or skin suture, do not do so until all liposuction is finished so that drainage can occur. Especially in anatomic lines such as the superpubic line, groin, etc., incision lines can be left open and will close with virtually no scarring and allow drainage.

POSTOP

Compression dressings applied to areas that have undergone blunt injury and aspiration are useful in controlling tissue fluid movement and hematoma formation and in occluding tunnels by apposition of the freshly abraded surfaces (Fig. 6).

Differences of opinion exist between those who use tape and those who are compression garments. Each method has its proponents and detractors: others take the middle ground and use both. As more sophisticated garments have become available from a variety of manufacturers, dependence on taping has lessened.

Immediately postoperative the patient is washed and ice packs are applied to the area. The author prefers to wrap some areas (e.g., abdomen, neck) with tape (french tape, Reston) for 2–3 days. Most areas will do well with one of the surgical garments now available. The patients wear these garments 24 hr a day for 5–7 days and then, depending on the area, 12–24 hr a day for the next 2–3 weeks. The patient can shower the next day but should be advised that the areas will drain for 24–48 hr. Sanitary napkins can be used over the incision sites, and towels can be used to sit on. Towels over a large plastic bag should be used in the car going home after surgery to collect the fluid and prevent staining.

Many patients take it easy for a day, but depending upon the number of areas treated and how they feel, they can usually return to work within 2–3 days. Most surgeons permit patients to enjoy nonjarring light exercise as soon as they feel up to it (e.g., stationary bicycle, walking.) Most do not allow patients to return to jarring activity such as aerobics, tennis, or jogging for 3 weeks postoperative. Patients often feel better when they wear the garments, which keep the area from moving around too, causing soreness. The tumescent technique causes much less bruising than was previously seen with other techniques. Ecchymosis generally disappears 2–3 weeks postoperatively and may not even occur with this technique.

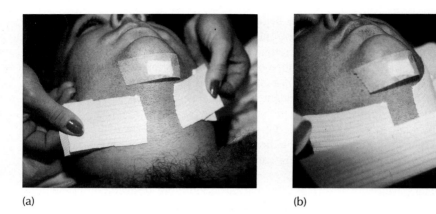

(a)   (b)

Figure 6 Postoperative dressing.

The author routinely uses IM Celestone postoperatively and prophylactic antibiotics. Antibiotics are started 2 days preoperatively and continued 5 days postoperatively. We call patients the night of surgery, and they are given the physician's and nurse's phone numbers. Patients are advised to watch their caloric intake, especially their intake of fat, and to begin an exercise program as soon as they feel up to it.

COMPLICATIONS

Few complications are seen with tumescent liposuction surgery. Several deaths have been connected to general and IV anesthesia. A death from fat embolism was reported, but the liposuction surgery had been combined with open abdominal lipectomy. The usual postoperative sequaelae may include dysesthesias in the area for a limited period of time, ecchymosis, and soreness.

Postoperative complications ranging from infection to development of hematomas or seromas, waviness, dimpling, cicatrical retraction, fat embolism, death, etc., are rarely seen. In the several thousand cases done by the author, the only complication seen was one seroma after removal of a huge lipoma the size of a large grapefruit. The end result was excellent.

When patients gain weight postoperatively, they gain it all over their bodies and no longer just in the focally unsightly area where surgical removal has occurred.

FOLLOW-UP VISITS

If there are no problems, the patient is seen at 2 days, 7 days, 1 month, 3 months, and 6 months postoperative. At the 3- and 6-month visits, photographs are taken so that the patient can follow his or her own improvement. It is amazing that patients who have lived with deformities for most of their lives cannot remember them 3 months later. It is important when the photographs are taken that patients also be weighed so that the surgeon can compare the weight with that taken before the procedure.

CONSIDERATIONS

Head and Neck

Submental adipose tissue may be removed with small diameter, spatula-type cannulas usually through a single small incision placed within the submental fold. Often this incision can hardly be seen a few days postoperative. If a patient has a larger deposit of fat on the neck, three incisions can be used: a submental incision and one behind each ear to criss-cross the area. Usually when the neck is done, the jowls are also done; in this area extra small cannulas are used very gently so as not to injure the marginal mandibular nerve. The skin pulls back nicely in this area. Removal of even a small deposit from the neck can take 10 years off a person's age (Figs. 7–11).

Occasionally the skin is so thin that it is advisable to have a neck lift. In patients who want a simpler procedure and understand its limitations, liposuction with a submental excision can be performed. The submental incision is made easier because the undermining has already been done by the preceding liposuction. An occasional patient may need to have the platysmal bands addressed (Fig. 12).

The neck is the one area where it is permissible to turn the cannula in all directions so as to get out as much as possible and to make as many tracts as possible so that the skin retracts. Usually the lipoaspiration from the neck is quite small ranging from 10 cc to 100 cc, yet the improvement may be astonishingly great. This is an easy procedure for the patient, and with tumescent anesthesia, there is often no bruising at all. The patient can go out 2 or 3 days later without any problem.

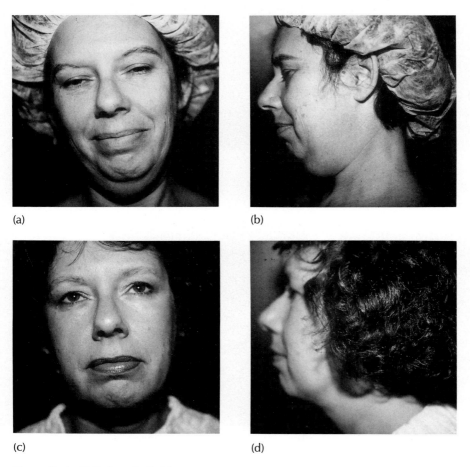

(a)

(b)

(c)

(d)

Figure 7 (a, b) Before; (c,d) After.

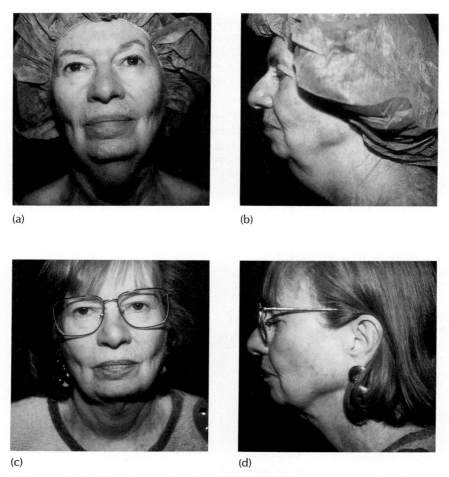

(a)   (b)

(c)   (d)

Figure 8   (a,b) Before liposuction. (c,d) After liposuction of neck.

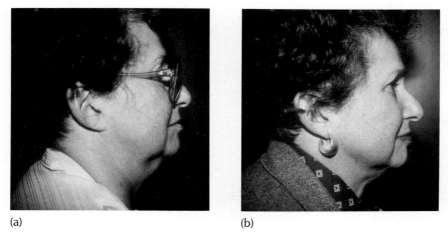

(a)   (b)

Figure 9   (a) Before liposuction. (b) After liposuction of neck.

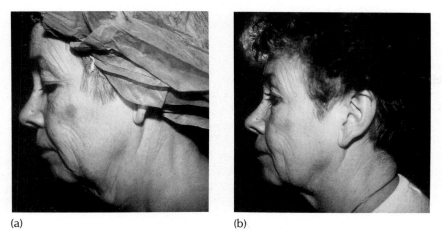

(a)   (b)

Figure 10   (a) Before liposuction. (b) After liposuction of neck.

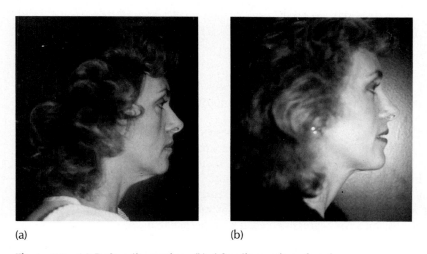

(a)   (b)

Figure 11   (a) Before liposuction. (b) After liposuction of neck.

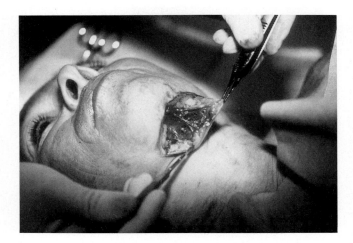

Figure 12   Excision of excess neck skin. Note tracks from liposuction.

When wrapping the neck, I usually tape the area for 2 days and then have the patient wear a chin guard. The initial pieces of tape are separated by 1 inch in the center of the neck so that there is less chance of getting vertical folds. These folds, if they occur, are temporary. Occasionally one does get some trauma to the nerve, but there has never been a report of permanent damage. I have seen a partial paralysis last for 2 months.

Liposuction, of course, is routinely used as an adjunct to rhytidectomy and, in fact, has changed the procedure and made it much easier to do. The principles of flap dissection and movement learned from suction-assisted rhytidectomy have been applied to the atraumatic elevation of various face and neck flaps needed in reconstructive surgery. Liposuction of the face should be done very carefully by an experienced operator, if at all. The results in this area can be disappointing and unattractive.

Upper Extremities

Many women accumulate fat in the upper arms as a result of heredity and/or obesity. It is important to do this area before the skin gets so loose that the liposuction results in unsightly, loosely hanging skin. In the usual patient with moderate or good skin turgor, an excellent result can be achieved through one incision above the elbow.

Torso

The "buffalo hump" or dowager deformity responds strikingly. One or two tiny incisions allowing the operator to criss-cross the cannula easily removes the loose and soft fat from this area (Fig. 13).

Adipose pseudogynecomastia responds beautifully to liposuction but is difficult to do (Fig. 14). The approach incision can be in the axilla. This is another area where the cannula may need to be turned upside down so that as much breast tissue as possible can be scraped out. This maneuver is done in the infraareolar and periareolar areas only. This procedure allows a patient to have vast improvement in the gynecomastic area without scarring and without loss of time from work. This is another area in which we want to remove as much as possible and also have the skin fibrose as much as possible. An aggressive cannula in the hands of an experienced operator gives the best results. Many patients with pseudogynecomastia have true gynecomastic tis-

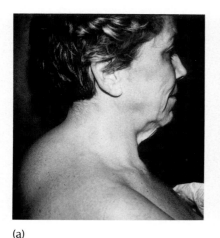   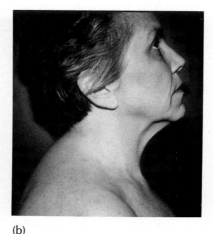

(a)   (b)

Figure 13   (a) "Buffalo hump." (b) After liposuction.

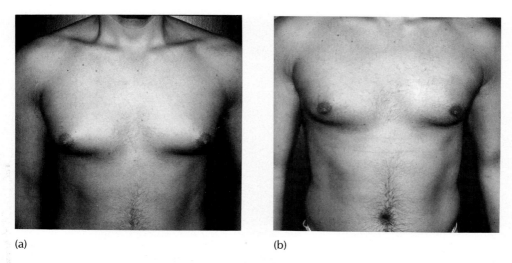

(a)   (b)

Figure 14   (a) Gynecomastia in male. (b) After liposuction.

sue in a subareolar location. An aggressive cannula can remove more of this tissue. Histologic examination of the aspirated subareolar would be appropriate.

Flanks

Flanks are the most common area in which men lay down fat (Figs. 15,16). This responds beautifully to liposuction surgery. Many of our patients are in wonderful shape and still have

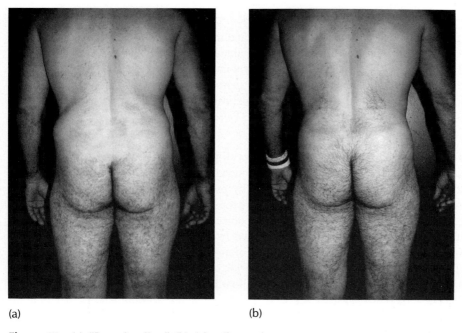

(a)   (b)

Figure 15   (a) "Love handles." (b) After liposuction.

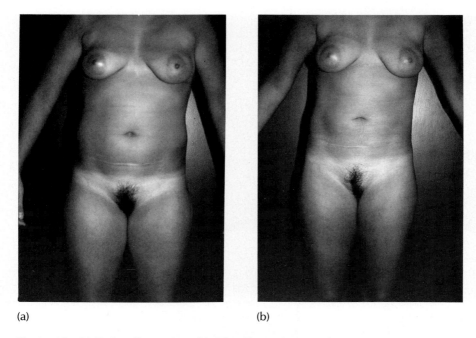

(a)   (b)

Figure 16   (a) Before liposuction. (b) After liposuction of waist.

this unsightly protrusion, which can hang over their waistbands. Fibrosis and retraction occur in this area and significant contour improvement results.

Back

The back is often done along with the flanks in men and the waist and hips in women. This area tends to be more fibrous and needs more aggressive cannulas. The waist and back area can often be approached from the incision used for the flanks, abdomen, or hips. At other times more direct approaches are necessary. The author likes to use an approach from a slight distance away rather than by direct entry into the middle of the adipose deposit.

Abdomen

This is one of the most common areas for liposuction (Figs. 17,18). The fat is soft and easy to remove and is found mainly in two locations: the rounded infraumbilical and periumbilical protuberance that extends laterally, and the more doughy protuberance extending from the costal margin downwards to meet the major abdominal fat deposit. Fat below and lateral to the umbilicus responds very well. The fat cells in the upper abdomen are arranged in large fibrous clumps that can be difficult to aspirate and should be aspirated from two tiny incisions directly adjacent to them so as not to break the fibrous banding that often occurs at the waist.

Usually the fat in the abdomen of women is anterior to the muscle, and thus is easily amenable to surgery. It is amazing how even an abdominal apron will pull back after liposuction surgery. Occasionally there are women whose skin is so loose due to pregnancies that in addition to doing liposuction surgery, a superpubic excision of skin can be done to give a nicer result. A very small number of people really do not benefit from liposuction and would be better off with an open lipectomy and repair of the rectus abdominus muscle. The "beer belly" fat occurs

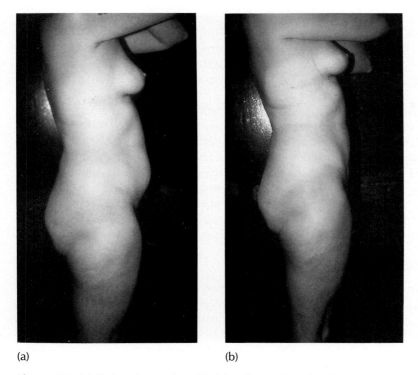

(a)   (b)

Figure 17   (a) Before liposuction. (b) After liposuction of abdomen.

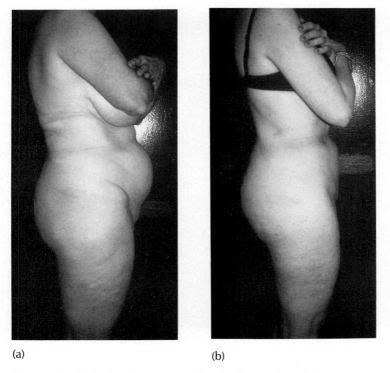

(a)   (b)

Figure 18   (a) Before liposuction. (b) After liposuction of abdomen.

in many men and lies behind the muscle, and, as such, one cannot remove it. This concern generally responds to diet and exercise.

It is important to rule out the possibility of an umbilical or ventral hernia. In addition the area around the umbilicus appears to be especially sensitive, and after the tumescent anesthetic is injected, the author often injects 10 cc of undiluted 1% lidocaine with epinephrine around the umbilicus and down the central line to the pubic area.

Multiple techniques have been used in the abdomen, including a grid pattern with 20–40 tiny incisions and injection of the tumescent solution and liposuction into each of these radially. I prefer to use three or five incisions for the lower abdomen and two for the upper abdomen. For the lower abdomen I like to hide the incisions one on either side of the superpubic fold and one above the umbilicus and/or one in each of the two lines extending out from the umbilicus. For the upper abdomen I like to do a tiny incision just laterally to each fat pad. If I am doing a large hip area as well, I may avoid the umbilical incisions and just put an incision laterally on each side of the abdomen from which I can reach the hips as well as the abdomen. The incisions always have to be geared to the patient and the areas that are being corrected.

Lateral Thighs ("Saddle Bags") and Buttocks

Along with the abdomen and neck, lateral thighs are the most common areas for which women request liposuction (Figs. 19–21). Often the hip is also involved in a "violin deformity." Both the hip and lateral thigh can be done using one incision between them. Moving the cannula vertically upward removes the fat in the hip area and vertically downward removes fat from the lateral thigh area. Criss-crossing the lateral thigh area from a second incision in the infragluteal region completes the procedure. Both of these incisions will suffice for the buttocks as well.

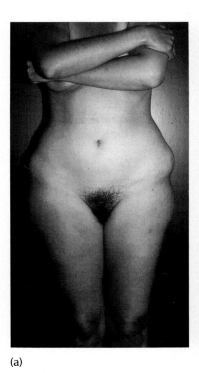 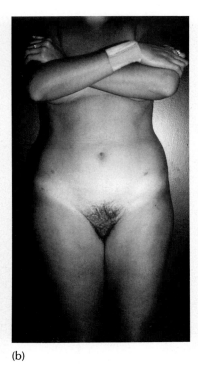

(a)   (b)

Figure 19   (a) "Violin deformity." (b) After liposuction of hips and lateral thighs.

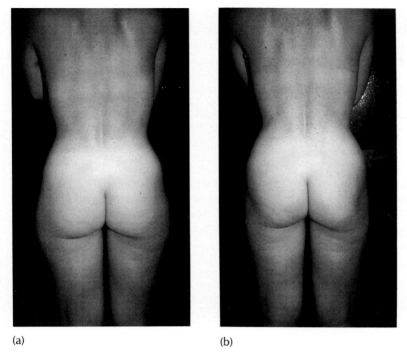

(a)   (b)

Figure 20   (a) Before liposuction. (b) After liposuction of lateral thighs.

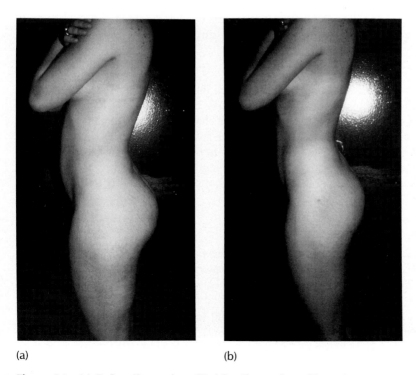

(a)   (b)

Figure 21   (a) Before liposuction. (b) After liposuction of buttocks.

Generally the lateral thigh has good skin turgor and responds very well. An excellent result can be achieved. Although the fibrous septae around the cellulite globules are sometimes broken, it is better to tell the patients that there will probably be no change. Adipose deposits in the lateral thigh can even occur in thin women and is usually inherited.

Circumferential Thigh Reduction

Circumferential thigh reduction is done from multiple incisions above the knee going around the entire thigh. Very large extremities can be reduced, but usually serial reductions are necessary.

Pubic Area

Both men and women may have undesirable deposits of fat in the pubic area. Although patients do not frequently complain about this area, when queried they may state the bulges are displeasing to them (especially when sitting). This fat is easily aspirated from any of the abdominal incisions, but some mons veneris softness should remain. Patients of both sexes should be forewarned of transient swelling and ecchymosis, which can be alarming.

Knees

Knees are easy to do and often can be done through one incision per knee. Small cannulas should be used, and one has to be careful not to do too much work just above the knee. Often the upper medial part of the calf is done as well to give a better contour.

Calves and Ankles

With the advent of the smaller Klein cannulas, liposuction surgery for calves and ankles has become easier. With the smaller cannulas multiple tiny incisions can be done with fat carefully sculpted from these areas. This is another area where the surgeon must be experienced.

Lipomas

The removal of even massive lipomas can be accomplished through very small incisions (Figs. 22,23). However, the fibrous stroma within the lipoma may be very difficult to remove. This is a much more difficult procedure in general, especially if the lipoma extends into the muscle, than removal of adipose tissue. After the mass of the lipoma has been removed, an excision must be done through the tiny incision area. The tissue will have to be teased out with counterpressure from the operator's fingers. It is very satisfying when the last bit of fibrous stroma and lipoma pop out of the small opening. This area must be taped with a pressure dressing and heals beautifully.

Fat Transplantation

There have been many attempts to transplant fat over the past century. The applications of liposuction surgery have been extended: fat-containing material has been extracted with both power and hand units. Physicians have then injected aspirant, with uncertain long-term success.

Greater longevity has been achieved by knowing which areas respond best to fat injections. Areas that are not great movement areas such as the lateral cheek or traumatic or surgical defects with loss of fat and lipodystrophy respond best with fat, often lasting for years. The past few years has also seen a great improvement in the longevity of fat injected for wrinkles such as nasolabial lines, etc. After being pushed through a sieve, the strained fat is injected. Many practitioners are freezing the fat and doing touch-up reinjection for several months following the

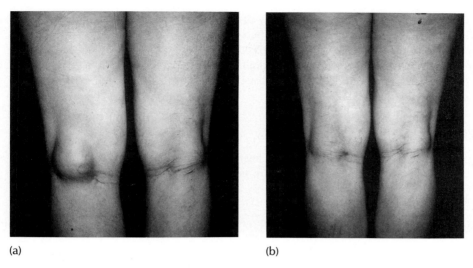

(a)   (b)

Figure 22 (a) Lipoma on knee. (b) After liposuction.

original harvesting and reinjection. Microlipoinjection has become a part of our therapeutic armamentarium and offers significant hope for the future.

TRAINING IN LIPOSUCTION SURGERY

For dermatologists embarking on a career of liposuction surgery, many pathways are open to them. Basic courses are being given by the American Society for Dermatologic Surgery, by the International Society for Dermatologic Surgery, by the American Society of Liposuction Surgery under the auspices of the American Academy of Cosmetic Surgery, and by members of the Tumescent Liposuction Council who gives courses under the auspices of the American Society

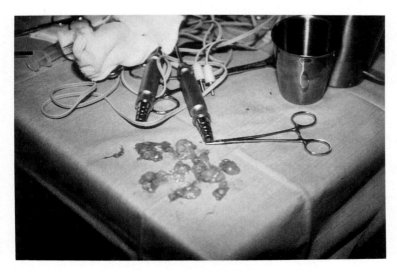

Figure 23 Lipoma in pieces after liposuction.

for Dermatologic Surgery. The American Academy of Dermatology has guidelines for liposuction surgery, and the Tumescent Liposuction Council puts out a newsletter several times a year with valuable tips and up-to-date instruction sheets. Acquaintance with a variety of experiences from different surgeons with varying approaches and philosophies is urged and encouraged.

Because the tumescent procedure has been proven to be safe and effective, this field will continue to expand.

ACKNOWLEDGMENTS

My thanks to Dr. Lawrence M. Field, who has been a mentor to many of us and who wrote this chapter for the first edition of this book. I am very grateful to him for all of his help and support.

BIBLIOGRAPHY

Am J Cosmet Surg. (Special liposuction issue.) 1986;1.

Asken SA. *Manual of Liposuction Surgery and Autologous Fat Transplantation Under Local Anesthesia.* 2nd ed. Irvine, CA, Keith C. Terry & Associates, 1986.

Coleman WP, III. The history of dermatologic liposuction. *Dermatol Clin* 1990;8:381.

Committee on Guidelines of Care. Guidelines of care for liposuction. *J Am Acad Dermatol* 1991;24:489.

Courtiss EH, Chouair RJ, Donelan MB. Large-volume suction lipectomy: An analysis of 108 patients. *Plast Reconstr Surg* 1992;89:1068.

Dillerud E. Suction lipoplasty: A report on complications, undesired results, and patient satisfaction based on 3511 procedures. *Plast Reconstr Surg* 1991;88:239.

Elam M, Fournier P. *Liposuction, The Franco-American Experience.* Beverly Hills, CA, Medical Aesthetics, Inc., 1986.

Field L, Narins R. Liposuction surgery. In *Skin Surgery.* 6th ed. E Epstein and E Epstein Jr, eds. Philadelphia, W.B. Saunders, 1987, pp. 370–378.

Field LM. Adjunctive liposurgical debulking and flap dissection in neck reconstruction. *J Dermatol Surg Oncol* 1986;12:917.

Field LM. The dermatologic surgeon and liposculpturing. In *Liposculpture: The Syringe Technique.* PF Fournier, ed. Paris, Arnette Blackwell, 1991, pp. 265–266.

Field LM. Liposuction surgery. A review. *J Dermatol Surg Oncol* 1984;10:530.

Fischer A, Fischer G. Revised techniques for cellulitis fat reduction in riding breeches deformity. *Bull Int Acad Cosmet Surg* 1977;2:40.

Fournier P. *Body Sculpturing Through Syringe Lipo-Extractions and Autologous Fat Re-Injection.* Solana Beach, CA, Samuel Rolf International, 1988.

Fournier P, Otteni F. Lipodissection in body sculpturing: The dry procedure. *Plast Reconstr Surg* 1983;72:598.

Fournier PF. *Liposculpture: The Syringe Technique.* Paris, Arnette Blackwell, 1991, p.163.

Hanke CW. Liposuction under local anesthesia (editorial). *J Dermatol Surg Oncol* 1989;15:12.

Hetter G. *Lipoplasty, The Theory and Practice of Blunt Suction Lipectomy.* Boston/Toronto, Little, Brown, 1984.

Illouz Y. Body contouring by lipolysis. A 5-year experience with over 3000 cases. *Plast Reconstr Surg* 1983;72:591.

Klein JA. Anesthesia for liposuction in dermatologic surgery. *J Dermatol Surg Oncol* 1988;14:1124–1132.

Klein JA. Peak plasma lidocaine levels are diminished and delayed twelve hours by tumescent technique for liposuction, permitting maximum safe lidocaine doses of 35 mg/kg. *J Dermatol Surg Oncol* 1990;

Klein JA. Tumescent liposuction: Totally by local anesthesia. In *Principles and Practice of Dermatological Surgery.* GP Lask, RI Moy, eds. New York, McGraw-Hill, 1993.

Klein JA. The tumescent technique: Anesthesia and modified liposuction technique. *Dermatol Clin* 1990;8:425.

Klein JA. The tumescent technique for liposuction surgery. *Am J Cosmet Surg* 1987;4:263.

Lillis PJ. Liposuction surgery under local anesthesia: Limited blood loss and minimal lidocaine absorption. *J Dermatol Surg Oncol* 1988;14:1145–1148.

Lillis PJ. The tumescent technique for liposuction surgery. *Dermatol Clin* 1990;8:439.

Lillis PJ, Coleman WP, III (eds.). Liposuction. *Dermatol Clin* 1990;8:381.

McKay W, Morris R, Mushlin P. Sodium bicarbonate attenuates pain on skin infiltration with lidocaine with our without epinephrine. *Anesth Analg* 1987;66:572.

Narins RS. Liposuction and anesthesia. *Dermatol Clin* 1990;8:421.

Narins RS. Liposuction of the face and neck. *Evaluation and Treatment of the Aging Face*. ML Elson, ed. 1994.

Newman J., Dolsky R. Liposuction surgery: History and development. *J Dermatol Surg Oncol* 1984;10:467.

Stegman S, Tromovitch T. Liposuction. In *Cosmetic Dermatologic Surgery*. Chicago, Year Book Medical Publishers, 1983, pp. 216–224.

Teimourian B. *Suction Lipectomy and Body Sculpturing*. St. Louis, C.V. Mosby, 1987.

75

Fat Transplantation and Autologous Collagen

Kevin S. Pinski and Henry H. Roenigk, Jr.
Northwestern University Medical School, Chicago, Illinois

Soft tissue augmentation with adipose tissue has been used clinically for many years. The more traditional approach has involved the placement of adipose tissue into the subcutis to correct cosmetic defects. More recently, constituents of this tissue have been processed into "autologous collagen" and utilized as a dermal filler substance.

FAT TRANSPLANTATION

History

Fat transplantation surgery began almost one century ago when, in 1893, Neuber reported on his technique of free fat transplantation. He utilized 1-cm pieces of free fat from the upper arm to reconstruct depressed facial defects. In 1911, Bruining was the first to report the technique of fat injections. He placed small pieces of fat into a syringe and by injecting this adipose tissue corrected postrhinoplasty deformities. Free fat transplants were then neglected because most surgeons preferred to use pedicle flaps, which preserved the blood supply to the fat thus making the outcome more predictable. In addition, artificial substances such as paraffin and silicone became available and were used to fill defects in the skin at that time. Peer reported a series of experiments in 1950 with autologous human fat transplants in which over 50% of the fat remained as a viable transplant one year following grafting. The current phase of fat transplantation began in 1976 when Fischer and Fischer performed fat extraction with the cellusuctiotome. Two years later Illouz introduced the simplified and safer method known today as liposuction using cannulas and suction. This has provided the cosmetic surgeon with an abundant supply of viable adipose tissue, which can be used to augment soft tissue deformities.

Technique

The physician should understand that autologous fat transplantation is really two procedures: extracting and injecting fat. Generally the quantity of fat needed for correcting facial defects is small, approximately 10–20 ml. The method used for harvesting the fat depends on how much is needed to correct the defect. Arbitrarily a volume of 20 ml is assigned to divide lipoextraction into micro and macro techniques.

Microlipoextraction

Microlipoextraction involves extracting and reimplanting adipose tissue by a closed technique. If less than 20 ml of fat are needed, a syringe and microextractor are the only instruments required. The microextractor can be a 14-gauge needle (Fig. 1) or a microcannula with a 2.1-mm diameter (Figs. 2 and 3).

Initially the donor site should be marked, and then under sterile conditions the fat is removed. Typical donor sites include the abdomen, buttocks, and thighs. It has been reported that the lateral thigh is the ideal donor site. The surgeon must respect the extracted tissue and minimize the hydraulic and chemical trauma. Several possibilities exist for anesthetizing the donor area: nerve block, local anesthesia, external cryanesthesia, or general anesthesia. The authors prefer local anesthesia with the tumescent technique.

After waiting 10–15 min for the maximum hemostatic effect of epinephrine, extract the fat with a 10- to 60-ml syringe using either a 1½ inch 14-gauge needle or a microcannula. The microcannula has a blunt distal end and a single aperture (Fig. 4). This is preferable to a 14-gauge needle, multiple port cannulas, or Cobra tip cannulas, which tend to retrieve more fibrous tissue and are more traumatic to the fat.

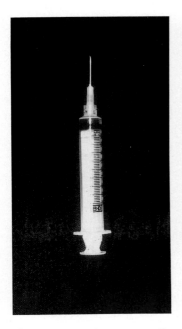   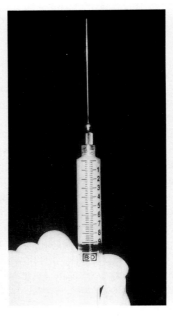   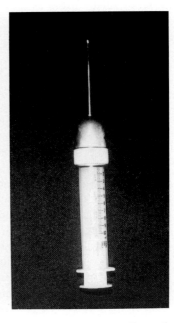

Figure 1 A 14-gauge needle attached to a 10-ml syringe.

Figure 2 A 2.1-mm luerlock microcannula attached to a 10-ml syringe.

Figure 3 A similar Tulip™ microcannula.

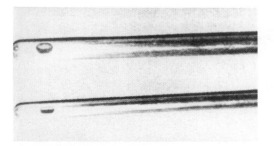

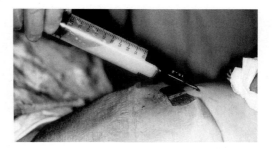

Figure 4 Close-up of microcannula apertures.

Figure 5 A sufficient vacuum is created within the syringe to aspirate fat.

It is important to fill the dead space in the syringe tip and cannula lumen in order to create the hydraulic action of the syringe vacuum. Fill the syringe with normal saline and then expel all but enough to fill the dead space in the cannula.

Next, a 2-mm incision is made in the skin with a No. 11 blade. Incision sites should be kept to a minimum as multiple incisions create an open atmosphere and diminish the benefits of a closed system. After the needle or the microcannula attached to the syringe is inserted into the fat, the plunger of the syringe is pulled to create a negative pressure. This relative vacuum will be sufficient to aspirate the fat as the needle is maneuvered back and forth within the fat (Fig. 5). During the entire procedure the skin is constantly palpated by the surgeon's free hand. The hand is held flat over the treated area, and the skin is pinched to feel the thickness of the fat.

The needle/cannula is moved back and forth five or six times in the same area, after which the maneuver is repeated in a radial fashion until sufficient fat has been aspirated. During the whole extraction the plunger will be kept in the same position. Several commercially available devices are specifically made to aid in maintaining the negative pressure of the syringe (Fig. 6).

Macrolipoextraction

Using a small syringe and a microextractor to harvest the fat becomes tedious when more than 20 ml of adipose tissue is needed for transplantation. A simple way to collect larger quantities of fat for transplantation is to use the first fat collected from the sterile tubing during liposuction before it enters the collection bottle (Fig. 7). When the sterile tube attached to the cannula is filled with fat, it is disconnected from the aspirating unit and emptied into the syringes to be used for injecting the fat.

It has been stated that any harvesting of fat with the suction pump as compared to the syringe is detrimental to adipocyte survival. When using a suction machine to obtain fat for transplantation, the vacuum pressure should be one half to two thirds that usually used for liposuction to avoid damaging the extracted fat. Others believe that the high negative suction pressure disrupts the fat tissue, allowing greater exposure of individual adipose sites, easier revascularization, and therefore better long-term survival rates and less volume loss. However, a recent experiment showed no difference in volume loss between particulate grafts (as obtained by liposuction) and whole grafts. The authors have previously published good long-term follow-up of several cases performed utilizing an aspiration unit for harvesting.

If performing macrolipoextraction, we prefer to use a sterile collecting filter (In-Line Collecting Set, Berkeley Medevices, Inc., Berkeley, CA), which collects the fat and allows fluid to pass to the aspirating unit (Fig. 8). This filter trap is placed between the cannula and the tube leading to the aspirating unit (Fig. 9).

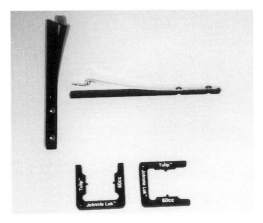

Figure 6 Devices that aid in keeping the syringe plunger withdrawn.

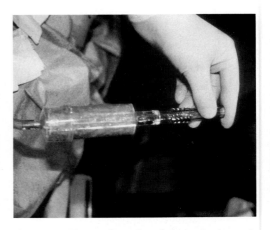

Figure 7 The suction tube of the aspirating unit can be used as a collecting device.

When the filter is filled with fat, the aspirating unit should be stopped and the collecting unit disconnected from the tube leading to the collecting bottle. The cannula is withdrawn last. This avoids a sudden increase in pressure within the system, which can force some of the fat through openings in the filter. The floor of the filter trap consists of a rubber plunger disc which, when pushed with the provided rod, empties the collected fat directly into a syringe.

The advantage of this unit is its ability to filter the fluid without excessive manipulation of fat. The collected fat may be washed by inserting the cannula into a container with lactated Ringer's or saline solution and letting the solution filter through the fat. Further drainage can be achieved by placing the Berkeley collecting device into a container for 10–15 min. This will allow the excess fluid to drain out of the filter trap and the fat will be of a better quality.

Treatment of the Collected Fat

When the extraction is complete, the filled syringe is capped and placed vertically in a test tube holder, plunger up. It should be allowed to stand for 10–15 min. This will cause separation, and the excess fluid (local anesthetic and blood) will accumulate in its dependent part, near the tip

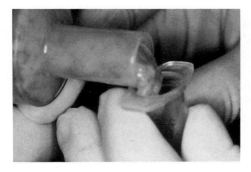

Figure 8 The In-Line Collecting Set.

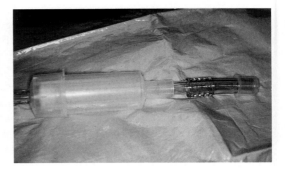

Figure 9 The collecting device attaches to a cannula at one end and the aspirating unit at the other.

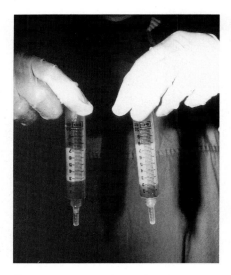

Figure 10 The aspirated fat will separate from anesthetic fluid and blood by gravitational pooling.

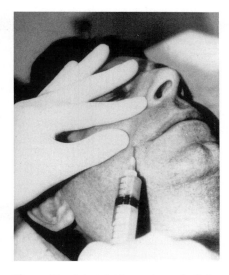

Figure 11 Inject fat in a retrograde fashion and away from orifices whenever possible.

(Fig. 10). This fluid should be expelled by removing the syringe cap and allowing it to drain. The syringe will also contain a turbid, pale yellow supranatant fluid from the broken adipocytes. This can be drained by removing the plunger and pouring it out.

If desired, the fat can be washed with either saline or lactated Ringer's solution, which seems to be more physiologically homeostatic for the extracted adipocytes. This isn't necessary if the tumescent technique of anesthesia is used at the donor site. In fact, excessive washing or manipulation of the fat cells may be detrimental to their survival.

Other methods of processing the harvested fat seem to decrease longevity of the transplanted tissue. Perfusing the cells with insulin increases resorption. Finally, centrifugation of collected fat completely destroys the cells, regardless of the centrifuge speed.

Reimplantation

Lipoinjection is typically performed with a 5- or 10-ml syringe and 16- or 18-gauge needle. It has been established that fat injected through a needle smaller than an 18-gauge needle is seriously damaged, as measured by nuclear, cellular, and globular morphology. This is confirmed by checking the biochemical integrity of the adipocyte as measured by glucose metabolism, fatty acid synthesis, and insulin stimulation. A 16-gauge needle seems to be the optimal size for transferring adipocytes. In addition, it does not scar the skin.

A small wheel of 1% Xylocaine is placed at each injection point in the dermis. Alternatively, one can use a regional nerve block to avoid tissue distortion. The injection needle is then directed into the anesthetized recipient sites.

The needle should be parallel with the surface of the skin, sliding just along the dermal subcutaneous junction, until it reaches its most distal point. As the needle is slowly withdrawn, the fat is injected in a retrograde fashion (Fig. 11). Thus, there is no need for subcutaneous tunneling and the possibility of an embolus is reduced. The defect is then injected in different areas until completely corrected. The injection of fat in different areas and levels ensures suffi-

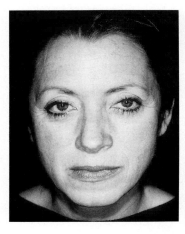 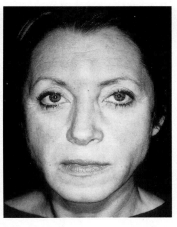

Figure 12 Before fat injections to glabellar and nasolabial/melolabial furrows.

Figure 13 Same patient immediately after fat injection. Note the overcorrection.

cient peripheral circulation around each graft to allow its incorporation in the surrounding tissue. Total control of fat deposition is maintained by applying manual pressure bilaterally along the edges of the defect. Lipoinjection should be continued until an overcorrection of 30% is achieved (Figs. 12,13). Occasionally a fibrous lobule of fat will block the entrance to the needle. Simply changing the needle is all that is required. Once the donor tissue is in place it should be gently molded into exact position.

Some ideal indications for lipoinjection are as follows:

1. Glabellar furrows: Typically less than 5 mm of fat are required here (Figs. 14,15). These furrows should be injected away from the eye to avoid intrusion of fat into the periorbital

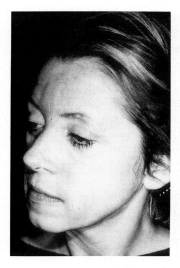 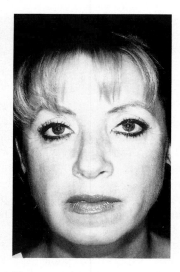

Figure 14 Immediately after fat injection, oblique view. Note the small marks left by the 16-gauge needle.

Figure 15 Two months after fat injection.

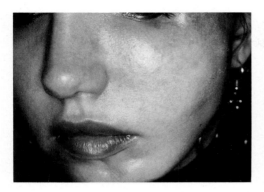

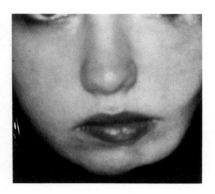

Figure 16 Melolabial folds and upper lip prior to fat injection.

Figure 17 Eight months after fat injection.

area. Marks left by the 16-gauge needle, if any, are not noticeable in the medial aspects of the eyebrows.

2. Nasolabial furrows/Melolabial furrows/Oral commissures: All three areas can be approached through the same entry point lateral to the commissures of the mouth (Figs. 16,17). Patients should be cautioned about excessive facial expressions and exertion for the first 12–24 hr postoperatively.

3. Lips: The same lateral entry points may be used. This will give the lips a full appearance and consequently diminish wrinkles. Perpendicular rhytides or "smoker's lines" will not be eradicated. This can also be used to evert the lips by injecting 4–5 ml of fat between the inner mucosa and muscular layers.

4. Cheeks: Whenever fat is injected into the face it should be directed away from orifices if possible. Cheeks can be augmented with lipoinjection (Figs. 18,19). Hollow cheeks and atrophic acne scars are amenable as well, but the scars should have associated atrophy of the subcutis (Figs. 20,21). If the scars are pitted or purely dermal defects, the chance of correction is unlikely.

5. Morphea/Lupus profundus: Both of these conditions respond quite well to lipoinjections (Fig. 22). However, the disease process should be inactive prior to beginning cosmetic correction. A biopsy may aid in documenting this.

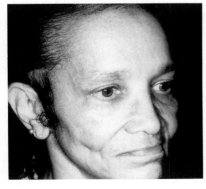

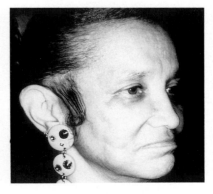

Figure 18 Before fat injection, oblique view.

Figure 19 Three months after fat injection.

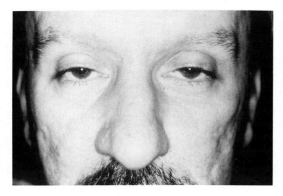

Figure 20 Atrophic acne scars of cheeks are amenable to correction with fat transplants.

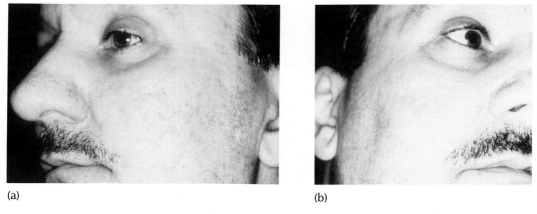

(a)   (b)

Figure 21 One year after fat injection. Note persistence of correction. (a) Oblique left; (b) oblique right.

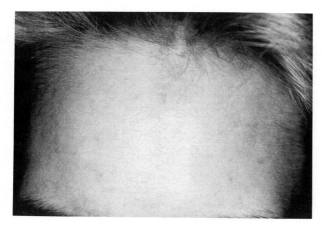

Figure 22 En coup de sabre morphea on central forehead 4 years after fat injection.

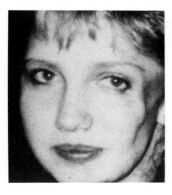 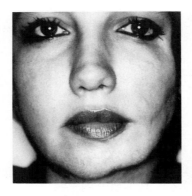

Figure 23   Facial hemiatrophy prior to treatment.

Figure 24   3 years after fat injection.

6. Facial hemiatrophy: Congenital defects such as facial hemiatrophy can be successfully treated (Figs. 23,24). However, as more fat is injected into one area, be careful to inject at different levels. The patient should be aware that several injections may be needed, usually 2–3 months apart.
7. Hands: Fat transplantation plays an integral role in hand rejuvenation. Transplanted fat provides thickness to an atrophic subcutaneous compartment, decreasing the prominence of blood vessels and tendons and giving the hands an overall plumper, younger appearance. The needle is inserted at the dorsal wrist crease and threaded along the tendon sheaths distally to each metacarpophalangeal joint. Approximately 5–10 ml are required for each hand. Overcorrection is not necessary as fat transplants tend to have less resorption here than elsewhere (Figs. 25,26).

Conclusions

Our experiences, like that of others, has shown few complications from the procedure of fat transplantation. Temporary swelling and very minor bruising at the recipient site and mild ten-

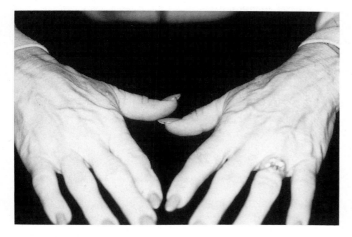

Figure 25   Senile lipoatrophy of the hands.

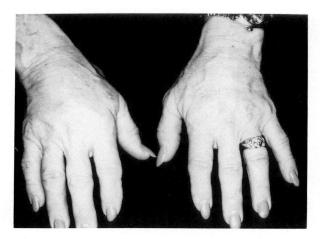

Figure 26 Six months after injection of 8 ml of adipose tissue to each hand.

derness at the door site have occurred. Thee has been a report of unilateral blindness following transplantation of autologous fat to the glabella. However, because of the large size of these particles, intravascular penetration of fat is a rare occurrence. It can be concluded that autologous fat transplantation is a safe and effective procedure.

Long-term results are still variable but are becoming more predictable as further follow-up studies are presented. One difficulty in evaluating results, as pointed out by Glogau, is the limitation of two-dimensional photography. The correction of subcutaneous defects is three dimensional and often subtle. It is difficult to translate results onto the printed page or photograph, even though the surgeon and patient may be able to appreciate improvement.

Survival rates for transplanted fat range from 30% to as much as 80%. Many clinical case reports have shown that a significant portion of the transplanted fat survives. Some have illustrated long-term survival at the time of reoperation or with the use of computed tomography or magnetic resonance imaging. However, most methods of assessing adipose tissue viability are performed on either a volumetric basis or from histologic study.

The current hypothesis regarding fat graft transfer supports the cell survival theory. The volume of fat, when surgically removed from the donor site, becomes ischemic. After transfer into the recipient site, some cells may die, some survive as adipocytes, and others dedifferentiate into preadipocyte cells. The preadipocyte cells, after recovery from the transfer process, can accumulate fat and mature into an adipocyte. Ultimately, the fat graft regains its blood supply from the periphery and those cells that have survived will remain and function. Those that die will be cleared and replaced by the normal process of fibrosis.

AUTOLOGOUS COLLAGEN

History

The concept of an ideal tissue for dermal augmentation has appealed to physicians for a number of years. Numerous substances have been used with varying records of success for thickening the dermis to eliminate wrinkles, creases, and scars. Some, like Zyderm collagen and Fibrel, have achieved commercial success. Others, like liquid silicone, have been well respected by physicians, but have been tainted by government regulations and questionable accusations and have not survived the competitive pharmaceutical marketplace.

Although Zyderm collagen and Fibrel have been used successfully for a number of years to improve dermal defects, there is a lingering dissatisfaction with the potential of these materials to cause allergic sensitization. Zyderm collagen is derived from bovine skin, whereas Fibril is obtained from porcine tissue. These foreign materials are antigenic in some individuals. Most of those allergic to these commercial fillers can be identified by the use of skin testing. However, some patients begin to react to these materials even after negative skin tests. Furthermore, there have been allegations of collagen diseases such as dermatomyositis produced by reactions to these foreign proteins.

An autologous source of collagen to augment dermal defects has been sought for the last 10 years. Fournier in Paris, and later Zocchi in Torino, used the term "autologous collagen" for processed fat cells that could be injected through a small gauge needle.

Fournier hypothesized that extracted adipose tissue consisted of intracellular fat contents, adipocyte cell walls, and intracellular fibrous septa. He added distilled water to the extracted fatty tissue and then froze the mixture. Thawing caused the adipocytes to rupture and led to the production of an oily and solid fraction. The oily fraction contained intracellular triglycerides, while the solid fraction consisted of cell walls and connective tissue. Decanting the oily fraction supposedly left collagen-rich autologous tissue as "autologous collagen." Fournier advocated freezing the unused portion for subsequent augmentation.

Zocchi, working with Founier and independently, is credited with the technique of preinjury of the donor site 10–12 days before harvesting the tissue. This theoretically initiated the wound-healing cascade, which Zocchi believed would increase the production of collagen in this tissue. After harvesting the fat by syringe, he recommended the use of ultrasound and centrifugation to separate the "autologous collagen" tissue. Because of the extra patient visit for preinjury and the cost of the commercial ultrasound device and special centrifuge, Zocchi's approach has not been widely adopted.

In the United States the use of autologous collagen has been minimal. Because the material is not as convenient as Zyderm collagen and requires a larger needle, it has gained popularity slowly. However, increased allegations of allergic sensitization and collagen disease associated with bovine collagen have scared many patients into requesting an autologous material for augmenting dermal defects.

Technique

The most efficient way to prepare autologous collagen from adipose tissue is to remove the fat using the microlipoextraction techniques described earlier in this chapter. This usually involves a 1.4- to 2.1-mm microcannula attached to a 60-ml syringe. Tumescent anesthesia is again preferred. The remainder of the harvesting procedure is similar to microlipoextraction, except that typically a greater volume of adipose tissue is removed. Any excess material not utilized during the initial injection can be frozen for future touch-up procedures.

After harvesting, the adipose tissue is ready to be processed into a substance suitable for dermal augmentation. The fat is transferred from a 60-ml syringe to a 5-ml syringe using a transfer adaptor device (Wells Johnson Co., Tucson, AZ). The 5-ml syringes are then placed into a centrifuge and spun at low rpm for 1 min. The infranate (anesthesia and blood) and supranate (triglycerides) are expelled, leaving a solid fraction containing fat cells, fibrous septa, and "autologous collagen." A 5-ml syringe containing this tissue is then attached to an empty 5-ml syringe by a dual lock device (Bernsco Surgical Supply, Inc., Seattle, WA) (Fig. 27). This device has a stopcock, which when maneuvered will progressively decrease the aperture between the two syringes. The material should be pushed back and forth approximately five to six times while

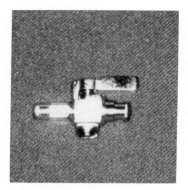

Figure 27 Dual luerlock device
for processing autologous collagen.

gradually diminishing the aperture. This will pulverize the tissue and create an emulsion. This
should be done again immediately prior to injection since the fat tends to harden and may be
difficult to pass through a small-gauge needle if left standing for 5 min or more.

Next the recipient site is anesthetized using field block local anesthesia. The dermal defect
should be carefully identified prior to this using a marking pen since the contour may be obliterated by infiltration of local anesthesia. Cryanesthesia is another alternative that avoids this
problem using a 5/8-inch 23- or 25-gauge needle (Lancet Point Needles, Bernsco Surgical Supply, Inc., Seattle, WA). Dermal wheels can be raised by injecting the autologous collagen directly into the lower dermis. This technique can be quite difficult to learn initially, and it may
take a number of procedures before the physician becomes comfortable with it. Once adequate
dermal augmentation has been achieved, the surgeon should then gently massage the area to
smooth out individual lumps so the entire defect is filled uniformly. Overcorrection is recommended since up to 50% of the augmentation may vanish within a few days after injection.

Conclusions

To date, very few complications have been reported with the use of fat-derived autologous collagen. Patients typically develop immediate erythema and swelling which may last for 2–3 days.
This can be minimized with the use of intramuscular steroids to reduce swelling. Postoperative
ice packing is also recommended to diminish bruising. Most patients can return to an active
lifestyle within 2 days after the treatment.

The longevity of fat-derived autologous collagen is variable. Just as with Zyderm collagen or
Fibril, the length of the correction varies from patient to patient. Histologically, the correction
is still present at 3 months. Longer histologic studies remain to be done. Clinically, correction
persists 9 months to 1 yr in most cases (Figs. 28–31).

Histologic studies reveal that the lipocytic autologous collagen consisted primarily of ruptured
adipocytes. Small amounts of collagen and elastic fibers were found in the processed fat. This
was also confirmed by electron microscopy (Fig. 32). Serial histologic assays revealed an intense inflammatory response after injection. This material was subsequently replaced by fibrosis and new collagen, which resulted in dramatic dermal thickening. In two patients biopsied 3
months after autologous collagen augmentation, there was a threefold increase in dermal thickness. The true autologous collagen was not that injected, but apparently that generated at the host
site.

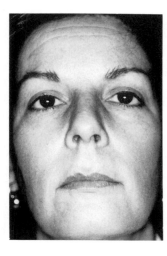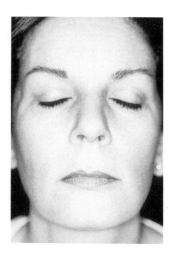

Figure 28,29 Pre- and 3 months postaugmentation of glabellar furrows, melolabial furrows, and lips with autologous collagen.

Laboratory analyses have also been performed on this material to determine its composition. Hydroxyproline assays were conducted to determine the percentage of collagen. The range was 1–4%, with a mean of 3%. This compares with 3.5% collagen weight by volume for Zyderm I. Western blot identified small amounts Type I, but primary Type III collagen. Serial bacterial and fungal cultures were negative for growth on previously harvested samples stored frozen for up to 6 months. At 8 months one sample grew *Staphylococcus aureus* and *Streptococcus epidermidis*. However, this occurred after prolonged thawing of the material.

The success of any technique for soft tissue augmentation depends on ease of use, safety, and clinical results. Lipocytic dermal augmentation or autologous collagen shows promise in all these areas. Although technically more difficult and time consuming to use than Zyplast or Fibrel, adipose tissue is available in larger quantities without appreciable additional effort. A 5-ml augmentation is not much more time consuming than a 1-ml augmentation. In addition, excess material can be stored for future touch-up procedures.

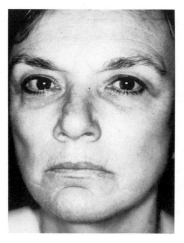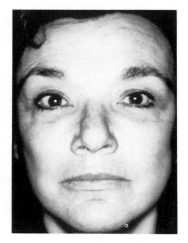

Figure 30,31 Pre- and 3 months postaugmentation of glabellar furrows, upper lip, and chin rhytides.

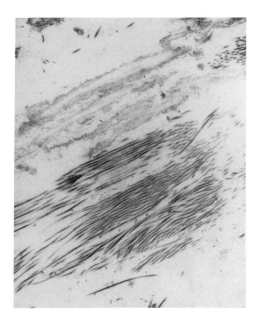

Figure 32   Electronmicroscopy of autologous collagen demonstrating intact collagen bundles and elastic fibers.

Because the tissue transplanted is autologous, there is no chance of an immune response to foreign tissue as with silicone, Fibrel, and Zyderm. The notion of a potential autoimmune reaction after lipocytic dermal augmentation must be considered, but this is neither consistent with modern immunologic theory, nor has it been observed in autologous transplantation of other human tissues. For soft tissue defects with dermal and subcutaneous components, autologous collagen is ideal. Some of the extracted fat can be injected, without mechanical processing, into the subcutaneous defect. The dermal component can then be augmented with processed fat as described here. The clinical results have been gratifying to date, especially in patients in whom a second touch-up procedure is performed after 2–4 weeks. The longevity appears to rival that of Zyplast and Fibrel. Apparently much of the improvement results from dermal thickening long after the transplanted tissue has involuted. This may be due to formation of new collagen at the site of injection.

BIBLIOGRAPHY

Asken S. Autologous fat transplantation: Micro and macro techniques. *Am J Cosmet Surg* 1978;4:111.

Asken S. Autologous fat transplantation. In *Dermatologic Surgery*. RK Roenigk, HH Roenigk, eds. New York, Marcel Dekker, 1989, pp. 1179–1213.

Billings E Jr., May JW Jr. Historical review and present status of free graft auto transplantation in plastic and reconstructive surgery. *Plast Reconstr Surg* 1989;83:368.

Broeckaert TJ. Contribution to a l'etude des greffes adipeueses. *Bull Acad R Med Belg* 1919;28:440.

Campbell G-Lem, Laudenslager, Newman J. The effect of mechanical stress on adipocyte morphology and metabolism. *Am J Cosmet Surg* 1987;4:

Chajchir A, Benzaquen I, Moretti E. Comparative experimental study of autologous adipose tissue processed by different techniques. *Aesth Plast Surg* 1993;17:113–115.

Clark ER, Clark EL. Microscopoic studies of the new formation of fat in living adult rabbits. *Am J Anat* 1940;67:255.

Coleman WP, Lawrence N, Sherman RN, Reed RJ, Pinski KS. Autologous collagen? Lipocytic dermal augmentation a histopathologic study. *J Dermatol Surg Oncol* 1993;19:1032–1040.

DeLustro F, Fries J, Kang A, et al. Immunity to injectable collagen and autoimmune disease: A summary of current understanding. *J Dermatol Surg Oncol* 1988;14(suppl):57–65.

Elson ML. The role of skin, testing in the use of collagen injectable materials. *J Dermatol Surg Oncol* 1989;15:301–303.

Eppley BL, Smith PG, Salove AM, et al. Experimental effects of graft revascularization and consistency on cervicofacial fat transplant survival. *J Oral Maxillofac Surg* 1990;48:54–62.

Fischer G. Autologous fat implantation for breast augmentation, Workshop on liposuction and autologous fat implant. Isola d'Elba, September 1986.

Fischer A, Fischer GM. Revised technique for cellulitis fat. Reduction in riding breeches deformity. *Bull Int Acad Cosmet Surg* 1977;2:40.

Fournier PF. *Collagen Autologue: Liposculpture ma Technique*. Paris, Arnette, 1989, pp. 227–229.

Glogau RG. Microliposuction. *Arch Dermatol* 1988;12:35.

Gurney CE. Studies on the fate of free transplants of fat. *Proc Staff Meet Mayo Clin* 1937;12:317.

Hochberg M. The cosmetic surgical procedures and connective tissue disease: The Cleopatra syndrome revisited. *Ann Int Med* 1993;118:981–982.

Horol HW, Feller AM, Biemer E. Technique for liposuction fat reimplantation and long-term volume evaluation by magnetic resonance imaging. *Am Plast Surg* 1991;26:248.

Hudson DA, Lambert EV, Bloch CE. Site selection for autotransplantation: Some observations. *Aesth Plast Surg* 1990;14:195.

Illouz-4-6. Communications at the Societe Francaise de Chirurgie Esthetique, June 1978 and 1979.

Illouz 4-6. L'Avnir de la reutilisation de la graisse apres liposuction. *Rev Chir Esthet Lang Franc* 1985;10.

Johnson G. Body contouring by macroinjection of autogenous fat. *Am J Cosmet Surg* 1987;4:103–109.

Klein JA. The tumescent technique for liposuction surgery. *Am J Cosmet Surg* 1987;4:263–267.

Lewis CM. The current status of autologous fat grafting. *Aesth Plast Surg* 1993;17:109–112.

Matsudo PKR, Toledo LS. Experience of injected fat grafting. *Aesth Plast Surg* 1988;12:35.

Neuber F. Fat grafting. *Cuir Kongr Verh Otsum Ges Chir* 1893;20:66.

Nguyen A, Pasyk KA, Bouvier TN, et al. Comparative study of survival of autologous adipose tissue taken and transplanted by different techniques. *Plast Reconstr Surg* 1990;85:378–387.

Orentreich D, Orentreich N. Injectable fluid silicone. In *Dermatologic Surgery*. RK Roenigk, HH Roenigk, eds. New York, Marcel Dekker, 1989.

Peer LA. Loss of weight and volume in human fat grafts. *Plast Reconstr Surg* 1950;5:217.

Pinski KS, Roenigk HH. Autologous fat transplantation: A long-term follow-up. *J Dermatol Surg Oncol* 1992;18:179–184.

Polsy Rl. Adipocyte survival. Presented at the Third Annual Scientific Meeting of the American Academy of Cosmetic Surgery and the American Society of Liposuction Surgery. Los Angeles, February 1987.

Sergott TJ, Limoli JP, Baldwin CM, et al. Human adjuvant disease, possible autoimmune disease after silicone implantation: A review of the literature, case studies and speculation for the future. *Plast Reconstr Surg* 1988;78:104–114.

Temourian B. Blindness following fat injections, correspondence and brief communications. *Plast Reconstr Surg* 1988;80:361.

Van RL, Bayliss CE, Roncari DA. Cytological and enzymological characterization of adult human adipocyte precursors in culture. *J Clin Invest* 1976;58:699.

Van RLR, Roncari DAK, Isolation of fat cell precursors from adult rat adipose tissue. *Cell Tissue Res* 1977;181:197.

Van Akkerveeken PF, Van de Kraan W, Muller JWT. The fate of the free fat graft. A prospective clinical study using CT scanning. *Spine* 1986;11:501.

Webster RC, Fuleihan NS, Hamdan US, et al. Injectable silicone; report of 17,000 facial treatments since 1962. *Am J Cosmet Surg* 1986;3:41–4.

Weisz GM, Gal A. Long-term survival of a fat free graft in the spinal canal. A 40 month postlaminectomy case report. *Clin Orthop* 1986;205:204.

Zocchi M. Melthode de production de collagene autologue par traitement du tissu graisseaux. *J Med Esthet Chir Dermatol* 1990;17:105–114.

76

Blepharoplasty and Brow Lifting

Robert S. Flowers
University of Hawaii School of Medicine and Plastic Surgery Center of the Pacific, Inc., Honolulu, Hawaii

Much has been written over the last 30 years about blepharoplasty, but there is very little in print to help the inexperienced or questing surgeon improve disappointing results (Fig. 1). The descriptions of surgical technique in most textbooks and essays on the subject do not reflect the modifications and methods used by those with the greatest expertise in the field. This is unfortunate because faulty procedure and methodology is being perpetuated.

Some months ago the author put his own thoughts on *traditional* blepharoplasty techniques into verse, and these lines sum up the thoughts conveyed in this chapter.

Resolute and committed we stand at the head
While the patient lies there on the surgical bed.
She looks rather calm, disguising her dread—
Having heard tales of some who suffered and bled.

Our energies blend with a touch of the hand,
Commending the work, that for months we had planned.
The fear that the patient had icily felt
Is a euphoric pool that was chemically melt.

With methylene blue and toothpick or quill
We mark the resection with long studied skill,
And fix in our minds what we hope to achieve—
The goal in which surgeons have come to believe.

"Take as much as we can from the upper eyelid."
Of all of that "extra," we'd like to be rid.
On the lower eyelids we raise up the skin,
Dissecting a flap, incredibly thin.

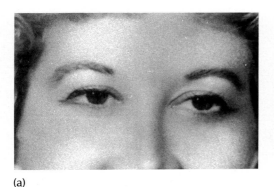
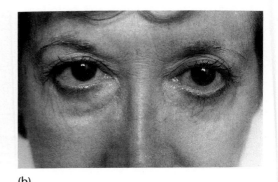

(a)   (b)

Figure 1 (a) Eyelids shown 10 years preoperatively. (b) Eyelids of same patient 10 years after blepha-roplasty. The operation was performed by another surgeon who followed traditional techniques advocated in most textbooks on cosmetic surgery.

We do an advancement, then rotate the flap—
Just like it's depicted in most textbook maps.
With the mouth opened wide, we decide what's excess
Taking a triangle of skin that's destined to bless

Some steel garbage pail . . . then we sew the wounds tight.
Next treat her with soaks, or a bandage overnight.
The next day we wince at the lids' downward pull
Could the textbooks we read have covered our lids with wool?

As the weeks pass to months, we try not to look.
Hoping all will be well, as it said in the book;
But the postoperative photos, shown in textbooks we read,
Look acceptable only—by tilting the head.

The fat we removed now seems imprecise,
And the patient's lagophthalmos just doesn't look nice
The excess skin's gone, but it cost us too much
There's a hood of tight skin, with the outer canthus in a clutch.

The upper lid's look strange, and the fold, less distinct;
The eyebrow's more ptotic; there's an incomplete blink;
The aperture's shortened; there's a new scleral show,
And the axis tilts down, but the patient may not know.

But those patients try hard to be pleasant and kind.
They dislike what they see, but are hard pressed to find
Precisely just what . . . it is that they see,
That register as eyes, "that just don't look like me."

If we're daring enough to carefully inspect
We'll find that the textbooks were just incorrect
And instead of our excelling, learning what our mentors wrote,
These techniques we "mastered" now have us by the throat.

So what must we do to improve on our aim
Neither give up our work, nor continue the same!

But rethink operations that don't turn out straight,
So lives are enhanced, and eyelids look great.

So let's look at our patients right straight in the eye
Which is tougher than the photos, which often can lie.
And be sure in our hearts, what we're doing is good—
That all eyelids operated, end up as they should! (Fig. 2).

The above lines delineate the tragedy of blepharoplasty and challenge us to improve upon the results of established and traditional techniques.

The surgeon who "cookbooks" technique in the orbital region is destined to produce dismal results. Unfortunately, these results can be photographically disguised by subtly tilting the head backwards for the postoperative picture. Thus true tragedy from the traditional operation is seldom recorded, although it may accompany the patient *through life*.

In a very simplistic way, it is possible to classify orbital surgery into two types: the good and the bad. Bad eyelid surgery involves the standardized, traditional, or cookbook approach to the eyelids. Good aesthetic orbital surgery involves careful analysis of the deformity and its causative factors, conceptualization of what would be aesthetically pleasing in the individual concerned, and skillful execution of an operation that is custom-designed to achieve maximum aesthetic improvement, done with an experienced awareness of the true long-term effects of each surgical maneuver.

Contemporary blepharoplasty is, in the truest sense, orbital surgery. It should never be misconstrued as simple skin surgery. This misconception has led to a great number of unfortunate results; we have failed to understand the intricacies, interrelationships, and the awesomely negative effect it can have on a life if less than expertly executed.

IMPORTANCE OF THE ORBITAL REGION

The orbital region is by far the most important aesthetic complex of the face. It is in this region that aging and weariness first show. It is where time, tissue elastosis, muscle hypertrophy, fat prominence, and tissue attenuation distort the features and leave the face with the appearance of grumpiness, agitation, dissipation, weariness, and other projected impressions. Indeed the public response is so consistent to this misperceived characterization that the hosts of these faces tend to become their often incorrectly characterized images.

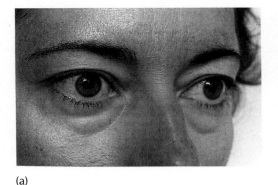

(a)

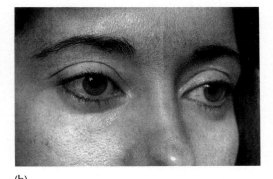

(b)

Figure 2 (a) Preoperative appearance of eyelids on young woman. (b) Postoperative eyelids shown at 4 years. This is the type of result that should, but unfortunately does not, accompany each blepharoplasty.

For some reason people generally tend to focus their dissatisfaction with physical aging on the neck and the lower face. This is done to the total denial of the changes that have occurred around the eyes, which are correctable with a great deal of permanency. The preponderance of improvement to be obtained in the face is usually found in the orbital region. It is this region from which we greet other people and greet ourselves in the mirror every day.

For the purpose of this chapter, the orbital region is divided into three categories: upper eyelids, lower eyelids, and brow. Before they are discussed, it is appropriate to devote some attention to the concept of what constitutes an attractive orbital region.

ORBITAL AESTHETICS

Although it is important that every person doing lid surgery have clearly defined criteria for the aesthetically pleasing eye (or orbital region), these criteria need not be rigid. It is important that we conceptualize what looks good, although we may consider that certain characteristics fit one face better than another. Thus the criteria may vary to a certain degree, particularly between different ethnic orbital racial groups and within each racial group. Although this chapter centers on the Caucasian eye, comment on the non-Caucasian eye is warranted. For instance, certain Asian eyes have such beautiful natural characteristics, with minimal or supratarsal fold, that it would be a shame to deeply invaginate such a lid. This contrasts with the desirability of lid folds for most Asian or Oriental eyes, even as they are present, at least to a small degree, in most people of East Asian ancestry (Fig. 3).

It is erroneous to assume that because we live in a predominantly Caucasian culture those features are most desired, and that this is the goal sought by all individuals requesting this change. It is generally a mistake to do anything that Caucasianizes the Oriental face. This is true in spite of the fixation of some Orientals that Caucasian lid folds (parallel to the lid margin or exposing more pretarsal eyelid medially) would enhance their good looks. Such alterations end up looking badly out of place.

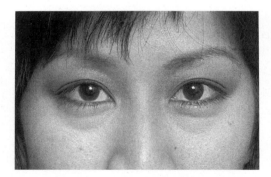

Figure 3 Naturally occurring lid folds in a young woman of East Asian ancestry. It is generally a mistake to attempt to do operations that Caucasianize Oriental lids.

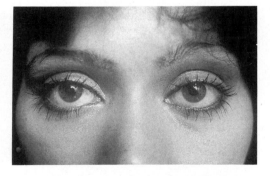

Figure 4 Attractive unoperated youthful eyelids with a prominent degree of scleral show. Such eyelids can sometimes be striking, but they give a saddened appearance. Such eyelids will not tolerate even 1 mm of additional scleral show. Also note the attractive contour of the upper lid with a generous pretarsal or "subfold" segment to the upper eyelid.

Yet today there is emerging a truly international standard of facial aesthetics. Moving gently in this direction can be advantageous so long as a person is not stripped of ethnic identity. The long-term "wearability" of facial alterations is far more important than what a patient may request at a given moment.

The aesthetically astute surgeon is always well advised to *avoid doing any operation that conflicts with his or her definition of enhancement of orbital aesthetics for any given patient.* A surgeon should never allow himself or herself to be backed into a compromising situation or have to explain, "I don't care for this result, but it's what the patient wanted." The chances are the patient will not want it for very long.

Assuming that standard operations or the simple removal of tissues that seem superfluous will lead to aesthetically pleasing results is ridiculous. In so doing there is little chance of fortuitously ending up with an aesthetically pleasing postoperative result. Therefore, we must conceptualize and then know how to produce surgically the conceptualized result.

Here are my personal preferences for the most beautiful orbital region. The characteristics need not be accepted by everyone, but it is essential that every surgeon have a concept of the most ideal characteristics for each given patient.

The first important feature of the attractive orbital region is a high degree of symmetry. Major problems that affect symmetry are unilateral lid ptosis; unilateral brow ptosis; and unilateral congenital, developmental, and traumatic deformity, including enucleations and inadequately repaired facial fractures. The second feature common to the aesthetically pleasing eye is a generous eyelid aperture in height and width but with limited scleral show. Both the intercanthal distance and the posture of the lid and the excursion of the upper lid, as well as the presence of lid heaviness and overhanding (pseudoblepharoptotic) skin, have an impact upon the apparent size of the aperture. The aperture size is also affected by the size and positioning of the globe and the prominence of the orbital rim. The most pleasing apertures have an almond shape, with the upper lid covering 2–3 mm of the iris. In certain instances a very slight lazy "S" configuration to the upper lid and even to the lower lid may be desirable, but there should not be too much lateral scleral show. When it does exist, especially when it is exaggerated laterally, youthful eyes may be striking (Fig. 4), but they generally take on a saddened appearance, like the cocker spaniel or hound dog look, because of the pronounced scleral show. This obviously works profoundly against orbital aesthetics.

There should be an upward tilt from medial to lateral of the line drawn between the medial and lateral canthus of the eye (Fig. 5). An exaggerated tilt is the secret of many of the world's greatest beauties. Traditional methods of make-up application are often designed to create an illusion of exaggerated medial-to-lateral tilt of this axis. This tilt adds exquisite beauty not only to the Caucasian eye but also to the Negroid and Oriental eye (Fig. 6).

There should be a crisp precise supratarsal lid fold. This fold should come closer to the lid margin nasally than it does laterally. It should reach its maximum divergence from the lid margin in the central portion of the lid and continue at that level across the entire lid (Fig. 7). The height between the lash line and the lid fold in the central portion of the eyelid should be no more than one fourth to one third of the vertical distance between the lid margin and the border of the resting eyebrow. Surgical scars should not be seen beyond the invaginated portion of the lid, except in the occasional elderly patient in whom exceptional redundancy mandates its existence. The fact that the lid fold comes closer to the lid margin nasally imparts to the eye an illusion of a greater medial-to-lateral tilt, an aesthetically pleasing characteristic, as mentioned above.

The unstyled eyelashes of the upper lid should be perpendicular to the long axis of the body. Lash eversion with exposure of the gray line of the upper lid can occur iatrogenically and as a

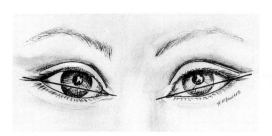

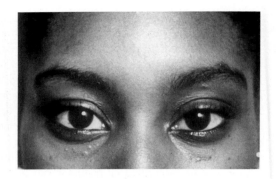

Figure 5 Desirable upward tilt of the line drawn between the medial and lateral canthus of the eye. Such a tilt is the source of beauty of many of the world's most famous eyes.

Figure 6 Beautiful upward tilt and Negroid eye.

result of exophthalmos. In both instances the lid and lash eversion gives the face an aura of surprise and harshness.

Epicanthal folds are, of course, characteristic of the Oriental race. They also appear sporadically in Caucasians and blacks (without Down syndrome), and they may occur asymmetrically. When excessively prominent, they give the eye a look of telecanthus and often internal strabismus (Fig. 8). Optimal aesthetics demand that epicanthal folds, when present, be subtle without concealing major portions of medially visualized sclera.

The eyebrow should be arched from medial to lateral, and the thickened brow skin or juxtabrow skin should not be hanging down onto the eyelid. There is no need for fixed creases on the forehead, caused by the involuntary contraction of the frontalis muscle, in order to move tissue out of the way to effect forward gaze. The orbital rim should not encroach on the lid fold lat-

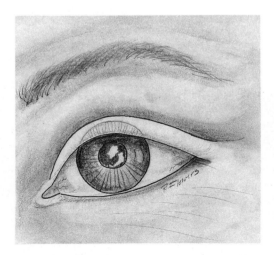

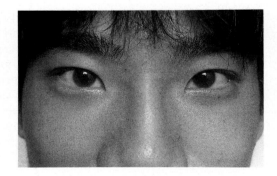

Figure 7 The optimal design of the upper lids for the best aesthetics.

Figure 8 Prominent epicanthal folds giving the eye the illusion of internal strabismus.

erally. In the area between the eyebrow, there should be no fixed frown or bulges at the location of the corrugator muscle.

Thus we can see that certain generalizations may be made about the aesthetically pleasing eye. The author has studied drawings and paintings extensively and was a student of facial structure prior to becoming a surgeon. Having continued that study, I am convinced that the above characteristics would enhance almost any face, but these criteria should not be inflicted on anyone else. Each surgeon must arrive at his or her own ideal criteria.

THE UPPER LID

Since the inception of aesthetic surgery of the orbital region, the principal method of repair has been the removal of as much skin as possible on the upper eyelid, often including large amounts of muscle. Indeed it has been said that "unless enough skin is reduced from the upper lid as to keep it from closing completely in the early postoperative period, not enough has been removed," or, equally absurd, "it is almost impossible to remove too much skin from the upper lid."

The extirpation of excessive quantities of tissue from the upper eyelid deprives that structure of its specialized skin, which is necessary for normal appearance and normal function. Instead of hoped-for improvement, deformity results and aesthetics are destroyed rather than created. Other severe conditions may also arise.

Heavy, unwieldy, juxtabrow skin delivered down onto the eyelid by these techniques neither looks good nor functions normally. Often the brow is lower than it was preoperatively (Fig. 9). The lid fold is usually less distinct, especially when the supratarsal crease has been resected together with the fibers connecting the region to the aponeurosis. It is not uncommon for the patient to have exposure problems after such traditional upper-lid blepharoplasties.

The common structural pathology in the upper half of the orbital region is due to a trilogy of deforming factors, the most important being brow ptosis, especially laterally. The second factor is attenuation or deficiency of the connections between the levator mechanism (the eye-opening mechanism) and the deeper layers of the skin. The third and least important factor is redundancy of the lid skin, which may or may not be present. Of course fat, if present, must be accurately

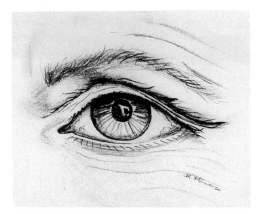

Figure 9 Note the postoperative brow appearance in a drawing of a patient in whom the surgeon had attempted to solve the problem of brow ptosis by excessive skin removal from the upper lid. This results in deformity, with a brow that is often lower than preoperatively. This may be accompanied by a lid lag with scleral show above the limbus on downward gaze, which is markedly worsened by restoring the brow to a normal position. Also see Figure 1.

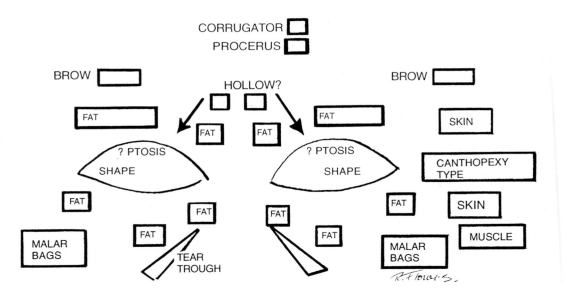

Figure 10 Characteristic map of planned procedures associated with blepharoplasty. Note that the fat has been quantitated in the central, medial, and lateral compartments of the lower lid and in the medial and lateral aspects of the upper lid. Fat must be assessed and quantitated accurately preoperatively, and the surgeon should resist all impulses to remove any amount other than that mapped preoperatively.

reduced. An accurate diagram planning its removal must be mapped out with the patient in a *vertical* position preoperatively (Fig. 10).

Too often, patients are seen after blepharoplasty for which an overenthusiastic surgeon has taken far more skin from the upper lid than was appropriate. The result commonly is lagophthalmos with failure of the lid to close adequately during sleep. The real difficulty comes when a surgeon recognizes primary deforming pathologic change as the ptotic brow and attempts to restore the brow to its physiological and properly functioning position. When this is stimulated by manually positioning the brow (Fig. 11), it becomes obvious that a severe degree of lagophthalmos will result, together with exposure problems, keratitis, and corneal ulcerations from an inadequate closure.

If, however, the trilogy of deforming factors is addressed with proper priority, there is restoration of the brow to its proper position and crisp invagination of the lid fold with secure attachments of the eye-opening mechanism, invaginating the skin when the eye is opened. This reduces skin removal to *only that amount truly redundant*. Minimal, if any, muscle resection is necessary. With this approach, the problem gets addressed in the same direction as the pathologic condition developed. Consequently, function is preserved, and the aesthetic appearance of the eye is greatly enhanced (Fig. 12).

Figure 13 shows the proper and improper skin incisions for upper-lid surgery. If a proper anchoring technique is used (Fig. 14), minimal, if any, skin need be resected. A small resection is usually adequate. It is best begun at a distance of the tarsus height, plus 2 mm above the lid margin, with the skin stretched uniformly tight. This distance will allow the free margin to reach comfortably down to attach to the upper margin of the tarsus without everting the lashes.

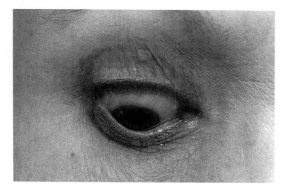

Figure 11 Manual restoration of the brow to its optimal position after blepharoplasty that has radically removed lid skin necessary for a normal functioning. A surgical correction of the ptotic brow in this patient (without placing skin grafts on the eyelid) will result in severe exposure problems.

These techniques should be used only by surgeons who are sufficiently familiar with orbital anatomy to be totally comfortable doing lid ptosis repairs.

If a surgeon insists on doing lid surgery without having the expertise to restore the crispness of supratarsal fold invagination, then he or she will be well advised to adhere to the following rules.

1. Do not resect the existing supratarsal fold; to do so without reconstructing skin to the lid opening mechanism will make the fold less distinct.
2. Take a conservative amount of skin from the upper lid, and *do not attempt to solve brow ptosis by upper-lid resection*. Be content to do a modest lid correction that will allow for the next step: brow positioning by someone comfortable with those operations. Excessive resection of eyelid skin ruins appearance and function and does nothing to help the primary offender, in most cases, brow ptosis.
3. Resect a small sliver of orbicularis muscle—no more than 2–3 mm wide. Do not tent it up when resecting, because the aponeurosis may be closely adherent to the muscle's undersurface. Because of its location, it may be inadvertently transected.

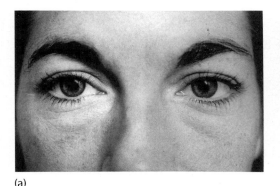
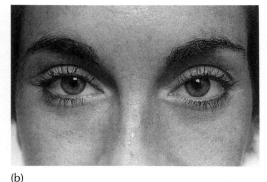

(a) (b)

Figure 12 Lid surgery in which a new fold has been created in conjunction with a large-flap brow positioning procedure, to which has been added a lateral canthopexy to tighten the laxity of the lower lid. Shown (a) preoperatively and (b) at 5 years after surgery.

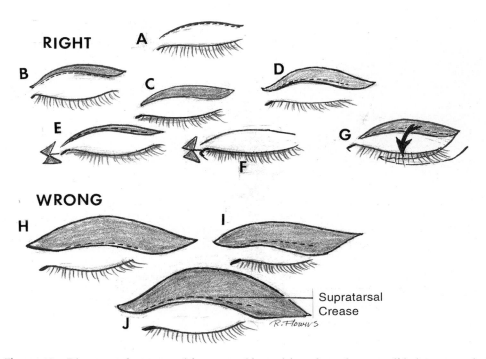

Figure 13 Diagrams of proper and improper skin excisions from the upper lid shown actual size. Broken line represents supratarsal crease. (A) Left upper lid incision without skin removal, to be used in patients without excess lid skin for fat removal and/or lid fold creation. (B) Lid with minimal skin excess, with minimal excision. The supratarsal fold should remain if a lid fold reconstruction is not to be done. (C) Skin excision where there is moderate redundancy. (D) Skin excision where there is considerable redundancy. The supratarsal fold is included, requiring creation of a new lid fold. (E) Typical Oriental lid repair combined with modified Uchida-type epicanthoplasty. (F) The same Oriental lid repair without skin excision. (G) An upper lid blepharoplasty; patient who has had previous lower lid blepharoplasty with excess skin removal laterally; this resulted in deformity. (Lowered lateral posture. Canthopexy usually is also required.) (H)Typical excessive skin excision from upper lid. (I) Typical excessive skin excision with upper angulation over the brow pad. (J) Excessive skin excision, combining removal of the supratarsal fold with excision crossing the supratarsal skin fold and the pretarsal skin bridge laterally.

4. Diagnose preoperatively whether there is bilateral or unilateral lid ptosis. Point out its existence to the patient preoperatively. Any preexisting ptosis will be at least temporarily worsened by blepharoplasty if it is not corrected. The best option, therefore, is to refer if the surgeon contemplating the operation is unable to correct this very common coexistence.

5. Brow ptosis should be corrected (see The Brow). If there is unilateral brow ptosis which *is not* and *will not subsequently be corrected*, resection of a little additional skin and muscle from the more ptotic side will add to the symmetry of the postoperative result.

Remember the age-old command in medicine, "First, do no harm." To proceed surgically in a direction that is likely to violate this rule is putting *desire to operate* before the *patient's wellbeing*. This is a breach of medical ethics and should be regarded as anathema by all practitioners.

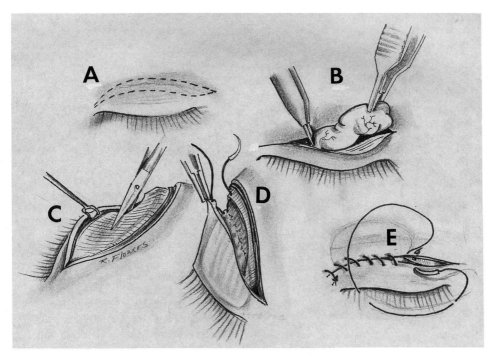

Figure 14 Author's technique of anchor blepharoplasty, for restoring the supratarsal lid fold. (A) Incisions designed with optimal medial epicanthoplasty. (B) Fat removed. (C) The pretarsal extension of the levator aponeurosis transected. (D) Dermis of pretarsal skin flap attached to the anterior or superior aspect of the tarsus and to the sectioned aponeurosis. (E) Aponeurosis is also incorporated into skin repair.

THE LOWER LID

Figure 15 shows the commonly performed lower-lid blepharoplasty. These triangular skin incisions are depicted in most illustrations on blepharoplasty technique. Such excisions invariably produce the results shown in Figure 16. There is scleral show, which is worse laterally. There is shortening of the aperture length with rounding of the lateral canthus, a lateral epicanthal fold from tension at the maximum height of the triangle of skin removal, and diagonal lines radiating from the lateral canthus toward the nasal ala. Unfortunately, the problem of attenuated tendons in the lower lid has been addressed by only the author and a small group of surgeons who are convinced of the real deformity. Most continue to remove deforming triangular sections of skin from the lower lid without solving the tonicity problem. When the tonicity *is* addressed, a wedge resection of the lid usually results, which diminishes the aperture size and fails to restore the lateral canthus to its normal and desirable position.

On the lower lid, the first important thing to realize is that *far too many lids are operated on*. This is because of incorrect diagnosis of excessive skin with the presence of lid lines. Deeply etched smile lines, often present only when the patient is smiling or partially smiling, are the leading complaint of patients concerned about lower lids, but they *are not relieved by blepharoplasty*. If this fact is adequately communicated to patients, many blepharoplasties would be avoided and much of this deformity averted. Most patients undergoing lower-lid blepharoplasties

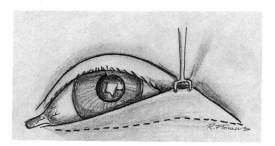

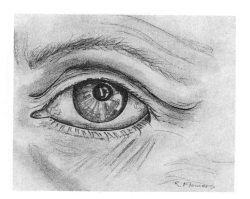

Figure 15 The commonly performed repair on the lower lid as suggested in most textbooks on cosmetic surgery or orbital or ophthalmic plastic surgery. Such triangular skin excisions should never be performed.

Figure 16 Drawing shows the characteristic results from triangular excision with upward lateral rotation of the lower lid skin flap. This commonly performed operation produces the following deformities: depressed posture of the lower lid margin, which is worse laterally; a shortening of the aperture length with rounding of the lateral canthus; a lateral epicanthal fold; and diagonal lines radiating from the lateral canthus down towards the nasal ala. Also see Figure 1.

end up with triangular resections that are usually inappropriate. The reason for this is the faulty surgical plan.

Patients are usually in the supine position during eyelid surgery when skin or skin muscle flaps get raised and assessed. When this is done, it invariably seems that there is more excess laterally than medially, even when assessed with the patient's mouth open. Neither this maneuver nor pressing on the globe simulates the drag of tissue on the lateral face when the patient is vertical. Because of this failure to reproduce vertical drag, the postoperative patient commonly ends up with a lower posture of the lateral third of the lower lid, *corresponding precisely to the triangle of skin or skin muscle excised* (Fig. 15). The upward lateral rotation of the skin of the lower lid results in a diagonal downward tug, resulting in a shortened rounded aperture, a lateral epicanthal fold produced at the gap of the greatest amount of skin excision, and diagonal lines running nasally from the lateral canthus across the lid. A marked, saddened eye results that carries the unfortunate stigma of looking "operated on" (Fig. 16).

Another effect of lower lid blepharoplasty is the tissue-paper–type crinkly wrinkling of the skin as a long-term result of raising skin flaps. This is unnecessary, since skin removal is often unnecessary. With the passage of years, there is attenuation of the lateral canthal tendon and perhaps the lid margin. The posture of the lid is thereby lowered, creating a mild scleral show that deposits additional skin onto the lower lid, which then appears deceptively excessive. Proper technique for these lids involves tightening and restoring the canthus to proper position by canthopexy, removing only skin that is truly excessive, if any (see Fig. 19).

Fat removal, when done, is characteristically inexact, leaving irregular protrusions, or depressions from excessive removal. *It would be far better that these lids remain uncorrected than that these deformities be created.*

77

Face-Lift Surgery: Principles and Variations

M. Eugene Tardy, Jr. and Mark Klingensmith
University of Illinois Medical Center and St. Joseph Hospital,
Chicago, Illinois

Oh! grief hath chang'd me since you saw me last;
And careful hours, with time's deform'd hand,
have written strange defeatures in my face.
                                    William Shakespeare

INTRODUCTION

As the human race increasingly searches for ways to delay the visible physical signs of aging, surgeons have responded to this trend by devising operations to predictably improve appearance. The face-lift operation, in the first half of the twentieth century, primarily emphasized undermining facial skin and lifting it under considerable tension. Advances in contemporary operations make it possible to reposition the muscle and fascia as well as the facial skin. In addition, removal or sculpturing of cervicofacial fat by direct excision or fat-suctioning techniques has become more credible and reliable in the past two decades. The variety of aesthetic facial procedures now available make substantial facial rejuvenation a safe and predictable option for properly selected, well-motivated patients (Fig. 1).

The face-lift operation, which refers to lifting and repositioning maneuvers to improve the appearance of the lower two thirds of the face and the neck, is at best a compromise with nature. A face lift, no matter how skillfully performed, will eventually deteriorate because of the inevitable decrease in skin elasticity and tone associated with aging along with the inexorable detrimental effects of constant gravitational pull. The surgeon's responsibility, recognizing this aesthetic shortfall, is to fashion the best lifting and repositioning procedure possible, consistent with the patient's wishes and anatomic limitations. Since the operation is completely elective, as few risks as possible should be taken to achieve the ultimate goal of the operation: a happy patient and proud surgeon. Heroic surgical attempts to achieve an extraordinary result must be balanced

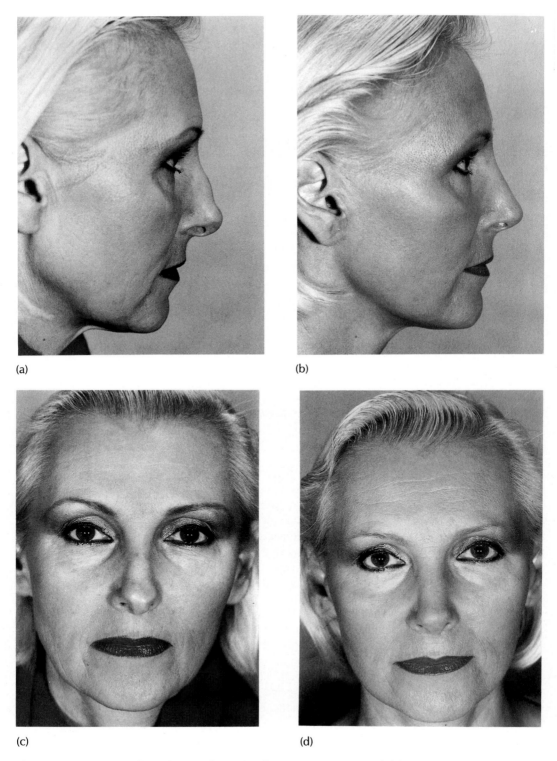

(a)

(b)

(c)

(d)

Figure 1 Suitable candidate for face lift (left) with result at one year (right).

with the risks, since any complication, no matter how insignificant, will be viewed with disenchantment.

The spectrum of procedures available for the effective amelioration of aging features has broadened considerably, due in large measure to techniques designed to tighten and reposition the underlying fascial network and muscular system of the face and neck. Improved immediate and long-term results are possible as more anatomic factors responsible for the aging appearance are being addressed and operations are individualized for each patient. The single most important factor responsible for favorable results remains *careful patient selection*, from both an anatomic and a psychological standpoint.

PROPER PATIENT SELECTION

No amount of surgical expertise can compensate for a poorly selected patient, a fact more true of the face-lift operation than any other (Fig. 2). When face-lift candidates are properly selected from both an anatomic and a psychological standpoint (Fig. 3), the surgery designed to ensure effective rejuvenation is straightforward and fundamental. It is axiomatic that even the most carefully selected patient from an anatomic aspect will be disappointed in even a superb surgical result if the operation is sought for the wrong psychological reasons.

Anatomic Considerations

Clearly the most successful face lifts result in patients for whom the aging process has not yet taken an overwhelming toll on the facial appearance. Chronologic age is an unreliable factor. Many diverse factors (genetic predisposition, sun damage, stress, etc.) influence the age at which a deteriorating facial appearance prompts patients to express concern.

From an anatomic standpoint, the ideal patient might be described as an attractive healthy female between the ages of 45 and 60. Retention of facial skin elasticity combined with a lack of severe solar or environmental skin damage is a favorable finding. The patient should not be overweight, especially when this results in excess deposits of fat in the facial and cervical areas. The facial skeleton should be angular and attractively developed, particularly in the malar, mandibular, and hyoid–thyroid complex areas. The facial skin and underlying soft tissue should be capable of sliding over the more static underlying facial skeletal features with relative ease when manipulated (Figs. 4, 5).

Although the above criteria constitute the most ideal candidates for face-lift surgery, other adjunctive aesthetic procedures (chin augmentation, submental fat removal, selective facial dermabrasion) may compensate for some anatomic shortcomings. A number of factors may render a patient a less than ideal candidate for surgery from an anatomic standpoint and thus limit the best surgical result. Overweight patients, particularly those with localized excessive accumulations of facial fat, severely limit the possibility for a favorable face lift result. A poorly developed, asymmetric, or inadequate facial skeleton, especially if associated with retrognathia and an inferiorly positioned hyoid complex (Fig. 6), is difficult to satisfactorily overcome surgically. Heavy nasolabial folds with deep creases, excessive jowling, and ptotic submandibular glands create significant surgical limitations. Fine or deep wrinkling of the facial and neck skin, permanently etched by sun and environmental exposures, is an unfavorable finding (Fig. 7). Caution is particularly advised with patients who smoke heavily or have significant health problems. Finally, the patient who has already undergone one or more poorly performed face lifts with widened scars, permanent skin damage, and hair loss has limited potential for improvement because of the anatomic damage now present.

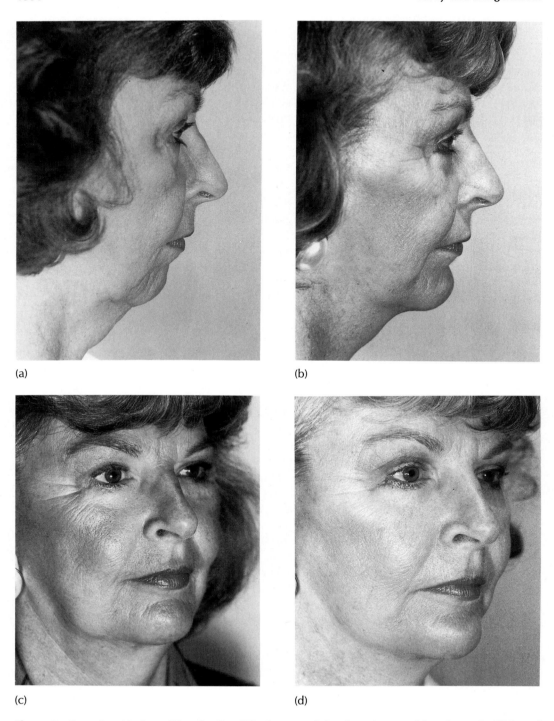

(a)

(b)

(c)

(d)

Figure 2   Less than ideal candidate for face lift whose result has been improved by virtue of addition of chin augmentation and submentoplasty to camouflage the low-lying hyoid and inadequate jawline.

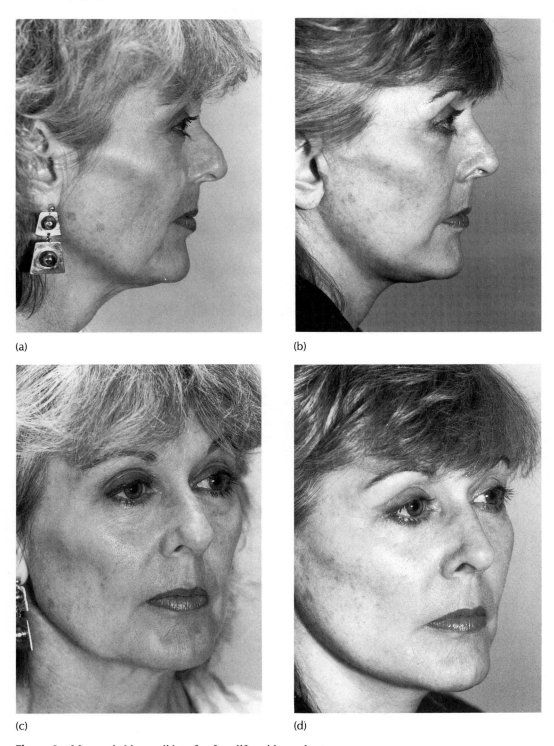

(a)

(b)

(c)

(d)

Figure 3 More suitable candidate for face lift, with result at one year.

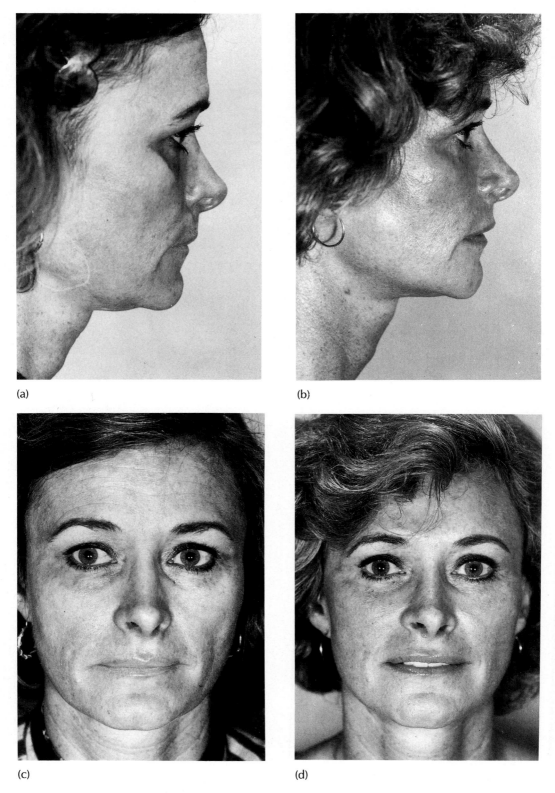

(a) (b)

(c) (d)

Figure 4 Frontal and lateral view of patient with excellent anatomic features for face-lift procedure.

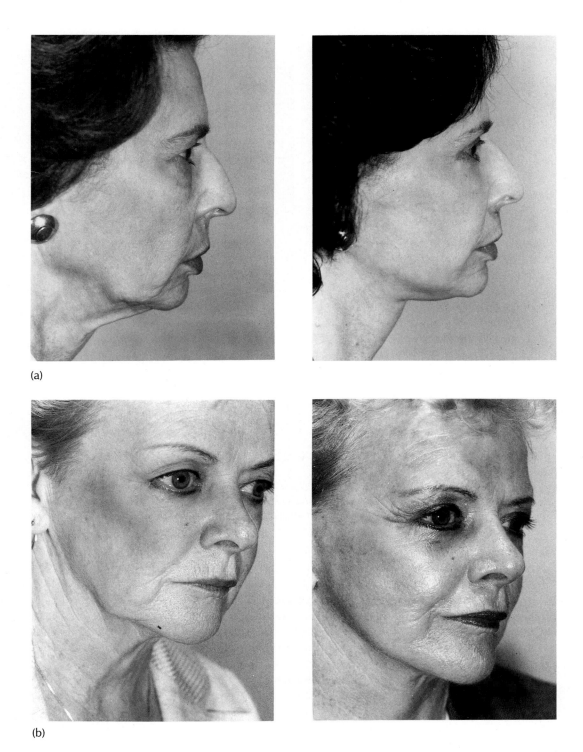

(a)

(b)

Figure 5 Ptotic, redundant facial skin and musculature should be capable of sliding easily over skeletal features unburdened by excess fat. Fine wrinkling and etching of skin are generally not correctable by contemporary face-lift techniques, being only improved but not removed by lifting procedures. Patients should be clearly advised that the apparent relief of fine wrinkling demonstrated by excessive upward lifting of facial tissues is not possible to achieve.

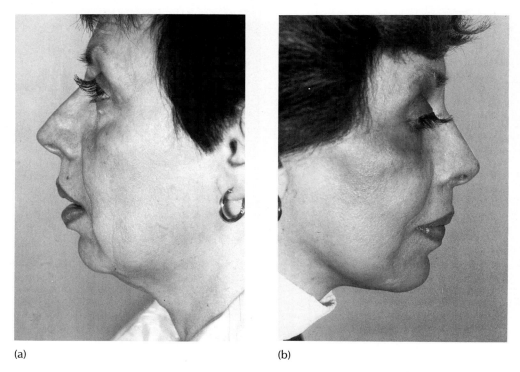

(a)   (b)

Figure 6 Less than ideal candidate for face lift because of retrognathia and low-lying hyoid complex. Excellent improvement is demonstrated at one year by virtue of addition of mentoplasty, submentoplasty, and rhinoplasty to the face-lift procedure. Improved facial balance is apparent.

It is clear that the single most important ingredient for a high level of success with face-lift procedures is accurate selection of the *most ideal anatomic candidates*. In such patients, not only is the immediate rejuvenation result as ideal as possible, but long-term retention of the improved appearance is more likely.

Psychological Considerations

All experienced aesthetic surgeons appreciate the critical importance and the extreme difficulty of selecting patients with appropriate motivation and expectations. Anatomic indications for a face-lift operation are easier to judge than the psychologic considerations. Surgical residents in training quickly and accurately learn the physical characteristics favorable for aesthetic surgical correction, but the experience and judgment to assess emotional motivations is less readily acquired. The experienced surgeon can predict the reasonable anatomic and aesthetic outcome of a surgical procedure; forecasting the patient's reaction to that outcome is an altogether different matter. A good surgical outcome does not always satisfy every patient. Since the fundamental endpoint of aesthetic surgery is a happy patient, every effort must be made to develop a "sixth sense" about patient expectations and motivation.

Being a good listener helps provide valuable insight into the many reasons why patients seek aesthetic surgery. Patients with particular personality disorders may not have a successful psychological outcome, despite a near perfect surgical result. Patients like those described in the following section have been encountered frequently enough over the past 20 years so that the

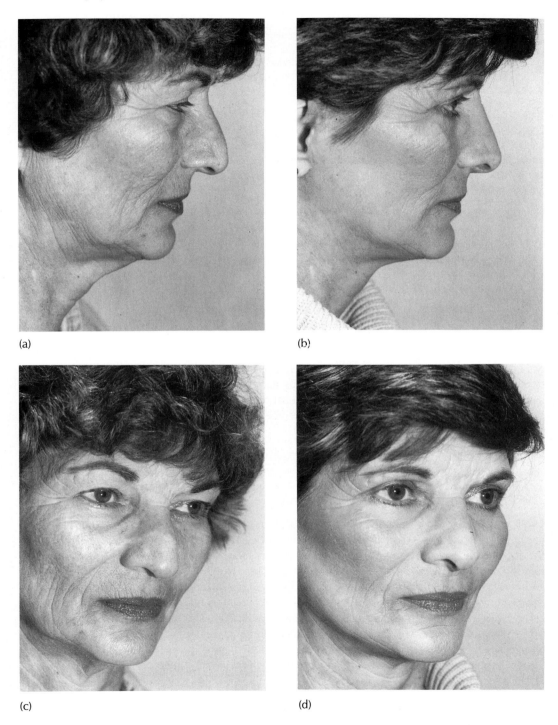

(a)

(b)

(c)

(d)

Figure 7 Excessive fine wrinkling and skin etching limit the result obtained from face-lift operations.

Table 1 Potential Problem Patients

1. The patient with unrealistic expectations
2. The obsessive-compulsive, perfectionistic patient
3. The "sudden whim" patient
4. The indecisive patient
5. The rude patient
6. The overflattering patient
7. The overly familiar patient
8. The unkempt patient
9. The patient with minimal or imagined deformity
10. The careless or poor historian
11. The "VIP" patient
12. The uncooperative patient
13. The overly talkative patient
14. The surgeon shopper
15. The depressed patient
16. The "plastic surgiholic"
17. The price haggler
18. The patient involved in litigation
19. The patient whom you or your staff dislikes

aesthetic surgeon should more closely evaluate them prior to surgery (Table 1). Although patients who fit into one or more of these groups may, upon further evaluation, be good surgical candidates with suitable motivations, many constitute entirely unsuitable patients. It is the surgeon's responsibility to exercise forbearance in the latter instance, either postponing or tactfully refusing a surgical procedure.

POTENTIAL PROBLEM PATIENTS

The Patient with Unrealistic Expectations

Often patients do not understand or may not wish to understand the *limitations* of aesthetic surgery. High expectations honed by mass media and current medical marketing hype imply that the surgeon can "remove" a scar or sculpt a "perfect face." On occasion patients produce magazine photographs of the highly angular, "chiseled" faces of photogenic models, expecting the surgeon to replicate that facial type. Such individuals fail to understand the limitations of their thick skin or coarse facial features.

In the same category are patients requesting a radical change that would appear disproportionate when balanced with other facial features. These patients may have their minds made up and do not wish to compromise their flawed expectations with gentle reason and surgical judgment. Common among these are surgeon shoppers, who seek out a surgeon willing to accept their unrealistic goals.

The Obsessive-Compulsive, Perfectionist Patient

These patients possess unrealistic expectations but exhibit several typical personality characteristics that differentiate them. Perfectionists are often immaculately dressed and groomed. Facial makeup and other cosmetic enhancements are liberally applied and typically overdone.

The perfectionist is often overly compulsive when arranging the initial consultation, sending detailed letters regarding their wishes, timing of office appointments and surgery, and even stipulating "ground rules" for the surgeon and staff to follow. Complaints about other surgeons who have treated the patient (usually "unsuccessfully") are often detailed or at least implied.

Overly perfectionistic patients frequently arrive with long, detailed (and at times unrealistic and inappropriate) questions and insist upon precise responses in advance of the natural interchange between the physician and patient that is the hallmark of the plastic surgery consultation. It is precisely because of their self-proclaimed need for a "perfect" surgical outcome that satisfaction with any surgical result is unlikely. Any slight imperfection or asymmetry will be magnified out of proportion with its importance postoperatively, followed by demands for immediate, and even repeated, revision surgery.

The "Sudden Whim" Patient

Some individuals who insist that surgery be performed immediately feel no need for routine systematic evaluation and surgical preparation. They impose an unrealistic time frame on the surgeon. These patients may be improperly motivated by the "sudden whim." Reasons for the expressed urgency for aesthetic surgery are often unclear and, if stated, are usually unrealistic, triggered by a friend's adverse comment or an abrupt life-style change. These patients can be identified through routine screening by the surgeon's office staff, since they demand appointments immediately, circumventing the orderly sequence of preoperative evaluation. Characteristically these patients have little patience with the surgeon's efforts to completely evaluate, discuss, and inform; instead they wish to schedule surgery immediately and show little concern for surgical hazards, complications, or even outcome. A search for some *significant* psychological event in such patients may often reveal a causal relationship.

THE INDECISIVE PATIENT

This patient characteristically requests the plastic surgical procedure but cannot clearly explain why. Typically the patient may seek several consecutive consultations and yet may remain uncertain whether a procedure should be done. Unsure of specific anatomic problems and desirable surgical outcome, the patient often prefers to allow the surgeon to make all of the decisions, imploring him to "just do whatever you think best" or stating "I'll just leave it up to you."

This category includes patients who may be seeking surgery at the behest of a relative, close friend, or in the case of actors, performers, and models, overzealous photographers and career advisors. Vagueness about what would make this patient happy is a characteristic hallmark, and surgery is sought precisely for the wrong reasons. Disenchantment and even depression may ensue when the requested surgery fails to bring happiness, favorable comment, and professional advancement. These patients typically schedule surgery, cancel, and reschedule, only to cancel again for obscure and indefinite reasons.

The Rude Patient

Although initially pleasant and deferential toward the surgeon as an authority figure, the rude and disrespectful patient usually is exposed by exhibiting an unpleasant, "pushy," and even demeaning form of behavior to the office or hospital staff. Unrealistic requests for preferential treatment may be made, with little regard for the rights and privileges of other patients. Playing by the rules of the game is usually outside the understanding of such patients, and impatience with "the system" is a common characteristic. These unpleasant traits are usually easy to discover during the evaluation process, as inappropriate, unpleasant behavior surfaces repeatedly.

The Overflattering Patient

The patient who excessively praises the surgeon's skills, reputation, and omnipotent surgical abilities sets a tempting trap for the surgeon unable to resist this false adulation. Delicate questioning may reveal the patient's previous visits to other colleagues with unsatisfactory consultations or even surgical outcomes. Demeaning comments may be expressed about other surgeons. Such patients may often travel great distances to "be treated by only the best" and may in reality possess little firsthand knowledge of the surgeon's actual skills and surgical results. Overflattering patients may be quick to turn on the surgeon if the surgical outcome is even slightly imperfect, replacing excessive praise with anger and outrage.

The Overly Familiar Patient

Typically such patients show little respect for the formal confines of the physician–patient relationship. An excessively familiar attitude is taken with both the office staff and the physicians. A first-name intimacy may be assumed inappropriately, and the term "Doc" is used repeatedly. Such patients may show little regard for the office furnishings, instruments, records, and accoutrements, helping themselves to whatever strikes their fancy. These inappropriate intimacies may extend to ingratiating or seductive behavior in order to gain favor or preferential treatment.

THE FACE-LIFT OPERATION

Patient Evaluation, Selection, and Preparation

Preparation for surgery begins, in a sense, even before the surgeon and patient meet. When a consultation is scheduled, the patient is sent an information packet containing generalized factual information about office procedures and a descriptive map to the office. This preconsultation of the patient is most invaluable. It sets a communicative tone for the doctor–patient relationship, emphasizing the importance and seriousness of aesthetic surgical procedures and the need for a team approach to solve the patient's problem. Moreover, written material allows the patient to formulate appropriate and accurate questions relating to specific operations. This information helps to clearly focus the first consultation in the office, fostering the efficient use of time, confirmed and expanded by the surgeon during initial consultation, and allowing more thorough informed consent. Patients uniformly appreciate this educational approach. Unquestionably, individuals who understand the surgical procedures as thoroughly as possible fare much better during and after the operation.

A short but precise medical history is elicited by the secretary during the initial phone interview. It is important to identify any medications being taken that might affect the outcome of surgery, particularly aspirin. Laboratory reports that substantiate the medical history and that might impact upon surgery are obtained prior to surgery.

The initial consultation by the surgeon is critical. Its fundamental purpose is to allow the surgeon to *listen* to the patient's concerns and wishes while assessing whether the request is realistic and properly formulated. This evaluation is of the utmost importance, since no matter how acceptable the patient may be from an anatomic standpoint, if expectations cannot be met surgically, even the most skillfully performed operation will likely fall short of fulfilling the patient's expressed or unexpressed expectations. It is useful to begin the consultation with *open-ended* questions that require more elaborate answers than "yes" or "no," such as "Mrs. Smith, what may I do for you today?" "What brings you in to see me today?" "How may I help you?" These short but precise questions draw the patient into a discussion of both anatomic and psychologic concerns which may impact upon the validity and appropriateness of the surgical request. As the dialogue develops, more specific queries can be formulated by the surgeon. A three-way mirror is helpful in pinpointing specific anatomic concerns. The surgeon must be certain that the patient discusses, as thoroughly and precisely as possible, his or her wishes and expectations. As the discussion begins to focus on specific patient requests, it is appropriate for the surgeon to point out anatomic areas that may be helped by surgery but had not been considered by the patient. It is inappropriate, however, for the surgeon to make suggestions until as much information as possible has been extracted from the patient. Frequently patients are not concerned about defects the surgeon might choose to correct.

The initial consultation may require a considerable amount of time to identify the factors necessary to schedule surgery. Therefore, surgeons practicing aesthetic surgery *must* schedule sufficient time for the initial consultation to achieve this goal. Face-lift candidates, in particular, require a greater investment of consultative time than patients undergoing other forms of cosmetic surgery. This time is well spent, particularly if the outcome of the in-depth initial consultation reveals that the patient is *not* an appropriate candidate for surgery.

As the evaluation continues and the surgeon develops a favorable judgment about the appropriateness of requested surgery, specific facts are discussed while the patient views his or her image in a three-way mirror. Approximate degrees of improvement (Fig. 8), as well as areas that will not be improved, are pointed out along with the location of all incisions. Ancillary procedures (chin augmentation, nasal tip elevation, submentoplasty) that may be of value in a given patient are discussed.

It is important to predict the results of an aesthetic procedure conservatively in order to appropriately shape the patient's expectations. Media hype and sensationalistic medical advertising tend to raise the level of expectation of patients unrealistically. Patients unwilling to accept

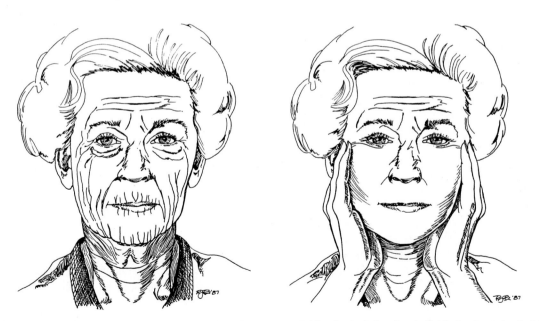

Figure 8 Demonstrations with a three-way mirror are useful in clearly informing individuals about the facial areas in need of improvement, areas that will not be corrected, the location of incisions, and approximate degrees of planned improvement. The apparent marked improvement created by strong manual lifting is seldom surgically possible.

the seriousness and major importance of aesthetic surgical procedures are poor candidates and should be tactfully discouraged from seeking such surgery.

Once the surgeon is assured that the patient's expectations can be met, a series of standard photographs are taken (Fig. 9). The anatomic and psychological assessment continues during the photography session since facial features often appear different when viewed through the confines of the portrait lens. Patients who are uncooperative during photography may be revealing aspects of their personality that make them unsuitable candidates for surgical care. A variety of views recorded on 2 × 2 35 mm Kodachrome slides is preferred, primarily because they accurately represent the patient's features and are easy to store and useful in teaching. Prints may be made in 30 sec, if needed, using the Polaroid or Vivitar slide-to-print copy units. Two exposures of each pose are taken and filed separately from the patient's medical record. One set is available for teaching or publishing, while the other identical set is strictly for archival value and never leaves the master file. It is usually advantageous for the surgeon to act as his or her own photographer; this assures uniformity and standardization. Special views can be taken if desired, and the investment of time (approximately 90 sec per patient) is well spent for the information gathered.

The preoperative education process continues with a detailed interview between the nurse specialist and the prospective patient. The value of these independent discussions cannot be overestimated, since patients (especially women) tend to relate in a highly personal manner to a sensitive, well-informed nurse who is able to discuss aesthetic surgery from a different perspective. Often the nurse becomes the patient's best friend and "ombudsman" before, during, and after surgery. The nurse fills a special need for patients who are understandably anxious about the procedure.

The nurse specialist, if a woman, can help place the procedure, and the events surrounding it, into perspective in a way uniquely possible with a female-to-female relationship. The discussion will revolve around an estimate of the time the procedure will take away from work and social activities, personal care of the face and hair, limitations to normal activities and exercise regimens, required laboratory studies, the type of anesthetic planned, immediate postoperative hospital and home care, and a wide variety of facts particular to the individual patient's needs.

All financial aspects of the surgery are reviewed by the nurse, and comprehensive consent forms for photography (Fig. 10) and the specific surgical procedures planned are further explained, signed, and witnessed (Fig. 11). Written preoperative and postoperative instructions, admission orders, and a preadmission information packet are provided at this meeting. The patient and any accompanying family or friends are once again given the opportunity to raise any and all questions relating to the surgery planned.

Finally, a second in-depth dialogue is held with the surgeon in a comfortable, nonclinical office setting where all specific details are again reviewed. The seriousness of the procedure as well as the potential complications are clearly outlined. Again the patient and family are encouraged to review any questions.

By this time, the patient has been given three separate opportunities to learn about and discuss the procedure with the surgeon and nurse specialist. This sequence provides the most complete understanding for the vast majority of patients. Each patient is encouraged to plan a sec-

---

Figure 9 Essential views of standard and uniform photographs obtained prior to surgery. Additional view of patient grimacing by forcibly pulling down the corners of the mouth is helpful in delineating the precise anatomy of the platysma muscle.

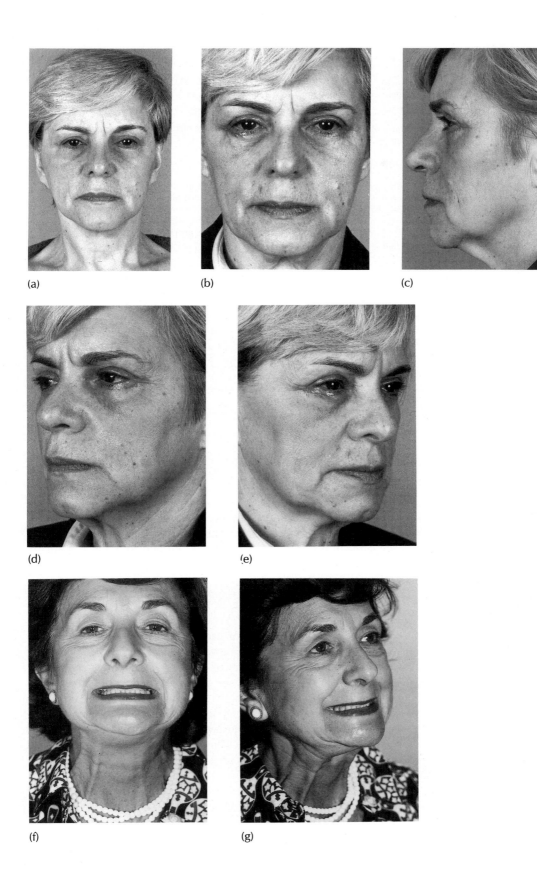

(a)

(b)

(c)

(d)

(e)

(f)

(g)

In connection with the medical services, which I am receiving from my physician, M. Eugene Tardy, Jr., M.D., I consent that photographs may be taken of me or parts of my body, under the following conditions:

A. The photographs may be taken only with the consent of my physician and under such conditions and at such time as may be approved by him.

B. The photographs shall be taken by my physician or by a photographer approved by my physician.

C. The photographs shall be used for medical records, and if in the judgement of my attending physician, medical research, education or science wil be benefitted by their use, such photographs and information relating to my case may be published and republished, either separately or in connection with each other, in professional journals or medical books, or used for any other purpose which he' may deem proper in the interest of medical education, knowledge, or research; provided, however, that it is specifically understood that in any such publication or use I shall not be identified by name.

D. The aforementioned photographs may be modified in any way that my physician, in his discretion, may consider desirable.

Patient's Signature: _____

If a minor or patient is unable to affix signature)
Authority to Sign Consent: (Type or Print)

_____   Witness: _____

Signed: _____   Address: _____

Relationship:_____   _____

Address: _____

_____

Figure 10   Photographic consent form.

ond follow-up visit before surgery in order to clarify any concerns and to further solidify the physician–patient relationship. In addition, each patient is encouraged to seek a second opinion from another qualified aesthetic surgeon if desired. This open and educational attitude is greatly appreciated by knowledgeable patients. The vast majority of intelligent patients who are acceptable candidates return to schedule their contemplated surgery.

Techniques of Face-Lift Surgery

Face lift is similar to rhinoplasty in that the procedure for each patient must be individualized based on individual anatomy. The aesthetic units of the face and neck are variably impacted by the aging process; therefore, the type, extent, and vectors of lift often differ for each patient. The temporal aesthetic unit does not require lifting in every patient; modifications in the incision and the extent of undermining are designed accordingly. The depth of the nasolabial folds and the degree of banding of the platysma muscle similarly influence the degree of undermining and management of the superficial musculoaponeurotic fascia. The distribution of localized fat deposits will dictate the need for regional fat removal. This discussion of the principles and technique most commonly employed by the author is an approach that has satisfied the needs and expectations of well-selected patients for two decades.

Patient Preparation

The patient is instructed to shampoo the head and neck area the night before and the morning of surgery with Phisohex. No other surgical prep solutions are used.

AUTHORIZATION AND INFORMED CONSENT

(Patient's Name)

1. I request and authorize M. Eugene Tardy, Jr., M.D. (the "Doctor") to perform an operation upon me (or my _____) entitled (description of procedure): _____

2. The nature and effects of the operation, the risks, ramifications, complications involved, as well as alternative methods of treatment, have been fully explained to me by the Doctor and I understand them.

3. I authorize the Doctor to perform any other procedure which he may deem desirable in attempting to improve the condition stated in paragraph 1 or any unhealthy or unforeseen condition that may be encountered during the operation.

4. I consent to the administration of anesthetics by the Doctor or under the direction of the physician responsible for this service. If an anesthesiologist assists in my surgery, I understand that the anesthesiologist will take full charge of the administration and maintenance of the anesthesia, and that this is an independent function of the surgery.

5. I have been thoroughly and completley advised that the object of the operation I have requested is primarily an improvement in appearance. Since I understand that the practice of medicine and surgery is not an exact science and therefore that no reputable surgeon can guarantee results, I acknowledge that imperfections might ensue and that the operative result may not live up to my expectations. I certify that no guarantees have been made by anyone regarding the operation(s) I have requested and authorized.

6. I understand that the two sides of the human body are not the same and can never be made the same.

7. I have been advised that part of this surgery is/maybe performed through external skin incisions which will leave permanent scars whose extent and location have been described to me. I have been advised that all scars may require up to a year or more to mature.

8. For the purpose of advancing medical education, I consent to the admittance of authorized observers to the operating room.

9. I give permission to M. Eugene Tardy, Jr., M.D. to take still or motion clinical photographs with the understanding that such photographs remain the property of the doctor. If, in the judgment of the Doctor, medical research, education or science will be benefitted by their use, such photographs, and related information may be published and republished in professional journals or medical books, or used for such publication or use. I shall not be identified by name.

10. I understand that if Dr. Tardy judges at any time that my surgery should be postponed or cancelled for any reason, he may do so.

11. I hereby authorize that the information furnished by Dr. Tardy by me during my diagnostic evaluation is correct.

12. I agree to follow the instructions given to me by Dr. Tardy to the best of my ability before, during and after my surgical procedure.

I certify that I have read the above authorization, that the explanations referred to therein were made to my satisfaction, and that I fully understand such explanations and the above authorization.

Signed _____

(Patient or person authorized to consent for patient)

Witness _____ Date _____

Figure 11 Surgical consent form.

The patient's color photographs are projected on a white dry-erase board in the operating room for reference and teaching during the procedure. The patient is seated upright to mark the face and neck prior to reclining on the operating table. Planned incisions, excess accumulations of fat, and cervical margins of the platysma muscle, if clearly evident, are also marked. By manually sliding the facial and cervical skin posterior and upward, the surgeon can judge clearly the most favorable vectors to lift and reposition, and these are marked accordingly with arrows. In men, the margins of the beard line are lightly marked. The hair is not shaved; rather it is moistened with saline and controlled with small hemostats.

The patient then reclines on the operating table, cushioned by an air mattress approximately half filled. The head of the table is elevated 20 degrees. The anesthesiologist begins an incremental intravenous infusion of Innovar supplemented from time to time with small doses of an ultra–short-acting barbiturate while the surgeon injects local anesthetic. This method of controlled, continuously monitored intravenous analgesia has proved most efficacious, being administered without a single serious complication in the past 20 years. Individualization of the incremental dosage is important, since there is a wide range of tolerance to medication, particularly potent narcotics and phenothiazines. This regimen is particularly well suited for face-lift surgery, since there is considerable postoperative amnesia, and intraoperative comfort is assured. Postoperative discomfort is minimized with the narcotic while the phenothiazine tends to counteract postoperative nausea and vomiting. This latter side effect should be assiduously avoided after face-lift surgery. Continuous monitoring of the patient's heart rate, blood pressure, electrocardiogram, body temperature, and general well-being is carried out during the operation.

Infiltration of lidocaine 1% with epinephrine 1:100,000 or 1:200,000 is first completed on the right side of the face. If other procedures are to be performed in addition to the face lift (blepharoplasty, submentoplasty, etc.), they are usually completed first, and local anesthesia of the face is delayed until approximately 15 min before the facial incisions are made. Local anesthesia is given in this incremental manner to avoid delivering a large bolus of lidocaine and epinephrine. The initial dose will metabolize partially before more is injected. Waiting 15 min after the injection before making the incision allows maximum vasoconstriction from the epinephrine for undermining and elevation. "Hydraulic infiltration" of the tissue, as recommended by some surgeons, is not employed by the author. Ballooning the tissues is not necessary when using the Shaw (hot) scalpel to directly visualize, dissect, and elevate the face-lift flap.

Incisions

Although the incisions for face-lift surgery are relatively standard, variations depend on whether the patient is male or female, the aesthetic units to be corrected, the distribution of hair and preferred hair style, the patient's wishes, and whether there are scars from a previous operation (Figs. 12–15). All incisions are done with a #15 scalpel blade. Undermining is done effectively and largely bloodlessly with the Shaw scalpel.

A small incision is initially made at the junction of the earlobe with the face; in men this incision is placed 2–3 mm below this junction to avoid lifting bearded skin onto the lobule. A single skin hook is placed in the incision for traction directed inferiorly. The auricle is placed on traction anteriorly with a temporary suture placed on the posterior surface of the ear. The *postauricular incision* is created on the posterior surface of the auricle approximately 3–5 mm above the auricular-mastoid junction. This allows the final scar to rest inconspicuously within this junction. The incision is carried upward to the intersection of the auricular helix with the oblique upward slant of the postauricular hairline (Fig. 16). This maneuver places the incision considerably cephalic to the traditional position of the horizontal scars and is located in the non–hair-bearing scalp, enhancing effective scar camouflage. As the incision swings posteriorly off the auricle to cross the indented auriculomastoid sulcus, an inferiorly directed dart is fash-

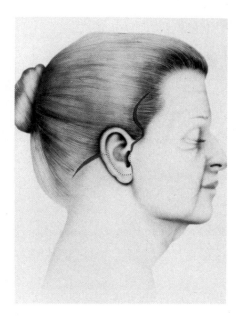

Figure 12 Incisions planned when temporal lift is to be included in the face-lift operation. Preauricular hair is preserved.

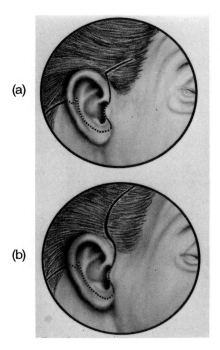

Figure 13 (a) Incision frequently chosen when temporal lift is not included in the face lift. (b) Alternative incision, which includes temporal life and is selected when preauricular hair is particularly abundant.

ioned (Fig. 16) to avoid the inevitable scar contracture that results when incisions traverse a significant concavity. The inferior point of the dart lies within the sulcus; the incision is then continued gently upward into the scalp hairline and carried obliquely posteriorly as far as is required to adequately develop the posterior flap. The posterior flap is undermined and completely developed before any further preauricular or temple incisions are created in order to minimize incisional bleeding.

The *temple incision* varies according to the anatomic needs and wishes of the patient. If the temporal unit is in need of lifting, the incision is begun at the junction of the superior helix with the temple and carried slightly posteriorly and upward within the hairline in a gently curved "C" configuration (Fig. 12). Undermining and elevation of the temporal unit will effectively tighten the temporal unit and lateral canthal and brow area but necessarily elevates the temporal hairline to a variable degree. If the temporal unit requires no elevation, then the temporal incision courses within the hairline from the superior helical junction obliquely anteriorly within the temporal hair approximately 30 degrees above the horizontal (Fig. 13a). This incision allows the removal of a triangle of hair-bearing skin to be excised after upward lifting of the face while preserving a substantial amount of sideburn hair.

The *preauricular incision* curves inferiorly from the superior helix junction into the supratragal notch, courses along or behind the crest of the tragus (except in men), and curves in front of the lobule to join the initial stab incision created at the lobular-facial junction (Figs. 12,13a). The

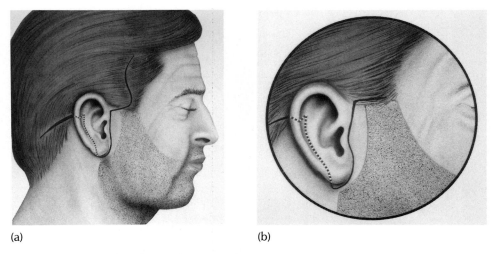

(a)   (b)

Figure 14 (a) Incision for face lift and temporal life in male patients. Sideburn is preserved. (b) Incision in male patient to preserve sideburn when temporal lift is not indicated.

retrotragal course of the face-lift incision is an effective method of camouflaging the incision (Fig. 17). Complications including anterior tragal displacement and blunting, described by some authors, may be avoided by fashioning a small flap of pretragal skin, carefully defatted, to fit without tension into the retrotragal incision. In men the incision differs, since the retrotragal incision is contraindicated because of the male beard. Therefore, the preauricular incision is positioned in a curvilinear fashion in preauricular creases, preserving at least 5 mm of non–hair-bearing skin in front of the auricle (Fig. 14).

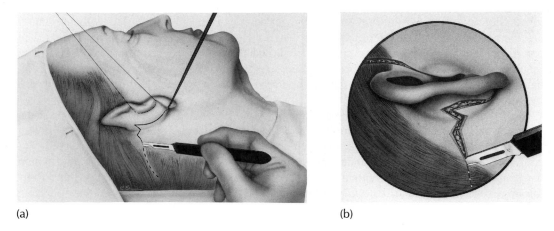

(a)   (b)

Figure 15 (a) Postauricular incision site on posterior surface of ear just above auriculomastoid sulcus and carried across non–hair-bearing skin into posterior scalp hairline. Exact height and angle of superior aspect of the incision depend upon the anatomy present. (b) To avoid the scar contracture common when any incision crosses a concavity, a dart is created in the posterior incision as it traverses the auriculomastoid sulcus.

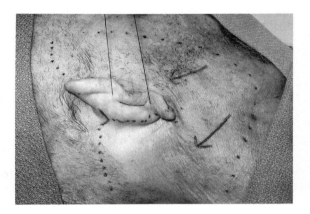

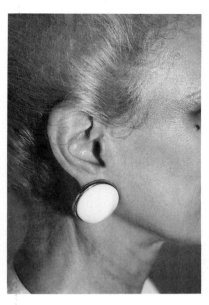

Figure 16 Typical postauricular incisions sited in cadaver specimen.

Figure 17 Example of excellent camouflage possible with retrotragal incision.

Flap Elevation and Undermining

Initially the posterior flap is undermined and elevated. The depth of dissection is quite superficial in this area, just deep to the hair follicles in the hair-bearing scalp and between the skin and the adherent dense fascia protecting the mastoid and sternocleidomastoid muscle. On the cheek, the flap is dissected within the subcutaneous fat above the fascia enveloping the parotid gland. In the temporal area, the level of undermining is deeper, proceeding largely with blunt dissection just above the level of the dense temporalis fascia.

Elevation of the posterior skin flap is best done with broad strokes of the Shaw scalpel, aided by dual skin hook traction on the flap at an angle vertical to the plane of the dissection (Fig. 18). The heated Shaw scalpel allows a near-bloodless dissection and the advantage of instant electrocoagulation of any vessels that do bleed. Direct vision surgery is tremendously facilitated in a dry surgical field. The thickness of the flap, which is of concern throughout the procedure, is thus more easily assessed. Since using the Shaw scalpel, the authors have noted a significant reduction in postoperative edema and ecchymosis due to minimal operative bleeding. The postoperative rebound vasodilation that occurs after the vasoconstrictive epinephrine effect has worn off is significantly negated. Since this instrument appears to seal the small vessels as it cuts, more rapid healing and return to normal activities result.

The postauricular skin is most adherent overlying the mastoid bone and the sternocleidomastoid muscle. It is not difficult, however, to sharply dissect the skin flap away from the muscle and the overlying great auricular nerve. The nerve may bifurcate or even trifurcate, and all branches should be carefully preserved to avoid sensory loss and potential painful neuromata. Dissection of the more anterior portion of the posterior flap is completed after division of the earlobe skin only from the flap. Bleeding can be avoided if the soft tissue mass medial to the lobule is not incised, limiting the dissection release to the skin only. This small detail may save several minutes and avoid the need for electrocautery in the lobule area. The tail of the parotid, which often

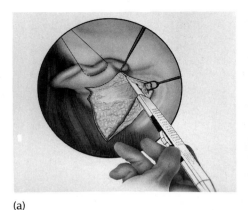

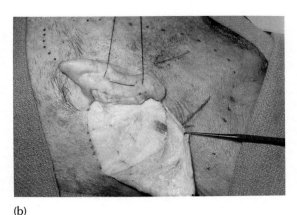

(a)   (b)

Figure 18 (a) Shaw scalpel dissection-elevation of the adherent posterior flap. (b) Elevated posterior flap with a small amount of fat remaining on the undersurface to preserve the subderma plexus blood supply. The sternocleidomastoid muscle is coming into view as the dissection proceeds anteriorly. Vertical traction on the flap from several different angles facilitates the knife dissection in a uniform plane.

adheres to the infralobular skin, should be identified and avoided. Typically the inferior and medial extent of elevation of the posterior flap ceases when the posterior border of the platysma muscle is encountered (Fig. 19). Meticulous hemostasis is ensured and attention turned to the temple and cheek flap elevation.

If indicated for optimum improvement, the temporal aesthetic unit may be elevated and tightened. Elevation proceeds with relative ease and little or no bleeding with blunt finger or instrument dissection under direct vision (Fig. 20). The proper plane of elevation is deeper under this flap, preserving the base of the hair follicles and traversing a natural loose areolar tissue plane over the fascia covering the temporalis muscle. The inferior aspect of this flap should not progress beyond the adherent tissue overlying the zygomatic arch in order to avoid placing the frontal branch of the facial nerve in jeopardy. The cheek flap and the temporal flap thus are not continuous, a safety measure that does not seem to limit the aesthetic result (Fig. 21).

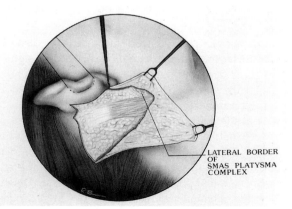

LATERAL BORDER
OF
SMAS PLATYSMA
COMPLEX

Figure 19 As dissection of the posterior flap continues anteriorly, the posterior edge of the platysma muscle, an important landmark, is encountered. The posterior extent of the edge of this muscle is variable.

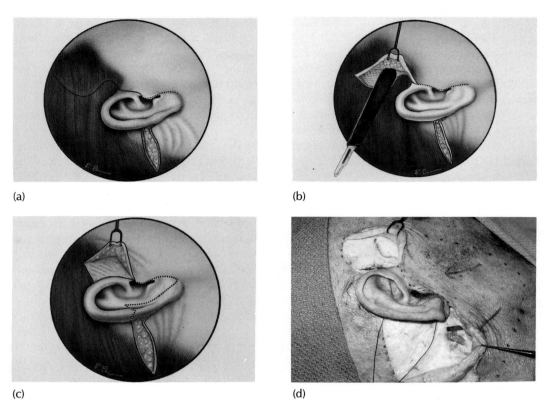

(a)

(b)

(c)

(d)

Figure 20 The temporal flap of the face-lift procedure may be elevated by blunt dissection after the incision is carried down to the level of the dense temporalis fascia. This plane is thus deeper than the immediate subcutaneous plane characteristic of the remainder of the face-lift flap dissection. Large preauricular and superficial temporal vessels may be encountered here, and should be avoided or suture ligated.

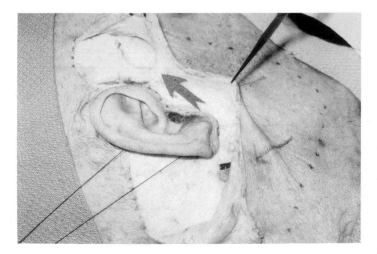

Figure 21 Arrow indicates bridge of tissue separating deeper temporal flap plane from the more superficial plane of the preauricular facial flap. Bringing these two planes into continuity may jeopardize the final nerve frontal branch.

If the temporal unit does not require elevation and tightening, the incision is then placed obliquely in the temporal hairline parallel to the hair follicles and the flap elevated under direct vision (Fig. 13a); it is ultimately brought into continuity with the elevated cheek flap. This flap should be created in the loose areolar tissue deep to the hair follicles. If the base of the hair follicles is visible on the undersurface of the hair-bearing flap, it is likely that their viability has been compromised. A generous venous network exists in the superior preauricular area; thus the surgeon should carefully avoid these vessels in his or her direct vision dissection or be prepared to ligate when indicated with absorbable sutures.

Elevation of the large facial cheek flap under direct vision is next accomplished with the Shaw scalpel (Fig. 22), preserving a thin layer of fat on the flap to protect the subdermal plexus. The fat has a characteristic cobblestone appearance immediately beneath the dermis; therefore, the appropriate thickness of the flap is easily determined. Light transluminated through the flap from the facial side helps gauge a uniform flap thickness. The cheek flap extends anteriorly well beyond the anterior border of the parotid gland (Fig. 23), but seldom beyond the nasolabial fold. Undermining is extended as planned preoperatively using skin hooks for traction on the anterior and posterior flaps. The two flaps are brought into continuity by dividing the bridge of subcutaneous tissue along the angle of the mandible (Fig. 24). It is important to appreciate that all undermining to this point has been *superficial* to the platysma muscle. Excessive fat is excised and meticulous hemostasis again ensured.

Once skin flap undermining and elevation is complete, a decision is made regarding management of the superficial musculoaponeurotic system (SMAS), fascia, and platysma muscle. Surgeons differ markedly in their preferences for management of the underlying musculocutaneous tissues of the facial skeleton. Logical anatomic arguments support the development of a separate SMAS-platysmal flap, suturing the tightened fascial flap (or split flaps) posteriorly to ostensibly improve both the amount and duration of improvement from the lift. Conversely, equally convincing arguments extol the virtues of *plication* or *imbrication* of the SMAS fascia without deeper undermining and separate SMAS flap elevation, citing greater safety. Both philosophies clearly have merit and should be thoroughly evaluated by every face-lift surgeon.

The author's philosophy embraces the middle ground on this issue. Clearly it is helpful to reposition and tighten the underlying musculoaponeurotic tissues of the face and neck to achieve superior results that resist gravitational deterioration. In approximately 80% of selected patients, the skin flaps are elevated as described above, followed by identification of the SMAS fascia and

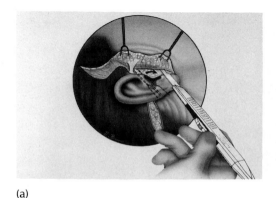

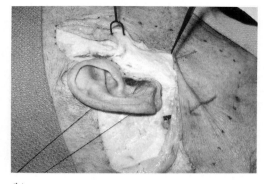

(a)   (b)

Figure 22   Shaw scalpel dissection of the large facial flap: (a) opened through a retrotragal incision in females; (b) a preauricular incision in males.

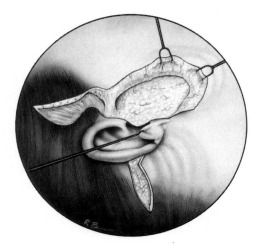

Figure 23 Continuation of elevation of the facial flap well beyond the anterior border of the parotid gland. The exact forward dissection of the flap will depend upon the individual anatomy encountered.

posterior platysma for tight posterior suture plication to the dense fascia overlying the mastoid, sternocleidomastoid, and parotid (Fig. 25). Eight to twelve 3-0 white Tevdek sutures are positioned to tightly suspend the fascia and muscle posteriorly and slightly cephalically (Fig. 26). This suspension rhytidectomy improves the immediate as well as long-lasting results. The favorable lifting effect is noted both on the facial and cervical tissues with no concomitant skin tension. This is one of the principal virtues of this procedure: the underlying tissue may be repositioned under considerable tension while the skin flaps may be sutured under no tension at all. In addition, the undermined subcutaneous tissue space is diminished significantly, which facilitates healing and diminishes the potential for postoperative bleeding.

In the remaining 20% of patients, definitive SMAS flaps are individually elevated, advanced and rotated posteriorly, trimmed, and permanently sutured in place (Figs. 27–29). Patients selected for this slightly more extensive procedure are those in whom SMAS plication alone is less effective in creating desired cervicofacial definition.

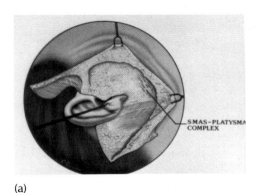

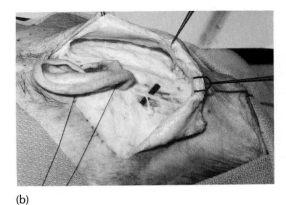

(a)   (b)

Figure 24 Anterior and posterior flaps brought into continuity, exposing the SMAS-platysmal muscle complex. The division of the great auricular nerve, carefully preserved, as highlighted with marker.

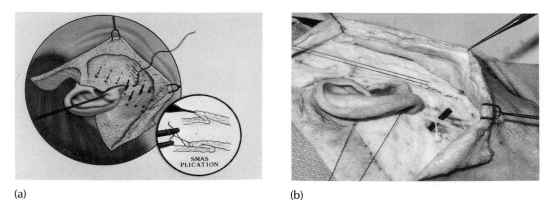

(a)   (b)

Figure 25 Identification of the SMAS-platysmal muscle complex in preparation for posterior suture plication. The relative mobility of this complex will determine how best to manage its posterior and cephalic replacement.

Once undermining of the flaps is complete and suture repositioning of the deeper tissues has created satisfactory support and lifting, the skin flaps are placed on traction and the vector factors of skin flap repositioning assessed (Fig. 30). If the flaps are rotated too cephalically, the sideburn and temporal hairline will be abnormally elevated. If the flap is simply advanced posteriorly with little or no upward rotation, then minimal lifting will be realized, particularly of the cheek and face. This represents one of the surgical compromises peculiar to the face-lift operation; the appropriate degree of both advancement and cephalic rotation is sought to provide the most improvement without distortion of the patient's hairline and facial features. Once the appropriate placement has been determined, the skin is positioned *under no tension* and is

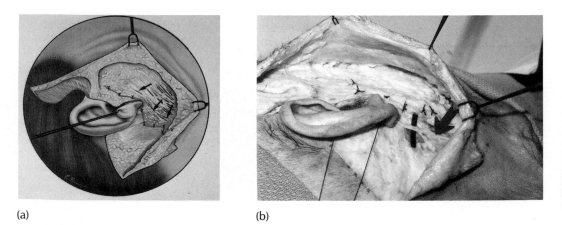

(a)   (b)

Figure 26 Plication of the SMAS-platysmal complex with nonabsorbable sutures, depicted here in black for emphasis (white 4–0 Tevdek is used). This maneuver exerts a strong lifting and repositioning vector force upon the face and neck tissues, allowing a strong and long-lasting lift, eliminating the majority of the subcutaneous dead space, and taking almost all tension off the repaired skin flaps.

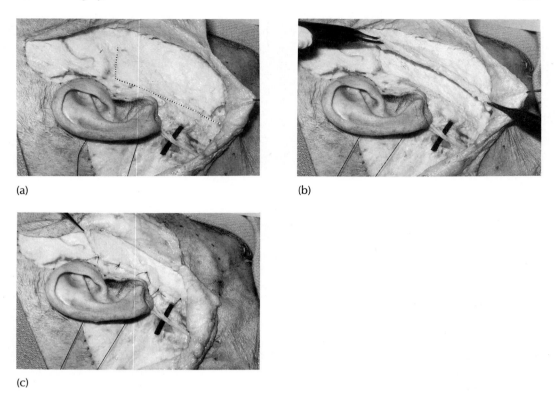

(a)

(b)

(c)

Figure 27 (a) Outline of incision to be made in SMAS fascia if separate SMAS flap is to be elevated and advanced. (b) SMAS flap elevated with blunt and sharp dissection. (c) Preauricular portion of SMAS flap advanced posteriorly, excess excised, and suture repair completed. Excessive cephalic portion of SMAS flap is ready for trimming and repair just below zygoma.

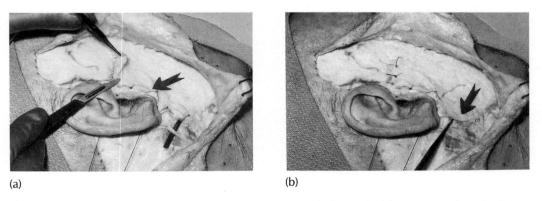

(a)

(b)

Figure 28 (a) SMAS may be divided into two flaps by fashioning an incision at approximately the ear-lobe (arrow) in order to exert an even greater pull posteriorly and cephalically. (b) Inferior segment of SMAS flap advanced posteriorward and sutured into place.

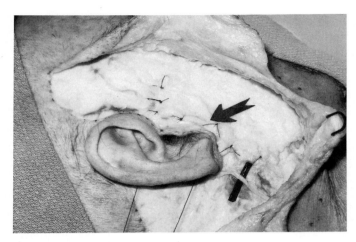

Figure 29 Repositioning and suture stabilization of deeper layers of face-lift operation now completed. Since all tension is borne by the SMAS-platysmal flap suture fixation, the skin flap may now be replaced without tension and redraping is efficiently carried out.

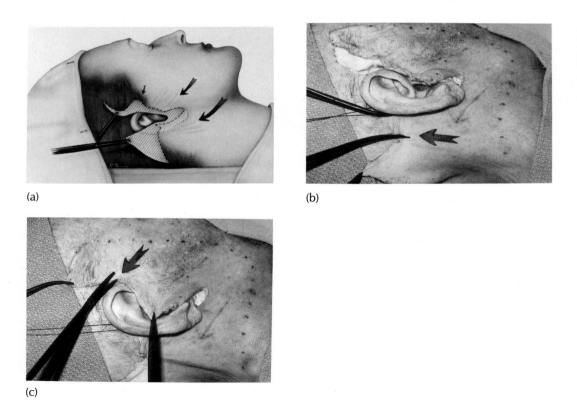

(a)

(b)

(c)

Figure 30 (a) Redraping of the skin flap without tension. The size of the arrow depicts the magnitude of lifting vector force gained into various areas of the face. (b) Tailoring of posterior flap without tension. (c) Tailoring of preauricular and temporal flaps without tension.

incised to the limits of the scalp incision in two places: at the junction of the scalp hairline with non–hair-bearing expanse of postauricular skin and just above the helix of the ear in the temple incision (Fig. 31). The flap is secured at each of these fixation points with a stainless steel surgical staple. The flap is again elevated for smoothness without tension. The midportion of the flap is then incised obliquely down the anterior aspect of the earlobe. Since the lobe has not been displaced by total excision from the underlying facial tissues, establishing the precise preoperative site of the lobular-facial junction is facilitated. A single key suture secures this newly created junction, which should rest comfortably in the "sling" or "hammock" of the newly positioned facial flaps to avoid downward displacement during healing. Lobular distortion following face lift can be significant and a cause for patient distress. If indicated or requested, the earlobe can be diminished or repositioned to achieve a more normal appearance.

The redundant skin in the hair-bearing portions of the flap is now excised, hemostasis ensured, and the skin edges apposed with surgical staples (Fig. 32). Because of the tension-reducing effect of the SMAS plication, the skin flaps may be gently approximated with *no* tension to facilitate healing with well-camouflaged fine scars. The majority of the skin in the immediate postauricular region is preserved in order to recreate the auriculomastoid sulcus (Figs. 33,34). Repair of the postauricular area precedes with 5–0 collagen catgut sutures, which require no removal. The curving transverse incision in the hairless skin from the auricle to the postauricular hairline, including the inferior dart created in the sulcus, may be closed with fine suture or skin adhesive tape (Fig. 34). Staples should not be placed in this hairless skin.

Before proceeding, time is now taken to infiltrate local anesthesia into the contralateral side of the face to allow a sufficient period for vasoconstriction. Careful attention is devoted to trimming and finely suturing the preauricular and retrotragal incision. A small flap of skin is now fashioned anteriorly to fit comfortably into the retrotragal incision (Fig. 35). The remainder of the anterior flap is assiduously tailored and defatted. Ideally the opposing edges of the skin should fall together easily and actually evert slightly to achieve the best scar possible. Closure ensues with a 6–0 black nylon or blue Prolene continuous suture (Fig. 36). A small Penrose drain is inserted into the postauricular incision and removed the next day. The wound margins are meticulously cleaned, and the author applies Neodecadron Ophthalmic ointment, Adaptic gauze, and moist 4 × 4 gauze fluffs supported with Kerlex gauze bandage applied circumferentially (Fig. 37). A tight bandage is unnecessary and undesirable.

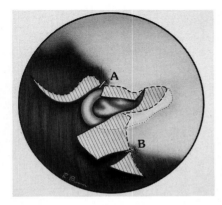

Figure 31 Location of key sutures (staples) A and B positioned before final tailoring of the skin flaps.

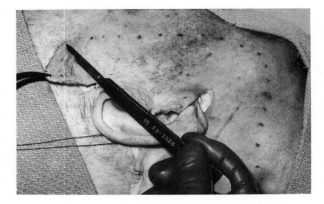

Figure 32 Redundant hair-bearing skin is excised and closed with stainless steel staples.

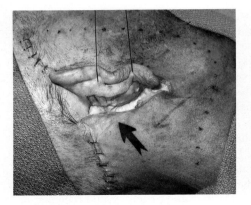

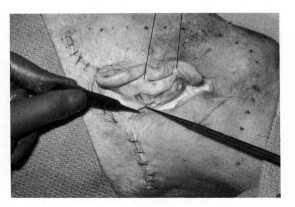

Figure 33 Rather than excising substantial skin in the immediate postauricular region, the skin is advanced anteriorly to recreate the depths of the auriculomastoid sulcus, thus avoiding blunting of this natural angle. Very little skin is excised in this area.

Figure 34 The curving transverse incision in the hairless skin from the auricle to the postauricular hairline, including the inferior dart created in the sulcus, is repaired with fine absorbable sutures.

Management of Platysmal Relaxation and Cervical Fat

Patients undergoing face-lift operations are uniformly concerned about improving the ptotic submental area. Aging in this area is characterized by relaxation and redundancy of the medial platysmal fibers, an accumulation of fat both superficial and deep to the platysmal decussation, and on occasion ptosis of the submandibular glands. The most favorable management of the medial cervical region depends on which of these factors must be surgically corrected. Except in the early stages of cervicofacial support loss, the platysmal muscle will require tightening and repositioning from both its lateral and medial aspects. Careful anatomic assessment will allow this to be determined prior to surgery.

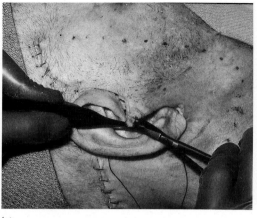

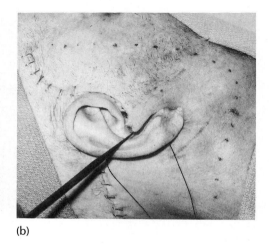

(a)   (b)

Figure 35 After defatting of the tragal flap, it is tailored to lie without tension over the tragus so that scar contracture during the postoperative period will not expose the retrotragal scar.

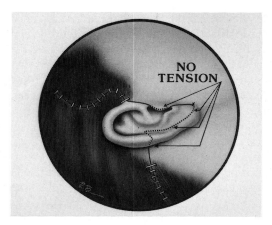

Figure 36 Final closure of the preauricular incision with 6–0 Prolene suture. No tension exists on the suture line, thus protecting the flap integrity and leading to improved scar camouflage.

If early ptotic changes with little or no medial platysmal banding and minimal submental fat accumulation exist, then incorporating posterior platysmal plication into the basic face-lift operation will satisfactorily improve cervical definition and contour. Unsightly vertical platysmal bands with excessive submental fat and skin require a direct approach to the area through a curvilinear incision placed in or slightly posterior to the submental crease. Submentoplasty is

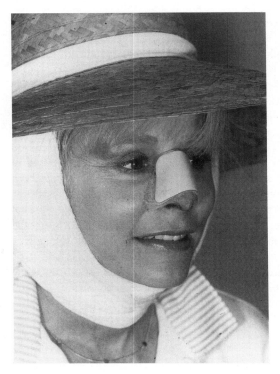

Figure 37 The supportive circumferential bandage useful in the early postoperative period may be effectively camouflaged with a light hat and scarf as worn by this patient.

ideally completed prior to beginning the face-lift operation before the facial skin and musculofacial flaps have been repositioned and tightened. In order to dissect in the neck under no tension and to excise or reposition the medial platysmal fibers precisely with direct vision, correcting the submental anatomy *before* the face-lift dissection facilitates submentoplasty. Firming this area first thus allows the repositioning of the face-lift flaps over a tightened and defatted submental and submandibular region. Extreme conservatism should be exercised in removing minimal submental skin in all but the most aged of patients. To create a defined cervicomental angle requires retropositioning excess submental skin into the angle, whereas overaggressive skin removal may result in insufficient submental skin to comfortably and smoothly cover this now-elongated area, creating blunting of the angle from the upper submental area to the midneck, a totally preventable but common sequela of overaggressive skin excision. Similarly, excision of a large triangle of submental skin and closure in a "T" configuration can lead to unsightly depressions, tissue bunching, and unacceptable scarring.

The preferred submental incision is made within or several millimeters posterior to the submental crease. The incision length will vary depending on the degree of exposure required for dissection, but should not be extended to the lateral mandible where advancement and rotation of the cervical flap might pull the lateral corners of the incision out of the submental area where it is visible. For patients who require modification of the medial platysma, direct vision excision and sculpture of the submental fat provides a superior, more reliable result despite validation of liposuction techniques in the submental area in younger patients. Direct access to the medial platysma is required. Dissection is facilitated with sharp scissors in a spreading and cutting manner with countertraction applied to the inferior margin of the submental incision. Fat superficial to the platysma is relatively bloodless except for a few penetrating vessels into the submental musculature. Fat beneath the platysma near the floor of the mouth is highly vascular and requires more delicate dissection with greater attention to hemostasis. Sufficient fat should be left on the submental skin flap (up to 1 cm) to avoid creating an unsightly submental depression which accentuates an early ptotic chin pad. Sculpture of the fat laterally to blend into the contours of the lateral mandible and cervical soft tissues requires some skill and experience. Ordinarily the thyroid cartilage represents the inferior extent of the fat excision where a feathering sculpturing may be required. Absolute hemostasis is critical, since a hematoma in the submental area will substantially prolong satisfactory healing.

Once fat sculpturing is complete and hemostasis ideal, the condition of the medial borders of the platysma may be evaluated and a treatment plan determined. The "hammock" effect caused by decussation and interdigitation of the medial platysmal fibers in the young is diminished in older patients, which results in deterioration of support and a variety of medial platysmal configurations. The fibers may have departed the midline with diminished or minimal decussations, they may hang in ptotic early folds along with their overlying skin, or thick prominent vertical bands may result in the typical "turkey gobbler" neck deformity. In the latter deformity, the medial vertical margins of the muscle and its investing fascia are resected and the upper free margins approximated with permanent sutures in the midline.

If thin ptotic cervical folds of muscle are present, the author prefers to create a transverse incision from medial to lateral partially through the body of the muscle approximately 4–6 cm inferior to its mandibular extent. Suture approximation of the upper submental platysmal fibers, in concert with the suture-fixation of the lateral SMAS-platysma complex, recreates a cervical sling critical to providing support to the more youthful appearing neck. The platysma is never completely divided transversely, since this maneuver often leads to an unsightly depression in the midneck as the two cut edges retract superiorly and inferiorly. Other complications associated with complete transverse muscle transection are loss of support of the submandibular triangle as well as possible pseudoparalysis of the lower lip.

The following instructions apply to patients who have undergone face lifts. Since no two patients are ever exactly alike in their surgical needs, type of surgery performed, or rate of healing, we may elect to individualize the following guidelines for each patient. In such instances, we will so instruct you. Otherwise, we *urge* you to follow the advice below very carefully, in order to accelerate your healing and maximize your surgical outcome.

1. Since you have just undergone a *major* surgical operation, use good common sense in the first 14 days after surgery in restricting your normal activities, exercise regimens, and any activity requiring heavy lifting or straining.

2. You may be up and around the day after surgery, but some natural fatigue may persist for 2–3 days due to the normal effects of the anesthesia and surgical procedures.

3. When you move, stand, or change positions, do so deliberately and carefully for the first 7 days. In turning your head, move the head and shoulders deliberately as a single unit.

4. You may eat a normal diet the day following surgery. In moderation, talking and smiling are perfectly acceptable.

5. Your head should be elevated on at least two pillows during sleep for the first 14 days in order to keep your head higher than your heart to help facilitate the resolution of swelling. Do not sleep face down, rather on your back or side.

6. DO NOT TAKE ANY ASPIRIN OR ASPIRIN-CONTAINING MEDICINES for 14 days, and then only on the advice of your personal physician. Other routinely taken medications may be taken as necessary.

7. Any unexplained development of pain, facial swelling, or fever should be reported to us immediately.

8. Some facial and neck swelling and bruising are normally present after face lifts, but the degree of each varies widely from patient to patient. Do not be concerned if you have more or less than others who have undergone the "same" operation. Generally, most patients appear quite socially acceptable within 10–14 days after surgery.

9. You may *gently* cleanse the incision lines twice daily with 3% hydrogen peroxide and cotton (or Q-tips). Apply the ointment provided *sparingly* twice daily to the incision lines in order to avoid excessive crusting of the incisions and to accelerate the reduction of incision redness. Do not apply any other ointment or medications unless we prescribe it.

10. You may *gently* shampoo your hair 72 hours after surgery, avoiding any strong rubbing or combing trauma to the incisions in the hair and around the ear. Do not blow dry for 5 days, and postpone any planned permanent waves or hair coloring for 4 weeks following surgery.

11. Your earlobes and portions of the face that have been lifted and repositioned will be slightly numb for several weeks; sensation will then return as healing progresses. Do not wear heavy or tight earrings for 6 weeks, and avoid prolonged exposure to extremely cold temperatures.

12. It is acceptable to do some light walking 72 hours after surgery. Jogging and light noncontact exercise should not be resumed until 3 weeks, and strenuous sports require 6 weeks of healing before being safely resumed.

13. Excessive exposure to sun (including suntanning parlors) in the first 3 weeks after surgery may result in prolonged facial swelling and injury to the skin. Thereafter, you should always protect your skin with a strong sunscreen containing PABA (para-aminobenzoic acid) in order to decrease the inevitable aging effects of sun on your skin.

14. Finally, it is *very important* to your well-being that you follow completely all instructions given you by this office, and that we check your progress regularly following surgery.

We greatly appreciate the confidence you have shown in us by allowing us to assist you in improving your appearance and health, and you may be assured of our very best efforts to achieve the most satisfactory surgical result possible for your particular individual anatomy and condition.

Figure 38 Patient Instructions Following Face-Lift Surgery

Postoperative Care

Attentive and sympathetic postoperative care of the face-lift patient shares equal importance with the operation itself. In the first few days following the operation, strong emotional support is necessary by the surgeon, the surgical staff, and family members in order to reinforce a positive patient attitude. Although most face-lift patients fare exceptionally well in this early postoperative period, particularly those who have been thoroughly prepared by the surgeon (Fig. 38), it is not uncommon for an occasional patient to encounter a transient period of mild depression. As facial ecchymosis and edema fades, mild depression routinely gives way to satisfaction in the vast majority of well-selected patients.

Anything other than mild discomfort is unusual in the early postoperative period. Pain is an infrequent complaint, which varies with the motivation and pain threshold of the patient. Mild non–aspirin-containing analgesics are ordinarily sufficient to ensure comfort in the first 48 hr. Significant pain should alert the surgeon to the possibility of expanding hematoma formation. No other special medications are given or appear to be useful. Prophylactic perioperative antibiotics are preferred by some surgeons; however, the author has not found their routine use necessary or advantageous.

All incisions are cleansed gently with hydrogen peroxide and kept moist with Neodecadrom Ophthalmic ointment twice daily during the first week after surgery. This prevents crusting over the incision sites and hastens resolution of redness. The supportive head bandage is changed the morning after surgery, and the small drains are removed. No bandages are required after 72 hr, and patients are encouraged to shower and gently shampoo at this time. The preauricular sutures and half of the staples are removed at 5–6 days; the remainder of the staples may be safely and painlessly removed at 10–14 days.

BIBLIOGRAPHY

Adamson JE, Toksu AE. Progress in rhytidectomy by platysma-SMAS rotation and elevation. *Plast Reconstr Surg* 1981;68:23.

Anderson JR. The tuck-up operation: A new technique of secondary rhytidectomy. *Arch Otolaryngol* 1975;101:739.

Aston SJ. Platysma muscle in rhytidoplasty. *Ann Plast Surg* 1979;3:529.

Baker DC. Complications of cervicofacial rhytidectomy. *Clin Plast Surg* 1983;10:543.

Baker DC, Conley J. Avoiding facial nerve injuries in rhytidectomy. *Plast Reconstr Surg* 1979;64:781.

Baker TJ, Gordon HL. Rhytidectomy in males. *Plast Reconstr Surg* 1969;44:218.

Baker TJ, Gordon HL. *Surgical Rejuvenation of the Face.* St. Louis, Mosby, 1985.

Connell BF. Cervical lift: Surgical correction of fat contour problems combined with full width platysma muscle flap. *Aesthet Plast Surg* 1978;1:355.

Courtiss EH. *Male Aesthetic Surgery.* St. Louis, Mosby, 1982.

Davis RA, et al. Surgical anatomy of the facial nerve and parotid gland based upon a study of 350 cervicofacial halves. *Surgery* 1956;102:385.

Dedo DD. A preoperative classification of the neck for cervicofacial rhytidectomy. *Laryngoscope* 1980;90:1894.

Dingman RO, Grabb WC. Surgical anatomy of the mandibular ramus of the facial nerve based on the dissection of 100 facial halves. *Plast Reconstr Surg* 1962;29:266.

Ellenbogen R. Pseudoparalysis of the mandibular branch of the facial nerve after platysmal face-lift operation. *Plast Reconstr Surg* 1979;63:364.

Fodor PB. Platysma-SMAS rhytidectomy. *Aesthet Plast Surg* 1982;6:173.

Goin MK, Burgoyne RW, Goin JW, et al. A prospective psychological study of 50 female facelift patients. *Plast Reconstr Surg* 1980;65:436.

Gonzalez-Ulloa M. Facial wrinkles: Integral elimination. *Plast Reconstr Surg* 1962;29:658.

Gordon HL. Rhytidectomy. *Clin Plast Surg* 1978;5:97.

Guerrero-Santos J, Espaillat L, Morales F. Muscular lift in cervical rhytidoplasty. *Plast Reconstr Surg* 1974;54:127.

Gurdin MM. Should the subcutaneous tissue be plicated in face lift? (letter to the editor). *Plast Reconstr Surg* 1975;55:84.

Hoffman S, Simon BE. Complications of submental lipectomy. *Plast Reconstr Surg* 1977;60:889.

Kamer FM. The two-stage concept of rhytidectomy. *Otolaryngol Head Neck Surg* 1979;87:915.

Lemmon M, Hamra ST. Skoog rhytidectomy: A five-year experience with 577 patients. *Plast Reconstr Surg* 1980;65:283.

McKinney P, Maywood BT. Camouflage of the postauricular scar in rhytidectomy. *Plast Reconstr Surg* 1982;69:352.

Mitz V, Peyronie M. The superficial musculoaponeurotic system (SMAS) in the parotid and cheek area. *Plast Reconstr Surg* 1976;58:80.

Rees TD. *Aesthetic Plastic Surgery*. Philadelphia, Saunders, 1980.

Rees TD, Aston SJ. A clinical evaluation of the results of submusculoaponeurotic dissection and fixation in face-lifts. *Plast Reconstr Surg* 1977;66:851.

Regnault P, Daniel RK. *Aesthetic Plastic Surgery*. Boston, Little, Brown, 1984.

Skoog T. *Plastic Surgery*. Philadelphia, Saunders, 1975.

Tardy ME, et al. *Surgery of the Aging Face*. Memphis, Richards Medical, 1981.

Tardy Me, et al. Surgical correction of facial deformities. In *Diseases of the Nose, Throat, and Ear*. Ballenger JJ, ed. Philadelphia, Lea & Febiger, 1977.

Tenta LT, Tardy ME, Pastorek NJ. Buccal lipectomy. In *Plastic and Reconstructive Surgery of the Face and Neck*. Conley J, Dickinson JT, eds. Stuttgart, Thieme, 1972, p. 22.

Tipton JB. Should the subcutaneous tissue be plicated in a facelift? *Plast Reconstr Surg* 1974;54:1.

Webster RC, Davidson TM, White MF, et al. Conservative face-lift surgery. *Arch Otolaryngol* 1976;102:657.

Webster RC, et al. Cosmetic platysmal surgery. *Facial Plast Surg* 1987;4:97.

Webster RL, Smith RC. *The Aging Face and Neck*. New York, Field, Rich, and Associates, 1985.

Index

RANDALL K. ROENIGK, M.D. is Professor of Dermatology at the Mayo Medical School and Consultant in dermatology specializing in dermatologic surgery and cutaneous oncology at the Mayo Clinic and Mayo Foundation, Rochester, Minnesota. Dr. Roenigk received the M.D. degree (1981) from Northwestern University Medical School, Chicago, Illinois.

HENRY H. ROENIGK, JR., M.D. is Professor of Dermatology at Northwestern University Medical School, Chicago, Illinois, specializing in clinical, dermatologic, and cosmetic surgery. Previously the Chairman of the Department of Dermatology at Northwestern University Medical School, Chicago, Illinois, and the Cleveland Clinic, Ohio, Dr. Roenigk is the coeditor (with Howard I. Maibach) of *Psoriasis, Second Edition* (Marcel Dekker, Inc.) and three other textbooks. He received the M.D. degree (1960) from Northwestern University Medical School, Chicago, Illinois.